Normal values

Haematology: full blood count (FBC)

Haemoglobin (Hb):		130–180 g/L (males), 115–165 g/L (females)
Mean cell volume (MCV):		80–96 fL
Packed cell volume (PCV) \ Haematocrit (Hct)		40–50% (males), 36–45% (females)
Mean corpuscular haemoglobin (MCH):		28–32 pg
Mean cell haemoglobin concentration (MCHC):		320–350 g/L
Reticulocytes:		25–85 × 10^9/L *or* 0.5–2.4%
Platelets:		150–400 × 10^9/L
White cell count (WCC):		4–11 × 10^9/L.
Differential WCC:	Neutrophils:	2.5–7.5 × 10^9/L
	Lymphocytes:	1.5–4.0 × 10^9/L
	Monocytes:	0.2–0.8 × 10^9/L
	Eosinophils:	0.04–0.44 × 10^9/L
	Basophils:	0.0–0.1 × 10^9/L

Coagulation screen

Prothrombin time (PT):	12–15 sec
Activated partial thromboplastin time (APTT):	40–50 sec
International normalized ratio (INR):	<0.9–1.2
Fibrinogen:	1.8–5.4 g/L
D-dimer	<0.5 mg/L (varies with assay used, e.g. ELISA/latex agglutination, etc.)

Biochemistry

Ions:	
Sodium (Na^+):	135–145 mmol/L
Potassium (K^+):	3.5–5.0 mmol/L
Chloride (Cl^-):	95–107 mmol/L
Bicarbonate (HCO_3^-):	20–28 mmol/L
Corrected calcium (Ca^{2+}):	2.2–2.6 mmol/L
Phosphate (PO^{4-}):	0.8–1.4 mmol/L
Copper (Cu^{2+}):	12–26 μmol/L
Caeruloplasmin:	200–350 mg/L
Magnesium (Mg^{2+}):	0.75–1.05 mmol/L
Anion gap:	12–16 mmol/L
	Calculated by: ($[Na^+] + [K^+]$) – ($[Cl^-] + [HCO_3^-]$)
Renal:	
Urea:	2.5–7.5 mmol/L
Creatinine:	60–110 μmol/L
Urate:	0.23–0.46 mmol/L (males), 0.19–0.36 mmol/L (females)
Plasma osmolality:	278–305 mosmol/kg
Hepatic:	
Total protein:	61–76 g/L
Albumin:	37–49 g/L
Total bilirubin:	1–22 μmol/L
Conjugated bilirubin:	0–3.4 μmol/L
Alanine aminotransferase (ALT):	5–35 U/L
Aspartate aminotransferase (AST):	1–31 U/L
Alkaline phosphatase (ALP):	45–105 U/L (over 14 years)
Gamma glutamyl tra[illegible]	[illegible] les)
Lactate dehydrogena[illegible]	[illegible]
Cardiac:	
Troponin I:	[illegible]
Troponin T:	[illegible]
High sensitivity Tn-T [illegible]	[illegible]
Borderline	[illegible]
Elevated	>52 ng/L
Others:	
Creatine kinase (CK):	24–195 U/L (males), 24–170 U/L (females)
Plasma lactate:	0.6–1.8 mmol/L
Fasting plasma glucose:	3.0–6.0 mmol/L
Haemoglobin A_1C (HbA_1C):	3.8–6.4%
Fructosamine:	<285 μmo/L
Serum amylase:	60–180 U/L
Lipids and lipoproteins:	
Cholesterol:	<5.2 mmol/L
LDL (low-density lipoprotein) cholesterol:	<3.36 mmol/L
HDL (high-density lipoprotein) cholesterol:	>1.55 mmol/L
Fasting serum triglyceride:	0.45–1.69 mmol/L

NB: These target levels vary depending on the patient's overall cardiovascular risk assessment.

Blood gases

(See respiratory chapters for further information)

H^+:	35–45 nmol/L
pH:	7.35–7.45
PaO_2:	10.6–12.6 kPa
$PaCO_2$:	4.7–6.0 kPa
Base excess:	±2 mmol/L

NB: 1 kPa = 7.6 mmHg. Atmospheric pressure is *c.* 100 kPa.

Urine

Glomerular filtration rate (GFR):	70–140 mL/min
Creatinine clearance (an estimate of GFR):	82–125 mL/min (males), 75–115 mL/min (females)
Total protein:	<150 mg/24 h
Albumin:	<30 mg/24 h
Albumin: creatinine ratio:	<3.5 mg/mmol (males), <2.5 mg/mmol (females)
Sodium:	100–250 mmol/24 h
Potassium:	14–120 mmol/24 h
Phosphate (inorganic):	15–50 mmol/24 h
Calcium:	2.5–7.5 mmol/24 h
Urobilinogen:	1.7–5.9 μmol/24 h
Osmolality:	350–1000 mosmol/kg
5-HT metabolite:	
5-Hydroxyindoleacetic acid (HIAA):	16–73 μmol/24 h
Catecholamine and metabolites:	
Noradrenaline (norepinephrine)	60–660 nmol/24 h
Adrenaline (epinephrine)	15–160 nmol/24 h
Metadrenaline (metanephrine):	0.03–0.695 μmol/mmol creatinine *or* <5.5 μmol/24 h
Hydroxymethylmandelic acid (HMMA)/ vanillomandelic acid (VMA):	16–48 μmol/24 h

NB: most centres are moving away from the measurement of VMA due to its poor relative sensitivity as compared to catecholamines and metadrenalines.

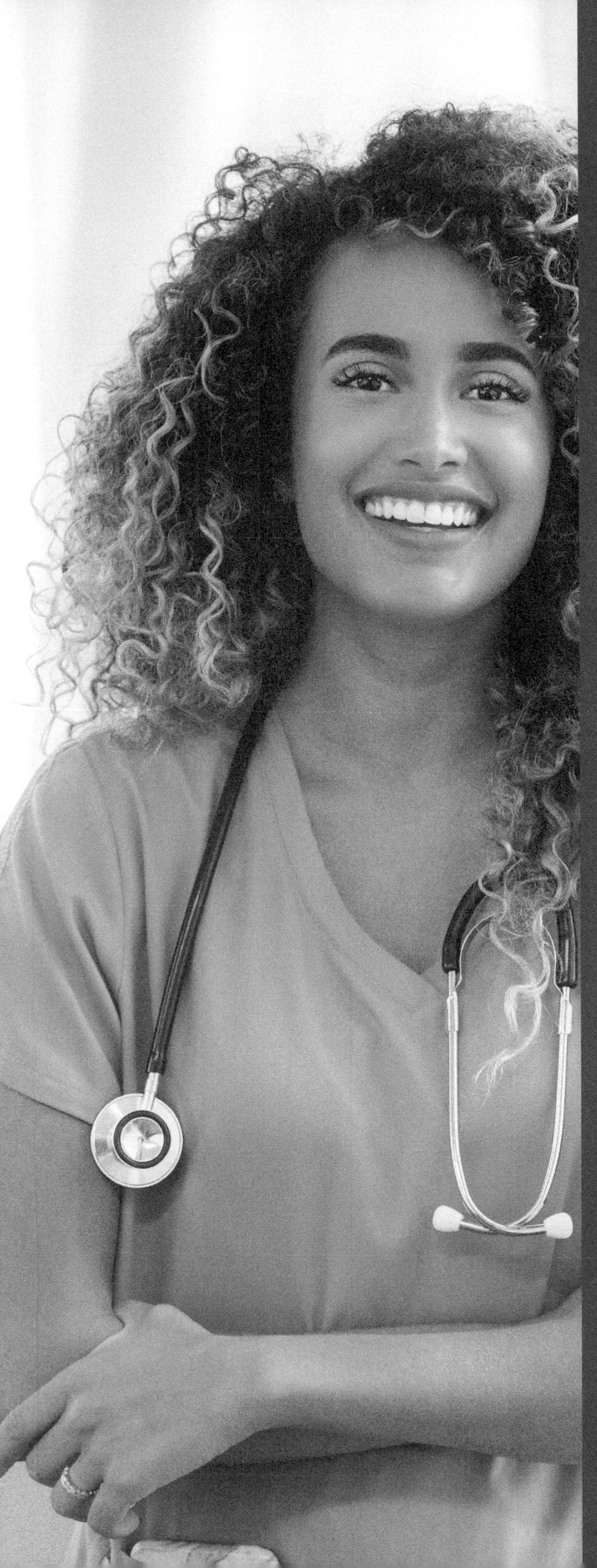

Medicine at a Glance

Fifth Edition

Edited by

Patrick Davey
Consultant Cardiologist
Northampton General Hospital
Northampton, UK

Alex Pitcher
Consultant Cardiologist
Oxford University Hospitals
Oxford, UK

WILEY Blackwell

This fifth edition first published 2024

Edition History
John Wiley & Sons, Ltd (4e, 2014); Blackwell Publishing Ltd (1e, 2002; 2e, 2006; 3e, 2010)

Registered Offices
John Wiley & Sons, Inc., 111 River Street, Hoboken, NJ 07030, USA
John Wiley & Sons Ltd, The Atrium, Southern Gate, Chichester, West Sussex, PO19 8SQ, UK

For details of our global editorial offices, customer services, and more information about Wiley products visit us at www.wiley.com.

Wiley also publishes its books in a variety of electronic formats and by print-on-demand. Some content that appears in standard print versions of this book may not be available in other formats.

Library of Congress Cataloging-in-Publication Data

Names: Davey, Patrick, editor. | Pitcher, Alex, editor.
Title: Medicine at a glance / edited by Patrick Davey, Pitcher, Alex.
Other titles: At a glance series (Oxford, England)
Description: Fifth edition. | Hoboken, NJ: Wiley-Blackwell, 2024. |
Series: At a glance | Includes bibliographical references and index.
Identifiers: LCCN 2022060475 (print) | LCCN 2022060476 (ebook) | ISBN 9781119430490 (paperback) | ISBN 9781119430438 (adobe pdf) | ISBN 9781119430445 (epub)
Subjects: MESH: Clinical Medicine | Handbook
Classification: LCC RC55 (print) | LCC RC55 (ebook) | NLM WB 39 | DDC 616–dc23/eng/20230328
LC record available at https://lccn.loc.gov/2022060475
LC ebook record available at https://lccn.loc.gov/2022060476

Cover Design: Wiley
Cover Image: © SDI Productions/E+/Getty Images

Set in 9.5/11.5 pt Minion Pro by Straive, Pondicherry, India

SKY10068377_022724

Contents

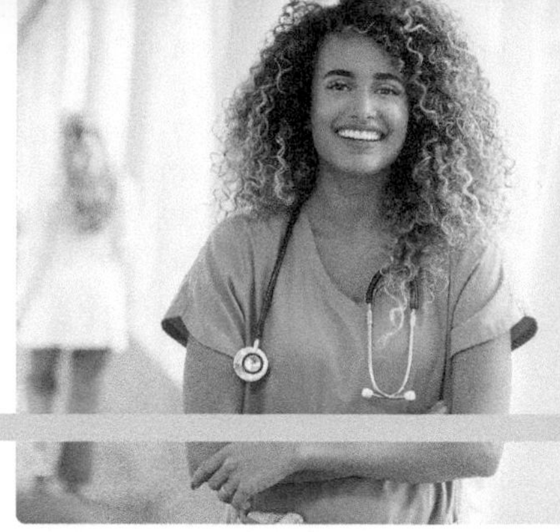

Ophthalmology

Rheumatology

Dermatology

Women's health

Other acute medical emergencies

Diseases and treatments at a glance 182

Cardiovascular disease

Respiratory disease

Gastroenterology

Renal medicine

Endocrinology

Infectious disease

Haematology

Oncology

Neurology

Rheumatology

Dermatology

Women's health

Miscellaneous

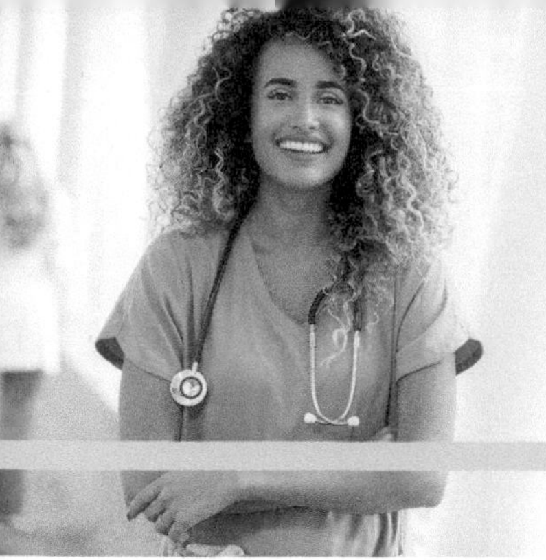

Contributors

Contributors to the fifth edition

Waseem Bakkour [Chapters 68–72, 221–229]
Consultant Dermatologist
University College London Hospitals
London, UK

Alka Bhide [Chapter 74]
Consultant Obstetrician and Gynaecologist, Urogynaecology Subspecialist
Imperial College Healthcare NHS Trust
London, UK

Chris Bunker [Chapters 68–72, 221–229]
Consultant Dermatologist and Professor of Dermatology
University College Hospitals
London, UK

Rajat Chowdhury [Chapters 197, 198]
Consultant Musculoskeletal Radiologist
Oxford University Hospitals
Oxford, UK

Patrick Davey [Chapters 1, 46]
Consultant Cardiologist
Northampton General Hospital
Northampton, UK

Suzanne Donnelly [Chapters 66, 67, 211–220]
Consultant Rheumatologist and Associate Dean (Medicine)
UCD and Mater Misericordiae University Hospital
Dublin, Ireland

Michael Dunn [Chapters 2, 3]
Associate Professor
Centre for Biomedical Ethics, National University of Singapore
Singapore

Charlotte Frise [Chapters 232–234]
Consultant Obstetric Physician
Queen Charlotte's and Chelsea Hospital
London, UK

Jonathan Gleadle [Chapters 4–9, 11, 34–36, 139–154]
Professor of Medicine
College of Medicine and Public Health, Flinders University
Adelaide, Australia

Adam Handel [Chapters 55–60, 62–64, 199–210]
Honorary Clinical Lecturer
Oxford University Hospitals
Oxford, UK

Deborah Hay [Chapters 50, 51, 53, 174–183]
Honorary Consultant Haematologist
Oxford University Hospitals
Oxford, UK

Ultan Healey [Chapters 155, 156]
Consultant Endocrinologist
Regional Hospital Mullingar
Mullingar, Ireland

Mark Juniper [Chapters 19–22, 97, 98, 101–104, 107–120]
Consultant Respiratory Physician
Great Western Hospital
Swindon, UK

Andrew Lewis [Chapters 13–18, 78, 81–96]
Clinical Lecturer in Cardiovascular Medicine
University of Oxford and Oxford University Hospitals
Oxford, UK

Josephine Lightowler [Chapters 75, 236–241]
Consultant Physician
Oxford University Hospitals
Oxford, UK

Emily Lord [Chapter 49]
Consultant in Genitourinary Medicine
Oxford University Hospitals
Oxford, UK

Mark Lythgoe [Chapters 54, 121, 136, 189–196]
Academic Clinical Fellow (Medical Oncology) and Pharmacist
Imperial College
London, UK

Alex Pitcher [Chapters 1, 184]
Consultant Cardiologist
Oxford University Hospitals
Oxford, UK

Susie Shapiro [Chapters 52, 185–188]
Associate Professor and Consultant Haematologist
Oxford University and Oxford University Hospitals
Oxford, UK

Tamsin Sleep [Chapters 61, 65]
Consultant Ophthalmologist
Torbay and South Devon NHS Trust
Torquay, UK

Gavin Spickett [Chapters 76, 77, 172, 173, 221]
Retired Consultant Immunologist
Royal Victoria Infirmary
Newcastle upon Tyne, UK

David Sprigings [Chapters 10, 79, 80]
Locum Consultant Cardiologist
Oxford University Hospitals
Oxford, UK

Jeremy Steele [Chapters 54, 121, 189–192, 196]
Consultant Medical Oncologist
St Bartholomew's Hospital
London, UK

Kevin Talbot [Chapters 55–60, 62–64, 199–210]
Professor of Neurology
University of Oxford
Oxford, UK

Laura Tookman [Chapters 54, 121, 136, 189–196]
Consultant Medical Oncologist
Imperial College Healthcare NHS Trust
London, UK

Helen Turner [Chapters 37–40, 157–163]
Consultant Endocrinologist
Oxford Centre for Diabetes, Endocrinology and Metabolism
Oxford University Hospitals
Oxford, UK

Gwilym Webb [Chapters 23–33, 122–135, 137, 138]
Consultant Hepatologist, Addenbrooke's Hospital
Cambridge University Hospitals NHS Foundation Trust
Cambridge, UK

Lisa Webber [Chapters 73, 230, 231]
Consultant Gynaecologist and Subspecialist in Reproductive Medicine, Imperial College Healthcare NHS Trust
London, UK

Matt Wise [Chapters 12, 99, 100, 105, 106, 235]
Consultant in Critical Care
University Hospital of Wales
Cardiff, UK

Charlie Woodrow [Chapters 41–45, 47, 48, 164–172, 242]
Consultant in Infectious Diseases and Acute General Medicine, Oxford University Hospitals
Oxford, UK

Sanaa Zayyan [Chapters 232–234]
Specialist Trainee in Obstetrics and Gynaecology
Oxford University Hospitals NHS Foundation Trust
Oxford, UK

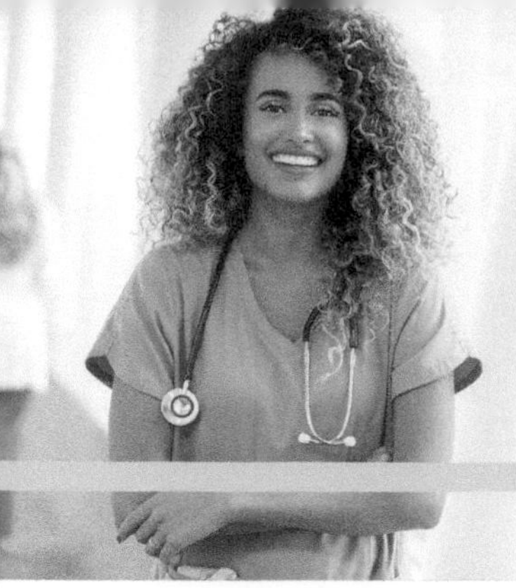

Preface

There are many challenges to studying medicine in the 2020s – the increasing complexity and subspecialization of the subject make it harder to learn, and the financial, regulatory and bureaucratic burdens are greater than ever in many countries. New exams are always being introduced, textbooks always seem to get longer, and online resources are almost infinite.

This textbook has been fully updated by active clinicians as we think medicine will be practised in 2030 and for years after and is particularly written with the next generation of doctors in mind. We focus on what is timeless in medicine as well as what is new. We lay out the key information you need to understand to get through exams, but more importantly, to understand what is happening to patients in the ward and in the clinic, and in the emergency department, across a double page, so you can see everything 'at a glance'.

We have a few thoughts which we would like you to reflect on as you study clinical medicine.

Doctors bring a huge breadth of skills to their interactions with patients – empathy, compassion, tact, knowledge, resilience, kindness, motor skills – but the most important one for most of us, and the one which you must learn first, is the ability to make a diagnosis. Novices (and even senior doctors), when encountering a new disease or clinical problem, are usually far too keen to know how to treat it, but the first step is to make an accurate and precise diagnosis. Great doctors make it look very easy but it rarely is, and learning to do it reliably takes many years of practice, reflection and humility.

However, that skill, once gained, is not easily lost, is of extreme value, and will help to avoid subjecting your patients in the future to much needless overinvestigation – and can be lifesaving.

So, how do doctors make a diagnosis? You need knowledge and skills. The most important skills are in history taking, examination and interpreting the results of tests, and then in integrating all this information – putting it all together.

It is important to remember that the history is an iterative process – it can and should often be repeated to clarify some important point that the clinician or patient has overlooked. The finding, for example, of an elevated mean cell volume on a full blood count will prompt the experienced clinician to retake the alcohol history; finding a long QT interval on the ECG will prompt a revisiting of the family history for any evidence of sudden cardiac death, even in remote family members, which might be of little significance had the ECG been normal.

There are three dangers to which we would like to draw your attention.

The first danger is sending a patient home with a diagnosis that is essentially a restatement of what they told you. For example, if a patient presents with chest pain, and you send them home with a so-called 'diagnosis' of 'chest pain? cause' (pronounced, apparently, 'chest pain query cause'), you have not made a diagnosis, you have simply restated to the patient (and the GP) the dilemma which they brought to you. This approach will from time to time result in missing a very dangerous diagnosis, and is usually the diagnosis made hours before a fatal aortic dissection finally ruptures. That condition is usually diagnosed by sudden-onset chest or back pain and is not extremely rare, can occur in young people, and should be considered in all cases of sudden-onset chest or back pain.

A second – almost opposite – problem is overprecision. Like people who give their weight to four decimal places, it is not a good idea to give a precise diagnosis when you really don't know what is happening. Some patients with chest pain elude diagnosis by even the most skilled diagnostician, so a diagnosis of 'chest pain of uncertain cause, but no evidence of ACS, PE or aortic dissection' is preferable to 'costochondritis' when there is no actual evidence that there is any costochondritis at all. These diagnostic inventions close off the mind of the next doctor and are not really honest.

A third problem is the 'exclusion' paradigm. It is not often possible to exclude anything in medicine. The CTPA does not exclude a pulmonary embolism; they will occasionally be missed by even experienced radiologists, or they might have been looking at the wrong CT – it has happened, we are sure. So we can only ever increase or decrease the probability of a diagnosis. This is a much more sophisticated way of thinking about diagnosis, and will serve you well when you move toward more difficult diagnoses.

One of us was taught to have five differential diagnoses for every case, and the other was taught to have three, but always including the most dangerous one. The point is not to think too narrowly at the beginning, or leap to the first diagnosis that comes to mind and assume that when that is supposedly 'excluded' all must be well – it may not be.

The key point is that you must carefully construct a differential diagnosis for each patient. Sometimes it will be obvious within a few minutes which is correct; sometimes the patient will actually have a problem list of a dozen or more diagnoses, especially in the frail elderly or in the critically ill.

The rewards of really understanding what is wrong with patients, using the clinical approach emphasized in this book, will repay you for the rest of your career, which, despite the challenges, remains one of the most satisfying students can choose.

We hope this book will give you just the right amount of detail you need to know to start you on your journey to becoming a brilliant diagnostician – an important part of being a great doctor.

Patrick Davey
Alex Pitcher
Oxford 2023

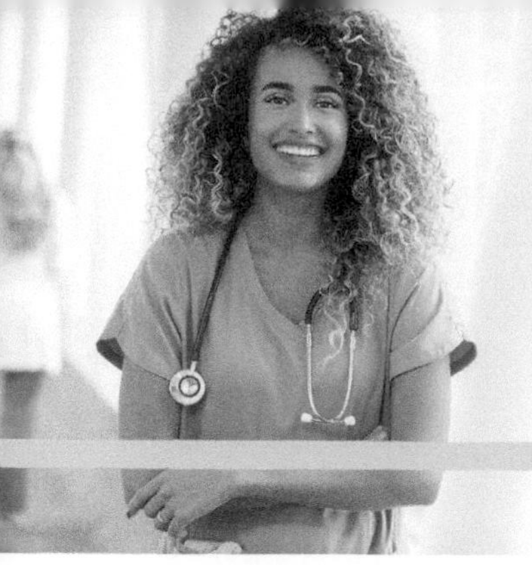

Acknowledgements

The editor, contributing authors and publishers would like to thank all those people who gave their time and expertise to advise us during the writing process of both this and previous editions. The specialist reviewers and medical students who reviewed material for the first edition were invaluable in shaping the final book and we would like to thank them unreservedly for their contribution. Thanks to Yassir Javaid for assistance with preparation of the cardiovascular MCQs. Patrick Davey dedicates this book to Anna Rathmell-Davey. Alex Pitcher dedicates this book to Olivia, Steve, Theo and Esther.

In addition, we would like to acknowledge the following individuals and companies for their kind permission to re-use material. Although the majority of the artwork in *Medicine at a Glance* is new, some tables and figures have been redrawn from other sources. The editor and publishers have made every effort to contact all the copyright holders to obtain their permission to reproduce copyright material. However, if any have been inadvertently overlooked, the publisher will be pleased to make the necessary arrangements at the first opportunity.

The editors and publisher would like to thank the following authors who contributed to previous editions:

Keith Channon, Arani Chandrakumar, Graham Collins, Peggy Frith, Daniel Glass, David Keeling, David Lalloo, Tim J. Littlewood, Grace McGeogh, Richard Penson, Anna Rathmell, Jeremy Shearman, Chin Whybrew, Paul Wordsworth

Books

Abraham, S., Kulkarni, K., Madhu, R. & Provan, D. The Hands-on Guide to Data Interpretation. Blackwell Publishing, Oxford, 2010.

Baran, R. & Dawber, R. Diseases of the Nails and their Management, 2nd edn. Blackwell Science, Oxford, 2001.

Baran, R., de Berker, D. & Dawber, R. Manual of Nail Disease and Surgery. Blackwell Science, Oxford, 1997.

Bourke, S. & Brewis, R. Lecture Notes on Respiratory Medicine, 5th edn. Blackwell Science, Oxford, 1998.

Champion, R.H., Burton, J.L. Burns, T. & Breathnach, S. (eds) Rook's Textbook of Dermatology, 6th edn. Blackwell Science, Oxford, 1998.

Chapel, H., Heaney, M., Misbah, S. & Snowden, N. Essentials of Clinical Immunology, 4th edn. Blackwell Science, Oxford, 1999.

Chowdhury, R, Wilson, I, Rofe, C & Lloyd-Jones, G. Radiology at a Glance. Wiley Blackwell, Oxford, 2010.

Gleadle, J. History and Examination at a Glance, 2nd edn. Wiley-Blackwell, Oxford, 2007.

Haslett, C., Boon, N., Colledge, N. et al. Davidson's Principles and Practice of Medicine, 18th edn. Churchill Livingstone, Edinburgh, 1999.

Hoffbrand, V., Moss, P. & Pettit, J. Essential Haematology, 4th edn. Blackwell Science, Oxford, 2001.

Howlett, D. & Ayers, B. The Hands-on Guide to Imaging. Blackwell Publishing, Oxford, 2004.

Hunter, J. & Savin, J. Clinical Dermatology, 2nd edn. Blackwell Science, Oxford, 1994.

Katona, C., Cooper, C. & Robertson, M. Psychiatry at a Glance, 4th edn. Wiley-Blackwell, Oxford, 2008.

Kumar, P. & Clark, M. (eds) Clinical Medicine, 4th edn. W.B. Saunders, Philadelphia, 1998.

Leach, R. Critical Care Medicine at a Glance. Blackwell Publishing, Oxford, 2004.

Mehta, A. & Hoffbrand, V. Haematology at a Glance. Blackwell Science, Oxford, 2000.

Munro, J. & Edwards, C. McLeod's Clinical Examination, 10th edn. Churchill Livingstone, Edinburgh, 2000.

Norwitz, E. & Schorge, J. Obstetrics and Gynecology at a Glance, 4th edn. Wiley Blackwell, Oxford, 2013.

Olver, J. & Cassidy, L. Ophthalmology at a Glance. Blackwell Publishing, Oxford, 2005.

Patel, P.R. Lecture Notes: Radiology, 2nd edn. Blackwell Publishing, Oxford, 2005.

Patton, K. Handbook for Anatomy and Physiology. Mosby, St Louis, 2000.

Rubenstein, E. & Federman, D.D. (eds) Scientific American Medicine, Wed MD Professional Publishing, 2003.

Sherlock, S. & Dooley, J. Diseases of the Liver and Biliary System, 11th edn. Blackwell Science, Oxford, 2002.

Warlow, C.P., Dennis, M.S., van Gijn, J. et al. (eds) Stroke: A Practical Guide, 2nd edn. Blackwell Science, Oxford, 2001.

Waye, J.D., Rex, D. & Williams, C. Colonoscopy: Principles and Practice. Blackwell Publishing, Oxford, 2003 (figures used are by Dr Michael Macari).

Weatherall, D. (ed.) Oxford Textbook of Medicine, 3rd edn. Oxford University Press, Oxford, 1995.

Journals

Hamm C.W. et al. ESC Guidelines for the management of acute coronary syndromes in patients presenting without persistent ST-segment elevation: The Task Force for the management of acute coronary syndromes (ACS) in patients presenting without persistent ST-segment elevation of the European Society of Cardiology (ESC). Eur Heart J 2011: 32(23): 2999–3054. doi:10.1093/eurheartj/ehr236. Reproduced with permission of Oxford University Press (UK) © European Society of Cardiology.

European Heart Rhythm Association et al. Guidelines for the management of atrial fibrillation: the Task Force for the Management of Atrial Fibrillation of the European Society of Cardiology (ESC). Eur Heart J 2010: 31(19): 2369–429. Reproduced with permission of Oxford University Press.

Langford, C. & Hoffman, G. Wegener's granulomatosis. Thorax 1999: 54; 629–37.

Soteriodes, E.S., Evans, J.C., Lanon, M.G. et al. Incidence and prognosis of syncope. New Engl J Med 2002: 347; 878–85.

Thadhani, R., Pascual, M. & Bonventre, J.V. Acute renal failure. N Engl J Med 1996: 334; 1448–60.

Other

Adult Advanced Life Support Guidelines. Resuscitation Council, 2010.

Special thanks to Dr Mansel Heaney for providing the cANCA figure for Chapter 147.

Nelson, M., Department of Medical Illustration and Photography, Chelsea and Westminster Hospital, London.

National Institute for Health and Care Excellence. CG 103 Delirium: diagnosis, prevention and management. London, 2010. NICE. Available from http://guidance.nice.org.uk/CG103. Reproduced with permission.

NEWS: standardising the assessment of acute illness severity in the NHS. Report of a working party. London, RCP, 2012. Reproduced with permission from the Royal College of Physicians. The chart is reproduced for reference only. For clinical use, please visit www.rcplondon.ac.uk/resources/national-early-warning-score-news where full-sized versions with instructions and guidance for use may be downloaded.

ONS: Cancer Statistics Registrations: Registrations of Cancers Diagnosed in 2001 England. ONS, Crown copyright, 2004.

World Health Organization. The World Health Report 2000: Health Systems: Improving Performance. Reproduced with permission of WHO.

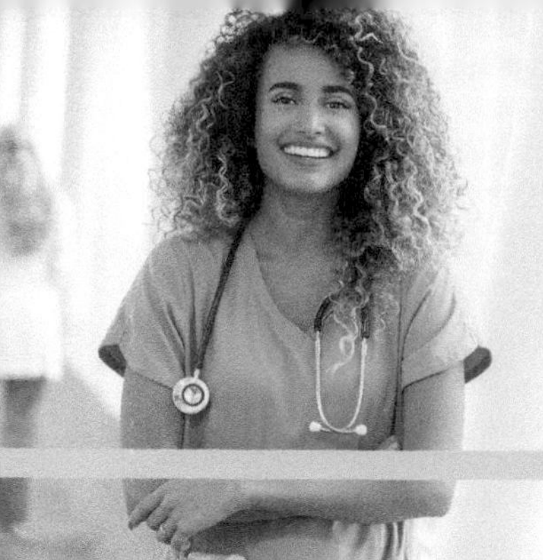

Abbreviations

AA	autoantibody
AAA	abdominal aortic aneurysm
Ab	antibody
ABC	airway, breathing and circulation
ABG	arterial blood gas
ABPA	allergic bronchopulmonary aspergillosis
AC	acromioclavicular
ACE	angiotensin-converting enzyme
ACS	acute coronary syndrome
ACTH	adrenocorticotrophic hormone
ADC	apparent diffusion coefficient
ADH	antidiuretic hormone
ADP	adenosine diphosphate
A&E	Accident and Emergency
AF	atrial fibrillation
AFB	acid-fast bacilli
Ag	antigen
AIDS	acquired immune deficiency syndrome
AIHA	autoimmune haemolytic anaemia
AION	anterior ischaemic optic neuropathy
AKI	acute kidney injury
ALL	acute lymphoid leukaemia
ALP	alkaline phosphatase
ALS	advanced life support
ALT	alanine transaminase
AMA	antimitochondrial antibody
AML	acute myeloid leukaemia
ANA	antinuclear antibody
ANCA	antineutrophil cytoplasmic antibody
ANF	antinuclear factor
Ao	aorta
APC	activated protein C
APKD	adult polycystic kidney disease
APS	antiphospholipid syndrome
APTT	activated partial thromboplastin time
AR	aortic regurgitation
ARB	angiotensin receptor blockers
ARDS	adult respiratory distress syndrome
ART	anti-retroviral therapy
AS	ankylosing spondylitis
ASD	atrial septal defect
ASO	antistreptolysin O
AST	aspartate transaminase
α_1-AT	α_1-antitrypsin
ATLL	adult T-cell lymphoma/leukaemia
ATN	acute tubular necrosis
ATP	adenosine triphosphate
AV	atrioventricular
AVNRT	atrioventricular nodal re-entrant tachycardia
AVRT	atrioventricular re-entrant tachycardia
AXR	abdominal X-ray
BAL	bronchoalveolar lavage
BBB	bundle branch block
BCC	basal cell carcinoma
BCE	basal cell epithelioma
BCG	bacilli Calmette–Guérin
bd	*bis die* (twice a day)
BDZ	benzodiazepine
BE	base excess
BLS	basic life support
BM	Boehringer Mannheim bedside testing stix
BMD	bone mineral density
BMI	body mass index
BMZ	basement membrane zone
BNF	*British National Formulary*
BOOP	bronchiolitis obliterans organizing pneumonia
BP	blood pressure
bpm	beats per minute
BRVO	branch retinal vein occlusion
CABG	coronary artery bypass graft
CAD	coronary artery disease
CAH	congenital adrenal hyperplasia
CAM	Confusion Assessment Method
cAMP	cyclic adenosine monophosphate

CBD	common bile duct
CBT	cognitive behavioural therapy
CCP	cyclic citrullinated peptide
CCU	coronary care unit
CF	cystic fibrosis
CFA	cryptogenic fibrosis alveolitis
CFS	chronic fatigue syndrome
CFTR	cystic fibrosis transmembrane conductance regulator
cGMP	cyclic guanosine monophosphate
CHAD	cold haemagglutinin disease
CHB	complete heart block
CHD	congenital heart disease
CHF	chronic heart failure
CHOP	cyclophosphamide, hydroxydaunorubicin, oncovin, prednisolone
CIDP	chronic idiopathic demyelinating polyneuropathy
CJD	Creutzfeldt–Jakob disease
CK	creatine kinase
CLD	chronic liver disease
CLL	chronic lymphoblastic leukaemia
CLO	*Campylobacter*-like organism test
CMC	carpometacarpal
CML	chronic myeloid leukaemia
CMV	cytomegalovirus
CNS	central nervous system
CO	carbon monoxide
CO_2	carbon dioxide
COPD	chronic obstructive pulmonary disease
COX	cyclo-oxygenase
CP	chest pain
CPAP	continuous positive airway pressure
CPK	creatine phosphokinase
CPR	cardiopulmonary resuscitation
CREST	calcinosis, Raynaud's, oesophagitis, sclerodactyly telangiectasia
CRF	chronic renal failure
CRH	corticotrophin-releasing hormone
CRP	C-reactive protein
CRT	cardiac resynchronization therapy
CRVO	central retinal vein occlusion
CS	Churg–Strauss; coronary sinus
CSF	cerebrospinal fluid
CT	computed tomography
CVA	cerebrovascular accident
CVID	common variable immunodeficiency
CVP	central venous pressure; cyclophosphamide, vincristine, prednisolone
CWP	coal worker's pneumoconiosis
CXR	chest X-ray
CYP	cytochrome P450
DAS	disease activity score
DC	direct current
DCIS	ductal carcinoma *in situ*
DCM	dilated cardiomyopathies
ddAVP	deamino-D-arginine vasopressin
DEXA	dual emission X-ray absorptiometry
DHEA	dehydroepiandrosterone
DHF/DSS	dengue haemorrhagic fever/dengue shock syndrome
DIC	disseminated intravascular coagulation
DIP	distal interphalangeal
DKA	diabetic ketoacidosis
DM	dermatomyositis, diabetes mellitus
DMARD	disease-modifying antirheumatic drug
DMSA	[^{99m}Tc] mercaptosuccinic acid
DNA	deoxyribonucleic acid
DNAR	'do not attempt resuscitation'
dsDNA	double-stranded DNA
DTPA	diethylene triamine penta-acetic acid
DU	duodenal ulcer
D&V	diarrhoea and vomiting
DVT	deep venous thrombosis
DWI	diffusion-weighted imaging
EAA	extrinsic allergic alveolitis
EBV	Epstein–Barr virus
ECG	electrocardiogram
ECT	electroconvulsant therapy
EDH	extradural haematoma
EEG	electroencephalograph
EGFR	epidermal growth factor receptor
ELISA	enzyme-linked immunosorbent assay
EM	electron microscopy
EMG	electromyography
EN	erythema nodosum
ENT	ear, nose, throat
ER	oestrogen receptor
ERA	enteric reactive arthritis
ERCP	endoscopic retrograde cholangiopancreatography
ESR	erythrocyte sedimentation rate
ESRF	end-stage renal failure
ETG	epidermal transglutaminase
EULAR	European League Against Rheumatism
EUS	endoscopic ultrasound
FAB	French–American–British

FBC full blood count
FDG fluorodeoxyglucose
FDP fibrin degradation product
FEV$_1$ forced expiratory volume in 1 second
FFA free fatty acid
FFP fresh frozen plasma
FLAIR fluid-attenuated inversion recovery sequences
FNA fine needle aspirate
FNAC fine needle aspiration cytology
FOB faecal occult blood
α-FP alpha fetoprotein
FRC functional residual capacity
FSGS focal segmental glomerulosclerosis
FSH follicle-stimulating hormone
FTD frontotemporal dementia
FUO fever of unknown origin
FVC forced vital capacity
GABA γ-aminobutyric acid
GBM glomerular basement membrane
GCS Glasgow Coma Score
GFR glomerular filtration rate
GH growth hormone
GI gastrointestinal
GIST gastrointestinal stromal tumour
GN glomerulonephritis
GnRH gonadotrophin-releasing hormone
GORD gastro-oesophageal reflux disease
Gp glycoprotein
GP general practitioner
G6PD glucose-6-phosphate dehydrogenase
GPA granulomatosis with polyangiitis
GPI glycosyl-phosphatidylinositol
γ-GT γ-glutamyl transferase
GTN glyceryl trinitrate
GU genitourinary
HAART highly active anti-retroviral therapy
HAE hereditary angioedema
HAIR-AN hyperandrogenism, insulin resistance and acanthosis nigricans
HAV hepatitis A virus
Hb haemoglobin
HBc hepatitis B core antigen
HBeAg hepatitis B e antigen
HBsAg hepatitis B surface antigen
HBV hepatitis B virus
HCC hepatocellular carcinoma
hCG human chorionic gonadotrophin
HCM hypertrophic cardiomyopathy
Hct haematocrit
HCV hepatitis C virus
HD Huntington's disease
HDL high-density lipoprotein
HER-2 human epidermal growth factor receptor 2
HHS hyperosmolar hyperglycaemic state
HHV human herpes virus
5-HIAA 5-hydroxyindoleacetic acid
HiB *Haemophilus influenzae* B
HIV human immunodeficiency virus
HLA human leukocyte antigen
HMG-CoA hydroxymethyl-glutaryl coenzyme A
HMMA hydroxymethylmandelic acid
HNF hepatocyte nuclear factor
HNPCC hereditary non-polyposis colon cancer
HPV human papillomavirus
HR heart rate
HRCT high-resolution computed tomography
HRT hormone replacement therapy
HSCT human stem cell transplantation
HSP Henoch–Schönlein purpura
HSV herpes simplex virus
5-HT 5-hydroxytryptamine (serotonin)
HTLV human T-cell leukaemia virus
HUS haemolytic uraemic syndrome
IBD inflammatory bowel disease
ICD implantable cardiovertor defibrillator
ICD-10 International Classification of Diseases version 10
ICH intracerebral haemorrhage
Ig immunoglobulin
IGF insulin-like growth factor
IHD ischaemic heart disease
IL interleukin
IM intramuscular
INR international normalized ratio
IP intrathoracic pressure
IPPV intermittent positive pressure ventilation
IRIS immune reconstitution inflammatory syndrome
ITP immune thrombocytopenic purpura
ITU intensive therapy unit
IUGR intrauterine fetal growth restriction
IV intravenous
IVC inferior vena cava
IVU intravenous urogram/ureography
JC John Cunningham virus
JVP jugular venous pressure
KCl potassium chloride
KOH potassium hydroxide

KS	Kaposi's sarcoma
LA	left atrium
LAD	left anterior descending
LBB	left bundle branch
LCA	leukocytoclastic angiitis
LCIS	lobular carcinoma *in situ*
LDH	lactate dehydrogenase
LDL	low-density lipoprotein
LFT	liver function test
LH	luteinizing hormone
LH-RH	luteinizing hormone-releasing hormone
LMN	lower motor neuron
LMNOP	lasix (diuresis), morphine, Na^{2+} and water restriction, oxygen and position upright
LMW	low molecular weight
LMWH	low-molecular-weight heparin
LN	lymph nodes
LP	lumbar puncture
LRP	lipoprotein related receptor protein
LSD	lysergic acid diethylamide
LTOT	long-term oxygen therapy
LTRA	leukotriene antagonists
LUQ	left upper quadrant
LV	left ventricle, left ventricular
LVH	left ventricular hypertrophy
MAC	*Mycobacterium avium-intracellulare* complex
MALDI	matrix-assisted laser desorption/ionization
MALT	mucosa-associated lymphoid tissue
MAO	monoamine oxidase inhibitors
MCA	middle cerebral artery
MCH	mean corpuscular haemoglobin
MCHC	mean cell haemoglobin concentration
MCP	metacarpophalangeal
M,C&S	microscopy, culture and sensitivity
MCV	mean cell volume
MDMA	3,4 methylenedioxymethamphetamine (ecstasy)
MDR	multidrug resistant
MDS	myelodysplastic syndrome
MDT	multidisciplinary team
ME	myalgic encephalomyelitis
MELAS	mitochondrial encephalopathy, lactic acidosis, stroke-like episodes
MEN	multiple endocrine neoplasia
MGUS	monoclonal gammopathy of uncertain significance
MHC	major histocompatibility complex
MI	myocardial infarction
MND	motor neuron disease
MODY	maturity-onset diabetes in the young
MR	mitral regurgitation
MRCP	magnetic resonance cholangiopancreatography
MRI	magnetic resonance imaging
MRSA	methicillin-resistant *Staphylococcus aureus*
MS	multiple sclerosis
MSA	multiple system atrophy
MSU	midstream urine
MTP	metatarsophalangeal
MUS	medically unexplained symptom
MV	mechanical ventilation
MVP	mitral valve prolapse
NaCl	sodium chloride
NADPH	reduced nicotinamide adenine dinucleotide phosphate
NEWS	NHS Early Warning Score
NF	nuclear factor
NG	nasogastric
NGU	non-gonococcal urethritis
NHL	non-Hodgkin's lymphoma
NHS	National Health Service
NICE	National Institute for Health and Care Excellence
NIV	non-invasive ventilation
NMO	neuromyelitis optica
NO	nitric oxide
NPV	negative pressure ventilation
NQMI	non-Q wave myocardial infarction
NSAID	non-steroidal anti-inflammatory drug
NYHA	New York Heart Association
OA	osteoarthritis
OCP	oral contraceptive pill
od	*omni die* (once a day)
OGD	oesophago-gastroduodenoscopy
OSA	obstructive sleep apnoea
PA	posteroanterior, pulmonary artery
PAN	polyarteritis nodosa
PARP	poly (adenosine diphosphate ribose) polymerase
PBC	primary biliary cirrhosis
PCI	percutaneous coronary intervention
PCOS	polycystic ovary syndrome
PCP	phencyclidine, *Pneumocystis carinii* (*jirovecii*) pneumonia
PCR	polymerase chain reaction
PCV	packed cell volume
PCWP	pulmonary capillary wedge pressure

PD	proton density
PDA	patent ductus arteriosus
PE	pulmonary embolism
PEEP	positive end-expiratory pressure
PEFR	peak expiratory flow rate
PEG	percutaneous endoscopic gastrostomy
PET	positron emission tomography
PGE_1	prostaglandin E_1
PID	pelvic inflammatory disease
PION	posterior ischaemic optic neuropathy
PIP	proximal interphalangeal
PKD	polycystic kidney disease
PM	polymyositis
PML	progressive multifocal leukoencephalopathy
PMR	polymyalgia rheumatica
PND	paroxysmal nocturnal dyspnoea
PNH	paroxysmal nocturnal haemoglobinuria
PNS	peripheral nervous system
PPI	proton pump inhibitor
PR	per rectum
PRL	prolactin
PrP	prion protein
PRV	polycythaemia rubra vera
PS	psychoactive substance
PSA	prostrate-specific antigen
PSC	primary sclerosing cholangitis
PT	prothrombin time
PTH	parathyroid hormone
PTHrP	parathyroid hormone-related protein
PTT	partial thromboplastin time
PUO	pyrexia of unknown origin
PUVA	psoralen and ultraviolet A
PVD	peripheral vascular disease
PVR	post-void residual
RA	rheumatoid arthritis, right atrium
RANK	receptor activator of nuclear factor κB
RANKL	receptor activator of nuclear factor κB ligand
RBB	right bundle branch
RBC	red blood cell
RE	reticuloendothelial
REM	rapid eye movement
RF	rheumatoid factor
RNA	ribonucleic acid
RNP	ribonucleic protein
RP	retinitis pigmentosa
rpm	respirations per minute
RR	respiratory rate
RTA	renal tubular acidosis
RUQ	right upper quadrant
RV	right ventricle, right ventricular
RVF	right ventricular failure
RVH	right ventricular hypertrophy
SA	sinoatrial
SACD	subacute combined degeneration of the cord
SAH	subarachnoid haemorrhage
SARA	sexually acquired reactive arthritis
SBE	subacute bacterial endocarditis
SCC	squamous cell carcinoma
SCID	severe combined immunodeficiency
SCLC	small cell lung cancer
SDH	subdural haematoma
SHBG	sex hormone-binding globulin
SIADH	syndrome of inappropriate antidiuretic hormone secretion
SIJ	sacro-iliac joint
SK	streptokinase
SLE	systemic lupus erythematosus
SMA	smooth muscle antibody
SOB	shortness of breath
SPECT	single photon emission computed tomography
SR	sinus rhythm
SRH	stigmata of recent haemorrhage
STD	sexually transmitted disease
STEMI	ST segment elevation myocardial infarction
SUA	serum uric acid
SUI	stress urinary incontinence
SVC	superior vena cava
SVT	supraventricular tachycardia
T_3	triiodothyronine
T_4	thyroxine
TACS	total anterior circulation syndrome
TB	tuberculosis
tds	*ter die sumendus* (3 times a day)
TED	thromboembolic
TGF	transforming growth factor
TIA	transient ischaemic attack
TIBC	total iron-binding capacity
TIH	tumour-induced hypercalcaemia
TIMP-1	tissue inhibitor of metalloproteinase 1
TIPSS	transjugular intrahepatic portosystemic stent shunt
TLC	total lung capacity
TMJ	temporomandibular joint
TNF	tumour necrosis factor
tPA	tissue plasminogen activator

TRUS	transrectal ultrasonography
TSH	thyroid-stimulating hormone
TT	thrombin time
TTP	thrombotic thrombocytopenic purpura
TURP	transurethral resection of the prostate
UC	ulcerative colitis
U&Es	urea and electrolytes
UFH	unfractionated heparin
UMN	upper motor neuron
URTI	upper respiratory tract infection
USS	ultrasound
UTI	urinary tract infection
UV	ultraviolet
UVB	ultraviolet B
VC	vital capacity
VDRL	venereal disease research laboratory
VEGF	vascular endothelium growth factor
VEP	visual evoked potential
VF	ventricular fibrillation
VIN	vulval intraepithelial neoplasia
VIP	vasoactive intestinal peptide
VLDL	very-low-density lipoprotein
VMA	vanillomandelic acid
$\dot{V}/\dot{Q}$	ventilation/perfusion
VSD	ventricular septal defect
VT	ventricular tachycardia
vWD	von Willebrand's disease
vWF	von Willebrand's factor
VZV	varicella-zoster virus
WCC	white cell count
WHO	World Health Organization
WoB	work of breathing
WPW	Wolff–Parkinson–White

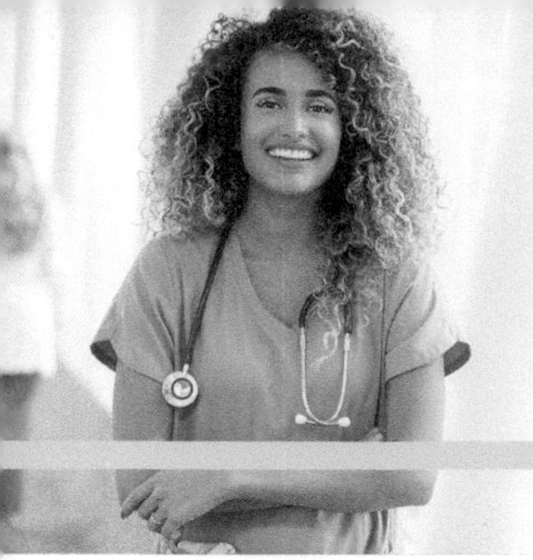

How to use your revision guide

Features contained within your textbook

The overview page gives a summary of the topics covered in each part.

Clinical presentations at a glance

Part 2

Each topic is presented in a double-page spread with clear, easy-to-follow diagrams supported by succinct explanatory text.

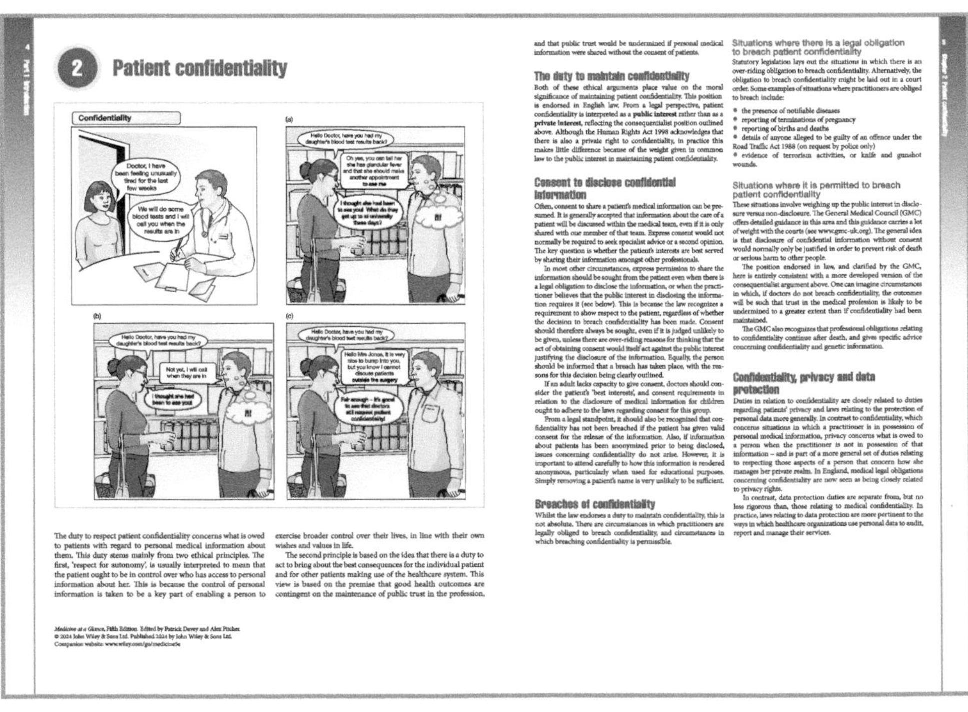

2 Patient confidentiality

The duty to respect patient confidentiality concerns what is owed to patients with regard to personal medical information about them. This duty stems mainly from two ethical principles. The first, 'respect for autonomy', is usually interpreted to mean that the patient ought to be in control over who has access to personal information about her. This is because the control of personal information is taken to be a key part of enabling a person to exercise broader control over their lives, in line with their own wishes and values in life.

The second principle is based on the idea that there is a duty to act to bring about the best consequences for the individual patient and for other patients making use of the healthcare system. This view is based on the premise that good health outcomes are contingent on the maintenance of public trust in the profession, and that public trust would be undermined if personal medical information were shared without the consent of patients.

Medicine at a Glance, Fifth Edition. Edited by Patrick Davey and Alex Pitcher.
© 2024 John Wiley & Sons Ltd. Published 2024 by John Wiley & Sons Ltd.
Companion website: www.wiley.com/go/medicine5e

The duty to maintain confidentiality

Both of these ethical arguments place value on the moral significance of maintaining patient confidentiality. This position is endorsed in English law. From a legal perspective, patient confidentiality is interpreted as a **public interest** rather than as a **private interest**, reflecting the consequentialist position outlined above. Although the Human Rights Act 1998 acknowledges that there is also a private right to confidentiality, in practice this makes little difference because of the weight given in common law to the public interest in maintaining patient confidentiality.

Consent to disclose confidential information

Often, consent to share a patient's medical information can be presumed. It is generally accepted that information about the care of a patient will be discussed within the medical team, even if it is only shared with one member of that team. Express consent would not normally be required to seek specialist advice or a second opinion. The key question is whether the patient's interests are best served by sharing their information amongst other professionals.

In most other circumstances, express permission to share the information should be sought from the patient even when there is a legal obligation to disclose the information, or when the practitioner believes that the public interest in disclosing the information requires it (see below). This is because the law recognizes a requirement to show respect to the patient, regardless of whether the decision to breach confidentiality has been made. Consent should therefore always be sought, even if it is judged unlikely to be given, unless there are over-riding reasons for thinking that the act of obtaining consent would itself act against the public interest justifying the disclosure of the information. Equally, the person should be informed that a breach has taken place, with the reasons for this decision being clearly outlined.

If an adult lacks capacity to give consent, doctors should consider the patient's 'best interests', and consent requirements in relation to the disclosure of medical information for children ought to adhere to the laws regarding consent for this group.

From a legal standpoint, it should also be recognized that confidentiality has not been breached if the patient has given valid consent for the release of the information. Also, if information about patients has been anonymized prior to being disclosed, issues concerning confidentiality do not arise. However, it is important to attend carefully to how this information is rendered anonymous, particularly when used for educational purposes. Simply removing a patient's name is very unlikely to be sufficient.

Breaches of confidentiality

Whilst the law endorses a duty to maintain confidentiality, this is not absolute. There are circumstances in which practitioners are legally obliged to breach confidentiality, and circumstances in which breaching confidentiality is permissible.

Situations where there is a legal obligation to breach patient confidentiality

Statutory legislation lays out the situations in which there is an over-riding obligation to breach confidentiality. Alternatively, the obligation to breach confidentiality might be laid out in a court order. Some examples of situations where practitioners are obliged to breach include:

- the presence of notifiable diseases
- reporting of terminations of pregnancy
- reporting of births and deaths
- details of anyone alleged to be guilty of an offence under the Road Traffic Act 1988 (on request by police only)
- evidence of terrorism activities, or knife and gunshot wounds.

Situations where it is permitted to breach patient confidentiality

These situations involve weighing up the public interest in disclosure versus non-disclosure. The General Medical Council (GMC) offers detailed guidance in this area and this guidance carries a lot of weight with the courts (see www.gmc-uk.org). The general idea is that disclosure of confidential information without consent would normally only be justified in order to prevent risk of death or serious harm to other people.

The position endorsed in law, and clarified by the GMC, here is entirely consistent with a more developed version of the consequentialist argument above. One can imagine circumstances in which, if doctors do not breach confidentiality, the outcomes will be such that trust in the medical profession is likely to be undermined to a greater extent than if confidentiality had been maintained.

The GMC also recognizes that professional obligations relating to confidentiality continue after death, and gives specific advice concerning confidentiality and genetic information.

Confidentiality, privacy and data protection

Duties in relation to confidentiality are closely related to duties regarding patients' privacy and laws relating to the protection of personal data more generally. In contrast to confidentiality, which concerns situations in which a practitioner is in possession of personal medical information, privacy concerns what is owed to a person when the practitioner is not in possession of that information – and is part of a more general set of duties relating to respecting those aspects of a person that concern how she manages her private realm. In England, medical legal obligations concerning confidentiality are now seen as being closely related to privacy rights.

In contrast, data protection duties are separate from, but no less rigorous than, those relating to medical confidentiality. In practice, laws relating to data protection are more pertinent to the ways in which healthcare organizations use personal data to audit, report and manage their services.

Your revision guide is full of **photographs, illustrations and tables.**

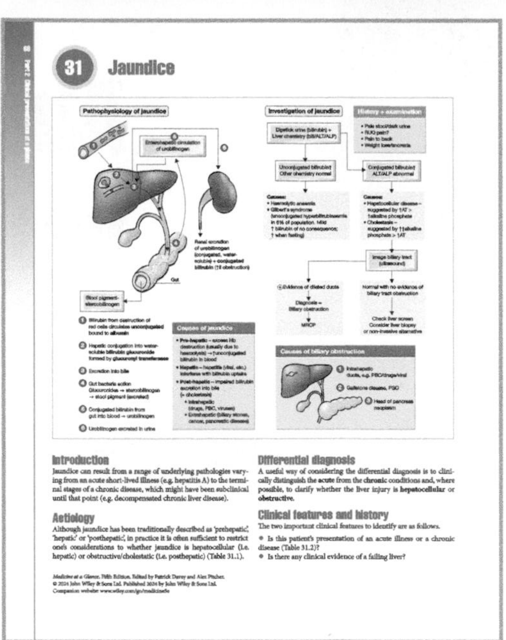

31 Jaundice

Introduction

Jaundice can result from a range of underlying pathologies varying from an acute short-lived illness (e.g. hepatitis A) to the terminal stages of a chronic disease, which might have been subclinical until that point (e.g. decompensated chronic liver disease).

Aetiology

Although jaundice has been traditionally described as 'prehepatic', 'hepatic' or 'posthepatic', in practice it is often sufficient to restrict one's considerations to whether jaundice is hepatocellular (i.e. hepatic) or obstructive/cholestatic (i.e. posthepatic) (Table 31.1).

Differential diagnosis

A useful way of considering the differential diagnosis is to clinically distinguish the **acute** from the **chronic** conditions and, where possible, to clarify whether the liver injury is **hepatocellular** or **obstructive.**

Clinical features and history

The two important clinical features to identify are as follows.

- Is this patient's presentation of an acute illness or a chronic disease (Table 31.2)?
- Is there any clinical evidence of a failing liver?

The website icon indicates that you can find accompanying resources on the book's companion website **www.wiley.com/go/medicine5e**

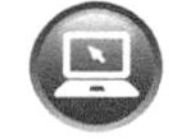

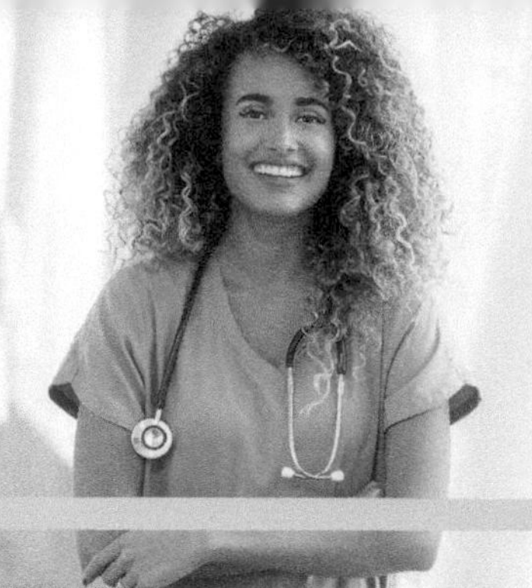

About the companion website

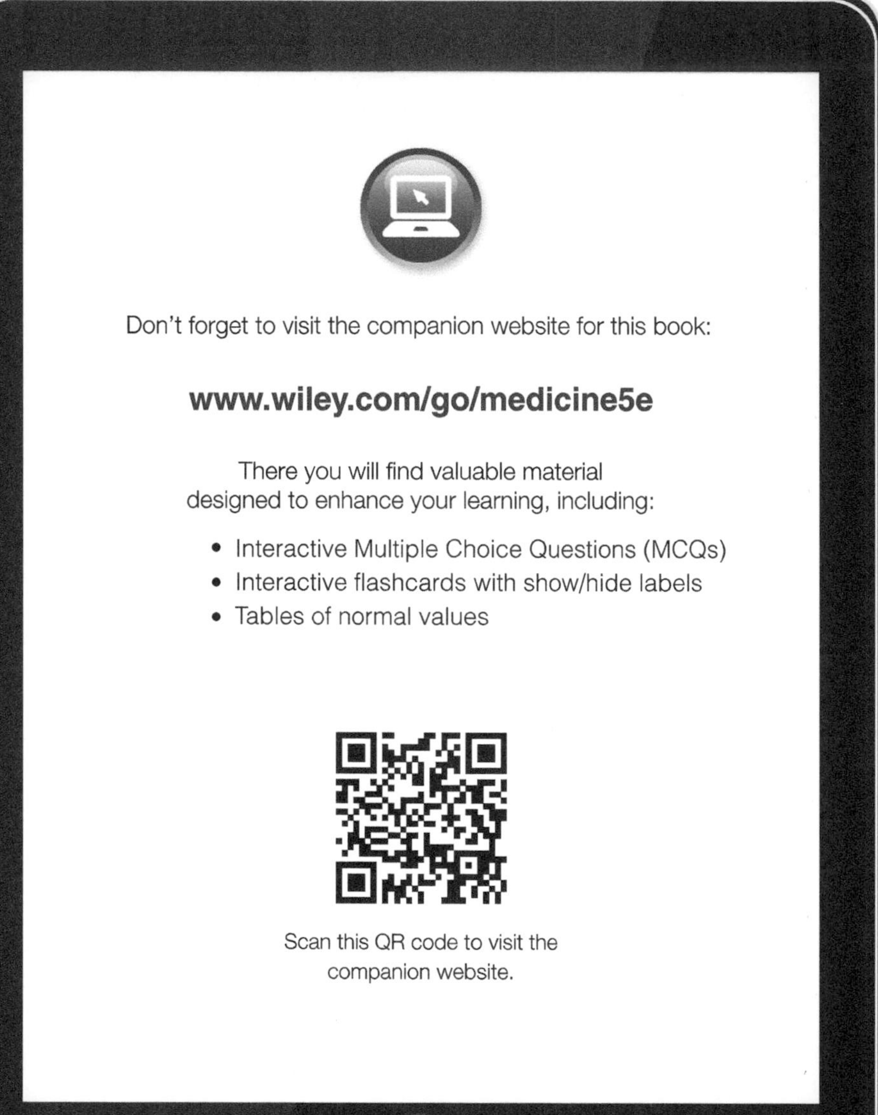

Don't forget to visit the companion website for this book:
www.wiley.com/go/medicine5e
There you will find valuable material designed to enhance your learning, including:
• Interactive Multiple Choice Questions (MCQs)
• Interactive flashcards with show/hide labels
• Tables of normal values
Scan this QR code to visit the companion website.

Introduction

Chapters

1 How to be a medical student

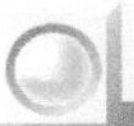

THE HIPPOCRATIC OATH

I SWEAR by Apollo the physician, and Aesculapius, and Health, and All-heal, and all the gods and goddesses, that, according to my ability and judgment, I will heed this oath and this stipulation to reckon him who taught me this Art equally dear to me as my parents, to share my substance with him, and relieve his necessities if required; to look upon his offspring in the same footing as my own brothers, and to teach them this Art, if they shall wish to learn it, without fee or stipulation; and that by precept, lecture, and every other mode of instruction, I will impart a knowledge of the Art to my own sons, and those of my teachers, and to disciples bound by a stipulation and oath according to the law of medicine, but to none other. I will follow that system of regimen which, according to my ability and judgment, I consider for the benefit of my patients, and abstain from whatever is deleterious and mischievous. I will give no deadly medicine to any one if asked, nor suggest any such counsel; and in like manner I will not give to a woman a pessary to produce abortion. With purity and with holiness I will pass my life and practise my Art. I will not cut persons laboring under the stone, but will leave this to be done by men who are practitioners of this work. Into whatever houses I enter, I will go into them for the benefit of the sick, and will abstain from every voluntary act of mischief and corruption; and, further from the seduction of females or males, of freemen and slaves. Whatever, in connection with my professional practice or not, in connection with it, I see or hear, in the life of men, which ought not to be spoken of abroad, I will not divulge, as reckoning that all such should be kept secret. While I continue to keep this oath unviolated, may it be granted to me to enjoy life and the practice of the art, respected by all men, in all times! But should I trespass and violate this oath, may the reverse be my lot.

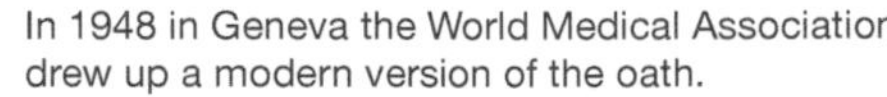

In 1948 in Geneva the World Medical Association drew up a modern version of the oath.

At the time of being admitted a member of the medical profession:
I solemnly pledge myself to consecrate my life to the service of humanity;
I will give my teachers the respect and gratitude which is their due;
I will practise my profession with conscience and dignity;
The health of my patient will be my first consideration;
I will respect the secrets which are confided in me, even after the patient has died;
I will maintain by all the means in my power, the honour and the noble traditions of the medical profession;
My colleagues will be my brothers;
I will not permit considerations of religion, nationality, race, party politics or social standing to intervene between my duty and my patient;
I will maintain the utmost respect for human life from the time of conception; even under threat
I will not use my medical knowledge contrary to the laws of humanity.
I make these promises solemnly, freely and upon my honour.

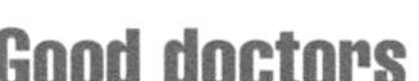

Good doctors

Medicine can seem a large and daunting subject, not only for reasons of intellectual rigour, but also because so many facts need to be learnt. In learning (and practising) medicine, it is vital to realize that facts alone are not enough! Good physicians have the following characteristics.

- A strong humanity, i.e. an interest in human beings.
- An interest in disease, its causation and treatment.
- An ability to communicate with patients, to obtain a correct and full understanding of their problems and, at the same time, to give accurate information sympathetically about the diagnosis, treatment and prognosis. Good physicians are non-judgemental, empathetic listeners.
- An ability to examine patients and elicit abnormal physical signs.
- An ability to marshal the facts into a coherent story and present them clearly to relevant parties, i.e. 'case' presentation of the history, examination and structured summary, a probable and differential diagnosis, with plans for further investigations, and treatment.
- An up-to-date knowledge base so that appropriate management (diagnosis + treatment) plans can be made.
- An ability to realize when knowledge/skills are deficient and an ability to learn in response to new knowledge, ideas, etc., from the best source available.
- An ability to acknowledge errors and learn from them. It is important to be open with patients and colleagues as soon as errors/misjudgements are recognized.
- Appropriate technical skills in diagnostic and therapeutic procedures.

Medicine at a Glance, Fifth Edition. Edited by Patrick Davey and Alex Pitcher.

Companion website: www.wiley.com/go/medicine5e

- An understanding of economic, social and cultural, political and healthcare systems so that the best possible help can be delivered to patients in the most timely fashion. If a deficiency in one or other of these systems damages patients, physicians should seek improvements.
- Excellent managerial and interpersonal skills, with personal, financial and intellectual probity.

Hippocratic oath and the modern perspective

High ethical and moral standards are an imperative for good practice – the Hippocratic oath and its modern successors aim to codify behaviour. They are guidelines to best behaviour, although medicine is more complex than implied by such phrases. However, regardless of phrasing, the implication that physicians should have the highest ethical, moral and technical standards stands. Society respects physicians, and consequently physicians face social as well as other penalties if performance is poor.

Healthcare systems

Healthcare systems are imperfect compromises among society's aspirations, wealth, humanity and individual needs (see Table 1.1). It is vital to understand how any system works, so that it can be used in a patient's best interests. If individual or organizational failure occurs, this should be highlighted to the appropriate responsible individuals, agencies or, rarely, the media.

Table 1.1 The three fundamental objectives of health systems.

- Improving the health of the population they serve
- Responding to people's expectations (including personal respect from the system to the patient)
- Providing financial protection against the costs of ill health

How to learn

Becoming a doctor means acquiring a set of skills, knowledge and values. How this is best done depends on the individual and the medical school. However, concentrating on one area/skill to the exclusion of others is counterproductive. Facts alone do not make a physician, and nor do learning or technical skills alone. It is the right combination of the above list that 'maketh the physician'. Students need to determine the right balance for themselves, bearing in mind their individual aptitudes and their medical school's doctrine. A reasonable approach is the 'patient-centred' one, approached in a 'problem-based' fashion, supplemented by dedicated learning sessions (e.g. seminars, lectures, etc.). Students should:

- see patients, so learning communication skills
- ascertain symptoms and signs, so learning clerking and examination skills
- formulate a diagnosis or differential diagnosis, so learning diagnostic skills. The first part of this book aims to aid in diagnosis, i.e. the turning of symptoms and signs into diseases with names
- present findings to attending physicians, so learning presentation skills
- formulate investigation and treatment plans, so refining diagnostic and therapeutic skills. The second part of this book aims to help here
- observe patients' progress, so determining whether the original diagnosis and therapy were correct. This feedback is an essential component in improving diagnostic and therapeutic skills.

Deficiencies in knowledge and technique are identified at each stage and corrected using information/skills training obtained from books and libraries, electronic resources, physicians, other healthcare professionals, patient groups, skills workshops, learning sessions, etc.

Some medical schools have a structured approach to this process, with substantial guidance at each stage; others are less formalized – which appeals more depends largely on you. Which is better is unclear.

How to behave on the wards

It is particularly important when performing ward work to:

- introduce yourself to the ward staff as well as the patient, so that they know who you are and why you are there
- respect patients' privacy, and their right to refuse to see you
- ask for consent before seeing a patient
- if you undress a patient to examine them, help them to dress again once you have finished
- be courteous to nurses and other members of staff (e.g. physiotherapists, ward cleaners, cooks, etc.) at all times
- be punctual in attending teaching sessions – you will find that your teachers, who are often busy clinicians, are often late; this is not deliberately done to infuriate you, rather it reflects how hectic their lives are. It is reasonable to wait for about 10 minutes before 'bleeping' to remind them of the session
- write in the notes: different medical schools have different policies on this. Often, however, senior medical students are expected to write in the notes. This is a legal document, so write legibly, never use pejorative phraseology, and sign your name, along with your status as student, legibly at the end. *Never* amend the record at a later time, unless you clearly identify who you are and when the alterations occurred
- enjoy yourself!

2 Patient confidentiality

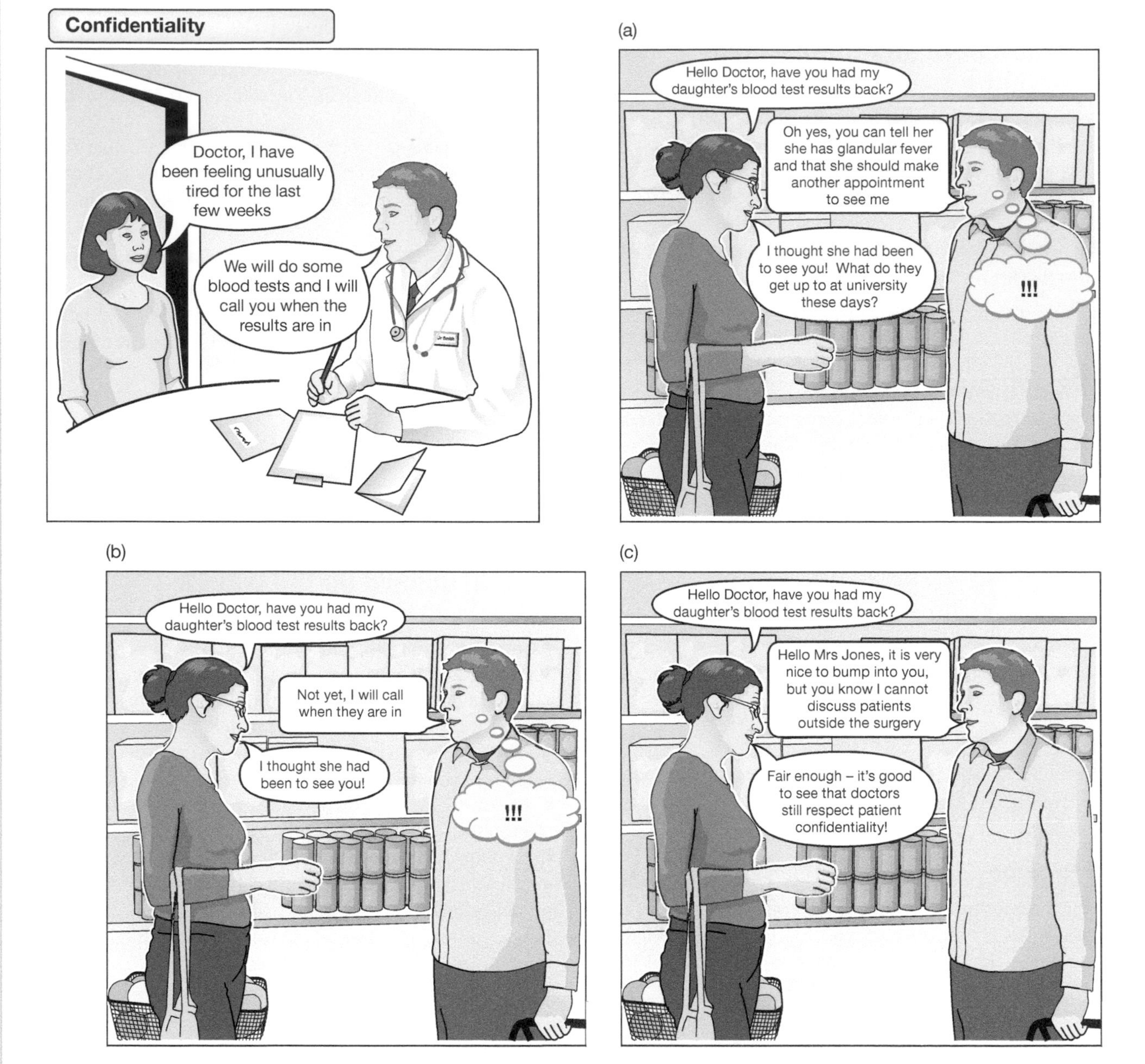
Confidentiality
Doctor, I have been feeling unusually tired for the last few weeks
We will do some blood tests and I will call you when the results are in
(a)
Hello Doctor, have you had my daughter's blood test results back?
Oh yes, you can tell her she has glandular fever and that she should make another appointment to see me
I thought she had been to see you! What do they get up to at university these days?
!!!
(b)
Hello Doctor, have you had my daughter's blood test results back?
Not yet, I will call when they are in
I thought she had been to see you!
!!!
(c)
Hello Doctor, have you had my daughter's blood test results back?
Hello Mrs Jones, it is very nice to bump into you, but you know I cannot discuss patients outside the surgery
Fair enough – it's good to see that doctors still respect patient confidentiality!

The duty to respect patient confidentiality concerns what is owed to patients with regard to personal medical information about them. This duty stems mainly from two ethical principles. The first, 'respect for autonomy', is usually interpreted to mean that the patient ought to be in control over who has access to personal information about her. This is because the control of personal information is taken to be a key part of enabling a person to exercise broader control over their lives, in line with their own wishes and values in life.

The second principle is based on the idea that there is a duty to act to bring about the best consequences for the individual patient and for other patients making use of the healthcare system. This view is based on the premise that good health outcomes are contingent on the maintenance of public trust in the profession,

Medicine at a Glance, Fifth Edition. Edited by Patrick Davey and Alex Pitcher.

Companion website: www.wiley.com/go/medicine5e

and that public trust would be undermined if personal medical information were shared without the consent of patients.

The duty to maintain confidentiality

Both of these ethical arguments place value on the moral significance of maintaining patient confidentiality. This position is endorsed in English law. From a legal perspective, patient confidentiality is interpreted as a **public interest** rather than as a **private interest**, reflecting the consequentialist position outlined above. Although the Human Rights Act 1998 acknowledges that there is also a private right to confidentiality, in practice this makes little difference because of the weight given in common law to the public interest in maintaining patient confidentiality.

Consent to disclose confidential information

Often, consent to share a patient's medical information can be presumed. It is generally accepted that information about the care of a patient will be discussed within the medical team, even if it is only shared with one member of that team. Express consent would not normally be required to seek specialist advice or a second opinion. The key question is whether the patient's interests are best served by sharing their information amongst other professionals.

In most other circumstances, express permission to share the information should be sought from the patient even when there is a legal obligation to disclose the information, or when the practitioner believes that the public interest in disclosing the information requires it (see below). This is because the law recognizes a requirement to show respect to the patient, regardless of whether the decision to breach confidentiality has been made. Consent should therefore always be sought, even if it is judged unlikely to be given, unless there are over-riding reasons for thinking that the act of obtaining consent would itself act against the public interest justifying the disclosure of the information. Equally, the person should be informed that a breach has taken place, with the reasons for this decision being clearly outlined.

If an adult lacks capacity to give consent, doctors should consider the patient's 'best interests', and consent requirements in relation to the disclosure of medical information for children ought to adhere to the laws regarding consent for this group.

From a legal standpoint, it should also be recognized that confidentiality has not been breached if the patient has given valid consent for the release of the information. Also, if information about patients has been anonymized prior to being disclosed, issues concerning confidentiality do not arise. However, it is important to attend carefully to how this information is rendered anonymous, particularly when used for educational purposes. Simply removing a patient's name is very unlikely to be sufficient.

Breaches of confidentiality

Whilst the law endorses a duty to maintain confidentiality, this is not absolute. There are circumstances in which practitioners are legally obliged to breach confidentiality, and circumstances in which breaching confidentiality is permissible.

Situations where there is a legal obligation to breach patient confidentiality

Statutory legislation lays out the situations in which there is an over-riding obligation to breach confidentiality. Alternatively, the obligation to breach confidentiality might be laid out in a court order. Some examples of situations where practitioners are obliged to breach include:

- the presence of notifiable diseases
- reporting of terminations of pregnancy
- reporting of births and deaths
- details of anyone alleged to be guilty of an offence under the Road Traffic Act 1988 (on request by police only)
- evidence of terrorism activities, or knife and gunshot wounds.

Situations where it is permitted to breach patient confidentiality

These situations involve weighing up the public interest in disclosure versus non-disclosure. The General Medical Council (GMC) offers detailed guidance in this area and this guidance carries a lot of weight with the courts (see www.gmc-uk.org). The general idea is that disclosure of confidential information without consent would normally only be justified in order to prevent risk of death or serious harm to other people.

The position endorsed in law, and clarified by the GMC, here is entirely consistent with a more developed version of the consequentialist argument above. One can imagine circumstances in which, if doctors do not breach confidentiality, the outcomes will be such that trust in the medical profession is likely to be undermined to a greater extent than if confidentiality had been maintained.

The GMC also recognizes that professional obligations relating to confidentiality continue after death, and gives specific advice concerning confidentiality and genetic information.

Confidentiality, privacy and data protection

Duties in relation to confidentiality are closely related to duties regarding patients' privacy and laws relating to the protection of personal data more generally. In contrast to confidentiality, which concerns situations in which a practitioner is in possession of personal medical information, privacy concerns what is owed to a person when the practitioner is not in possession of that information – and is part of a more general set of duties relating to respecting those aspects of a person that concern how she manages her private realm. In England, medical legal obligations concerning confidentiality are now seen as being closely related to privacy rights.

In contrast, data protection duties are separate from, but no less rigorous than, those relating to medical confidentiality. In practice, laws relating to data protection are more pertinent to the ways in which healthcare organizations use personal data to audit, report and manage their services.

3 Consent

Information contained in a typical consent form

Patient details on a Patient identifier/label

Patient identifier/label

Name of proposed procedure or course of treatment (include brief explanation if medical term not clear) ....

Statement of health professional (to be filled in by health professional with appropriate knowledge of proposed procedure, as specified in consent policy)

I have explained the procedure to the patient. In particular, I have explained:

The intended benefits ....

Serious or frequently occurring risks ....

Any extra procedures which may become necessary during the procedure

☐ blood transfusion ....

☐ other procedure (please specify) ....

I have also discussed what the procedure is likely to involve, the benefits and risks of any available alternative treatments (including no treatment) and any particular concerns of this patient.

☐ The following leaflet/tape has been provided ....

This procedure will involve:

☐ general and/or regional anaesthesia ☐ local anaesthesia ☐ sedation

Signed:.................................... Date ....
Name (PRINT) .... Job title....................................

Contact details (if patient wishes to discuss options later) ....

Statement of interpreter (where appropriate)

I have interpreted the information above to the patient to the best of my ability and in a way in which I believe s/he can understand.

Signed .... Date ....
Name (PRINT) ....

Top copy accepted by patient: yes/no (please ring)

Patient identifier/label

Statement of patient

Please read this form carefully. If your treatment has been planned in advance, you should already have your own copy of page 2 which describes the benefits and risks of the proposed treatment. If not, you will be offered a copy now. If you have any further questions, do ask – we are here to help you. You have the right to change your mind at any time, including after you have signed this form.

I agree to the procedure or course of treatment described on this form.

I understand that you cannot give me a guarantee that a particular person will perform the procedure. The person will, however, have appropriate experience.

I understand that I will have the opportunity to discuss the details of anaesthesia with an anaesthetist before the procedure, unless the urgency of my situation prevents this. (This only applies to patients having general or regional anaesthesia.)

I understand that any procedure in addition to those described on this form will only be carried out if it is necessary to save my life or to prevent serious harm to my health.

I have been told about additional procedures which may become necessary during my treatment. I have listed below any procedures **which I do not wish to be carried out** without further discussion..

Patient's signature.................................... Date ....
Name (PRINT) ....

A witness should sign below if the patient is unable to sign but has indicated his or her consent. Young people/children may also like a parent to sign here (see notes).

Signature .... Date ....
Name (PRINT) ....

Confirmation of consent (to be completed by a health professional when the patient is admitted for the procedure, if the patient has signed the form in advance)

On behalf of the team treating the patient, I have confirmed with the patient that s/he has no further questions and wishes the procedure to go ahead.

Signed:.................................... Date ....
Name (PRINT) .... Job title....................................

Important notes: (tick if applicable)

☐ See also advance directive/living will (e.g. Jehovah's Witness form)

☐ Patient has withdrawn consent (ask patient to sign /date here)....................................

In modern healthcare, it is acknowledged that patient consent is required before any medical intervention is carried out. Consent provides the means for patients to authorize treatment, in a way that reflects and respects their own values and commitments in life. In this sense, the practice of consent stems from the ethical concept of autonomy: the ability to exercise control over our own lives, and the value of this.

Valid consent has been conceptualized in medical ethics and English law around three criteria.

1 That the patient has been **informed** as to the purpose, nature, risks and benefits of the medical procedure.

2 That the patient is **competent** (has capacity) to understand this information.

Medicine at a Glance, Fifth Edition. Edited by Patrick Davey and Alex Pitcher.

Companion website: www.wiley.com/go/medicine5e

3 That the patient has given voluntary **consent**, i.e. the patient has not been coerced.

In English law, a patient who is informed, competent and making a voluntary decision can give or withhold consent for any medical treatment, even if this leads to their death.

The consent form is a standard mechanism used in healthcare to document and evidence the choice a patient is making – a choice, of course, that a patient could change at any point prior to the intervention being initiated.

For patients to be validly informed in legal terms, they should be given general information about the purpose and nature of the proposed course of action. Failure to do this could result in the patient making a claim for **battery** (touching a person without consent).

In order to protect themselves from an action in **negligence**, doctors must also provide information about material risks associated with the intervention, and information about any reasonable alternatives. In England, doctors are now required to consider what the 'reasonable person in the patient's position' would expect to know, given the nature of the procedure, the risks, benefits and alternatives associated with it. They are also expected to consider the 'particular patient' in front of them, and how her values, beliefs or preferences point towards disclosing certain information and withholding other information.

The General Medical Council offers detailed guidance on consent aimed at doctors. This guidance has recently been reviewed in 2020, with the new version titled 'Decision making and consent'. This guidance stresses, in particular, the importance of doctors establishing a patient-centric dialogue that enables the exchange of meaningful personal information and facilitates shared decision making.

Mental capacity and consent

It is common for doctors to encounter situations in which, for various reasons, an adult patient will be unable to give consent to medical treatment due to lack of mental capacity.

The Mental Capacity Act 2005 (MCA) outlines the procedures for determining capacity and how to act when a patient over the age of 16 lacks the capacity to make her own decisions. All adult patients are presumed to have capacity, unless there is evidence to prove that they do not. Under the MCA (Part 1 Section 3(1)), a person lacks capacity if she has 'an impairment of, or disturbance in the functioning of, mind or brain', and because of this impairment or disturbance she is unable to:

- **understand** the information relevant to the decision, *or*
- **retain** that information, *or*
- **use or weigh** that information as part of the process of making the decision, *or*
- **communicate** her decision (by any means).

If a patient is shown to lack capacity, then those caring for her must attempt to enhance her capacity insofar as this is practical. Note that '**capacity**' here refers to the ability of the patient to make one or more specific decisions. In addition, a patient does not lack capacity simply because she makes an unwise decision.

Under the MCA, patients who lack capacity (and have not appointed a Lasting Power of Attorney or made an Advance Decision to Refuse Treatment – see below) should be treated in their 'best interests' (Part 1 Section 4). The MCA specifies some factors that should be taken into account when making a decision about best interests, which are sensitive to the person's past and present wishes, beliefs, feelings and values.

A Lasting Power of Attorney can be appointed by a person who currently has capacity to make medical and non-medical decisions on her behalf at a future time when she no longer has capacity. The Act also allows Advance Decisions to Refuse Treatment (ADRT) to be made by persons aged 18 or over who have capacity. These authorize treatment to be withheld at a future time when they lack capacity. An ADRT can relate to life-sustaining treatment if it is in writing, is specific to that effect, and if it is appropriately signed and witnessed.

In Scotland, although the approach to determining capacity and treatment of those without capacity is similar, the legal criteria differ in some important ways, as outlined in the Adults with Incapacity (Scotland) Act 2000.

Consent and children

When faced with the need to make a decision about medical care or treatment concerning a child aged less than 18 years, it is important to remember that in an emergency situation when the child and/or those with parental responsibility cannot or will not give consent, the medical professional should normally act to prevent death or serious harm to the patient. This is because, under the Children Act 1989 in English law, the child's welfare is 'paramount'.

Children aged 16 or 17 years are presumed to have capacity to consent to medical treatment unless it can be shown otherwise. Those with parental responsibility (usually the parents) can also give consent. If valid consent for the relevant procedure has been given either by the child or by any person with parental responsibility, then the doctor has consent to proceed. Doctors (and those with parental responsibility) have a legal obligation to act in ways that advance a child's welfare. If neither the child patient nor a person with parental responsibility provides consent, and the doctor judges that without treatment the child will come to serious harm or die, then permission for the treatment to be given should be sought from the courts.

Children aged less than 16 are presumed not to have capacity to consent unless they demonstrate that they are 'Gillick competent', i.e. have reached a level of intelligence and understanding sufficient to understand what is being proposed. Again, a person with parental responsibility can also give consent. The legal position for refusal of treatment by Gillick-competent children is the same as for competent 16 or 17 year olds.

Consent should be obtained from at least one person with parental responsibility for children below the age of 16 who are not Gillick competent. If no-one with parental responsibility gives consent and failure to carry out the procedure would compromise the child's welfare, then doctors should apply to the court for a 'specific issue order'. As outlined above, however, in an emergency doctors should act immediately to save the child from the risk of death or serious harm.

4 Relationship with the patient

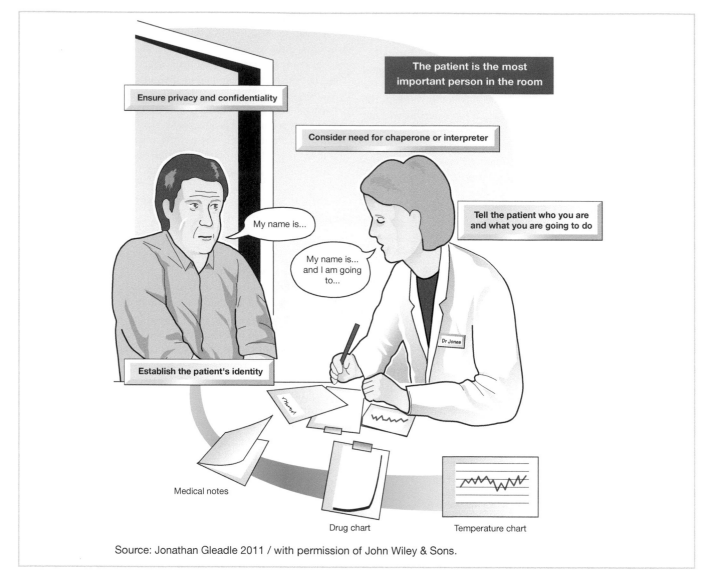

Source: Jonathan Gleadle 2011 / with permission of John Wiley & Sons.

Your relationship with your patient is the key determinant of your effectiveness as a clinician. Why is this? You need the patient to give you *all* the information necessary for diagnosis. You must then communicate this decision and any uncertainty surrounding it to the patient in language they understand, and you must convince them that the treatment you recommend is appropriate and effective. None of this will occur unless you have established an effective relationship with your patient. This is true for patients you see only once or twice, for those that you might see a score of times during an admission or over 30 or more years.

Different patients require different techniques to develop relationships; with some you can be informal and quite chatty, with others you may need to be more formal, and keep to the point; some appreciate humour and others find it unprofessional. Develop your style, but modify it for individual patients.

So, how do you develop such a relationship? In many ways, though some tips include the following.

- Listen to your patient, let them do the talking, albeit guided by yourself to elaborate on certain areas and to move on from others.
- Engage in eye contact.
- Appropriate use of non-verbal gestures, such as smiling.
- Minimize the chance of interruptions and other distractions (such as phones going off or staring endlessly at a computer screen).
- Dress appropriately; in years gone by, most patients expected consultants to wear suits. This era has largely passed – consultants

Medicine at a Glance, Fifth Edition. Edited by Patrick Davey and Alex Pitcher.

Companion website: www.wiley.com/go/medicine5e

attending patients in the middle of the night often wear jeans, so do adjust your attire according to the setting and time. However, you should be certain you and your clothes are smart and clean, and that you follow the dress code of your institute (in the UK National Health Service, this includes no jewellery and only short-sleeved shirts), which is recommended to minimize your risk of transmitting hospital-acquired infection.

When meeting a patient, establish their identity unequivocally (ask for their full name and confirm with their name band, ask for their date of birth, address, etc.) and be certain that all records, notes, test results, etc. refer to that patient, as results can sometimes find their way into the wrong patient's notes. Similarly, ensure the patient knows who you are and what your role is. If you are a medical student, ensure that the patient understands that and gives their permission for you to talk to them.

Often you may wish to shake their hand and say 'My name is Dr Davey and you are . . . ?' Or 'Your name is . . .?', 'Your date of birth is . . .?', 'Your address is . . .?' Tell them your name, your title and job and what you are about to do. For example:

> *'I am Dr Davey, a consultant specializing in heart medicine, and I've been asked to try and work out whether your heart is working properly. I'm going to spend about half an hour talking to you about your medical problems, and then I'll examine you thoroughly. After that I'll explain to you what I think the matter is and what we need to do to help you.'*

Or you could say, 'I am Patrick Davey, a medical student, and I'd like to ask you some questions about your illness if I may'. Even if you've met several times before, it's worth reminding the patient of your identity: 'Hello, Mrs Glance, Dr Davey again . . .'

Always be polite, be respectful and be clear. Remember the patient may be feeling anxious, unwell, embarrassed, scared or in pain. If you detect these emotions, ask the patient to elaborate on their fears – unless you know what is really worrying them, you will not have a satisfactory consultation.

You should be gathering information and observing the patient as soon as you meet them: history taking and examination are not distinct, sequential processes, they are ongoing. Your best clues to the presence of thyroid disease, acromegaly, Cushing syndrome, alcohol dependency and many other conditions are gleaned from the patient's appearance in the first few seconds of the consultation, so start thinking diagnostically the moment you see the patient, not just at certain times in the consultation.

Sequence of the consultation

Although your diagnostic processes will be working continuously throughout the consultation, the usual order is history, examination, explanation to the patient about their illness and then, crucially, to ask the patient if they have questions they wish to address. Effective communication is a two-way process, so ensure the patient has the opportunity to question, reframe, discuss their worries and perspective.

Privacy

Ensure that there is privacy (this is not always easy in busy hospital wards: make sure curtains are properly closed; see if the examination room is free).

Language

Establish whether the patient is fluent in the language you intend to use and, if not, arrange for an interpreter to be present or at least a telephone interpreter. Often a family member will be willing to interpret, but this may subtly distort the history and there may be issues with confidentiality, so you should establish that the patient is happy to discuss their problems via this relative. In the UK, the NHS has issued a guideline stating that relatives should not be used as interpreters as patients may not then divulge key information, for example about abuse that has a particular cultural context. Accordingly, in the UK, use alternatives such as hired translators or other members of staff.

There may be other barriers to good communication which need to be considered, including impaired hearing or sight, overwhelming anxiety, clouded consciousness, pain and intellectual impairment.

Relatives, friends and chaperones

Establish who else is with the patient, their relationship with the patient and whether the patient wishes for them to be present during the consultation. Ask if the patient wishes for a chaperone to be present during the examination; this may be appropriate in any case.

Remember that **the patient is the most important person in the room**! Remember that all information you gain from your patient or anyone else is **confidential**. This means that information about the patient should only be discussed with other professionals involved in the care of that patient. You must ensure that patient discussions or records cannot be overheard or accessed by others.

Some guidelines for the use of chaperones

- A chaperone is a third person, (usually) of the same sex as the patient and (usually) a health professional (not a relative).
- When asking a patient if they would like a chaperone to be present, ensure they know what you mean; for example, 'We often ask another member of staff to be present during this examination, would you like us to have someone else present?'
- If either the patient or the doctor/medical student wishes a chaperone to be present then the examination should not be carried out without one.
- Record the presence of a chaperone in the notes – **this is vital if you are to fully protect yourself medicolegally**.
- A chaperone *must* be present for intimate examinations by doctors or students examining patients of the opposite sex (vaginal, rectal, genitalia and female breast examination), and offered for any intimate examinations of either gender.

Hand washing and hospital-acquired infection

In modern healthcare systems, there is considerable and appropriate concern about hospital-acquired infection; the hands of staff are the most common vehicles by which micro-organisms are transmitted between patients and hand washing is the single most important measure in infection control. So, always ensure your hands are washed, whether using alcoholic rubs or medicated soap is less important than that the hands are actually washed. Hands should be washed before and after each patient contact, and also between wards.

You should also ensure that you minimize the risk of your clothes transmitting infection by not wearing jewellery, long-sleeved shirts or a tie, and ensuring that your stethoscope is disinfected regularly. The use of personal protective equipment (PPE) may make communication more challenging but a smile and eye contact are still important and possible.

5 History of presenting complaint

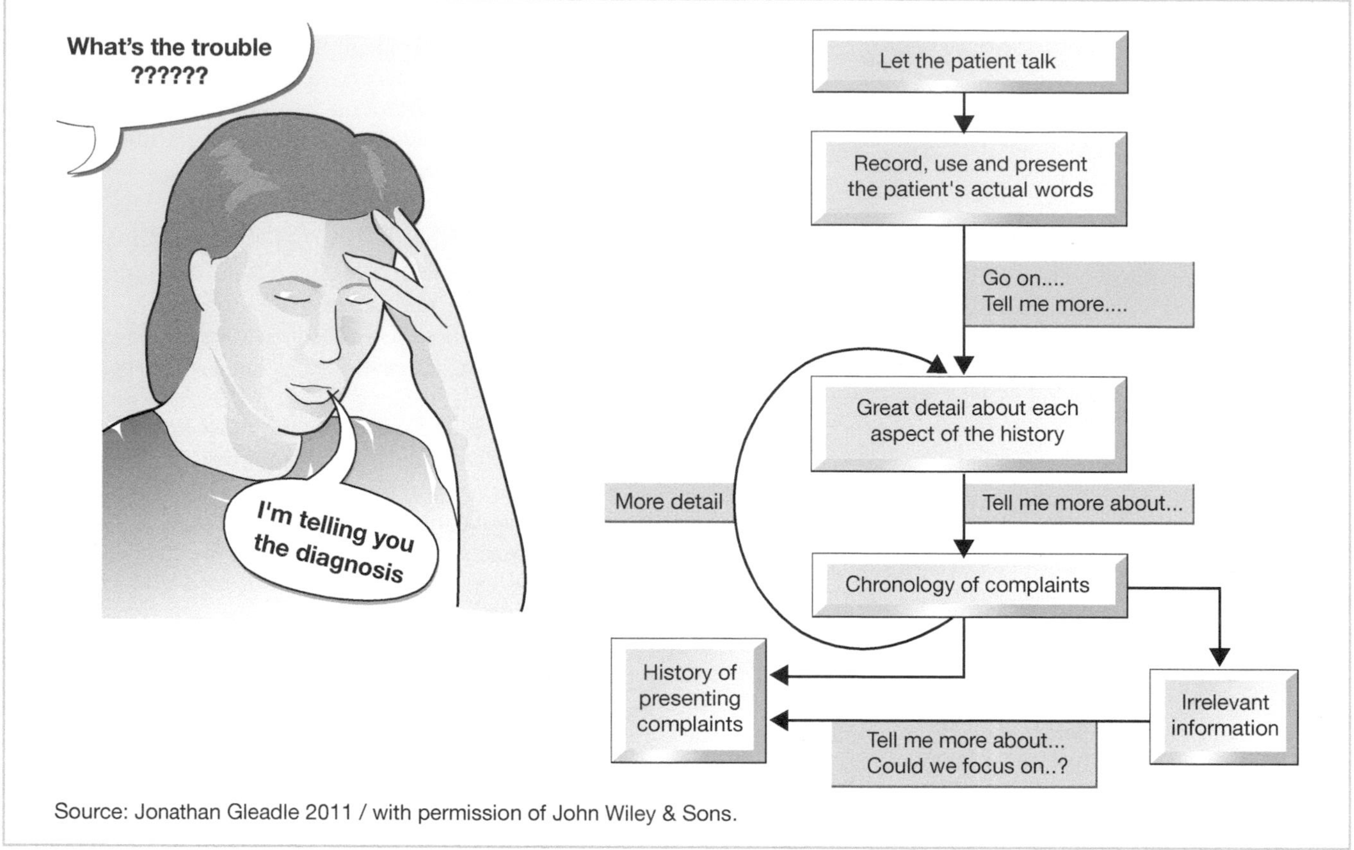

Source: Jonathan Gleadle 2011 / with permission of John Wiley & Sons.

The history of the presenting complaint is the most important part of the history and examination. It provides the information necessary to create the differential diagnosis and also provides vital insight into the features of the complaints most important to the patient. It should usually receive most time during a consultation.

The history obtained should be recorded and presented in the patient's own words, and not be masked by medical phrases such as 'dyspnoea', 'myocardial infarction', etc., which may disguise the true nature of the complaint and important nuances. As you listen to the presenting complaint, continually ask yourself 'What does this tell me about the diagnosis?'. Remember, it is the patient's problems that you are trying to understand and record in order to establish diagnoses and to understand the effects of the problems on the patient and how you can help address them. Do not force or overinterpret what the patient says to fit into a particular diagnosis or symptom, nor simply record what the patient reports other doctors have said.

If a clear history cannot be obtained from the patient then the history should be sought from relatives, friends or other witnesses. It may be appropriate to seek corroboration of features of the history, such as alcohol consumption or details of a collapse, always bearing in mind the principles of medical confidentiality.

Let the patient talk

The presenting complaint should be obtained by allowing the patient to talk without interruption, if possible. This may be initiated by asking an open question such as:

- 'Why have you come to see me today?'
- 'What's the problem?'
- 'Tell me what's been happening'.
- 'Tell me what seems to be the trouble.'
- 'How long have you been ill for, and what have you noticed over this time?'

Medicine at a Glance, Fifth Edition. Edited by Patrick Davey and Alex Pitcher.

Companion website: www.wiley.com/go/medicine5e

The patient should always be allowed to talk for as long as possible without interruption. Small interjections such as 'Go on' or 'Tell me more' may help produce more information from a reticent patient.

It may be possible to enable patients to elaborate on areas of particular medical interest. One way to do this is to repeat the last phrase that a patient has voiced in a questioning way. For example, to 'I'm finding breathing more difficult' you could respond 'Breathing more difficult?' or 'Tell me more' or 'Tell me more about your breathing'.

More specific questioning

After this, open questions should be addressed to reveal more detail about particular aspects of the history. For example, 'Tell me more about the pain', 'Tell me in more detail about your tiredness' or 'You've said that you've been feeling tired?'.

More direct questions can then be addressed to gain information about the chronology and other detail of the complaints; for example, 'When exactly did you first notice the breathlessness?', 'Which came first, the chest pain or the breathlessness?' or 'What exactly were you doing when the breathlessness came on?'. Sometimes patients find it difficult to accurately recall chronology – in this situation, establish when the patient was last completely well, as this will often tell you for how long they have been ill.

Directed questions can then be addressed to establish diagnostically important features about the complaints; for example, 'What was the pain like?', 'Was the pain sharp, heavy or burning?', 'What made the pain worse?', 'Did breathing affect the pain?' or 'What about breathing in deeply?'.

Other aspects of the history (e.g. past medical history or social history) relevant to the presenting complaint, although they are conventionally analysed separately, commonly arise during discussion of the presenting complaint and can receive detailed attention at this point.

In some settings, such as during resuscitation of a very ill patient, very focused or abbreviated questioning may be appropriate.

Premorbid functional status

It is *crucial* to ascertain this. This information is essential in managing the patient, and also for conveying the patient's history to colleagues. This is because:

- usually, you aim to restore a patient's health to that immediately prior to an illness – knowing their premorbid state means that you know what you are aiming to achieve
- functional status is a most important predictor for life expectancy. If a patient's premorbid functional status is poor, or they are very frail, then the premorbid life expectancy is usually not good. This information can then be factored into how intensively you should investigate and treat their current illness.

There are many ways to convey premorbid functional status – a good empirical method is to find out how far a patient can walk unaided in one go at a normal pace (e.g. 5 miles, quarter of a mile), if they are housebound or using a Zimmer frame for mobility, etc. It is also important to ascertain what symptom limits them. You can do this by asking:

- 'How far can you usually walk?'
- 'What stops you walking further?'
- 'How do the symptoms interfere with your life (with walking, working, sleeping, etc.)?'
- 'What things would you like to do that you can't? What stops you?'

If the person is housebound, ask about mobility within the home, and what carers are needed to support their life (e.g. how many carers are needed to get them up in the morning, wash them, etc.).

Patients' understanding of their illness

You should ask the patient what they think is wrong with them and how the problems have affected them (e.g. ability to work, mood, etc.) and their family.

Focus on the main problems

Some patients devote considerable attention to aspects of their illness that are not helpful in achieving a diagnosis or to understanding the patient and their problems. It may be necessary to interject and divert discussion with phrases such as, 'Could you tell me more about your chest pain?' or 'Could we focus on why you came to the doctor's surgery this time?'. Sometimes there may be a very long list of different complaints in which case the patient should be asked to focus on each in turn. Keep in mind the main problems and direct the history accordingly, and for each symptom, obtain and record a precise history.

Summarize your findings

Perhaps the most important aspect to establishing the presenting complaint is to summarize your understanding of the history to the patient, and to ask if you have got it exactly right. You could also ask 'What have I missed?', 'What else should I know about?'.

Past medical history, drugs and allergies

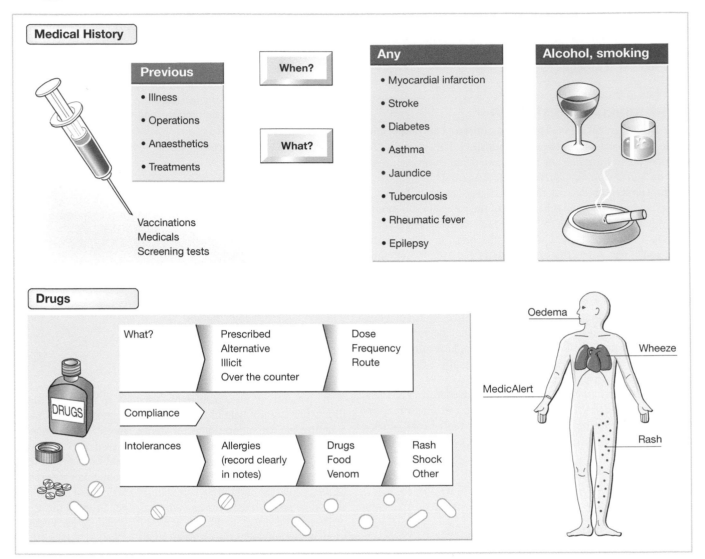

Medical History

Previous
- Illness
- Operations
- Anaesthetics
- Treatments

When?

What?

Vaccinations
Medicals
Screening tests

Any
- Myocardial infarction
- Stroke
- Diabetes
- Asthma
- Jaundice
- Tuberculosis
- Rheumatic fever
- Epilepsy

Alcohol, smoking

Drugs

DRUGS

What? → Prescribed, Alternative, Illicit, Over the counter → Dose, Frequency, Route

Compliance

Intolerances → Allergies (record clearly in notes) → Drugs, Food, Venom → Rash, Shock, Other

Oedema
Wheeze
MedicAlert
Rash

Past medical history

The past medical history is a vital part of the history. It is important to record in detail all previous medical problems and their treatment in chronological order. You could ask:

- 'What illnesses have you had?'
- 'What operations have you had?'
- 'Have you ever been in hospital?'
- 'When did you last feel completely well?'

If major diagnoses have been previously made, always ask for the information that corroborates this. For example, patients often mention they have been diagnosed as having angina; establish which symptoms led to this diagnosis (do you think they indicate angina?), who made the diagnosis (clearly, a cardiologist should be the most reliable in making a diagnosis of angina due to coronary artery disease) and what tests were done to confirm or refute the diagnosis. Specifically in this situation, ask if they have had a coronary angiogram, and if so what the result was, as many patients with normal coronary arteries still believe that the diagnosis of angina made prior to angiography stands regardless of the normality of the angiogram. What is true for coronary heart disease is also true for all other major diagnoses; always ask who made the diagnosis and how it was proved.

Medicine at a Glance, Fifth Edition. Edited by Patrick Davey and Alex Pitcher.

Companion website: www.wiley.com/go/medicine5e

Ask if there were any problems with operations or anaesthetics, and, if so, what they were. You might turn up a bleeding tendency or an intolerance to particular anaesthetic agents.

If not already discussed in relation to the presenting complaint, specific aspects of the past medical history may need to be enquired about. For example, ask about previous chest pain (angina) in a patient presenting with severe chest pain.

It is conventional to record the occurrence of specific common illnesses, in particular jaundice, anaemia, tuberculosis, rheumatic fever, diabetes mellitus, bronchitis, myocardial infarction, stroke, epilepsy, asthma and problems with anaesthesia.

The patient should also be asked about vaccinations, medicals, screening tests (e.g. cervical smear) and pregnancies. You could ask what other doctors, specialists, nurses, allied health practitioners the patient is seeing.

Drug history

- What medication is the patient taking?
- What medication is prescribed and what other remedies are they taking (e.g. herbal remedies, 'over-the-counter' tablets)? Ask to see the actual medication and/or the prescription list.
- Do not forget to ask about injections (e.g. insulin), topical treatments and inhalers as patients may not consider them to be drugs.
- Don't forget oral contraception (patients often do) and other hormone-containing long-acting contraception such as implants.
- What recreational drugs do they or have they taken? It is usually best to come straight out with this question and not 'beat around the bush'. Ask 'Have you ever used any non-prescription drugs?' or 'What other drugs do you take?'. If the answer is yes, find out what sort, how frequently and how it was taken, e.g. nasally (cocaine), orally or intravenously. If the latter, find out if they shared needles.
- What is the patient's likely concordance with prescribed medication? It is not always easy to know how to assess this. You can ask the patient if you feel they will answer truthfully (clearly, the overwhelming majority of patients). You might ask 'How often do you miss or forget a tablet?'. You can find out from their general practitioner how often they renew their prescription. You can ask relatives, who are an extremely useful source of information (always bear in mind the rules on confidentiality).
- Is there supervision? For example, does a relative or the district nurse supervise drug taking? Is a 'dose-it' box used?
- What medication has the patient been intolerant of and why?

Allergies

It is vital to obtain an accurate and detailed description of the patient's allergic responses to drugs and other potential allergens. The patient should be asked if they are allergic to anything. They should be asked specifically whether they are allergic to any antibiotics, including penicillin. It is also important to elicit the precise nature of the allergy. Was there true allergy with a full-blown anaphylactic shock, an erythematous rash or an urticarial rash, or did the patient only feel nausea or experience another drug side-effect? Many patients label the latter as an allergy, whereas often this is a component of the illness for which they were taking the antibiotic.

Other important allergies may exist to foodstuffs, such as nuts, or to bee or wasp stings.

It is also important to elicit other intolerances, such as side-effects, to medication. This is particularly true for drugs used to treat hypertension. If you establish an intolerance, ask what symptoms they noticed, and whether they were present before taking the drug or after they stopped (in which case it is unlikely to actually reflect a genuine reaction to that drug).

Ensure allergies are clearly recorded in notes, drug charts and, if appropriate, MedicAlert bracelets.

Smoking

Does the patient smoke or have they ever? If so, what type and how many, for how long? Cigarettes, vapes, pipe or cigar? Tobacco, cannabis? Have any relatives suffered smoking-related complications (e.g. heart attacks, lung diseases, malignancy)? Establish what the patient's attitude is to giving up; often patients are misinformed about the actual risk of smoking, and giving them the facts, in a polite, digestible manner, helps support them in giving up. Have they tried to stop before and what supports were tried?

Alcohol

Does the patient drink alcohol? If so, what type of alcohol? How many units and how often? People find it very easy to underestimate their alcohol consumption, so it is often helpful to draw up a list of exactly how much they drink and when. If they stay at home drinking, ask how much beer and how many bottles of wine and spirits (and what size) they buy each week.

Are there/have there been problems with alcohol dependence? There are many ways to assess this, but the CAGE questionnaire is useful.

- Have you ever felt you should *C*ut back?
- Have you ever been *A*ngry when your alcohol intake is commented on?
- Have you ever felt *G*uilty about the amount you drink?
- Have you ever needed an *E*ye-opener (alcoholic drink first thing in the morning)?

Scores of 2 or more are fairly strongly associated with an alcohol problem.

7 Family and social history

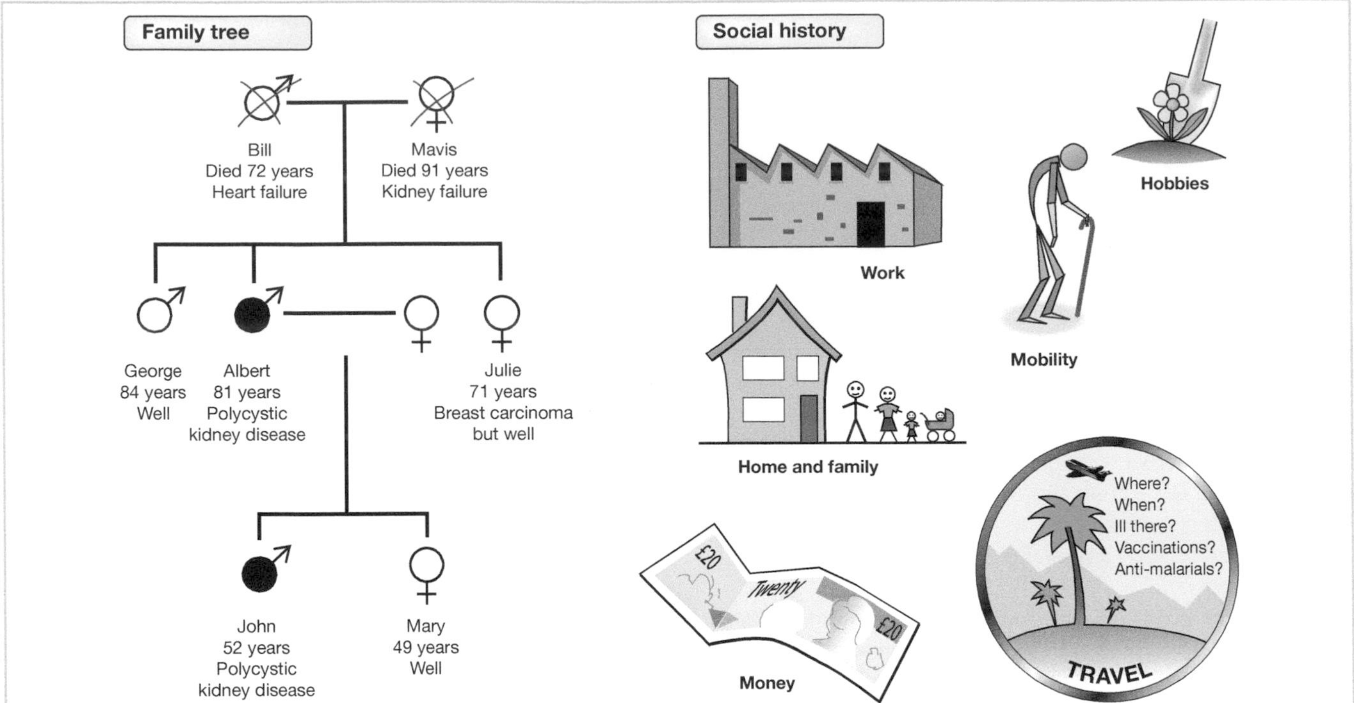

Family history

It is important to establish the diseases that have affected relatives given the strong genetic contribution to many diseases.

- 'What relatives do you have?'
- 'Are your parents still alive? If not, how old were they when they died? What did they die from? Did they suffer from any significant illnesses?'
- 'Have you any siblings, children or grandchildren?'
- 'Are there any diseases that run in the family?' (In rare genetic conditions, consider the possibility of consanguinity; you can construct a family tree.)
- 'Are there any illnesses that 'run in the family'?'

Social history

It is vital to understand the patient's background and the effect of their illnesses on their life and their family. Furthermore, the social determinants of health are non-medical factors that profoundly shape the occurrence and impact of illness and health outcomes. These determinants include income, education, unemployment and job insecurity, housing, childhood development, access to affordable, quality health services, gender and discrimination.

Particular occupations are at risk of certain illnesses so a full occupational history is important. The following questions should be asked.

- 'What is your job? What does that actually involve doing?'
- 'What other jobs have you done?'
- 'Who do you live with? Is your partner well? Who else is at home? What sort of place do you live in?'
- 'Do you have any financial difficulties? What things can't you afford?'
- 'Who does the shopping, washing, cleaning, bathing, etc.?'
- 'What have your illnesses prevented you doing?'
- 'How has it affected your spouse, partner, family?'
- 'Do you get out of the house much? What is your mobility like? Do you use any walking aids? How far can you walk? Do you have stairs at home?'
- 'What are your hobbies? What else do you enjoy doing?
- 'What help do you get at home? Do you have a home help or 'meals-on-wheels'? What modifications have been made to the house?'
- 'Do you have pets? Are they well?'

Travel history

Consider the following questions when taking a travel history from a patient.

- 'Have you been abroad? Where? When?'
- 'Where did you stop *en route*?'
- 'Where did you visit? Was it rural or urban?'
- 'Did you stay in hotels, camps, etc.?'
- 'Were you well whilst there?'
- 'Did you have specific vaccinations? Have you taken antimalarial prophylaxis? If so, what and for how long?'

Medicine at a Glance, Fifth Edition. Edited by Patrick Davey and Alex Pitcher.

Companion website: www.wiley.com/go/medicine5e

8 Functional enquiry

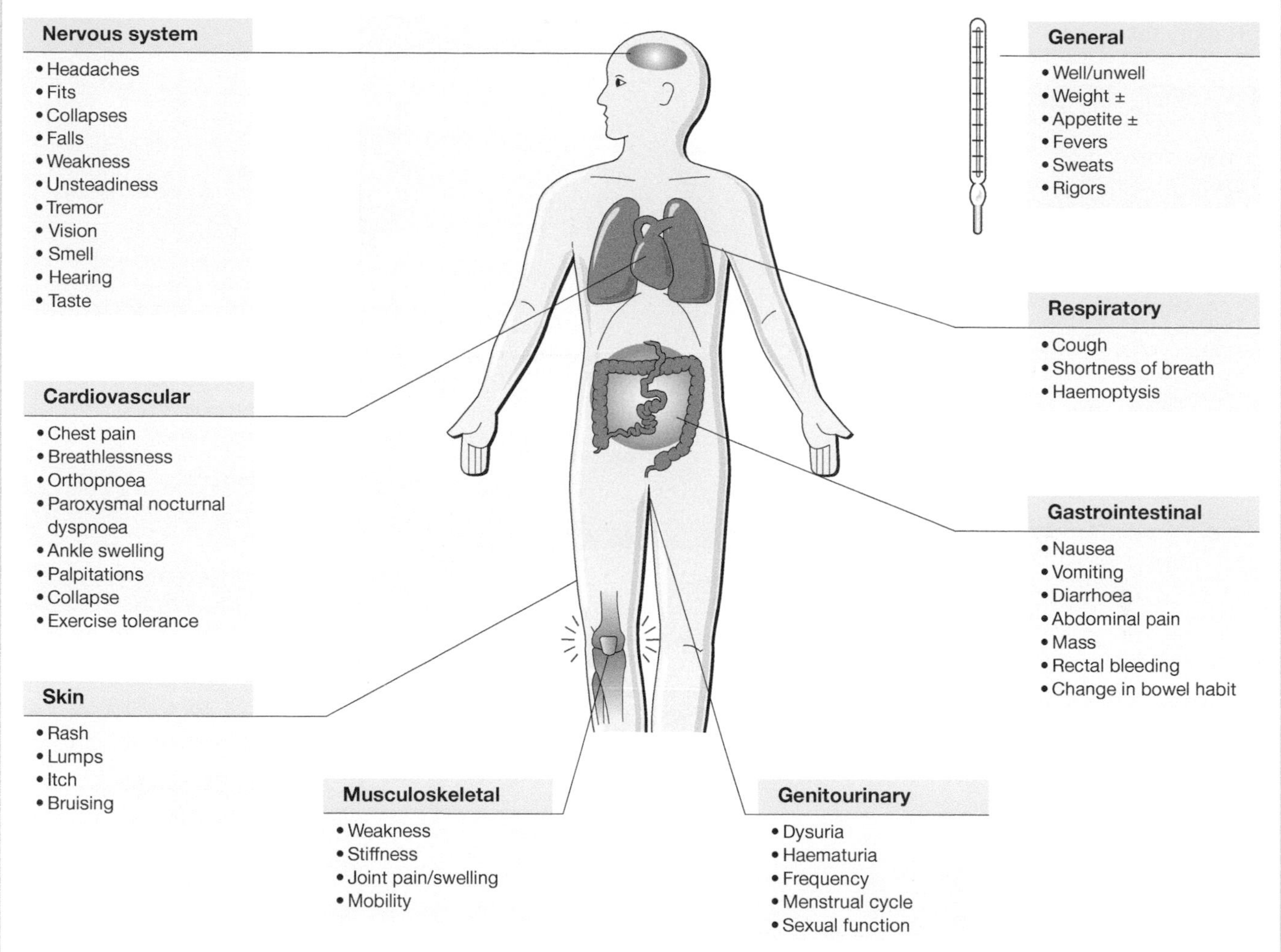

This part of the history is designed to elicit any symptoms that have not been obtained from the patient in the history of the presenting complaint. There are obviously a huge number of questions that can be asked. In any given clinical situation, these questions will need to be focused depending on the nature of the presenting complaint. The discovery of abnormalities on examination or after investigation may lead to the necessity for further directed questioning. Ask about the symptoms in the figure above.

Two of the most important aspects of the functional enquiry are:

1 to establish the exercise capacity of the patient – how far they can walk unaided in one go (flat and hills), and what are the symptoms that stop them. *If you only ask one question, ask this one!*
2 to ascertain whether the patient has a systemic illness, the usual manifestations of which are feeling unwell (malaise), loss of appetite and weight loss.

Other general questions that may be appropriate are asking about heat or cold intolerance (thyroid disorders) or whether there has been any recent injury or falls.

You should specifically ask about breathlessness, on effort and at night, wheeze and chest pain. Also, ask about pains anywhere. Ask whether the patient has brought up blood (coughing, vomiting), or passed blood in their urine and stool. Do not forget the sexual and gynaecological history: length of the menstrual cycle, period duration, whether periods are heavy, number of pregnancies, age of menarche and menopause.

Ask if the patient has any other symptoms or concerns that have not yet been discussed, e.g. 'Is there anything else bothering you?', 'Do you have any other worries about your health?', 'What things can't you do?'.

Medicine at a Glance, Fifth Edition. Edited by Patrick Davey and Alex Pitcher.

Companion website: www.wiley.com/go/medicine5e

9 Basic clinical skills

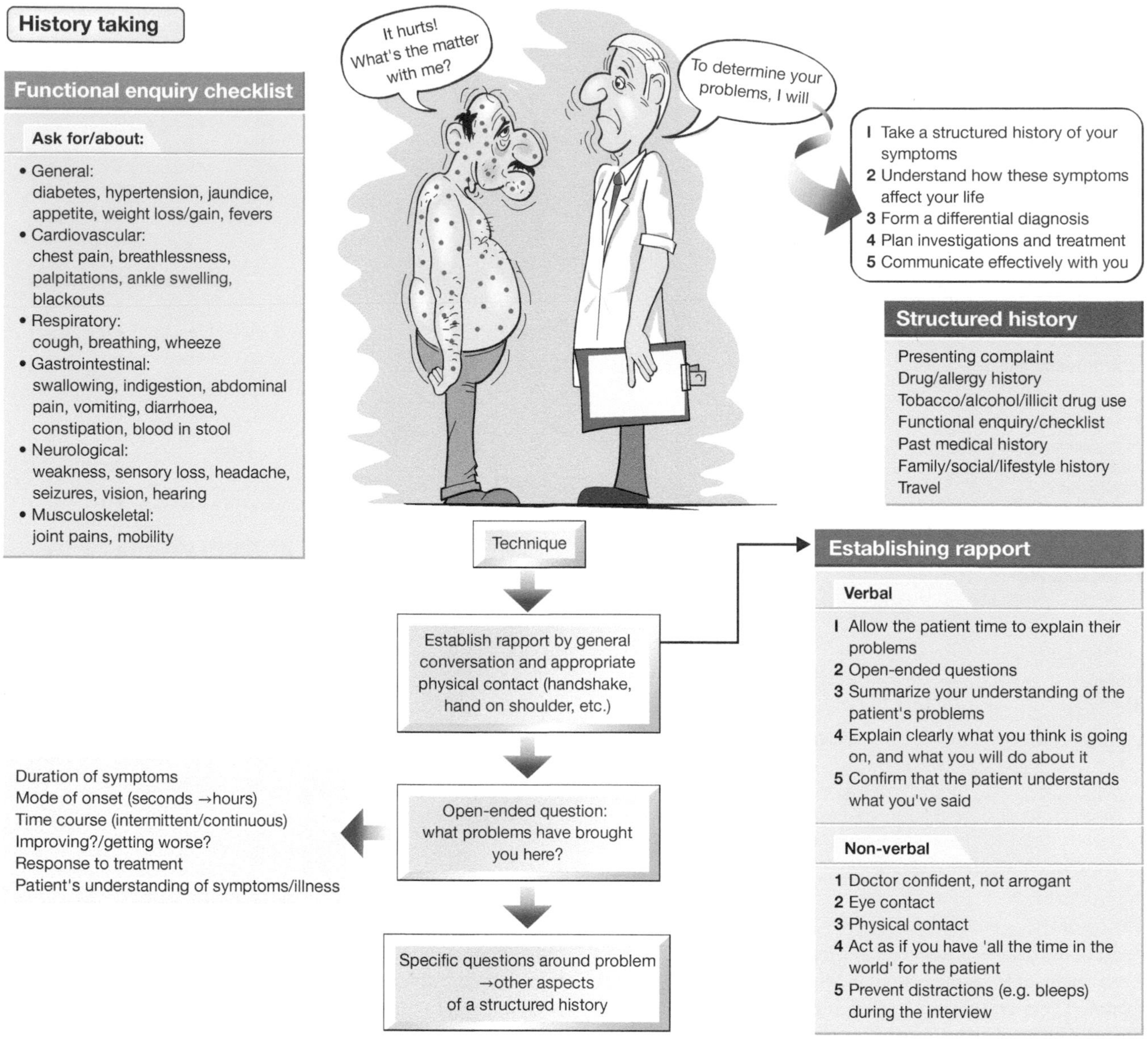

History taking

Functional enquiry checklist

Ask for/about:

- General:
  diabetes, hypertension, jaundice, appetite, weight loss/gain, fevers
- Cardiovascular:
  chest pain, breathlessness, palpitations, ankle swelling, blackouts
- Respiratory:
  cough, breathing, wheeze
- Gastrointestinal:
  swallowing, indigestion, abdominal pain, vomiting, diarrhoea, constipation, blood in stool
- Neurological:
  weakness, sensory loss, headache, seizures, vision, hearing
- Musculoskeletal:
  joint pains, mobility

It hurts! What's the matter with me?
To determine your problems, I will

1 Take a structured history of your symptoms
2 Understand how these symptoms affect your life
3 Form a differential diagnosis
4 Plan investigations and treatment
5 Communicate effectively with you

Structured history

Presenting complaint
Drug/allergy history
Tobacco/alcohol/illicit drug use
Functional enquiry/checklist
Past medical history
Family/social/lifestyle history
Travel

Technique

↓

Establish rapport by general conversation and appropriate physical contact (handshake, hand on shoulder, etc.)

↓

Open-ended question: what problems have brought you here?

→ Duration of symptoms
Mode of onset (seconds →hours)
Time course (intermittent/continuous)
Improving?/getting worse?
Response to treatment
Patient's understanding of symptoms/illness

↓

Specific questions around problem →other aspects of a structured history

Establishing rapport

Verbal

1 Allow the patient time to explain their problems
2 Open-ended questions
3 Summarize your understanding of the patient's problems
4 Explain clearly what you think is going on, and what you will do about it
5 Confirm that the patient understands what you've said

Non-verbal

1 Doctor confident, not arrogant
2 Eye contact
3 Physical contact
4 Act as if you have 'all the time in the world' for the patient
5 Prevent distractions (e.g. bleeps) during the interview

Source: Joy Sigmon.

Clinical assessment of the patient

Taking the history and performing a physical examination, the twin components of clinical assessment, are skills we will deploy perhaps 100 000 times during a medical career, so it pays to make them as effective as possible. They have as their goal the answers to these questions.

- *What is the clinical problem to be addressed, and what is its context?* The clinical problem is typically a symptom (the presenting or chief complaint), but could be an abnormal finding on screening, such as high blood pressure, or a concerning family history. The context refers to the circumstances in which the problem has arisen. Elements that are always relevant in framing the context

Medicine at a Glance, Fifth Edition. Edited by Patrick Davey and Alex Pitcher.

Companion website: www.wiley.com/go/medicine5e

include the age and sex of the patient, the time course of the problem, and any long-term health conditions.

- *What is the impact of the problem on the patient as a person?* For example, are they able to carry out the activities of daily living, to work, to look after their family?
- *What is the differential diagnosis?* The differential diagnosis is a shortlist of the possible causes of the problem in its context. For example, acute breathlessness in a 64-year-old man, presenting two weeks after right hemicolectomy for colon cancer, could be due to pulmonary embolism, pneumonia or heart failure. Differential diagnosis is the hinge between gathering information and planning management; how to formulate a differential diagnosis is discussed below.
- *What should I do next?* This will include seeking further clinical information at the bedside, choosing diagnostic tests and deciding if immediate treatment is needed.

Your clinical assessment must be adapted to the situation. If the patient has evidence of critical illness, for example, a reduced level of consciousness or respiratory distress, then you should assess the patient using the ABCDE approach (Table 9.1) while taking a focused history, and seek help.

The approach to history taking and examination that follows assumes that your patient is in a physiologically stable state, and does not require immediate medical care.

Taking the history

Begin with some friendly words of introduction, and then ask an open-ended question (e.g. 'Could you tell me what led to your coming into hospital?'). Listen to the patient's story, taking notes if needed as the patient talks. After a few minutes of listening, you will usually need to clarify points in the history with the intelligent use of questions. This applies particularly to complaints such as weakness, dizziness, blackouts, collapse and indigestion – words that may be applied to a number of different symptoms. Cover all the important areas (Table 9.2) so that you have a complete picture. In some situations, for example if the patient has impaired memory, you may need to supplement the patient's account with information gained from family members or carers (the collateral history).

'Getting the story straight' is a crucial part of history taking; it is the process of summarizing the information you have gathered and shaping it into a coherent account of what has happened to the patient. A clear chronology of events is the key to understanding causal relationships.

Having taken the history, you should make a note of the major problems identified, mentally or on paper, and form a provisional differential diagnosis which will help focus your examination. This need only be at the level of the body region, physiological system or category of disease (such as sepsis or cancer) that could be involved. Don't perform the physical examination on 'autopilot', but rather adjust it in the light of the history and ongoing examination findings. Be prepared to interrupt the examination to ask further questions if needed. For example, if you find an enlarged spleen, you should extend the history taking to ask about fever, weight loss, night sweats and any previous diagnosis of haematological or liver disease, and examine carefully for lymphadenopathy, hepatomegaly and the presence of ascites.

Table 9.1 Examination of the patient with suspected critical illness using the ABCDE approach

System	Observation	Signs of critical illness
Airway	Airway patency	Abnormal voice Inspiratory stridor Coughing and choking
Breathing	Is there respiratory distress?	Respiratory distress is characterized by dyspnoea, tachypnoea, the ability to speak only in short sentences or single words, agitation and sweating
	Respiratory rate[a]	Respiratory rate ≤8 or ≥25/min
	Arterial oxygen saturation[a]	SaO_2 ≤90%
Circulation	Heart rate[a]	≤40 or ≥131/min
	Blood pressure[a]	Systolic blood pressure ≤90 or ≥220 mmHg
	Organ perfusion	Cool or mottled skin with capillary refill time >2 s Agitation or reduced conscious level Oliguria
Disability	Conscious level[a]	Reduced conscious level: the patient does not respond to voice
	Mental state[a]	New confusion
	Blood glucose	<4 mmol/l with signs of hypoglycaemia (sweating, abnormal behaviour, reduced conscious level, seizures)
Exposure	Core temperature[a]	≤35 or >38°C, with signs of organ dysfunction
	Systematic examination	Clinical features such as purpuric rash, abdominal tenderness, limb ischaemia

[a] These observations are combined in the UK National Early Warning Score, version 2 (NEWS2).

Examination of the patient

Before examining the patient, you must obtain his or her consent, and ensure that privacy and dignity will be maintained during the examination. A chaperone, ideally of the same sex as the patient, should be present when you are examining a patient of the opposite sex. For intimate examinations – that is, examination of the female breasts, the external genitalia of both sexes, vaginal examination and anorectal examination – the chaperone must be a nurse or doctor, you should have the permission of a doctor with responsibility for care of the patient to carry out this element of the examination, and the patient should confirm consent. Include the name and designation of the chaperone in the medical record.

For most patients, you should examine in detail the system or systems relevant to the clinical problem, and also perform a rapid but thorough general examination. One approach is to perform a general examination by region

Table 9.2 Taking the history: areas to be covered

The patient as a person	**The presenting problem and its context** **Other active medical problems and long-term health conditions**	**Analysis of symptoms**	**Functional capacity and exercise tolerance**
Age and gender Racial heritage Living arrangements Important relationships Occupation Functional capacity: the patient's ability to carry out the activities of daily living Exercise tolerance Need for care or services The patient's concerns, expectations and wishes	Establish the problem and its context (the circumstances in which the problem has arisen, the date and mode of onset [abrupt / gradual], and time course [constant/intermittent; getting better/getting worse/ staying the same]) Establish other active medical problems and long-term conditions: all issues that affect the patient's current health or require treatment or monitoring	Establish the symptoms related to the presenting problem Screen for symptoms in other systems (the systems review or functional enquiry) Analysis of pain: S – site O – onset (date and mode) C – character R – radiation A – associated symptoms T – timing: pattern, frequency, duration, time course E – exacerbating/relieving factors, response to treatment S – severity (1-10/10)	If appropriate, ask about activities of daily living: • the patient's ability to move from one position to another and walk independently • to feed themselves • to select appropriate clothes and put these on • to bathe and groom themselves and to maintain dental hygiene, nail and hair care • to control bladder and bowel function • to get to and from the toilet, use it appropriately, and maintain personal hygiene Establish exercise tolerance: how far can the patient walk on the flat without stopping? What limits exercise? Has exercise tolerance changed, and if so, over what time?
Medications, adverse drug reactions, allergies, medical equipment, devices and dressings	**Past history/inactive medical problems**	**Family history**	**Social history and occupational history**
Establish: • prescribed medications • over-the-counter medications • Complementary and alternative medicine products • Dietary supplements Have there been any adverse drug reactions (allergies or intolerances)? Does the patient have any allergies? Record allergens, dates and reactions Does the patient use any medical equipment, devices or dressings?	Record under these headings, with dates: • medical • surgical • obstetric-gynaecological (gravida is the number of pregnancies a woman has had; para is the number of completed pregnancies beyond 20 weeks gestation, whether viable or non-viable) • bone fractures and other significant injuries • psychiatric What immunizations has the patient received?	Take a three-generation family history: establish the age, race/ ethnicity, health or cause of death of parents, siblings and children Has any family member had a similar medical problem?	Establish: • lifestyle, including frequency of exercise • diet • tobacco use • alcohol use (units consumed per week) • use of other substances, if relevant If relevant: • travel history • sexual history • pets and contact with animals Occupational history 'Which job do you do now? Which job did you do before that? Which job have you done the longest?'

(e.g. hands–arms–head–neck–chest–abdomen–legs–feet) and then complete a detailed examination of the relevant system or systems.

Before you lay hands on the patient, it pays dividends to make a general survey. Does the patient look well or ill and, if ill, in what way? Endocrine disorders (such as hypothyroidism) are easily missed unless you make a point of thinking of them. A checklist for the general examination is in Table 9.3.

It is important to learn and practise a rapid screening neurological and musculoskeletal examination, to use when disease in these systems is not suspected. The following is one approach that can be used.

Table 9.3 Checklist for the general examination

Element	Comment
Appearance	Does the patient appear well, acutely unwell or chronically unwell? Are they comfortable at rest? Are they in pain?
Conscious level and mental state	Is the patient alert? Are they lucid or confused? The conscious level can be graded clinically using the simple four-point AVPU scale (A, alert; V, responds to voice; P, responds to painful stimuli; U, unresponsive). The mental state examination should include assessment of attention, orientation and memory (e.g. by using the 4AT Test, Table 79.2, p. 173)
Physiological observations	All hospital inpatients, and all patients presenting to the emergency department, should have measurement of pulse rate, blood pressure, respiratory rate, arterial oxygen saturation and body temperature, and assessment of their conscious level and mental state (see Table 9.1)
Nutritional state	Measure the height and weight and calculate the body mass index: the body mass index (BMI) is the weight in kilograms divided by the square of the height in metres. A BMI of <18.5 signifies underweight, 18.5–<25 normal weight, 25–<30 overweight and ≥30 obesity
Muscle mass	Loss of skeletal muscle mass (sarcopenia) is an important prognostic feature of diseases such as cancer, heart failure and chronic obstructive pulmonary disease, and is a key element of the frailty syndrome of old age
Presence or absence of specific important signs	
Pallor	Conjunctival pallor is typically present when the haemoglobin is <100 g/l. Anaemia may be due to decreased production of red cells, haemolysis or blood loss
Cyanosis	Central cyanosis (affecting the lips and tongue) is usually detectable when arterial oxygen saturation is <90%, unless anaemia is present; however, it is an unreliable sign and, where possible, always check oxygen saturation with pulse oximetry. Central cyanosis may be due to respiratory failure or right-to-left shunt
Jaundice	Jaundice is detectable when plasma bilirubin concentration is >40–50 micromol/l: consider prehepatic, hepatic and posthepatic (obstructive) causes
Finger clubbing	Causes include intrathoracic neoplasms and infection, cyanotic congenital heart disease and inflammatory bowel disease
Lymphadenopathy	Check cervical, supraclavicular, epitrochlear, axillary and inguinal regions. Assess the number, size, mobility, consistency and tenderness of enlarged lymph nodes
Abnormalities of the skin, nails and subcutaneous tissues	These may include rash, pigmentation, surgical and other scars, purpura, bruising, lumps and ulceration

- Inspect the hands, for wasting of the intrinsic muscles and joint abnormalities, test the power of finger abduction, and check light touch sensation over the hands – gently stroke the skin and ask the patient if this feels normal and equal on both sides.
- Ask the patient to hold the arms outstretched with palms down and fingers abducted, and to make piano-playing movements (upper motor neuron lesions cause the movements to be performed more slowly or clumsily), then to turn the palms up and maintain the posture with the eyes closed (upper motor neuron lesions cause the arm to drift downwards and into pronation).
- Put the wrist, elbow and shoulder joints through their range of movement (to assess muscle tone and detect restriction of joint movement) and test the power of shoulder abduction (proximal limb weakness is a feature of myopathies). Ask the patient to put the hands behind the head with the elbows back (to assess the glenohumeral, acromioclavicular and sternoclavicular joints). Check the finger–nose test.
- Check cervical spine movements (ask the patient to touch the ear on to the shoulder).
- Check visual acuity, fields, eye movements and pupils and examine the fundi.
- Put the hip, knee and ankle joints through their range of movement (including rotation of the hip joint with the knee flexed, to assess muscle tone and detect restriction of joint movement); test the power of hip flexion.
- Inspect the feet: test the power of ankle dorsiflexion. Check light touch sensation over the feet – gently stroke the skin and ask the patient if this feels normal and equal on both sides. Check the heel–knee–shin test; test the tendon reflexes and plantar responses.
- Observe the patient standing, walking and turning.

Formulating a differential diagnosis

After our first encounter with a new patient, we often can't say for certain what specific disease is the cause of the problem. Indeed, if we fix on a single diagnosis at this stage, there is a good chance that we will be wrong, and misdiagnosis may carry a penalty for the patient if it delays the correct treatment. Our aim, rather, is to generate a shortlist (3–5 items) of possible causes, which can be expressed at the level of clinical syndrome (such as heart failure) or pathophysiology, as well as specific diseases. For example, if our patient is a 57-year-old woman with progressive exertional breathlessness over the course of six months, the differential diagnosis could include anaemia, respiratory, cardiovascular or neuromuscular disease, or a combination of these. Maintaining a broad-brush approach early in the diagnostic process, and considering a range of possibilities, helps us avoid the trap of accepting the first diagnosis which seems to fit the facts without considering better alternatives.

Differential diagnosis is a challenge when you are starting out in medicine. However, it is generally the case that the problem that led the patient to seek medical attention reflects an important manifestation of their disease, and often the best place to start the diagnostic process is with the presenting complaint. Several approaches to this are possible. Your analysis can be carried out by:

- *the anatomy of a body region*: this works well for the symptom of pain or the finding of a mass.
- *physiological system*: this is applicable to complaints that relate to disorders of function, such as breathlessness or muscular weakness.
- *category of disease*: this can be combined with your analysis by anatomy or physiology. The mode of onset, time course and duration of symptoms are valuable clues to the underlying pathophysiology. The onset of symptoms over seconds or minutes is characteristic of vascular disease, epilepsy or arrhythmia; over hours or days, of infection; over weeks or months, of autoimmune inflammation or neoplasia; and over months or years, of degenerative disease.

The differential diagnosis can be generated from this analysis, from discussion with colleagues, from reading the medical literature, and from the internet – a Google search is often a fruitful way of expanding the differential diagnosis, particularly when there is a cluster of definite abnormalities. Suggestions from the patient and their family as to the diagnosis can sometimes be very helpful, and should always be considered seriously.

Most symptoms can reflect a broad range of diseases, from the self-limiting to the life-threatening. Our differential diagnosis should therefore include the most serious causes of a problem, obviously if there are features pointing to these, but also if they cannot be excluded on clinical grounds. Acute chest pain, for example, is often due to gastro-oesophageal reflux or benign musculoskeletal disease, but acute coronary syndrome, pulmonary embolism and aortic dissection are also possibilities, and as we proceed with history taking and examination, we should test the findings in our patient against the characteristics of these diseases.

Co-ordinating diagnosis with safe care of the patient

Occasionally, you can make the right diagnosis immediately and with confidence. However, often the diagnosis is unclear, and the tests required to rule in or rule out possible serious diagnoses are not available (e.g. because it is the middle of the night) or take too long to come back (e.g. blood culture). In this situation, you must treat what is probable, and also what might be dangerous, while data collection continues.

Correction of abnormal physiology is crucial in those with life-threatening disease (e.g. volume replacement in severe gastrointestinal bleeding). Immediate empirical treatment may be needed for diseases that are dangerous and rapidly progressive (e.g. empirical antibiotic therapy in suspected bacterial meningitis, before lumbar puncture). For patients seen in clinic, with a history which does not suggest major disease and with reassuring findings on examination, observation over time (with or without further investigation) can be the right course.

Presenting the case

The cardinal virtues here are brevity, clarity and enthusiasm. Your presentation should last under five minutes. If your listener wants more detail, they will ask for it. Always include the age and occupation of the patient in your opening remarks. Do not mention the sex and racial heritage of the patient if you are presenting the case in their presence.

Begin with a short summary of the patient's problems and any long-term health conditions. You should then deal, in turn, with information gained from the history, the relevant findings on examination, your differential diagnosis and your plan of action. Be prepared to answer the following questions.

- What do you think is the most likely diagnosis? How well does this diagnosis explain the significant positive and negative findings? Does it provide a plausible mechanism to link them, and account for the time course of events?
- What other diagnoses should we consider? What are the most serious causes of this clinical problem? Which of these do we need to include in the differential diagnosis of this patient?
- What should we do next? What additional information could we gain from further history taking and examination? What diagnostic tests should be done?
- Is any immediate treatment needed?
- What should we say to the patient and their family?

10 Principles of examination

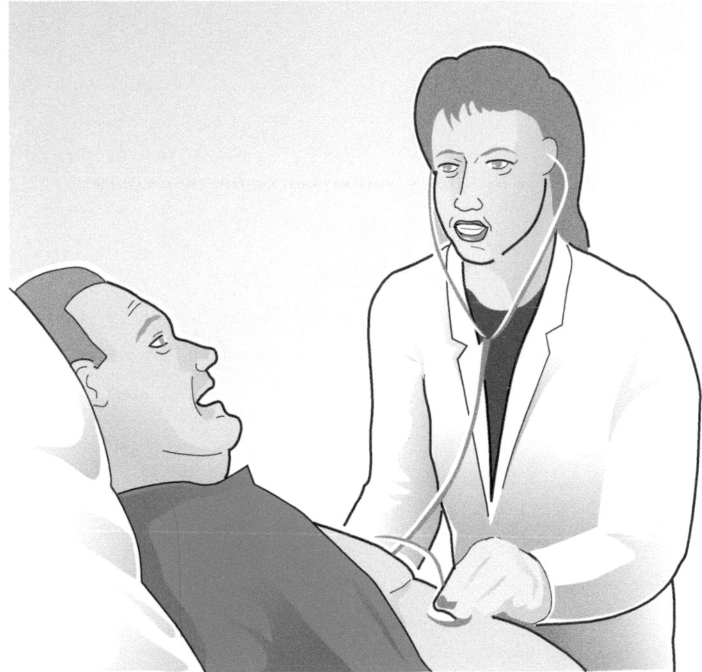

Ensure
Patient's comfort, privacy, confidentiality
Presence of chaperone if appropriate

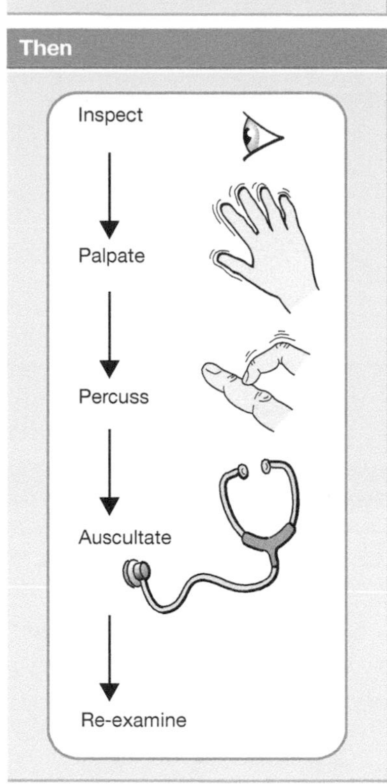

Source: Jonathan Gleadle 2011 / with permission of John Wiley & Sons.

Explain to the patient what you plan to do. Ensure they are comfortable and warm and that there is privacy. Use all your senses: sight, hearing, smell and touch.

Inspect

Stand back. Look at the whole patient. Ensure there is adequate lighting.

- Look around the bed for other 'clues' (e.g. oxygen mask, nebulizer, sputum pot, walking stick, vomit bowl).
- Ensure the patient is adequately exposed (with privacy and comfort) and correctly positioned to permit a full examination.
- Look carefully and thoroughly. Are there any glaring abnormalities (e.g. lumps, unconsciousness, jaundice, cyanosis)? Are there any subtle abnormalities (e.g. pallor, fasciculations)?
- Look with specific manoeuvres, such as coughing, breathing or movement.

Palpate

Seek the patient's permission and explain what you are going to do. Ask whether there is any pain or tenderness. Begin the examination lightly and gently, looking at the patient's face for signs of apprehension, discomfort or pain, and then use firmer pressure. Define any abnormalities carefully, perhaps with measurement. Check if there are thrills.

Percuss

Percuss, comparing sides. Listen and 'feel' for any differences. Ensure that this does not cause pain or discomfort.

Auscultate

Ensure the stethoscope is functioning and take time to listen. Consider the positioning of the patient to optimize sounds; for example, sitting forward and listening in expiration for aortic regurgitation.

If abnormalities are found at any stage, try to compare them with the 'normal'; for example, compare the percussion note over equivalent areas of the chest.

Record findings

Record findings accurately, measure any abnormality and consider photographic documentation of visible abnormalities such as a rash or leg ulcer.

Medicine at a Glance, Fifth Edition. Edited by Patrick Davey and Alex Pitcher.

Companion website: www.wiley.com/go/medicine5e

11 Is the patient ill?

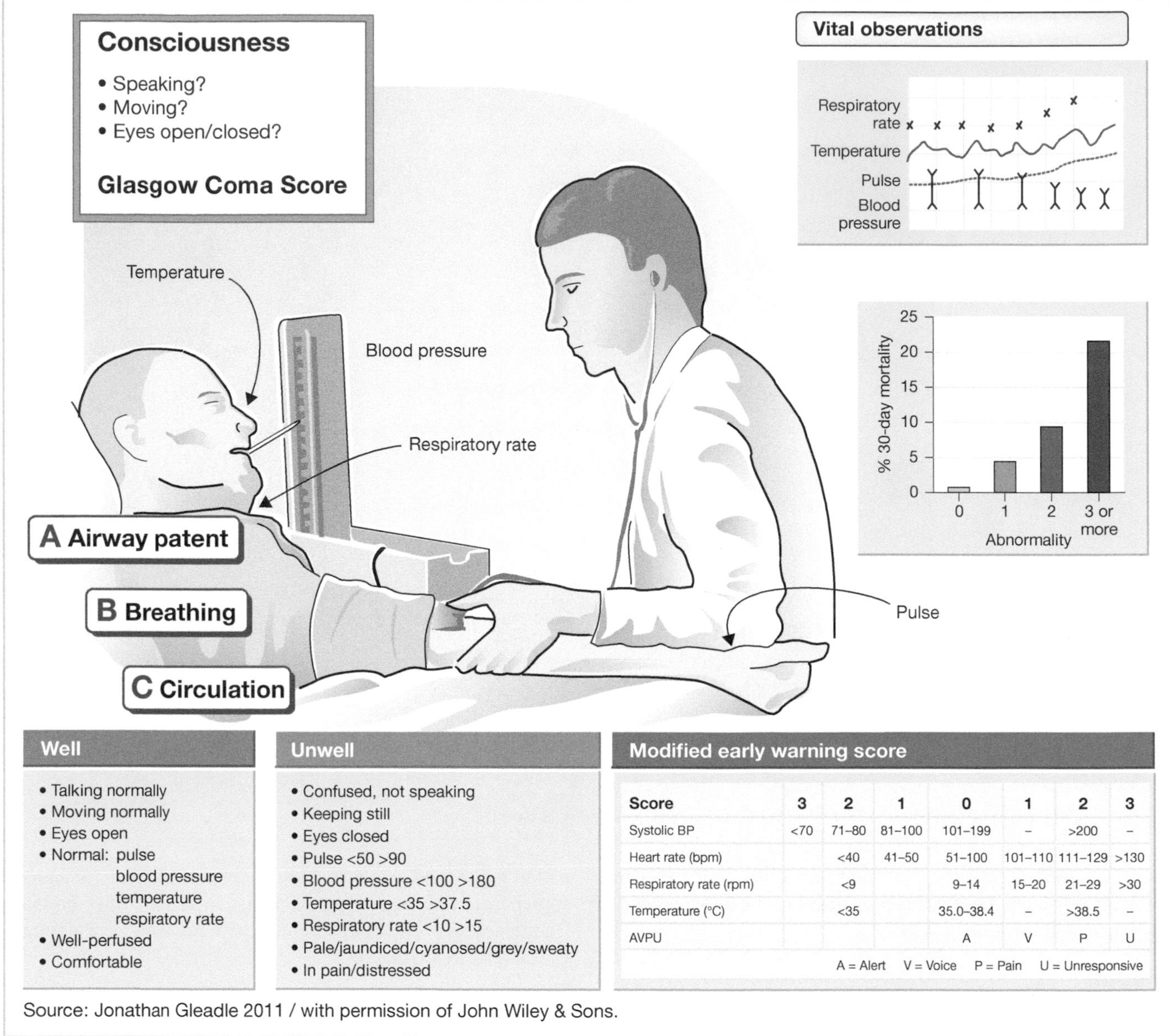

Score	3	2	1	0	1	2	3
Systolic BP	<70	71–80	81–100	101–199	–	>200	–
Heart rate (bpm)		<40	41–50	51–100	101–110	111–129	>130
Respiratory rate (rpm)		<9		9–14	15–20	21–29	>30
Temperature (°C)		<35		35.0–38.4	–	>38.5	–
AVPU				A	V	P	U

A = Alert V = Voice P = Pain U = Unresponsive

Source: Jonathan Gleadle 2011 / with permission of John Wiley & Sons.

One of the most important skills a doctor can gain is the recognition that a patient is ill. The definition of 'being ill' or 'being sick' is different in hospital medicine when compared to primary care, or from what patients mean by this phrase.

- Patients mean they feel unwell, or, in other words, experience malaise; most inflammatory illnesses cause this and, in primary care, most of these are benign and self-limiting, with a low mortality risk. This definition is not what doctors mean by the phrase.
- In primary care, the phrase usually implies a need for immediate hospital admission; mortality risk exists but is relatively low, probably around 2–5%.
- In hospital, the phrase 'being ill' means that the patient has a high chance of early death or disability. This is largely what most hospital doctors mean when they say a patient is ill – they think the patient has an appreciable chance of dying, and dying really quite soon.

So, being ill in hospital inevitably leads to the activation of many resources, including specialist wards (coronary care,

Medicine at a Glance, Fifth Edition. Edited by Patrick Davey and Alex Pitcher.

Companion website: www.wiley.com/go/medicine5e

high-dependency unit, critical care), specialist clinicians, and often expensive out-of-hours investigations and treatment. This complex array of therapies is applied to improve an otherwise poor outcome. It is therefore really important, where possible, to diagnose the severity of a patient's illness accurately, so that ill patients can benefit from such resources, avoiding the inappropriate use of these expensive resources, and so that patients and relatives can be prepared for the possibility of a poor outcome. **If you think a patient is acutely and seriously ill, get help immediately from other doctors and nurses.**

There are several features that experienced clinicians notice instantly as signs that a patient is seriously ill.

Clues from the history

There are many clues in the history to pick up on – for example, acute severe breathlessness following a long plane journey is likely to constitute a life-threatening pulmonary embolus; or a patient who has just had a very sudden onset of the most severe headache they have ever experienced may have had a critical subarachnoid haemorrhage. In other words, many clinicians will know a patient is ill before they have even seen them!

Laboratory clues

Some patients may have immediately life-threatening illness without any abnormal findings (e.g. severe hyperkalaemia); always check laboratory results on *all* patients shortly after admission in case this applies to your apparently healthy patient.

Observational clues

Experienced nurses and clinicians may also feel that a patient is seriously ill without being able to identify objective abnormalities. Patients who are seriously ill often look ill; picking up on this is an acquired skill, and experienced clinicians are amalgamating information from the history and examination in reaching this diagnosis.

Clues from the charts

However, perhaps the most important means of picking up on sickness is from the vital signs, the observations of pulse, blood pressure, temperature, respiratory rate and conscious level. These data can then be picked up in 'early warning scores' (see the figure at the start of this chapter), firstly on the early warning score itself and secondly on the relationship between the score and mortality.

Assessment of ill patients

Once you think a patient is ill, go through the following ABC checklist to further assess the patient – this list will essentially tell you that the patient's lungs, cardiovascular system and brain are, at least for the time being, functioning.

- **A for airway.** Is the airway patent? Is the patient breathing easily and talking comfortably? Is there stridor?
- **B for breathing.** Is the patient breathing slowly or rapidly? Noisily? With difficulty, such that they are unable to talk because of breathlessness? Check the respiratory rate and the pattern of breathing – for example, are there periods of deep breathing lasting half a minute or so interspersed with almost absent breathing, so-called Cheyne–Stokes respiration (found in brainstem lesions and heart failure)? Is there wheeze, and are the accessory muscles being used?
- **C for circulation.** Check there is adequate circulation – are the peripheries warm or cold, is there peripheral (poor cardiac output or vasoconstricted) or central (arterial hypoxaemia) cyanosis? Is the pulse volume low, and what is the heart rate? What is the blood pressure, and is there a postural drop (suggests hypovolaemia)?

General findings

- Is the patient comfortable or uncomfortable?
- What is the patient's colour? Is the patient pale (anaemia or shock)?
- What is the temperature? Is the patient pyrexial? Hypothermic?
- Is the patient blue (cyanosed)?
- Is the patient grey (combination of cyanosis and pallor)?
- Is the patient clammy (sweaty and poor perfusion)?
- Is the patient sweaty?
- Is the patient in pain? Grimacing? Appearing abnormally still?
- Is the patient moving normally, restless or paralysed?

Consciousness

The level of consciousness is well assessed using the Glasgow Coma Score (GCS); if significantly impaired, is there abnormal posture, e.g. abnormal extension of limbs (decerebrate) or abnormal flexion of arms (decorticate)? If the Glasgow Coma Score is normal, further assessment of brain function can be picked up by the following.

- Is the patient confused? If so, use the Mini-Mental State Score.
- How does the patient engage with you? Can they talk, smile, make eye contact and answer questions appropriately (are they drowsy, but not actually confused)?

In any patient, significant changes in these observations may indicate serious deterioration.

12 The critically ill patient

The key features of the clinical assessment of the critically ill patient

Clinical Assessment
Airway
Breathing
Circulation
Disability (neurological status)
Exposure (full patient examination)

Review of notes/charts of physiological variables and trends

Simple scales have the advantage that they are easier for inexperienced health-care workers to use and show less interobserver variability than more complicated scales like the Glasgow Coma Score (see Chapter 80)

Simple Assessment of Conscious Level (AVPU, ACDU)			
A	**A**lert	**A**	**A**lert
V	Responds to **V**oice	**C**	**C**onfused
P	Responds to **P**ain	**D**	**D**rowsy
U	**U**nresponsive	**U**	**U**nresponsive

Recognition of the critically ill patient

The severity of illness and associated patient morbidity and mortality varies widely between individuals (and demographics such as age, frailty and co-morbid illness, such as diabetes, heart failure, etc., are all crucial). However, when approaching a potentially sick patient, as in all other patients, taking a history, performing an examination and ordering appropriate investigations are essential in order to make the correct diagnosis and to institute appropriate therapy.

The management of critically ill patients outside the intensive therapy unit (ITU) is often suboptimal, predominantly because there has been a failure to recognize the severity of the patient's illness. Sometimes critical illness is obvious from the end of the bed. Often, however, critical illness is recognized by alterations in key physiological variables rather than 'just' by the patient 'looking' sick.

Maintenance of adequate airway, breathing and circulation is a prerequisite for survival. Accordingly, simple physiological observations such as heart rate (HR), systolic blood pressure (BP), oxygen saturations, respiratory rate (RR), level of consciousness, urine output and temperature define inpatient mortality. Mortality can be directly correlated with the number of abnormalities, rising from 0.7% (30-day mortality) with none, 4.4% with one, 9.2% with two, to 21.3% with three or more.

Many patients who suffer a cardiorespiratory arrest or are admitted to intensive care have a documented decline in these physiological variables prior to these events, which often goes unrecognized. It is therefore important to have a system for recognizing critically ill patients, ensuring sufficient monitoring takes place in a designated area, instituting appropriate therapy and calling for additional help or expertise if required. In some cases it might be the realization that the patient is in the process of dying and that their symptoms should be palliated.

Examination of the critically ill patient

As the patient is examined, specific immediate life-saving therapies or investigations may be initiated, such as a chest drain in a patient with a tension pneumothorax, before other parts of the examination are undertaken. Adequate monitoring in an appropriate area also needs to be ensured. If the patient is being seen for the first time, a full assessment of the notes needs to be undertaken.

Dysfunction of the airway, breathing or circulation can lead to immediate death and so the patient assessment should focus on these systems.

Airway

Obstruction of the airway is an emergency and unless rectified, leads to rapid hypoxia and death within minutes. It is therefore pointless making an examination of the circulation in a hypotensive patient with an obstructed airway; indeed, the hypotension may be the consequence of airway obstruction.

- **Complete airway obstruction** leads to paradoxical chest and abdominal movements so that the chest moves in and the abdomen out on inspiration (as opposed to both moving out in normal

Medicine at a Glance, Fifth Edition. Edited by Patrick Davey and Alex Pitcher.

Companion website: www.wiley.com/go/medicine5e

Observation chart for NEWS

NEWS key	FULL NAME	
0 1 2 3	DATE OF BIRTH	DATE OF ADMISSION

Parameter	Row	Score
	DATE	
	TIME	
A+B Respirations Breaths/min	≥25	3
	21–24	2
	18–20	
	15–17	
	12–14	
	9–11	1
	≤8	3
A+B SpO$_2$ Scale 1 Oxygen saturation (%)	≥96	
	94–95	1
	92–93	2
	≤91	3
SpO$_2$ Scale 2† Oxygen saturation (%) Use Scale 2 if target range is 88–92%, eg in hypercapnic respiratory failure	≥97 on O_2	3
	95–96 on O_2	2
	93–94 on O_2	1
	≥93 on air	
	88–92	
†ONLY use Scale 2 under the direction of a qualified clinician	86–87	1
	84–85	2
	≤83%	3
Air or oxygen?	A=Air	
	O_2 L/min	2
	Device	
C Blood pressure mmHg Score uses systolic BP only	≥220	3
	201–219	
	181–200	
	161–180	
	141–160	
	121–140	
	111–120	
	101–110	1
	91–100	2
	81–90	3
	71–80	3
	61–70	3
	51–60	3
	≤50	3
C Pulse Beats/min	≥131	3
	121–130	2
	111–120	2
	101–110	1
	91–100	1
	81–90	
	71–80	
	61–70	
	51–60	
	41–50	1
	31–40	3
	≤30	3
D Consciousness Score for NEW onset of confusion (no score if chronic)	Alert	
	Confusion	3
	V	3
	P	3
	U	3
E Temperature °C	≥39.1°	2
	38.1–39.0°	1
	37.1–38.0°	
	36.1–37.0°	
	35.1–36.0°	1
	≤35.0°	3
NEWS TOTAL		
	Monitoring frequency	
	Escalation of care Y/N	
	Initials	

Clinical response to the NEWS trigger thresholds

NEW score	Frequency of monitoring	Clinical response
0	Minimum 12 hourly	• Continue routine NEWS monitoring
Total 1–4	Minimum 4–6 hourly	• Inform registered nurse, who must assess the patient • Registered nurse decides whether increased frequency of monitoring and/or escalation of care is required
3 in single parameter	Minimum 1 hourly	• Registered nurse to inform medical team caring for the patient, who will review and decide whether escalation of care is necessary
Total 5 or more Urgent response threshold	Minimum 1 hourly	• Registered nurse to immediately inform the medical team caring for the patient • Registered nurse to request urgent assessment by a clinician or team with core competencies in the care of acutely ill patients • Provide clinical care in an environment with monitoring facilities
Total 7 or more Emergency response threshold	Continuous monitoring of vital signs	• Registered nurse to immediately inform the medical team caring for the patient – this should be at least at specialist registrar level • Emergency assessment by a team with critical care competencies, including practitioner(s) with advanced airway management skills • Consider transfer of care to a level 2 or 3 clinical care facility, ie higher-dependency unit or ICU • Clinical care in an environment with monitoring facilities

NEWS thresholds and triggers

NEW score	Clinical risk	Response
Aggregate score 0–4	Low	Ward-based response
Red score Score of 3 in any individual parameter	Low–medium	Urgent ward-based response*
Aggregate score 5–6	Medium	Key threshold for urgent response*
Aggregate score 7 or more	High	Urgent or emergency response**

* Response by a clinician or team with competence in the assessment and treatment of acutely ill patients and in recognising when the escalation of care to a critical care team is appropriate.

**The response team must also include staff with critical care skills, including airway management.

Source: Reproduced with permission from the Royal College of Physicians. This chart is reproduced here for reference only. For clinical use, please visit www.rcplondon.ac.uk/resources/national-early-warning-score-news where full-sized versions with instructions and guidance for use may be downloaded breathing) and vice versa on expiration. Accessory muscle use and a tracheal tug are present. No movement of air is present at the mouth either audibly or by feeling with a hand at the patient's mouth.

- **Partial airway obstruction** leads to noisy breathing with detectable movement of air at the mouth. Stridor indicates obstruction at the larynx or above, while snoring often occurs when the tongue obstructs the pharynx.

In the majority of patients, simple measures resolve airway obstruction. Blood, vomit, secretions or foreign bodies may be removed by suction. If consciousness is impaired, loss of muscle tone causes the tongue to fall back and obstruct. A chin lift or jaw thrust opens the airway; occasionally an airway adjunct such as an oropharyngeal (Guedel) or nasopharyngeal airway is required. If these simple methods fail then endotracheal intubation or *rarely* a surgical cricothyroidotomy is required. The use of airway adjuncts, endotracheal intubation or surgical airways should only be undertaken by appropriately trained staff. These techniques may cause vomiting or laryngospasm if performed by inadequately trained individuals, potentially transforming a partially occluded airway to one that is completely obstructed.

Breathing

Visual examination is extremely informative, with respiratory rate being one of the most important observations. A rate <8 or >20 per minute should alert the examiner to severe illness. Tachypnoea is the most common physiological abnormality in critical illness so great care should be taken to record respiratory rate accurately. Expansion of the chest should be compared bilaterally, as well as depth, abdominal breathing, accessory muscle use and tracheal tugging (respiratory pattern). Abnormal expansion usually accompanies underlying disease (collapse, consolidation, effusion, pneumothorax).

The inspired oxygen concentration should be noted and oxygen saturations on pulse oximetry recorded (cyanosis is often a late sign); if indicated, a blood gas is performed. The latter provides information on adequacy of ventilation ($PaCO_2$) and oxygenation (PaO_2 and A-a gradient). Respiratory acidosis (pH <7.3, PCO_2 >6.0 kPa) or failure of oxygenation (SaO_2 <90% or PaO_2 <8 kPa on high-flow oxygen) requires urgent intervention. Treatment is discussed in Chapters 99, 105 and 106 – all critically ill patients need oxygen saturations maintained above 90%.

Circulation

Important parameters of the circulatory examination are blood pressure, pulse, capillary refill, limb temperature, urine output and level of consciousness. A 'normal' blood pressure may represent hypotension in some patients and it is therefore useful to know the patient's usual pressure. Hypotension may also be a late sign when homeostatic mechanisms fail to compensate and is usually preceded by an abnormal pulse (often tachycardia). Normal capillary refill is less than 2 seconds and prolongation suggests inadequate tissue perfusion. However, this sign is less reliable in elderly patients where normal capillary refill may exceed 2 seconds. An arterial blood gas may be indicated and show metabolic acidosis with a raised lactate if the circulation is inadequate (base excess more than −4 or lactate >2 mmol/L). Treatment of circulatory abnormalities is discussed in Chapters 18 and 235.

Disability

Neurological status is assessed by examining the pupils and the level of consciousness (Glasgow Coma Score [GCS] or simple scales such as AVPU or ACDU). Hypoglycaemia should be excluded in all sick patients.

Exposure

A general examination should be made with particular attention to drains and wound sites. The temperature should be recorded.

Examination of critically ill patients' charts

It is important to examine the patient's charts, which record physiological variables of blood pressure, pulse, temperature, respiratory rate, oxygen saturations, consciousness level and urine output over time. While the absolute values are important, *equal value is attached to the trends and response to treatment.* As emphasized earlier, the number of physiological abnormalities defines mortality. Earlier recognition of patient deterioration would be expected to prevent unexpected cardiac arrests and admissions to intensive care. Many hospitals now utilize severity triggers or modified early warning scoring systems in combination with medical emergency or outreach teams. Some disease-specific scoring systems that define severity of illness and mortality are also in common use and incorporate physiological variables; examples include the CURB-65 (community-acquired pneumonia) and Rockall (upper gastrointestinal bleeding) scores.

The Royal College of Physicians has recommended a standardized NHS Early Warning Score (NEWS2) be used in all NHS hospitals.

Admission to intensive care

This is a key decision in the management of the sick patient; clearly, patients who will benefit from ITU should go there, whereas those who won't shouldn't. However, discriminating between these two groups reliably is often not possible, and will require judgement. Obtaining patients' and relatives' views of ITU, in the light of data on outcomes, is crucial to the decision to admit to ITU. Most ITU admissions should be the consequence of discussions between the consultant looking after the patient and the consultant intensivist.

Treatment of the critically sick patient

This is covered in other chapters. Often, the crucial question is 'how much treatment', rather than 'what sort of treatment'. This aspect requires great judgement and excellent communication skills; indeed, in this area perhaps more than any other, the ability to know when to discontinue therapy, when not to escalate treatment, and when to implement terminal care at just the right stage are what defines clinical excellence. As relatives often have inappropriately high expectations about the outcome of intensive care therapy, it is important to be realistic (and kind) at all times.

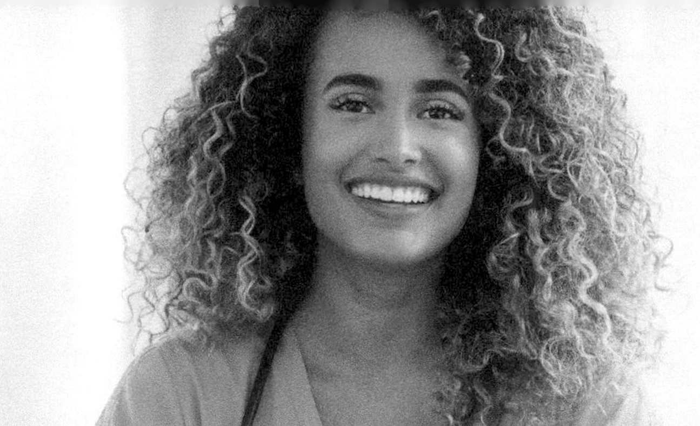

Chapters

Clinical presentations at a glance

13 Chest pain

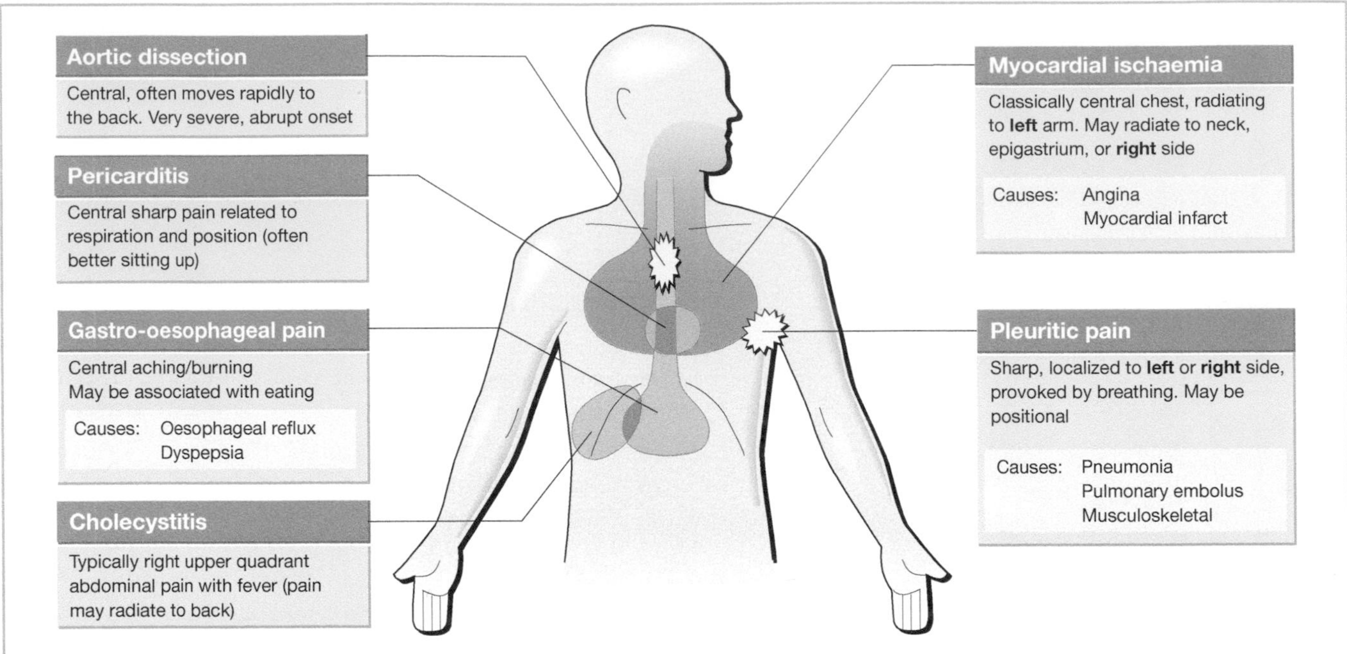
Aortic dissection
Central, often moves rapidly to the back. Very severe, abrupt onset
Pericarditis
Central sharp pain related to respiration and position (often better sitting up)
Gastro-oesophageal pain
Central aching/burning
May be associated with eating
Causes: Oesophageal reflux
Dyspepsia
Cholecystitis
Typically right upper quadrant abdominal pain with fever (pain may radiate to back)
Myocardial ischaemia
Classically central chest, radiating to left arm. May radiate to neck, epigastrium, or right side
Causes: Angina
Myocardial infarct
Pleuritic pain
Sharp, localized to left or right side, provoked by breathing. May be positional
Causes: Pneumonia
Pulmonary embolus
Musculoskeletal

Determining the cause of chest pain is a common clinical problem which can present a diagnostic challenge. The greatest concern is usually whether the pain relates to heart disease. This thought dominates the clinical and investigative approach. Most pains are diagnosed by a full history, sometimes aided by the clinical examination.

The diagnostic approach involves determining the nature of the pain, how long it has been present, typical provoking and relieving factors, and the presence of risk factors for heart/lung disease. For patients who are well, you should always carry out the full diagnostic process in a thoughtful and methodical manner – history, then examination, then simple investigations, followed by synthesizing the differential diagnosis so as to guide special investigations. However, some patients with chest pain are sick, indeed sometimes on the edge of death; in such sick patients you will have to act quickly, amalgamating the history with the examination, while simultaneously working with others to organize chest X-rays, computed tomography (CT) scans, echocardiography, immediate cath lab access, etc. Tailor your approach to the sickness of the patient.

In the reasonably healthy patient, once a diagnosis has been suggested by the history, perform the physical examination, both to try and obtain data to support the diagnosis (though this is often not forthcoming) and also to exclude other serious illness. Though a full examination should be carried out, the key aspects are to determine the following.

- Is the patient well? If not (see Chapter 12), you must rapidly work out why and start appropriate therapy as soon as possible.
- What is the haemodynamic status and oxygenation? Check skin perfusion (warm or cold), capillary refill time, heart rate, blood pressure and oxygen saturation; if there is any major upset, you must reach a diagnosis quickly and intervene.
- Is there evidence of heart failure (see Chapter 87), especially tachycardia, raised JVP, third heart sound and bibasal pulmonary crepitations?
- Are there features of pulmonary embolus – particularly breathlessness, tachypnoea, increased heart rate and hypoxia – in the absence of lung signs indicating an alternative pathology (e.g. of infection, failure or chronic obstructive pulmonary disease [COPD])? Regardless of how certain you are about the diagnosis, always actively think whether pulmonary embolus could be a component of the illness.
- Are there features suggesting lung sepsis, such as fever, increased heart rate, tachypnoea and areas of bronchial breathing?
- Are there features suggesting that major risk factors for coronary disease are present – old age, high BMI (suggesting the metabolic syndrome, the triad of hypertension, diabetes and increased abdominal girth), evidence of smoking (a lined face, nicotine-stained hands, smell of tobacco smoke on clothes), evidence of hyperlipidaemia (look for cholesterol deposits in extensor tendons and around the eyes)?

Medicine at a Glance, Fifth Edition. Edited by Patrick Davey and Alex Pitcher.

Companion website: www.wiley.com/go/medicine5e

- Is there any evidence of vascular disease? Examine all peripheral pulses and listen for bruits over the major arteries, particularly the carotids and femorals.
- Are there features of any important co-morbid illness, such as COPD, dementia, immobility or frailty that will impact on the diagnostic process and influence treatment?

Assimilate all the key historical and examination features so that you have a clear view of what has happened to the patient, what the likely diagnosis is, and what you are going to do about it.

The diagnostic process for chronic chest pain versus acute chest pain differs significantly, in that for chronic chest pain (by which is meant pain that is reasonably long standing, e.g. present for more than eight weeks, and has not changed in nature recently), the main diagnostic condition to consider is stable effort angina which, while there can be risks associated with this, is on the whole a condition with a low chance of very early death. This means that, for most patients, outpatient assessment is appropriate. In acute chest pain, by which is meant chest pain that has been present either for only a few hours or up to a few weeks, the greatest concern is that the cause is immediately life-threatening, either myocardial infarction of one form or another, or another potentially life-threatening diagnosis such as pulmonary embolism or aortic dissection. While most patients with chronic chest pain can safely be managed on an outpatient basis, many patients with acute chest pain need at least a period of in-hospital assessment, to rule out immediately dangerous conditions.

Diagnostic assessment of acute chest pain

The process is the same as for any other diagnostic process, except that the condition is so common that most hospitals have well-established protocols which you should follow. However your hospital approaches this problem, we suggest that the aim of the process should be four-fold.

1 Always ***reach either a diagnosis or differential diagnosis using your own skills***: do not be distracted by protocols into ceasing your thought process and slipping into a syndromic diagnosis, e.g. 'troponin-negative chest pain', which is not a diagnosis (and includes many serious illnesses), or 'troponin-positive chest pain' (which includes at least three major and quite different diagnoses, including acute coronary syndrome [ACS], pulmonary embolism [PE] and renal failure). Always strive to reach a clear diagnosis.

2 Regardless of what has just been said, you must actively consider and exclude an ACS; often this is ***entirely possible*** on the basis of the exact symptoms (see below) combined with a knowledge of the pretest probability of coronary disease (which is heavily influenced by demographics [age, sex] and risk factors), with only the simplest tests, e.g. an ECG. Sometimes you will feel that you cannot exclude an ACS by these simple means, and you will need some extra investigations – most protocols rely on the fact that most (though crucially not all) patients with an ACS will have (or will develop over a short period of time) an abnormal ECG and/or a rise in a highly selective biomarker of cardiac damage called troponin. How long patients need to be observed while having sequential ECGs and troponins varies according to the troponin assay used, but with modern highly sensitive troponin assays, the time period is commonly 1–3 hours, while with older, less sensitive troponin assays closer to 12 hours is required.

3 You must also actively consider and exclude a pulmonary embolus; how this is done depends on the situation. For patients with low probability symptoms, heart rate, oxygen saturation and an ECG are usually sufficient. Remember that the most common ECG sign of a PE is not the commonly taught S1Q3T3 changes; rather, for almost all patients the most common sign is tachycardia alone, with the underlying ECG being otherwise unremarkable. For higher risk patients, these data, along with a blood gas, chest X-ray and D-dimer, may well be required. A small number will need specific radiology imaging. Regardless of how you exclude a PE, always think PE and in your mind exclude it.

4 Always consider and exclude aortic dissection; this immediately life-threatening illness is commonly diagnosed later, largely as doctors do not consider it. Furthermore, if you have made the mistake of slipping into the sloppy habit of labelling patients syndromically (e.g. troponin-negative chest pain), you too will miss this diagnosis, as patients can have unremarkable ECGs and troponins. The clues, as ever, are in the history (see below) and examination. If you have any doubt as to whether dissection is present, order an immediate CT aortogram. The take-home message, however, is that you will never diagnose aortic dissection in time to save your patient unless you routinely think in all patients with chest pain whether this could be the diagnosis.

All patients seen in emergency departments with chest pain must have a full history, examination (including oxygen saturation), chest X-ray and ECG as a bare minimum.

Typical myocardial ischaemic pain (cardiac pain)

Myocardial ischaemia is a clinical diagnosis, made on the history and supported by finding risk factors for atheromatous coronary disease (see Chapter 84). There are two forms of ischaemic chest pain: angina and myocardial infarction.

Angina

Typical angina is a heavy pain or discomfort felt retrosternally, which may radiate to the neck, and is often associated with heaviness in the left arm. Some patients have atypical symptoms, such as shortness of breath or pain in unusual places (e.g. the right chest, shoulder blade), although isolated left-sided chest/submammary pain is rarely angina. It has been reported that women and people of black and minority ethnic extraction may be more likely to describe angina in different ways.

A key diagnostic feature is the **relationship of symptoms to effort**. For genuine angina, whatever its location, pain is reliably brought on by effort and relieved within 1–2 minutes of rest.

Angina is described clinically as stable, crescendo or unstable. In **stable angina**, symptoms are only provoked by effort and readily relieved by rest. In **crescendo angina**, the amount of effort required to provoke symptoms decreases rapidly over several weeks, although symptoms do not occur at rest. In **unstable angina**, symptoms come on unpredictably, either with minimal exertion or at rest.

Angina is usually the result of ischaemic heart disease, although it may be caused by:

- aortic stenosis, the signs of which are a slow rising pulse (a difficult sign to elicit reliably), a praecordial thrill (only in a few) and a loud ejection systolic murmur, often best heard in the mid-left sternal edge (quiet if left ventricular function is poor, or if the patient is gravely unwell from heart failure)

- severe pulmonary hypertension, suggested by a left parasternal lift and a loud second heart sound (a very difficult sign to ascertain reliably).

In those with coronary artery disease, the occurrence of crescendo or unstable angina means that the underlying coronary obstruction has increased, usually because of thrombus formation. This is associated with a greatly increased risk of myocardial infarction. Most patients with crescendo or unstable angina should be admitted immediately to hospital.

Myocardial infarction (Table 13.1)

Acute myocardial infarction (MI) pain typically comes on over a few minutes. Although feeling identical to angina, it is often very severe, and differs from angina in lasting 20 minutes or more and not being relieved by nitrates. Sweating, nausea and vomiting are very common and when present, increase the chance that symptoms are caused by a myocardial infarct rather than angina.

Aortic dissection

Aortic dissection pain is usually unheralded and of abrupt (instantaneous) onset (unlike MI pain which evolves over minutes), is very severe. The location of the pain reflects the site of origin of the dissection and the spread of the pain reflects the propagation of the dissection plane along the aorta. Thus, classically, dissection of the ascending aorta starts in the anterior chest and rapidly (in less than a few minutes) moves into the neck and then the back. Dissections originating in the aortic arch start as neck pain, and those in the descending thoracic aorta as interscapular or shoulder pain.

Pleuritic pain

Pleuritic pain is defined as a 'sharp', 'catching' chest pain, exacerbated by respiration, particularly extreme inspiration. When severe, patients breathe shallowly to avoid pain. There are two causes.

Table 13.1 Clinical features altering the probability of myocardial infarction (MI)

Substantial increase in probability (>2-fold increase in risk)

- Radiation to right arm/shoulder
- Radiation to both arms/shoulders
- Associated with exertion
- Radiation to left arm
- Associated sweating

Small increase in probability (<2-fold increase in risk)

- Associated with nausea and/or vomiting
- Worse than previous angina or the same as previous MI
- Described as a pressure

Small decrease in the chance of MI (probability reduction 50% or less)

- Inframammary location
- Not associated with exertion

Substantial decrease in the chance of MI (probability reduction more than 50%)

- Described as pleuritic
- Described as positional
- Described as sharp
- Reproduced with palpation

- **Pleural pain**: this is 'pleurisy' localized to one side of the chest, but not position dependent. A pleural rub may be heard. Achieving a diagnosis depends on defining the associated symptoms and signs. Pleurisy occurs with pneumonia (fever, cough, tachypnoea, bronchial breathing), pulmonary embolus (breathlessness, tachycardia, cyanosis, no bronchial breathing) and pneumothorax (absent breath sounds).
- **Pericardial pain**: as with pleurisy, pericardial pain is worse on deep inspiration but unlike pleurisy, it is located in the centre

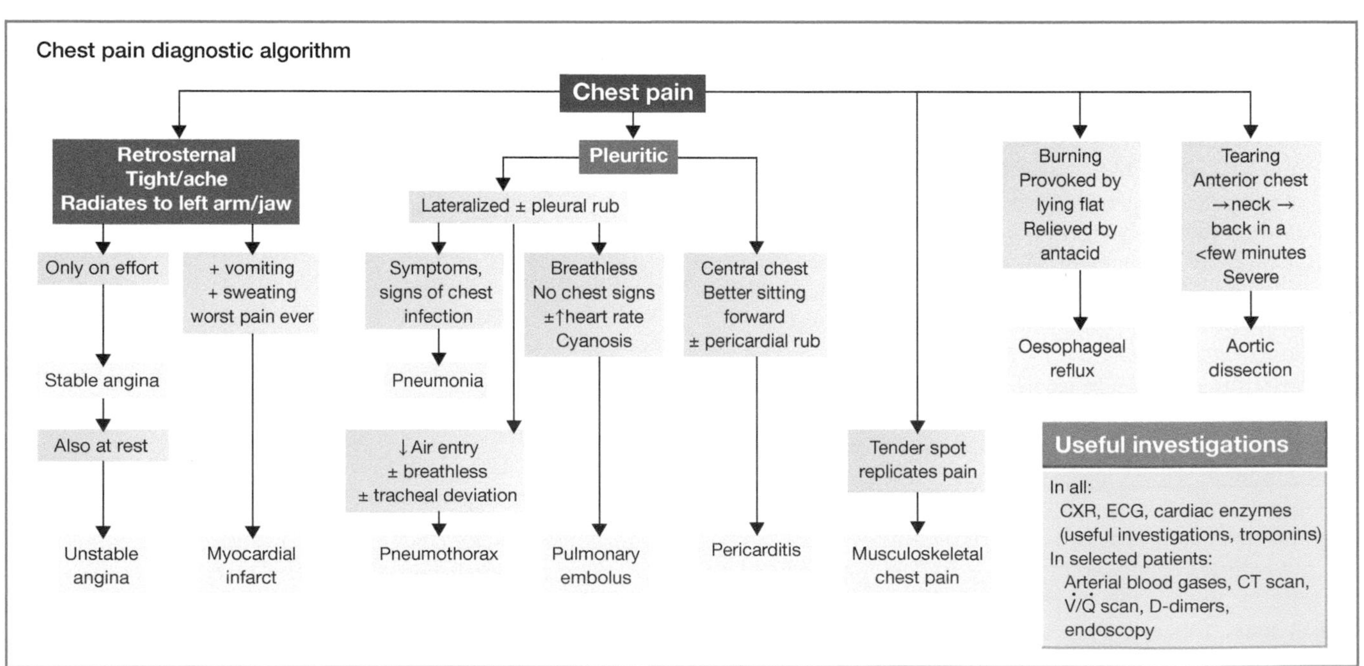

of the chest, is positional in nature and typically is worse lying down and relieved by sitting. A pericardial rub may be heard on auscultation, which may be positional, quite localized or intermittent. Pericarditis occurs with viral infections, post MI and in autoimmune diseases.

Note that these factors can all alter the probability of myocardial infarction, but that none mean that an infarct either must have occurred or could not have occurred. Always use all the information available to reach this diagnosis.

Musculoskeletal chest pain

This is very common. There may be a history of physical injury or unusual exertion, although this is found surprisingly infrequently. Pain is provoked by arm/chest movement and lasts many hours. Although pains may be exacerbated by effort, rest does not reliably relieve them. Examination may show localized tenderness. This diagnosis should be considered only once more serious diagnoses have been excluded, because chest wall pain and coronary disease may co-exist.

Gastro-oesophageal pain

Several different gastrointestinal pains can cause diagnostic confusion with cardiac pain.

- **Oesophageal reflux** causes a retrosternal burning, travelling from the epigastrium upwards. There may be frequent belching, odynophagia or, if a stricture has occurred, dysphagia. Reflux is particularly frequent in obese individuals who smoke, just the population in whom coronary disease is found!
- **Oesophageal spasm**, often provoked by oesophageal reflux, can be very difficult to distinguish from cardiac pain, because it causes a retrosternal tightness/heaviness which may be severe. It may, however, be relieved by liquid antacids (e.g. milk) or cold drinks.

The key to the diagnosis of gastrointestinal pain is its clear relationship with food, and the absence of a relationship between the onset of the pain and exertion. Confusingly, some oesophageal reflux (and spasm) can be provoked by exercise, although such pain often resolves only slowly on resting. This can lead to diagnostic confusion with angina – if the risk of coronary artery disease is high, a cardiac origin to the pain should be actively excluded.

Gall bladder disease

Classic biliary colic is felt in the epigastrium and cholecystitis in the right upper quadrant of the abdomen. However, biliary disease may also be felt in the chest and confused with angina. Typically, attacks of pain are intermittent, unrelated to exertion and may be severe. Eating certain particularly fatty foods can precipitate them. It is more common in women than in men, and is diagnosed on ultrasonography and by the exclusion of anginal syndromes.

14 Oedema

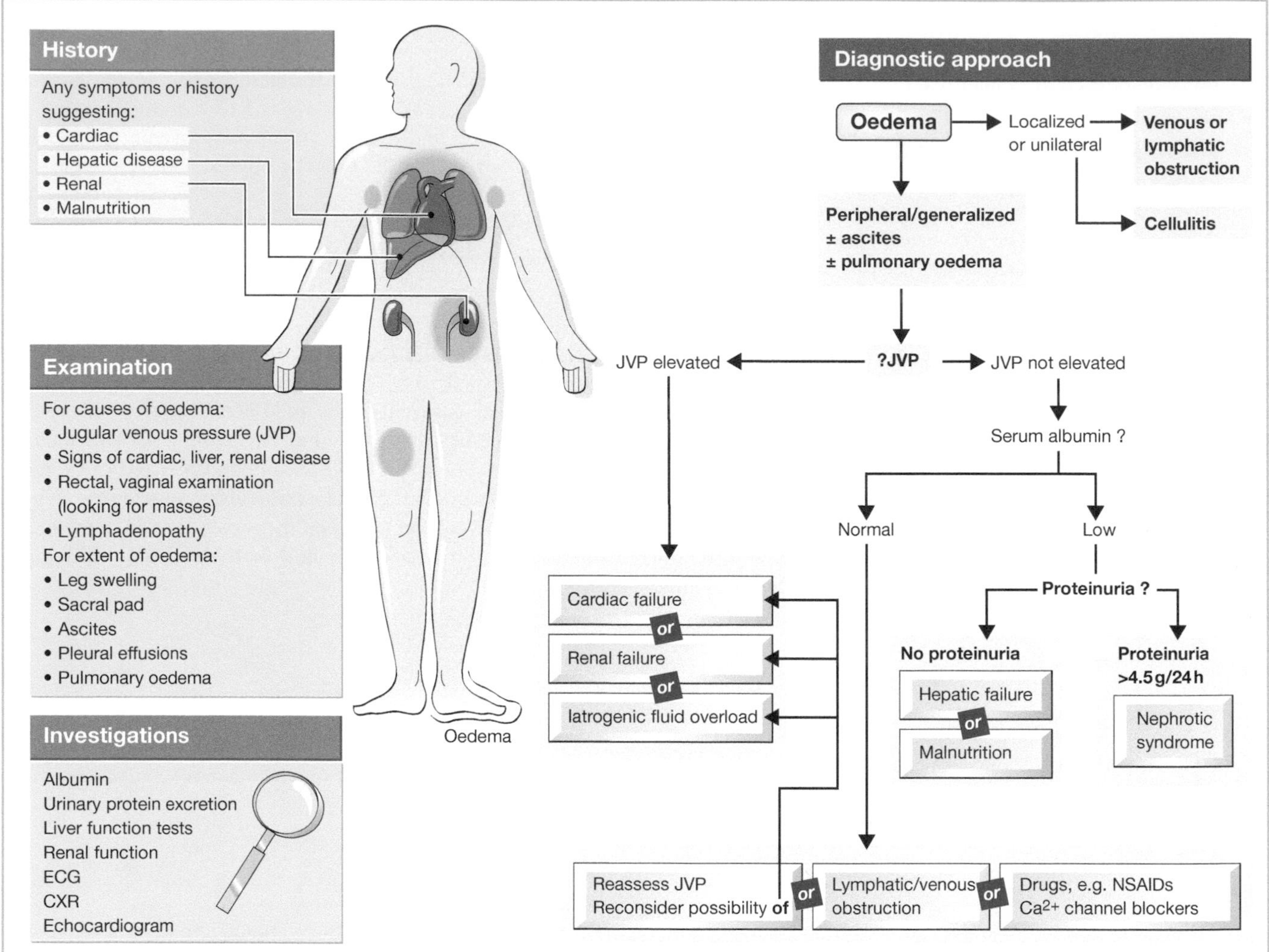

Oedema ('an abnormal build-up of fluid in the tissues') can be a presenting feature of many serious medical conditions, notably congestive heart failure, liver failure, malnutrition and the nephrotic syndrome. Peripheral oedema can also result from venous or lymphatic obstruction or from excessive administration of salt and water. Medications including non-steroidal anti-inflammatory drugs (NSAIDs) and calcium channel blockers can be associated with peripheral oedema.

Presentation

Patients present complaining of swelling of the legs. In severe cases, oedema extends to cause abdominal swelling (from ascites), sacral oedema, pleural effusions, pulmonary oedema and even facial swelling. Oedema is often, although not always, posturally dependent, and in bed-bound individuals it may be confined to the sacrum.

Medicine at a Glance, Fifth Edition. Edited by Patrick Davey and Alex Pitcher.

Companion website: www.wiley.com/go/medicine5e

Diagnosis

Accurate history taking is vital. Symptoms and signs of cardiac, liver and renal disease should be sought. Two questions are the key to the diagnosis: 'Is the oedema unilateral or bilateral? Is the venous pressure raised or not?' (Table 14.1). It is also important to determine whether oedema is present in other sites. Oedema diffusely affecting the whole body suggests a low serum albumin, or 'leaky' capillaries, rather than heart failure.

Bilateral leg oedema

In bilateral leg oedema, key clues to the diagnosis lie in determining whether the venous pressure is elevated and whether there are signs of liver disease, severe immobility or malnourishment.

- **Heart failure**: leg oedema occurs from right-sided heart failure and is always associated with a high jugular venous pressure (JVP). Hepatomegaly is often seen, as are signs of underlying

Table 14.1 Causes of oedema

Bilateral oedema

- Congestive cardiac failure
- Hepatic failure
- Renal failure
- Nephrotic syndrome
- Malnutrition
- Immobility
- Drugs (NSAIDs, calcium channel blockers)

Unilateral oedema

- Lymphatic obstruction
- Venous obstruction (usually deep vein thrombosis [DVT]; rarely, external compression)
- Venous valve incompetence from previous DVT
- Cellulitis
- Ruptured Baker's cyst
- Localized immobility, e.g. hemiparesis

cardiac pathology. If the oedema is mild in the legs but severe in the abdomen, the rare diagnosis of pericardial constriction should be considered.

- **Liver failure**: leg oedema is caused by a low serum albumin (usually <20 g/dl). There may be signs of chronic liver disease, such as spider naevi, leuconychia, gynaecomastia, dilated abdominal veins indicating portal hypertension, and bruises (impaired liver synthetic function). The JVP is not elevated. In severe chronic liver disease (e.g. cirrhosis), liver enzyme tests may be only mildly disturbed, although the prothrombin time is often prolonged (>20 s). In acute liver failure, the patient is usually very unwell, cerebral disturbance is prominent and liver function tests are usually grossly abnormal.
- **Renal failure**: oedema is caused by either a low serum albumin (nephrotic syndrome, where the urine is frothy and contains 3–4+ of protein on dipstick testing; confirmatory tests include estimation of serum albumin [usually <30 g/dl], urinary protein [usually >4 g/24 h] and serum creatinine and urea) or an inability to excrete fluid (nephritic syndrome, associated with hypertension, haematuria and low urine output).
- **General immobility**: the patient is usually elderly, and obviously immobile from general infirmity or cerebrovascular disease. The JVP is down, and there are no signs of liver or renal disease.
- **Malnutrition**: any chronic illness may be associated with a catabolic state and a degree of malnutrition that can be severe enough to depress serum albumin and cause leg oedema.
- **Inferior vena cava (IVC) compression**: rarely, bilateral leg oedema can be caused by compression of the IVC. This can be diagnosed by ultrasonographic studies of the abdomen, using colour flow Doppler to determine blood flow and computed tomography (CT), and occurs:
  - in extreme obesity
  - in severe (tense) ascites from whatever cause
  - with extensive venous thrombosis in the IVC, such as occurs in malignancy, or as a complication of the nephrotic syndrome.

Unilateral leg oedema

A one-sided leg swelling is likely to have a local underlying cause, such as the following.

- A **deep venous thrombosis** in the leg causes a slow onset (more than a few hours) of unilateral leg pain, swelling, skin warmth and possibly tenderness in the calves and along the veins, particularly the great saphenous vein. As symptoms/signs are unreliable for diagnosis, all patients with suspected DVT should undergo definitive investigations (vein ultrasonography or venography) and be examined for complicating pulmonary embolisms (see Chapter 92).
- **Ruptured Baker's cyst**: a Baker's cyst is a knee joint bursa that juts into the popliteal fossa and usually occurs in rheumatoid arthritis. It may rupture and cause sudden-onset leg pain and calf swelling. Ultrasonography is diagnostic.
- **Cellulitis** consists of an intense, spreading skin erythema, sometimes well demarcated, occasionally tracking up the line of the lymphatics. It is often very painful and is associated with a temperature and raised erythrocyte sedimentation rate, C-reactive protein and white cell count. The organism is usually one of the staphylococci or streptococci species, and is occasionally grown from blood cultures, although rarely from skin swabs.
- **Lymphatic obstruction** results in a 'woody' form of unilateral oedema, sometimes described as 'non-pitting'. It is very rare in the West, and when found is usually the result of carcinomatous invasion and obliteration of the draining lymph nodes, e.g. in metastatic melanoma. In Africa, lymph obstruction is very common, often bilateral and caused by filarial infestation.
- **Pelvic tumours** can unilaterally compress veins, causing unilateral oedema.
- **Localized immobility** can cause unilateral leg oedema, e.g. long-standing hemiparesis.

Investigations

These vary depending on the features established by the history and examination, but determination of serum albumin, urinary protein loss, liver function tests, creatinine, electrocardiogram (ECG), chest X-ray (CXR) and echocardiography are often appropriate.

Treatment

Therapy is directed at correcting the underlying cause. In bilateral oedema, diuretics are often used to promote salt and water excretion, although their use should be balanced against the risk of hypovolaemia and worsening renal function, postural hypotension and falls. Several different classes of diuretic agent are used (Table 14.2). The use of a loop diuretic in combination with a thiazide can produce a pronounced diuretic effect that is useful in resistant oedema. Spironolactone, a competitive aldosterone antagonist, produces a mild natriuresis and potassium retention, and is utilized in conditions with secondary hyperaldosteronism such as liver cirrhosis with ascites. Spironolactone and amiloride are 'potassium-sparing' diuretics, in contrast to the loop and thiazide diuretics which promote potassium depletion.

Table 14.2 Diuretics used in treating oedema

Class	Example	Diuretic potency	Na^+/K^+ lowering potential
Thiazide	Bendroflumethiazide	+	++/+
Loop	Furosemide (frusemide)	+++	+/+++
K^+ sparing	Amiloride	±	±/0
	Spironolactone	±	±/0

15 Palpitations

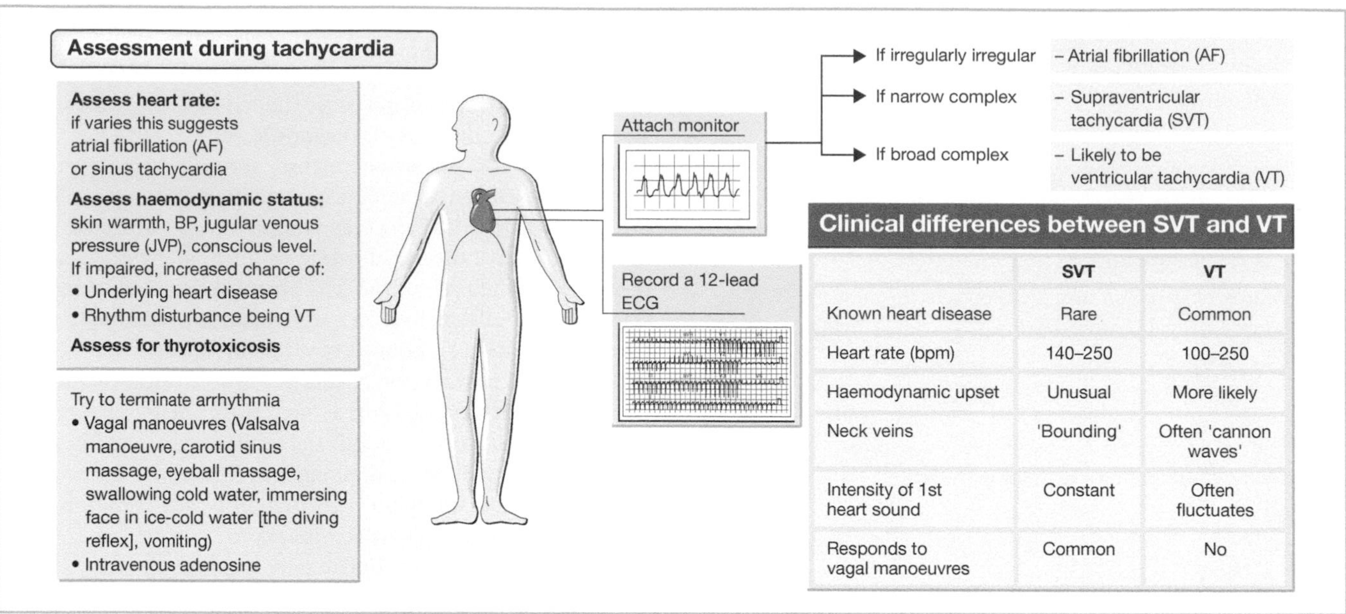
Assessment during tachycardia
Assess heart rate:
if varies this suggests
atrial fibrillation (AF)
or sinus tachycardia
Assess haemodynamic status:
skin warmth, BP, jugular venous
pressure (JVP), conscious level.
If impaired, increased chance of:
• Underlying heart disease
• Rhythm disturbance being VT
Assess for thyrotoxicosis
Try to terminate arrhythmia
• Vagal manoeuvres (Valsalva manoeuvre, carotid sinus massage, eyeball massage, swallowing cold water, immersing face in ice-cold water [the diving reflex], vomiting)
• Intravenous adenosine
Attach monitor
Record a 12-lead ECG
If irregularly irregular - Atrial fibrillation (AF)
If narrow complex - Supraventricular tachycardia (SVT)
If broad complex - Likely to be ventricular tachycardia (VT)
Clinical differences between SVT and VT

	SVT	VT
Known heart disease	Rare	Common
Heart rate (bpm)	140–250	100–250
Haemodynamic upset	Unusual	More likely
Neck veins	'Bounding'	Often 'cannon waves'
Intensity of 1st heart sound	Constant	Often fluctuates
Responds to vagal manoeuvres	Common	No

Palpitations are an awareness of the heart beat, due to an abnormal appreciation of the normal heart beat, from ventricular ectopic beats or from a tachyarrhythmia (bradyarrhythmias only very rarely cause palpitations). To gain clues as to the diagnosis, it is helpful to establish the speed of onset (instantaneous or over several minutes) and the rate and rhythm (ask the patient to tap out the palpitations using their hand).

1 **Palpitation with sinus tachycardia**: here the heart rhythm is normal, but the heart beats more rapidly and strongly than usual. This can occur with exercise, fear or psychological distress (e.g. anxiety). The diagnosis is suggested by a characteristic history; palpitations start and stop over many minutes, unlike tachyarrhythmias which start (and stop) rapidly. There is often a background of anxiety (work, relationship stress, etc.). Vagal manoeuvres are unhelpful and syncope never occurs.

Causes of a sinus tachycardia include:

- physiological: exercise, anxiety
- common pathologies: sepsis/fever, pain, heart failure, respiratory distress, haemodynamic compromise, anaemia; thyrotoxicosis
- rare pathologies: phaeochromocytoma, sinus node re-entrant or atrial tachycardia – suggested by 'fixed' heart rate on ambulatory monitoring. The syndrome of inappropriate sinus tachycardia is rare and is a diagnosis of exclusion.

2 **Tachyarrhythmia-associated palpitations**: here the heart beats more quickly than usual as a result of a tachyarrhythmia or extra beats. The characteristic history of a genuine tachyarrhythmia is of sudden (i.e. instantaneous) onset and fast palpitations, which last for a very clearly defined period of time (usually minutes rather than hours) and may (although not reliably) stop as suddenly as they started. Anxiety may occur, but does so during, not before, an attack. Vagal manoeuvres are helpful for supraventricular arrhythmias, and there is often a history of prior heart disease in ventricular arrhythmias. Syncope may occur. After the event, patients may pass abnormally large volumes of urine due to natriuretic peptide release. A number of different tachyarrhythmias have additional characteristic features.

- **Supraventricular tachycardia (SVT)**: most commonly either atrioventricular re-entrant tachycardia (AVRT) or AVNRT (AV nodal re-entrant tachycardia). These often start during the teenage years and tend to lead to rapid, sustained palpitation. Syncope is very unusual. Postevent polyuria, from atrial natriuretic factor release resulting from atrial stretching during the attack, may occur.
- **Atrial fibrillation**: characteristically the palpitations are felt 'all over the place' or are 'irregularly irregular'. Syncope is very rare (unless the patient has a very fast ventricular response to the atrial fibrillation) but, as this arrhythmia occurs in those with heart disease, breathlessness resulting from associated heart failure is common.
- **Ventricular tachycardia (VT)**: patients are often although not always known to have heart disease. Syncope is common in those with underlying heart disease, although not universal and VT can occur in structurally normal hearts. Vagal manoeuvres are unhelpful.
- **Ventricular ectopic beats/extrasystoles**: patients usually do not feel the extrasystole, but feel the postextrasystolic beat, which is of increased contraction. They thus feel that the heart misses a beat, then 'restarts' with a thump. Patients often say that they are 'worried that their heart may not restart'.

The single most helpful investigation in palpitations is an electrocardiogram (ECG) recorded during symptoms, and the aim of investigation should be to obtain this. For lengthy attacks, this is straightforward. If short-lived, then a 24-hour Holter monitor may be useful if symptoms occur frequently (every 24–48 h). For infrequent attacks, a variety of electronic recorders are available which the patient can apply during the episode, and increasingly include a range of wearable devices, many of which are commercially available.

Whatever the cause of the palpitation, patients with a structurally normal heart, a reassuring family history and no syncope generally have a good prognosis, whereas patients with impaired ventricular function or other red flags, including an adverse family history or abnormal resting ECG, generally mandate more aggressive investigation and treatment.

16 The painful leg

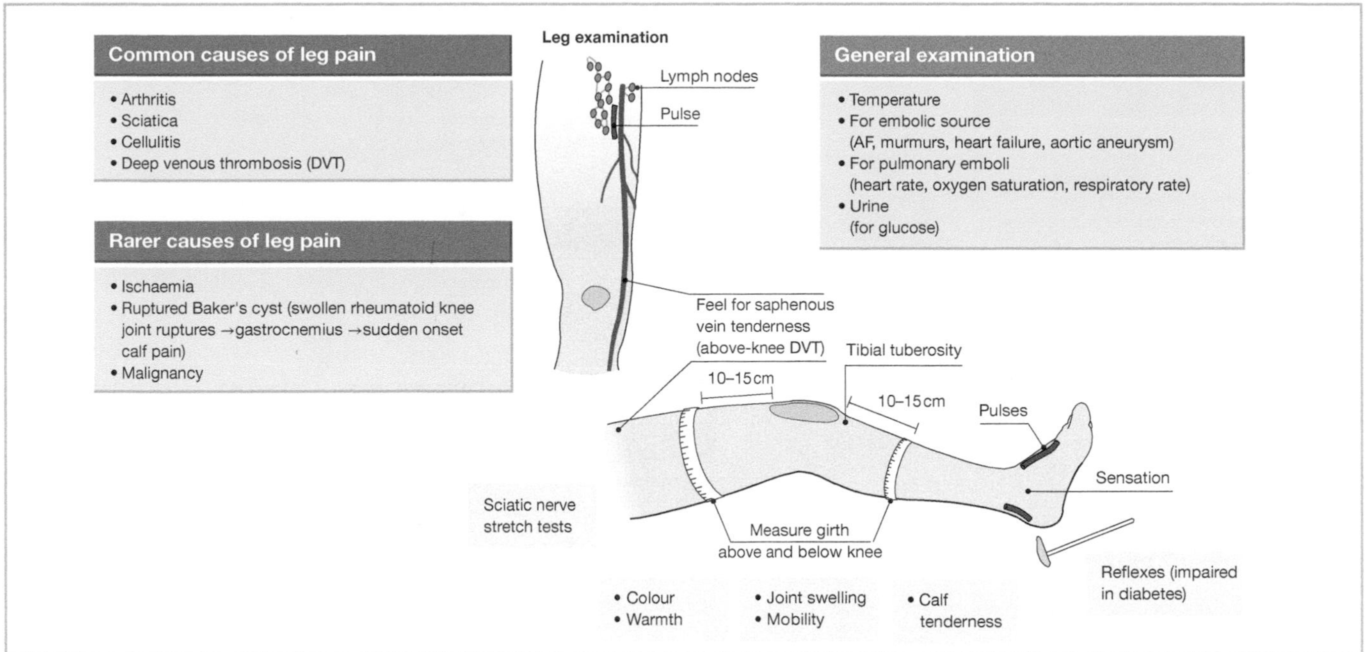

Common causes of leg pain
• Arthritis
• Sciatica
• Cellulitis
• Deep venous thrombosis (DVT)
Rarer causes of leg pain
• Ischaemia
• Ruptured Baker's cyst (swollen rheumatoid knee joint ruptures →gastrocnemius →sudden onset calf pain)
• Malignancy
Leg examination
Lymph nodes
Pulse
General examination
• Temperature
• For embolic source (AF, murmurs, heart failure, aortic aneurysm)
• For pulmonary emboli (heart rate, oxygen saturation, respiratory rate)
• Urine (for glucose)
Feel for saphenous vein tenderness (above-knee DVT)
Tibial tuberosity
10–15 cm
10–15 cm
Pulses
Sensation
Sciatic nerve stretch tests
Measure girth above and below knee
Reflexes (impaired in diabetes)
• Colour
• Warmth
• Joint swelling
• Mobility
• Calf tenderness

As for all symptoms, a clear description of the site, nature and duration of pain, with provoking and relieving factors, along with a careful examination, is usually sufficient to establish the diagnosis. The following are the common causes of leg pain.

- **Deep venous thrombosis (DVT)**: patients notice a gradually increasing (over hours) unilateral calf (more rarely thigh) ache and often calf (or thigh) swelling. Absence of leg swelling does *not* exclude a DVT, although the greater the swelling, the more likely it is. Normal D-dimer levels effectively exclude the diagnosis. Those with raised D-dimers should go on to have definitive imaging: ultrasonography as the default with venography reserved for indeterminate cases. The risk of pulmonary embolism (PE) is lower for below-knee and higher for above-knee DVTs. All patients may need anticoagulation to relieve symptoms. DVTs may indicate a procoagulant state (see Chapter 190), either genetic or acquired. The incidence of recurrent DVTs/PEs is 10% per annum (i.e. 20% after two years, 50% after five years, etc.). If there is a clear precipitating factor for the DVT (e.g. recent surgery and immobility), it can be described as provoked and anticoagulation for a defined period of time (usually three months) recommended. If there is no clear precipitant, the DVT is considered unprovoked and long-term anticoagulation is recommended.
- **Cellulitis** (see Chapter 228).
- **Arterial disease**: chronic arterial insufficiency presents with **intermittent claudication** – pains felt in the calves and/or the buttocks, brought on by exercise and rapidly relieved by rest (i.e. in less than 1 min). Examination shows reduced or absent arterial pulses, findings confirmed by Doppler measurements. Patients with **critical ischaemia** have pain at rest. Hanging the leg over the edge of the bed relieves symptoms (gravity improves perfusing pressure). **Acute leg ischaemia** presents as a painful leg, and examination shows absent pulses and a bluish discoloration. Causes include ***in situ* thrombosis** (usually in long-standing claudication) or arterial embolus, from the heart (consider recent myocardial infarction, atrial fibrillation [AF] or mitral stenosis) or a diseased aorta (e.g. abdominal aortic aneurysm; much more rarely from aortic dissection). Doppler measurements and angiography (invasive, CT or MRI) are diagnostic. Treatment is immediate anticoagulation, and removal of any embolic clot (which should be sent for histology, because a few are embolized atrial myxomas or lung tumours) using a Fogarty catheter, arterial reconstructive surgery or amputation, along with diagnosis and treatment of any cardiac problem.
- **Leg ulcers** (see Chapter 71).
- **Arthritis**: symptoms have often been present for months or years. Pain is usually (not always) localized to the affected joint and worse on joint movement or weight bearing, although hip osteoarthritis may cause sufficient nocturnal pain to wake the patient. Septic arthritis presents acutely with systemic symptoms (fever, malaise, shivers) and a hot, red, swollen joint with painful, globally restricted movements. Joint aspiration is diagnostic (see Chapter 215).
- **Nerve root compression**, especially sciatic nerve compression from a prolapsed intervertebral disc ('sciatica'), is common – pain characteristically radiates all the way down the back of the leg (see Chapter 209).

Medicine at a Glance, Fifth Edition. Edited by Patrick Davey and Alex Pitcher.

Companion website: www.wiley.com/go/medicine5e

17 Heart murmurs

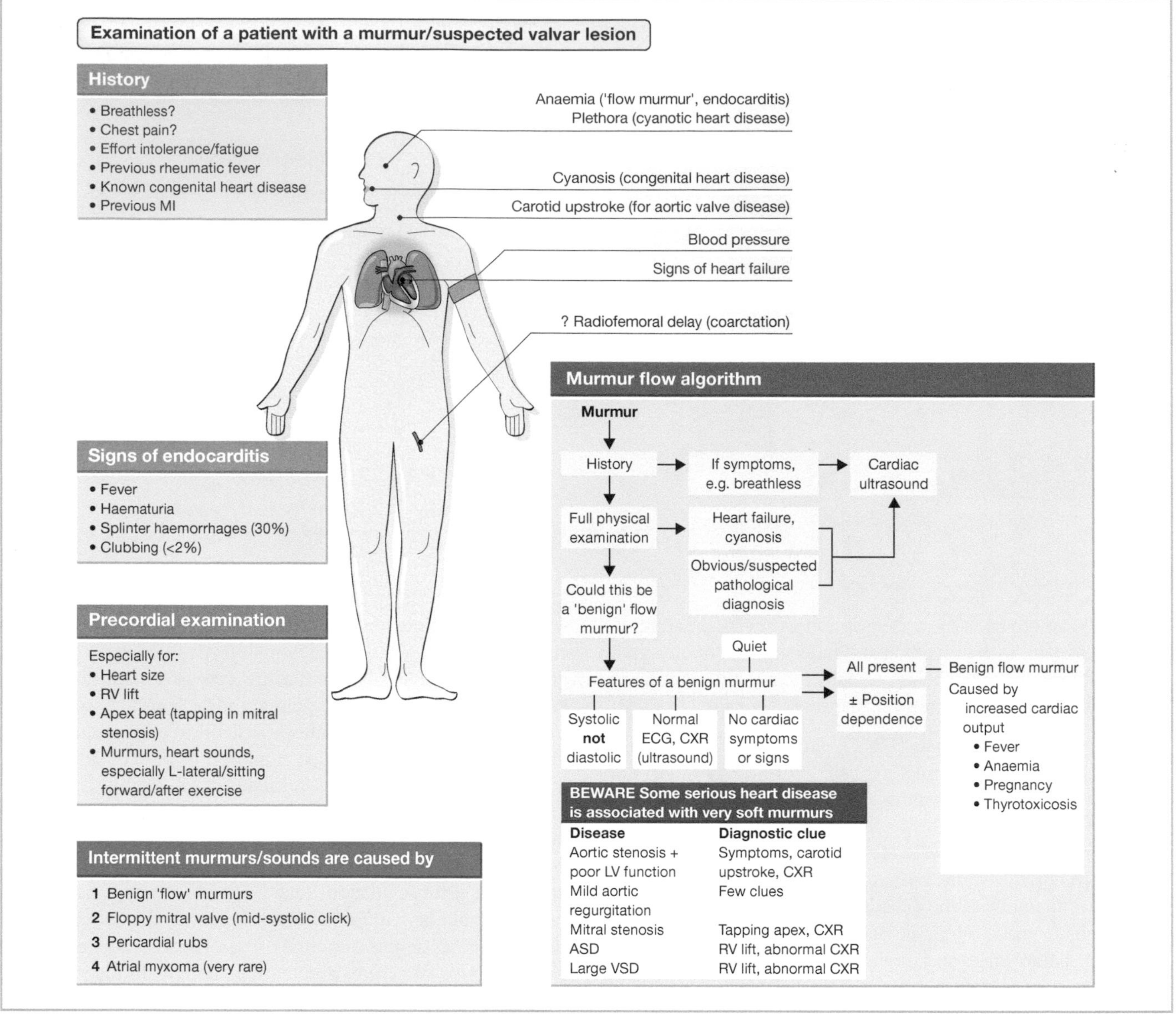

Disease	Diagnostic clue
Aortic stenosis + poor LV function	Symptoms, carotid upstroke, CXR
Mild aortic regurgitation	Few clues
Mitral stenosis	Tapping apex, CXR
ASD	RV lift, abnormal CXR
Large VSD	RV lift, abnormal CXR

Murmurs are commonly found on routine physical examination. Although some are benign and do not arise from important cardiovascular disease ('flow murmur'), occasionally they are important clues to the presence of heart disease, such as valvular disease, left ventricular (LV) dysfunction (leading to functional mitral regurgitation), intracardiac shunts (atrial septal defect [ASD] and ventricular septal defect [VSD]). Very occasionally, other malformations, such as an arteriovenous malformation or coarctation of the aorta, are responsible for murmurs.

Valvular heart disease is common, important and in most cases associated with murmurs. The characteristics of a murmur depend on the flow velocity, the nature and size of the orifice, and the direction of the flow.

As a rule, narrow or stenosed atrioventricular (AV) valves cause diastolic murmurs, and leaking AV valves cause systolic murmurs; the reverse is true for the pulmonary and aortic valves. Murmurs radiate in the direction of the blood flow across the diseased valve (e.g. aortic stenosis murmurs radiate to the neck, and mitral regurgitation caused by anterior mitral leaflet prolapse radiates to the back). The intensity of a murmur is directly proportional to the pressure gradient and the size of the orifice, unless ventricular function is compromised.

Chronic scarring and calcification make a valve orifice smaller (stenosis), whereas destructive disease processes (e.g. endocarditis, vasculitis, degeneration) make a valve incompetent (regurgitation). Stenosis of a valve causes pressure overload on the cardiac

Medicine at a Glance, Fifth Edition. Edited by Patrick Davey and Alex Pitcher.

Companion website: www.wiley.com/go/medicine5e

chamber pumping blood through the valve; regurgitation results in volume overload to compensate for the leak.

Aetiology of valvar lesions

- **Degenerative valve disease**: acquired calcific aortic stenosis is the most common example of a degenerative lesion. Myxomatous degeneration of the mitral valve leads to destruction of leaflets and chordal rupture.
- **Infection**: endocarditis causes destruction of the valve structure and valvar regurgitation.
- **Prosthetic**: artificial valves may degenerate (biological prostheses calcify or develop pannus) or leak as a result of valve dysfunction or dehiscence of the surgical sutures (paraprosthetic leak). Endocarditis is especially high risk with prosthetic valves.
- **Congenital**: increasingly common as those with congenital heart disease survive longer, as a result of better childhood surgery and medicines. The most common adult presentation of a congenital valve lesion is that of a bicuspid aortic valve, which may be asymptomatic for many years, but can predispose to both aortic stenosis and regurgitation.
- **Rheumatic fever** causes scarring, thickening and calcification of valves over subsequent decades. Affects mitral more than aortic valves. Common in elderly people and in developing countries, but rare in developed countries.

Investigations

- **Chest X-ray** (CXR): shows shape of the heart and suggests chamber enlargement.
- **Electrocardiogram** (ECG): may reveal atrial fibrillation, left atrial enlargement (mitral valve disease) or LV hypertrophy (aortic valve disease).
- **Echocardiography**: this is the most important investigation in (suspected) valvular heart disease, and is used to assess cardiac chamber size and function, valve morphology and opening. Doppler echocardiography measures blood flow velocity, which is then used to calculate pressure gradients across narrow valves and the severity of regurgitation from leaky valves. Colour Doppler turns echo signals from turbulent blood flow into a two-dimensional colour picture, and is particularly useful for assessing valvular leaks. Standard cardiac transthoracic echocardiography with modern equipment produces high-quality images and (usually) sufficient information. Transoesophageal echocardiography (an ultrasound probe is placed in the oesophagus) produces high-resolution images of the heart, because there are no intervening structures (unlike the ribs and lungs for transthoracic echocardiography) and is particularly useful when transthoracic images are inadequate, for left atrial or mitral valve pathology, or for prosthetic valves. Cross-sectional imaging, including CT and MRI, has a growing role in the assessment of valvular heart disease, and for planning intervention.
- **Cardiac catheterization**: enables accurate direct measurement of pressure in the cardiac chambers. Non-invasive imaging has essentially replaced cardiac catheterization as a routine investigation for diagnosis of valvular heart disease. However, coronary angiography may still be used to diagnose concomitant coronary artery disease when surgery is being considered.

Treatment

The general principles underlying the treatment of all patients with valvar disease involve the following.

- **Monitor for symptoms** that indicate a need for surgery. It is important to realize that a valve lesion alone is not an indication for valve replacement because many patients live for decades with medically treated valvular disease.
- **Document left ventricular function**, which if it deteriorates may, even in the absence of symptoms, indicate a need for surgery.
- **Maintain left ventricular function**, e.g. using angiotensin-converting enzyme (ACE) inhibitor therapy in regurgitant lesions where valve intervention is not planned or is deferred.
- **Slow progression** of the stenosis/regurgitant leak, e.g. using antihypertensive therapy in the aortic regurgitation associated with hypertension.
- **Treat any complicating rhythm disturbances**, e.g. atrial fibrillation is a common rhythm disturbance in all forms of valvular heart disease, and can be treated using digoxin and β-blockers to control the ventricular response.
- **Prevent complications** such as endocarditis, e.g. using prophylactic antibiotics, when procedures with a risk of bacterial translocation, such as dental work, are carried out (Table 17.1).
- **Prevent systemic thromboembolism**, e.g. using anticoagulants in atrial fibrillation.

Valve intervention

Indications for valve intervention vary, but generally include intrusive symptoms (breathlessness, exercise limitation) or deterioration in ventricular function occurring in the absence of symptoms (e.g. as in mitral regurgitation).

Contemporary valve intervention includes a wide range of surgical and minimally invasive percutaneous options.

- **Surgical valve replacement** is performed by opening the chest, removing the old valve and implanting a prosthetic valve. Surgical prostheses include **mechanical** valves (usually a composite of metal and other synthetic materials), which require lifelong anticoagulation to prevent thromboembolism but are highly durable. The second form of prosthesis is a valve from an animal (**xenograft**) or human (**homograft**). No long-term anticoagulation is needed because the thromboembolic risk is lower and they have good haemodynamic function, although they are less durable, and may last only 10–15 years or less. Transcatheter aortic valve implantation has become a compelling alternative to surgical aortic valve replacement in many patients, especially for those with aortic stenosis at increased surgical risk, though less is known about the very long-term durability of transcatheter valves versus surgical valves.
- **Valve repair** is possible in many regurgitant valve lesions, and is especially favoured for mitral regurgitation with suitable anatomy. Percutaneous treatment options for regurgitant lesions include edge-to-edge repair using clips, again most commonly used for (functional) mitral regurgitation. Transcatheter options for replacing regurgitant valves are also emerging.
- **Valvuloplasty** is most commonly performed using a percutaneous approach to deliver a balloon for mitral stenosis with suitable anatomy but can also be used for aortic or pulmonary stenosis in certain cases.

Table 17.1 Cardiac conditions at higher risk of developing infective endocarditis

- Prosthetic heart valve
- Complex cyanotic congenital heart diseases
- Surgically constructed systemic or pulmonary conduits
- Acquired valvular heart disease
- Mitral valve prolapse with valvular regurgitation or severe valve thickening
- Non-cyanotic congenital heart disease (except for secundum-type ASD)
- Hypertrophic cardiomyopathy
- Previous endocarditis

Indications for endocarditis prophylaxis using antibiotics prior to surgery vary.

18 Shock

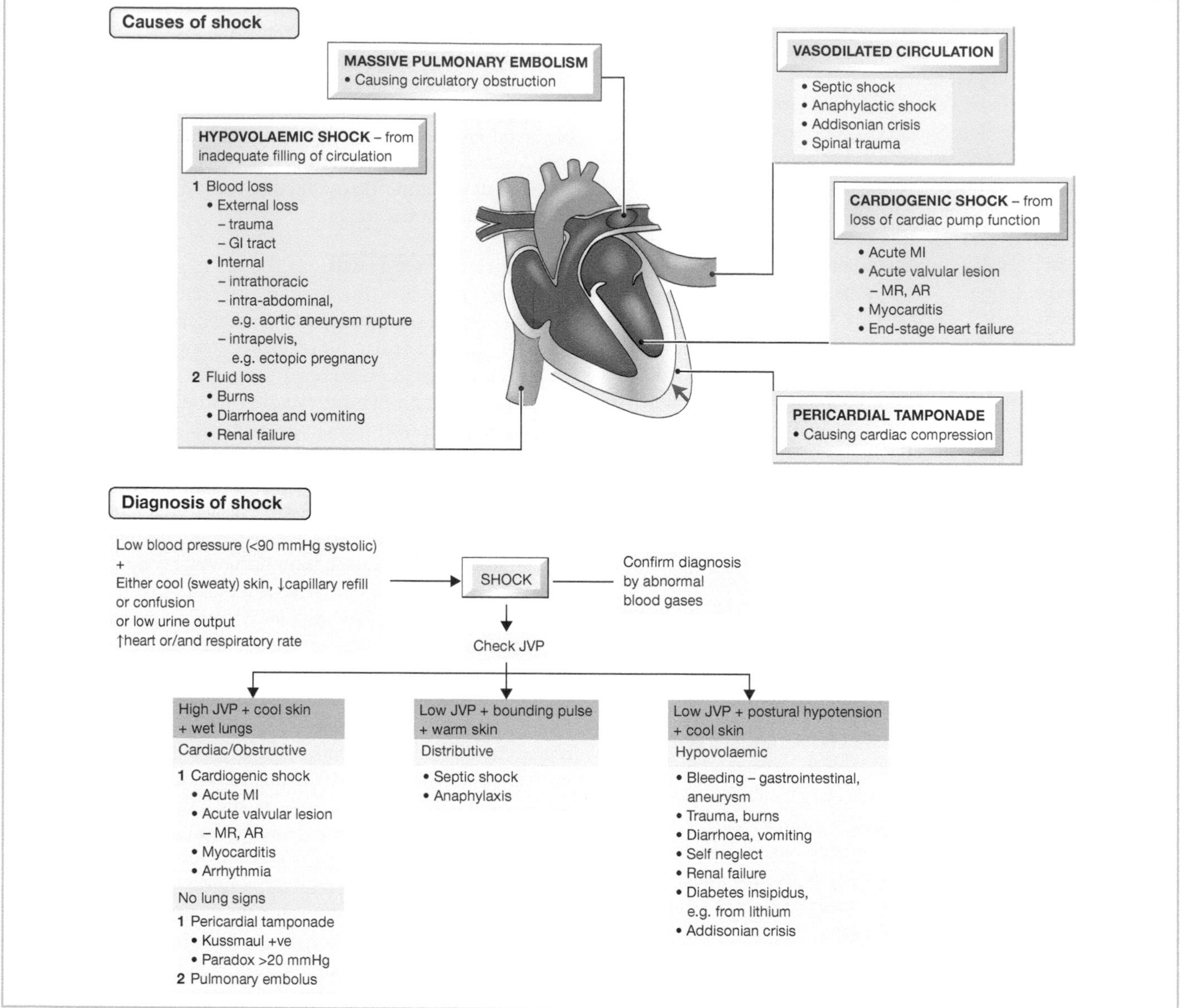

Shock is characterized by hypoperfusion and subsequent tissue hypoxia, leading to a switch from aerobic to anaerobic metabolism and lactic acidosis. All forms of shock have a high mortality and it is therefore important to make an early diagnosis and institute aggressive treatment. The following types of shock have been characterized.

- **Cardiogenic**: ventricular (usually left) pump failure (myocardial infarction [MI], acute valve dysfunction, acute ventricular septal defect, arrhythmia).
- **Hypovolaemic**: loss of circulating volume with normal cardiac function (trauma, gastrointestinal [GI] bleed, pancreatitis, severe diarrhoea, burns).
- **Distributive**: reduced systemic vascular resistance with normal cardiac function (sepsis, anaphylaxis, addisonian crisis, spinal trauma).
- **Obstructive shock**: impaired ventricular filling or obstruction of outflow tract (pulmonary embolism [PE], tension pneumothorax, cardiac tamponade).

Clearly, more than one form of shock may be present in the same patient. Frequently, myocardial depression occurs in the latter stages of other shock states such as sepsis or hypovolaemia, especially if severe acidosis is present.

Successful outcome depends on early diagnosis and treatment. In some patients, the cause may be obvious; for example in a

Medicine at a Glance, Fifth Edition. Edited by Patrick Davey and Alex Pitcher.

Companion website: www.wiley.com/go/medicine5e

patient with acute MI or tension pneumothorax; however, in other cases it may be more subtle, as in massive PE or acute mitral regurgitation (MR). **Tissue hypoperfusion is the hallmark of shock but no single sign or investigation is diagnostic on its own**. Clinical signs of shock such as hypotension, reduced central venous pressure, oliguria and confusion tend to be late features when homeostatic mechanisms can no longer compensate. Tachypnoea, tachycardia, reduced capillary refill and lactic acidosis often occur at a much earlier stage, but are very non-specific.

There is an extremely poor correlation between direct measurement of cardiac output and clinicians' ability to estimate whether it is low, normal or high. It is therefore crucial to be able to recognize the acute severely ill patient, consider a diagnosis of shock and institute appropriate investigations early.

Useful investigations in diagnosis and management

- **Electrocardiogram** (ECG): MI (ST elevation), pericardial tamponade (low voltage), PE ($S_1Q_3T_3$, which is rare, right axis deviation, right bundle branch block).
- **Chest X-ray**: pulmonary oedema in cardiogenic shock, enlarged cardiac silhouette (massive PE, cardiac tamponade), tension pneumothorax.
- **Echocardiogram**: cardiogenic shock due to pump dysfunction (MI, myocarditis), acute valve lesions (colour flow Doppler), PE (pulmonary hypertension, right ventricular dysfunction, clot in transit), pericardial tamponade (effusion and right ventricular collapse in systole), hypovolaemia (left ventricle chamber size).
- **Arterial blood gases**: raised lactate and base deficit, as a consequence of tissue hypoperfusion and anaerobic metabolism, correlate with both severity of shock and mortality. These may be abnormal before hypotension, oliguria or confusion are present. Serial measurements are useful in assessing adequacy of treatment.
- **Central ($ScvO_2$) or mixed venous ($SmvO_2$) oxygen saturations**: true mixed venous saturations (from a pulmonary artery catheter) are 10–15% lower than central mixed venous saturations because of the addition of highly deoxygenated blood from the cardiac veins at the level of the right atrium. When oxygen extraction exceeds delivery, such as in cardiogenic shock, venous saturations are low ($ScvO_2$ <70%). However, in septic shock, saturations may be normal or elevated because cells are unable to extract the delivered oxygen, or low if there is myocardial depression.
- **Blood tests.**
  - Haematology: full blood count (haemorrhage, sepsis/disseminated intravascular coagulation [DIC]), coagulation (haemorrhage and sepsis/DIC), cross-match (haemorrhage).
  - Biochemistry: electrolytes: low sodium and raised potassium (Addison), raised urea (GI haemorrhage, severe diarrhoea); **amylase (pancreatitis)**.
  - Blood cultures: to isolate the organism in septic shock and tailor subsequent antibiotic choice.

General principles of management

Resuscitation should be prompt, as should measures specific to the underlying diagnosis, such as the insertion of a chest drain in tension pneumothorax. However, general principles of resuscitation should not be forgotten. There must be adequate vascular access, the airway should be patent, oxygen applied if hypoxic and adequate ventilation ensured.

Monitoring

Whether or not mechanical ventilation is required, the patient should be managed in a critical care area with appropriate monitoring and nursing. A minimum requirement is for ECG, pulse oximetry, respiratory rate, central venous pressure, Glasgow Coma Score (GCS), urine output and blood pressure to be monitored. The latter should be continuous through an arterial catheter as both fluid and vasoactive drugs may be required. Furthermore, an arterial line will enable serial measurements of pH, lactate and base deficit to be performed, which help to guide treatment. Additional haemodynamic monitoring is desirable, either in the form of a pulmonary artery catheter (their use is uncommon in the UK outside cardiothoracic centres) or monitoring of cardiac output.

Supportive treatment

With the exception of cardiogenic shock, intravenous fluid is used in most forms of shock. This may be in the form of crystalloid or colloid (blood products in trauma or haemorrhage); however, many UK physicians favour lactated Ringer's solution. Colloids containing starch are associated with an increased risk of death and renal failure in septic shock. Fluid should be given rapidly after assessment of intravascular status and the response to a challenge assessed (see Chapter 237). Large-volume resuscitation with NaCl-rich fluid may itself cause a metabolic (hyperchloraemic) acidosis.

Mechanical ventilation may be required because of either a primary respiratory problem or the inability to protect the airway (GCS <8). The metabolic demand of breathing increases 10-fold in shock and uses one-fifth of cardiac output. Mechanical ventilation therefore reduces metabolic demand, but positive thoracic pressures can have adverse haemodynamic effects if the patient is hypovolaemic.

Renal replacement therapy in the form of haemofiltration may be required if there is anuria, hyperkalaemia, unresolving acidosis or resistant fluid overload (cardiogenic shock).

Following optimization of intravascular volume, vasoactive drugs may be required to ensure an adequate cardiac output and blood pressure. Inotropes such as adrenaline (epinephrine), dobutamine, dopamine or milrinone may be used in low cardiac output states, while vasoconstrictors such as noradrenaline (norepinephrine) are used in forms of distributive shock with low systemic vascular resistance, including sepsis.

Specific treatments

- **Cardiogenic**: inotropes, thrombolytics and/or angioplasty, intra-aortic balloon pump, haemofiltration (fluid removal), surgery (MI, acute valve lesion), mechanical circulatory support (e.g. ventricular assist device).
- **Hypovolaemic**: fluids, blood products.
- **Distributive.**
  - Sepsis: fluid, vasoconstrictors (noradrenaline ± vasopressin), steroids, antibiotics, inotropes if reduced cardiac output ($ScvO_2$ <70%).
  - Anaphylaxis/Addison: steroids.
- **Obstructive**: cardiac tamponade (pericardial drain), tension pneumothorax (chest drain), PE (thrombolysis, embolectomy).

19 Breathlessness, cough and haemoptysis

Cough

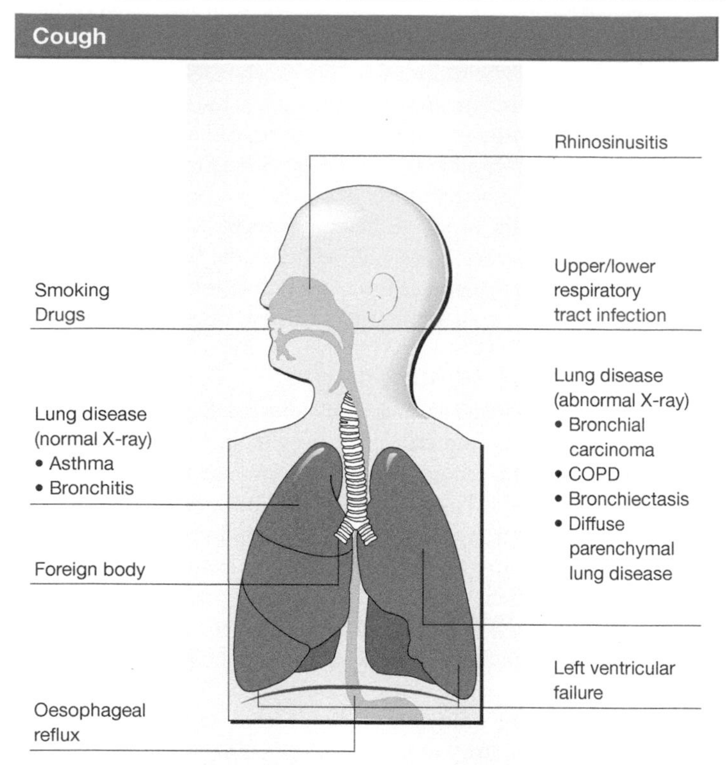

Haemoptysis

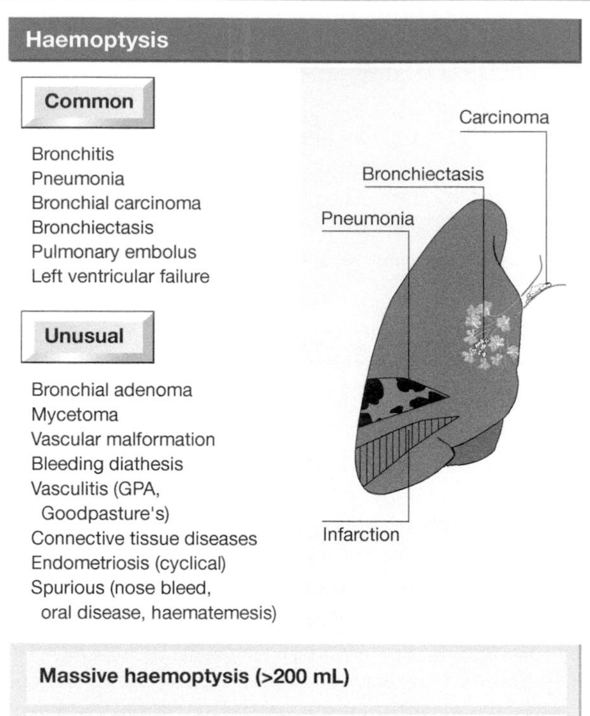

Common

Bronchitis
Pneumonia
Bronchial carcinoma
Bronchiectasis
Pulmonary embolus
Left ventricular failure

Unusual

Bronchial adenoma
Mycetoma
Vascular malformation
Bleeding diathesis
Vasculitis (GPA, Goodpasture's)
Connective tissue diseases
Endometriosis (cyclical)
Spurious (nose bleed, oral disease, haematemesis)

Massive haemoptysis (>200 mL)

- TB
- Bronchiectasis
- Mycetoma

Breathlessness

NYHA grade*

Unlimited effort capacity I

Breathless on severe exercise II

Breathless on mild exercise III

Breathless at rest IV

Recurrent
Asthma
Psychogenic
Exacerbation of COPD | Usually on a background of deteriorating breathlessness
Pulmonary oedema

Threshold for symptoms
Slow onset ⟶ adaptive response + greater tolerance of any symptoms

Mins–hours
Asthma
Pneumothorax
Pulmonary embolism
Pulmonary oedema
Respiratory infection
Psychogenic

Weeks–months
Pleural effusion
Pericardial effusion
Pulmonary fibrosis
Lung cancer
Recurrent pulmonary emboli
Cardiac failure
Neuromuscular disease
Anaemia
Physical deconditioning (from any illness)

Years
COPD
Pneumoconiosis

*NYHA grade = New York Heart Association – usually used for heart failure, can be used for any breathlessness

Medicine at a Glance, Fifth Edition. Edited by Patrick Davey and Alex Pitcher.

Companion website: www.wiley.com/go/medicine5e

Breathlessness

Breathlessness is 'an awareness of the act of breathing' and is a common and frightening symptom. The common causes of breathlessness are listed in Table 19.1.

The rate of onset and the pattern of breathlessness (dyspnoea) may be helpful diagnostically. The characteristic history in some of the different diseases causing breathlessness is outlined below.

Heart failure

- Dyspnoea is not associated with wheeze, a characteristic differentiating it from chronic obstructive pulmonary disease (COPD) (unless 'cardiac asthma', bronchospasm provoked by pulmonary oedema, is present). Symptoms from the underlying heart disease also occur.
- In **mild heart failure**, breathlessness occurs only on effort.
- In **more advanced heart failure**, breathlessness also occurs on lying flat (**orthopnoea**), promptly (<5–10 min) improved by sitting or standing. When severe, this is called **paroxysmal nocturnal dyspnoea**. There is often ankle oedema – better in the morning, worse at night.

Airway disease

This results in a wheeze when breathless.

- In **COPD**, breathlessness on effort slowly progresses over years (often >5 years). Patients often also have **chronic bronchitis** (productive morning cough >3 months/year for two years in succession).

Table 19.1 Common causes of breathlessness

	Acute breathlessness at rest	Chronic breathlessness on effort
Cardiovascular	Left ventricular failure Acute pulmonary emboli *Mitral stenosis*	Chronic heart failure 'Angina-equivalent' breathlessness Chronic pulmonary emboli
Respiratory	Acute severe asthma	Chronic obstructive pulmonary disease (COPD)
	Acute exacerbation of COPD	Pleural effusion
	Pneumonia Pneumothorax Adult respiratory distress syndrome Acute anaphylaxis *Inhaled foreign body*	*Interstitial lung disease* Bronchial cancer *Lymphangitis carcinomatosis*
Other	Psychogenic hyperventilation Fever *Metabolic acidosis* *Neurological disease*	Physical deconditioning Obesity Anaemia *Neurological disease*

Rarer causes are in *italics*.
Source: Based on Table 4.5 in *Davidson's Principles and Practice of Medicine*, 18th edn, Churchill Livingstone, Edinburgh, 1999.

- In **asthma**, symptoms vary, usually with no symptoms between attacks. Wheezing may be provoked by exercise, pollen (and thus be seasonal), drugs (especially aspirin or β-blockers) or emotion. Symptoms may be worse at night, when a dry cough may occur. Nocturnal symptoms in asthma, unlike those in heart failure, improve slowly (>30 min) or not at all on sitting/standing.

Respiratory tract infections

Fever and a productive cough are characteristic of respiratory tract infections; sore throat occurs in upper respiratory tract infections. In pneumonia, constitutional upset (fever and malaise) is common and pleuritic chest pain may occur.

Pulmonary embolus

Pulmonary embolus presents with sudden-onset (i.e. instantaneous) breathlessness, in those predisposed (immobile, obese, oral contraceptive pill, postoperative, cancer). Pleuritic chest pain may occur.

Pneumothorax

Pneumothorax presents with sudden-onset chest pain, often pleuritic in nature, with breathlessness. The diagnosis is made from the physical examination and chest X-ray.

Lung parenchymal disease

Lung parenchymal disease (interstitial pneumonitis/fibrosis) presents with progressive breathlessness on effort and, with advanced disease, at rest without associated wheeze. Breathlessness, unlike in heart failure, is not strongly dependent on posture. The examination and chest X-ray are often diagnostic.

Obesity

If severe, obesity can cause breathlessness, both on effort and on lying (orthopnoea, caused by diaphragmatic splinting). Pulmonary embolism, heart failure and obstructive sleep apnoea are all more common in obese individuals.

Physical deconditioning

Physical deconditioning is a potent cause of breathlessness, and often exacerbates breathlessness resulting from other causes. Importantly, most pathological dyspnoea is improved to some extent by physical conditioning. This is helpful therapeutically (rehabilitation).

Rarer causes of breathlessness

There are two much rarer causes of breathlessness.

- **'Angina-equivalent' breathlessness**: angina (especially in people with diabetes) is sometimes experienced as breathlessness rather than chest pain. This is usually caused by severe coronary artery disease.
- **Respiratory failure**: can result from neuromuscular disease, such as motor neuron disease, or be related to obesity (Pickwickian syndrome). Physical examination usually reveals the cause and blood gases show type II respiratory failure (see Chapter 98).

Psychological causes for breathlessness

Breathlessness for 'psychogenic' reasons may also occur (**hyperventilation**). The patient complains that they are 'unable to fill the chest'. Breathlessness at rest is suggestive. Associated perioral tingling is a specific symptom. Patients can be helped by physiotherapy exercises. **Beware**: many patients breathless from organic disease are frightened and appear anxious. Assume that breathlessness within a hospital is the result of organic disease unless there is incontrovertible evidence to the contrary.

Classification of severity of breathlessness

Although there are many ways of classifying the severity of chronic breathlessness (e.g. blood gases, lung volumes, peak oxygen uptake, etc.), the most useful is the **exercise capacity** of the patient at their usual pace, without stopping, e.g. is the patient able to walk 50 m, quarter of a mile or several miles? This is the key parameter in understanding the impact of the disease and the severity/extent of the underlying pathology.

Physical examination

The following are diagnostically helpful clues in severe breathlessness. In patients with effort breathlessness alone, the signs may be subtle and diagnosis rests on the history and investigations.

- **Skin warmth**: in cardiac dyspnoea (left ventricular [LV] failure, large pulmonary embolus, pericardial effusion), the skin is cool and may be sweaty, whereas in COPD most patients have warm skin with a 'bounding' pulse. A fever may indicate a respiratory tract infection.
- **Heart rate**: severe breathlessness from any cause increases the heart rate. In both LV failure and asthma, it can be used as a 'minute-to-minute' guide to the severity of the condition and the effect of treatment.
- **Heart rhythm**.
- **Blood pressure** (BP) itself is rarely diagnostically helpful, but paradox (the difference between inspiratory and expiratory systolic BP: normally <5 mmHg) is. It is increased in asthma, in severe cases to 15–20 mmHg, and in pericardial effusion (>20 mmHg).
- **Mucous membranes** for pallor (**anaemia**) and for blueness (**cyanosis**). Patients severely breathless as a result of organic disease are usually centrally cyanosed when breathing air. If not, consider pericardial effusion, anxiety or metabolic acidosis.
- **Jugular venous pressure** (JVP) is a key sign. It is raised in:
  - heart failure: the most common cause
  - advanced COPD (cor pulmonale), when the right heart has failed
  - large pulmonary emboli.

  If the JVP is not raised, the breathlessness is less likely to be caused by heart failure, although a normal JVP does not rule out *pure* LV failure.
- **Precordial cardiac examination** may demonstrate a large heart or abnormal LV impulse in most cases of heart failure or a left parasternal lift from right ventricular hypertrophy (in advanced cardiac failure, cor pulmonale and pulmonary embolus). A third heart sound is universal in LV failure, and its absence when breathless suggests that heart failure is not present. Diagnostic murmurs may be heard.
- **Chest examination**.
  - Respiratory rate is increased in most patients who are breathless at rest, although not in respiratory failure resulting from neuromuscular disease (which is rare). A rise in respiratory rate is the most important and often the first sign of any acute illness.
  - 'Hyperinflation': a decreased sternal notch-to-trachea distance ('barrel chest') indicates air trapping in the lungs, usually resulting from airway disease (COPD or acute asthma).
  - 'Stony dull' resonance to percussion occurs in pleural effusions.
  - Wheeze (see Chapter 20).
  - **Crepitations**, if 'wet', are often caused by infection (e.g. pneumonia) or fluid (e.g. heart failure), and if 'dry' often indicate pulmonary fibrosis.
  - Bronchial breathing indicates consolidation (usually pneumonia).

Investigations

Investigations are directed towards the most likely cause but always include:

- **chest X-ray**
- **electrocardiogram (ECG)**
- **spirometry**
- **haemoglobin.**

The following tests help in specific situations.

- **Blood gases**: usually at rest, sometimes on exercise.
- More detailed **lung function tests**, including lung volumes and measures of gas exchange (e.g. carbon monoxide transfer factor).
- **Computed tomography (CT)**: spiral CT with contrast (CT pulmonary angiography) is helpful for diagnosis of pulmonary emboli, and high-resolution thin-cut CT for many interstitial lung diseases. Expiratory cuts can reveal gas trapping due to small airways disease.
- **Ventilation/perfusion (V/Q)** (scan to diagnose a pulmonary embolus), though many units now are switching to **CT pulmonary angiograms**, as they not only diagnose/exclude pulmonary emboli but can show other relevant diseases, such as emphysema.
- **Cardiac ultrasonography**.
- **Brain natriuretic peptide** is a small peptide molecule that, despite its name, is released by the atria in response to stretch. A normal level means that symptoms are most unlikely to be due to heart failure; a very raised level means that symptoms are likely to be due to heart failure. A mild or moderate rise means that symptoms *could* be due to heart failure. In other words, this test is most useful in *excluding* heart failure. It is also useful in following the response to treatment in those *known* to have heart failure.

The following tests are occasionally helpful.

- **Cardiopulmonary exercise testing**: used before major surgery to assess fitness for anaesthesia and to investigate breathlessness with no clinical clues as to the cause.
- **Exercise ECG** to determine whether myocardial ischaemia is present, and to document exercise capacity objectively.
- **Cardiac catheterization**: to measure intracardiac pressures and perform coronary angiography.

Treatment

Treatment is for the underlying condition (see relevant chapters). General advice should encourage physical fitness. Hyperventilation is treated by reassurance and relaxed breathing exercises.

Cough

'A reflex forced expiration against an initially closed glottis.' The explosive expiration is a protective mechanism, clearing the lung of harmful substances.

Key points

- Upper respiratory tract infection is by far the most common cause.
- If the chest X-ray is normal, 90% of patients with chronic cough (lasting >6 weeks) have asthma, gastro-oesophageal reflux disease (GORD) or rhinosinusitis. Empirical treatment for these conditions is often helpful because cough may be the only symptom and they may co-exist.
- Persistent cough in a smoker raises the possibility of bronchial carcinoma.

Epidemiology

- Extremely common.
- Prevalence is between 5% and 40%.
- May indicate serious underlying pathology but commonly of little significance, not warranting investigation.

Differential diagnosis

Acute cough (<3 weeks)

- Viral upper respiratory infection: most common cause is associated sore throat/rhinitis.
- Other acute infections: pneumonia and infective exacerbations of COPD.
- Foreign body: history of choking and sudden onset.

Chronic cough (>6 weeks)

- Bronchial carcinoma: smoker, weight loss, haemoptysis.
- Asthma: atopy, wheeze, shortness of breath, nocturnal symptoms, variable peak flow.
- GORD: heartburn, symptoms on change of posture, often absent at night.
- Rhinosinusitis: headache, nasal blockage, postnasal drip.
- Bronchiectasis: clubbing, copious mucus production, wheeze.
- Diffuse parenchymal lung disease: clubbing, breathlessness.
- Drugs: β-blockers, angiotensin-converting enzyme (ACE) inhibitors.
- Smoking: 50% of those who smoke >20/day have a persistent cough.

Investigations

A new cough lasting >6 weeks is more likely to be caused by serious disease requiring investigation and treatment. The clinical features often suggest the diagnosis, such as interstitial lung disease, COPD or bronchiectasis.

- **Chest X-ray**: if the cough is chronic or the patient is a smoker, this may reveal infection, neoplasm or diffuse lung disease.
- **Spirometry** to diagnose airflow obstruction (peak flow monitoring may be useful in assessing asthma).
- **CT** is used to stage tumours or to diagnose diffuse lung disease.
- **Bronchoscopy** is used to remove a foreign body or for tissue diagnosis of tumours.
- **Oesophageal pH monitoring** is occasionally used to diagnose reflux disease.

In patients with a chronic cough and normal X-ray, sequential empirical treatment with inhaled steroids, antireflux treatment and treatment for rhinosinusitis will provide a 'cure' in a significant percentage of patients.

Haemoptysis

Haemoptysis is the coughing of blood from the lungs.

Causes

Minor haemoptysis is common, often related to respiratory tract infection. This resolves quickly and requires no further investigation. Haemoptysis that persists is more likely to indicate underlying serious pathology. Patients should have a chest X-ray and many will need CT, bronchoscopy and a specialist respiratory opinion.

Clinical approach

Haemoptysis persisting for more than 2 weeks should be investigated (Table 19.2). A history of smoking (past or present) raises the possibility of lung carcinoma and all patients aged over 40 who smoke should be assumed to have lung cancer until investigation proves otherwise. Serious pathology is more common with increasing age. Associated symptoms or clinical signs may point towards a specific diagnosis.

Routine investigations

- **Plain chest X-ray**, blood count (for anaemia from bleeding or chronic disease), clotting profile.
- **Renal biochemistry** because some diseases produce pulmonary haemorrhage and renal failure – so-called 'pulmonary-renal syndromes', e.g. Goodpasture disease, granulomatosis with polyangiitis (GPA; formerly known as Wegener's granulomatosis).
- **Liver biochemistry** for evidence of metastatic disease.
- **Special investigations** include high-resolution CT (HRCT) of the chest and bronchoscopy. These together achieve a diagnosis in >90% of patients.

Management

The key is to find the underlying diagnosis and treat appropriately, or to exclude serious disease. Most haemoptysis is minor or self-limiting, although on occasions bleeding can be severe and uncontrolled.

- **Coagulopathy** should be corrected if present. Antifibrinolytic drugs may help.
- In massive haemoptysis, **bronchoscopy** allows identification and local treatment of the bleeding point.
- **Radiological embolization** or **lung resection** may be necessary in life-threatening haemorrhage.

Table 19.2 Causes of haemoptysis

Very common	Uncommon
Bronchitis Pneumonia	Bronchial adenoma Mycetoma
Common	**Rare**
Bronchial carcinoma Bronchiectasis Pulmonary embolus Spurious (nose bleed, oral disease, haematemesis)	Vascular malformation Bleeding diathesis Vasculitis (GPA, Goodpasture disease) Connective tissue diseases Endometriosis (cyclical)

20 Wheeze (stridor)

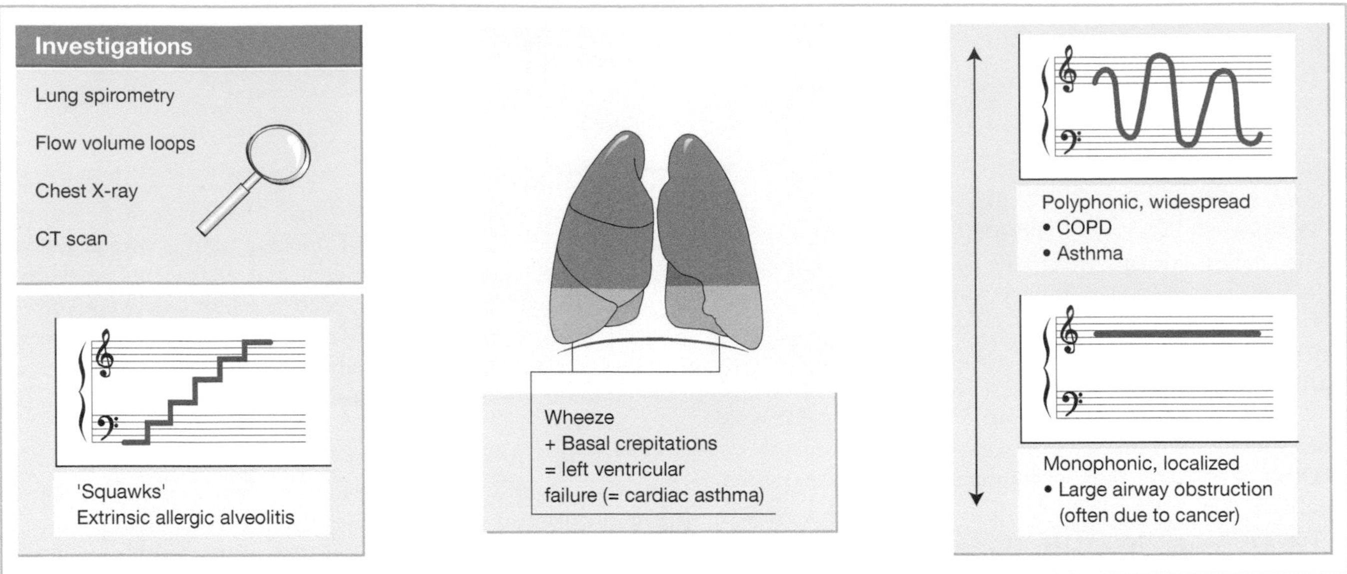

Wheeze is a prolonged sound caused by airway narrowing with apposition of the airway walls. The sound is produced by vibration of airway walls and adjacent tissues. As the airways are generally narrower on expiration, wheeze is more pronounced during the expiratory phase. There are a number of causes of wheeze (Table 20.1).

Wheeze can be divided according to the timing in the respiratory cycle and the actual sound produced (a single note or multiple notes of different pitches).

- **Polyphonic wheeze**: the most common type of wheeze typical of COPD and asthma. Multiple simultaneous different pitched sounds occur during expiration and imply diffuse disease of different-sized airways.
- **Fixed monophonic wheeze**: a note of single pitch resulting from localized narrowing of a single airway. The sound does not change with coughing and particularly raises the possibility of bronchial carcinoma (see also stridor).
- **Sequential inspiratory wheeze**: otherwise known as 'squawks', caused by vibration after the opening of a previously collapsed airway; they are typical of hypersensitivity pneumonitis.
- **Stridor**: low-pitched monophonic wheeze heard on inspiration and implying local obstruction to the extrathoracic airways (which tend to collapse on inspiration). Often implies carcinoma or foreign body in the major airways.

Table 20.1 Causes of wheeze

• Asthma
• Chronic obstructive pulmonary disease (COPD)
• Bronchiectasis
• Large airway obstruction
• Pulmonary oedema

Investigations

The cause of most wheezes is readily apparent on clinical grounds, and using straightforward tests such as chest X-ray and simple lung function tests. Occasionally, diagnostic difficulty occurs; in these situations, flow–volume loops may be helpful, as may computed tomography (CT) and cardiac ultrasonography.

Medicine at a Glance, Fifth Edition. Edited by Patrick Davey and Alex Pitcher.

Companion website: www.wiley.com/go/medicine5e

21 Pleural effusion

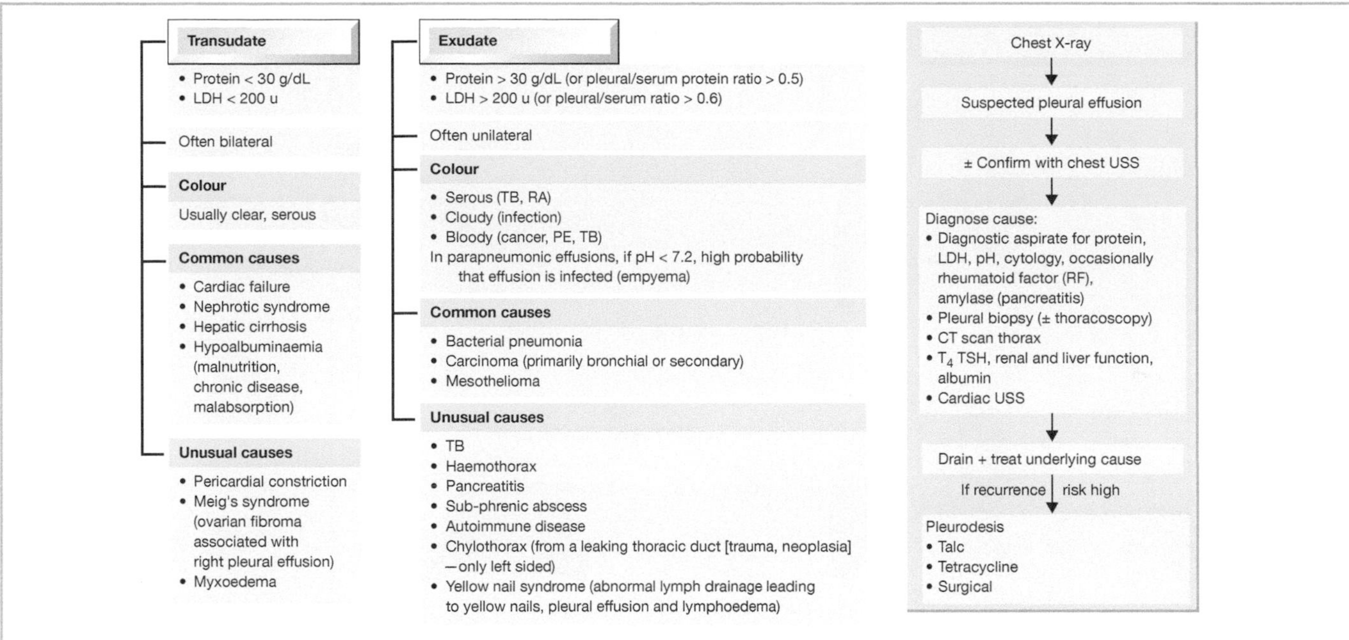

Definition

A collection of fluid in the pleural space. If the effusion is infected, it is called an 'empyema'. If it relates to pneumonia, it is called a 'parapneumonic effusion'.

Introduction

Pleural effusion is a common problem. The normal parietal pleura produces fluid which is reabsorbed by the visceral pleura. Either excessive fluid production (e.g. as a result of inflammation) or impaired reabsorption leads to an accumulation of fluid. An effusion needs to be at least moderate in size before it produces symptoms of shortness of breath.

Clinical approach

The most common presentation is with breathlessness. Pleural inflammation may cause pain and large effusions may cause cough. The clinical signs are of reduced expansion, stony dullness and reduced breath sounds and vocal resonance. Effusions ≤500 ml are difficult to detect clinically. The chest X-ray will show blunting of the costophrenic angle in small collections and more extensive change in the presence of larger effusions. Large effusions are more commonly the result of malignancy. Bilateral effusions are suggestive of heart failure as the cause, though heart failure can also commonly cause an isolated right pleural effusion. Ultrasound is used to confirm the presence of fluid and to ensure a safe approach when samples are taken for analysis.

Investigations

The main distinction to make in determining the cause of an effusion is between high and low protein content, i.e. exudates versus transudates.

If pleural infection is suspected, the pH of fluid should be measured (pH ≤ 7.2 suggests complicated parapneumonic effusion or empyema, which will only resolve with pleural drainage). Fluid should also be sent for biochemistry (lactate dehydrogenase [LDH] – high in rheumatoid effusions and exudates – and protein estimation), microbiology for culture, and cytology. For unilateral effusions, CT scanning is used to look for a cause.

Management

Treatment of the underlying condition, particularly for transudates.

- **Therapeutic large-volume aspiration** will improve symptoms. Formal drainage with intercostal tubes is often necessary with large effusions. Ultrasound guidance is recommended.
- In malignant and other recurrent effusions, **regular drainage** can be achieved by inserting an indwelling pleural catheter (IPC). Use of an IPC has now largely superseded pleurodesis (introduction of a substance, usually talc, via a drain to stick the two layers of pleura together and prevent reaccumulation) in these patients.
- **Thoracoscopy** (under local or general anaesthetic) may be useful in some patients to provide access to the pleura for guided biopsies and subsequent pleurodesis.

Medicine at a Glance, Fifth Edition. Edited by Patrick Davey and Alex Pitcher.

Companion website: www.wiley.com/go/medicine5e

22 Pneumothorax

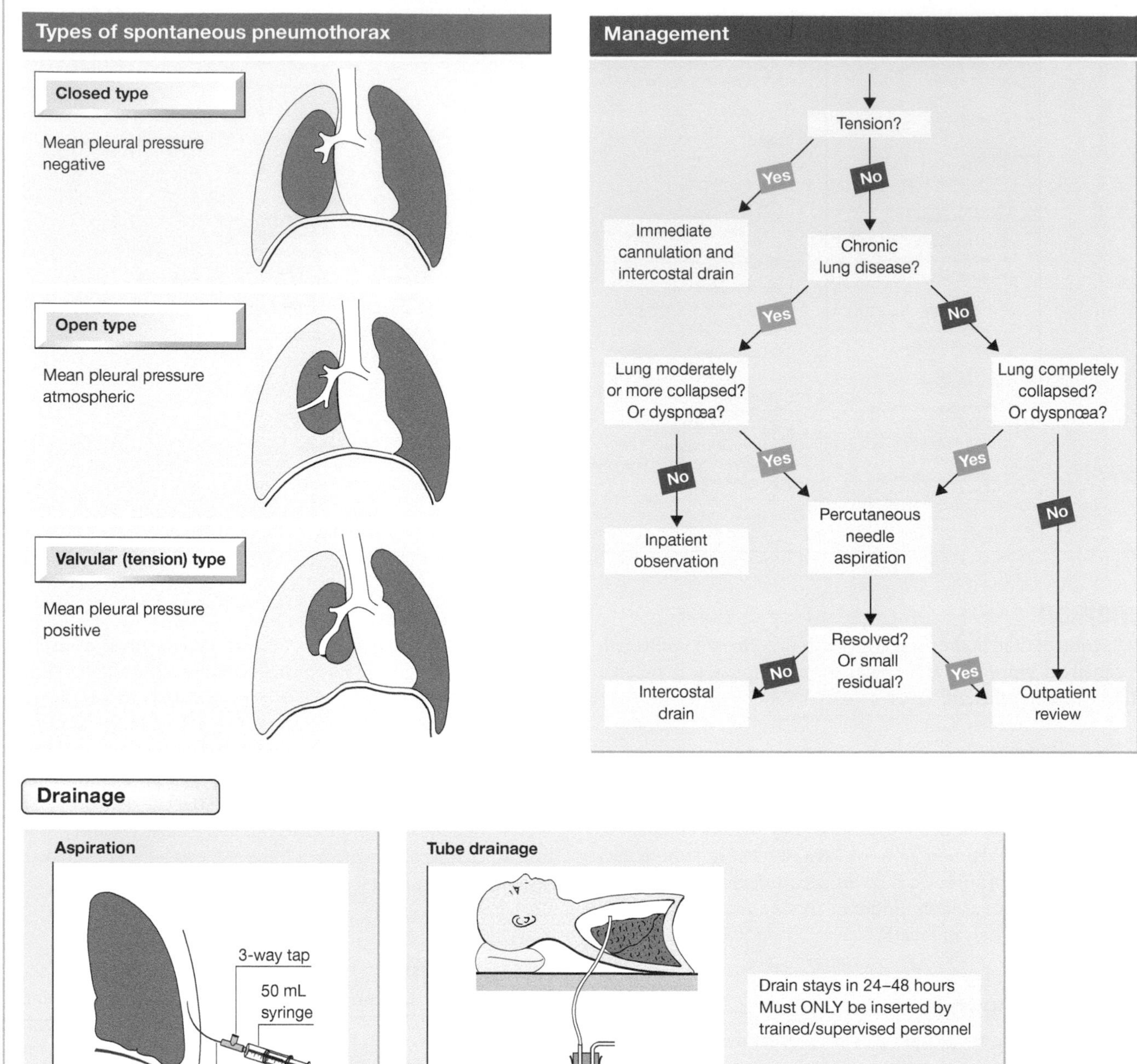

Medicine at a Glance, Fifth Edition. Edited by Patrick Davey and Alex Pitcher.

Companion website: www.wiley.com/go/medicine5e

Definition

The presence of free gas in the pleural space.

Epidemiology

The incidence is 10/100 000 adults per year, males > females, and sometimes runs in families. Taller individuals are more prone to primary spontaneous pneumothorax.

Aetiology

- **Primary spontaneous pneumothorax**: implies normal underlying lungs and is caused by rupture of a pleural 'bleb'.
- **Secondary spontaneous pneumothorax** occurs in association with lung disease (chronic obstructive pulmonary disease [COPD], pneumonia, etc.). Rupture of the visceral pleura results in communication between the airway and pleural space.
- **Traumatic**, such as stab wounds or following rib fractures. Also after lung biopsy.

Pathophysiology

The effects of a pneumothorax depend on whether the pleural leak persists or not.

- **'Closed' pneumothorax**: the leak closes as the lung deflates so the amount of air escaping into the pleural space is limited, pleural pressure remains negative and slow resolution will occur even without treatment.
- **'Open' pneumothorax** occurs when persistent communication between the airway and pleural space develops (bronchopleural fistula), seen as a persistent bubbling of the chest drain. The lung cannot re-expand and there is a risk of infection developing by transmission of organisms via the airway into the pleural space.
- **A tension pneumothorax** occurs when the leak remains open but acts as a one-way valve between the airway and pleural space. The volume of gas in the pleural space progressively increases and the pressure increases above atmospheric, causing compression of both lungs and the heart and mediastinal shift. Cardiac filling and cardiac output decrease. The patient can become extremely unwell and die unless treated urgently.

Clinical features

- **Small pneumothorax** may be asymptomatic.
- **Medium/large pneumothorax**: sudden onset of chest pain with shortness of breath is the most common presentation. There is hyperresonance with reduced expansion and reduced breath sounds.
- **Subcutaneous emphysema**, felt as a crackling feeling in the skin, can occur if there is communication between the pleural space and the skin and subcutaneous tissues. Dramatic facial swelling and airway compromise may occur.
- **Tension pneumothorax** results in pronounced dyspnoea, tracheal deviation, tachycardia and hypotension.

Investigations

- **Chest X-ray** is diagnostic. Mediastinal deviation suggests the presence of tension. The X-ray will also show the presence of any underlying lung diseases.
- **Oxygen saturation** should be measured – usually normal unless there is underlying lung disease.
- **Ultrasonography** or **computed tomography** are both superior to the plain chest X-ray for detection of small pneumothoraces and are often used after percutaneous lung biopsy.

Management

- **Drainage (aspiration or tube)** is not required for small (virtually) asymptomatic primary spontaneous pneumothoraces, but is in all symptomatic patients (initial trial of aspiration is often appropriate). Those with underlying lung disease are at greater risk of complications and should be treated as inpatients. Tension pneumothorax is a medical emergency and requires immediate treatment.
- **Surgical treatment**, with pleural abrasion or pleurectomy to obliterate the pleural space, is used for pneumothoraces not resolving after tube drainage and for recurrent pneumothoraces.
- **Aeroplane travel**: patients with pneumothorax should not fly for three months because the pressure changes lead to expansion of any gas left in the pleural space and so to a tension pneumothorax.

Prognosis

With adequate drainage, even in the presence of underlying lung disease, resolution can almost always be achieved. After primary spontaneous pneumothorax, 30% of patients have a further episode within five years. After a second episode, the recurrence rate rises above 50% and surgical pleurodesis is therefore usually recommended. Recurrence is extremely unusual following pleurodesis.

23 Unintentional weight loss

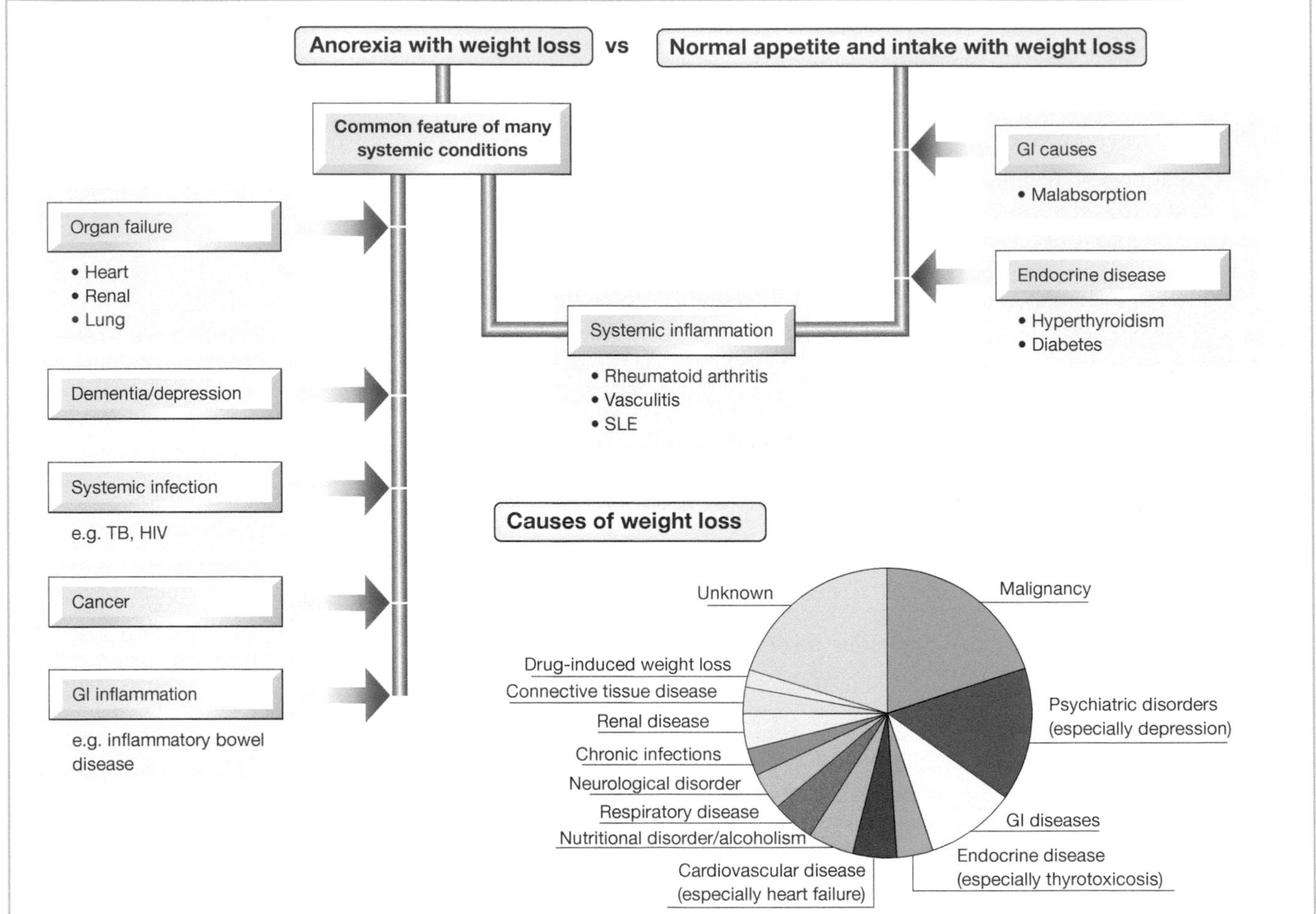

Overall approach

Weight loss is a non-specific symptom, which might relate to a gastrointestinal (GI) condition or to a systemic pathology. It may represent the presentation of a behavioural or psychiatric problem.

Epidemiology

Unintentional weight loss is common, affecting up to 8% of elderly patients who seek healthcare. Severe and rapid weight loss (≥7.5% of usual body weight lost in ≤6 months) is relatively unusual.

Differential diagnosis

See figure above.

Consequences of weight loss

- Unintentional weight loss is associated with increased morbidity and mortality.
- Some of the increased mortality seen in those who unintentionally lose weight is due to the underlying disease process.
- Some of the morbidity and mortality in those with weight loss is due directly to the consequences of malnutrition on vital structures. Skeletal muscle mass may decline rapidly (sarcopenia) leading to loss of mobility and increased number of falls, which in turn may lead to fractures.

Clinical features

The most important task is to establish the **cause** of the weight loss. It is usually possible on the basis of history, examination and some elemental tests to distinguish between the following.

- **Dietary insufficiency**: poor diet is not infrequently the cause of weight loss; a full dietary assessment should be carried out; beware, however, as poor diet by itself does not rule out organic disease. It is crucial to determine why the diet is poor: is it due to loss of appetite (which may relate to inflammatory disease including cancer, to depression, to dementia, etc.) or is it due to social factors (poverty, alcoholism, etc.)?

Medicine at a Glance, Fifth Edition. Edited by Patrick Davey and Alex Pitcher.

Companion website: www.wiley.com/go/medicine5e

- **Malabsorption**: often a good question to ask patients with weight loss is whether their appetite is preserved; anorexia and subsequent weight loss often relates to inflammatory disease, whereas weight loss in the presence of a good appetite can relate to malabsorption, thyrotoxicosis, etc.
- **In systemic inflammatory disease ('consumption')**: although the term *consumption* is historically associated with tuberculosis (TB), any infective, inflammatory or malignant disease can cause weight loss. Similarly, weight loss is a feature of the endstages of other disease processes such as dementia, heart failure and chronic obstructive pulmonary disease, and features of these should be sought.

History

Important questions to be answered concern the following.

- Try and quantify the weight loss; if weights have not been measured, ask about trouser fit/belt tightening.
- Ask about appetite.
- Ask about gastrointestinal symptoms, e.g. dysphagia, change in bowel habit including the advent of steatorrhoea suggestive of fat malabsorption, nausea and vomiting, rectal bleeding.
- Fever, night sweats, headache (non-specific but ~intracranial tumour, temporal arteritis).
- Muscle weakness (may suggest polymyalgia rheumatica).
- Mood and sleep symptoms of depression (diurnal mood variation, early wakening, anhedonia, etc.).
- Smoking increases the risk of most neoplasms (particularly lung and pancreas) as well as Crohn's disease; smoking cessation is often associated with the presentation of ulcerative colitis.
- Ask about family history of cancer.
- Alcohol abuse is associated with weight loss.
- Travel history and contact with TB, etc.
- Sexual history and other risks for human immunodeficiency virus (HIV), e.g. intravenous drug use.
- Endocrine symptoms, e.g. those of thyrotoxicosis.
- If a psychiatric component is suspected, ask about perception of weight loss and body image and purging behaviours.

Examination

Look specifically for the following.

- Fever and potentially signs of deep infection such as those of endocarditis.
- Signs of endocrine disease, e.g. thyroid or adrenal insufficiency.
- Signs of malnutrition (leuconychia, cheilitis, glossitis, scurvy, pellagra) and objective evidence of weight loss (loose skin, fat and/or muscle loss); record the weight.
- Lymphadenopathy: generalized as well as Troisier's sign (enlarged left supraclavicular [Virchow's] node suggesting intra-abdominal malignancy).
- Breast examination.
- Abnormalities in respiratory or abdominal examination indicating infection or malignancy.

Investigations

These should be targeted to specific clinical suspicions raised by the history to determine both the cause and the consequence of weight loss.

- **Blood tests**: full blood count (FBC) and raised inflammatory markers (erythrocyte sedimentation rate [ESR]/C-reactive protein [CRP]) often provide non-specific evidence for a worrying cause for weight loss. Also urea and electrolytes (U&Es), liver chemistry and albumin, Ca^{2+}, vitamin B_{12}, folate (B_9), thyroid function, serological testing for coeliac disease, and HIV test. HbA1c, iron studies, cortisol; consider blood cultures.
- **Chest X-ray**: indicated in all patients regardless of respiratory symptoms (for TB, mediastinal lymphadenopathy, metastases, primary or secondary lung carcinoma).
- **Urine dipstick examination**: for haematuria and glycosuria.
- **Upper gastrointestinal endoscopy**: indicated regardless of upper GI symptoms. Distal duodenal biopsies should be taken if coeliac disease is suspected.
- **Computed tomography** (CT) of the abdomen and pelvis with intravenous ± gastrointestinal contrast: pancreatic or ovarian carcinoma is a frequent cause of anorexia and weight loss. If a chest X-ray is not performed, the chest should also be imaged.
- **Faecal elastase/chymotrypsin** for pancreatic exocrine insufficiency.
- **Nutritional assessment** and observation of weight stability on clinic scales are useful where investigations fail to identify a specific cause.

Management

Treat the underlying cause (see relevant sections elsewhere). Food supplements may have a role. If no diagnosis is reached and weight loss continues, try these next steps.

- **Repeat baseline investigations**: 'blind' CT (i.e. without clinical pointers) of the abdomen and pelvis (occasionally of the chest) often leads to a diagnosis, or at least excludes many neoplastic lesions.
- **Trial of nutritional support** (sip feeds, nasogastric tube feeding): weight gain with nutritional support makes sinister causes of weight loss less likely.
- **Therapeutic trials**: in a few elderly patients with elevated inflammatory indices, an empirical trial of steroids is justifiable although a response is not very discriminatory. If the clinical suspicion of TB is high, empirical antituberculous treatment is occasionally justified.

24 Constipation and change in bowel habit

Causes of constipation

Common

General

- Dehydration
- Slow transit/dysmotility
- Neurodegenerative/Parkinson's disease

Intraluminal defects

- Inadequate dietary fibre

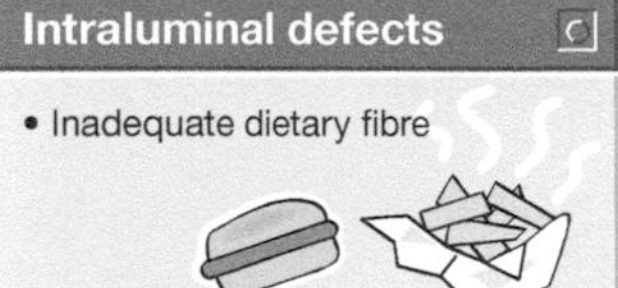

Common/general

- Dehydration
- Slow transit/dysmotility
- Neurodegenerative/Parkinson's disease

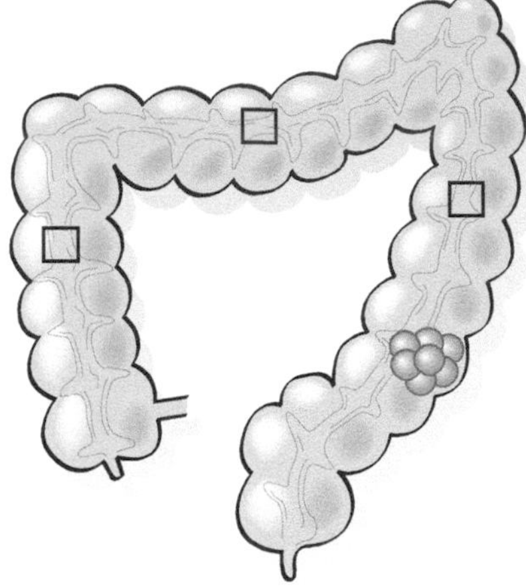

Rare

Metabolic

- Hypothyroidism
- Hypercalcaemia

Drugs

- Opiates
- Antidepressants
- Verapamil and other Ca^{2+} channel blockers
- Many others

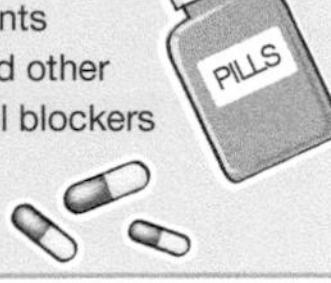

Neoplasia

- Colon cancer
- Rectal cancer

Colonic imaging

Barium enema

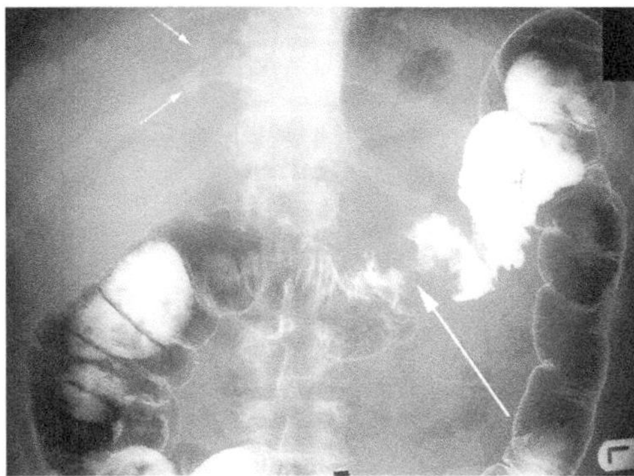

Film from double contrast barium enema in a patient with a large transverse colon carcinoma (see arrow). There is irregular stricturing of the bowel with shouldering apparent. Note lung metastases at lung base (small arrows).

Conventional colonoscopy

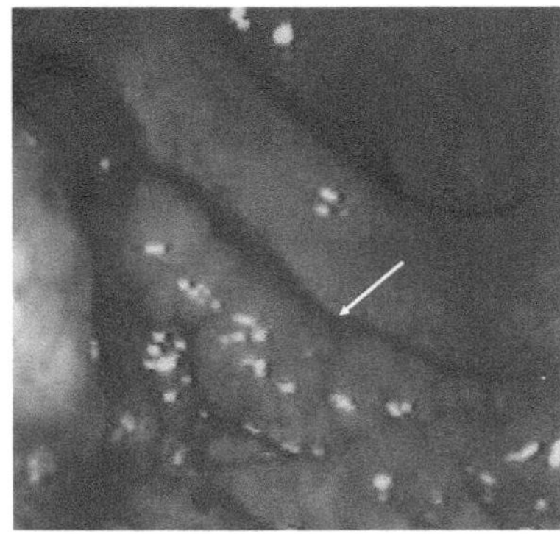

View from conventional colonoscopy confirms irregular morphology of the wall of the rectum. Histological analysis revealed villous adenocarcinoma. Occasionally, very large amounts of fluid are present using a polyethylene glycol preparation and despite supine and prone imaging the entire colonic surface may not be seen.

Virtual colonoscopy

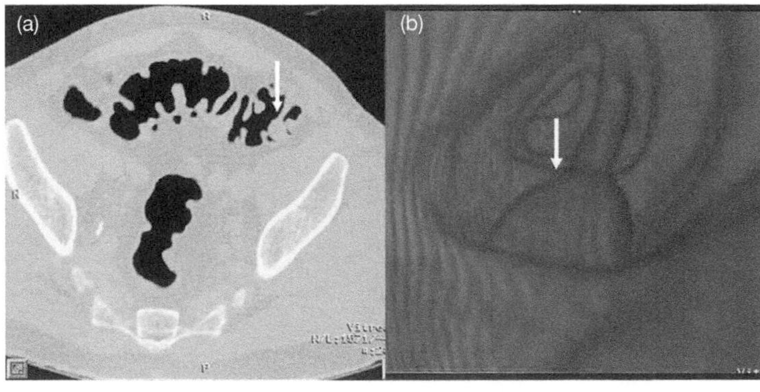

Patient who was unwilling to have conventional colonoscopy. Axial image (a) shows pedunculated polyp (arrow) in sigmoid. Endoluminal image (b) confirms 13mm pedunculated polyp on a stalk (arrow) in the sigmoid colon. When the patient was told of the abnormality he immediately requested endoscopy for removal of the lesion.

Reproduced with permission of Michael Macari

Medicine at a Glance, Fifth Edition. Edited by Patrick Davey and Alex Pitcher.

Companion website: www.wiley.com/go/medicine5e

Table 24.1 Differential diagnosis of constipation

Common
• Idiopathic/dietary
• Drugs, e.g. opioid pain killers, antidepressants, calcium channel antagonists, antiemetics
• Irritable bowel syndrome
• Dehydration
Uncommon
• Colorectal neoplasia
• Hypothyroidism
• Hypercalcaemia
Rare
• Hirschsprung disease and other dysmotility disorders

Chronic constipation

Frequency of defecation varies enormously between individuals and in response to dietary and other environmental changes. Patients are often referred when their bowel frequency/habit changes. Although in many circumstances the clinical fear might be the presence of colonic malignancy, benign and functional causes are still more common (Table 24.1).

Overall approach

It is important to ascertain the exact nature of the patient's problem (i.e. consistency, frequency or both). Does the patient harbour concerns about cancer or are they troubled by symptoms?

Clinical features

A clear history is paramount. Important questions include the following.

- Over what time period has the patient been constipated? Often a problem dates back many years and many over-the-counter remedies have been tried (often with varying success).
- What exactly is the problem? Has the nature of the problem changed or has the problem become more significantly inconvenient, i.e. needing regular aperients or manual evacuation?
- Past medical history and particularly obstetric history in women: pelvic trauma during protracted labour or assisted delivery may present at a later date with defecatory problems.
- Has there been any rectal bleeding? This may be due to an innocent cause (e.g. haemorrhoids) but may raise considerable anxiety on a background of constipation.
- Dietary history is very important. Patients often take too little regular dietary fibre (e.g. bran) and fluids.
- Drug history: opioids, calcium antagonist, anticholinergics, calcium-containing antacids, iron supplements.

Examination and investigations

This may be unrewarding but a thorough physical examination, including rectal examination (with consideration of anal sensation and tone), is important in providing reassurance.

- **Blood tests**: full blood count (FBC) with additional tests guided by symptoms and of low yield in isolated constipation.
- **Colonic imaging where there are features of concern**: computed tomography (CT) colonography is more useful than colonoscopy in symptomatic constipation. It delineates colonic length and diameter and excludes colorectal neoplasia.
- **Anorectal physiology and defecating proctography**: in patients with abnormal examination, high risk for abnormal defecation or not responding to laxative regimes.
- **Transit studies**: in selected cases the passage of radio-opaque markers may distinguish 'slow transit' from problems of the pelvic floor.

Management

Management depends largely on the patient's view of the problem and correction of any specific causes that may have been found on investigation.

Reassurance

If the major concern was colorectal cancer, normal investigations may be sufficient.

Diet and hydration

In those with troublesome symptoms, the first line of treatment is to optimize the patient's intake of fibre and fluids, and to trial stopping contributory medications.

Laxatives

- **Stimulant laxatives** (e.g. senna): in general, their use should be limited to short-term constipation (such as that associated with hospitalization). Some patients with chronic constipation may come to depend on stimulants. Senna is available over the counter. Prucalopride, a $5HT_4$ agonist, may be useful in refractory chronic constipation; a similar drug is the guanylate cyclase 2C agonist linaclotide.
- **Bulk-forming laxatives** (e.g. Fybogel®, Isogel®): these agents are quite safe but they may exacerbate symptomatic bloating.
- **Osmotic laxatives** (e.g. Movicol®, magnesium sulfate): these are generally well tolerated and should be considered first-line treatment. Many of these agents are available over the counter (e.g. Milk of Magnesia®, Epsom salts). Although lactulose is effectively an osmotic laxative, it is of limited benefit and may cause inconvenient colic and wind.

Surgery

In very resistant/recalcitrant cases, surgical intervention (e.g. subtotal colectomy) may be necessary to restore quality of life.

Change in bowel habit in older patients

In the older patient, a change in a previously stable bowel habit will often raise specific concerns about the development of colorectal cancer. The following are particular features of the history suggestive of a significant underlying pathology.

- Anorexia and/or weight loss.
- Nocturnal diarrhoea or pain disturbing sleep.
- Rectal bleeding.

Examination

Although often unrewarding, a full physical examination is mandatory. In particular, lymphadenopathy, abdominal masses and organomegaly should be sought, and careful rectal examination performed.

Management

Evidence of serious underlying disease is sought from an FBC, ESR, iron indices, liver chemistry, thyroid function and serum calcium; any abnormality here warrants further investigation. Colonoscopy or CT colonography is required to exclude colorectal cancer.

American Gastroenterological Association Medical Position Statement: guidelines on constipation. Gastroenterology 2000;119:1761–1766.

25 Diarrhoea: acute and chronic

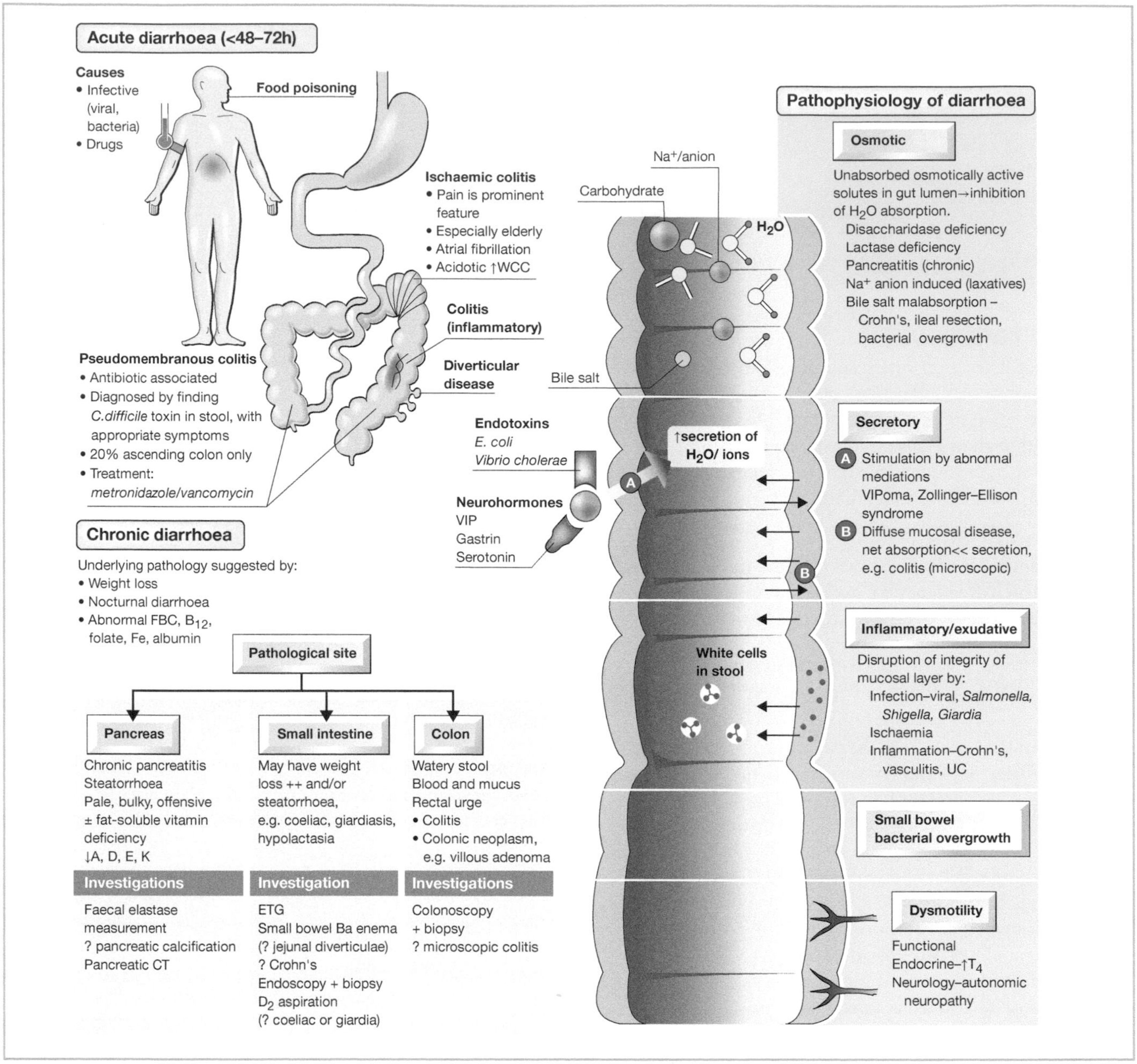

Acute diarrhoea (<48–72h)

Causes
- Infective (viral, bacteria)
- Drugs

Food poisoning

Ischaemic colitis
- Pain is prominent feature
- Especially elderly
- Atrial fibrillation
- Acidotic ↑WCC

Colitis (inflammatory)

Diverticular disease

Pseudomembranous colitis
- Antibiotic associated
- Diagnosed by finding *C.difficile* toxin in stool, with appropriate symptoms
- 20% ascending colon only
- Treatment: *metronidazole/vancomycin*

Chronic diarrhoea

Underlying pathology suggested by:
- Weight loss
- Nocturnal diarrhoea
- Abnormal FBC, B_{12}, folate, Fe, albumin

Pathological site

Pancreas	Small intestine	Colon
Chronic pancreatitis Steatorrhoea Pale, bulky, offensive ± fat-soluble vitamin deficiency ↓A, D, E, K	May have weight loss ++ and/or steatorrhoea, e.g. coeliac, giardiasis, hypolactasia	Watery stool Blood and mucus Rectal urge • Colitis • Colonic neoplasm, e.g. villous adenoma
Investigations	**Investigation**	**Investigations**
Faecal elastase measurement ? pancreatic calcification Pancreatic CT	ETG Small bowel Ba enema (? jejunal diverticulae) ? Crohn's Endoscopy + biopsy D_2 aspiration (? coeliac or giardia)	Colonoscopy + biopsy ? microscopic colitis

Pathophysiology of diarrhoea

Na+/anion
Carbohydrate
H_2O
Bile salt

Osmotic

Unabsorbed osmotically active solutes in gut lumen→inhibition of H_2O absorption.
Disaccharidase deficiency
Lactase deficiency
Pancreatitis (chronic)
Na^+ anion induced (laxatives)
Bile salt malabsorption – Crohn's, ileal resection, bacterial overgrowth

Endotoxins
E. coli
Vibrio cholerae

Neurohormones
VIP
Gastrin
Serotonin

↑secretion of H_2O/ ions

Secretory

(A) Stimulation by abnormal mediations
VIPoma, Zollinger–Ellison syndrome
(B) Diffuse mucosal disease, net absorption<< secretion, e.g. colitis (microscopic)

White cells in stool

Inflammatory/exudative

Disruption of integrity of mucosal layer by:
Infection–viral, *Salmonella, Shigella, Giardia*
Ischaemia
Inflammation–Crohn's, vasculitis, UC

Small bowel bacterial overgrowth

Dysmotility

Functional
Endocrine–↑T_4
Neurology–autonomic neuropathy

Acute diarrhoea

Overall approach

Most acute (<48–72 h) diarrhoea is infective and may be viral or related to bacterial gastrointestinal infection acquired in food. Other intestinal pathologies (particularly pseudomembranous colitis) may also present acutely. The differential diagnosis is as follows.

- **Common**: viral (more commonly associated with vomiting), acute bacterial (commonly 'food poisoning'); colitis; *Clostridium difficile* toxin-related diarrhoea. Drug side-effects.
- **Uncommon**: inflammatory bowel disease; ischaemic colitis; diverticular change.
- **Rare**: colon cancer.

Clinical features

See figure above.

History

- Travel, contacts, take-away/restaurant food, sexual history.
- Recent medications: *C. difficile* toxin-related diarrhoea is common two days to one month after broad-spectrum antibiotics (particularly cephalosporins and clindamycin) in the infirm elderly patient.

Medicine at a Glance, Fifth Edition. Edited by Patrick Davey and Alex Pitcher.

Companion website: www.wiley.com/go/medicine5e

- Bleeding is more suggestive of specific aetiological agents such as *Campylobacter* spp., *Shigella* spp. or enterohaemorrhagic *E. coli*, or alternatively of inflammatory colitis.

Examination

The state of hydration should be determined; even young patients may be considerably volume depleted on admission, with tachycardia and postural hypotension, and may require intravenous saline. Fever generally suggests an infective cause, but may be present in severe colitis. Markers of chronic disease (clubbing, koilonychia, leuconychia, mouth ulcers, weight loss) may reflect an underlying chronic inflammatory bowel disease. Abdominal examination may reveal non-specific tenderness. Sigmoidoscopy and rectal biopsy may be useful although these might not discriminate between the various causes.

Investigations

- **Blood tests**: full blood count (FBC); anaemia or thrombocytosis raises the suspicion of a chronic underlying pathology. A low albumin is a good marker of severity of illness but is non-specific.
- **Stool culture** (and/or PCR which is becoming first line in many centres) may identify the responsible organism. *C. difficile* bacteria are found in 5% of normal individuals; diagnosis therefore requires appropriate symptoms in the presence of the toxin rather than the organism alone.
- **Plain abdominal X-ray**: may show features of acute colitis (see Chapter 128). Dilation of the colon in *C. difficile* diarrhoea is ominous and may mandate colectomy.

Management

- **Rehydration**: the initial management involves giving parenteral or enteral rehydration.
- **Treat the underlying cause.**
  - Steroids might be indicated if investigations reveal an underlying inflammatory bowel disease.
  - Antibiotics may be indicated in some acute bacterial infections.
  - Oral vancomycin and/or metronidazole are typically used first line for pseudomembranous colitis in conjunction with stopping causative antibiotics and proton pump inhibitors where possible. Relapse occurs in up to 20% and is typically treated with a longer course of oral vancomycin. Other antibiotic regimens, including fidaxomicin or tigecycline, may be used second line, and faecal transplantation is also used.

Chronic diarrhoea

Overall approach

Most infectious forms of diarrhoea resolve within 2–3 weeks and any diarrhoea that lasts longer than this warrants further investigation. In the outpatient clinic, it is important to distinguish diarrhoea from rectal 'frequency' where the number of defecations per day is increased in the absence of an increase in stool weight.

The differential diagnosis is as follows.

- **Common**: inflammatory bowel disease, coeliac disease, giardiasis, drugs (e.g. proton pump inhibitors); factitious, e.g. laxative misuse; irritable bowel syndrome.
- **Uncommon**: hypolactasia, colonic neoplasms (including villous adenomas), thyrotoxicosis; bile acid malabsorption, pancreatic insufficiency, small bowel intestinal overgrowth.
- **Rare**: endocrine tumours (e.g. Zollinger–Ellison syndrome, which results from a gastrin-secreting tumour).

Clinical features

In difficult cases, it may be important to confirm that the patient has true diarrhoea (by stool weights) and not a functional bowel disorder (see Chapter 138). The features suggesting pathological diarrhoea include nocturnal diarrhoea, unintentional weight loss and mouth ulcers.

History

The clinical history may give clues about whether the predominant pathology is colonic, small intestinal or pancreatic.

- **Colonic diarrhoea**: watery stool often with blood and mucus. May be associated with urgency of defecation.
- **Small intestinal diarrhoea**: may have features of steatorrhoea (pale, bulky stools that are difficult to flush away) and weight loss.
- **Exocrine pancreatic insufficiency**: steatorrhoea and weight loss are the hallmarks of pancreatic insufficiency. In addition, the patient may describe pancreatic pain, which is epigastric (often radiating through to the back) associated with fatty food intolerance.
- **Gall bladder surgery** is associated with bile acid malabsorption.
- **Gastrointestinal surgery** may be associated with malabsorption or small bowel intestinal overgrowth.
- Excessive consumption of non-absorbable sugars, e.g. sweeteners, can cause diarrhoea.

Examination

- **General appearance**: determine whether the patient looks well or not. If possible, corroborate a history of weight loss (loose clothes or skin, belt notches, etc.).
- **Physical signs of malabsorption**: nail changes such as koilonychia and leuconychia; signs in the tongue and mouth of glossitis, cheilitis and ulcers.
- **Abdominal examination**: this should include rectal examination.

Investigations

Investigations should be chosen depending on the most likely diagnosis on clinical grounds.

- **Blood tests**: FBC, erythrocyte sedimentation rate and biochemistry, particularly for serum albumin, vitamin B_{12} and folate; thyroid function; coeliac serology.
- **Stool microscopy and culture** (×3): negative cultures do not exclude giardiasis; many institutions require a specific request to examine for ova, cysts and parasites.
- **Faecal elastase (or faecal chymotrypsin)** will be low in exocrine pancreatic insufficiency.
- **Upper gastrointestinal endoscopy and duodenal biopsy**: to exclude coeliac disease and giardiasis.
- **Colonoscopy and biopsies**: lower gastrointestinal endoscopy has the advantage over contrast radiology in that, even if the mucosa looks normal, biopsies might reveal a microscopic colitis (e.g. lymphocytic colitis, collagenous colitis).
- Although now rarely performed, **hydrogen breath tests** can confirm a suspicion of hypolactasia (lactose breath test) or small bowel bacterial overgrowth (lactulose breath test), which may also be suggested by low serum B_{12} and high serum folate.
- **Small bowel imaging** (e.g. CT or magnetic resonance enterography): may show jejunal diverticula *or* intestinal strictures (e.g. Crohn's disease) that might act as a substrate for bacterial overgrowth.
- **Twenty-four-hour stool weights** (repeated when fasting): although this often appears low on the list of investigations, it remains the most useful way of distinguishing osmotic diarrhoea from a secretory one.
- **Fasting gut hormones**: if a hormone-secreting tumour is suspected, fasting hormone levels should be measured, usually with chromogranin A as first line. If gastrin levels are measured, proton pump inhibitors must be stopped.
- **SeHCAT radionucleotide scanning** to assess bile acid retention can diagnose bile acid malabsorption.

Management

Treat the specific cause (see relevant sections).

Arasaradnam, R.P., Brown, S., Forbes, A., et al. Guidelines for the investigation of chronic diarrhoea in adults: British Society of Gastroenterology, 3rd edition. Gut 2018;67:1380–1399.

26 Vomiting and intestinal obstruction

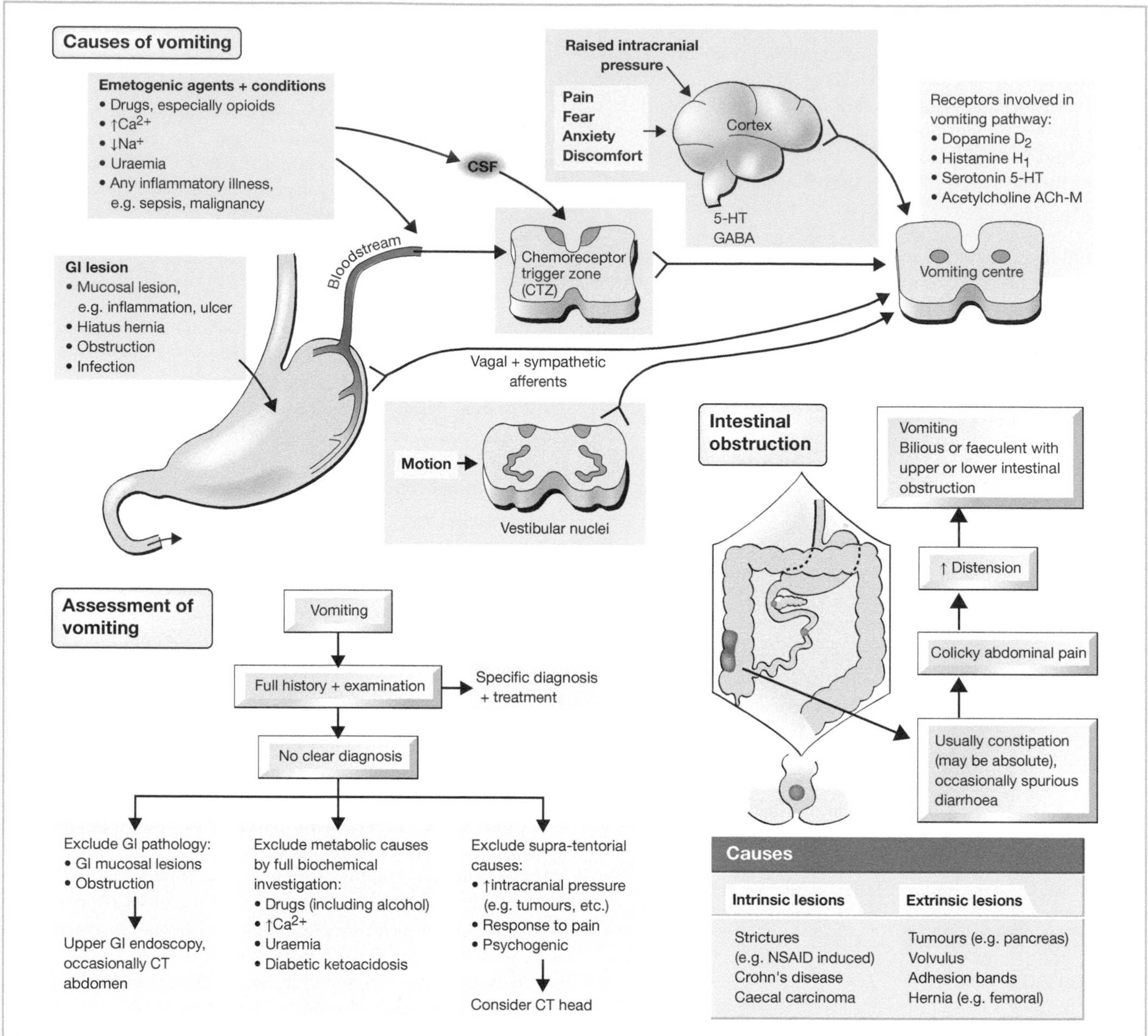

Intestinal obstruction

Overall approach

The first step in the assessment of vomiting is to consider whether or not there is intestinal obstruction. Intestinal obstruction can be caused by the following.

- **Intrinsic factors.**
  - Gastrointestinal (GI) neoplasia, e.g. gastric or colonic carcinoma.
  - Crohn's disease.
  - Strictures, e.g. postsurgical; ischaemia; other, including non-steroidal anti-inflammatory drugs (NSAIDs).
- **Extrinsic factors.**
  - Tumour, e.g. pancreas.
  - Incarcerated hernia.
  - Adhesion bands secondary to previous surgery.
  - Volvulus.
- **Pseudo-obstruction**: paralytic ileus/motility disorders.

Medicine at a Glance, Fifth Edition. Edited by Patrick Davey and Alex Pitcher.

Companion website: www.wiley.com/go/medicine5e

Clinical features

Key clinical features indicating that vomiting is caused by intestinal obstruction are, first, the presence of colicky abdominal pain and, second, a change in bowel habit (ranging from diarrhoea to absolute constipation).

History

- Ask about the duration of symptoms, anorexia and weight loss (suggests progressive pathology).
- Site of pain (see Chapter 30).
- A sudden onset of pain and vomiting implies a physical/mechanical cause.
- Previous intestinal illness or operations.

Examination

General

Observe the general appearance and presence of lymphadenopathy. It is vital to determine the fluid status of the patient from skin turgor, pulse rate, blood pressure (including postural drop) and urine output.

Abdominal examination

- Scars from previous surgery raise the possibility of obstruction caused by adhesions.
- Abdominal distension may be present. Absent bowel sounds suggest paralytic ileus (pseudo-obstruction), whereas in most other cases of obstruction, bowel sounds are increased. A succussion splash suggests gastric outflow obstruction.
- Tenderness and rebound suggest peritonitis (i.e. perforation).
- Palpable inflammatory or neoplastic masses.
- Rectal examination.

Investigations

- **Blood tests**: full blood count (FBC)/erythrocyte sedimentation rate (ESR) and biochemistry are indicated, partly to determine the effect of vomiting/obstruction on potassium and renal function.
- **Abdominal X-ray**: usually shows features of intestinal obstruction (i.e. dilated fluid-filled loops of bowel) and on occasion may suggest the level of the obstruction (e.g. air absent from the rectum).
- **Upper gastrointestinal endoscopy**: if gastric outflow obstruction is suspected. Beware the risk of aspiration of intestinal contents.
- **Abdominal computed tomography** (CT) with contrast after discussion with radiologist and surgical team.

Initial management

- **Nil by mouth**: gut rest is probably the best way to relieve symptoms. A large-bore nasogastric tube (Ryle's tube/Levin tube) helps to drain obstructed intestinal contents and in cases of protracted large-volume vomiting is imperative in preventing aspiration.
- **Intravenous fluids**: patients may be significantly volume depleted/dehydrated on admission and require substantial fluid resuscitation.
- Avoid opiate analgesia when possible (as this further inhibits intestinal motility).
- Electrolyte replacement is important.
- Antiperistaltic drugs should be stopped.
- Gastrograffin by mouth or by nasogastric tube is often used conservatively initially.

Subsequent management

In cases that do not resolve with conservative management, a laparotomy may be necessary even before a definitive diagnosis has been achieved.

Chronic vomiting

Overall approach

In the absence of evidence of mechanical obstruction, other causes of vomiting should be considered.

- **Metabolic**.
  - Hypercalcaemia.
  - Hypoadrenalism (Addison disease).
- **Inflammatory disease**.
  - Visceral inflammation, e.g. pancreatitis.
  - Remote infection, e.g. pneumonia.
- **Drugs**.
  - Cytotoxics.
  - Analgesics (especially opioids).
  - Antibiotics.
- **Neurogenic**.
  - Intracranial tumours.
  - Vestibulocochlear disease.
  - Psychogenic.
- **GI causes**.
  - Obstruction.
  - Gastroenteritis.

History

Ask specifically about:

- duration of symptoms, and whether the problem is getting worse
- drugs, including those bought over the counter
- headache or other features of raised intracranial pressure
- unusual foods, restaurants, travel
- hearing, balance.

Examination

- **General**: check overall appearance and the presence of any relevant pathology. State of hydration, particularly postural blood pressure.
- **Abdominal examination**: usually unrewarding but may reveal signs of intestinal obstruction.

Investigations

- **Blood tests**: FBC, CRP and biochemistry, including renal and liver chemistry, sodium, potassium and calcium, amylase.
- **Cortisol**: short Synacthen test if hypoadrenalism is suspected.
- **Chest X-ray**: for infection (including aspiration pneumonia), neoplasm.
- **Upper GI endoscopy** is usually indicated in patients with persistent vomiting when no other cause is found.
- **Small bowel imaging or fluoroscopy**: may be indicated in difficult cases to exclude occult subacute obstruction.
- **CT or magnetic resonance imaging scan of the head**: indicated when no other pathology is identified.

Management

- Treat the underlying cause.
- Empirical treatment with antiemetics may be necessary if physical/mechanical obstruction has been excluded. Domperidone does not cross the blood–brain barrier and is useful for long-term 'as needed' treatment although there are concerns about QT prolongation with chronic use. Other agents (e.g. metoclopramide, prochlorperazine) are increasingly being replaced by centrally acting serotonin antagonists (e.g. ondansetron).

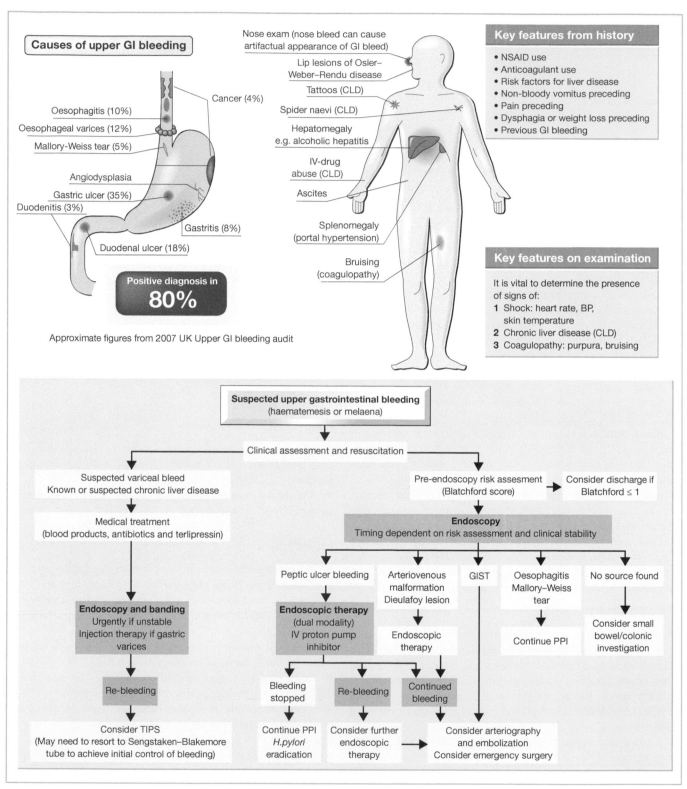

Haematemesis and melaena

Causes of upper GI bleeding

- Cancer (4%)
- Oesophagitis (10%)
- Oesophageal varices (12%)
- Mallory-Weiss tear (5%)
- Angiodysplasia
- Gastric ulcer (35%)
- Duodenitis (3%)
- Gastritis (8%)
- Duodenal ulcer (18%)

Positive diagnosis in 80%

Approximate figures from 2007 UK Upper GI bleeding audit

- Nose exam (nose bleed can cause artifactual appearance of GI bleed)
- Lip lesions of Osler–Weber–Rendu disease
- Tattoos (CLD)
- Spider naevi (CLD)
- Hepatomegaly e.g. alcoholic hepatitis
- IV-drug abuse (CLD)
- Ascites
- Splenomegaly (portal hypertension)
- Bruising (coagulopathy)

Key features from history

- NSAID use
- Anticoagulant use
- Risk factors for liver disease
- Non-bloody vomitus preceding
- Pain preceding
- Dysphagia or weight loss preceding
- Previous GI bleeding

Key features on examination

It is vital to determine the presence of signs of:

1. Shock: heart rate, BP, skin temperature
2. Chronic liver disease (CLD)
3. Coagulopathy: purpura, bruising

Suspected upper gastrointestinal bleeding (haematemesis or melaena)

→ Clinical assessment and resuscitation

→ Suspected variceal bleed: Known or suspected chronic liver disease
→ Medical treatment (blood products, antibiotics and terlipressin)
→ **Endoscopy and banding**: Urgently if unstable; Injection therapy if gastric varices
→ Re-bleeding
→ Consider TIPS (May need to resort to Sengstaken–Blakemore tube to achieve initial control of bleeding)

→ Pre-endoscopy risk assesment (Blatchford score) → Consider discharge if Blatchford ≤ 1
→ **Endoscopy**: Timing dependent on risk assessment and clinical stability

- Peptic ulcer bleeding → **Endoscopic therapy** (dual modality) IV proton pump inhibitor
  - → Bleeding stopped → Continue PPI *H.pylori* eradication
  - → Re-bleeding → Consider further endoscopic therapy → Consider arteriography and embolization; Consider emergency surgery
  - → Continued bleeding → Consider arteriography and embolization; Consider emergency surgery
- Arteriovenous malformation, Dieulafoy lesion → Endoscopic therapy → Continued bleeding
- GIST → Consider arteriography and embolization; Consider emergency surgery
- Oesophagitis, Mallory–Weiss tear → Continue PPI
- No source found → Consider small bowel/colonic investigation

Medicine at a Glance, Fifth Edition. Edited by Patrick Davey and Alex Pitcher.

Companion website: www.wiley.com/go/medicine5e

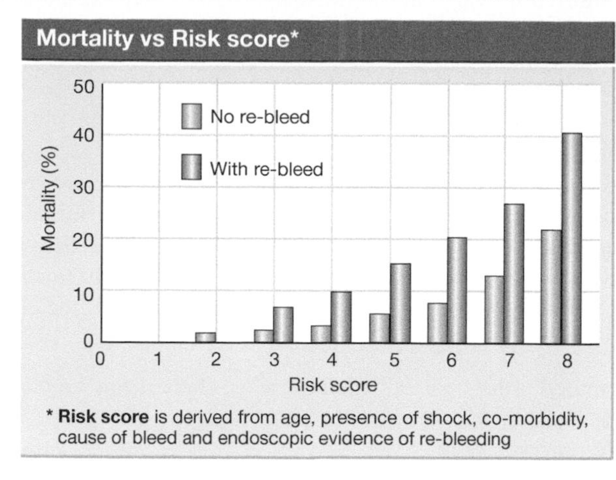

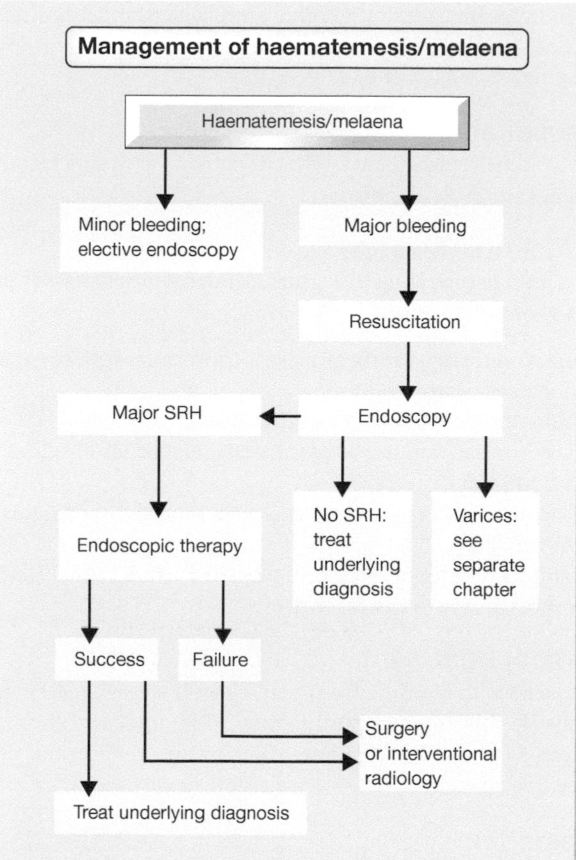

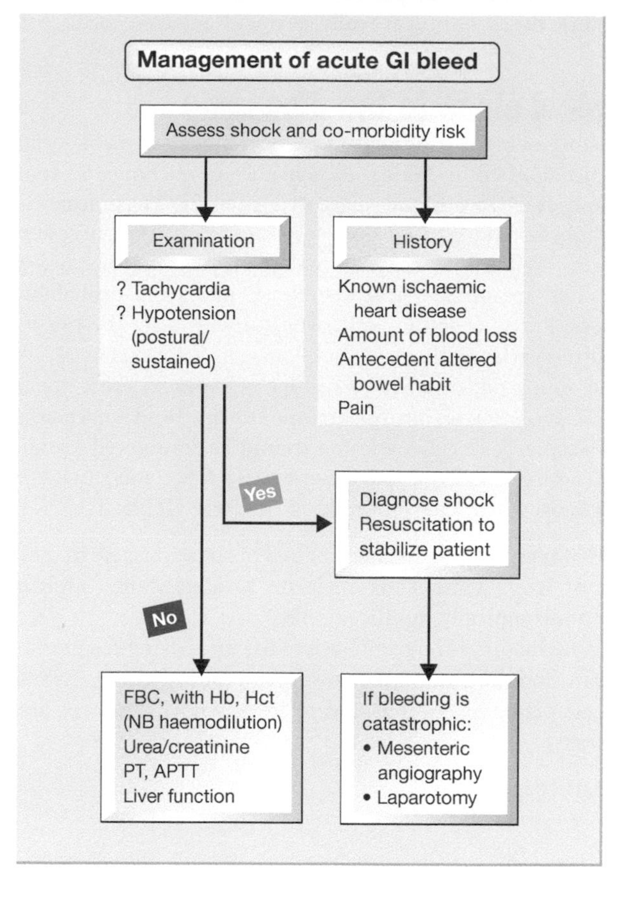

Immediate treatment

1 IV access: 2 large bore IV lines
2 Fluid (blood)
3 Endoscopy <12 h or sooner if continued bleeding

Introduction

- **Haematemesis** refers to the vomiting of blood. Blood may be fresh (clots or bright red liquid) or altered by intestinal acid and enzymes, appearing brown and likened to 'coffee grounds'. Vomiting a small amount of altered blood is often a non-specific feature of protracted retching and does not always reflect a significant upper gastrointestinal (GI) haemorrhage.
- **Melaena** refers to a loose, tarry, jet-black stool, with a deeply offensive smell, which sticks to the pan and indicates brisk upper GI haemorrhage with digestion of the blood in the intestine. Solid dark stool that tests positive for occult blood may indicate intestinal bleeding but is *not* melaena.

Differential diagnosis

- **Common**: peptic ulcer (duodenal, gastric); Mallory–Weiss tear; gastritis, duodenitis, oesophagitis.
- **Uncommon**: oesophageal varices/portal hypertensive gastropathy.
- **Rare**: upper GI malignancy – including gastrointestinal stromal tumours (GISTs).

- **Very rare**: angiodysplasia (including a Dieulafoy lesion); aortoenteric fistula only ever really seen with infected aortic grafts.

Clinical clues to the diagnosis

A history of indigestion may make peptic ulcer more likely but its absence does not exclude this. A history of retching and vomitus initially free from blood suggests a Mallory–Weiss tear. Heavy alcohol consumption suggests gastritis (30–40%) or occasionally varices. Weight loss suggests malignancy. Severe bleeding with clots and treatment-refractory shock raises the probability of varices. Previous abdominal aortic surgery raises the possibility of aortoenteric fistula.

In young patients with a history of repeated brisk upper GI bleeding (often with haemodynamic collapse) and 'unremarkable' endoscopies, a Dieulafoy lesion should be considered (a submucosal artery, usually on the lesser gastric curve and situated near the cardia, which intermittently causes large GI bleeds).

- **History**: postural dizziness or loss of consciousness in the context of haematemesis or melaena is significant, implying a 'haemodynamically significant bleed'.
- **Drug history** is relevant both to the underlying diagnosis (e.g. aspirin and non-steroidal anti-inflammatory drugs [NSAIDs] suggest peptic ulceration) and to treatment (β-blockers, anticoagulants).

- **Anticoagulation**.

Examination

General

- General appearance: is the patient cool and clammy, indicating significant peripheral vasoconstriction?
- Pulse and blood pressure (BP), including postural drop. Documentation of the severity of shock is vitally important.
- Signs of chronic liver disease.
- Signs of neoplasia: lymphadenopathy, organomegaly, weight loss.

Abdominal

This may be uninformative. Epigastric tenderness is most often non-specific. Hepatosplenomegaly and/or abdominal ascites raise the possibility of portal hypertension and therefore varices.

Predictors of mortality

A number of factors have now been defined as predicting mortality from upper GI bleeding and these form the basis of clinical risk assessment tools (Table 27.1). The Blatchford score is based upon initial observations and blood test results, whereas the Rockall score incorporates endoscopic finding in predicting risk.

Investigations

- **Blood tests**: full blood count (FBC) and cross-match.
- **Urea and creatinine**: a raised urea relative to creatinine (i.e. raised urea/creatinine ratio) is present in significant upper GI haemorrhage and reflects the protein load of fresh blood within the gut, as well as dehydration ('pre-renal' uraemia, see Chapter 150).
- **K^+**: this may be disproportionately high as a result of absorption from blood in the small bowel.
- **Clotting** should be checked.
- **Endoscopy**: will establish the diagnosis and may allow immediate endoscopic treatment. It also provides prognostic information (i.e. identification of stigmata of recent haemorrhage [SRH]).

Management

All cases should be managed in conjunction with an experienced endoscopist and GI surgeons. If the patient has had abdominal aortic surgery, a vascular surgeon should be consulted. Episodes of rebleeding after admission (as suggested by further haematemesis, melaena, cardiovascular instability or fall in haemoglobin) have a worse prognosis.

- Limited transfusion is beneficial when there is not haemodynamic instability; aim for ≥70^g/l haemoglobin.
- PPI intravenously.
- Tranexamic acid has previously been recommended but is ineffective.
- Aspirin should not be stopped.
- Consider reversal of anticoagulants.
- Minimize interruption to other antiplatelets/anticoagulation.
- Consider discharge without endoscopy if risk score is low at the outset, e.g. Glasgow Blatchford 0.

Resuscitation

Early volume replacement is vital in patients with shock and coexistent cardiovascular disease.

Endoscopic therapy

In addition to providing a diagnosis, endoscopy also allows treatment to bleeding lesions.

- Injection therapy: adrenaline for peptic ulcers with stigmata of recent haemorrhage.
- Endoscopic clipping of bleeding vessels.
- Heater probe and argon plasma coagulation of bleeding vessels, tumours and ulcers.
- If treating ulcers, two or more therapeutic modalities are recommended.
- Band ligation of oesophageal varices; cyanoacrylate (glue) or thrombin therapy to gastric varices.

Medical treatment

In patients with bleeding from peptic ulcers showing SRH, intravenous (IV) proton pump inhibitors (PPIs) increase intragastric pH leading to clot stabilization, which in turn reduces the risk of rebleeding episodes.

Rebleeding

Any evidence of rebleeding after initial therapy carries a poor prognosis and should be addressed by either repeated endoscopic therapy or surgery.

Angiography and interventional radiology

Interventional radiology may gain control of bleeding uncontrolled at endoscopy. Placing endoscopic clips may be useful to guide the radiologists.

Surgery

Although surgery is less common now than in the days before the development of endoscopy, it remains a vital treatment. Surgical intervention should be considered in individuals not responding to

Table 27.1 Clinical risk assessment tools: the Blatchford and Rockall scores

Blatchford score system	**Score**	**Rockall score system**	**Score**			
Blood urea (mmol/l)			0	1	2	3
>6.5 <8.0	2	Age	<60	60–79	>80	
>8.0 <10.0	3	Shock	'No shock' BP>100 Pulse<100	'Tachycardia' BP>100 Pulse>100	'Hypotension' BP <100	
>10.0 <25	4					
>25	6	Co-morbidity	No major co-morbidity		Cardiac failure, ischaemic heart disease	Renal failure, liver failure, disseminated malignancy
Haemoglobin (g/l, men)						
>120 <130	1					
>100 <120	3	Diagnosis	Mallory–Weiss tear, no lesion identified	All other diagnoses	Upper GI malignancy	
<100	6					
Haemoglobin (g/l, women)						
>100 <120	1	Major SRH	None, or dark spot only		Blood in upper GI tract, adherent clot, visible or spurting vessel	
<100	6					
Systolic blood pressure (mmHg)						
100–109	1					
90–99	2					
<90	3					
Other markers						
Pulse >100	1					
Presentation with melaena	1					
Presentation with syncope	2					
Hepatic disease	2					
Cardiac failure	2					

Higher scores are associated with higher risk of further bleeding and death.
SRH, stigmata of recent haemorrhage.

resuscitation, those with a clinically significant rebleed and those in whom endoscopy has failed or is not feasible. Early consultation with the surgical team always facilitates subsequent management.

- NICE Clinical Guideline 141. Acute upper GI bleeding in over-16s: management. www.nice.org.uk/guidance/cg141
- Hearnshaw, S.A., Logan, R.F.A., Lowe, D., Travis, S.P.L., Murphy, M.F., Palmer, K.R. Acute upper gastrointestinal bleeding in the UK: patient characteristics, diagnoses and outcomes in the 2007 UK audit. Gut 2011;60(10):1327–1335.
- Gralnek, I., Dumonceau, J.M., Kuipers, E.J., et al. Diagnosis and management of non-variceal upper gastrointestinal hemorrhage: European Society of Gastrointestinal Endoscopy (ESGE) Guideline. Endoscopy 2015;47:a1–46.

28 Rectal bleeding

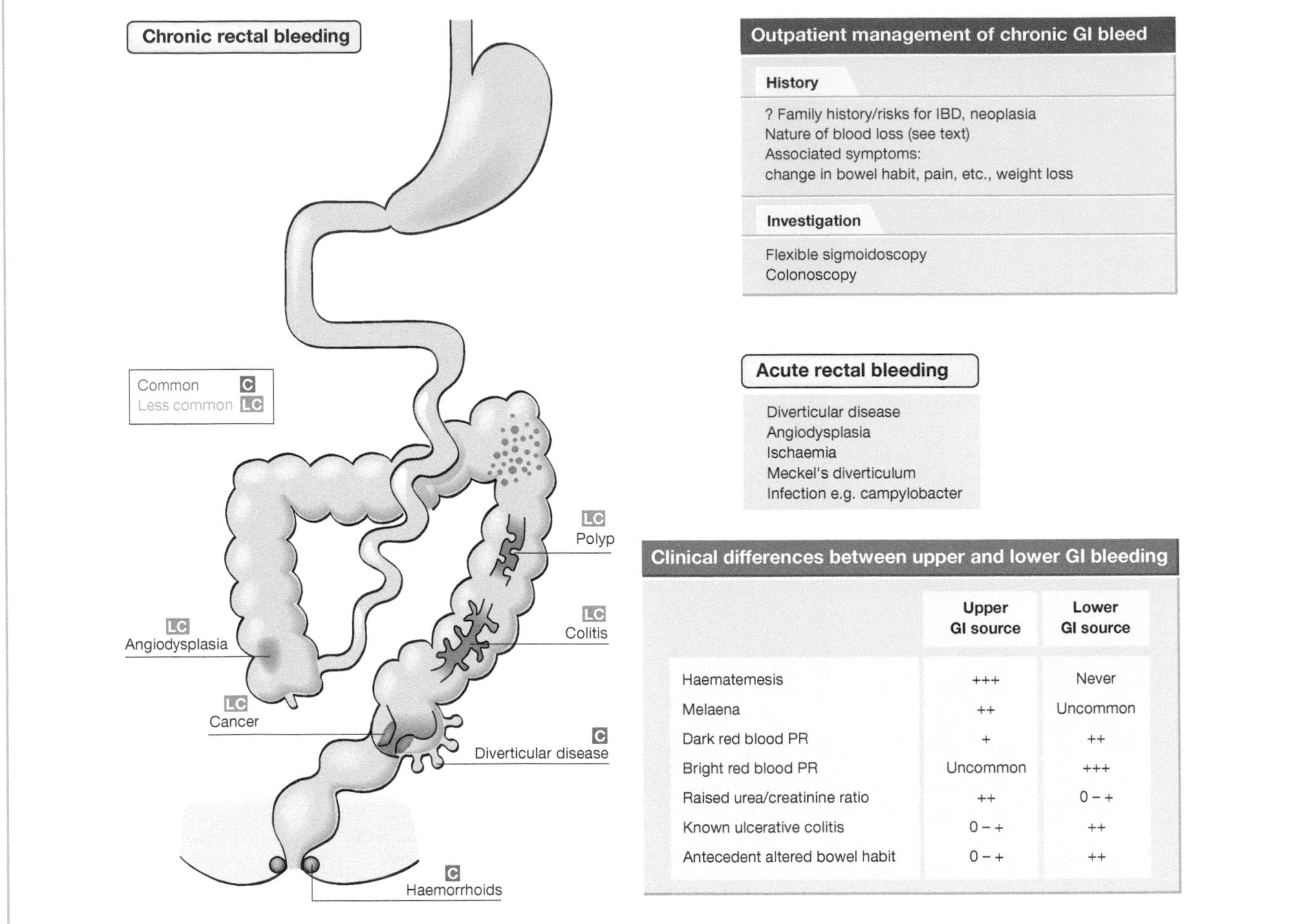

	Upper GI source	Lower GI source
Haematemesis	+++	Never
Melaena	++	Uncommon
Dark red blood PR	+	++
Bright red blood PR	Uncommon	+++
Raised urea/creatinine ratio	++	0 – +
Known ulcerative colitis	0 – +	++
Antecedent altered bowel habit	0 – +	++

Distinguish between acute, heavy or lower gastrointestinal (GI) haemorrhage and chronic, persistent, small-volume rectal bleeding. The term *haematochezia* is used, primarily in North America, to describe rectal bleeding.

Acute lower GI haemorrhage

Sudden large-volume rectal bleeding most commonly presents in elderly people as a clinical emergency with varying degrees of cardiovascular compromise.

Differential diagnosis (Table 28.1)

The common underlying causes are age-related and although they are often in themselves benign, the presence of significant co-morbidity (e.g. ischaemic heart disease) in this group of patients contributes to a significant mortality.

Table 28.1 Differential diagnosis of acute lower GI haemorrhage

Common

- Diverticular disease
- Colonic angiodysplasia
- Ischaemic colitis

Uncommon

- Distal colon/rectal carcinoma
- Inflammatory bowel disease
- Meckel diverticulum

Clinical features

It can be a challenge to distinguish proximal colonic bleeding from a brisk upper GI bleed. The passage of red blood per rectum (PR) is unlikely to be from an upper GI source. Likewise, the passage of classic melaena (jet-black, tarry, smelly) indicates an upper GI tract lesion. The problem arises when blood appears to be neither one nor the other, when upper and lower GI tract investigations are needed.

Medicine at a Glance, Fifth Edition. Edited by Patrick Davey and Alex Pitcher.

Companion website: www.wiley.com/go/medicine5e

History

- **Nature of the bleeding**: was it black 'like tar' (i.e. melaena) or black 'like bramble jelly' (i.e. arising from the colon)?
- **Onset**: most commonly the onset of bleeding is sudden, although it is important to elicit whether there had been an antecedent change in bowel habit, which may indicate a colonic neoplasm or colitis.
- **Abdominal pain**: mild colicky pain is a non-specific finding; severe *sudden* pain suggests intestinal ischaemia (i.e. ischaemic colitis).
- **Significant co-morbidity**: the recognition of significant co-morbidity is important in guiding resuscitation and specific interventions.

Examination

- **State of circulation** (pulse, postural blood pressure): any degree of shock must be recognized early and corrected (see below).
- **Abdominal examination**: the absence of a palpable **mass** in the abdomen does not exclude a malignant underlying cause.
- A **bruit** may rarely be heard, indicating mesenteric atheroma and potentially ischaemia.
- **Rectal examination** may identify a low rectal cancer and may be useful in clinically distinguishing lower from upper GI bleeding (melaena = upper).

Risk scoring

The Oakland score predicts safe discharge to allow outpatient investigation. The score includes variables based on age, sex, previous admission, rectal examination, heart rate, blood pressure and haemoglobin.

Investigations

- **Blood tests**: a full blood count (FBC) should be taken, although in acute GI bleeding haemodilution takes several hours, so the haemoglobin level may underestimate the severity of the bleed. A clotting profile should be checked if the patient is on anticoagulants or if there are clinical indications of chronic liver disease.
- **Group & screen**: cross-match if shock is present on admission or if there is significant anaemia. A raised urea/creatinine ratio may indicate an upper, not lower, GI source. An elevated lactate may suggest ischaemia.
- **Lower GI endoscopy**: once resuscitation has been completed and preferably after the acute bleed has subsided. The timing and extent of the endoscopy (i.e. colonoscopy vs flexible sigmoidoscopy) must be determined on individual clinical grounds. Computed tomography (CT) colonography may be necessary if the upper limit of bleeding is not identified or if total endoscopic examination is prevented by technical limitations (e.g. severe diverticular change, ischaemia, stricture).
- **Upper GI endoscopy**: usually at the time of sigmoidoscopy/colonoscopy for formal exclusion of a significant upper GI pathology.
- **Mesenteric angiography**: in persistent heavy colonic bleeding (≥2 ml/min) angiography can identify areas of angiodysplasia or a bleeding vessel that can be embolized. Often initial angiography is performed using CT.

Management

- **Resuscitation**: early correction of shock is vital.
- **Cessation or reversal of anticoagulant medication**: whilst considering the indications for these medications.
- **Treat specific pathology**: in most circumstances, colonic bleeding will, at least temporarily, cease, allowing for diagnostic investigations.
- **Laparotomy**: in catastrophic bleeding, a laparotomy, if possible with on-table colonoscopy, and occasionally a 'blind' colectomy may be necessary.

Chronic rectal bleeding

Overall approach

The recurrent/persistent passage of blood PR may present at any age and, in most situations, can be managed as an outpatient.

Differential diagnosis

Although the most common cause of rectal bleeding is benign, appropriate investigations are always indicated in order to make an early diagnosis of colorectal cancer. The differential diagnosis is: **common**: haemorrhoids ('piles' in common parlance), colorectal neoplasia (polyps, cancer) – more common in the elderly; distal colitis or proctitis; **rare**: solitary rectal ulcer, rectal varices, radiation enteritis, e.g. after prostate radiotherapy.

History

The history (particularly the appearance of the blood) often suggests the site of bleeding.

- Bright red 'like tomato ketchup' or dark red 'like bramble jelly' blood suggest, respectively, lower and upper colonic pathology.
- Blood only on the toilet paper and the surface of the stool strongly suggests 'piles' as the source. Blood mixed throughout the stool suggests that the pathology is higher up.
- A change in bowel habit may suggest an underlying neoplasm or colitis.
- Bright red bleeding, with mucus discharge, urge and a sense of incomplete emptying (otherwise known as tenesmus), suggest proctitis.
- A family history of colorectal cancer increases the probability (and worry) of this disease.

Examination

Abdominal examination should include the identification of any masses or palpable organomegaly and rectal examination for detection of low rectal tumours. *All* patients should at some point undergo lower gastrointestinal endoscopic evaluation to exclude colorectal polyps/cancer and colitis; haemorrhoids may also be confirmed at the same examination.

Investigations

- **Blood tests**: FBC, inflammatory markers, iron indices – iron deficiency anaemia should not be ascribed to haemorrhoids unless there has been careful exclusion of other potential sources.
- **Lower GI endoscopy**: flexible sigmoidoscopy after an enema should provide good views of the colon as far as the splenic flexure. Total colonoscopy requires full bowel preparation and is indicated when a proximal colonic neoplasm is suspected clinically, from iron deficiency or the presence of distal colonic polyps.
- **CT colonography** is an alternative to total colonoscopy. This requires full bowel preparation and inflation of the colon with air or CO_2. This technique does not yet have an equivalent sensitivity to colonoscopy and most abnormalities require further evaluation (i.e. colonoscopy). A sigmoidoscopic examination should be performed in addition to exclude a low rectal neoplasm, which might otherwise be missed on the scan.

Management

- **Treat specific pathology**: see relevant chapters.
- **Haemorrhoids**: often advice on diet and defecatory habits is sufficient to control symptoms. Injection sclerotherapy, banding and excision may be necessary in some circumstances.

29 Dysphagia

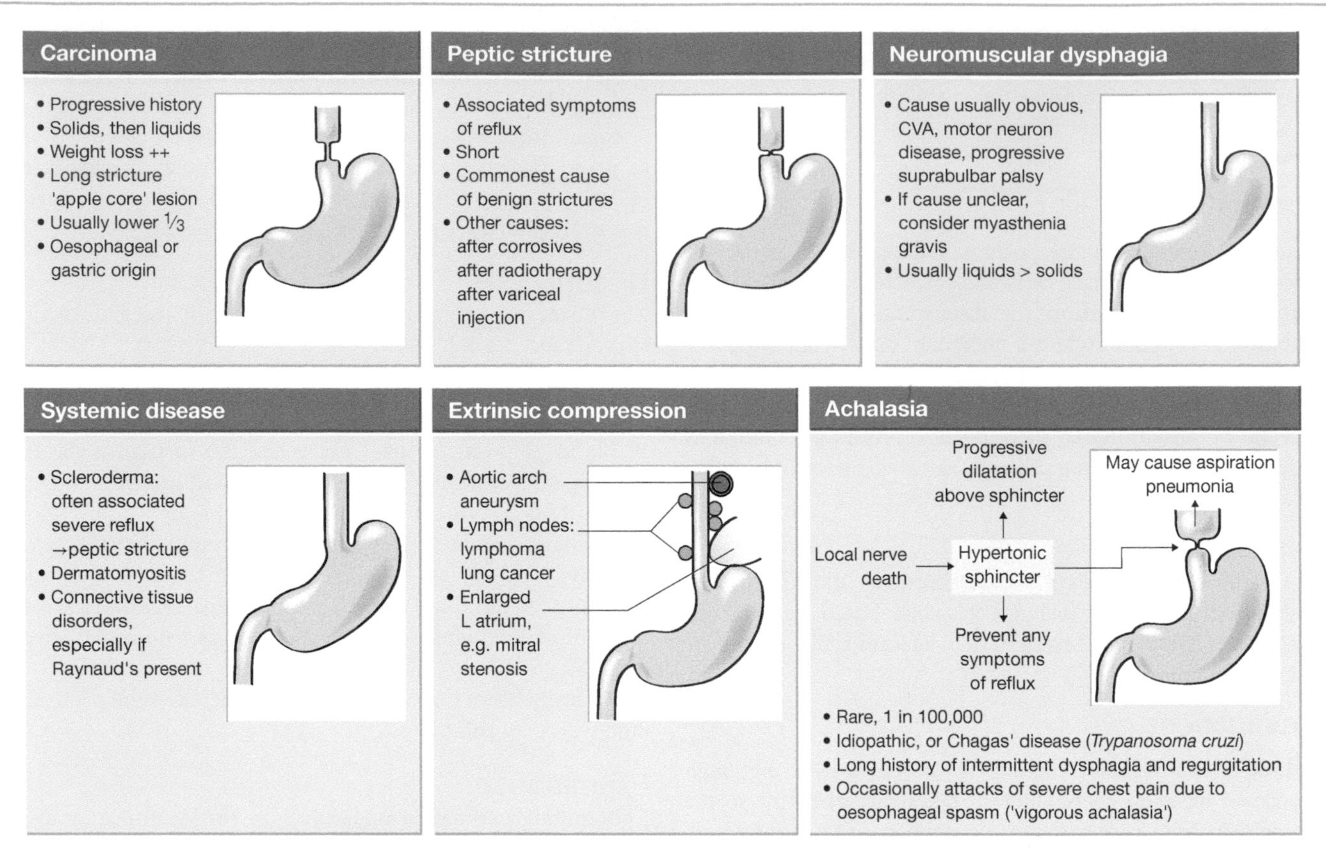

Carcinoma
• Progressive history
• Solids, then liquids
• Weight loss ++
• Long stricture 'apple core' lesion
• Usually lower 1/3
• Oesophageal or gastric origin
Peptic stricture
• Associated symptoms of reflux
• Short
• Commonest cause of benign strictures
• Other causes: after corrosives after radiotherapy after variceal injection
Neuromuscular dysphagia
• Cause usually obvious, CVA, motor neuron disease, progressive suprabulbar palsy
• If cause unclear, consider myasthenia gravis
• Usually liquids > solids
Systemic disease
• Scleroderma: often associated severe reflux →peptic stricture
• Dermatomyositis
• Connective tissue disorders, especially if Raynaud's present
Extrinsic compression
• Aortic arch aneurysm
• Lymph nodes: lymphoma lung cancer
• Enlarged L atrium, e.g. mitral stenosis
Achalasia
Progressive dilatation above sphincter
May cause aspiration pneumonia
Local nerve death
Hypertonic sphincter
Prevent any symptoms of reflux
• Rare, 1 in 100,000
• Idiopathic, or Chagas' disease (Trypanosoma cruzi)
• Long history of intermittent dysphagia and regurgitation
• Occasionally attacks of severe chest pain due to oesophageal spasm ('vigorous achalasia')

Introduction

Dysphagia relates to difficulty in swallowing which in turn implies oesophageal obstruction. Odynophagia relates to painful swallowing. Globus refers to a patient's description of a sensation 'like a lump in the throat' – this is quite distinct and should not be confused with dysphagia.

Differential diagnosis

See Table 29.1.

Clinical features

Dysphagia is an ominous and frightening symptom and should be investigated at the earliest opportunity.

History

The duration of symptoms and associated heartburn/dyspepsia are useful clinical clues. Progressive symptoms and weight loss are ominous features.

Examination

Examination is often unrewarding. Check for anaemia, weight loss and lymphadenopathy (including Virchow's node behind the head of the left clavicle, indicative of metastatic upper gastrointestinal [GI] cancer).

Investigations

- **General investigations** include a full blood count and CRP, liver function tests and calcium. A chest X-ray may show either a primary or a secondary lung neoplasia.
- **Endoscopy**: upper GI endoscopy must be performed with great care but allows definitive diagnosis through biopsy and immediate treatment (oesophageal dilatation, placement of stent).
- **Contrast swallow:** fluoroscopic assessment of liquid radio-opaque material such as barium allows assessment for dysmotility and for silent aspiration.
- **Other specific tests** (manometry, pH monitoring, computed tomography) are indicated depending on the results of the above. See sections on reflux and oesophageal carcinoma (Chapters 123 and 135).

Medicine at a Glance, Fifth Edition. Edited by Patrick Davey and Alex Pitcher.

Companion website: www.wiley.com/go/medicine5e

Table 29.1 Differential diagnosis of dysphagia

Common

- Oesophageal carcinoma
- Gastric cancer at the cardia
- Oesophagitis and peptic stricture

Uncommon

- Diffuse oesophageal spasm (intermittent symptoms associated with pain)

Rare

- Achalasia
- Eosinophilic oesophagitis: can only be diagnosed by taking biopsies of distal oesophagus

Management

- **Peptic stricture**: strictures associated with reflux oesophagitis occasionally require endoscopic dilatation. Recurrence may be reduced by treatment with proton pump inhibitors.
- **Oesophageal carcinoma**: see Chapter 135.
- **Achalasia**: there are a range of treatments for achalasia. Cardiomyotomy (Heller's operation) remains the definitive procedure and can now be performed laparoscopically. Forced pneumatic dilation is an alternative for patients in whom surgery is not possible, as is infiltration with botulinum toxin.
- **Oesophageal dysmotility**: reassurance after exclusion of a malignant underlying cause for the symptoms often helps patients with oesophageal spasm, together with simple advice about diet and nutrition. Calcium antagonists and nitrates have no role.
- **Eosinophilic oesophagitis**: this condition may be diagnosed on oesophageal biopsy. Treatments include exclusion diets and corticosteroids.
- **Neuromuscular dysphagia**: see below.
- **Extrinsic compression** is treated according to the underlying cause.
- **Systemic diseases** producing dysphagia are managed similarly. Scleroderma may produce severe symptoms of reflux, requiring high-dose proton pump inhibition.

Neuromuscular dysphagia

Dysphagia to liquids may occur in motor neuron disease and is an important finding in stroke (it occurs in some 50–70% of stroke patients). Aspiration of food in stroke patients is a crucial mechanism contributing to pneumonia, which itself accounts for some 20–40% of stroke-related deaths.

Neurological disease may interfere with any of the three phases of swallowing.

- The **oral phase**, where food is prepared for swallowing (usually by chewing) and then propelled into the oropharynx (the oral propulsive phase): paralysis of the cranial nerve supplying the tongue, or interference with the cerebellar mechanisms controlling the tongue, may lead to impairment of this phase.
- The **pharyngeal phase**, where food is propelled into the oesophagus, by a complex series of reflex events, involving cranial nerves IX–XII.
- The **oesophageal phase**, where the bolus of food is propelled down the oesophagus by peristaltic motion.

Clinical features

The features of dysphagia in stroke patients include coughing when eating/drinking, recurrent chest infections, weight loss with food avoidance and dehydration. As dysphagia is so frequent in stroke patients, it is crucial to assess swallowing as part of the acute assessment of a stroke. Until this has been done, the patient should be 'nil by mouth'.

Examination

Swallowing assessment consists of a full neurological examination, with some additional features.

- Assess cranial nerves V, VII–XII.
- Observe jaw movement, mastication, tongue strength and mobility.
- Test the individual functions of the mouth.
- Test for the gag reflex.
- Assess how strong the cough is, as this determines how good the lung is at protecting against infection.
- If the functions of the mouth are intact, ask the patient to swallow; while doing so, place three fingers on the larynx and assess how it moves during the swallow.
- If all the above are intact, assess how the patient swallows a small amount of water.

If swallowing is impaired, then the patient should not be fed orally; for the very short run, intravenous fluids are appropriate. If swallowing is not satisfactory after a few days, feeding should occur via a nasogastric tube. If swallowing remains impaired after 2–3 weeks, consideration should be given to percutaneous endoscopic gastrostomy (PEG) feeding.

Prognosis

Most patients who have acutely impaired swallowing due to a stroke have recovered by 6 months – a small proportion need ongoing PEG feeding.

30 Abdominal pain and dyspepsia

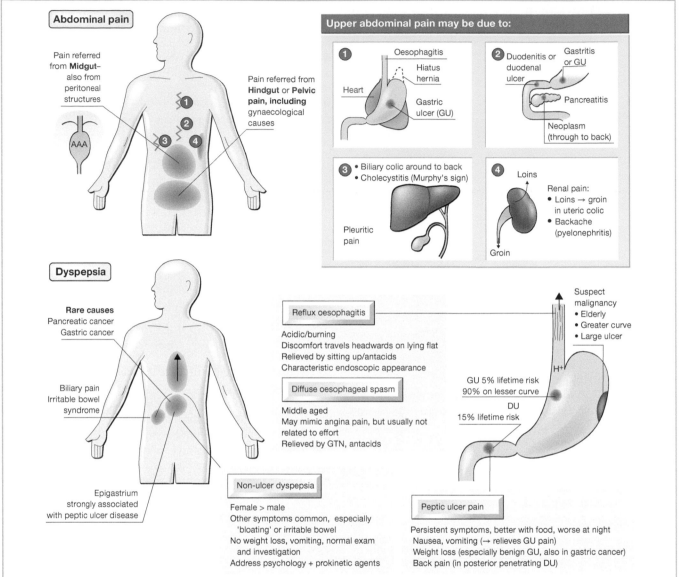

Abdominal pain

Pain referred from **Midgut**– also from peritoneal structures

Pain referred from **Hindgut** or **Pelvic pain, including** gynaecological causes

AAA

Upper abdominal pain may be due to:

1 Oesophagitis; Hiatus hernia; Heart; Gastric ulcer (GU)

2 Duodenitis or duodenal ulcer; Gastritis or GU; Pancreatitis; Neoplasm (through to back)

3 • Biliary colic around to back • Cholecystitis (Murphy's sign); Pleuritic pain

4 Loins; Groin; Renal pain: • Loins → groin in uteric colic • Backache (pyelonephritis)

Dyspepsia

Rare causes Pancreatic cancer Gastric cancer

Biliary pain Irritable bowel syndrome

Epigastrium strongly associated with peptic ulcer disease

Reflux oesophagitis: Acidic/burning; Discomfort travels headwards on lying flat; Relieved by sitting up/antacids; Characteristic endoscopic appearance

Diffuse oesophageal spasm: Middle aged; May mimic angina pain, but usually not related to effort; Relieved by GTN, antacids

Non-ulcer dyspepsia: Female > male; Other symptoms common, especially 'bloating' or irritable bowel; No weight loss, vomiting, normal exam and investigation; Address psychology + prokinetic agents

Suspect malignancy • Elderly • Greater curve • Large ulcer

H^+

GU 5% lifetime risk 90% on lesser curve

DU 15% lifetime risk

Peptic ulcer pain: Persistent symptoms, better with food, worse at night; Nausea, vomiting (→ relieves GU pain); Weight loss (especially benign GU, also in gastric cancer); Back pain (in posterior penetrating DU)

Abdominal pain

A very careful history is critical to formulate a differential diagnosis. Pains usually come from within an organ (midline pain, not often localized to the affected viscus) or from irritation of the peritoneal lining (localized to the site of the inflamed viscus). Patients in pain are often frightened. Patience and perseverance in history taking are rewarded with an earlier and more accurate diagnosis.

History

This is critical to the assessment as physical signs might be limited. Consider the SQITAS questions: *S*ite, *Q*uality, *I*nitiating factors, *T*ime course, *A*lleviating factors, as*S*ociated symptoms.

Certain patterns point to specific sources of pain although there is considerable overlap.

- **Oesophageal pain** has two forms: 'heartburn' relates to acidic sensations and is commonly related to reflux. Oesophageal spasm usually manifests as a tightening felt in the chest, and is sometimes indistinguishable from cardiac pain with radiation into the neck.
- **Biliary pain** (biliary tree and gall bladder) is felt in the epigastrium and sometimes the right upper quadrant. It is colicky in nature. Ask about features of cholestasis (pale stools, dark urine,

Medicine at a Glance, Fifth Edition. Edited by Patrick Davey and Alex Pitcher.

Companion website: www.wiley.com/go/medicine5e

jaundice). Pain from the liver itself is unusual, although it may occur in hepatitis, hepatic metastases or right heart failure as a persistent right upper quadrant discomfort from hepatic capsular distension.

- **Pancreatic pain** is usually epigastric and typically radiates through to the back. Common precipitants include fatty foods and alcohol.
- **Foregut (gastroduodenal) pain** tends to be acidic (dyspeptic) and situated in the epigastrium. This will be influenced by eating – acid/dyspeptic symptoms may be relieved whilst obstructive/irritative symptoms may be exacerbated.
- **Midgut (small intestinal) pain** is usually colicky and situated periumbilically. It is often associated with bloating, nausea and vomiting.
- **Hindgut (colonic) pain** is usually colicky and experienced below the umbilicus. Other features may include a change in bowel habit and rectal bleeding. Remember that carcinoma of the caecum is more likely to lead to subacute *small* bowel obstruction than colonic dysfunction.
- **Peritonitic pain** is more localized because the parietal peritoneum has a rich sensory innervation. The classic example of this is evolving appendicitis. Initially, the pain is periumbilical and colicky, relating to an inflamed midgut viscus. As inflammation progresses, there is local peritonism with persistent pain and tenderness in the right iliac fossa. This may progress to perforation and generalized peritonitis with severe global abdominal pain if left untreated.
- **Loin pain** tends *not* to be related to gastrointestinal (GI) tract pathology but is more likely to arise from the kidneys and ureters or to be mechanical and related to the lumbar spine.

Other features of the history

It is useful to determine whether the current pain represents an acute problem or a manifestation of a chronic underlying condition (possibly subclinical until then). Previous GI problems or operations suggest an exacerbation of an old problem. Anorexia and weight loss suggest serious pathology.

Examination

General

Look at general appearance, including jaundice. Assess the circulatory state. Look for markers of chronic disease.

Abdominal

- Areas of tenderness: ask the patient to point to where the pain is maximal. Look for peritonism: guarding and more importantly rebound tenderness.
- Masses, including organomegaly.

Investigations

- **Blood tests**: full blood count (FBC), C-reactive protein, renal function tests; liver biochemistry, calcium; amylase and/or lipase.
- **Abdominal X-ray**: may show intestinal obstruction, vascular calcification (raising the possibility of ischaemia), loss of psoas outline (implying retroperitoneal pathology), and areas of absent gas pattern (bowel loops displaced by a mass). Look for features of a pneumoperitoneum (e.g. Wriggler's sign).
- **Erect chest X-ray**: look for the presence of air under the diaphragm.
- **Abdominal ultrasonography**: excellent for the biliary and renal tracts. Less good for imaging the pancreas and retroperitoneal structures and less sensitive in obese individuals.
- **Abdominal computed tomography** (CT) with intravenous and with or without oral contrast is the investigation of choice for otherwise unexplained abdominal pain that is of concern.
- **Endoscopy**: allows assessment for ulceration and inflammation that may cause abdominal pain.

Management

General measures

- Rest the gut: parenteral rehydration.
- Analgesia: gut-related pain is relatively resistant to simple analgesics. Opioids are effective but are limited by side-effects (nausea, constipation, etc.). Antispasmodics (mebeverine, buscopan) might be more effective.
- Treat the underlying cause.

No cause identified

If no cause for persistent pain is identified, a diagnostic laparoscopy/laparotomy is occasionally required. Consider several diagnoses.

- Functional GI disorders.
- Munchausen syndrome: have a very high index of suspicion when patients not resident to the locality present with severe abdominal pain without convincing clinical or investigative abnormalities.
- There may be stigmata of multiple previous operations. Very rarely, myocardial ischaemia presents as upper abdominal pain.
- Rare diseases such as porphyria and familial Mediterranean fever.

Dyspepsia

Dyspepsia refers to symptoms originating from the upper GI tract. These may relate to eating or drinking and include 'heartburn' and 'indigestion' (pain, usually 'acidic', in the upper abdomen/lower chest, as well as 'bloating', anorexia and vomiting). The most common underlying mechanism is gastro-oesophageal reflux. The figure shows the differential diagnosis of dyspepsia.

History and examination

Symptoms have often been present for some years. Lifestyle factors (smoking, alcohol, weight, 'stress') are relevant for reflux. Although many patients fear that cancer might account for their long-standing symptoms, this is a rare cause of dyspepsia. However, dysphagia and/or weight loss require urgent investigation. Physical examination is usually unrewarding, but may suggest neoplasia (weight loss, lymph nodes, abdominal masses). Abdominal obesity predisposes to reflux.

Investigations

Investigations should exclude serious pathology, principally gastric cancer, as well as establish the diagnosis. In many, the cancer risk is low and empirical treatment without endoscopy may be adequate.

- **Blood tests**: a normal FBC and ESR help to exclude serious pathology. Positive *Helicobacter pylori* serology might suggest peptic ulcer disease but does not exclude an upper GI malignancy.
- **Endoscopy**: the definitive test for most serious upper GI pathologies (oesophagitis, Barrett epithelium, peptic ulcer disease). Antral biopsy and urease test for *H. pylori* (CLO test) – see Chapter 124.
- **Barium swallow/meal**: now largely surpassed by endoscopy.

Management

- Treat the underlying cause (see Chapters 123 and 124).
- Treat the symptoms (see Chapters 123 and 124).

31 Jaundice

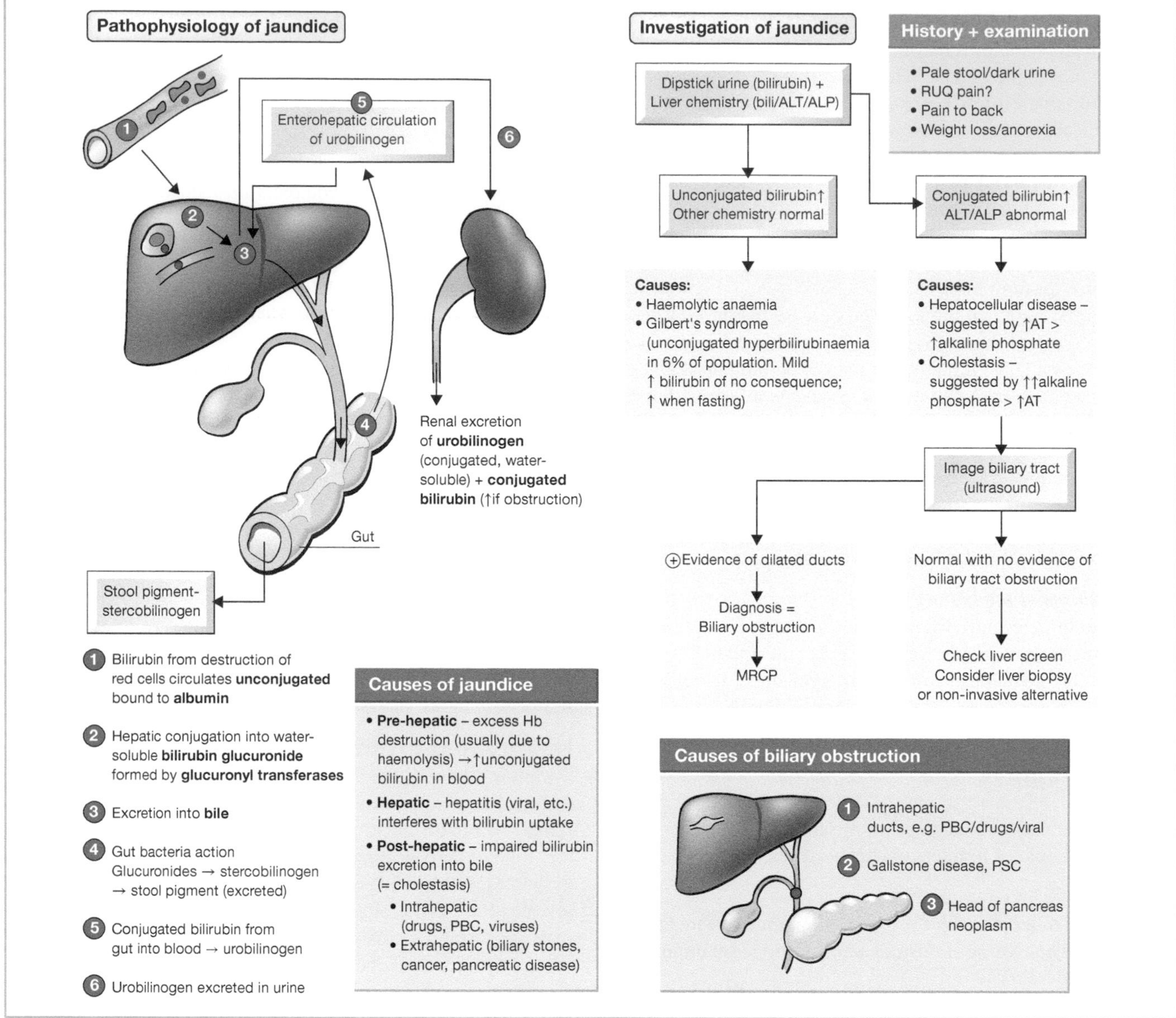

Pathophysiology of jaundice
Enterohepatic circulation of urobilinogen
Renal excretion of **urobilinogen** (conjugated, water-soluble) + **conjugated bilirubin** (↑if obstruction)
Gut
Stool pigment-stercobilinogen
1 Bilirubin from destruction of red cells circulates **unconjugated** bound to **albumin**
2 Hepatic conjugation into water-soluble **bilirubin glucuronide** formed by **glucuronyl transferases**
3 Excretion into **bile**
4 Gut bacteria action Glucuronides → stercobilinogen → stool pigment (excreted)
5 Conjugated bilirubin from gut into blood → urobilinogen
6 Urobilinogen excreted in urine
Causes of jaundice
• **Pre-hepatic** – excess Hb destruction (usually due to haemolysis) →↑unconjugated bilirubin in blood
• **Hepatic** – hepatitis (viral, etc.) interferes with bilirubin uptake
• **Post-hepatic** – impaired bilirubin excretion into bile (= cholestasis)
• Intrahepatic (drugs, PBC, viruses)
• Extrahepatic (biliary stones, cancer, pancreatic disease)
Investigation of jaundice
History + examination
• Pale stool/dark urine
• RUQ pain?
• Pain to back
• Weight loss/anorexia
Dipstick urine (bilirubin) + Liver chemistry (bili/ALT/ALP)
Unconjugated bilirubin↑ Other chemistry normal
Conjugated bilirubin↑ ALT/ALP abnormal
Causes:
• Haemolytic anaemia
• Gilbert's syndrome (unconjugated hyperbilirubinaemia in 6% of population. Mild ↑ bilirubin of no consequence; ↑ when fasting)
Causes:
• Hepatocellular disease – suggested by ↑AT > ↑alkaline phosphate
• Cholestasis – suggested by ↑↑alkaline phosphate > ↑AT
Image biliary tract (ultrasound)
⊕Evidence of dilated ducts
Diagnosis = Biliary obstruction
MRCP
Normal with no evidence of biliary tract obstruction
Check liver screen
Consider liver biopsy or non-invasive alternative
Causes of biliary obstruction
1 Intrahepatic ducts, e.g. PBC/drugs/viral
2 Gallstone disease, PSC
3 Head of pancreas neoplasm

Introduction

Jaundice can result from a range of underlying pathologies varying from an acute short-lived illness (e.g. hepatitis A) to the terminal stages of a chronic disease, which might have been subclinical until that point (e.g. decompensated chronic liver disease).

Aetiology

Although jaundice has been traditionally described as 'prehepatic', 'hepatic' or 'posthepatic', in practice it is often sufficient to restrict one's considerations to whether jaundice is hepatocellular (i.e. hepatic) or obstructive/cholestatic (i.e. posthepatic) (Table 31.1).

Differential diagnosis

A useful way of considering the differential diagnosis is to clinically distinguish the **acute** from the **chronic** conditions and, where possible, to clarify whether the liver injury is **hepatocellular** or **obstructive**.

Clinical features and history

The two important clinical features to identify are as follows.

- Is this patient's presentation of an acute illness or a chronic disease (Table 31.2)?
- Is there any clinical evidence of a failing liver?

Medicine at a Glance, Fifth Edition. Edited by Patrick Davey and Alex Pitcher.

Companion website: www.wiley.com/go/medicine5e

Table 31.1 Aetiology of jaundice

	Acute	Chronic
Hepatocellular	Acute hepatitis: viral hepatitis, drug reactions, Budd–Chiari syndrome	Chronic liver disease: hepatitis B and C, alcohol related, autoimmune hepatitis, haemochromatosis
Cholestatic	Biliary obstruction: 2° biliary disease	Chronic biliary disease: Primary biliary cholangitis
	Pancreatitis	Primary sclerosing cirrhosis
	Pancreatobiliary carcinoma	
	Metastasis	

Table 31.2 Differences between acute and chronic disease underlying jaundice

	Acute	Chronic
Preceding ill health	0	0 to ++
Skin signs of chronic liver disease	0	0 to ++
Encephalopathy	0 to +	+ to +++
Ascites	0 to +	++
Varices at endoscopy	0	++
Splenomegaly at ultrasound	0	++
Laboratory tests:		
Mean corpuscular volume	→	↑
Urea	→	↓
Albumin	→ or ↓	↓ to ↓↓
Prothrombin time	→ or ↑	↑ to ↑↑

These questions can often be answered from a careful history/

- What is the duration of the illness and was the patient unwell before the jaundice developed? This is often very revealing and may suggest a long period of subclinical ill health before the jaundice.
- Are there clinical features of cholestasis? Pale stools, dark urine and pruritus?
- Has the patient experienced any pain? Pain and cholestasis should be considered to be related to gallstones until proved otherwise. The presence of fever and rigors strongly suggests cholangitis (biliary tract infection) as the diagnosis.
- Are there risk factors for chronic liver disease? Alcohol – seek corroborative evidence. Travel/contacts – any favoured sexual practices? Intravenous drug use – ask specifically.
- Are there any features of liver failure? Hepatic encephalopathy (this may be overt or more subtle with reversal of sleep pattern, reduced attention span, daytime somnolence, constructional dyspraxia)?

Examination

The depth of the jaundice does not actually matter as much as recognizing features of a failing liver and determining whether there is chronic liver disease.

Recognition of liver failure

Encephalopathy is the clinical hallmark of liver failure. Any degree of confusion/delirium in a jaundiced patient should be considered a manifestation of encephalopathy. The specific clinical sign to seek is the metabolic flap (or asterixis). Other bedside measures of encephalopathy include a constructional dyspraxia (e.g. drawing a five-pointed star) or the trail test (i.e. a join-the-dots test against the clock).

Features of chronic liver disease

Typically, features of chronic liver disease are considered to be the peripheral stigmata such as palmar erythema, Dupuytren contracture, spider naevi and gynaecomastia. In practice, the clinical features of portal hypertension, such as ascites and splenomegaly, often represent 'harder' physical signs.

Investigations

- **Blood tests**: full blood count; a macrocytosis, thrombocytopenia or low urea may indicate chronic liver disease. Hyponatraemia (not caused by diuretics) is a poor prognostic sign.
- **Liver blood tests**: a low albumin may be non-specific. The transaminases give a clue as to whether the jaundice is predominantly hepatocellular (aspartate transaminase [AST] or alanine transaminase [ALT] > alkaline phosphatase) or cholestatic (alkaline phosphatase or γ-glutamyl transferase [γ-GT] > AST), although the picture is often 'mixed'. Normal transaminase activities suggest the less common conditions of haemolysis or the very common Gilbert syndrome (affecting up to 5% of some populations).
- **Viral hepatitis serology**: hepatitis A IgM is diagnostic of acute hepatitis A. Acute hepatitis B is typified by HBsAg (hepatitis B surface antigen) and detection of hepatitis B DNA. Hepatitis C rarely causes an acute hepatitis but is an increasing cause of chronic liver disease. It is important to consider hepatitis e virus IgM (and IgG) – hepatitis E is now the most common cause of infectious jaundice in parts of Europe. In acute hepatitis, consider CMV and EBV.
- **Autoantibody profile and immunoglobulin** (Ig): antinuclear, antimitochondrial, anti-smooth muscle, anti-liver–kidney microsomal antibodies and serum IgG, IgA and IgM.
- **Liver ultrasonography**: this may help in consolidating a clinical diagnosis. It may show focal liver abnormalities such as metastatic deposits, liver abscesses or vascular abnormalities. It might show evidence of biliary obstruction (i.e. dilated bile ducts) and possibly the underlying cause (e.g. gallstones, pancreatic cancer).
- In chronic liver disease, consider iron overload (ferritin), α1-antitrypsin deficiency (blood α1-antitrypsin quantification), and Wilson disease (copper studies).
- **Magnetic resonance cholangiopancreatography** (MRCP) and **endoscopic ultrasound** (EUS): increasingly, such non-invasive methods are used to delineate biliary anatomy as a prelude to endoscopic intervention.
- **Endoscopic retrograde cholangiopancreatography** (ERCP): if there is good evidence of biliary obstruction, ERCP remains the definitive test in determining whether the obstruction is intraluminal (i.e. gallstones in the common bile duct) or extraluminal (e.g. malignant stricture from carcinoma of the pancreas). It may also allow relief of the obstruction.
- **Liver biopsy**: liver histology remains the definitive investigation for hepatocellular jaundice and also, in some cases, cholestatic jaundice (e.g. primary biliary cirrhosis [PBC], drug-induced intrahepatic cholestasis). The absolute indications vary.

Management

The management of patients with jaundice depends on the underlying cause and whether there are clinical features of liver failure. Jaundice itself does not necessarily require hospital admission – many of the underlying conditions and associated complications do.

32 Abdominal mass

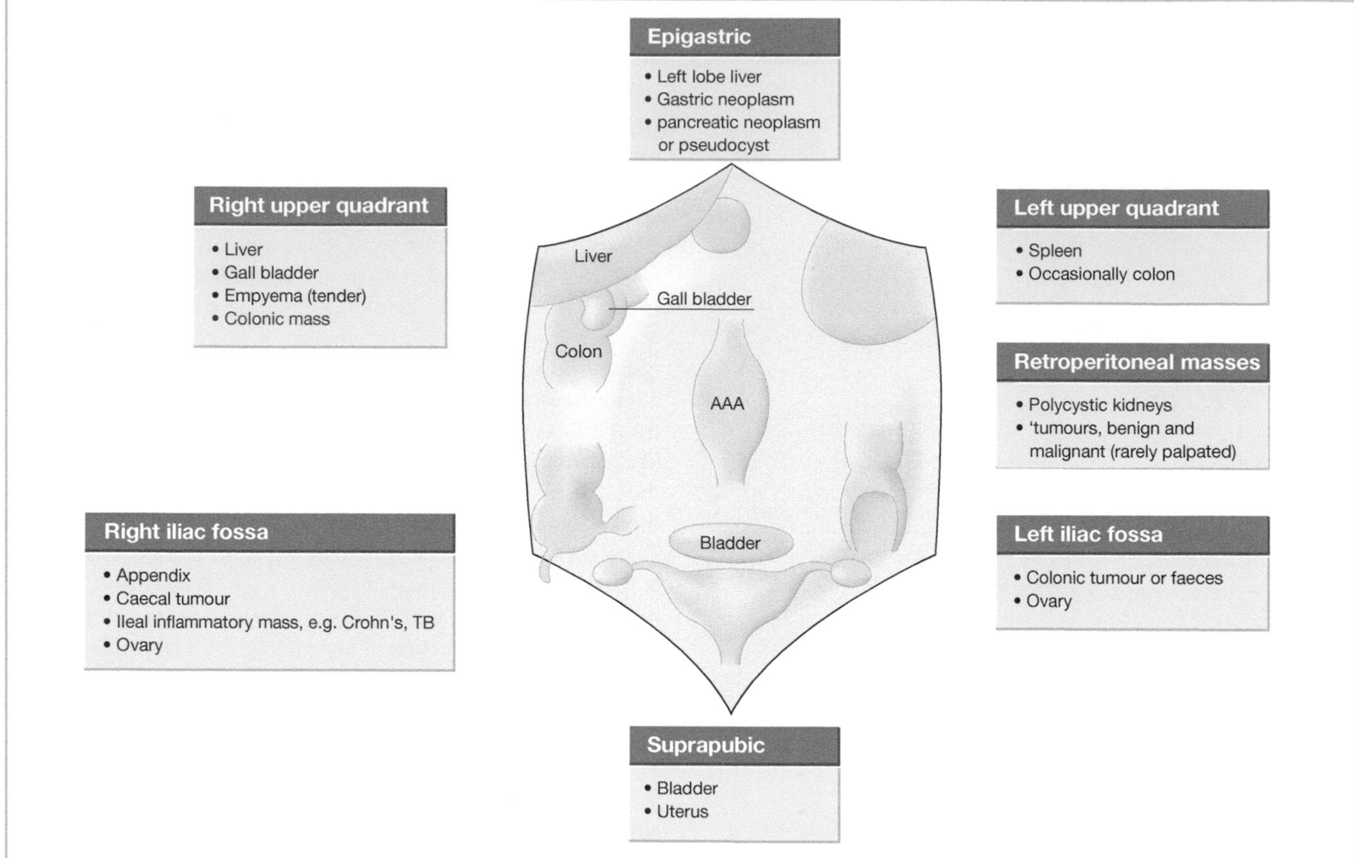

Epigastric
• Left lobe liver
• Gastric neoplasm
• pancreatic neoplasm or pseudocyst
Right upper quadrant
• Liver
• Gall bladder
• Empyema (tender)
• Colonic mass
Left upper quadrant
• Spleen
• Occasionally colon
Retroperitoneal masses
• Polycystic kidneys
• 'tumours, benign and malignant (rarely palpated)
Right iliac fossa
• Appendix
• Caecal tumour
• Ileal inflammatory mass, e.g. Crohn's, TB
• Ovary
Left iliac fossa
• Colonic tumour or faeces
• Ovary
Suprapubic
• Bladder
• Uterus
Liver
Gall bladder
Colon
AAA
Bladder

It is uncommon for patients to present solely with a palpable abdominal mass. Usually there are other clinical features such as weight loss or pain, or a change in bowel habit.

Clues as to the nature of the mass may be derived from movement with respiration (liver, gall bladder, spleen) or percussion note (ascites or gaseous distension).

Differential diagnosis

The differential diagnosis depends largely on the position of the mass (see the figure).

Investigations

- **Blood tests**: full blood count, erythrocyte sedimentation rate – anaemia, thrombocytosis and raised inflammatory markers suggest an underlying chronic disease process. Biochemistry – abnormal liver blood tests likewise suggest malignancy. The role of tumour markers (e.g. carcinoembryonic antigen, CA19–9, α-fetoprotein) in the diagnosis of malignancy is limited. CA-125 is, however, included in UK guidelines for women with abdominal bloating; many centres use α-fetoprotein surveillance in patients with cirrhosis. Their value is greater in monitoring response to treatment and identification of disease relapse.
- **Urinalysis/pregnancy test**.
- **Ultrasonography**: this is very useful as a first-line investigation but has now been largely superseded by abdominal computed tomography (CT). The utility of ultrasound is reduced in the obese.
- **CT scan**: very useful for characterization of retroperitoneal masses and probably more sensitive in identifying intra-abdominal lymphadenopathy. As CT relies on defining tissue planes (i.e. solid tissue against fat), it is less sensitive in very thin individuals. Intravenous with or without oral contrast increases diagnostic yield.
- **Biopsy/aspiration**: if there is doubt about the nature of an intra-abdominal mass, it is usually possible to aspirate cells for cytology or take a percutaneous biopsy under ultrasonic or CT guidance.
- **Laparoscopy/laparotomy**: if the nature of a mass remains obscure, the definitive approach is ultimately a laparotomy and excision. Such interventions are unlikely to be undertaken without shared care with surgeons, radiologists and pathologists through a multidisciplinary team (MDT).

Medicine at a Glance, Fifth Edition. Edited by Patrick Davey and Alex Pitcher.

Companion website: www.wiley.com/go/medicine5e

33 Ascites

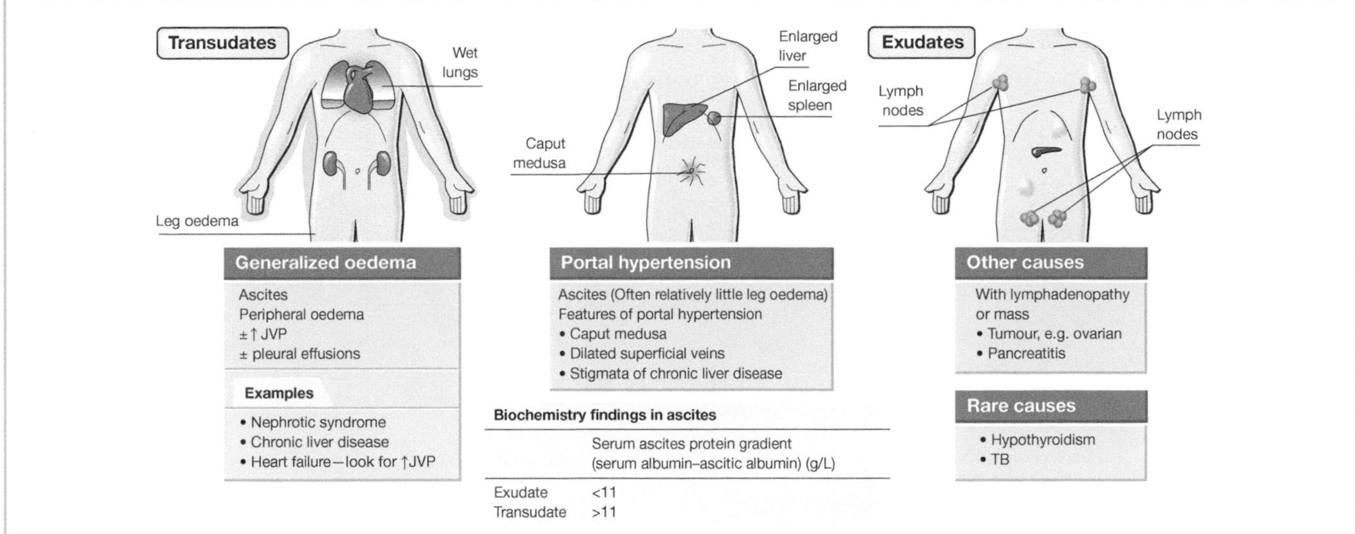

Biochemistry findings in ascites

	Serum ascites protein gradient (serum albumin–ascitic albumin) (g/L)
Exudate	<11
Transudate	>11

The pathological accumulation of fluid within the abdominal peritoneal cavity. It frequently reflects the presentation of a chronic disease process that may have been subclinical until that point.

As with other fluid collections, ascites is clinically classified as being either an exudate or a transudate, primarily according to the difference between the serum and ascites albumin (serum-ascites albumin gradient; SAAG).

- **Exudative ascites** has a low SAAG content and occurs with inflammatory (e.g. infective, pancreatitis) or malignant processes.
- **Transudative ascites** has a high SAAG and occurs in cirrhosis as a result of portal hypertension and alterations in renal sodium clearance.

The differential diagnosis usually lies between decompensated chronic liver disease and intra-abdominal malignancy. Other conditions with ascites are heart failure, constrictive pericarditis, nephrotic syndrome, pancreatitis and tuberculosis (TB).

Clinical features and investigations

There are few features in the history and examination that confidently distinguish between the late presentation of liver disease and malignancy. Notwithstanding this, any historical factor pointing to a liver disease is important. Gross ascites may be evident on inspection with pronounced distension of the abdomen, often with eversion of the umbilicus. Lesser degrees of ascites can be demonstrated clinically by eliciting 'shifting dullness'. Helpful investigations include the following.

- **Examination of the ascitic fluid**: for albumin and protein, cell count, bacterial culture and cytology for malignant cells. Ascites may be straw-coloured in cirrhosis, bloody in malignancy and cloudy in infection. A leucocyte count of more than >250 polymorphs/ml in transudative ascites is considered diagnostic of bacterial peritonitis regardless of whether or not organisms are cultured. Cytology (large volume and fresh specimen) may be diagnostic of malignancy. Pancreatic disease may present with ascites, and if suspected, ascitic amylase should be measured.
- **Ultrasonography of the abdomen**: to confirm ascites, to measure liver size (small in cirrhosis), signs of portal hypertension (splenomegaly) and patency of the portal and hepatic veins (to exclude hepatic vein thrombosis and Budd–Chiari syndrome), for finding focal abnormalities (e.g. disseminated malignancy) and for the diagnosis of intra-abdominal tumours (e.g. ovarian). **Abdominal CT** may reveal a primary malignant process.
- **Other blood tests**: biochemistry and liver blood tests looking for markers of liver cirrhosis (low albumin, hyperbilirubinaemia, elevated liver enzymes, low platelets, etc.). Tumour markers if malignancy is suspected (especially α-fetoprotein for hepatocellular carcinoma, CA125 for ovarian carcinoma).

Management

Exudative ascites

Treat the underlying cause. **Malignant ascites**: treat underlying malignancy (commonly ovarian). Therapeutic paracentesis is often needed for symptomatic relief.

Transudative ascites

Treat the underlying cause, and consider the following factors.

- Fluid and salt restriction: fluid restriction to ≤1–1.5 l/day and a 'no added salt' diet may be sufficient.
- Diuretics: usually aldosterone antagonist (e.g. spironolactone) ± loop diuretic (furosemide/frusemide).
- Therapeutic paracentesis for resistant ascites (not responding to diuretic therapy) or refractory (with unacceptable drug side-effects – hyponatraemia, encephalopathy, etc.).
- Very low protein ascites in cirrhosis is an indication for prophylactic antibiotics to reduce subsequent spontaneous bacterial peritonitis; similarly, prophylactic antibiotics are indicated after an episode of spontaneous bacterial peritonitis.
- In selected cases, an indwelling ascitic drain, transjugular intrahepatic portosystemic shunt (TIPS) or liver transplantation may be indicated.

Medicine at a Glance, Fifth Edition. Edited by Patrick Davey and Alex Pitcher.

Companion website: www.wiley.com/go/medicine5e

34 Polyuria and oliguria

Urinary retention

Urinary tract infection

Drugs

Spinal cord damage
- Trauma
- Tumour
- Multiple sclerosis

Pelvic tumour/mass
- Pregnancy
- Fibroids
- Tumour

Prostatic hypertrophy

Prostatic cancer

Urethral stricture

Oliguria

↑ ADH release
- Postoperatively
- Due to pain and nausea

Intravascular volume depletion
- Diarrhoea, vomiting
- Fever (sweating)
- Haemorrhage
- Inadequate fluid replacement

Inadequate cardiac output
- Heart failure
- PE
- Cardiac tamponade

Urinary retention

Acute renal failure:
- Drugs
- ATN from prolonged hypotension
- Other causes see Chapter 150

Sepsis

Signs of dehydration

Early
- Postural hypotension

Later
- ↑Heart rate
- ↓BP

Advanced
- Peripheral cyanosis
- Poor capillary return

Polyuria

Cranial diabetes insipidus
↓↓ ADH release due to:
- Head injury
- Tumours

Excess oral intake (psychogenic polydipsia)

Excess IV fluids

Osmotic diuresis —uncontrolled diabetes mellitus

Renal causes:
- Renal failure—especially tubular disease → lack of concentrating ability
- Nephrogenic diabetes insipidus: Ca^{2+}, Li^{+} toxicity

Investigations (water deprivation test)

	Urine osmolality (mOsm/kg H_2O)	
	Following water deprivation	Following exogenous vasopressin
Normal	>750*	>750
Central diabetes insipidus	<300	>750
Nephrogenic diabetes insipidus	<300	300–500*
Primary polydipsia	>500*	>500

* little or no increase

Water deprivation test – only performed in hospital. Patients denied fluids until 3–5% body weight is lost

Polyuria

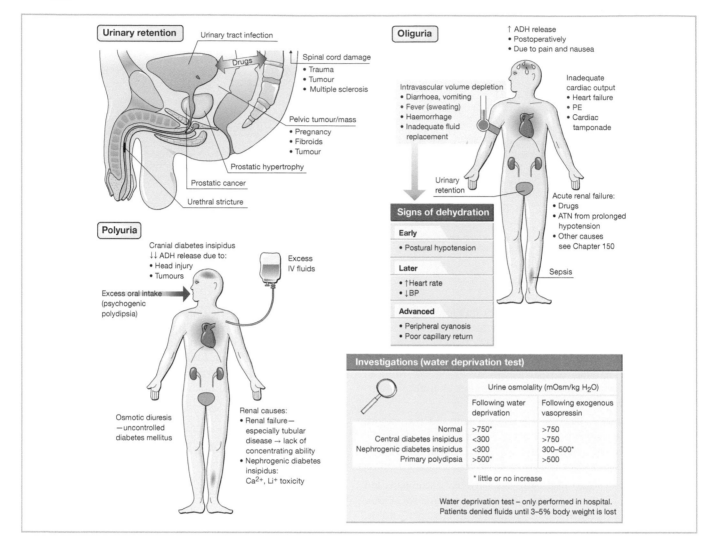

Polyuria is an excessive urine volume, usually ≥3 l/day, and may be accompanied by the symptoms of frequency, nocturia, thirst and polydipsia. A presentation with polyuria requires careful investigation as it may be caused by serious underlying disease.

Many conditions can produce polyuria, of which the most common is **diabetes mellitus**, in which increased concentrations of glucose have an osmotic diuretic effect. The causes may be grouped as follows.

1 Excess intake of fluid (primary polydipsia), often associated with psychological disturbance leading to compulsive water drinking. Very rarely, hypothalamic lesions lead to primary polydipsia.
2 An increase in tubular solute load, as with urea in chronic renal failure or glucose from hyperglycaemia caused by diabetes mellitus.
3 Disordered medullary concentration gradient as a consequence of medullary disease (see Chapter 149) or in hypercalcaemia.
4 A reduction in antidiuretic hormone (ADH or vasopressin) production (diabetes insipidus), after trauma to the head, or tumours or infections of the hypothalamus or pituitary (cranial diabetes insipidus).
5 Conditions in which the tubular response to ADH is impaired. These conditions are termed 'nephrogenic diabetes insipidus' and include hypercalcaemia, chronic potassium depletion, lithium toxicity and a rare inherited insensitivity to ADH with X-linked recessive inheritance (due to mutations in the ADH receptor, V2) or autosomal inheritance with mutations affecting the aquaporin-2 water channel.
6 After relief of urinary tract obstruction, such as insertion of a catheter to relieve bladder outlet obstruction by a hypertrophied prostate.

In a patient with polyuria, the history may provide the diagnosis. If blood glucose is normal, creatinine, calcium and potassium should be determined. If diabetes insipidus is suspected, then a

Medicine at a Glance, Fifth Edition. Edited by Patrick Davey and Alex Pitcher.

Companion website: www.wiley.com/go/medicine5e

water deprivation test should be undertaken with caution; the patient must not become excessively dehydrated. A water deprivation test involves the restriction of water intake until a 3–5% weight loss has been achieved. Measurements of urinary osmolality and change in urinary osmolality in response to exogenous vasopressin will help establish the diagnosis.

It is important to correct any major water deficit and then to treat the underlying cause. Cranial diabetes insipidus can be treated by the intranasal administration of the vasopressin analogue desmopressin.

Oliguria in the hospital setting

Oliguria is defined as a urine output of less than 0.5^ml/kg weight/h. Many patients in hospital develop a reduced urinary output, particularly postoperative or in severely ill individuals. It often forms part of the triggers for observation charts for the early detection of patient deterioration. Urine output is a sensitive indicator of fluid status and haemodynamic adequacy. It is particularly important because oliguria may progress to acute kidney injury (AKI). Pain and nausea are very potent stimuli of ADH secretion. In managing the oliguric patient, information can be acquired from the history, examination and investigations. The central issues are whether or not the patient is replete with fluid and excluding urinary retention.

An accurate **history** of fluid intake and output should be obtained. Fluid balance and daily weight charts should be examined; loss of fluid from haemorrhage, diarrhoea, sweating, vomiting, drains and insensible losses all need to be considered. The presence of nausea, pain and thirst should be elicited. Symptoms suggesting urinary retention should be elicited and a urinary catheter passed if there is any doubt.

Examination should include palpation and percussion for a bladder. Signs suggesting fluid depletion or overload should be sought. The signs of fluid depletion include tachycardia, hypotension and, most importantly, postural hypotension, while other signs can include dry mucous membranes, reduced skin turgor, cool peripheries and contracted peripheral veins. Signs of fluid overload can include orthopnoea, tachypnoea, peripheral oedema, pulmonary oedema, elevated jugular venous pressure (JVP) and hypertension. A central venous line provides a direct measurement of central venous pressure (CVP) if the fluid status is uncertain.

Investigations and management

Fluid depletion can be accompanied by elevations in haematocrit, serum albumin and creatinine (with urea often disproportionately raised), whereas in fluid overload a chest X-ray may reveal pulmonary oedema. In the oliguric patient, a urinary catheter should be passed or, if present, flushed to exclude blockage. If the situation suggests fluid depletion then intravenous (IV) fluid (often normal saline) should be given. Replacement fluid should be administered until postural hypotension has been abolished and the JVP or CVP is normal. If there is evidence of haemorrhage, then a blood transfusion may be necessary; the source of blood loss should be identified and treated, and clotting times determined. If the patient appears replete with fluid then other causes of shock need to be considered, such as sepsis, myocardial infarction and pulmonary embolism (PE), and other causes of acute renal failure considered (Table 34.1). An urgent renal tract ultrasound should be requested, to look for signs of renal tract obstruction (e.g. hydronephrosis), and also to check kidney size (small in long-standing disease).

It is particularly important to avoid agents that may jeopardize renal perfusion (e.g. NSAIDs, ACE inhibitors), which could be nephrotoxic (e.g. gentamicin) or accumulate in renal failure (e.g. digoxin).

Urinary retention

Acute urinary retention is a sudden inability to pass urine, usually accompanied by pain, the sensation of bladder fullness and a distended bladder. **Chronic urinary retention** is the presence of an enlarged bladder often without difficulty in micturition, and accompanied by frequency, overflow incontinence, bladder distension and sometimes renal failure. Causes can be grouped into those affecting the lumen of the urethra or the urethral wall, compression of the urethra or neurological dysfunction. Urinary tract infection or pain may precipitate retention. Urinary retention is common in elderly men due to benign prostatic hyperplasia or, more rarely, prostate carcinoma; in young adults, serious neurological causes may be responsible and require careful investigation. Rectal examination is crucial to assess both the prostate and anal tone and sensation. In women, urinary obstruction is more likely to be neurological or gynaecological in origin than urological. Once retention is relieved, anticipate the possibility of postobstructive diuresis.

Table 34.1 Typical urine findings in conditions that cause acute renal failure

Condition	Dipstick test	Sediment analysis	Urine osmolality (mOsm/kg)	Fractional excretion of sodium[a] (%)
Prerenal failure	Trace or no proteinuria	A few hyaline casts possible	>500	<1
Renal failure				
Tubular injury ischaemia	Mild-to-moderate proteinuria	Pigmented granular casts	<350	>1
Nephrotoxins	Mild-to-moderate proteinuria	Pigmented granular casts	<350	>1
Acute interstitial nephritis	Mild-to-moderate proteinuria; haemoglobin; leucocytes	White cells and white cell casts; eosinophils and eosinophil casts; red cells	<350	>1
Acute glomerulonephritis	Moderate-to-severe proteinuria; haemoglobin	Red cells and red cell casts; red cells can be dysmorphic	>500	<1
Postrenal failure	Trace or no proteinuria; can have haemoglobin, leucocytes	Crystals, red cells and white cells possible	<350	>1

[a] Fractional excretion of sodium (FENa) = (UNa × PCr)/(PNa × UCr) × 100, where Cr is creatinine, Na is sodium, P is plasma and U is urine.
Data from Thadhani et al. 1996.

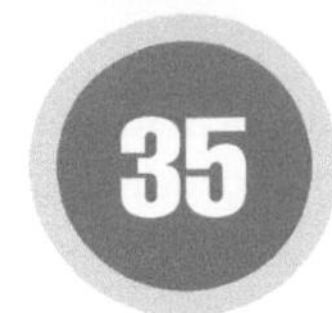

35 Dysuria, frequency and urgency

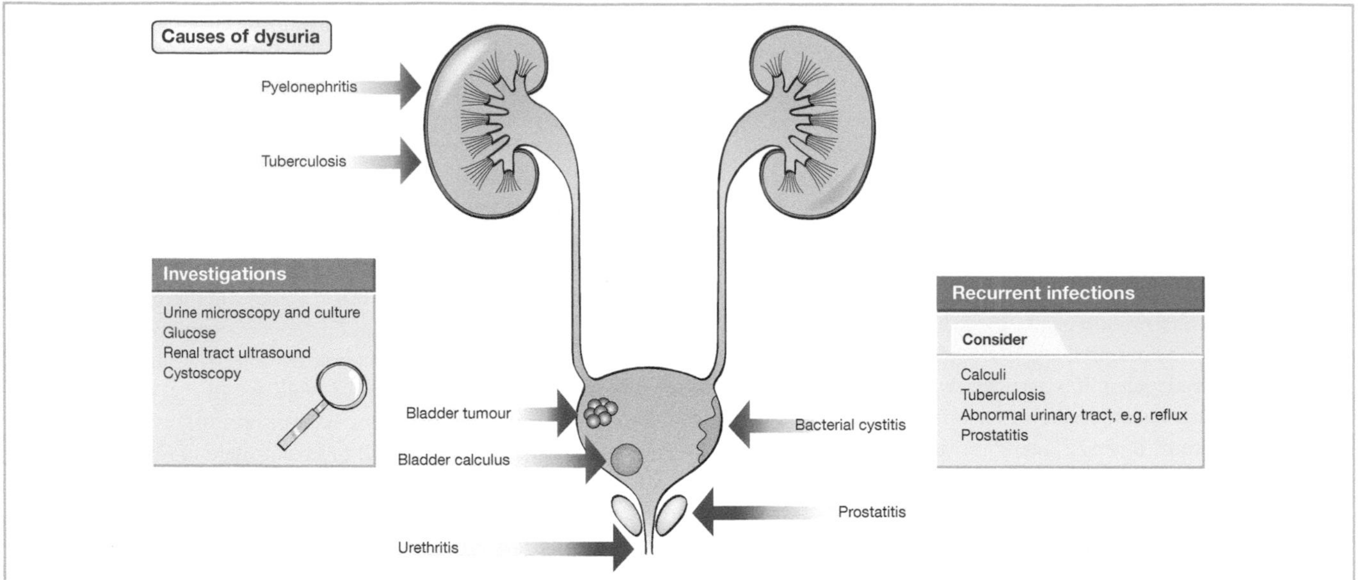

Dysuria is painful micturition. Urinary frequency is the increased frequency of the passage of urine. Urgency is an uncontrollable desire to micturate. In adults, the most common cause is urinary tract infection (UTI), a very common diagnosis in both general practice and hospital patients.

Urinary tract infection is commonly looked for in elderly patients (or children) who present with confusion or general deterioration but asymptomatic bacteriuria is common and may not be the underlying cause. It is particularly important in all UTIs to ensure that there is pyuria accompanying any bacterial growth from urine, because imperfectly sterile urine collections are common. Bacteriuria is likely to be of clinical significance only when accompanied by pyuria (i.e. >100 000 white cells/ml).

Acute pyelonephritis

Urinary tract infection involving the upper urinary tract has systemic features such as fever, which may be very high (>39 °C), rigors, malaise, anorexia and flank pain, in addition to the symptoms of dysuria, frequency and urgency. Predispositions include calculi, reflux, obstruction and a neurogenic bladder. Pyelonephritis in an obstructed kidney requires urgent medical attention because of the irreversible loss of renal function that may occur.

The key to diagnosis is the microscopy and culture of urine and blood cultures. There should be pyuria (i.e. >100 000 white cells/ml), bacteriuria and often microscopic or even macroscopic haematuria.

Acute cystitis

Urinary tract infection confined to the urinary tract is commonly called acute cystitis. It is more common in women and coliforms are the most common infecting organisms.

- *Escherichia coli* (90% of outpatients, 50% of inpatients).
- *Proteus* and *Klebsiella* species (5% of outpatients, 20% of inpatients).
- Enterococci (2% of outpatients, 7% of inpatients).
- *Pseudomonas* species (0.5% of outpatients, 6% of inpatients).

The symptoms may include dysuria, suprapubic discomfort, frequency, urgency, incontinence and microscopic haematuria. Diagnosis, as in pyelonephritis, requires the growth of a pathogenic organism from a midstream specimen of urine, in a quantity sufficient to cause disease, defined as ≥100 000 colony-forming units/ml.

Urethritis

This is a condition characterized by dysuria and meatal discharge, and is most commonly caused by sexually transmitted diseases such as gonococci or *Chlamydia* species.

Investigations

The microscopy and culture of urine are critical in the management of patients suspected of having a UTI. Urine dipsticks can suggest the possibility of bacterial infection if there are leucocytes present and/or nitrites. Other important investigations, particularly with recurrent infections, may include urine or blood glucose, ultrasonography of the renal tract, plain X-rays of the kidney, ureters and bladder, urography or cystoscopy. In recurrent infection, obstruction, prostatitis, renal calculi, diabetes mellitus and bladder dysfunction are potential causes.

Other causes of dysuria, other than acute bacterial infection, are bladder calculi, bladder tumours and tuberculosis (suggested by sterile pyuria in a patient at risk of tuberculosis).

Medicine at a Glance, Fifth Edition. Edited by Patrick Davey and Alex Pitcher.

Companion website: www.wiley.com/go/medicine5e

36 Haematuria

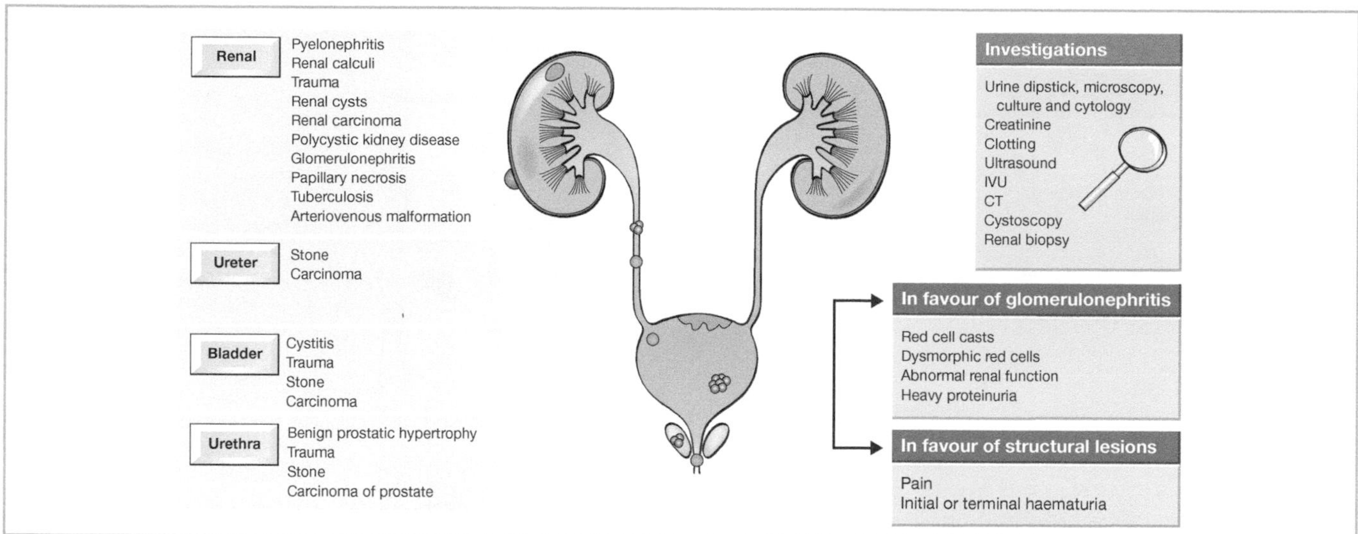

Blood can appear in the urine from pathology at any site in the urinary tract. Even small quantities of blood can produce a significantly pink or red coloration in the urine (although this should not be confused with ingested substances that discolour the urine, such as beetroot or rifampicin antibiotic). The small amount of blood found occasionally in urine from patients with glomerulonephritis can make it 'smoky' in appearance. Urinary dipsticks are very sensitive to even a very few red cells in the urine. False-positive dipstick tests for blood can be obtained with the presence of free haemoglobin or myoglobin in the urine and by contamination from menstruation. Haematuria can be confirmed by finding more than three red blood cells per high power field of spun urine.

Macroscopic (frank blood) haematuria definitely requires investigation because it may be the first presentation of a carcinoma of the renal tract or a serious renal disorder. The continuing presence of microscopic haematuria (present on dipstick and seen on microscopy) should prompt consideration of the presence of renal disease (is there proteinuria, abnormal creatinine, hypertension?) or a structural lesion of the renal tract but can be detected in a large proportion of asymptomatic normal individuals (from 1% of young adults to 10% in the elderly).

History and examination

The **history** should include the timing of haematuria in the urinary stream; blood on commencing urination suggests a urethral cause, whereas terminal haematuria suggests a bladder or prostatic cause. The presence of painful urination suggests a urinary tract infection or calculus. Episodes of trauma should be sought, as should systemic features that might indicate a disseminated malignancy or a vasculitis.

The **examination** must include palpation for abdominal masses, which might represent renal tumours or cysts, a rectal examination for prostatic malignancy and measurement of blood pressure.

Investigations

Once the presence of haematuria has been established, urinary microscopy may indicate whether the source is likely to be glomerular or from elsewhere in the urinary tract. Red blood cells of glomerular origin tend to be dysmorphic and may be accompanied by red cell casts and significant proteinuria. Glomerular disease can affect renal function (see Chapter 146) which should be assessed with plasma creatinine, and is often accompanied by proteinuria. Abnormal urine cytology can suggest the presence of a urinary tract malignancy. If a structural lesion of the renal tract is suspected, imaging can be undertaken with plain radiography looking for radio-opaque calculi (although only a small minority of stones are visible on plain X-ray); ultrasonography looking for renal masses or bladder lesions; intravenous or CT urography (IVU), particularly looking for filling defects within the urinary tract; and cross-sectional imaging with computed tomography (CT) or magnetic resonance imaging (MRI). (Remember to be cautious with iodinated contrast media in patients with renal impairment because of the increased risk of contrast nephropathy and the rare skin disorder nephrogenic systemic fibrosis that can be associated with gadolinium.)

If these investigations fail to demonstrate a cause for the haematuria, a cystoscopy should be performed. If a renal source of the haematuria is suspected (usually because there is proteinuria or biochemical evidence of renal impairment), a renal biopsy may be undertaken which could reveal a glomerulonephritis. The most common renal cause of microscopic or macroscopic haematuria is IgA nephropathy. In this condition, the haematuria commonly follows a sore throat. Macroscopic haematuria can be seen in other glomerulonephritides occurring in Goodpasture syndrome and ANCA-associated vasculitis. Bleeding disorders are a very unusual cause of haematuria but should be considered if the patient has other sites of abnormal blood loss.

Medicine at a Glance, Fifth Edition. Edited by Patrick Davey and Alex Pitcher.

Companion website: www.wiley.com/go/medicine5e

37 Sweating, flushing and thyroid swellings

Sweating

Causes

Common
- Anxiety
- Primary dermatological condition
- Self-limiting infections

Rare
- Endocrine disease
- Cardiac disease
- Chronic inflammatory/neoplastic conditions

Sweating

↓

Duration? → Long duration suggests a benign diagnosis

↓

Associated symptoms/signs? — Yes → **Clues to serious disease**
- Weight loss/gain
- Altered bowel habit
- Pain
- Syncope or near syncope
- Palpitations
  - Anxiety preceding palpitations = anxiety disorder
  - Palpitations preceding anxiety = tachyarrhythmia
- Fever

No ↓

Anxiety disorder
1° dermatological condition
– inflammatory
– excess sweat production

Flushing

Most cases relate to emotion or the menopause

Skin disease
- Acne
- Rosacea
- Photosensitive dermatosis

Drugs
- Alcohol
- Ca^{2+} channel blockers

Food
- Scombroid poisoning

Menopausal flushes
- Affects 80% of females
- Due to oestrogen decline, not absence
- Heat → (1 minute) warmth + sweat upper body ↑ skin temp (3°C) + ↓ core temp (0.3°C)

Rare causes
- Medullary thyroid cancer
- Systemic mastocytosis

Neuroendocrine tumours
Secrete biologically active substances → portal vein
Destroyed by 1st pass hepatic metabolism. Liver secondaries bypass this protection, producing the **carcinoid syndrome**
- Flushing: paroxysmal → fixed
- Watery diarrhoea + abdominal pain
- Right-sided heart valve lesions

Neuroendocrine tumours arise from **neuroendocrine cells** which:
- Mostly arise in small bowel
- 10% present as appendicitis

Thyroid swellings

Isolated nodule
- 'Colloid cyst'
- Functioning adenoma
- Cancer:
  pain
  rapid enlargement
  local lymphadenopathy

Multiple nodules throughout both lobes
- I_2 deficiency
- Autoimmune disease
- Multinodular goitre

Diffuse enlargement
- Graves' disease
  – overlying bruit
- Viral thyroiditis – tender

Investigations

- Thyroid function test (?hyper-/hypo-function)
- Fine needle aspiration cytology
- ^{131}I scan: if 'hot' (i.e. functioning) – very unlikely to be cancer
- Ultrasound (?microcalcification, hypoechoicity for malignancy)

Complications of a multinodular goitre

Compression of:
- Trachea
- Oesophagus
- Pemberton's sign (venous engorgement when both arms elevated due to SVC obstruction)

Recurrent laryngeal nerve palsy (rarely benign)

Retrosternal extension

Medicine at a Glance, Fifth Edition. Edited by Patrick Davey and Alex Pitcher.

Companion website: www.wiley.com/go/medicine5e

Sweating

Sweating is a very common problem, but is very rarely serious. The crucial diagnostic features are how long the problem has been present (the longer it has been there, the more benign the underlying process); the presence of any associated symptoms (isolated sweating is rarely serious, and usually indicates a dermatological hypersecretory response rather than any underlying disease process); and whether there is anxiety during the episode (anxiety normally indicates a panic disorder; very rarely, it indicates an underlying phaeochromocytoma).

Differential diagnosis

The most common causes are an anxiety state or a primary dermatological condition. Rarely, other disease processes are responsible.

- **Endocrine disease**: thyrotoxicosis, acromegaly, phaeochromocytoma, hypoglycaemia (sweating several hours after last eating, relieved by food), hypogonadism (particularly menopausal).
- **Cardiovascular disease**: paroxysmal tachyarrhythmias cause paroxysmal sweating, although it is very rare for palpitations not to be felt during the event. Very poor left ventricular function causes sweating on effort, as does marked physical deconditioning.
- **Pain**: if severe enough, pain induces sweating. Some individuals sweat with mild pain.
- **Inflammatory disease**: including cancer (lymphoma or other malignancies) and chronic infection, which may cause sweats, particularly at night (see Chapter 45).
- **Gustatory sweating**: due to autonomic dysfunction.

Investigations

The aim of any investigation is to exclude serious diagnoses.

- **Laboratory tests**: thyroid-stimulating hormone (TSH); inflammatory markers; insulin-like growth factor 1 and oral glucose tolerance test (for acromegaly); urinary metanephrines and plasma metanephrines (for phaeochromocytoma), fasting glucose and insulin (for hypoglycaemia), follicle-stimulating hormone (FSH)/oestradiol testosterone (for hypogonadism); blood film ± marrow, CRP and immunoglobulins.
- **Other tests**: very rarely, a 24-hour electrocardiogram (ECG) recording (for arrhythmias) may be indicated.

Management

Treatment is for the underlying cause. If no cause is found, cleanliness, antiperspirants and physical conditioning are recommended. Botulinum A injections may help. Occasionally, local excision of sweat glands is indicated.

Flushing

Flushing is very common. The usual causes are emotions in youth. Diseases that may have flushing as a prominent component include the following.

- **Primary dermatological disease**, especially photodermatosis (see Chapter 72), including autoimmune (systemic lupus erythematosus), metabolic (porphyria), plant-related (especially hogweed) and drug-induced (especially amiodarone); rosacea.
- **Drugs**: alcohol (especially in those deficient in alcohol dehydrogenase or on disulfiram – Antabuse®) and calcium channel blockers commonly cause flushing, as do spicy foods, food allergy and toxin ingestion.
- **Hypogonadism**: most commonly menopause-related (see Chapter 165).
- **Neuroendocrine tumours**: rare tumours, most commonly located in the small bowel and the lung. They may be associated with secretion of hormones and biochemically active substances (principally 5-hydroxytryptamine [5-HT or serotonin], but also bradykinin, histamine and other peptides) into the systemic circulation, causing paroxysmal flushing which later becomes fixed, with abdominal pain (cramps) and watery diarrhoea – the carcinoid syndrome. Right-sided valve lesions (tricuspid regurgitation or pulmonary stenosis) occur in 50%. The diagnosis is confirmed by finding hepatic metastasis on liver ultrasound examination and elevated chromogranin A associated with high levels of 5-HT metabolites, particularly 5-hydroxyindoleacetic acid (5-HIAA) in the urine. Management is surgical excision if possible. Octreotide and other long-acting somatostatin analogues that inhibit the release of many gut peptides are very useful in controlling symptoms. Hepatic embolization, α-interferon, chemotherapy and therapy with radiolabelled somatostatin analogues and radiolabelled peptides, e.g. Lu-DOTATATE, are also useful. The tumour is often remarkably slow growing and some patients live for many years.
- **Medullary thyroid carcinoma**: this rare tumour can present with a neck mass, as Cushing's syndrome or intractable diarrhoea. However, it can also produce a carcinoid-like syndrome. Of the tumours, 75% are sporadic in elderly individuals, but 25% relate to genetic cancer syndromes – familial medullary thyroid cancer or multiple endocrine neoplasia (MEN2).
- **Systemic mastocytosis**: overproliferation of mast cells. May be associated with myeloproliferative disorders or lymphomas. Intermittent release of histamine occurs, causing a syndrome much like scombroid poisoning (see below). Hepatosplenomegaly, portal hypertension and malabsorption also occur.
- **Scombroid poisoning**: histamine is produced by certain bacteria (e.g. *Proteus morgani*) acting to decompose the flesh of scombroid (e.g. tuna, mackerel) or non-scombroid (e.g. sardine, pilchard) fish. Symptoms occur four hours after ingestion: flushing, urticarial itching, conjunctival suffusion, abdominal colic; vomiting and diarrhoea may also occur. Treatment is supportive, antihistamines may help, and symptoms disappear after several hours.

Investigations

Investigation is indicated only if unusual features are present, suggestive of underlying disease. Laboratory tests include FSH testosterone/oestradiol, urinary 5-HIAA for carcinoid syndrome; and calcitonin, serum mast cell tryptase, bone marrow and urinary analysis for histamine excretion in suspected mastocytosis.

Management

Treatment is of the underlying cause.

Thyroid swellings

Thyroid nodules occur in 5% population, (F : M – 5 : 1) and may relate to a thyroid goitre (euthyroid or hypothyroid), benign adenoma (associated with hyperthyroidism) or malignancy (2% of goitres). Cancer is suggested by hard consistency associated with lymph node enlargement, known radiation exposure, a family history or voice change (resulting from recurrent laryngeal nerve palsy). Goitres and cancer can cause tracheal (stridor) or oesophageal (dysphagia) compression.

Investigations

Investigation of any thyroid swelling should include the following.

- Thyroid status (TSH).
- Fine needle aspiration cytology (FNAC) in outpatients is diagnostic in the majority of cases, and may exclude malignancy, diagnose malignancy or be suspicious of malignancy. Surgical excision is indicated in the latter two categories.
- Ultrasonography of the thyroid gland: hypoechoicity and microcalcification are suspicious if nodules are found; radionuclide scanning may be indicated – cancer appears as a 'cold' nodule. FNAC is indicated for cold nodules to determine whether cancer is present.
- Spirometry and ENT assessment if breathing problems/voice change.

Management

Cancer is treated with surgical excision, thyroxine (to suppress TSH, which otherwise promotes tumour growth) and radioactive iodine in hormonally active diseases. Drug treatment may be given (anaplastic or iodine resistant) with tyrosine kinase inhibitors.

Specific thyroid cancers

These account for <1% of all cancers, and affect women more than men, most commonly aged 40–50 years. Exposure to irradiation, particularly at a young age, leads to increased risk. There are five types.

1 **Papillary** is the most common thyroid cancer, accounting for >80%; it affects those aged 30–50 years, spreads via the lymphatics and usually has a good prognosis.
2 **Follicular** accounts for 10% of thyroid cancers, usually in those aged 40–50 years; it has a haematogenous spread and usually a good prognosis.

Differentiated thyroid cancer (papillary and follicular thyroid cancers) are treated according to risk (very low to high risk) with surgery (lobectomy/thyroidectomy), +/- postoperative thyroxine to suppress TSH ± radioiodine ablation of the thyroid remnant.

3 **Anaplastic** is an undifferentiated thyroid cancer accounting for <5%; it affects those aged 60–80 years and spreads haematogenously. It has a poor prognosis; the treatment is thyroidectomy ± chemotherapy (tyrosine kinase inhibitors) ± radiotherapy.
4 **Medullary** cancer (also, see above for flushing) arises from C cells of the thyroid, and accounts for 5–10% of all thyroid cancer. It is usually familial (MEN-2, RET proto-oncogene) and is treated by thyroidectomy with central compartment neck dissection, and tyrosine kinase inhibitors if progression/metastasis.
5 **Lymphoma** is a rare cancer, associated with Hashimoto thyroiditis, or systemic non-Hodgkin lymphoma, treated with radio- and chemotherapy.

38 Obesity

Obesity

Secondary Causes

Genetic polymorphisms
Accounts for 30–60% of variation in weight

Diseases < 1% of cases
- Cushing's
- Hypothyroidism
- Polycystic ovary syndrome
- Hypothalamic disease
- Genetic disorders, e.g. Prader–Willi syndrome

Environment
- Lack of exercise
- Easy access to food
- High alcohol intake
- Drugs (tricyclics, haloperidol, steroids)
- Poverty

Consequences of obesity

Stroke
Depression
Obstructive sleep apnoea (OSA)
Breathlessness
Restrictive defect → type II respiratory failure
Hypertension
Gallstones
Hiatus hernia
Ischaemic heart disease
Oligomenorrhoea
Hypogonadism
Pregnancy morbidity
Type II diabetes
Deep vein thrombosis, varicose veins
Osteoarthitis knee/hip

Increased risk of cancer
- Colorectal
- Gynaecological (breast, ovary, uterus)
- Prostate
- Pancreas
- Liver
- Multiple myeloma

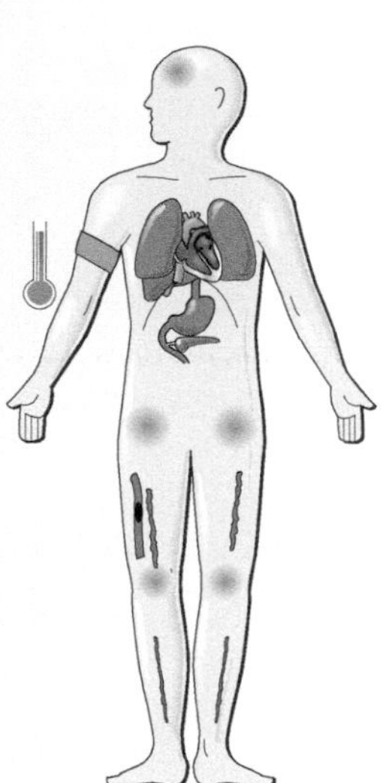

Patterns of obesity

	Centripetal	Visceral
Waist-hip ratio	♂ >1.0 ♀ >0.9	♂<0.85 ♀ <0.75
	• Easier to lose weight • Men • Stress, cigarette smoking	• Harder to lose weight • Women
	Stronger link with mortality	

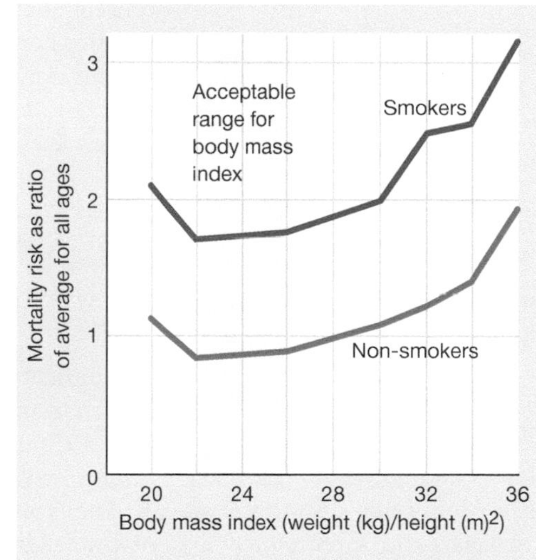

Treatment

1. Energy intake restriction and exercise
2. Orlistat (BMI >28 kg/m^2 with risk factors; BMI >30 kg/m^2 if no risk factors)
3. Surgery BMI >30 with diabetes; BMI >35 with complications of obesity

135–200% ideal weight – very low calorie diet ± drugs

30 kg/m^2 and DM, or BMI >35 and/or comorbidity ideal weight – surgery

Losing even small amounts → substantial improvement in BP, IHD + diabetes

Medicine at a Glance, Fifth Edition. Edited by Patrick Davey and Alex Pitcher.

Companion website: www.wiley.com/go/medicine5e

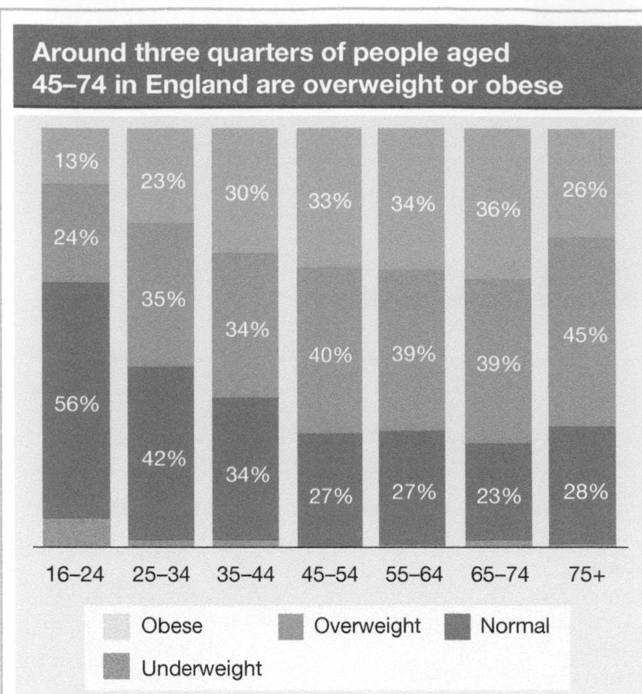

Table 38.1 Multiple endocrine and neurological events involved in the regulation of body weight

	Afferent signals ↓ appetite or ↑ energy expenditure	Afferent signals ↑ appetite or ↓ energy expenditure
Gastrointestinal tract	Glucagon, cholecystokinin, glucagon-like peptide 1, peptide YY, oxyntomodulin, glucose	Ghrelin, opioids, neurotensin, growth hormone-releasing hormone, somatostatin
Endocrine system	Adrenaline (β-adrenergic effect), oestrogens	Adrenaline (α-adrenergic effect)
Adipose tissue	Leptin	
Peripheral nervous system	Noradrenaline (β-adrenergic effect)	Noradrenaline (α-adrenergic effect)
Central nervous system	Dopamine, γ-aminobutyric acid, serotonin, cholecystokinin	Galanin, opioids, growth hormone-releasing hormone, somatostatin

Definition

Obesity is defined as an excess of body fat, sufficient to adversely affect health, and is measured using body mass index or fat distribution; body mass index (BMI) >30 kg/m^2 (BMI = weight (kg)/[height^2 (m^2)]); healthy = 18.5–24.9; overweight = 25–29.9; obese >30, extreme obesity >40. Central obesity measured by waist circumference (>102 cm in men, >88 cm in women) is more directly linked to metabolic and cardiovascular risk.

Epidemiology

The prevalence of obesity has doubled in the last decade and is now 27% in the UK adult population.

Aetiopathogenesis of 'simple obesity'

- **Genetic**: genetic effects are complex and polygenic (e.g. FTO gene) with a heritability of 30–60%. Monogenic disorders, e.g. leptin deficiency/resistance, and melanocortin 4 receptor deficiency are very rare.
- **Environment**: readily available high-fat, energy-rich diet, often cheaper hence role of poverty, associated with a sedentary lifestyle and positive energy balance.
- **Neuroendocrine**: ghrelin (released from the fundus of the stomach) increases food intake via hypothalamic neuropeptide Y release. Neuropeptide Y (hypothalamic hormone that stimulates appetite) and leptin (peptide hormone synthesized in adipose tissue which acts in the hypothalamus to suppress food intake and energy expenditure), in association with other neurotransmitters, regulate energy balance, though multiple other pathways are also involved such as bile acids and gut bacteria (Table 38.1).

These afferent signals act on hypothalamic tracts, involving ghrelin, noradrenaline, serotonin, neuropeptide Y, melanocyte-concentrating hormone, glucagon-like peptide I, corticotropin-releasing hormone, orexin A and oxytocin.

The hypothalamic tracts effect changes via the sympathetic nervous system, parasympathetic nervous system and thyroid hormones. These systems then affect energy intake and expenditure.

Assessment of the obese patient

The clinical assessment of the obese patient involves the following factors.

- **Confirmation of obesity** from the BMI and assessment of the pattern of body fat distribution: centripetal obesity (waist : hip ratio >0.9 in women, >1.0 in men) is associated with increased cardiovascular risk.
- **Time course of obesity**: whether the obesity is long-standing or new (suggests secondary cause if sudden onset), any previous treatment for obesity and the family history. Explanation of obesity may also be sought by reference to eating habits and physical activity.
- **Secondary causes**: very rare but should be considered if in recent (less than several) years there has been unexplained weight gain and/or if there are abnormal physical signs or biochemical tests. Underlying pathology may include Cushing syndrome (24 h urinary free cortisol, overnight 1 mg dexamethasone suppression test), hypothyroidism (thyroid-stimulating hormone), hypothalamic disorder (uncontrolled appetite) (MRI hypothalamus), Prader–Willi syndrome (deletion of part of the long arm of chromosome 15, resulting in hypogonadism and obesity) or Lawrence–Moon–Biedl syndrome.

- **Overall cardiovascular risk assessment**: from fasting glucose, lipid profile, LFTs and other standard risk factors (age, sex, blood pressure [BP], smoking status, alcohol consumption) and presence of vascular disease.

Complications

- **Metabolic complications**: hyperinsulinaemia and insulin resistance ± impaired glucose tolerance/diabetes mellitus; hypertension; ischaemic heart disease (IHD) (four-fold risk if BMI >29); cerebrovascular disease; hyperlipidaemia.
- **Hepatic complications**: obesity can lead to non-alcoholic fatty liver disease (NAFLD), which can produce a hepatitis, and eventually lead to cirrhosis. Gallstones may occur.
- **Physical problems**: osteoarthritis, varicose veins, hernias (both hiatal hernia and abdominal hernias), obstructive sleep apnoea (see Chapter 98), operative complications, hirsutism.
- **Increased cancer risk**: breast, ovary, endometrium, prostate, cervix, bowel.
- Depression.

Management

Severely obese individuals need treatment to improve prognosis, improve self-image and minimize symptoms, particularly those arising from physical problems. In men, being 10% overweight increases death rates by 13%, and being 20% overweight by 25%.

Behavioural modifications

Behavioural modifications include dietary modification (low fat, high protein and low glycaemic), dietary restriction, increased exercise and stopping smoking. Alcohol intake should be minimized. Behavioural therapy, e.g. goal setting, social support and cognitive therapy are helpful.

Drugs

- **Fat absorption inhibitor**: orlistat inhibits pancreatic lipase, so reducing fat absorption (side-effect – steatorrhoea).
- **POMC hypothalamic stimulation**: naltrexone/bupropion (side-effects – headache and dizziness).
- **Appetite suppressants**: Semaglutide (GLP-1 agonist) suppresses appetite (side-effects – nausea, diarrhoea and constipation).

The following drugs have been withdrawn.

- Sibutramine (centrally acting serotonin and noradrenaline [norepinephrine] reuptake inhibitor); withdrawn because of hypertension and tachycardia.
- Rimonabant (cannabinoid type 1 receptor antagonist reduces appetite); withdrawn because of side-effects – depression and risk of suicide.
- Amphetamine derivatives (dexfenfluramine, fenfluramine) suppress appetite but have been withdrawn as a result of side-effects (cardiac valvulopathy).

Weight loss (bariatric) surgery (BMI >30 kg/m^2 in diabetes, >35 kg/m^2 if other co-morbidity and no diabetes)

Usually performed laparascopically; gastric band, sleeve gastrectomy and adjustable gastric banding. Complications include nutritional deficiency, renal stones and psychological sequelae. Sudden profound weight loss has its own complications, including liver dysfunction and QT interval prolongation, which may predispose to an arrhythmic death.

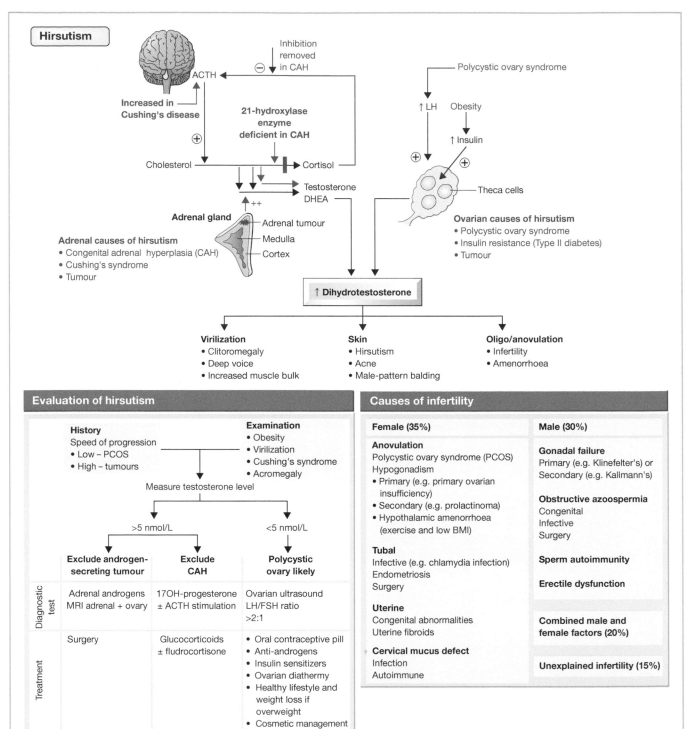

Hirsutism and infertility

Hirsutism

Inhibition removed in CAH

ACTH

Polycystic ovary syndrome

Increased in Cushing's disease

21-hydroxylase enzyme deficient in CAH

↑ LH

Obesity

↑ Insulin

Cholesterol

Cortisol

Testosterone

DHEA

++

Theca cells

Adrenal gland

Adrenal tumour

Medulla

Cortex

Adrenal causes of hirsutism

- Congenital adrenal hyperplasia (CAH)
- Cushing's syndrome
- Tumour

Ovarian causes of hirsutism

- Polycystic ovary syndrome
- Insulin resistance (Type II diabetes)
- Tumour

↑ Dihydrotestosterone

Virilization

- Clitoromegaly
- Deep voice
- Increased muscle bulk

Skin

- Hirsutism
- Acne
- Male-pattern balding

Oligo/anovulation

- Infertility
- Amenorrhoea

Evaluation of hirsutism

History
Speed of progression
- Low – PCOS
- High – tumours

Examination
- Obesity
- Virilization
- Cushing's syndrome
- Acromegaly

Measure testosterone level

>5 nmol/L → Exclude androgen-secreting tumour; Exclude CAH

<5 nmol/L → Polycystic ovary likely

	Exclude androgen-secreting tumour	Exclude CAH	Polycystic ovary likely
Diagnostic test	Adrenal androgens MRI adrenal + ovary	17OH-progesterone ± ACTH stimulation	Ovarian ultrasound LH/FSH ratio >2:1
Treatment	Surgery	Glucocorticoids ± fludrocortisone	• Oral contraceptive pill • Anti-androgens • Insulin sensitizers • Ovarian diathermy • Healthy lifestyle and weight loss if overweight • Cosmetic management

Causes of infertility

Female (35%)	Male (30%)
Anovulation Polycystic ovary syndrome (PCOS) Hypogonadism • Primary (e.g. primary ovarian insufficiency) • Secondary (e.g. prolactinoma) • Hypothalamic amenorrhoea (exercise and low BMI)	**Gonadal failure** Primary (e.g. Klinefelter's) or Secondary (e.g. Kallmann's)
Tubal Infective (e.g. chlamydia infection) Endometriosis Surgery	**Obstructive azoospermia** Congenital Infective Surgery
Uterine Congenital abnormalities Uterine fibroids	**Sperm autoimmunity** **Erectile dysfunction**
Cervical mucus defect Infection Autoimmune	**Combined male and female factors (20%)** **Unexplained infertility (15%)**

Medicine at a Glance, Fifth Edition. Edited by Patrick Davey and Alex Pitcher.

Companion website: www.wiley.com/go/medicine5e

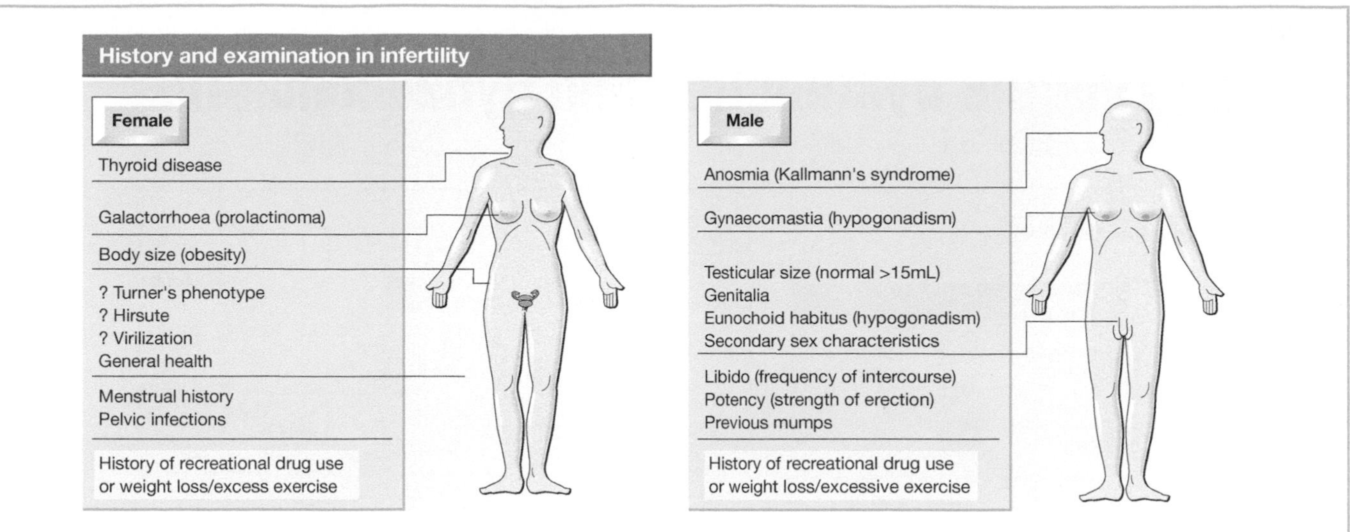

Hirsutism

Hirsutism is common, affects 5% of premenopausal women and usually does not indicate a serious underlying illness. It is defined as excess hair growth in women due to increased androgen production or skin sensitivity. Hair growth follows a male pattern, being predominantly facial (moustache or beard), thoracic and abdominal. Male-pattern baldness may develop. Serious disease should be suspected in thin women, in rapidly progressive hirsutism, in treatment-resistant hypertension or with severe menstrual disruption. If other features of virilization are present (clitoromegaly, deep voice, male muscle pattern), investigations for androgen-secreting tumours are mandatory.

The principal causes of hirsutism are listed below, although it is important to realize that hirsutism is often only a minor feature of these conditions.

- **Obesity** is commonly associated with mild hirsutism. Insulin resistance increases virilization. Acanthosis nigricans occurs in morbidly obese individuals.
- **Polycystic ovary syndrome** (PCOS) affects 10% of women, commonly causing hirsutism. Sufferers often have oligomenorrhoea, obesity and mild virilization (male-pattern hair growth and loss, with acne).
- **Familial or idiopathic hirsutism**, usually in those of Mediterranean descent.
- **Drugs**, particularly androgenic steroids in athletes.
- **Cushing syndrome** (<1% of cases): patients rarely present with hirsutism and more common physical signs are of thin skin, proximal myopathy and (new and progressive) central obesity.
- **Congenital adrenal hyperplasia** (CAH) is a rare cause of hirsutism (there are 4000 CAH patients in the UK), and is usually caused by deficiency of 21-hydroxylase – the enzyme responsible for degrading progesterone (via intermediate metabolites) to corticosterone, cortisol and aldosterone. 17-Hydroxyprogesterone accumulates, is turned into androstenedione and, in turn, to testosterone. While classic CAH is diagnosed in infancy because of cortisol deficiency and salt wasting, non-classic CAH is diagnosed later due to excess androgens. High 17-hydroxyprogesterone levels are found, particularly with synacthen (adrenocorticotrophic hormone [ACTH]) stimulation. Treatment is with glucocorticoid and mineralocorticoid replacement in classic CAH. Non-classic CAH can be treated as for PCOS but occasionally low dose glucocorticoids are used.
- **Androgen-secreting tumour**: <1% of cases; can arise from the ovary or the adrenals.

The diagnostic approach is to pick up clues from the history and examination (particularly of marked virilization) and to measure luteinizing hormone (LH)/follicle-stimulating hormone (FSH) and androgen levels. Testosterone levels of >5 nmol/l (i.e. significant elevation) imply that a diagnosis of PCOS is unlikely and that of an androgen-secreting tumour or CAH more likely. These need to be formally excluded by hormonal assessment, including stimulation tests and imaging.

Treatment of hirsutism (other than that for the underlying cause)

Weight loss, cosmetic approaches (topical acne treatment, waxing, electrolysis and laser), combined oral contraceptive pill (OCP), specifically Dianette® (an OCP containing the antiandrogen cyproterone acetate), are useful. Androgen receptor blockers (e.g. spironolactone and cyproterone acetate), usually combined with an OCP, are effective. Insulin-sensitizing drugs (metformin).

Infertility

Infertility is defined as failure of pregnancy after one year of unprotected intercourse. It affects 10–15% of couples.

Investigation of male and female partners is needed for diagnosis. In men, the first investigation is semen analysis: normal sperm motility and numbers exclude the man from further investigation. If abnormal sperm are found, FSH and testosterone are measured to investigate the possibility of gonadal failure. If such investigations are normal, then the possibility of obstruction to the spermatic tract should be considered. In the female, midluteal progesterone is measured. Normal levels (>30 pmol/l) imply normal gonadal function. The problem may then be mechanical and laparoscopy for tubal patency is undertaken. Abnormally low progesterone suggests lack of ovulation, e.g. premature ovarian failure or PCOS.

Management

Treatment is for the underlying cause where possible. For anovulation, clomiphene (selective estrogen receptor modulator [SERM]), letrozole (aromatase inhibitor) gonadotrophin-releasing hormone or gonadotrophins are used in low FSH cases (success rate 50–80%), and oocyte donation for raised FSH cases (50% success rate).

Complex stimulatory regimens are needed in male pituitary failure. For tubal or obstructive azoospermia, reconstructive surgery is occasionally possible and for oligospermia, intracytoplasmic sperm injections (success rate 20% per cycle). Unexplained infertility may respond to *in vitro* fertilization (25% success rate/cycle, though rates are much lower in women aged over 40 years).

Erectile dysfunction and gynaecomastia

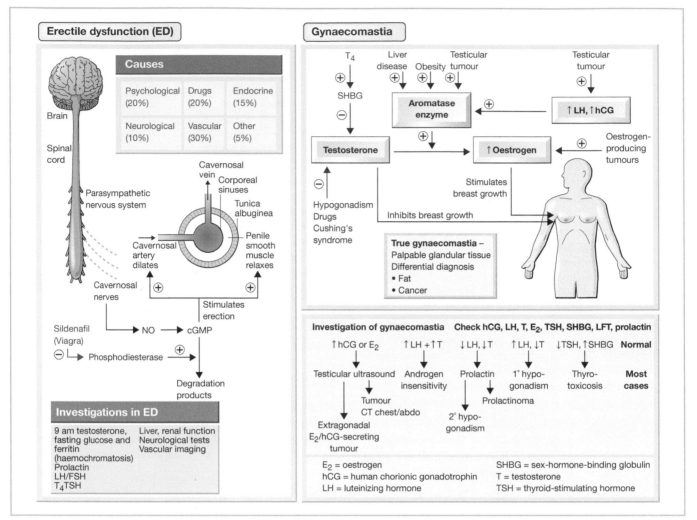

Erectile dysfunction (ED)

Brain
Spinal cord
Parasympathetic nervous system
Cavernosal nerves

Causes

Psychological (20%)	Drugs (20%)	Endocrine (15%)
Neurological (10%)	Vascular (30%)	Other (5%)

Cavernosal vein
Corporeal sinuses
Tunica albuginea
Cavernosal artery dilates
Penile smooth muscle relaxes
Stimulates erection
Sildenafil (Viagra)
NO → cGMP
Phosphodiesterase
Degradation products

Investigations in ED

9 am testosterone, fasting glucose and ferritin (haemochromatosis)
Prolactin
LH/FSH
T_4TSH
Liver, renal function
Neurological tests
Vascular imaging

Gynaecomastia

T_4
SHBG
Liver disease
Obesity
Testicular tumour
Aromatase enzyme
↑LH, ↑hCG
Testosterone
↑Oestrogen
Oestrogen-producing tumours
Stimulates breast growth
Inhibits breast growth
Hypogonadism
Drugs
Cushing's syndrome

True gynaecomastia – Palpable glandular tissue
Differential diagnosis
- Fat
- Cancer

Investigation of gynaecomastia **Check hCG, LH, T, E_2, TSH, SHBG, LFT, prolactin**

- ↑hCG or E_2 → Testicular ultrasound → Tumour, CT chest/abdo; → Extragonadal E_2/hCG-secreting tumour
- ↑LH + ↑T → Androgen insensitivity
- ↓LH, ↓T → Prolactin → Prolactinoma; → 2° hypogonadism
- ↑LH, ↓T → 1° hypogonadism
- ↓TSH, ↑SHBG → Thyrotoxicosis
- **Normal** → **Most cases**

E_2 = oestrogen
hCG = human chorionic gonadotrophin
LH = luteinizing hormone
SHBG = sex-hormone-binding globulin
T = testosterone
TSH = thyroid-stimulating hormone

Erectile dysfunction

The normal erection is produced by vasoconstriction of the venous outflow from the penis, resulting in blood distending the corpus cavernosa of the penis. Venous vasoconstriction is the result of activation of sacral autonomic nerves raising levels of venous cyclic adenosine monophosphate (cAMP). Interference with the arterial supply, autonomic nervous system or sex drive (libido) impairs erectile success. Erectile dysfunction (impotence) is defined as an inability to achieve an erection sufficient for sexual intercourse. It affects 10% of males and becomes more common in older age.

Causes include the following.

- **Drugs** commonly underlie or exacerbate erectile failure. Particularly important ones are β-blockers, calcium channel blockers and psychotropic agents.
- **Recreational substances**: alcohol, marijuana.
- **Psychological problems**: very common; may cause erectile failure in its own right or complicate a pre-existing medical problem. Impotence is usually variable in severity and morning erections are unaffected.
- **Endocrine disorders**: 30–60% of people with diabetes of six years' standing develop some degree of erectile failure, as a result of both neuropathy and vascular disease. Thyroid dysfunction can also impair libido and potency. Androgen deficiency underlies 20% of cases of impotence seen in endocrinology outpatients. Libido is reduced in hypogonadal males.
- **Vasculogenic**: peripheral arterial insufficiency involving the terminal aorta is a very common cause for erectile dysfunction. Penis venous insufficiency is, however, a very rare cause of impotence.
- **Neurogenic**: many neurological diseases can be associated with impotence, either directly through damage to the mechanisms involved in erection and ejaculation, or indirectly through psychological mechanisms. Particularly important causes include damage to the sacral nerves, as can occur with radical prostate or pelvic surgery.

Medicine at a Glance, Fifth Edition. Edited by Patrick Davey and Alex Pitcher.

Companion website: www.wiley.com/go/medicine5e

- **Other diseases**: structural penile abnormalities such as Peyronie disease (which results in a curved penis) and microphallus may cause erectile dysfunction. Any chronic debilitating disease can also cause impotence.

Diagnosis

The key is to diagnose any underlying disease, which may require specific therapy. Absence of early morning erections is a good clue to the presence of underlying organic disease. Symptoms and signs of hypogonadism must be carefully sought (gynaecomastia, decrease in body hair, fatigue, testicular shrinkage, premature osteoporosis). Arterial disease and the factors closely associated with it should be sought (intermittent claudication, presence of diabetes, hypertension or smoking, presence of foot and leg pulses). General health needs to be assessed, particularly whether liver, renal or neurological disease is present.

Treatment

Any underlying disease should be treated and any causative drug withdrawn.

- **Androgen treatment** if hypogonadal.
- Oral **phosphodiesterase 5 inhibitors** (sildenafil [Viagra®], vardenafil, tadalafil): inhibit penile phosphodiesterase type 5 and enhance the normal erectile response to sexual stimulation. Contraindicated in recent myocardial infarction/cerebrovascular accident, hypotension, severe heart failure and treatment with nitrates (profound hypotension can occur).
- **Intracavernous prostaglandin E_1 (PGE_1) injection**: potent vasoconstrictor when injected into the penile venous circulation or intraurethral, preventing venous efflux, so producing erections. Erections may be persistent and painful (priapism).
- **Vacuum devices**: these work but are cosmetically unattractive.
- **Penile prosthesis**: surgically implanted prosthetic devices can stiffen, or mechanically inflate, the penis; they are useful when other forms of treatment are ineffective, undesirable or contraindicated.
- **Psychosexual counselling**.

Gynaecomastia

This is palpable enlargement of the male breast glandular tissue. It affects 30% of men aged <30 years and 50% aged >45 years. It rarely indicates serious underlying disease but if the patient is thin, enlargement is rapid or painful and in particular if the glandular tissue is >5 cm, underlying disease should be suspected. Causes include the following.

- **Physiological**: puberty (transient in up to 50%).
- **Obesity**: probably the most common cause. Increased peripheral conversion of testosterone to oestrogen by the aromatase enzyme promotes breast growth.
- **Drugs**: a common cause – digoxin, cimetidine, spironolactone, antiandrogens, alcohol, marijuana, antiretroviral drugs, etc.
- **Hyperprolactinaemia**: high prolactin levels induce secondary hypogonadism, depressing testosterone levels and allowing for unopposed oestrogen action on the breast.
- **Hypogonadism (primary or secondary)**: suspect if libido is reduced with erectile dysfunction.
- **Systemic disease**: liver cirrhosis, chronic renal failure (relative oestradiol excess), malnutrition.
- **Underlying hormone-secreting tumour**: accounts for 3% of cases of gynaecomastia seen in the endocrine service. The tumour may be testicular (human chorionic gonadotrophin [hCG], oestradiol or aromatase producing), adrenal (oestradiol producing) or ectopic secretion from, e.g., lung/gastrointestinal cancer producing hCG.
- Breast cancer, which is rare (0.1% breast cancer), may need to be excluded if the breast tissue is hard.

Treatment

Treat underlying disorder when present, and change drug treatment if possible. Treatment is mainly by reassurance, withdrawal of the offending drug and advice on weight reduction. Drug treatment (anti-oestrogens [tamoxifen or clomiphene] or aromatase inhibitors) may be helpful; all are unapproved apart from danazol. Surgical resection is occasionally used.

41 Principles of infection

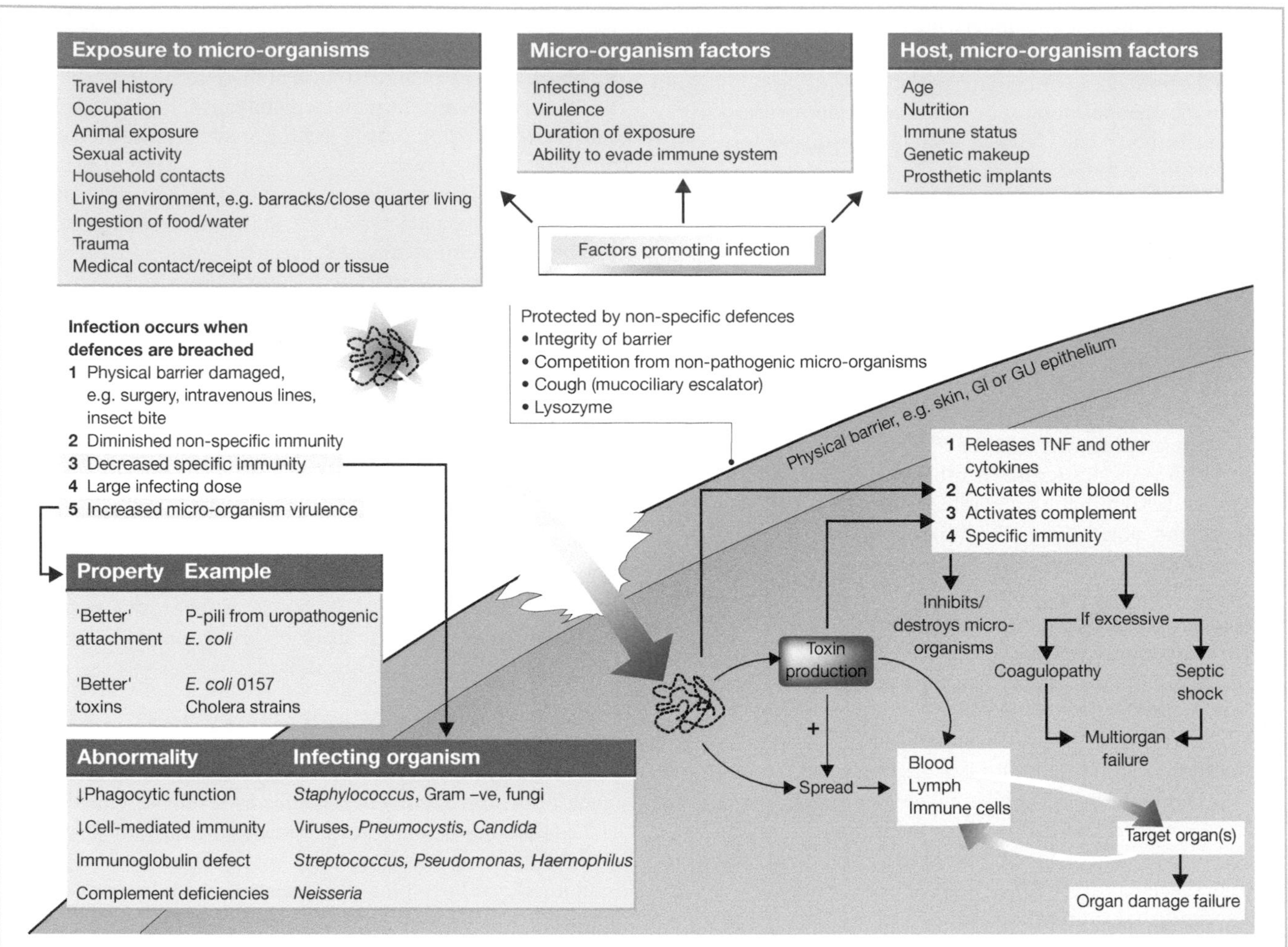

Property	Example
'Better' attachment	P-pili from uropathogenic *E. coli*
'Better' toxins	*E. coli* 0157 Cholera strains

Abnormality	Infecting organism
↓Phagocytic function	*Staphylococcus*, Gram –ve, fungi
↓Cell-mediated immunity	Viruses, *Pneumocystis, Candida*
Immunoglobulin defect	*Streptococcus, Pseudomonas, Haemophilus*
Complement deficiencies	*Neisseria*

The scope of infectious disease

Despite antimicrobial agents being available for an increasing range of organisms, infectious disease remains a significant cause of morbidity and mortality because of the emergence and spread of new agents (e.g. COVID-19) and antimicrobial resistance, the persistence of infections once considered controlled, e.g. tuberculosis (TB) and syphilis, and wider societal issues, including poverty and conflict. In resource-rich settings, infections associated with immunosuppression and prosthetic material form an increasing proportion of infectious disease problems and awareness of the distinct way in which these infections manifest is important at all levels of the health system.

Principles of managing infection

Emergency services in resource-rich settings are generally set up to detect and treat 'classic' bacterial infections, including sepsis, as well as acute viral infections (coronaviruses, flu, RSV). However, the diagnosis of less common forms of bacterial infection (e.g. endocarditis) or infections with less familiar presenting features (e.g. tuberculosis, PCP) remains a significant challenge. A high index of suspicion for these specific infections is needed to avoid delay in diagnosis and instigation of appropriate management.

Host and microbial factors leading to infection

Exposure

- Particular behaviour leading to pathogen exposure.
- Prevalence of infection in a community.

Breakdown in barriers

- **Physical barriers**: breaks in skin and mucosa can lead to entry of micro-organisms; urinary catheters or intravenous lines are iatrogenic examples.
- **Chemical barriers**: for example, proton pump inhibitors reduce stomach acid, increasing the risk of *C. difficile* infection.
- **Loss of physical mechanisms expelling bacteria**: for example, urine and bile flow are impaired by stones or strictures.
- Loss of **competition** from commensal flora following antibiotics leading to pathogenic microbe colonisation e.g. *Candida*.

Presence of prosthetic material

This can lead to the development of biofilm-associated infection; a biofilm is an assembly of surface-associated microbial cells, enclosed in an extracellular matrix.

Immunosuppression (see Chapters 172 and 173)

A growing proportion of the population are immunosuppressed to some degree by virtue of acquired diseases or their treatment.

Other forms of vulnerability

A wide range of illnesses predispose to infection, or severe consequences of infection, without being directly immunosuppressive, e.g. neurological illness (multiple sclerosis, myasthenia gravis). Any illness leading to loss of sensation or impaired blood supply, e.g. the foot in diabetes mellitus.

Microbial factors

Disease may arise via the following pathways.

- **Endogenous infection**, i.e. micro-organisms that exist on mucosal surfaces or are present in the body as a latent infection. Endogenously acquired infections have become progressively more important in developed countries as the proportion of immunocompromised people in the population has grown.
- **Exogenous infection** from the environment. *Direct* exogenous transmission occurs from contact with, or droplet transmission from, an infected host or source (such as soil). *Indirect* infection may be vector-borne, air-borne or result from transmission via infected blood, blood products or organs.

Disease production

Pathogens have evolved strategies to make transmission and establishment in a host more efficient. Different strategies may be utilized by micro-organisms at different points in the establishment of an infection; the following are examples.

- **Mucosal contact**: attachment to epithelial surfaces may be crucial for pathogenesis.
  - Non-specific interactions occur between the hydrophilic bacterial cell surface and the lipophilic endothelial cell surface.
  - Specific interactions also exist. Some strains of *Escherichia coli* have hair-like structures, called P-pili, which adhere to a specific glycolipid receptor on the cell surface of the urothelium (the endothelium lining the urinary tract), contributing to their potential to cause urinary tract infection. Influenza virus attaches to cells via the haemagglutinin antigen.
- **Invasion**: pathogens cause damage by invading deeper tissues, either through breaks in the skin or mucosal surface or via specific invasion mechanisms.
  - Schistosomal cerceriae are able to penetrate intact skin and subsequently enter the circulation.
  - Enteropathogens utilize a number of different mechanisms to adhere to and then interact with the M cell, leading to transport, invasion and multiplication.
  - *Neisseria meningitidis*, and the measles virus, are able to penetrate epithelium.
- **Immune evasion**: some pathogens produce enzymes or have surface components, which bind or inhibit secretory IgA on mucosal surfaces.
  - The polysaccharide capsule of bacteria such as *Streptococcus pneumoniae* or *Haemophilus influenzae* type B helps to resist phagocytosis.
  - *Leishmania*, *Mycobacterium* or *Salmonella* species are able to survive and multiply within macrophages.
- **Toxin production** is important in the pathogenesis of some diseases.
  - Cholera toxin activates the adenyl cyclase mechanisms of host intestinal cells, thus producing the excretion of large amounts of fluid and electrolytes. The production of toxin transforms asymptomatic carriage of *Clostridium difficile* into a disease-causing pathogen.
  - The lipopolysaccharide of Gram-negative bacteria (endotoxin) partly underlies the sepsis syndrome.

Potential clinical consequences of infection

Acute consequences

- Cytokine effects: fever, malaise, anorexia, catabolic state, increased white cells and platelets, acute phase response with increased acute phase proteins.
- Circulatory failure (see Chapter 18).
- Disseminated intravascular coagulation.
- Organ damage and failure from shock (e.g. renal failure), direct invasion (e.g. pneumonia producing respiratory failure) or by multiple mechanisms (e.g. adult respiratory distress syndrome).
- Stroke (endocarditis or other endovascular infection)

Chronic consequences

- Muscle wasting and weight loss.
- Anaemia of chronic disease: see Chapter 175.
- Permanent organ destruction: e.g. liver cirrhosis from chronic hepatitis, left ventricular failure after viral myocarditis, permanent paralysis following polio.
- Postinfective phenomena: e.g. lactose intolerance after gastrointestinal (GI) infection.

Autoimmune phenomena

- Generalized syndromes: e.g. poststreptococcal phenomena, such as rheumatic fever.
- System-specific: the following are examples.
  - Neurological: Guillain–Barré syndrome after a viral infection, cerebellar syndromes after chickenpox.
  - Haematological: haemolytic anaemia after *Mycoplasma* infection.
  - Rheumatological: arthritis after gut or urinary tract infection in genetically predisposed individuals.
  - Dermatological: scarlet fever (rash after streptococcal infection).

Prevention of infection

1) Avoidance of exposure to, or contact with, pathogen via altered behaviour. 2) Public health measures such as sanitation. 3) Infection control within healthcare settings. 4) Prophylactic measures: presurgery antibiotics before invasive procedures. 5) Before inducing immunosuppression: treatment of latent TB before transplant. 6) After exposure to potential pathogen: postexposure HIV drugs. 7) Immunization, with one of the following: Live attenuated or killed organisms, or components of microbes, or altered toxins, or within RNA/DNA vaccines.

Treatment of infection

- Symptomatic support: antipyretics, maintenance of hydration.
- Antimicrobials: either empirical or targeted to identified micro-organisms.
- Removal of sources of infection: e.g. draining of abscesses or removal of infected lines.
- Adjunctive therapy: circulatory and vital organ support in sepsis.
- Immunomodulatory treatment: e.g. COVID-19, acute bacterial meningitis, TB meningitis.
- Many infections (particularly viral) are self-limiting and do not need specific treatment.

Investigation of suspected infection

Infective process suggested by:

1. Specific regional syndromes, often pain + fever + specific symptoms
2. Generalized syndromes = unwell + fever ± shock ± haemostatic failure

Helpful tests in suspected infection

1. **Full blood count** (FBC): to look for changes in white cell counts
2. **CRP** and **ESR**. Assess degree of acute inflammatory response:
   - ESR
   - C-reactive protein: acute phase protein with short half-life, rises briskly, falls quickly; particularly useful for assessing response to treatment
3. Tests to assess effect of infection: LFTs, clotting tests, renal function
4. Determination of organism: microscopy/culture/histology of appropriate samples or serological diagnosis
5. Imaging to assess site or extent of infection

Useful imaging

CT head scan
- Brain abscess
- Otogenic abscess

CT chest
- Lymph nodes
- Parenchymal disease

USS heart
- Endocarditis
- Pericardial effusion

USS abdomen
- Subphrenic abscess
- Renal abscess
- Pancreatic abscess

MRI
- Spine-related infection
- Other bones/joint infection

Chest X-ray
- Pneumonia
- Empyema

CT abdomen
- Occult abscesses
- Lymph nodes
- Splenic infarcts associated with endocarditis

CT pelvis
- Prostatic abscess

Diagnosis

Rests on proving presence of pathogenic organisms + appropriate clinical presentation.

1. Identification of organism
   - Light microscopy, e.g. Ziehl–Neelson stain for TB
   - Electron microscopy—useful for many viruses
   - Biopsy specimen
2. Identification of microbial antigen
   - e.g. PCR of CSF for viral, bacterial Ag
3. Culture of organism
   - Plating out (various media/ biochemical reactions)
   - Cytopathic effect (viruses)
   - Xenodiagnosis (infection of sterile animal, e.g. trypanosomiasis)
4. Immunological response
   - Antibody response, usually detection of IgM, or rise in IgG titre over time
   - Skin response to antigen, e.g. Mantoux test (TB)

Highly suggestive findings

If organisms are not found, findings highly suggestive of infection are:

1. Classic radiological findings (e.g. 'halo' sign in aspergilloma)
2. Response to specific treatment (e.g. anti-TB treatment)

The initial history and examination usually indicate the most appropriate investigation. In a febrile patient with no obvious source of infection, useful investigations include a full blood count (FBC), C-reactive protein (CRP) or erythrocyte sedimentation rate (ESR), liver function tests (LFTs), blood cultures, urine examination and a chest X-ray.

Full blood count

- **Normochromic/normocytic anaemia** occurs in many chronic infections.
- **Raised neutrophil count** or toxic granulation suggests bacterial sepsis.
- **Raised lymphocyte count**: occurs in many viral infections and some bacterial disorders, e.g. typhoid and brucellosis. Atypical lymphocytes suggest Epstein–Barr virus (EBV) or cytomegalovirus (CMV) infection.
- **Low neutrophil count**: iatrogenic immunosuppression or infection with typhoid, brucellosis or rickettsial disease. Bad prognostic indicator in severe sepsis.
- **Low lymphocyte count:** occurs with a wide range of acute infections, with viruses the most common agents; if chronic, consider human immunodeficiency virus (HIV) in particular.
- **Low platelet count**: Very common in malaria and dengue fever in particular. May reflect disseminated intravascular coagulation in severe sepsis.
- **Eosinophilia** may occur in schistosomiasis and tissue invasion by other parasites.

CRP and ESR

The CRP rises within 4–8 hours after the onset of infection and has a half-life in the circulation of around 18 hours (although clearance may be slower with renal impairment). It tends to rise later than the neutrophil count in bacterial sepsis. CRP levels are useful in following the response to treatment and are particularly useful when empirical antibiotics have been given (i.e. to treat a suspected rather than proven infection). CRP levels tend to be relatively lower in patients with chronic liver disease due to impaired synthetic function.

The ESR is the rate at which red cells settle through plasma. It is dependent on age, sex, serum immunoglobulins, especially IgM, acute phase proteins such as fibrinogen, and the shape and nature of the red cell membrane. It increases with age (the normal ESR is $<[age/2] + 10$). The ESR is elevated in most infections, but does not reliably discriminate between infective and inflammatory conditions and rises only slowly (over 2 weeks). It is possible to have an acute infection and a normal ESR.

The two tests are not interchangeable. ESR gives an average of inflammation over the preceding 2–3 weeks, while the CRP gives the picture over the preceding 8 hours. ESR is elevated in untreated HIV (because of polyclonal gammopathy) and active SLE, whereas CRP in these conditions is normal, unless there is super-added infection.

Liver function tests

Abnormalities in liver function suggest either local infective processes (hepatitis, hepatic abscesses, biliary sepsis) or systemic or disseminated infections. Unrelated causes such as medication or alcohol can change liver function so further evidence is needed to define specific infection. A rapid fall in albumin indicates a significant acute phase response.

Microscopy

Direct microscopy of clinical samples allows rapid identification of micro-organisms. Wet preparations are used for urine examination or the detection of parasites in the stool.

Fixed stained preparations

- **Gram staining**: the size, morphology (cocci or bacilli) and staining characteristics (Gram positive or negative) of bacteria give a clue to their species, but definitive identification is rarely possible. Commensal or contaminant organisms in samples make interpretation of microscopy difficult. Microscopy is most useful for samples from normally sterile sites, e.g. cerebrospinal fluid (CSF), joints, etc.
- Specific stains are used to identify some micro-organisms, e.g. Ziehl–Neelsen stain for mycobacteria or Giemsa for parasites such as malaria on a blood slide.

Viruses cannot be identified on standard microscopy and although electron microscopy can be used to identify some species, improvements in molecular technology in recent years mean that microscopy has largely been superseded by the polymerase chain reaction (PCR) in clinical practice.

Culture

Culture is the definitive diagnostic method for most bacteria and fungi. Samples are cultured on growth media, whose composition and incubation conditions are varied to isolate particular micro-organisms selectively. Organisms are identified by colonial morphology, growth on specific media and in certain conditions, and by biochemical reactions. The use of antibiotic discs on culture plates allows determination of antibiotic sensitivity. These traditional methods are now complemented by molecular techniques, which are used in many laboratories for identification and sensitivity testing.

Contamination of cultures with normal flora, such as non-pathogenic mouth organisms in sputum samples, may make detection of pathogens more difficult.

Blood cultures may identify bacteraemia resulting from infection in many different sites of the body. Repeated blood cultures are necessary to detect organisms that do not grow readily or to determine the significance of an initial isolation of a potential contaminating organism. It is rare to need more than three sets of blood cultures. Blood cultures should ideally be taken before starting antibiotics.

In stable patients where there is diagnostic doubt, it is sometimes appropriate to stop all antibiotics and re-culture all potentially infected sites, e.g. blood, etc.

Serology

Some organisms, particularly viruses, are difficult to identify. Serology measures the host immunological response to an infection. The presence of IgM antibodies is diagnostic of recent infection, while high IgG levels indicate past infection. Serology is particularly useful in hepatitis or glandular fever.

Histology

Infection can sometimes be diagnosed only by seeing specific pathological features on examination of tissue. These features include:

- inclusion bodies suggesting infections such as CMV
- granulomas: associated with a number of different infections, including tuberculosis (TB)
- demonstration of fungi in tissues by the use of specific stains. Tissue biopsy may sometimes be the only way of making a diagnosis in difficult cases.

Molecular methods

Molecular techniques are becoming increasingly important.

- **PCR** uses genetic probes to recognize and amplify the nucleic acid from specific viruses or bacteria that are difficult to culture. Multiple organisms can be detected via commercial 'platform' systems, e.g. throat swabs can be tested for likely respiratory viruses such as influenza, parainfluenza, coronavirus and RSV; CSF samples can be tested for bacterial and viral causes of meningitis. Quantification is also possible and may guide treatment, e.g. in hepatitis B or CMV infection. PCR is also used for the rapid detection of resistance conferred by specific genes in organisms such as *Mycobacterium tuberculosis*.
- **Lateral flow devices** are rapid, single-sample tests that identify proteins associated with particular infections. Their simplicity allows use far from medical facilities; the diagnosis of malaria is more commonly made via lateral flow than microscopy. Their utility was demonstrated in the COVID-19 pandemic. Urine *Legionella* antigen is useful for Legionnaire's disease, although not 100% sensitive.
- **Computerized identification**: use of matrix-assisted laser desorption/ionization (MALDI) combined with mass spectrometry has led to faster microbiological identification. Once a colony has grown, the signature from ionization of the organism is compared with a database of known organisms. Automated systems now use colorimetry to compare the growth of unknown organisms against a battery of different antibiotics. They decrease the time it takes from culture to identification of its species and antibiotic susceptibility to just a few hours, and are highly accurate.

Imaging

- **Chest X-rays** can show focal lesions, which are undetectable clinically, and are mandatory in those suspected of having an infection in whom the source is not readily apparent.
- **Abdominal and pelvic ultrasonography** may detect hepatic lesions, identify abdominal nodes and locate intra-abdominal or pelvic abscesses as a source of fever or bacteraemia.
- **Computed tomography** (CT) scans examine all regions of the body in a search for, or to delineate the extent of, infection. They are a useful early investigation in febrile patients with presumed but unidentified infections, and may identify a source in patients who are bacteraemic with gastrointestinal pathogens. CT also allows for diagnostic sampling and therapeutic drainage.
- **Magnetic resonance imaging** (MRI) is used in the diagnosis of soft tissue and bony/joint infections. X-rays may identify bone changes from long-standing infection but MRI is more sensitive.
- **Nuclear imaging**: white cell scans are rarely useful because they do not distinguish acute inflammation from infection, nor detect chronic low-grade infections caused by parasites, viruses, mycobacteria or fungi. They are sometimes helpful in identification of the site of pyogenic inflammation.
- **Positron emission tomography** is functional imaging using a radiolabelled glucose (fluorodeoxyglucose [FDG]) which is taken up by metabolically active tissues. This information is then mapped onto a CT done simultaneously. Its main use is for identification of metastases but it can occasionally help in fevers of unknown origin and occult sources of infection.
- **Cardiac ultrasonography** in suspected bacterial endocarditis, to look for vegetations and assess valve function. In bacteraemia/septicaemia by *Staphylococcus aureus*, early cardiac ultrasonography is mandatory to identify features of endocarditis. Transoesophageal study is more sensitive than the transthoracic approach, especially where echo windows are suboptimal (see Chapter 93).

43 An approach to the patient with fever of short duration

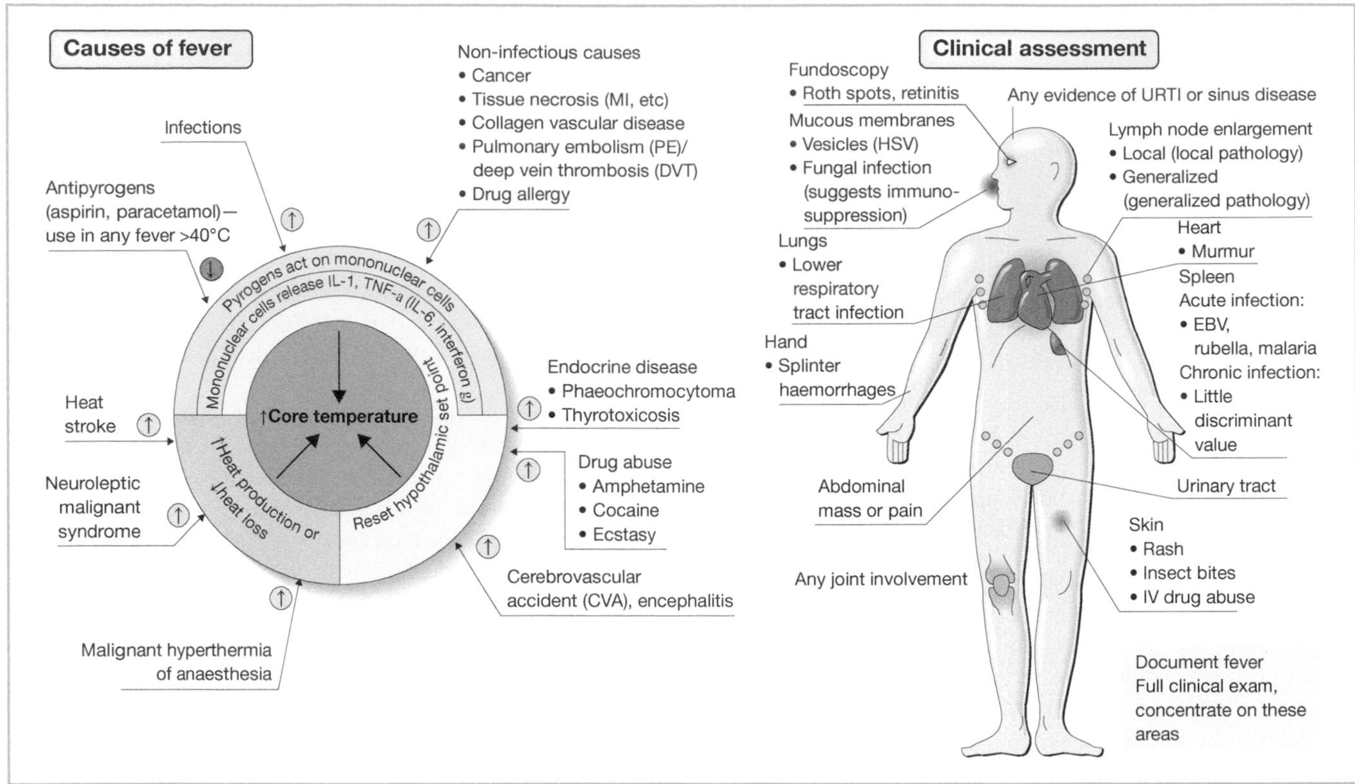

Fever

Fever is a physiological response where the body temperature is increased due to re-setting of the normal hypothalamic set point. Normal body temperature varies considerably between individuals (oral range, 36.0–37.7 °C) and varies diurnally (peaks in evening, troughs in early morning).

Fever is a strong clue to infection but it can be absent, even with significant infection, in patients who are frail, immunosuppressed or have fallen and been on the floor for a significant period. In overwhelming sepsis, the temperature can be normal or even low (a poor prognostic sign).

Hyperthermia

Hyperthermia is an elevated body temperature above the hypothalamic set point. It occurs when there is excessive heat production, reduced heat loss or hypothalamic damage. Temperatures >41 °C are rarely the result of infections and usually imply loss of thermoregulation.

Pathogenesis of fever

Fever is produced by the effect of exogenous pyrogens which trigger cytokine and prostaglandin release. Infectious agents and their breakdown products or toxins are the most common triggers of fever. Other molecules, such as immune complexes and lymphocyte products, can also elicit a febrile response. These are the basis of fever in malignancy, drug reactions and connective tissue disorders.

Assessment of the patient with fever

Firstly – could it be sepsis (severe infection with worsening organ function)?

This concern is addressed by rapid assessment of vital signs, alertness and overall appearance (?cyanosis, rash), and whether carers/relatives are concerned. If sepsis is suspected, the patient should rapidly receive intravenous antibiotics (after blood cultures),

Medicine at a Glance, Fifth Edition. Edited by Patrick Davey and Alex Pitcher.

Companion website: www.wiley.com/go/medicine5e

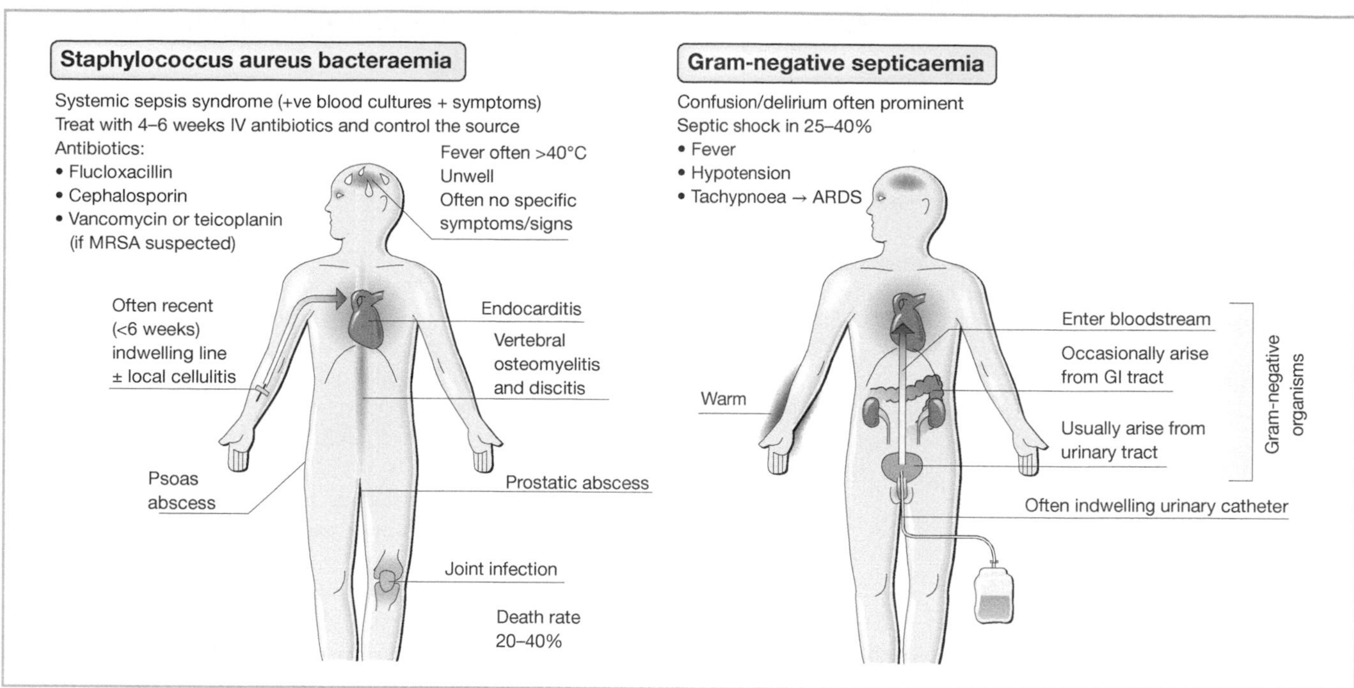

oxygen and intravenous fluid, alongside appropriate monitoring. In the UK, these actions are termed the 'Sepsis 6' and should be carried out within an hour of presentation. Evidence of organ dysfunction (kidney, lung, etc.) suggests urgent need for intensive care (mechanical ventilation, blood pressure support). See also Chapter 164.

It is always worth remembering that younger patients with no co-morbidities, and therefore a large physiological reserve, may only present to hospital with life-threatening sepsis, or downstream complications of infections such as endocarditis.

Comprehensive history and examination are essential for establishing the site and type of infection and its mode of acquisition.

History of presenting complaint

- Symptoms arising from a particular organ are usually reliable guides to the site of infection. Non-specific symptoms (e.g. fever, muscular aches) may occur in generalized infection (septicaemia, viraemia).
- Duration (acute vs chronic) and fever pattern may provide diagnostic clues.
- Rigors are uncommon in non-infective causes of fever and are often seen with urinary/biliary tract sepsis and cellulitis as well as malaria.
- Weight loss occurs in most chronic infections (notably tuberculosis, endocarditis, intra-abdominal abscesses).

Exposure history

This involves exploring all possible exposures resulting from the patient's home circumstances, occupation, leisure and travel (see Chapter 45). Inhalation of soil or compost dust, and use of an air humidifier are risk factors for Legionnaire's disease while recreational or occupational exposure to fresh water or sewage can lead to leptospirosis. It is important to ask about pets (focusing on scratches and bites or licking of broken skin) as well as exposure to farm or wild animals (including birds).

In patients with recent travel, there may be a history of bites from specific vectors (mosquitoes, ticks, flies) or noteworthy leisure activities (hiking, caving). Other areas of enquiry should include diet (?consumption of raw or undercooked meat, unpasteurized milk products) as well as sexual history and injection of intravenous drugs.

Drug history

Patients receiving chemotherapy may have neutropenic sepsis and require urgent broad-spectrum antibiotics (after blood cultures but before other investigations; see Chapter 42). Patients on transplant immunosuppressants, 'biologics' such as rituximab, or cytotoxics such as cyclophosphamide are susceptible to more severe infections as well as opportunistic infections, requiring a high index of suspicion (e.g. PCP, CMV). Chronic opiate use is associated with increased incidence of severe infection, and may lead to reduced awareness of symptoms. It is also important to ask about recreational drugs; in addition, tri-iodothyronine taken in a body-building programme can cause fever and tachycardia.

Recently prescribed medication and herbal or traditional remedies may occasionally cause fever. Previous antimicrobial treatment may modify clinical presentation or make isolation of an organism difficult.

Past medical history

- Does the patient have a long-term condition predisposing to infection (see Chapter 172)?
- **Immunosuppressive** conditions include HIV, chronic leukaemia (CLL, CML) and immunosuppressive medication (associated with transplant, immune-mediated inflammatory disorder or cancer).
- In **vulnerable groups** the nature of infection and its severity can be harder to recognize in people with learning disability or dementia. Patients with reduced sensation (e.g. spina bifida, spinal cord injury) may have no localizing symptoms and severe

illnesses such as appendicitis or musculoskeletal infection may only be recognized late, with severe consequences. Lymphoedema predisposes to cellulitis which can initially present with fever without obvious skin manifestations.

- Does the patient have a **prosthetic implant**, vascular line or urinary catheter? Infection of prosthetic valves, pacemakers, joints, CSF shunts, etc. may not present in the same way as infections in native structures.
- Immunization and transfusion history are relevant when considering respiratory viruses, travel-related infection and blood-borne viruses.

Family history

If close contacts have also been unwell recently, this may suggest person-to-person transmission. History of infection in family may also suggest hereditary immune defects.

Examination

A comprehensive clinical examination is also vital not only to provide information on where infection is established but also to understand the portal of entry (e.g. skin breaks, dentition). While examination should naturally take into account diagnoses suggested by the history, symptoms can sometimes be subtle or non-localized (e.g. endocarditis) so certain items of the examination should always be carried out.

Investigations

Routine investigations, discussed in detail in Chapter 42, include the following.

- Blood cultures: critical in suspected sepsis (prior to antibiotics), or where initial clinical assessment and immediate investigations have failed to identify a clear site of infection such as pneumonia or urinary tract infection (making endocarditis or deep-seated infection more likely).
- Midstream urine cultures (see also Chapter 154); note that positive cultures from long-term urinary catheters usually identify colonizing, not infecting, organisms.
- FBC, renal and liver function, lactate, glucose, CRP.
- Chest X-ray.
- Throat swab (see Chapter 42).
- Serological tests (HIV testing should be undertaken routinely in all patients presenting with fever).
- According to clinical progress and results of the above, ultrasonography and cross-sectional imaging via CT; these can also be used to guide aspiration/biopsy of abscesses or abnormal organs.
- Most positive blood cultures 'flag' within 24 hours. *Staphylococcus aureus* and Gram-negative rods make up a relatively high proportion of positive cultures; if either is found, the patient should be carefully re-evaluated clinically and via imaging to assess the likely source. For most other positive cultures, the organism identified often provides a strong clue to the site of infection, e.g. *Enterococcus* and viridans streptococci suggest endocarditis, β-haemolytic streptococci suggest throat or soft tissue infection.
- If clinical assessment and early investigations do not reveal a cause, take a wide view. Stop all unnecessary drugs, culture all possible sites frequently, and consider causes of fever other than infection.

Non-infective causes of fever in acutely unwell patients

- **Alcohol withdrawal, drug abuse** (amphetamines, ecstasy, cocaine)
- **Status epilepticus**
- **Phaeochromocytoma** and **thyrotoxicosis** (endogenous or via exogenous thyroid
- **Neuroleptic malignant syndrome**: a rare idiosyncratic reaction to antipsychotic agents, promoted by intercurrent illness or dehydration
- **Heat stroke**: a result of exercise and/or when individuals are unable to lose heat sufficiently quickly; associated with dehydration, alcohol misuse and psychotropic medications. Patients present with sudden-onset delirium, rapidly progressing to coma. Core temperature is >41°C; sweating may or may not be present. Extreme tachycardia and hyperventilation are common. Pulmonary oedema with shock and multiorgan failure occurs in advanced cases. The diagnosis is clinical, supported by finding elevated muscle enzymes. Treatment involves removing the patient from the hot environment and giving cool fluids, either sprayed on the skin to encourage heat loss or given intravenously. Specific organ support may be needed.

Infective causes

Staphylococcus aureus

Patients are usually acutely unwell with high fevers and rigors. The mortality rate is 20–30%. Proven staphylococcal bacteraemia requires prolonged (2–6 weeks) intravenous (IV) antibiotic therapy to prevent metastatic infection, especially acute bacterial endocarditis and bone/joint infections, or pulmonary, cerebral and spinal/paraspinal abscesses.

Repeated blood cultures ('clearance' cultures) are required to prove that the organism has disappeared from the bloodstream. Persisting blood culture positivity despite appropriate antibiotic therapy indicates an ongoing source of infection and necessitates urgent and thorough imaging to detect the source and intervention to remove/control it (see Chapter 42).

Gram-negative organisms, particularly *Escherichia coli*, *Pseudomonas* and *Klebsiella* species

These usually arise from the urinary or gastrointestinal (GI) tracts. Around 25–40% of Gram-negative bacteraemias are associated with shock, with a mortality rate of 25%. In addition to fever, chills and hypotension, the earliest sign is often tachypnoea and adult respiratory distress syndrome (ARDS) may develop (see Chapter 120). Mental signs (confusion, delirium) may be prominent. Therapy involves antibiotics, supportive measures, and identification and drainage of any collection.

Specific conditions that should not be missed

These conditions (Table 43.1) should be considered *proactively*. Patients with these conditions do not present with classic 'sepsis' – indeed patients suffering from them can 'look well' – and so a high index of suspicion is needed to diagnose them early.

Table 43.1 Conditions to be considered proactively.

Infection	Clinical clues	Key investigations	Notes
Infective endocarditis	Continuous fever in the absence of clear focus, heart murmur	Blood cultures	With high suspicion, consider admission to allow repeated blood cultures, even if the patient looks well
PCP	Subacute, steadily worsening respiratory symptoms (cough, breathlessness on exertion), weight loss	HIV testing CT chest Bronchoscopy	Start PCP treatment if it is suspected, before awaiting confirmation from respiratory samples
TB meningitis	Subacute onset of headache and fever, epidemiological risk of TB	Lumbar puncture (usually after CT brain)	
HSV keratitis	Painful red eye with reduced visual acuity, immunosuppression	Slit-lamp examination	
Diabetic foot infection	Diabetes, peripheral neuropathy	Early discussion with podiatry, vascular/orthopaedic surgery	
Necrotizing fasciitis	Portal of entry, immunosuppression	Early discussion with plastic surgery	

44 Healthcare-associated infections

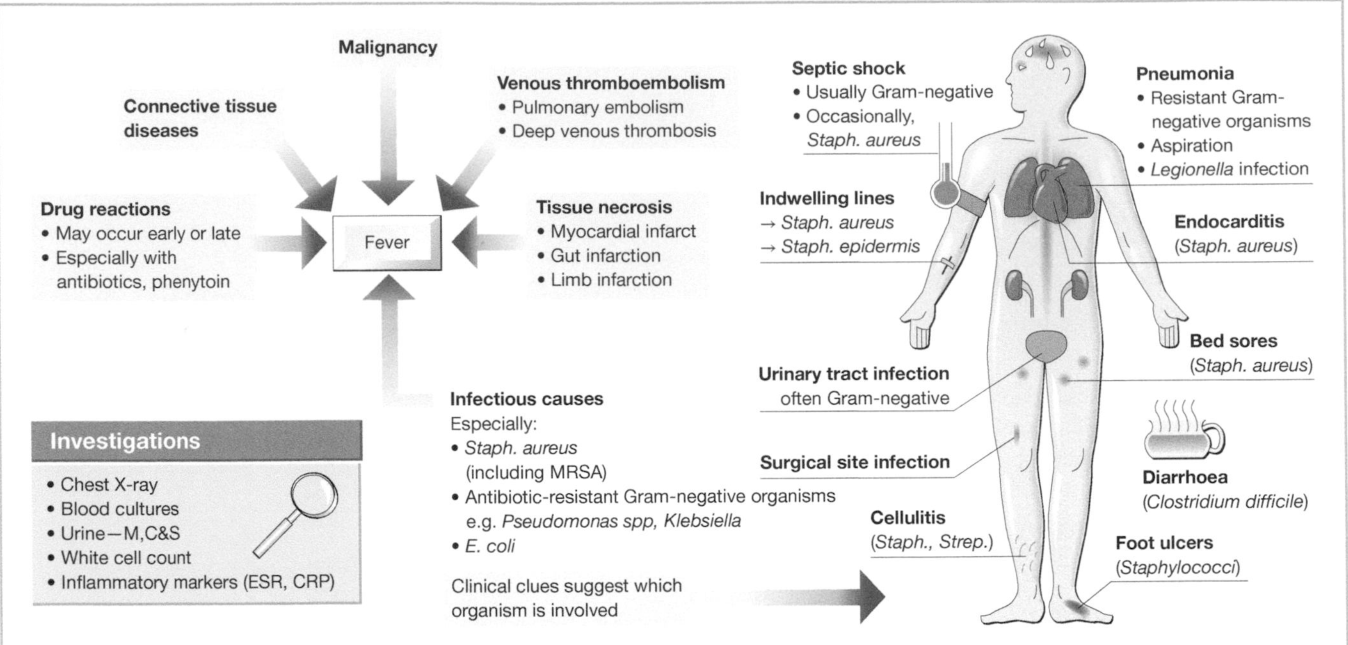

Healthcare-associated infections (HCAIs) (also termed nosocomial) are infections occurring in a healthcare setting that were not present prior to a patient entering that care setting. In the UK, the incidence of HCAI in acute hospitals is around 5%, resulting in several hundred thousand HCAIs each year and thousands of deaths. Important factors underlying this figure are:

- treatments or underlying conditions associated with decreased immunity
- procedures and care interfering with the body's natural defences, e.g. surgical procedures, intravascular lines, urinary catheters, endotracheal tubes
- prolonged or repeated admissions
- exposure to specific infectious agents (e.g. respiratory viruses, *C. difficile*)
- initial or previous treatment with antibiotics; this selects for organisms that are more challenging to eradicate because they are resistant or associated with devices (see below).

Nosocomial fever

This may be infectious or non-infectious in origin.

Common infections in hospital patients

- **Respiratory tract** including COVID-19, influenza and hospital-acquired pneumonia. Prolonged ventilation on ICU is associated with pneumonia caused by a wide range of bacterial pathogens and fungi (*Candida* and *Aspergillus* spp.).
- **Urinary tract** infection, often catheter-associated, with Gram-negative organisms.
- **Intravascular line infection** with bacteraemia or candidaemia. Complications such as septic thrombophlebitis or endocarditis or metastatic infection may occur. With some positive blood cultures (e.g. coagulase-negative staphylococci) it is important to determine if the isolate is a true pathogen or skin flora; repeated blood cultures growing one organism suggest a true infection. Alongside antibiotic administration, removal of infected catheters is a priority (achieving 'source control'), but precious semi-permanent lines (e.g. dialysis, Hickman lines) can sometimes be 'salvaged' with antibiotics if the patient is stable, the organism is amenable and there is no evidence of tunnel/exit site infection.
- **Surgical wound** or intra-abdominal sepsis (may not always present with obvious signs).
- ***Clostridium difficile* diarrhoea**: this carries a significant mortality and prolongs hospital stay by up to 20 days. Those most commonly affected are:
    - the immunosuppressed and the elderly
    - those treated with broad-spectrum antibiotics, particularly cephalosporins
    - patients taking proton pump inhibitors.
- Diagnosis is by finding *C. difficile* toxin in the stool. Treatment is fluids and oral vancomycin or metronidazole; 10–20% relapse after treatment.

Medicine at a Glance, Fifth Edition. Edited by Patrick Davey and Alex Pitcher.

Companion website: www.wiley.com/go/medicine5e

- **Norovirus** with vomiting and diarrhoea: treatment is supportive but effective case recognition and isolation are important to protect other vulnerable patients in healthcare settings.

Common non-infectious causes

- Drug fever.
- Venous thromboembolism (deep venous thrombosis or pulmonary embolism), resolving haematoma.
- Myocardial infarction and infarction of other tissue (particularly intestinal).
- Local hypothalamic damage: cerebrovascular accidents, head injury, encephalitis and hypothalamic surgery.

Clinical assessment

- Assessment of immune status.
- History of recent surgical or invasive procedures.
- Examination of lines and catheters.
- Check on new medications and antibiotic therapy.
- Crucial investigations: white cell count, chest X-ray, urinalysis, urine and blood cultures. Other tests are determined by clinical findings. If diarrhoea is present, *C. difficile* toxin should be assayed.

Significant infection can occur in the absence of fever, particularly in elderly patients or those with renal or hepatic disease. Infection should be considered in any patient with changes in clinical state (pulse, blood pressure, mental state).

Antimicrobial resistance (AMR)

Use of antibiotics leads to selection of organisms that are intrinsically resistant to commonly used antimicrobials or acquire resistance through genetic mechanisms. Patients may acquire such infections following their own treatment or from other patients. These infections are more challenging to treat (see Table 44.1), and infection control measures to screen for and isolate 'carriers' are vital to prevent spread within healthcare settings.

Common AMR infections include the following.

- Methicillin-resistant *S. aureus* (MRSA): no more virulent than methicillin-sensitive strains of *S. aureus* (MSSA), but treatment is more complex. Asymptomatic MRSA skin colonization can be treated via topical decontamination.
- Extended-spectrum β-lactamase (ESBL)-producing bacteria: resistant to most penicillins and cephalosporins so treatment commonly requires carbapenems (e.g. ertapenem, meropenem).
- Carbapenemase-expressing Enterobacteriaceae (CPE): relatively less common but very challenging to treat if deep-seated infection becomes established.

Fever in the neutropenic patient

This is common after chemotherapy for haematological or other malignancies. It is defined as a temperature of greater than 38°C or any symptoms and/or signs of sepsis, in a person with an absolute neutrophil count of 0.5 x 10^9/L or lower. Infection is only proven in 50–60% of patients. Drug- and transfusion-related fevers should be considered. The likelihood and seriousness of infection are increased by the duration and severity of neutropenia.

Special attention should be paid to the common sites of infection: skin, lungs, perioral and pharynx, and perianal area.

Signs of inflammation may be subtle; the absence of neutrophils means that the inflammatory response is blunted. Classic signs of infection (e.g. erythema and induration or an infiltrate on a chest X-ray) may not occur. Bacteraemia may occur in the absence of an obvious source.

Profound or prolonged neutropenia and fever unresponsive to broad-spectrum antibiotics for more than one week increase the likelihood of fungal infection.

Empirical antibiotic regimens are required in all febrile neutropenic patients as a result of the high mortality in this group. Monotherapy (meropenem) or dual therapy (aminoglycoside and antipseudomonal penicillin) is equally effective.

Vancomycin should be considered in the MRSA-colonized patient, if serious line-related sepsis is suspected, or if prophylaxis against Gram-negative organisms has been used (e.g. ciprofloxacin).

If there is no response, consider:

- changing antibiotics (e.g. adding vancomycin)
- further investigation for rarer causes of fever (herpes simplex virus, cytomegalovirus, *Toxoplasma* spp.)
- adding antifungal therapy, particularly if no response by 5–7 days
- using drugs to increase white cell numbers such as growth colony-stimulating factor.

Table 44.1 Simplified 'antibiogram' showing typical antimicrobial activity against common HCAIs.

	MSSA	MRSA	Enterobacteriaceae (*E. coli, Klebsiella*)	ESBL	CPE	Pseudomonas
Co-amoxiclav, ceftriaxone	+	–	+	–	–	–
Vancomycin	+	+	–	–	–	–
Ertapenem	+	–	+	+	–	–
Meropenem, piperacillin-tazobactam	+	–	+	+	–	+

45 Fever of unknown origin

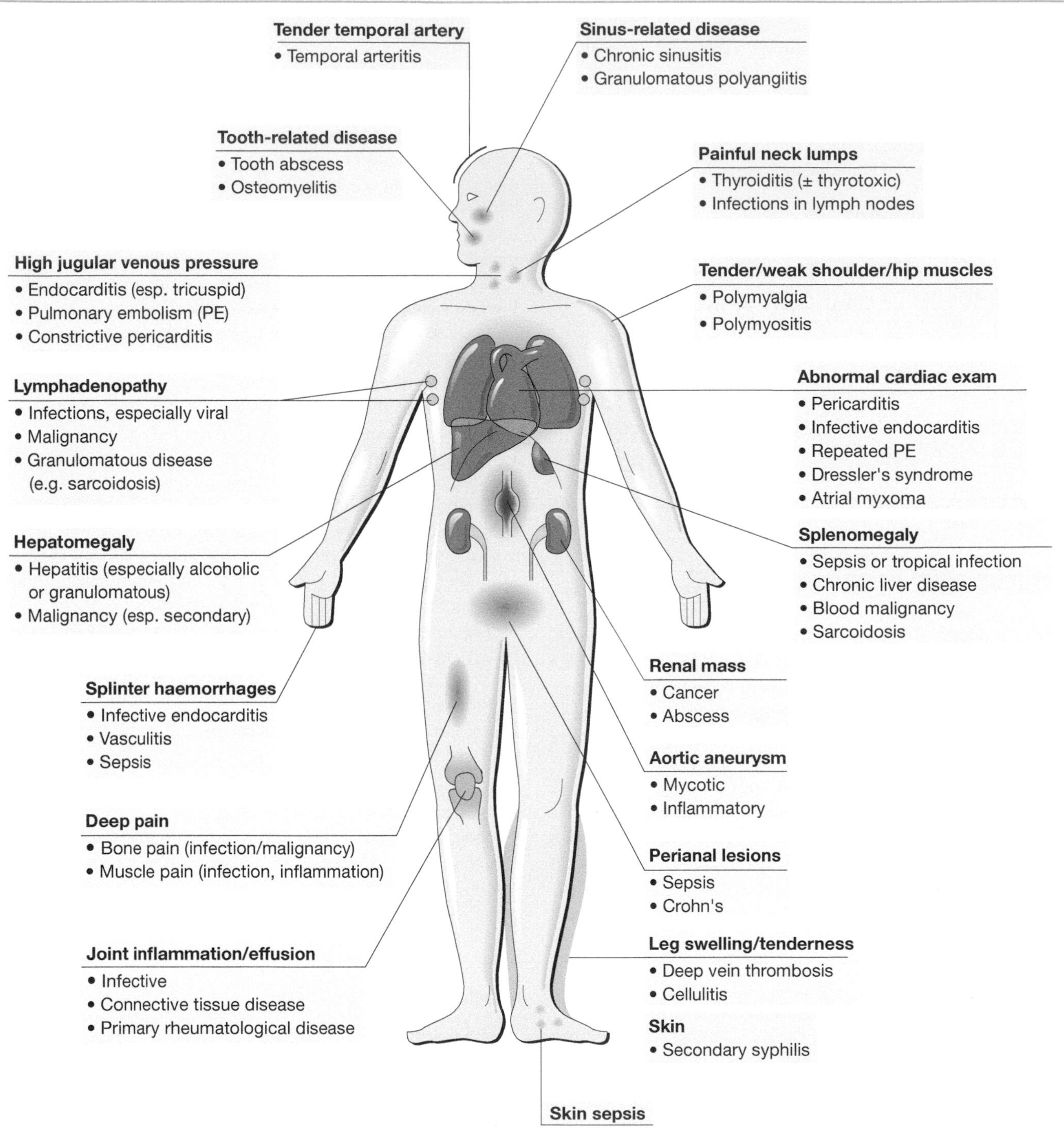

Medicine at a Glance, Fifth Edition. Edited by Patrick Davey and Alex Pitcher.

Companion website: www.wiley.com/go/medicine5e

Most patients presenting with fever have a short-lived acute illness, which is rapidly diagnosed. Persisting fever in the face of initial negative investigations is termed 'fever (pyrexia) of unknown origin' (FUO). The classic definition of this is a fever of >38.3 °C persisting without diagnosis for three weeks including one week's investigation in hospital. Most clinicians have modified this definition in the face of an increasing number of immunocompromised hosts and more rapid diagnostic facilities. Practically, patients with unexplained fever can be divided into categories defined by their immune status.

- Classic FUO (community acquired).
- FUO in hospital patients (see Chapter 44).
- FUO in neutropenic and immunosuppressed patients (see Chapter 44).
- FUO in HIV patients (see Chapter 47).

Classic fever of unknown origin

This may be caused by many different processes (Table 45.1).

- Infections (25–50%).
- Neoplasms (10–30%).
- Connective tissue/collagen vascular diseases (10–25%).
- Miscellaneous (10–20%).
- Undiagnosed (10–25%).

The relative contribution of different categories depends on the geographical location and the age of the patient: infections are more important in the developing world; neoplasia and connective tissue disorders become more important with increasing age.

Infections

Many different infections are implicated in FUO, but consider:

- systemic infections that are difficult to diagnose, e.g. disseminated mycobacterial disease, culture-negative endocarditis

Table 45.1 The most common causes of FUO.

Infections
• Abscess
• Mycobacteria
• Endocarditis
Neoplasms
• Lymphoma
• Solid tumours (gastrointestinal tract, liver, renal cell, sarcoma)
• Leukaemias
• Other haematological tumours
Connective tissue disease
• Temporal arteritis/polymyalgia rheumatica
• Polyarteritis nodosa
• Systemic lupus erythematosus
• Adult Still disease

- localized infections and abscesses where the normal inflammatory or immune response is not able to clear organisms, but the diagnosis is difficult because bacteraemia may not occur.

Neoplasms

The majority of neoplasms producing FUO are haematological: fever may precede the appearance of lymphadenopathy in lymphoma. In older patients, consider solid tumours, particularly occult gastrointestinal-related neoplasms, such as in the pancreas. In women, ovarian cancer should be excluded.

Connective tissue diseases

Adult Still's disease, the most common cause, is essentially a diagnosis of exclusion. It typically causes myalgia, lymphadenopathy and splenomegaly in addition to fever. In elderly patients, temporal arteritis/polymyalgia rheumatica and associated large vessel vasculitis and sometimes aortitis are common, accounting for up to 20% of FUO presentations, but classic temporal artery tenderness and an extremely high erythrocyte sedimentation rate (ESR) do not always occur. A PET CT can be considered. If other investigations have not been productive, a temporal artery ultrasound or temporal artery biopsy should be considered.

Miscellaneous

- Drug fever: can occur with many drugs, particularly antibiotics and anticonvulsants. Eosinophilia and a rash are suggestive of the diagnosis.
- Pulmonary embolism (PE): occasionally, repeated PEs cause fever. Breathlessness with a clear chest X-ray should raise the possibility, which can be pursued with a CT pulmonary angiogram scan or a $\dot{V}/\dot{Q}$ (ventilation/perfusion) scan. The lactate dehydrogenase is often raised in this situation.
- Abnormal liver function tests may reflect a hepatological process, but may also be a non-specific response to systemic disease, particularly sepsis.
- Habitual hyperthermia: the hypothalamic set point may be high – exaggerated diurnal variations in temperature may occur. This is of no pathological significance.
- Rare genetic syndromes including familial Mediterranean fever. A family history may give clues, as may chronicity with complete recovery between episodes.
- Factitious fever, either as a result of inaccurate measurement or associated with psychiatric disorder.

Approach to diagnosis

A comprehensive history and examination are crucial. Establish whether a fever is truly present (a significant proportion of patients have no documented fever at all). The fever pattern may occasionally help. Look for signs accompanying the fever (flushing, sweats, tachycardia, etc.). Determine whether the patient is unwell and whether stable or deteriorating. Stop all non-essential drugs.

Investigations (see Chapter 42 for details)

Bloods: ESR and/or C-reactive protein (CRP), renal and liver function including albumin, serial blood cultures (off antibiotics), HIV and syphilis serology, immunoglobulins and autoantibody screen (antineutrophil cytoplasmic antibody, antinuclear antibody, rheumatoid factor, complement). Specific blood cultures for brucellosis, other fastidious organisms and mycobacteria should be taken according to epidemiological risk.

Urinalysis: microscopic haematuria might suggest glomerulonephritis (potentially associated with infective endocarditis) or renal cell carcinoma, while sterile pyuria suggests tuberculosis, in which case send early morning urine samples for mycobacterial culture, particularly if there is a significant epidemiological risk of tuberculosis.

Imaging: Contrast-enhanced CT scan of the chest, abdomen and pelvis, even in the absence of localizing features, is increasingly used early in the diagnostic process as it may demonstrate occult abscesses and lymph nodes, silent infarcts of the spleen and kidney (relevant to the diagnosis of endocarditis) or evidence of malignancy.

CT PET scanning is useful in diagnosis of large-vessel vasculitis and a range of occult processes. Patients need to be mobile.

Echocardiography to look for vegetations or pericardial abnormalities; if transthoracic echocardiography is unrevealing, a transoesophageal study should be considered.

Tissue biopsy should be aggressively pursued, especially if any organ-specific abnormality is identified. Liver, skin, temporal artery, lymph node and bone marrow biopsy can all be helpful. Imaging can guide the choice of site for deep lymph node biopsy via radiological or (occasionally) laparoscopic approaches. Care should be taken not to place all tissue samples in formalin (for histology) but reserve a portion for microbiological (mycobacterial and fungal) culture in parallel. The presence of granulomas on histology indicates the need for special stains for mycobacteria and fungi. TB-PCR on samples can provide relatively rapid diagnosis (see Chapter 170).

CT brain and lumbar puncture (if any neurological symptoms, including headache) with molecular testing of CSF if there is a significant degree of meningitis.

Diagnostic trials of therapy

- **Antibiotics**: broad-spectrum antibiotics may be indicated if the patient is deteriorating or culture-negative endocarditis is suspected.
- **Antimycobacterial therapy**: a trial of anti-tuberculosis (anti-TB) therapy, after obtaining appropriate specimens for culture, can be justified if the clinical suspicion is high because TB culture confirmation may take several weeks. Defervescence and an increase in weight are good signs of response to anti-TB therapy. Some anti-TB drugs have broad-spectrum antibacterial activity.
- **Corticosteroids**: treatment should only be commenced with the involvement of a relevant specialist physician, typically a rheumatologist. Rapid improvement is expected in temporal arteritis/polymyalgia rheumatica syndrome and adult-onset Still's disease. Systematic efforts must have been made to exclude infection and malignancy via the above investigations, and the fever and ESR/CRP response followed. An initial response does not always prove a non-infectious aetiology; steroid therapy will blunt fevers caused by some infections and may improve systemic symptoms resulting from malignancy and many other conditions.

In 5–15% of patients, no cause is found despite extensive investigation. Undiagnosed patients who remain well (no weight loss, stable albumin levels) can be observed. The outcome in this group is extremely good; fever will often spontaneously remit.

46 Fever and rash

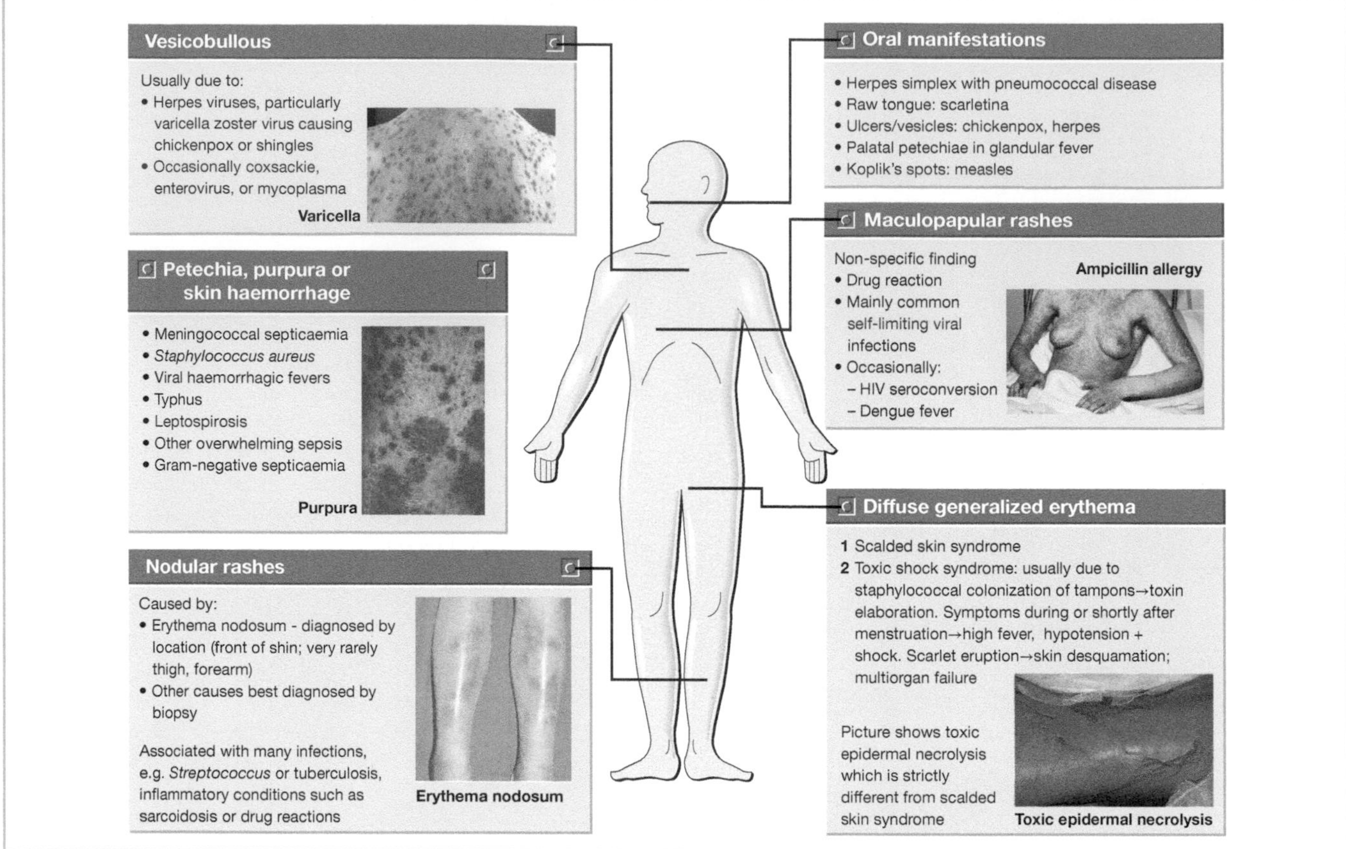
Vesicobullous
Usually due to:
• Herpes viruses, particularly varicella zoster virus causing chickenpox or shingles
• Occasionally coxsackie, enterovirus, or mycoplasma
Varicella
Petechia, purpura or skin haemorrhage
• Meningococcal septicaemia
• Staphylococcus aureus
• Viral haemorrhagic fevers
• Typhus
• Leptospirosis
• Other overwhelming sepsis
• Gram-negative septicaemia
Purpura
Nodular rashes
Caused by:
• Erythema nodosum - diagnosed by location (front of shin; very rarely thigh, forearm)
• Other causes best diagnosed by biopsy
Associated with many infections, e.g. Streptococcus or tuberculosis, inflammatory conditions such as sarcoidosis or drug reactions
Erythema nodosum
Oral manifestations
• Herpes simplex with pneumococcal disease
• Raw tongue: scarletina
• Ulcers/vesicles: chickenpox, herpes
• Palatal petechiae in glandular fever
• Koplik's spots: measles
Maculopapular rashes
Non-specific finding
• Drug reaction
• Mainly common self-limiting viral infections
• Occasionally:
– HIV seroconversion
– Dengue fever
Ampicillin allergy
Diffuse generalized erythema
1 Scalded skin syndrome
2 Toxic shock syndrome: usually due to staphylococcal colonization of tampons→toxin elaboration. Symptoms during or shortly after menstruation→high fever, hypotension + shock. Scarlet eruption→skin desquamation; multiorgan failure
Picture shows toxic epidermal necrolysis which is strictly different from scalded skin syndrome
Toxic epidermal necrolysis

Patients with fever and a rash are challenging; it is vital to identify those with acute bacterial sepsis who require prompt antimicrobial therapy. Although fever and a rash are most commonly caused by an infection, other processes produce similar clinical syndromes.

- Drug reactions.
- Vasculitis (see Chapter 220).

Some rashes are instantly recognizable; others require a systematic approach for diagnosis. Atypical features of a common disease (e.g. appearance modified by an impaired host immune system) are more likely than rare diseases. Factors that are helpful in diagnosis include:

- time relationship of fever to rash
- drug history
- the presence of mucosal lesions or conjunctivitis, lymphadenopathy or hepatosplenomegaly, arthropathy.

In addition to standard investigations and blood cultures, the following may be helpful.

- Aspiration of lesions allows Gram smear and culture of organisms in meningococcal, staphylococcal, pseudomonal or systemic fungal infections.
- Punch biopsy may reveal organisms, particularly in fungal infections, or demonstrate specific histological features.
- Polymerase chain reaction (PCR) of body fluids for identification of viruses, including:
  - vesicle fluid: herpes simplex and zoster infection
  - blood: acute viraemias including viral haemorrhagic fevers
  - urine: measles
  - stool: enterovirus.

Diffuse erythema

Diffuse erythema is the term given to a widespread reddening of the skin. Scarlet fever, caused by a group A streptococci, used to be a common cause of a diffuse blanching erythema. Drug eruptions are currently an important cause of fever with diffuse erythema. Important infective causes that should be excluded include the following.

- **Toxic shock syndrome**, caused by *Staphylococcus* or *Streptococcus* spp., produces generalized erythema, and later desquamation with multiorgan involvement.
- **Scalded skin syndrome** in children, from staphylococcal toxin, produces diffuse erythema, bulla formation and exfoliation.

Vesiculo-bullous rashes

Vesicles are small fluid-filled blisters, whereas bullae are larger fluid-filled blisters. Varicella zoster infection has two manifestations with vesiculo-bullous rashes.

Medicine at a Glance, Fifth Edition. Edited by Patrick Davey and Alex Pitcher.

Companion website: www.wiley.com/go/medicine5e

- **Varicella** (chickenpox): vesicles produced on a halo of erythema, initially clear and then cloudy. There is successive cropping.
- **Zoster** (shingles): a dermatomal distribution is found, initially maculopapular, then vesicles, bullae and crusting. The rash may be preceded by pain in the same area. Lesions outside the affected dermatome occur in 5% of the immunocompetent and in the immunocompromised.

Rarer causes of vesiculo-bullous rashes are as follows.

- **Disseminated herpes simplex**: may occur from labial/genital lesions with considerable systemic upset in those with eczema or those who are immunocompromised.
- **Hand–foot–mouth** (Coxsackie virus or enteroviruses): small vesicles in the mouth, and on the hands and feet.
- **Bullous erythema multiforma**: classically *Mycoplasma* and herpes simplex infections; many other agents implicated.
- **Staphylococcal infections**: bullous impetigo.

Petechial–purpuric rashes

Bleeding into the skin has a number of terms – petechiae are small bleeds into the skin, <1–2 mm in diameter, whereas purpura describes larger areas of bleeding into the skin (>2 mm in diameter). Skin bleeds larger than about 4 mm are termed ecchymoses.

The key purpuric rash to diagnose in acutely sick patients is **meningococcaemia**, which produces a spectrum of rashes from isolated petechiae to multiple purpuric lesions, confluent over the body, associated with complete haemostatic failure and a very high mortality. **Gonococcaemia** typically produces pustular lesions and arthritis, and more rarely mild purpuric rashes; haemostatic failure is unusual and mortality is very low.

Other causes of petechial-purpuric rashes include the following.

- **Staphylococcal endocarditis**: petechiae and purpura may occur, usually immune complex mediated – a 'vasculitic rash'.
- **Disseminated intravascular coagulation** occurs in many severe infections – an important diagnostic clue is spontaneous haemorrhage from old venepuncture sites.
- **Leptospirosis**: conjunctival haemorrhage is common but skin haemorrhage only occasionally develops in those patients who are very unwell.
- **Viral haemorrhagic fevers**: haemorrhages may occur in Lassa, Ebola and Marburg and yellow fever; these patients are very unwell, often jaundiced and very likely to die.
- Petechiae are common in severe dengue infection (**dengue haemorrhagic fever**).

Maculopapular rashes

Macular rashes can be seen but cannot be felt, i.e. they do not cause any bumps on the skin. The individual spots are usually small, often only a few millimetres in diameter. Papular rashes can be seen and felt, i.e. there are spots a few millimetres in diameter, which cause raised lumps on the skin surface. These rashes are extremely common and can be produced by many pathogens.

Viral infections

These are the most common cause. Although **rubella** (German measles) and **measles** both produce rashes starting on the face, spreading to the trunk, they differ in that, in rubella, the rash is of discrete pink macules, whereas in measles it is maculopapular with lesions (Koplik spots) in the mouth. Other common childhood viral rashes are the result of **enteroviruses** (diarrhoea and a rash) and **parvovirus** ('slapped cheeks' syndrome). Rarer causes include:

- **acute human immunodeficiency virus (HIV) infection**: macules, papules or urticaria
- **dengue** (uncomplicated): classically, a transitory rash followed by generalized maculopapular rash in the second febrile phase.

Rickettsial infections

Maculopapular rashes occur in most rickettsial infections, and an eschar (focal necrosis at the site of the antecedent tick bite) is present in infection by some species.

Mycoplasma and chlamydial infections

These infections may cause maculopapular rashes.

Bacterial infections/spirochaetal

- **Secondary syphilis**: macules that may become papular or pustular. There are erosions on the oral mucosa and condylomata lata in intertriginous areas.
- **Leptospirosis**: macules, papules or petechiae occur.
- **Meningococcaemia**: initial lesions may be macules before classic petechiae/purpura.

Nodular lesions

Nodular lesions are seen and can be very easily felt – they differ from papules in that they are larger (and often far fewer in number).

The most common nodular lesion is erythema nodosum (EN), an inflammation of small blood vessels in the deep dermis (a panniculitis), usually on the anterior aspect of the lower leg. EN is often preceded or accompanied by systemic upset (fever and malaise) and sometimes with arthralgia. Lesions never scar and normally heal within 2–3 weeks – much longer and other diagnoses should be sought. Common causes for EN in the UK are streptococcal infections, sarcoidosis, inflammatory bowel disease. Worldwide causes commonly include tuberculosis (TB) and leprosy and, rarely, *Yersinia* spp., hepatitis C, *Histoplasma* and *Coccidioides* spp.

Other nodular rashes are caused by:

- **disseminated fungal infections**, usually in immunocompromised individuals, most commonly with *Candida*, *Histoplasma* or *Cryptococcus* spp.
- **mycobacterial disease**: nodular rashes occur occasionally in disseminated TB or atypical mycobacteria.

Other rashes/lesions of importance

- **Typhoid** characteristically results in rose spots (pink papules on the abdomen).
- **Lyme disease** produces a diagnostic lesion (erythema chronicum migrans); the initial macule develops into large, flat, ring-like lesions.
- ***Pseudomonas aeruginosa*** can cause ecthyma gangrenosum (erythema surrounded by haemorrhages and necrosis) in neutropenic patients.
- **Necrotizing fasciitis**: mild/minimal skin inflammation with pain out of keeping with the clinical signs or rapidly developing skin inflammation should make one consider this diagnosis; it needs urgent management.

Unusual rashes in tropical disease

- **Cutaneous larva migrans**: caused by larvae of the dog or cat hookworm migrating through the skin, resulting in raised, scaly, erythematous serpiginous lesions in skin that is in contact with ground or sand.
- **Calabar swellings**: transient, non-erythematous, pruritic, subcutaneous swellings found in loiasis.
- **Onchocerciasis**: nodules and pruritic papules or urticaria.
- **Strongyloides infection**: urticaria and 'larva currens' (evanescent urticarial wheals).

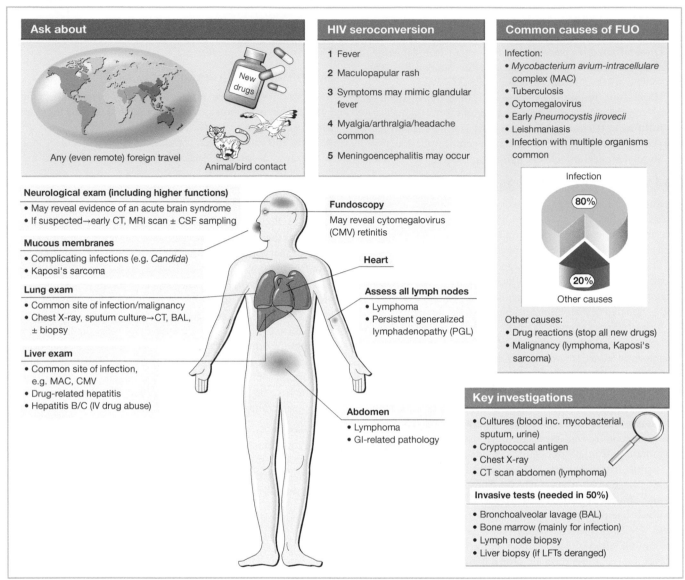

47 Fever in HIV-infected patients

Ask about

Any (even remote) foreign travel

New drugs

Animal/bird contact

HIV seroconversion

1 Fever
2 Maculopapular rash
3 Symptoms may mimic glandular fever
4 Myalgia/arthralgia/headache common
5 Meningoencephalitis may occur

Common causes of FUO

Infection:
- *Mycobacterium avium-intracellulare* complex (MAC)
- Tuberculosis
- Cytomegalovirus
- Early *Pneumocystis jirovecii*
- Leishmaniasis
- Infection with multiple organisms common

Infection 80%
Other causes 20%

Other causes:
- Drug reactions (stop all new drugs)
- Malignancy (lymphoma, Kaposi's sarcoma)

Neurological exam (including higher functions)
- May reveal evidence of an acute brain syndrome
- If suspected→early CT, MRI scan ± CSF sampling

Mucous membranes
- Complicating infections (e.g. *Candida*)
- Kaposi's sarcoma

Lung exam
- Common site of infection/malignancy
- Chest X-ray, sputum culture→CT, BAL, ± biopsy

Liver exam
- Common site of infection, e.g. MAC, CMV
- Drug-related hepatitis
- Hepatitis B/C (IV drug abuse)

Fundoscopy
May reveal cytomegalovirus (CMV) retinitis

Heart

Assess all lymph nodes
- Lymphoma
- Persistent generalized lymphadenopathy (PGL)

Abdomen
- Lymphoma
- GI-related pathology

Key investigations

- Cultures (blood inc. mycobacterial, sputum, urine)
- Cryptococcal antigen
- Chest X-ray
- CT scan abdomen (lymphoma)

Invasive tests (needed in 50%)
- Bronchoalveolar lavage (BAL)
- Bone marrow (mainly for infection)
- Lymph node biopsy
- Liver biopsy (if LFTs deranged)

Fever is common in human immunodeficiency virus (HIV) infections.

- **Early HIV infection**: fever is a common feature of an acute HIV seroconversion reaction. Appropriate testing should be undertaken in patients who present with a fever especially if they have risk factors for HIV infection.
- **Fever in established HIV infection**: fever occurs frequently in all patients with reduced CD4 counts; up to half of patients will present with fever at some point. The source of fever is often obvious on initial investigation and is most commonly the result of either standard or opportunistic infections associated with HIV infection, e.g. bacterial or *Pneumocystis* pneumonia (PCP). However, fever may be difficult to diagnose, particularly in late disease where CD4 counts are extremely low (<50 cells/ml).

Fever of unknown origin (FUO) in HIV-infected patients has been defined as fever >38.3 °C lasting more than four days in hospital or four weeks in outpatients without diagnosis. This usually reflects:

- systemic infection with few localizing signs or symptoms, e.g. *Mycobacterium avium-intracellulare* complex (MAC) infection
- initial stages of an infective process before organ-related signs, e.g. *Pneumocystis jirovecii*, leishmaniasis or cytomegalovirus (CMV) infection

Medicine at a Glance, Fifth Edition. Edited by Patrick Davey and Alex Pitcher.

Companion website: www.wiley.com/go/medicine5e

Table 47.1 Most common infections causing FUO in advanced HIV infection.

- *Mycobacterium avium-intracellulare* complex (MAC)
- *Mycobacterium tuberculosis*
- *Pneumocystis jirovecii* infection (PCP)
- Cytomegalovirus (CMV) end organ disease
- Histoplasmosis
- Leishmaniasis
- HIV infection itself (debated by some)

- a drug reaction: common because of the increased predisposition to drug reactions in HIV and the polypharmacy often associated with the disease
- malignancy, most commonly lymphoma, occasionally Kaposi sarcoma.

In contrast to FUO in other hosts, over 80% of patients will have an infection (see Table 47.1) and up to 20% will have more than one cause for their fever.

History

It is important to assess the stage of HIV infection and degree of immunosuppression, normally measured by the CD4 T-cell count. In earlier stages of HIV with higher CD4 counts (>500 cells/mm^3), infections are usually caused by common organisms and are more easily diagnosed. The profound immunosuppression of advanced HIV disease (CD4 cell counts <100 cells/mm^3) means that fever may be caused by unusual organisms or recrudescence of a previously latent infection. A history of potential exposure to such organisms is crucial. Close note should also be taken of the following factors.

- Periods of time spent overseas: this increases the likelihood of infections such as tuberculosis (TB) or histoplasmosis.
- Travel abroad, even if in the distant past: Mediterranean travel is associated with risks of visceral leishmaniasis. Talaromycosis (formerly known as penicillinosis) is specific to patients who have spent time in the Far East.
- Contact with animals or birds.
- Prophylactic regimens with co-trimoxazole reduce the chance of, but do not exclude, the diagnosis of conditions such as PCP or toxoplasmosis.
- Pre-existing serology for *Toxoplasma* spp. and CMV.
- Recent commencement of antiretroviral drugs. Immune reconstitution inflammatory syndromes (IRIS) occur as the immune system improves and an inflammatory response occurs to a previously treated or subclinical infection. IRIS most commonly occurs as the CD4 count starts to rise in the first weeks/months after beginning antiretroviral treatment.

Examination

This should include particularly:

- skin and mucosal membranes
- lungs
- examination of the dilated fundi for evidence of CMV retinitis
- examination of the lymph nodes
- assessment of hepatomegaly or splenomegaly.

Few clinical or biochemical findings are specific for a particular disease process; for example, abnormal liver function may be found in drug reactions, lymphoma or MAC, and lymph node enlargement may occur in MAC or lymphoma. However, abnormalities warrant further investigation.

Diagnosis

Discontinuing drugs, particularly ones started recently, and watching the fever response may be helpful. Routine cultures should be performed but several specific investigations may be helpful.

Non-invasive methods

- Chest X-ray (CXR).
- Urine, stool and regular blood cultures.
- Mycobacterial and fungal blood cultures: particularly looking for MAC; 60–80% sensitivity using modern techniques.
- Serum cryptococcal antigen.
- CMV viral load by polymerase chain reaction (PCR).
- Examination of induced sputum; diagnosis of PCP in asymptomatic patients, *Mycobacterium tuberculosis* and atypical mycobacteria and other respiratory pathogens. However, this is associated with infection control risks which have reduced its use in recent years.
- Computed tomography (CT) of the abdomen: may show retroperitoneal lymph nodes or masses.

Invasive methods

These are required in up to 50%.

- Bronchoscopy with bronchoalveolar lavage (BAL), in which small aliquots of saline are flushed in and out of the lung, collecting inflammatory cells and organisms from there. Organisms can be identified by culture or specific stains.
- Bone marrow examination: useful for MAC culture and diagnosis of intracellular organisms, e.g. *Histoplasma* spp., cryptococci, leishmaniasis and lymphoma.
- Lymph node biopsy of enlarged nodes: diagnosis of lymphoma or TB. PCR on the sample can be undertaken to detect *Mycobacterim tuberculosis* complex (and if positive, rifampicin sensitivity). Surgical excision of lymph nodes may be necessary if biopsy is inconclusive or the node cannot be easily reached.
- Liver biopsy: if there is evidence of liver enzyme abnormality that persists after stopping drug therapy.
- Skin biopsies of unusual rashes should be cultured to exclude fungal diseases.
- Lumbar puncture should be considered if there is altered mentation or neurological function.

Management

Diagnosis is eventually made in about 80% of cases and appropriate therapy can be instituted. Failure of response should lead to searches for other causes because of the high prevalence of multiple conditions. Empirical therapy is sometimes necessary, particularly in very advanced HIV with <50 CD4 cells/mm^3 when MAC and disseminated histoplasmosis are common but cannot always be demonstrated.

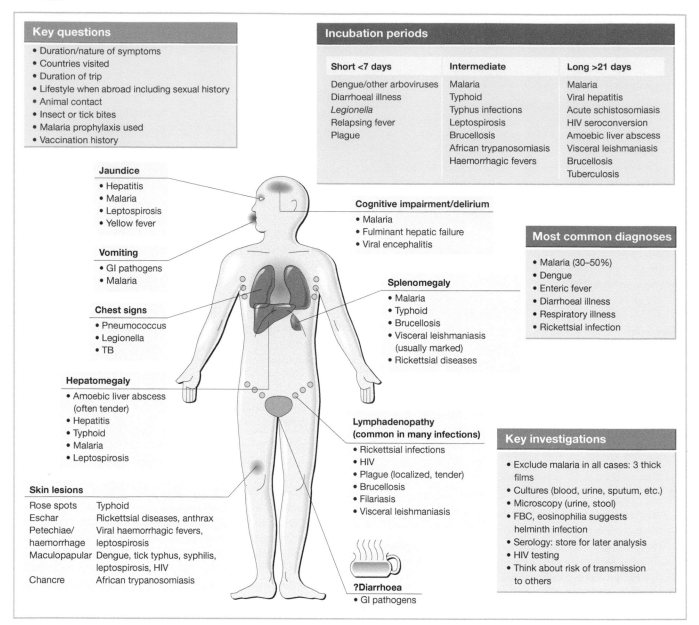

48 Fever in the returned traveller

Key questions

- Duration/nature of symptoms
- Countries visited
- Duration of trip
- Lifestyle when abroad including sexual history
- Animal contact
- Insect or tick bites
- Malaria prophylaxis used
- Vaccination history

Incubation periods

Short <7 days	Intermediate	Long >21 days
Dengue/other arboviruses	Malaria	Malaria
Diarrhoeal illness	Typhoid	Viral hepatitis
Legionella	Typhus infections	Acute schistosomiasis
Relapsing fever	Leptospirosis	HIV seroconversion
Plague	Brucellosis	Amoebic liver abscess
	African trypanosomiasis	Visceral leishmaniasis
	Haemorrhagic fevers	Brucellosis
		Tuberculosis

Jaundice
- Hepatitis
- Malaria
- Leptospirosis
- Yellow fever

Vomiting
- GI pathogens
- Malaria

Chest signs
- Pneumococcus
- Legionella
- TB

Hepatomegaly
- Amoebic liver abscess (often tender)
- Hepatitis
- Typhoid
- Malaria
- Leptospirosis

Skin lesions

Rose spots	Typhoid
Eschar	Rickettsial diseases, anthrax
Petechiae/ haemorrhage	Viral haemorrhagic fevers, leptospirosis
Maculopapular	Dengue, tick typhus, syphilis, leptospirosis, HIV
Chancre	African trypanosomiasis

Cognitive impairment/delirium
- Malaria
- Fulminant hepatic failure
- Viral encephalitis

Splenomegaly
- Malaria
- Typhoid
- Brucellosis
- Visceral leishmaniasis (usually marked)
- Rickettsial diseases

Lymphadenopathy (common in many infections)
- Rickettsial infections
- HIV
- Plague (localized, tender)
- Brucellosis
- Filariasis
- Visceral leishmaniasis

?Diarrhoea
- GI pathogens

Most common diagnoses
- Malaria (30–50%)
- Dengue
- Enteric fever
- Diarrhoeal illness
- Respiratory illness
- Rickettsial infection

Key investigations
- Exclude malaria in all cases: 3 thick films
- Cultures (blood, urine, sputum, etc.)
- Microscopy (urine, stool)
- FBC, eosinophilia suggests helminth infection
- Serology: store for later analysis
- HIV testing
- Think about risk of transmission to others

Incidence

Around 10% of international travellers seek medical attention while visiting low-income countries or after return home, with fever a common symptom. Many of these fevers are not caused by exotic pathogens but reflect standard viral, urinary tract or respiratory infections although significant tropical pathogens, particularly malaria, need to be excluded. It is also important to think of potential non-infectious causes, particularly in the elderly.

Early on in any assessment, it is important to consider whether the patient may be carrying a high-consequence infectious disease (e.g. viral haemorrhagic fever) that may be transmissible to others (see below).

Most common imported infections

- Malaria (see Chapter 169).
- Diarrhoeal illness (see Chapter 25).

Medicine at a Glance, Fifth Edition. Edited by Patrick Davey and Alex Pitcher.

Companion website: www.wiley.com/go/medicine5e

- Respiratory illness (see Chapters 107 and 108).
- Dengue (see Chapter 171).
- Enteric fever (typhoid or paratyphoid – see Chapter 171).
- Rickettsial infections (see Chapter 171).

Up to a quarter of fevers settle spontaneously and are undiagnosed.

Diagnosis

Assessing the immune status of the traveller is important. Although most travellers are healthy, increasing numbers of elderly or immunocompromised people are travelling abroad. These individuals may be at particular risk of certain infections. In addition to the presenting symptoms, the history should focus on the time course of the illness, which can include or exclude certain infections on the basis of the incubation period, and on activity and behaviour that can determine potential exposure to pathogens.

Important questions

- What symptoms did you have while away?
- Where exactly did you go and when? Ask the patient to write down a list of all relevant places and dates. Names of countries alone are not adequate – the risk of a specific infection can vary considerably within a country (e.g. malaria risk is negligible in Nairobi but considerable on the Kenyan coast). Patients may themselves be aware of specific risks in the area they visited.
- What did you do? Business, tourism (hiking in rural areas, swimming in fresh water) or living with local people? Visits to friends and relatives, or aid work, are associated with a higher risk of acquiring malaria and enteric fever.
- Were you bitten by any insects/arthropods? A range of rickettsial 'typhus' infections are acquired via **tick bites** (tick typhus in Africa, spotted fevers in Europe and USA) while scrub typhus is acquired from mites found in rural areas of Asia and northern Australia. Considering these infections is important because they are insensitive to penicillins but respond rapidly to doxycycline. The protozoal infection human African trypanosomiasis is acquired following the bite of the tsetse fly, in tourists typically during visits to East/Southern African game parks.
- Look back to previous (as well as most recent) trips as some conditions have long incubation illnesses, e.g. amoebic liver abscess.
- Full immunization history (appropriate vaccination reduces but does not exclude the chance of a specific infection).
- Malaria prophylaxis and adherence (and whether prophylaxis was appropriate for area visited).
- Food and water history (enteric infections, hepatitis, exotic parasites). Consuming unpasteurized dairy products is a risk factor for brucellosis.
- Freshwater exposure (schistosomiasis, leptospirosis).
- Sexual activity.
- Illness in fellow travellers (possible single source exposure) or contact with potentially infected individuals (particularly for health workers with potential exposure to viral haemorrhagic fevers).
- Animal bites or contact (rabies, brucellosis, histoplasmosis – bats in caves). Subsequent health of animal is particularly important for assessing rabies risk. Cats as well as dogs can carry rabies.

Important features of examination

- Physical signs are often rather non-specific.
- Establishing fever and sometimes pattern (biphasic in dengue, tertian in untreated malaria).
- Presence of rash, mosquito bites or ticks. Searching for eschars (necrotic lesions at the site of previous tick bites) necessitates careful examination – they may often be found in skin crevices or under waistbands or straps of underwear.
- Jaundice.
- Hepatosplenomegaly and lymphadenopathy.

Important investigations (guided by symptoms)

- Routine screening tests including blood cultures, chest X-ray, urine dipstick and culture.
- Malaria slide (at least three thick films if malaria is possible). Rapid diagnostic tests are now used by many laboratories.
- Consider HIV test and sexual screen if sexually active while away.
- Stool examination for ova, cysts and parasites, and culture.
- Look for eosinophilia (schistosomiasis, filariasis, liver flukes).
- Serology for dengue and other arboviruses, rickettsial diseases and brucellosis. Store serum for later serology if the diagnosis is uncertain.
- If the patient was admitted to hospital while travelling, undertake screens for MRSA and CPE (see Chapter 44).

Management

Two major immediate aims should be:

1 to exclude malaria: one of the most common conditions and by far the most potentially dangerous
2 to consider whether this may be a 'high-consequence' infection, i.e. an acute infectious disease with a high fatality rate that lacks effective prophylaxis/treatment and which can spread within community and healthcare settings. The main agents at the time of writing are viral haemorrhagic fevers, such as Ebola, and the Middle Eastern respiratory syndrome (MERS) virus. If there is any suspicion of these conditions, an infectious disease specialist should be consulted immediately.

Treatment of specific conditions is covered later in this book. Some conditions should be treated on clinical grounds alone as serological confirmation can take several weeks, or may not even be possible at all. If there are typical symptoms of a rickettsial infection (eschar, lymphadenopathy or maculopapular rash), such as seen in African tick bite fever or scrub typhus, then an empirical course of doxycycline should be given, alongside specialist infection input. When considering empirical antibiotic therapy in the absence of culture confirmation, patterns of antibiotic resistance in the visited country must be considered – this is particularly important for diseases such as enteric fever and TB.

Vaginal discharge and urethritis in men

Vaginal discharge

Table 49.1 History and management of most common causes of vaginal discharge.

	Physiological	Bacterial vaginosis	*Candida*	*Trichomonas* (TV)
Patient description	'Normal for me – varies with my menstrual cycle'	'A fishy-smelling watery discharge'	'A thick itchy discharge, looks like "cottage cheese", my vulva feels sore'	'A thin greenish discharge which is irritating' NB: may be asymptomatic
Examination	Small amount of white discharge	• Normal vulva and vagina • Thin, malodorous grey discharge	• Vulval erythema, inflammation and sometimes fissures • White, thick discharge	• Vulval inflammation • Inflamed 'strawberry cervix' • Profuse yellow/green frothy discharge
PH	<4.5	>5	<4.5	>5
Microscopy	• Normal epithelial cells • Gram-positive lactobacilli	• Few/absent lactobacilli • Clue cells present • Anaerobic bacteria	• Blastospores • Pseudo-hyphae • Neutrophils	• Motile trichomonads (wet slide – not Gram stained)
Investigations	Exclude STI if risk (STIs can be asymptomatic)	Exclude STI	• Exclude STI • Consider differentials (e.g. genital dermatoses)	• Nucleic acid amplification test (NAAT) for TV • Test for other STIs
Management	Nil	Metronidazole	• Oral fluconazole • Clotrimazole pessary	Metronidazole

Table 49.2 Red flag symptoms in women with abnormal vaginal discharge.

Abnormal vaginal bleeding	Intermenstrual or postcoital bleeding can indicate cervicitis (caused by infections such as chlamydia and gonorrhea (CT/GC)) or cervical/uterine pathology
Pelvic pain or dyspareunia	Pelvic inflammatory disease (PID) can be caused by STIs or other bacteria and is characterized by lower abdominal pain, especially during sex. Cervicitis may be seen, and adnexal tenderness and cervical excitation elicited on bimanual palpation
Vaginal soreness/ irritation	After excluding infection, dermatological causes (e.g. lichen planus and postmenopausal vulvovaginal atrophy) should be considered

Definition

Normal physiological vaginal discharge is usually white or clear, non-offensive and varies with the menstrual cycle, being thick and sticky apart from during ovulation, when it becomes clear and stretchy to facilitate the passage of sperm. Interruption to the menstrual cycle, due to pregnancy, menopause or the use of hormonal contraception, may also affect vaginal discharge.

An abnormal discharge can be characterized by a change in colour, consistency, volume or odour. It is important to identify other symptoms, such as itch, soreness, pelvic pain and intermenstrual or postcoital bleeding, which will help guide appropriate investigations.

Aetiology

Abnormal vaginal discharge can be caused by infections that are sexually transmitted, but there are also other causes to consider; see Table 49.3.

Table 49.3 Causes of vaginal discharge.

	Cause
Infective (non-sexually transmitted)	Bacterial vaginosis *Candida*
Infective (sexually transmitted infections [STIs])	*Chlamydia trachomatis* (CT) *Neisseria gonorrhoeae* (GC) *Trichomonas vaginalis* (TV)
	Herpes simplex virus (HSV) *Mycoplasma genitalium* (MG)
Non-infective	Foreign bodies (e.g., retained tampons, condoms) Physical irritation (e.g., soaps, douching, sanitary wear). Atrophic vaginitis (associated with menopause) Genital dermatoses Cervical polyps and ectopy Genital tract malignancy Fistulae

History

A detailed history should be taken, including a sexual history, washing practices, sanitary wear and hormonal status. Women considered at 'increased risk' of STIs may have the following attributes: aged <25years, report a new sexual partner (or >1 in last 12 months), have a history of previous STI.

However, in symptomatic women, an STI screen should be offered as a routine investigation, regardless of the documented history. If assumptions about risk are made, infections will be missed.

Box 49.1 How to ask about sex

It is often hard to ask about sex. A helpful phrase can be: 'In order to exclude all causes of your symptoms I just need to ask some routine questions about sex, and sexual practice. Can I check when was the last time you had any sexual contact, of any kind with anyone?'.

Examination

In all new presentations of abnormal vaginal discharge, a full examination should be carried out, including:

- comprehensive assessment of the genital and perineal skin
- speculum examination
- bimanual palpation (if pelvic pain or dyspareunia described).

Investigations

Investigations should be guided by the clinical history and examination, but may include the following.

- **Microscopy:** high vaginal swab specimen – Gram stained and evaluated using light field microscopy.
- **pH**: of vaginal discharge.
- **STI screening:** CT/GC/TV – consider MG.
- ***Candida* culture and sensitivities:** especially if recurrent *Candida*.
- **Cervical cytology:** if indicated by history or from examination.
- **Skin biopsy:** if dermatological condition suspected.

Table 49.1 summarizes the history, examination and investigations for the most common causes of vaginal discharge.

Although most causes of vaginal discharge are simple and relatively easy to treat, some presentations may indicate a more serious condition, for instance as shown in Table 49.2.

Management

Treatment of the underlying cause is key and should be guided by the history, investigations and history of previous treatment response.

Urethritis in men

Definition

Urethritis, or inflammation of the urethra, is a multifactorial condition, sexually acquired in most (but not all) cases. Urethritis is usually defined as either:

- gonococcal urethritis (due to *Neisseria gonorrhoeae* [GC])
- non-gonococcal urethritis (NGU).

Aetiology

Table 49.4 highlights the most common organisms isolated in those diagnosed with NGU. An infective cause may not be found, and symptoms may be secondary to irritants, foreign bodies and some inflammatory diseases.

Table 49.4 Micro-organisms isolated in non-gonococcal urethritis.

Micro-organism	Prevalence
Chlamydia trachomatis (CT)	11–50%
Mycoplasma genitalium (MG)	6–50%
Ureaplasma urealyticum	11–26%
Trichomonas vaginitis (TV)	1–20%
Adenoviruses	2–4%
Herpes simplex virus (HSV)	2–3%

History

- A full history, including a sexual history is important (see Box 49.1). Ask about condom use.
- Ascertain time of onset, duration, and exacerbating/relieving factors.
- Enquire about associated symptoms (see Box 49.2).

Box 49.2 Associated Symptoms

1) Dysuria: If associated with frequency, urge, nocturia, consider urinary pathogens; 2) Urethral discharge: a) gonococcal urethritis can be copious, purulent, yellow/cream in colour b) NGU: usually clear and smaller volume; 3) Penile irritation; 4) Urethral discomfort

Examination

Examine all the external genitalia.

- Note the colour/quantity of urethral discharge.
- Examine the testes and epididymis for pain/swelling.
- Check the foreskin and glans for any erythema or inflammation.

Investigations

- **Microscopy:** a Gram-stained sample taken from the anterior urethra is examined under the microscope. Patients should not pass urine for at least 1 hour prior to examination.
  - **GC urethritis**: presence of intracellular Gram-negative diplococci (in symptomatic men, sensitivity is 90–95%).
  - **NGU**: >5 polymorphs (PMNLs) per high-power (×1000) microscopic field (and no GC).
- **GC culture**: taken from urethral swab (important given antibiotic resistance).
- **Nucleic acid amplification tests (NAATs)**: for CT/GC (urine sample – posturethral samples).
- **Urine dipstick**: leukocytes alone common in NGU.
- **Urine culture**: if indicated by urine dip (nitrites, leukocytes, protein, blood) or symptoms.
- **Other**: consider testing for *Mycoplasma genitalium* if recurrent or persistent symptoms.

Complications

- 1) Epididymo-orchitis. 2) Sexually acquired reactive arthritis/Reiter syndrome (<1%). 3) Rarely, disseminated gonococcal infection (skin lesions, joint swelling).

Treatment

- Patients should be advised to abstain from sexual intercourse until 14 days after the start of treatment, and until symptoms have resolved. Screening and treatment of sexual partners is important (even if STI screen is negative). Treatment is 1) for NGU, Doxycycline or Azithromycin 2) for GC urethritis: first line – IM ceftriaxone (treatment is guided by antimicrobial sensitivities).

50 Anaemia

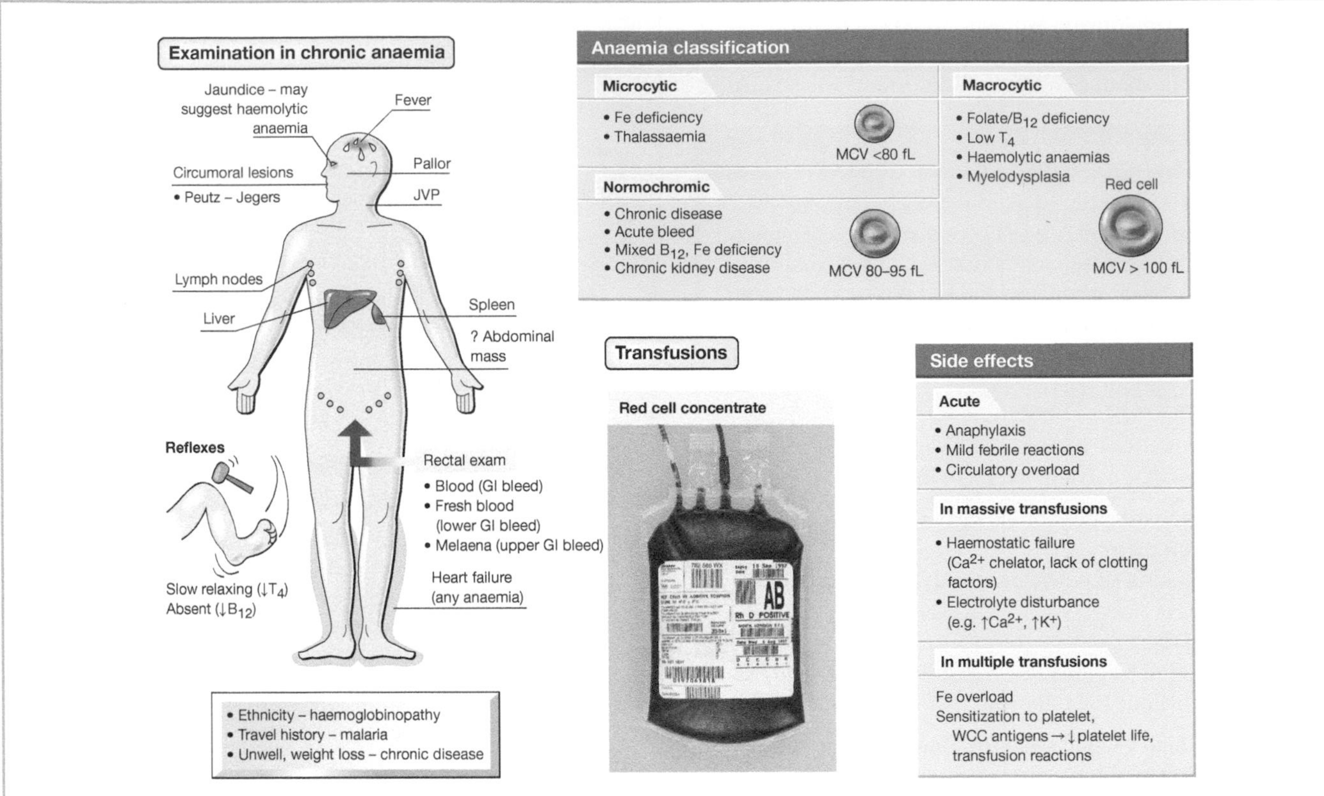

Anaemia is present when a patient's haemoglobin is more than two standard deviations below the age- and sex-matched mean – in practical terms, below the normal range for a given laboratory. It may reflect a primary haematological disorder, but is also a sensitive marker for a variety of non-haematological diseases.

Clinical features

Symptoms depend on the nature of the underlying pathology as well as on the severity and speed of onset of the anaemia. Mild anaemia often causes no symptoms, and anaemia of insidious onset, even if profound, may also be relatively well tolerated by the patient. In more severe or rapid-onset anaemia, the following may occur.

- Fatigue.
- Peripheral oedema, e.g. swollen feet.
- Breathlessness: particularly if heart or lung disease is present. Anaemia is one cause of decompensation in chronic heart failure.
- Angina, if there is underlying coronary disease, which may have been undetected before the anaemia.

The physical examination in anaemia is usually unremarkable; there may be pallor, though this is neither a sensitive nor specific finding, and a systolic 'flow' murmur is common. In addition, there may be evidence of the underlying pathology (e.g. splenomegaly in some forms of chronic haemolysis).

Classification

Anaemia is not a diagnosis in itself, and its underlying cause must always be sought. There are two main mechanisms for classifying anaemia in order to establish its underlying cause: a morphological classification based on red cell size, and a dynamic or functional classification based on bone marrow activity, represented by reticulocyte count.

Morphological classification

- **Microcytic anaemia**: the red cells are smaller than normal (microcytic) and contain less haemoglobin than normal (hypochromic). The two most common causes are iron deficiency anaemia and thalassaemia trait.
- **Normochromic anaemia**: causes include the 'anaemia of chronic disease' which arises in response to raised hepcidin levels caused by chronic inflammation. This may be seen in chronic infections, e.g. tuberculosis (TB) and osteomyelitis, inflammatory diseases such as rheumatoid arthritis and connective tissue disorders, and malignant disease. Hepcidin (levels are increased by chronic inflammation) prevents iron absorption from the gut, and limits mobilization of iron stores from the reticuloendothelial system; with increasing duration, the normocytic picture of the anaemia of chronic disease can become increasingly microcytic. Erythropoietin deficiency,

Medicine at a Glance, Fifth Edition. Edited by Patrick Davey and Alex Pitcher.

Companion website: www.wiley.com/go/medicine5e

common in chronic renal impairment, causes the anaemia of chronic kidney disease which is also typically normocytic.

- **Macrocytic anaemia**: the red cells are larger than normal. Common causes include the following.
  - Vitamin B_{12} or folate deficiency.
  - Cytotoxic drug treatment, e.g. azathioprine or cyclophosphamide.
  - Myelodysplasia (see Chapter 185).
  - Haemolytic anaemias – predominantly because of the associated reticulocytosis, since reticulocytes are larger than mature red cells.
  - Hypothyroidism: can cause either a normocytic or a macrocytic anaemia.
  - Liver disease and alcohol excess result in a macrocytosis, but not usually anaemia, unless there is coincidental bleeding or haematinic deficiency.

Macrocytic anaemias can be further described as either megaloblastic (B_{12} and folate deficiency, cytotoxic drug treatments) or normoblastic (haemolysis, thyroid dysfunction and liver disease.

Functional classification

- **Low reticulocyte count**: this suggests that the bone marrow is unable to respond adequately to anaemia, perhaps because of deficiencies in the key components required for erythropoiesis (e.g. iron, vitamin B_{12}, folate), because of inadequate erythropoietin stimulation (anaemia of chronic kidney disease) or because the bone marrow is infiltrated by non-haemopoietic tissue (e.g. metastatic disease or fibrosis).
- **High reticulocyte count**: a reticulocytosis suggests there is bone marrow capacity to respond to anaemia, and this is typically seen in acute haemorrhage and the haemolytic anaemias. Patients with haematinic deficiency anaemia who are given supplementation will also develop a reticulocytosis.

Investigations

The clinical features and morphological characteristics of the red cells determine further investigations (see diagram of red cell morphology, Chapter 186), but the following tests are frequently helpful.

- **Haematinic status** (ferritin, iron, transferrin, serum vitamin B_{12} and folate): iron status should be evaluated in micro- or normocytic anaemias, and vitamin B_{12}/folate status in macrocytic anaemias. Haematinic deficiency may be seen even when another cause for anaemia is clear (e.g. folate deficiency in haemolytic anaemia, iron deficiency in colon cancer, etc.). Once haematinic deficiency is found, the specific cause of this deficiency (malnutrition, malabsorption, excessive losses, etc.) should always be determined.
- **Blood film**: this is often diagnostic in primary haematological disease as well as in many systemic diseases. It is therefore mandatory in all patients with anaemia that has not been diagnosed by other investigations. Discussion with the haematologist often speeds up the diagnostic process.
- **Blood count**: the rest of the blood count may also provide useful information in the investigation of anaemia. Significant neutropenia and thrombocytopenia in conjunction with anaemia raises the likelihood of an underlying primary bone marrow disease (e.g. myelodysplasia or acute leukaemia). A raised neutrophil count or platelet count may support the suspicion of infection or inflammation, or may suggest a myeloproliferative disorder; while a persistent raised lymphocyte count may suggest a lymphoproliferative disease.
- **Other investigations** important in some patients with anaemia include:
  - renal and liver biochemistry, to diagnose underlying organ-specific disease
  - markers of inflammation (erythrocyte sedimentation rate or C-reactive protein) which are often raised in anaemia of chronic disease, e.g. disseminated malignancy, sepsis or vasculitis
  - thyroid status
  - blood cultures – useful if sepsis is suspected
  - bone marrow examination: this is often helpful and should be discussed with a haematologist if less invasive investigations have failed to reach a diagnosis.

Treatment

Treatment of anaemia involves management of the underlying disease. Where this is not possible, optimization of haematinic availability is essential, and patients may also benefit from blood transfusion or treatment with recombinant erythropoietin.

Blood transfusion

Donor and recipient need to be blood group 'matched' for successful transfusion.

- **The ABO system**: the A and B genes encode enzymes transforming a cell membrane glycoprotein (substance H) into either A or B antigens. Individuals possess either two A or two B genes (AA or BB), one of each (AB), one copy of either A or B (AO, BO) or neither (O). There are naturally occurring IgM antibodies to the antigen that an individual does not possess (i.e. anti-B if AA or AO, and anti-A if BB or BO). To avoid transfusion reactions, patients must receive blood either similar to their own group or from a group 'O' donor (sometimes incorrectly termed a 'universal donor').
- **The Rh system** comprises three allelic sets of genes: cC; D (Rh positive) and no D (Rh negative); and eE.
- **Other systems**: these include the Kell, Duffy, Jka and MNS blood groups, though there are very many more of clinical significance.

Complications of blood transfusion

- **Transfusion reactions** are relatively uncommon, with the majority of complications in transfusion practice arising because the wrong blood product has been administered to the wrong patient (i.e. administrative error). The most serious reactions include an acute intravascular haemolytic reaction, due to ABO incompatibility, and acute anaphylaxis (e.g. due to plasma product administration to an IgA-deficient patient). Delayed transfusion reactions can also occur, with immune haemolysis of the transfused red cells as a consequence of previous alloimmunization.
- **Transfusion-associated circulatory overload (TACO)** can result in pulmonary oedema, especially in those with pre-existing cardiac compromise.
- **Transfusion-related acute lung injury (TRALI)** is an uncommon but serious complication occurring 1–6 hours after transfusion, especially of plasma products. It is thought to be a consequence of transfusion of antibodies to HLA, or the neutrophil antigens. A capillary leak syndrome develops, leading to pulmonary oedema and respiratory distress. A chest X-ray reveals widespread interstitial infiltrates. Treatment is supportive.
- **Iron overload** is problematic for those receiving multiple transfusions (e.g. patients with transfusion-dependent thalassaemia), and necessitates iron chelation therapy.
- **Viral transmission** is avoided in many countries by robust screening strategies for human immunodeficiency virus (HIV) and hepatitis B or C, but blood services must be alert to the potential risk posed by emerging pathogens.
- **Transfusion-associated graft-versus-host disease**: this is a rare condition in which lymphocytes from the donor blood survive in the blood transfusion recipient, and recognize the recipient as being 'foreign'. This typically occurs only if the transfusion recipient is heavily immunosuppressed. The clinical consequences include a rash, diarrhoea and biochemical evidence of liver damage, usually early after transfusion. The illness has a high mortality, but can be avoided by gamma irradiation of blood products for severely immunocompromised patients.

51 Clinical approach to lymphadenopathy and splenomegaly

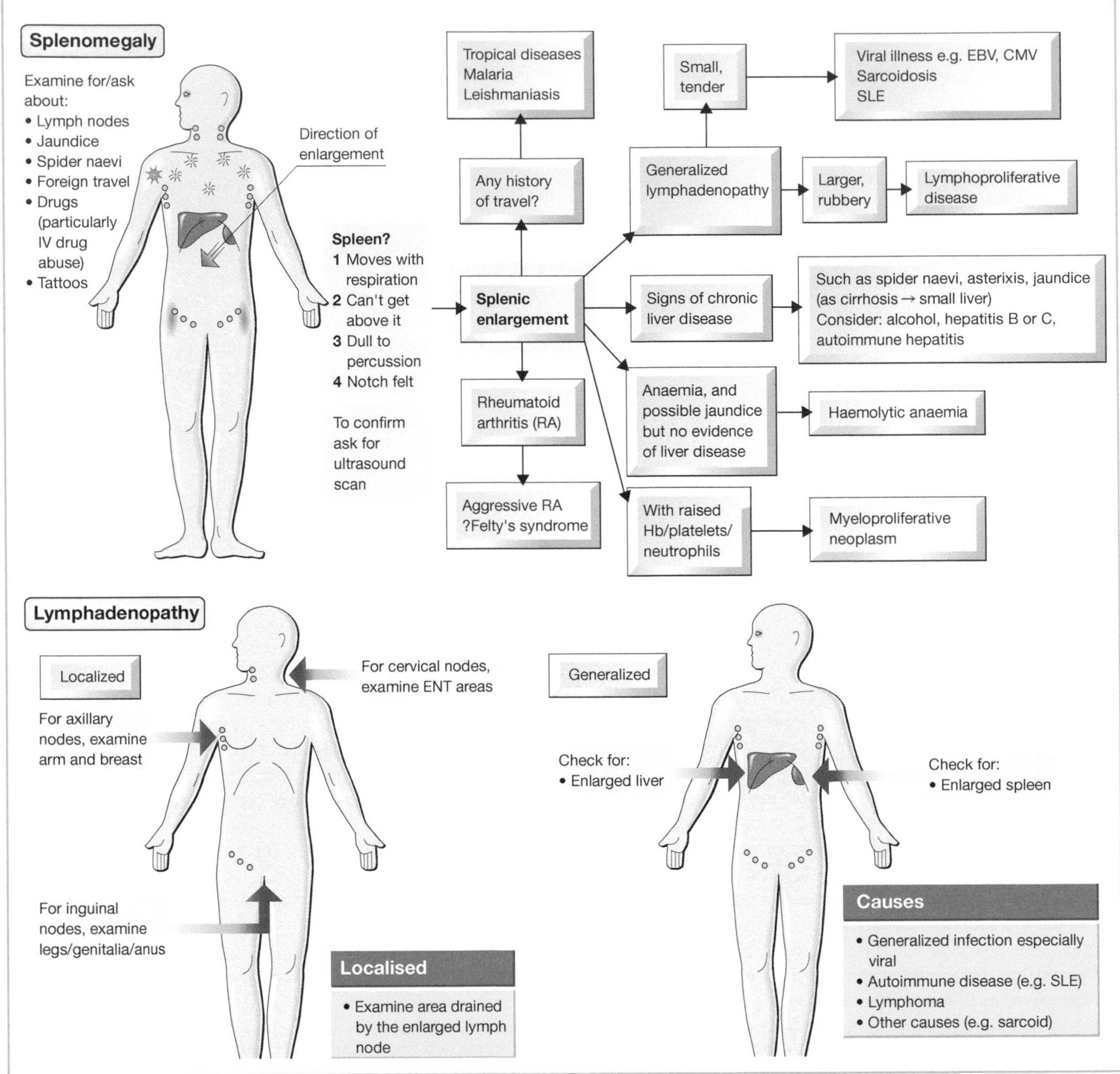

Lymphadenopathy

Local lymphadenopathy often relates to local infection or malignancy, whereas generalized lymphadenopathy has a wider differential diagnosis, including the following.

- **Infections**: viral, spirochaetal, rickettsial or protozoal.
- **Inflammatory disorders**, such as autoimmune conditions, particularly systemic lupus erythematosus (SLE). Sarcoidosis can also cause diffuse lymphadenopathy.
- **Malignancy**, i.e. the lymphoproliferative diseases.
- **Dermatopathic**: diffuse skin disease such as eczema which can cause widespread, small-volume lymphadenopathy.

Medicine at a Glance, Fifth Edition. Edited by Patrick Davey and Alex Pitcher.

Companion website: www.wiley.com/go/medicine5e

History and examination

The history and examination should focus on possible sites or sources of infection resulting in lymphadenopathy, the presence of inflammatory or connective tissue diseases such as rheumatoid arthritis (RA), SLE, or the symptoms of weight loss, long-lasting malaise or sweats, which might indicate a malignant disease. On examination, lymph node size and texture give some clues.

- Bulky, hard nodes are suggestive of malignant disease.
- Soft, mobile, tender nodes suggest infection.

However, these features can be misleading and it is unwise to make a judgement solely on these findings. It is vital to examine the area drained by the lymph node thoroughly, if necessary using radiological techniques, e.g. mammography for axillary lymph nodes.

Investigations

A full blood count (FBC), erythrocyte sedimentation rate (ESR), liver function tests and C-reactive protein estimation are useful screening tests. Other investigations (e.g. cross-sectional imaging by computed tomography [CT]) should be tailored to the clinical situation. A biopsy should be undertaken if there is any suspicion of malignancy causing lymph node enlargement. A fine needle aspirate (FNA) may be misleading, and core biopsy is likely to be required for diagnosis, especially of lymphoproliferative diseases.

Splenomegaly

The differential diagnosis for a mass in the left upper quadrant includes renal or colonic masses and, less commonly, a mass of abdominal lymph nodes. Ultrasonography or CT scan can confirm that the mass is a spleen. The spleen needs to enlarge three-fold before it can be palpated. Thus, a palpable spleen is always pathological and should prompt investigations to establish the cause.

The differential diagnosis of splenomegaly includes the following.

- Infections: e.g. infectious mononucleosis and malaria.
- Lymphoproliferative diseases.
- Myeloproliferative diseases: particularly chronic myeloid leukaemia (CML) and myelofibrosis.
- Haemolytic anaemias, especially when chronic (e.g. hereditary spherocytosis).
- Portal hypertension complicating cirrhosis, or much more rarely without cirrhosis (e.g. portal vein thrombosis, schistosomiasis).
- Autoimmune disease, e.g. SLE.
- Other rarer causes such as sarcoidosis or Gaucher disease.

The history and physical signs in addition to the splenomegaly often give a strong pointer towards the correct diagnosis.

- Viral infection, often Epstein–Barr virus (EBV) or cytomegalovirus (CMV): several days of flu-like symptoms, sore throat and generalized lymphadenopathy, often with mild hepatomegaly.
- Liver cirrhosis: features of chronic liver disease may be noted (see Chapter 133) and, unlike the above disorders, the liver is often small and therefore impalpable.
- Lymphoma: general malaise, weight loss, sometimes night sweats, bulky lymphadenopathy and hepatomegaly.

Investigations

An FBC and film are helpful.

- **Myeloproliferative disorder**: the haemoglobin is high in polycythaemia vera, the white cell count (WCC) (both mature and immature granulocytes) is high in CML and the platelet count is high in essential thrombocythaemia.
- **Myelofibrosis**: where the bone marrow is replaced by fibrous tissue. Haematopoiesis occurs in extramedullary sites, including the spleen, resulting in massive splenomegaly. The peripheral blood shows leucoerythroblastic features (see Chapter 186) along with misshapen red cells.
- **Haemolytic anaemia**: the blood count shows anaemia and polychromasia (reflecting increased reticulocytes). Other abnormalities (such as spherocytes) may be present depending on the underlying cause of the haemolysis.
- **Viral infection**: reactive lymphocytes in the blood suggest a viral infection.
- **Liver disease**: target cells and a macrocytosis are often seen in liver disease.
- **Lymphoproliferative disease**: the blood count and film of patients with any form of lymphoma may be normal or nonspecifically abnormal; however, in some causes such as chronic lymphocytic leukaemia, there will be a circulating lymphocytosis.

Additional investigations, including lymph node or bone marrow biopsy, are sometimes necessary for diagnosis. A diagnostic splenectomy is very rarely necessary, but may be considered in persistent undiagnosed splenomegaly despite full investigation. However, cross-sectional imaging (e.g. PET-CT) of the abdomen/thorax often reveals either the diagnosis or lymphadenopathy suitable for percutaneous biopsy. In young patients with unexplained splenomegaly, white cell enzymes may be assayed to look for Gaucher disease – a rare but treatable condition.

Complications

Splenomegaly itself is usually asymptomatic, although there may be discomfort in the left upper quadrant. Occasionally splenomegaly is complicated by the following.

- **Infarction**, resulting in a 'pleuritic' pain over the spleen. The differential diagnosis is from other causes of pleurisy (see Chapter 13).
- **Rupture**: a pathologically enlarged spleen may rupture more easily, causing abdominal pain and circulatory collapse. Thus, the differential diagnosis of anyone with splenomegaly who becomes hypotensive includes splenic rupture, requiring emergency assessment.
- **Hypersplenism**: spleens pool blood in proportion to their size. A normal spleen pools 2% of the blood volume; a very large spleen may pool ≥20% of the blood volume, which may result in anaemia, thrombocytopenia (especially in portal hypertension) or even pancytopenia (see Chapter 177). Diagnosis is by exclusion.

Patients in whom splenic function is compromised, or who are post-splenectomy, are susceptible to overwhelming bacterial infection by encapsulated organisms (e.g. *Pneumococcus*, *Meningococcus*, *Haemophilus influenzae*). Such patients should receive immunization and life-long prophylactic penicillin (or alternative in penicillin-sensitive patients).

52 The patient with abnormal bleeding or bruising

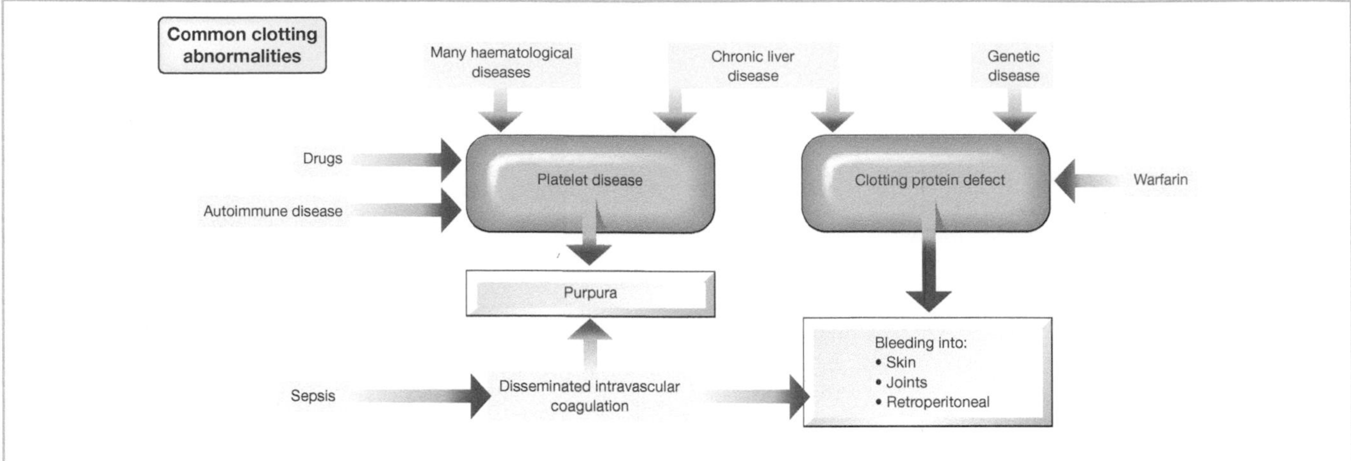

The key to assessing a bleeding/bruising problem lies in the history and in particular whether the bleeding has been life-long or is new.

- **Life-long bleeding** suggests an inherited disease, confirmed by ascertaining the bleeding response to remote haemostatic challenges (e.g. operations, dental extractions or postpartum bleeding). The family history and mode of inheritance should be determined (e.g. X-linked for haemophilia A and B).
- **New-onset bleeding** suggests an acquired problem. This often relates to medical problems, either covert (e.g. hypothyroidism) or overt (e.g. septicaemia, disseminated intravascular coagulation, medications such as antiplatelets and anticoagulants).

It can often be difficult to assess the severity of bleeding, and objective findings such as iron deficiency anaemia or the need for a blood transfusion should be recorded. A full drug history must always be taken – aspirin and non-steroidal anti-inflammatory drugs are the most common causes of platelet dysfunction. Other drugs may cause marrow aplasia (see Chapter 179).

Examination

The main purpose of the physical examination is to exclude any underlying medical disease (e.g. sepsis, leukaemia, etc.) and determine the consequences of bleeding (e.g. haemarthroses, gastrointestinal blood loss), which in themselves need specific treatment. Any bleeding pattern present should be determined because this relates to the underlying defect.

- In **platelet defects** (quantitative or qualitative), purpura/petechiae are common; other manifestations include epistaxes and, in women, menorrhagia.
- In contrast, in **coagulation factor deficiency** (e.g. haemophilia), bleeding is usually into muscles or joints.

Investigations

First-line investigations (the 'basic clotting screen') include the following.

- **Full blood count**: particularly the platelet count; the haemoglobin and white cell count provide important clues to the presence of marrow aplasia or leukaemia.
- **Coagulation screen**: a prothrombin time (prolonged when any of factors II, V, VII, X or fibrinogen are deficient/inhibited), activated partial thromboplastin time (prolonged if any of factors II, V, VIII, IX, X, XI, XII or fibrinogen are deficient/inhibited). Some coagulation screens include a thrombin time (prolonged when fibrinogen is deficient, when fibrinogen polymerization is inhibited by fibrin degradation products or if heparin is present). If a prolonged clotting time is found, adding normal plasma (which contains all clotting factors) allows differentiation between bleeding caused by clotting factor deficiency (coagulation corrects) and that caused by inhibition (coagulation does not correct). A common inhibitor is the lupus anticoagulant (see Chapter 190), which paradoxically is associated with a procoagulant state rather than with bleeding.
- **Factor VIII, von Willebrand factor (VWF) activity and VWF antigen** particularly when inherited disorders are suspected.
- **Bleeding time/PFA 100**: after a skin cut 1 mm deep and 1 cm long, prolonged bleeding occurs with deficient or defective platelets. This bleeding time test has poor sensitivity and specificity and is no longer recommended; it has largely been replaced as a screening test by *in vitro* alternatives, such as the PFA 100 test. Abnormalities can be further investigated by *in vitro* tests of platelet function including lumiaggregation and measuring platelet nucleotides (these tests require specialized haemostasis laboratories).

If a patient has a markedly abnormal bleeding history then even if basic coagulation screening tests are normal, the patient should be referred to a specialist haemostasis centre for clinical assessment, consideration of platelet function tests and additional coagulation factor tests. Of note, factor XIII deficiency is a rare autosomal recessive bleeding disorder that does not affect screening tests, so it should be considered when there is a good history and first-line tests are negative, especially if there is parental consanguinity.

Treatment

This depends on the underlying cause. Specific treatments are outlined in Chapters 187 and 188.

Medicine at a Glance, Fifth Edition. Edited by Patrick Davey and Alex Pitcher.

Companion website: www.wiley.com/go/medicine5e

53 Leukopenia

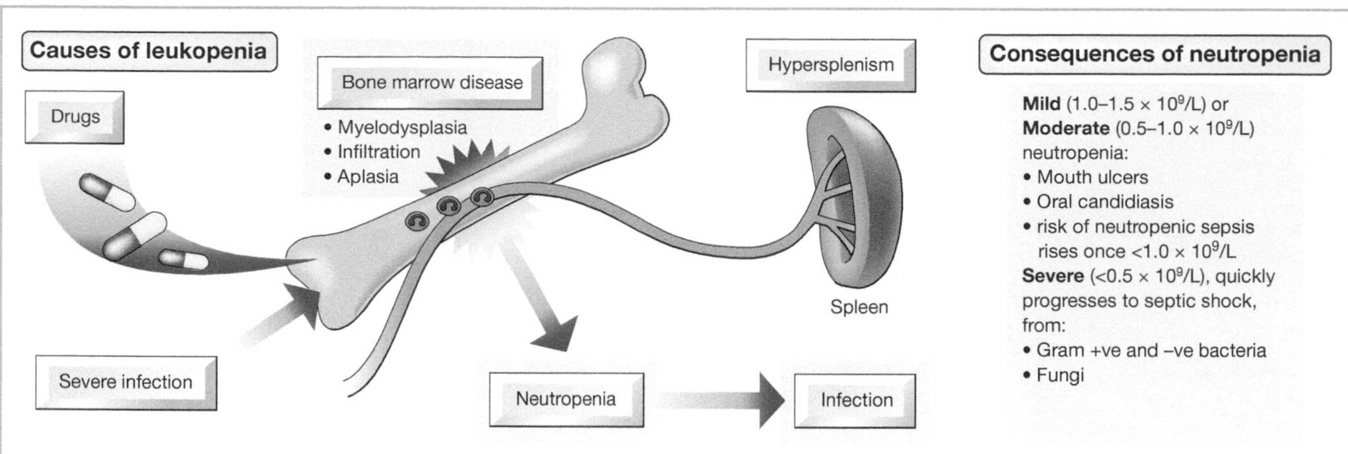

A decrease in the number of circulating white cells (leukopenia) is common, and may indicate serious disease needing immediate diagnosis and treatment. Any further assessment requires an understanding of the type of white cells affected.

Neutropenia

Neutropenia means decreased circulating neutrophils (total count ≤2.0 × 10^9 neutrophils/l). In extreme cases there may be no circulating neutrophils – called agranulocytosis.

There are many causes of neutropenia.

- **Ethnic origin**: a mild neutropenia is more common in people of Afro-Caribbean ethnicity than in White individuals. This is of no clinical significance and not associated with an increased risk of infection.
- **Drug-induced neutropenia** is common, and may result in a selective decrease in neutrophils (e.g. carbimazole), or a more general bone marrow depression, a pancytopenia. Examples of the latter include cytotoxic chemotherapy, rheumatological drugs including sulfasalazine and some non-steroidal anti-inflammatory drugs. Many other drugs have been implicated.
- **Myelodysplastic syndrome**: this clonal disorder of the bone marrow is a precursor to acute myeloid leukaemia and may cause an isolated neutropenia or more general mild but progressive pancytopenia (see Chapter 183).
- **Severe infection** can cause neutropenia, as in pneumococcal pneumonia with complicating septicaemia, where the low white cell count is associated with a worse prognosis. Viral infections likewise can depress neutrophil counts.
- **Bone marrow infiltration**, particularly from haematological malignancy. Usually affects all cell lines (pancytopenia) (see Chapter 177).
- **Bone marrow failure** results in pancytopenia, e.g. aplastic anaemia.
- **Hypersplenism** (see Chapter 51).
- **Autoimmune neutropenia.**
- Very rare causes include **cyclical neutropenia**.

Consequences of neutropenia

Most patients with mild/moderate neutropenia (counts 1.0–2.0 × 10^9/l) have no symptoms. However, the lower the count, the greater the risk of infection (neutropenic sepsis); this risk becomes significant when counts are below 0.5 × 10^9/l and very significant below 0.1 × 10^9/l.

- Mouth ulceration is common in sustained neutropenia.
- Infection can occur very rapidly (i.e. within hours) and become overwhelming, producing severe septic shock (see Chapter 18).
- Organisms may be 'typical' pathogenic bacteria (e.g. *Staphylococcus aureus*, pathogenic streptococci, Gram-negative bacilli), although other organisms are also commonly implicated.

Treatment

- Treatment for neutropenic sepsis involves establishing which organism is responsible (blood cultures), providing circulatory support (fluids, sometimes vasoconstrictors in an intensive care setting) and, most importantly, giving broad-spectrum antibiotics without delay.
- Treatment with granulocyte colony-stimulating factor may sometimes help to shorten a period of neutropenia, depending on the cause (e.g. especially chemotherapy-induced neutropenia).
- The underlying cause of neutropenia must be established, and a bone marrow examination may be required.

Lymphopenia

A significant decrease in the number of circulating lymphocytes is less common than neutropenia. Causes other than haematological malignancy (and its treatment) include:

- drugs (e.g. corticosteroids)
- autoimmune disease, such as systemic lupus erythematosus
- lymphoproliferative disease
- viral infections, either acute (e.g. Epstein–Barr virus, severe acute respiratory syndrome coronavirus 2 and cytomegalovirus) or chronic (e.g. human immunodeficiency virus)

Medicine at a Glance, Fifth Edition. Edited by Patrick Davey and Alex Pitcher.

Companion website: www.wiley.com/go/medicine5e

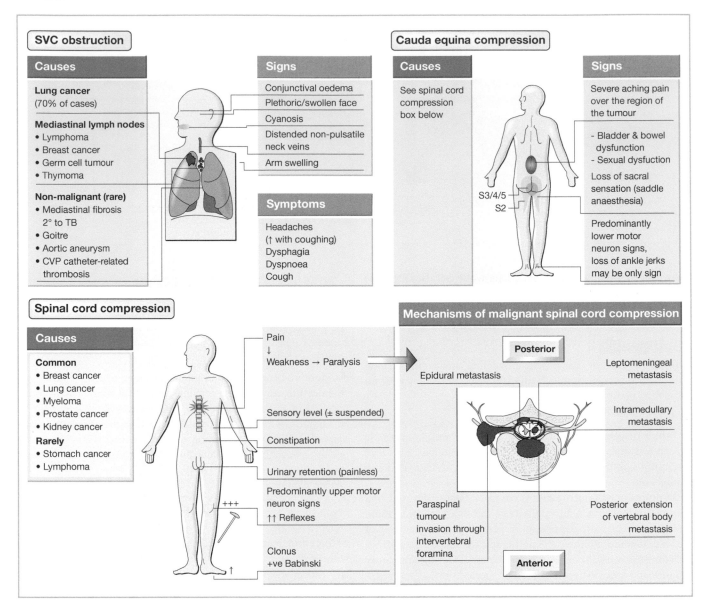

Oncological emergencies

SVC obstruction

Causes

Lung cancer
(70% of cases)

Mediastinal lymph nodes
- Lymphoma
- Breast cancer
- Germ cell tumour
- Thymoma

Non-malignant (rare)
- Mediastinal fibrosis 2° to TB
- Goitre
- Aortic aneurysm
- CVP catheter-related thrombosis

Signs

Conjunctival oedema
Plethoric/swollen face
Cyanosis
Distended non-pulsatile neck veins
Arm swelling

Symptoms

Headaches (↑ with coughing)
Dysphagia
Dyspnoea
Cough

Cauda equina compression

Causes

See spinal cord compression box below

Signs

Severe aching pain over the region of the tumour
- Bladder & bowel dysfunction
- Sexual dysfuction

Loss of sacral sensation (saddle anaesthesia)
Predominantly lower motor neuron signs, loss of ankle jerks may be only sign

S3/4/5
S2

Spinal cord compression

Causes

Common
- Breast cancer
- Lung cancer
- Myeloma
- Prostate cancer
- Kidney cancer

Rarely
- Stomach cancer
- Lymphoma

Pain
↓
Weakness → Paralysis
Sensory level (± suspended)
Constipation
Urinary retention (painless)
Predominantly upper motor neuron signs
↑↑ Reflexes
+++
Clonus
+ve Babinski
↑

Mechanisms of malignant spinal cord compression

Posterior
Epidural metastasis
Leptomeningeal metastasis
Intramedullary metastasis
Paraspinal tumour invasion through intervertebral foramina
Posterior extension of vertebral body metastasis
Anterior

Superior vena caval obstruction

This is a clinical syndrome arising from obstruction of blood flow through the superior vena cava (SVC). This thin-walled vessel may be compressed, invaded or thrombosed.

Aetiology

- **Malignant** (usually): from malignant lymph nodes compressing or invading the SVC. Lung cancer is responsible for 70% of SVC obstruction. Other less common causes include lymphoma and breast cancer.
- **Non-malignant** (rarely): mediastinal goitre, aortic aneurysm, iatrogenic (e.g. thrombosis from indwelling central venous catheters), and mediastinal fibrosis (histoplasmosis/tuberculosis).

Clinical features

Symptoms arise from the increase in venous pressure in the jugular and subclavian veins, and from the local effects of a mediastinal or bronchial tumour; they comprise dyspnoea, facial/arm swelling, headaches (worse on coughing) or head fullness, cough or dysphagia. Signs include non-pulsatile distension of the neck

Medicine at a Glance, Fifth Edition. Edited by Patrick Davey and Alex Pitcher.

Companion website: www.wiley.com/go/medicine5e

and chest wall veins, oedema of the face, neck and arms, plethoric facies, dilated veins over the upper chest wall, cyanosis, tachypnoea, vocal cord paresis and conjunctival oedema (chemosis). SVC obstruction may occasionally present as a medical emergency with life-threatening symptoms (central airway obstruction, laryngeal oedema, cerebral oedema). These patients require stabilization, and urgent referral to a specialized oncology team for urgent treatment.

Investigations

Previously, patients with SVC obstruction received immediate radiotherapy, but modern oncological therapy now makes histological diagnosis vital.

Immediate investigations include:

- chest X-ray: Typical findings include superior mediastinal widening, pleural effusions, right hilar mass
- CT (with contrast) to confirm diagnosis of SVC obstruction.

Further imaging (for example, CT abdomen and pelvis [and head], or PET-CT) may be required to assess the extent of disease and guide appropriate investigations to obtain a diagnosis. Investigations to obtain a diagnosis may include tumour markers (including LDH, β-HCG, AFP), sputum cytology, bone marrow examination, bronchoscopy, mediastinoscopy/thoracotomy and image-guided biopsy (often CT guided).

Management and prognosis

Bed rest with head elevated, oxygen and high-dose steroids (however, if SVCO is the first presentation of malignancy, steroids may affect the interpretation of biopsies and may not be advisable; discuss with oncology team).

Additional therapy depends on aetiology and severity of symptoms.

- **Malignant disease**.
  - Stent insertion – rapid symptomatic relief (should be discussed with interventional radiology/cardiothoracics). Anticoagulation is then required.
  - Chemotherapy for chemotherapy-sensitive tumours (e.g. small cell lung cancer [SCLC], lymphoma and germ cell tumours).
  - Radiotherapy.
- **Thrombotic SVC obstruction**: remove the local precipitant of thrombosis (SVC catheter) and consider thrombolysis and anticoagulation. Surgery (bypassing the blocked SVC) is rarely indicated and is reserved for non-malignant cases refractory to other therapies.
- **Non-malignant causes** can be treated by percutaneous angioplasty and wire stent insertion.

Patients with SVC obstruction from non-SCLC often live <6 months. Presentation with SVC obstruction does not affect the prognosis in patients with lymphoma or SCLC. Those with non-malignant causes of the syndrome live much longer – reported average being nine years.

Malignant spinal cord compression

Malignant spinal cord compression is the second most common neurological complication of malignancy after cerebral metastases. It can be the initial manifestation of malignancy and often arises in the preterminal phase of the illness. Spinal cord compression can occur in many malignancies but breast, prostate, lung cancer and myeloma are the most common.

Pathophysiology, aetiology and clinical features

In adults, the tip of the spinal cord usually lies at the L1 vertebral level; below this level, the lumbosacral nerve roots form the cauda equina. The pathophysiology of cauda equina compression is similar to the more rostral compression but the clinical signs may differ.

The spinal cord and its nerve roots are most commonly compressed anteriorly by posterior extension of haematogenously spread metastases in the vertebral body, extending into the epidural space or through vertebral body collapse. The cord may also be compromised by extension of a paraspinal tumour through the intervertebral foramina, which can occur without evidence of bony involvement. Damage is principally mediated by disruption of small vessel circulation, which is precipitated by changes in pressure within the spinal canal. There may be multiple metastases causing cord compression at different levels. See the figure for the aetiology. Most patients are known to have malignancy but spinal cord compression is the first manifestation of cancer in 10–20%.

The thoracic spine is the most common site of compression, followed by the lumbosacral and cervical regions.

Symptoms and signs of spinal cord compression

- **Pain**: this is the most common symptom; it may predate neurological signs. Constant, dull, aching pain that prevents sleep. Pain may radiate laterally, and is worse on movement (flexion) or increases with thoracic pressure (sneezing, straining). The involved vertebrae may be tender to percussion.
- **Weakness**: particularly to the proximal muscles of the lower limbs in an upper motor neuron pattern, although the exact distribution of power loss depends on the site of compression. Deep tendon reflexes are increased and the plantar response is extensor.
- **Sensory loss/paraesthesiae**: ascending to or just below the level of the relevant dermatome at the level of compression (suspended level).
- **Ataxia**: loss of proprioception (posterior columns).
- **Urinary retention and constipation**: late symptoms of autonomic dysfunction.

Clinical signs of cauda equina compression include pain; weakness (lower motor neuron pattern of lower limb weakness); ankle jerks may be lost and Babinski reflex may be negative; sensory loss (sacral anaesthesia may be present); and urinary retention and constipation.

Investigations

Malignant spinal cord compression is a medical emergency and mandates urgent investigation, i.e. within 24 hours of symptom onset.

- **Whole-spine magnetic resonance imaging** is the investigation of choice. It defines the exact location and disease extent. The whole spine must be examined as multiple sites of compression can occur.
- CT-guided **percutaneous biopsy** may be considered if the primary is unknown.

Management

- All patients with suspected cord or cauda equina compression require a full examination, including a complete neurological exam assessing power, tone, sensation (including assessment of saddle anaesthesia), reflexes and a rectal examination to assess anal tone and sensation.

- Analgesia and prophylactic anticoagulation (if no contraindications).
- Patients should be nursed flat with neutral spinal alignment (log rolling); if cervical lesion is present, may also require immobilization in a hard collar.
- **High-dose corticosteroids** (for example, 16 mg dexamethasone immediately followed by 8 mg dexamethasone twice a day 8am and 12pm with gastric protection, e.g. omeprazole) may improve symptoms and outcome.
- **Surgery**: all patients with spinal cord compression should be discussed with the neurosurgeons. Surgery carries significant morbidity and mortality, but has a role in those without a diagnosis, those with a single level of compression and those with spinal instability. Surgery may also be useful in patients with progression of neurological deficit during radiotherapy, compression in a previously irradiated area or in radioresistant disease, and may be associated with better outcome.
- **Radiotherapy** to debulk the tumour is the treatment of choice in those with radiosensitive tumours, if not considered to be surgical candidates, or following surgical decompression. It may improve pain and increase muscle power, but paraplegia is reversed in only 10–15% of patients. The radiation field includes two vertebrae either side of the site of compression (the site of frequent recurrence).
- **Chemotherapy**: cytotoxic chemotherapy is the treatment of choice in children with chemosensitive tumours, and in adults with chemosensitive disease (radiotherapy may also be given with chemotherapy).
- **Physiotherapy** is crucial to maximize any return of function.

Prognosis

The three main predictors of outcome are:

1 **pretreatment neurological status**: 80% of those ambulant at diagnosis remain so with urgent treatment. Paraplegia is reversed in <15% of cases

2 **speed of onset of neurological deficit**: disease progressing gradually is more likely to be reversible

3 **tumour type**: radiation- and chemotherapy-sensitive disease responds faster and better to treatment. Radioresistant tumours have poor outcomes.

Some patients presenting with malignant spinal cord compression will not achieve ambulation. They are often preterminally ill and face the loss of independence that confinement to a wheelchair brings. Maximizing physical and psychological support in this situation is an important part of the holistic treatment these patients should receive.

For **hypercalcaemia** see Chapter 162. For **fever with neutropenia** see Chapter 53.

Tumour lysis syndrome

Tumour lysis syndrome (TLS) is caused by rapid lysis of tumour cells resulting in the release of large amounts of intracellular contents into the circulation. It is characterized by high urate, high phosphate, high potassium, low calcium and the potential to develop acute renal impairment, cardiac arrhythmias and seizures. It most often occurs shortly after the start of anti-cancer therapy although it can also be the result of large tumour burdens with high proliferative rates. TLS is most commonly associated with haematological malignancies (lymphoma and acute lymphoblastic leukaemia) but it can also occur with solid tumours, such as germ cell tumours.

Management

- Identify high-risk patients pretreatment and treat prophylactically with allopurinol (reduces uric acid formation) or rasburicase (recombinant urate oxidase, metabolizes uric acid – important to check G6PD status before use).
- Investigations: regular monitoring of bloods including urea and electrolytes, uric acid, calcium, LDH and phosphate.
- Management of tumour lysis includes IV rehydration with close fluid balance. Renal/ITU advice should be sought and early consideration of renal dialysis. Correction of metabolic abnormalities, especially hyperkalaemia. Intravenous rasburicase should be considered to help clear uric acid.

Introduction to neurological diagnosis 1: Neuroepidemiology

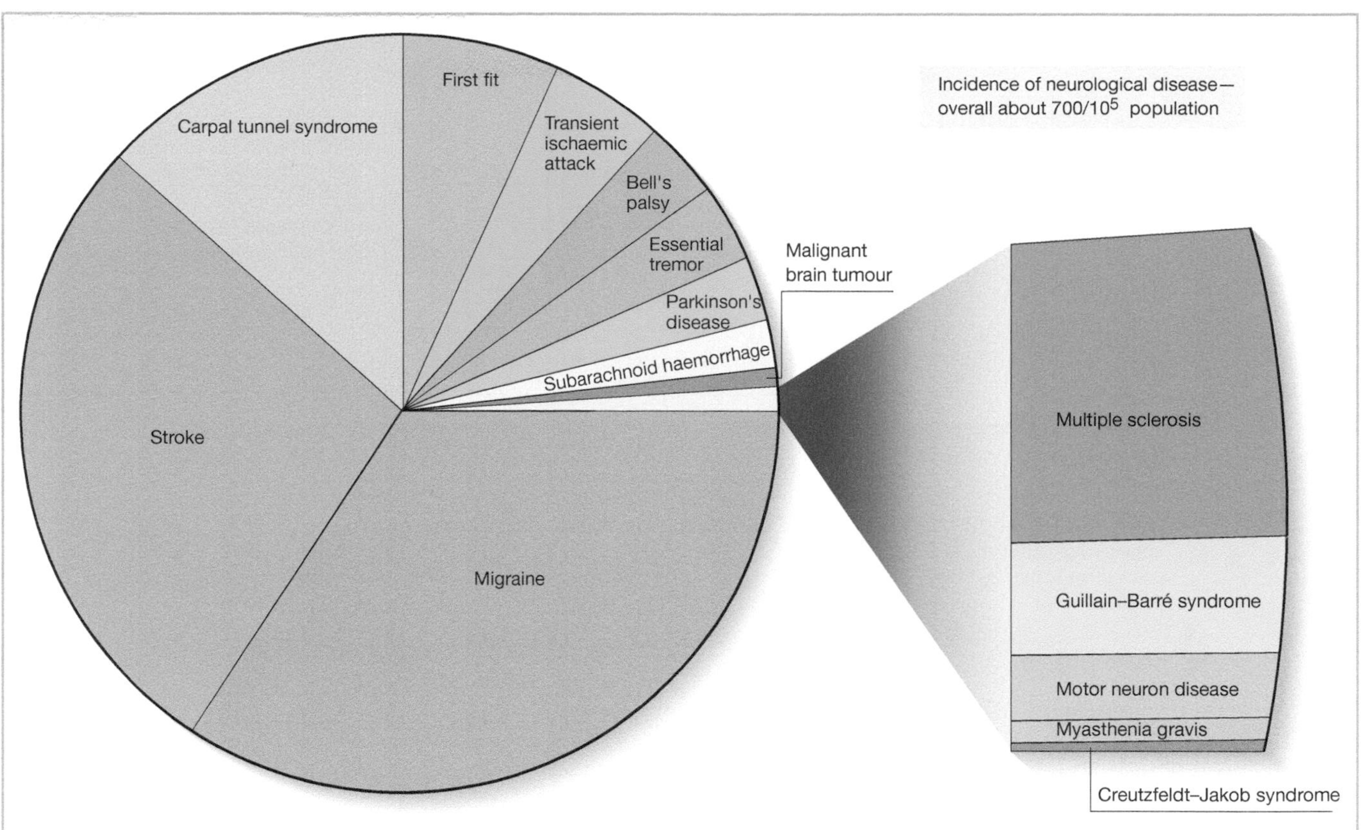

One of the difficulties in learning neurology is that there are apparently a bewildering number of possible conditions and diagnosis for each clinical syndrome, e.g. there are hundreds of different causes of peripheral neuropathy. Therefore, a sensible diagnostician bases the likelihood of a certain diagnosis on the prior probability, or incidence, of that condition. As many conditions are rare, it is reasonable to express this as cases per 100 000 population per year.

It will be strikingly apparent from Table 55.1 that the incidence of conditions in general practice is very different from that in a neurology clinic. Although a consultant neurologist (there are one per 75 000 people in the UK) will see a patient with a first fit in virtually every clinic, a GP may only see one such patient a year. It is also important to remember that it may be the *prevalence* of a disorder that gives a true indication of its impact on society as a whole. For example, multiple sclerosis and Parkinson's disease are disorders that do not significantly shorten lifespan in most patients, but last for decades, and therefore they have a high prevalence and impose a high burden on health and social care systems. It will also be immediately apparent that neurology teaching tends to overemphasize rare conditions that many students may never see again.

Table 55.1 Incidence of neurological conditions in the general population

Condition	Migraine	Stroke	Carpal tunnel syndrome	First fit	Transient ischaemic attack	Bell palsy	Essential tremor	Parkinson's disease	Subarachnoid haemorrhage	Malignant brain tumour	Multiple sclerosis	Guillain-Barré syndrome	Motor neuron disease	Myasthenia gravis	Creutzfeldt-Jakob disease
Annual incidence per 100 000 population	250	200	50	50	35	25	25	20	15	5	5	2	1	0.4	0.1
Time between each new case for a GP	10 weeks	12 weeks	6 months	1 year	17 months	2 years	2 years	2.5 years	3.3 years	10 years	10 years	25 years	33 years	125 years	500 years

Source: Warlow C.P. et al. 2001. Reproduced with permission of John Wiley & Sons.

Medicine at a Glance, Fifth Edition. Edited by Patrick Davey and Alex Pitcher.

Companion website: www.wiley.com/go/medicine5e

56 Introduction to neurological diagnosis 2

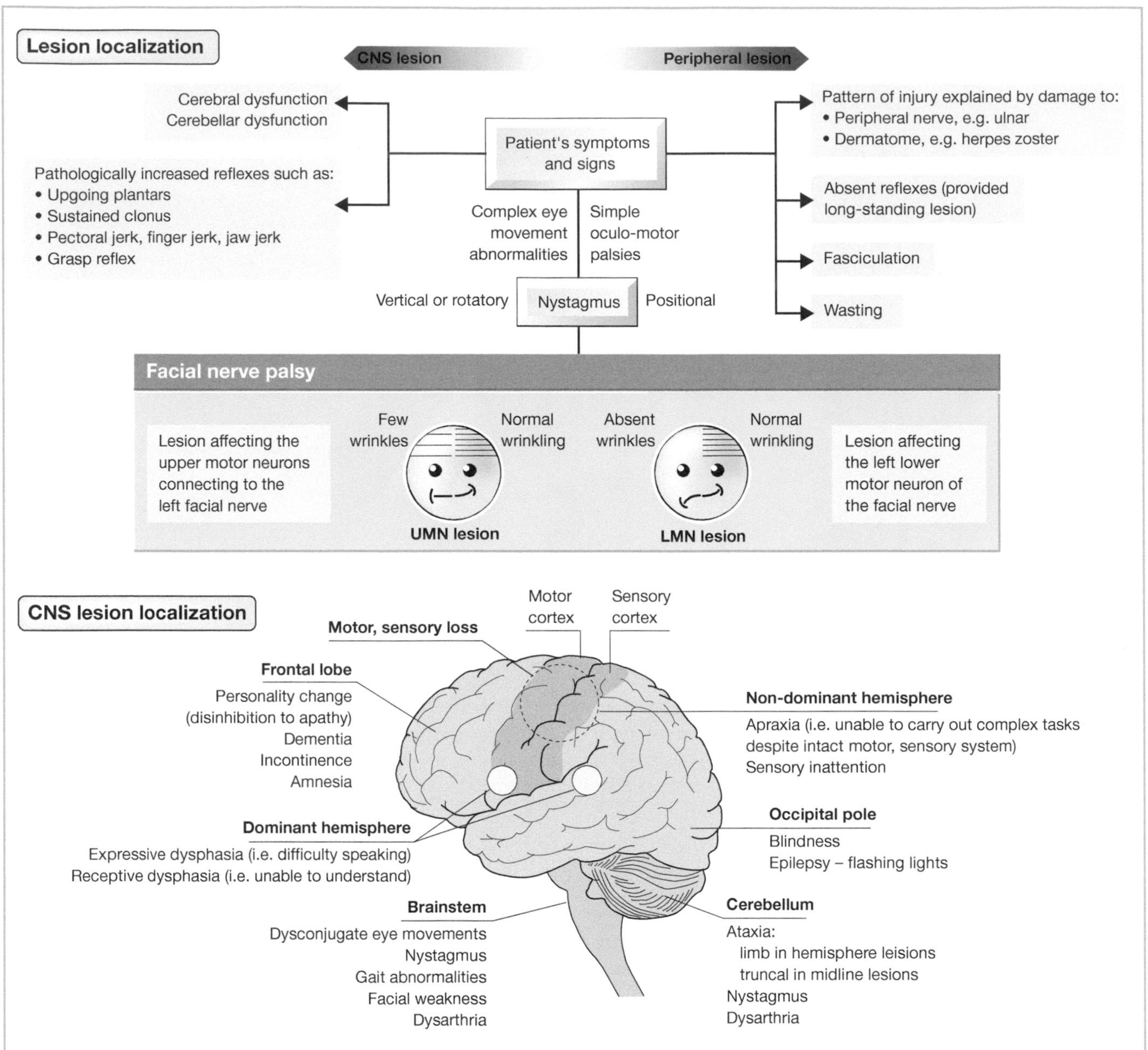

There are many different neurological diseases and it is not always possible to make a firm diagnosis from a particular set of signs and symptoms. For example, there are numerous causes of ataxia – the combination of peripheral neuropathy and ataxia only narrows this down but still leaves a range of possible underlying diagnoses. Neurologists therefore make an anatomical diagnosis followed by an aetiological or pathological diagnosis.

In addition to acquired diseases, there are many inherited conditions involving the nervous system. Individually, these are rare, but collectively they form an important proportion of the burden of neurological disease. Partly, this is because a high proportion of the 20 000 genes in the human genome are expressed in the nervous system. Mutation of these genes may be devastating but not lethal, allowing the survival of individuals with genetic disease.

Medicine at a Glance, Fifth Edition. Edited by Patrick Davey and Alex Pitcher.

Companion website: www.wiley.com/go/medicine5e

Furthermore, most cells of the central nervous system (CNS) are non-dividing and there is little capacity for regeneration. Therefore, the brain is susceptible to the accumulation of damaged protein with ageing and progressive neurodegenerative diseases become an increasing problem as the population ages.

Six steps to neurological diagnosis

1 Knowledge of neuroepidemiology (see Chapter 55). The prior probability of an individual diagnosis depends on the age of the patient and other factors.
2 A neurological diagnosis always depends most of all on a good history, without which the neurological examination and subsequent investigations will be difficult to interpret. Many common neurological diseases are frequently associated with normal scans (e.g. headache, primary epilepsies, many neurodegenerative diseases).
3 Perform a standard, simple examination on every patient. Extend this examination in particular situations.
4 Synthesize the history and examination to decide whether the problem is in the peripheral nervous system (including the muscles) or the CNS, of psychiatric origin, or not due to nervous system disease at all.
5 Only then can you draw up a differential diagnosis, taking into account the location of the problem (brain, spinal cord, nerve, muscle), the onset and progression of symptoms, and the age of the patient.
6 Perform special investigations to confirm your diagnostic hypothesis.

Lesion localization

In clinical practice, the key distinction in lesion localization is between the central and the peripheral nervous system (PNS). In diagnostic terms, this is far more important than whether the lesion is in a specific brain region.

Cerebral hemispheres

The extent of neurological dysfunction is affected by individual variation, the tempo and nature of the pathological process and cortical plasticity. Hemispheric lesions cause less motor and sensory dysfunction than lesions of equivalent volume in lower structures, and show a less consistent relationship between dysfunction and lesion localization than in the brainstem, spinal cord or PNS.

- **Contralateral hemianaesthesia** arises from damage to the cortical sensory area or from damage to thalamocortical connections. It is usually incomplete because somatosensory function is partially represented in both hemispheres.
- **Hemiplegia** may be caused by:
  - lesions of the contralateral primary motor cortex (when conscious level is also often decreased)
  - the descending motor tracts in the corona radiata or the posterior limb of the internal capsule (when conscious level is usually normal)
  - the brainstem (rarely), when there are usually associated cranial nerve signs
  - the ipsilateral spinal cord if there is a lesion discretely affecting one side. Accompanying sensory disturbance is usual.
- **Bilateral weakness** is unlikely to be the result of a single lesion of the cerebral cortex, except in the context of coma, because the motor pathways for each side of the body are in separate cerebral hemispheres. An extraordinarily rare exception of a single cortical lesion causing bilateral weakness is a midline parasagittal meningioma.
- **Language dominance** is in the left hemisphere in 98% of people (including 60% of left-handed individuals). This is important in deciding whether a lesion is in the left hemisphere.
- **Expressive (Broca) dysphasia** is caused by lesions of the dominant frontal lobe; patients show a marked decrease in verbal fluency but normal comprehension.
- **Receptive (Wernicke) dysphasia** is the result of dominant temporal lobe lesions; it is characterized by fluent speech with frequent paraphrasic errors (use of the wrong word) and poor comprehension. Mixed expressive and receptive dysphasia is common.
- **Disorders of spatial awareness**, including neglect, are more common in right posterior hemisphere (parietal) disease.
- **Immediate memory** is dependent on the functional integrity of both hippocampi, which lie adjacent to the temporal lobes. These structures are affected in herpes encephalitis and anoxia (e.g. after cardiac arrest or carbon monoxide poisoning).
- **Executive function** (planning, impulse control, etc.) is probably a diffuse brain function, but selective disorders of executive control have some localizing value for lesions of the frontal lobes.

Cerebellum

The cerebellum functions as a modulator of motor learning and execution to facilitate the smooth integration of movement. Anatomically, it is divided into the midline vermis and two hemispheres. The vascular supply of the cerebellum is from the vertebrobasilar system via the posterior inferior cerebellar artery, the anterior inferior cerebellar artery and the superior cerebellar artery.

- Lesions of the vermis cause **truncal ataxia**; lesions of the hemispheres cause **limb ataxia**.
- **Ocular features** of cerebellar disease are usually prominent and include nystagmus, broken smooth pursuit, slow (hypometric) saccadic movement and ocular dysmetria (saccadic overshoot).
- **Cerebellar tremor** is a kinetic tremor with exacerbation at the end of movement, underlining the function of the cerebellum in damping movement.
- Other signs of cerebellar disturbance are **gait ataxia** and **dysarthria**. The latter is characteristically a disorder of loss of prosody with monotonous, slurred speech.

Brainstem

The brainstem consists of the midbrain, pons and medulla oblongata. There is a concentration of anatomically important structures in a small area, so most lesions of the brainstem are complex.

- Typical features of brainstem disease are nystagmus and disorders of conjugate gaze, vertigo, facial weakness, dysarthria, gait disturbance and ataxia. All these can occur as a result of disease in other sites, but the constellation together suggests a brainstem origin.
- Most eponymous vascular brainstem syndromes are rarely seen in pure form – precise localization has been greatly aided by magnetic resonance imaging and angiography.

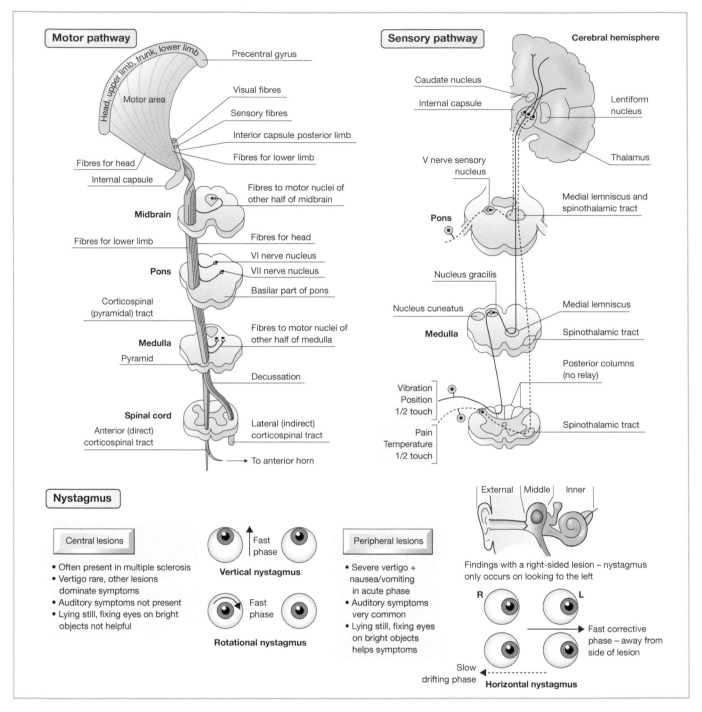

57 Introduction to neurological diagnosis 3

Motor pathway

Head, upper limb, trunk, lower limb
Precentral gyrus
Motor area
Visual fibres
Sensory fibres
Interior capsule posterior limb
Fibres for lower limb
Fibres for head
Internal capsule
Fibres to motor nuclei of other half of midbrain
Midbrain
Fibres for lower limb
Fibres for head
VI nerve nucleus
Pons
VII nerve nucleus
Basilar part of pons
Corticospinal (pyramidal) tract
Fibres to motor nuclei of other half of medulla
Medulla
Pyramid
Decussation
Spinal cord
Anterior (direct) corticospinal tract
Lateral (indirect) corticospinal tract
To anterior horn

Sensory pathway

Cerebral hemisphere
Caudate nucleus
Internal capsule
Lentiform nucleus
Thalamus
V nerve sensory nucleus
Medial lemniscus and spinothalamic tract
Pons
Nucleus gracilis
Nucleus cuneatus
Medial lemniscus
Medulla
Spinothalamic tract
Posterior columns (no relay)
Vibration
Position
1/2 touch
Pain
Temperature
1/2 touch
Spinothalamic tract

Nystagmus

Central lesions

- Often present in multiple sclerosis
- Vertigo rare, other lesions dominate symptoms
- Auditory symptoms not present
- Lying still, fixing eyes on bright objects not helpful

Fast phase
Vertical nystagmus
Fast phase
Rotational nystagmus

Peripheral lesions

- Severe vertigo + nausea/vomiting in acute phase
- Auditory symptoms very common
- Lying still, fixing eyes on bright objects helps symptoms

External
Middle
Inner

Findings with a right-sided lesion – nystagmus only occurs on looking to the left

R
L
Fast corrective phase – away from side of lesion
Slow drifting phase
Horizontal nystagmus

Eye movements

Virtually every region of the brain has some influence on the control of conjugate gaze. Voluntary gaze centres in the frontal lobes and parietal cortex initiate volitional eye movement. These send descending pathways to the brainstem nuclei, which receive influences from the cerebellum and basal ganglia, and the ascending influences from the spinal cord. There are important internuclear connections. Thus disorders of conjugate gaze may be:

Medicine at a Glance, Fifth Edition. Edited by Patrick Davey and Alex Pitcher.

Companion website: www.wiley.com/go/medicine5e

- supranuclear
- internuclear (see Chapter 60)
- nuclear.

Eye movements are also affected by disease of the extraocular muscles and the structures of the orbit, and damage to the peripheral segments of cranial nerves III, IV and VI. Examination of eye movements is thus far more than simply the examination of cranial nerves III, IV and VI. It should be directed at describing the abnormality without assumptions about whether the lesion is in the nerve, the brainstem or higher up. Common patterns of abnormality in conjugate gaze are described in Chapters 60 and 61. Nystagmus should be described as:

- occurring in the primary position (the midline)
- or occurring on horizontal or vertical gaze.

In practice, it is often difficult to localize nystagmus and it is best to consider it in the context of the rest of the history and examination, before deciding if it is arising from peripheral structures (the labyrinth), the brainstem or the cerebellum. The slow phase of nystagmus is the 'pathological' component and the fast phase is corrective.

- **Peripheral (vestibular) nystagmus** is typically associated with severe symptoms of dysequilibrium, nausea and vomiting, and is often unilateral. The fast phase is away from the lesion because the vestibular apparatus functions to stimulate eye movement towards the contralateral side.
- **Central nystagmus**: ipsilateral structures in the brainstem maintain horizontal gaze. Thus, the pathological drift of the eye (the slow phase of nystagmus) is away from the lesion, with a corrective (fast) phase towards the affected side of the brainstem in central nystagmus. Furthermore, central lesions are often bilateral.
- **Cerebellar nystagmus** is similar in that it is probably mediated by cerebellar–brainstem connections.

Spinal cord

The spinal cord is a small structure <1.5 cm in diameter. There is no anatomical boundary between each side, and many pathological processes are therefore bilateral.

The vascular supply to the spinal cord is of clinical relevance. A single spinal artery supplies the anterior portion of the cord, leaving it vulnerable to ischaemic damage (see Chapter 209), whereas the posterior part of the cord has a rich anastomotic supply (from posterior spinal arteries).

Weakness caused by spinal cord disease is therefore usually bilateral and associated with a motor and sensory level. At the level of the lesion, there are lower motor neuron (LMN) signs as evidenced by diminished tendon reflexes and weakness; below the lesion, there are upper motor neuron (UMN) signs, and above the lesion the limbs are normal.

Descending tracts from the motor cortex travel as the lateral corticospinal tract before synapsing on LMNs in the ventral horns. These cells receive descending influences from the basal ganglia, red nucleus and vestibular apparatus. LMNs thus serve as a final common pathway for motor function.

The ascending sensory pathways can be divided into:

- spinothalamic tracts, which carry pain and temperature in the contralateral lateral spinothalamic tract and light touch in the ventral spinothalamic tract to synapse in the thalamus
- gracile and cuneate fasciculi, which carry joint position sense, kinaesthetic sense, two-point discrimination and light touch on the ipsilateral posterior columns to synapse in the medullary nuclei and on to the thalamus
- spinocerebellar tracts.

The vertebral level is not the same as the spinal cord level – the cord ends at L1, so it is safe to perform a lumbar puncture in adults in L2/3, L3/4 and L4/5 spaces.

The cord terminates in the conus medullaris and the cauda equina. Conus lesions are characterized by sphincter dysfunction, sensory loss in the perineum and loss of ankle jerks. Cauda equina lesions can involve the same functions, but sphincter disturbance is a late feature and symptoms and signs are usually asymmetrical.

Nerve roots

The identification of lesions at specific spinal root levels requires knowledge of dermatomes and myotomes.

- Root disease is characterized by radicular pain, and sensory and motor dysfunction.
- Particular diseases (e.g. herpes zoster and Guillain–Barré syndrome) have a predilection for nerve roots.
- The most common levels for intervertebral disc prolapse are between the sixth and seventh vertebrae in the cervical region (C7 root compression) and between the fourth and fifth vertebrae in the lumbar region (L5 root compression).
- The effects of root compression at various levels are as follows.
    - C5: weakness of shoulder abduction (deltoid) and forearm flexion (biceps), sensory loss on the lateral aspect of the arm and loss of the biceps jerk.
    - C6: weakness of forearm flexion, finger and wrist extension, loss of the biceps jerk, sensory loss on the lateral surface of the forearm and first and second digits.
    - C7: loss of the triceps reflex, weakness of elbow extension and wrist extension and flexion, sensory loss in the third and fourth digits.
    - C8: weakness and wasting of intrinsic hand muscles, sensory loss in the fifth digit and the medial forearm; there may be an ipsilateral Horner syndrome.
    - T1: wasting of the small muscles of the hand and ipsilateral Horner syndrome.
    - L4: weakness of knee extension, loss of the knee jerk and wasting of quadriceps.
    - L5: weakness of knee flexion, ankle dorsiflexion and plantarflexion.
    - S1: loss of the ankle jerk, weakness of dorsiflexion of the great toe.

Lesion localization in peripheral nerve and muscle

See Chapters 209, 210 and 211.

Common neurological symptoms

'Waddling' gait

Difficulty walking upstairs

Difficulty reaching up

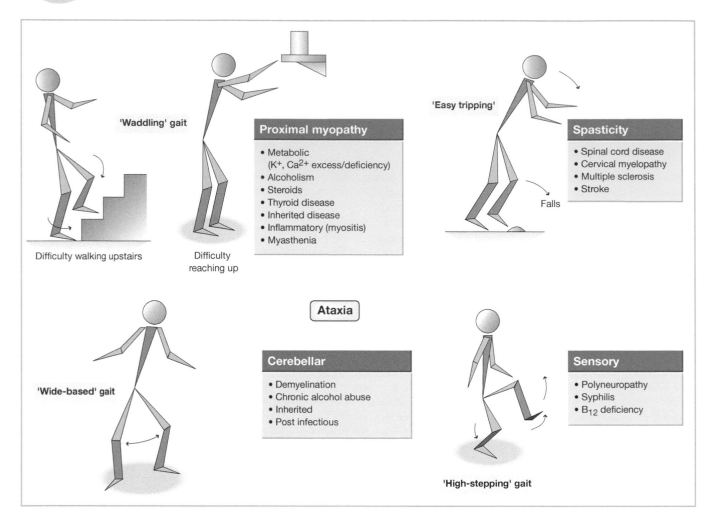

Proximal myopathy

- Metabolic (K^+, Ca^{2+} excess/deficiency)
- Alcoholism
- Steroids
- Thyroid disease
- Inherited disease
- Inflammatory (myositis)
- Myasthenia

'Easy tripping'

Falls

Spasticity

- Spinal cord disease
- Cervical myelopathy
- Multiple sclerosis
- Stroke

Ataxia

'Wide-based' gait

Cerebellar

- Demyelination
- Chronic alcohol abuse
- Inherited
- Post infectious

'High-stepping' gait

Sensory

- Polyneuropathy
- Syphilis
- B_{12} deficiency

Difficulty walking

Both neurological and non-neurological diseases, e.g. joint disease, can cause difficulty in walking. Analysing gait problems in elderly people carries particular difficulties in interpretation and is complicated by:

- multiple co-morbidities
- age-related changes in musculoskeletal function
- joint disease
- underlying cerebrovascular disease
- postural hypotension (see Chapter 64)
- fear of falling.

A full neurological and rheumatological history and examination are necessary to place all of these contributory factors in context. The most important part of the assessment is to see the patient walking. Invaluable information is obtained by watching the patient get up from the waiting room chair and walk into the consulting room.

Patterns of gait disturbance

Bear in mind that classic gait patterns may be present in their pure form only in advanced disease. Frequently, a non-specific or mixed gait abnormality is observed.

- **Peripheral neuropathies.**
  - Motor nerve damage: foot drop occurs with a 'high-stepping' gait.
  - Sensory (proprioceptive) nerve damage: ataxia and sometimes a 'stamping' gait develop.
- **Muscle disease** usually causes proximal muscle weakness and a 'waddling' gait.
- **Spinal cord or upper motor neuron damage**: the earliest symptom is 'easy tripping up' or difficulty walking on rough ground. Subsequently, the leg(s) drag. Examination shows a narrow-based gait and brisk reflexes, often with clonus. The gait is described as being 'stiff', and 'spastic scissoring' together of the legs sometimes occurs.
- **Cerebellar disease** causes a wide-based, staggering gait (termed 'ataxic'). Midline cerebellar lesions may cause gait ataxia with relatively few signs in the limbs. For causes of ataxia, see next section.

Medicine at a Glance, Fifth Edition. Edited by Patrick Davey and Alex Pitcher.

Companion website: www.wiley.com/go/medicine5e

- **Hemispheric damage** causes a contralateral hemiplegic gait, with the contralateral arm held in flexion. In walking, the leg is swung outwards and forwards, in a circular motion – a movement termed 'circumduction'.
- The earliest feature of **Parkinson's disease** is an asymmetrical loss of arm swing. Later, a stooped posture with shuffling footsteps develops. The gait may be 'festinant', which means that there is a tendency to hurry, and turning is slow, resulting in instability.
- **Diffuse vascular disease** causes a variety of gait disturbances, including a form of lower body parkinsonism with a wide-based gait and small steps termed 'marche à petit pas'.
- **Gait apraxia** is an inability to carry out complex tasks, such as walking, as a result of damage to the part of the brain that integrates complex motor function. The gait is disordered and the patient is apparently unable to initiate steps, but individual actions, e.g. making cycling motions on a bed, remain intact. It occurs in a number of different cortical diseases, including diffuse vascular disease and also normal pressure hydrocephalus.
- **Dizziness**: see section below on dizziness.
- **Loss of balance**: may relate to inner ear disease (often either continuous or episodic), cerebellar disease, dorsal column loss or peripheral sensory or motor neuropathy.

Differential diagnosis of ataxia

Ataxia is defined as inco-ordination of complex movement, such as walking in a straight line. Anatomically, ataxia is caused by the following.

- **Lesions of the cerebellum** ('cerebellar ataxia'): wide-based gait, falling to the side of the lesion. A 'kinetic' or intention tremor (brought out by the 'finger–nose' test) is usually present.
- **Disorders of proprioception** ('sensory ataxia') caused by polyneuropathies (see Chapter 211) or lesions of the dorsal columns (classically, as in subacute combined degeneration due to vitamin B_{12} deficiency or in tabes dorsalis, causing a 'high stepping' or broad-based gait).

The causes of ataxia are legion and include the following.

- Drugs: anticonvulsants, alcohol, benzodiazepines.
- Multiple sclerosis.
- Cerebellar lesions: tumours or vascular insults.
- Degenerative disease: multiple system atrophy.
- Inherited disease: Friedreich ataxia, spinocerebellar ataxias.
- Metabolic: vitamin B_{12} deficiency, heavy metal poisoning.
- Parainfectious (more common in children): chickenpox, glandular fever, *Mycoplasma* infection, psittacosis and legionellosis.
- Paraneoplastic cerebellar degeneration.

Dizziness

This extremely common problem causes considerable misery to patients, although it rarely has a serious underlying cause. First, establish what is meant by 'dizziness' because this word is used to express a large range of subjective feelings, from presyncope or faintness, through vertigo to an odd light-headedness. It is crucial to define the symptom accurately. Although it is always better to let the patient use their own words and unwise to put

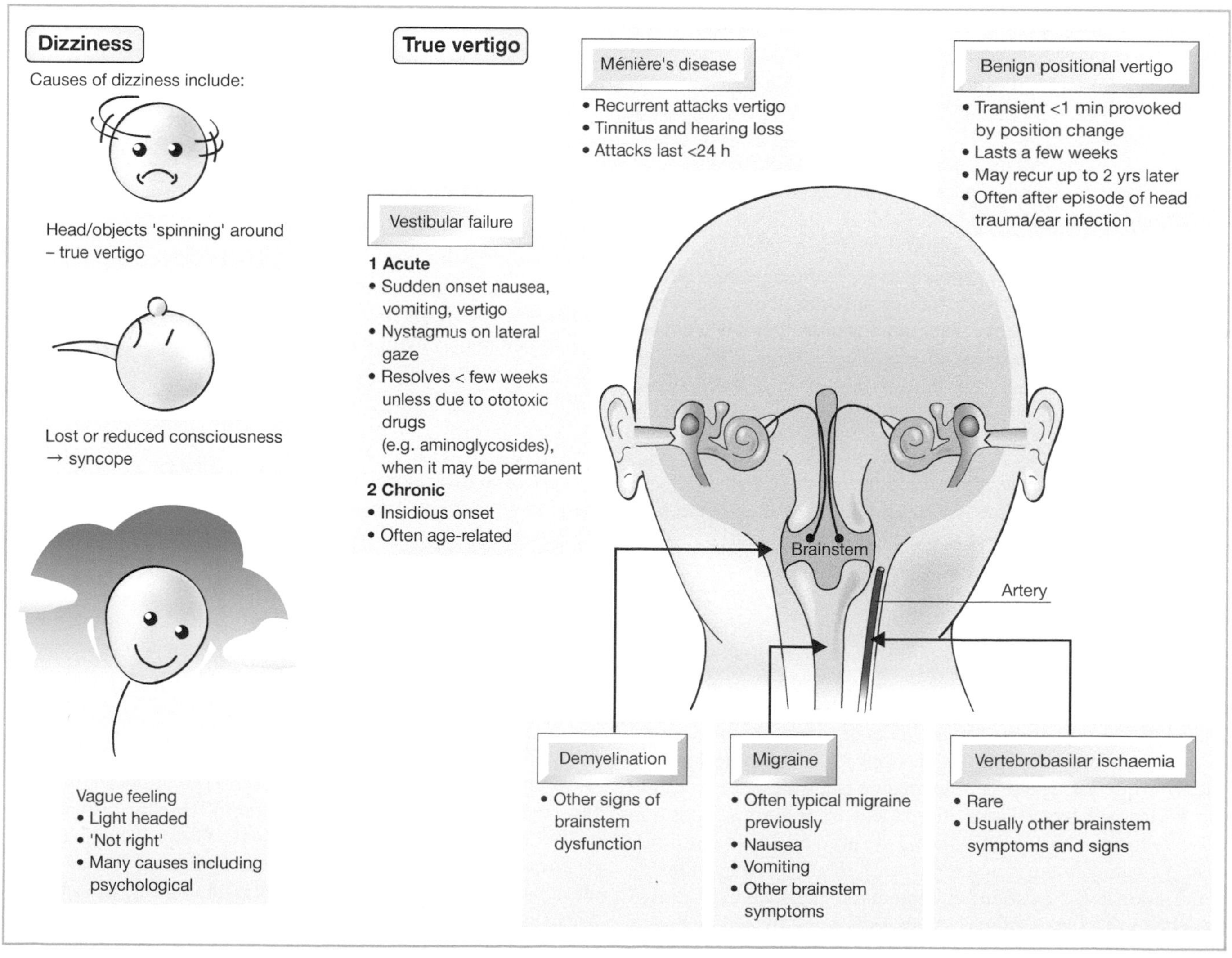
Dizziness
Causes of dizziness include:
Head/objects 'spinning' around – true vertigo
Lost or reduced consciousness → syncope
Vague feeling
• Light headed
• 'Not right'
• Many causes including psychological
True vertigo
Ménière's disease
• Recurrent attacks vertigo
• Tinnitus and hearing loss
• Attacks last <24 h
Benign positional vertigo
• Transient <1 min provoked by position change
• Lasts a few weeks
• May recur up to 2 yrs later
• Often after episode of head trauma/ear infection
Vestibular failure
1 Acute
• Sudden onset nausea, vomiting, vertigo
• Nystagmus on lateral gaze
• Resolves < few weeks unless due to ototoxic drugs (e.g. aminoglycosides), when it may be permanent
2 Chronic
• Insidious onset
• Often age-related
Brainstem
Artery
Demyelination
• Other signs of brainstem dysfunction
Migraine
• Often typical migraine previously
• Nausea
• Vomiting
• Other brainstem symptoms
Vertebrobasilar ischaemia
• Rare
• Usually other brainstem symptoms and signs

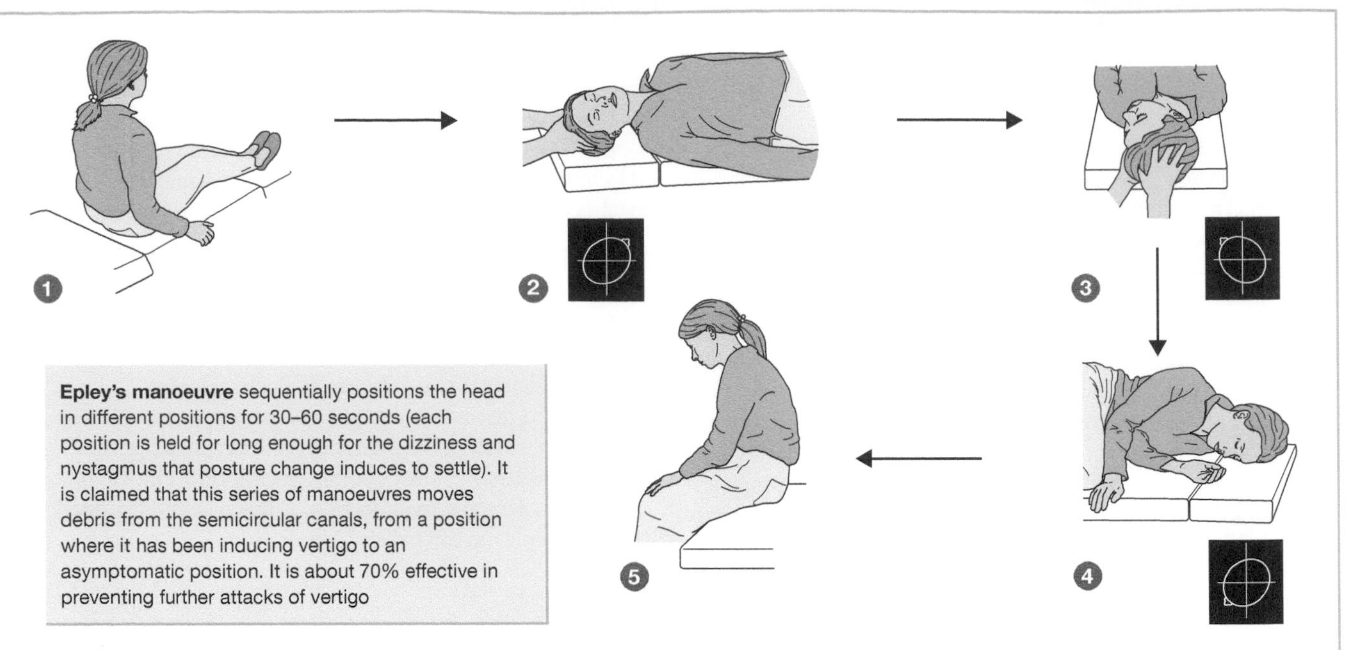

Epley's manoeuvre sequentially positions the head in different positions for 30–60 seconds (each position is held for long enough for the dizziness and nystagmus that posture change induces to settle). It is claimed that this series of manoeuvres moves debris from the semicircular canals, from a position where it has been inducing vertigo to an asymptomatic position. It is about 70% effective in preventing further attacks of vertigo

words into patients' mouths, some people have such difficulty describing this symptom that it may be appropriate cautiously to offer some possibilities.

- Do you feel as if you are going to faint? This symptom is likely to represent presyncope (see Chapter 64).
- Do objects in your vision such as furniture or pictures on the wall actually move around or do you feel as if you are moving? Suggests true vertigo, caused by peripheral pathology affecting the inner ear or cranial nerve VIII, or central pathology affecting the brainstem.
- Do you just have a vague feeling all the time of light-headedness? May represent a variety of problems ranging from hyperventilation through to tension headache. This is sometimes called psychophysical dizziness. It is uncommon to find a clear diagnosis.
- What other symptoms are present? Tinnitus with deafness suggests inner ear pathology. Nausea and vomiting suggest vestibular or brainstem disease. Diplopia suggests brainstem disease. For ataxia, see earlier section.
- What provokes symptoms? If head movement provokes symptoms, then vestibular disease is likely. Provocation on standing suggests postural hypotension.

Once the nature of the symptom has been established, a physical examination should be directed at excluding cardiac arrhythmia or postural hypotension. Then a specific neurological examination should look for evidence of cerebellar and brainstem disease.

Peripheral causes of vertigo

- **Benign paroxysmal positional vertigo** causes recurrent attacks of transient (lasting seconds) dizziness and vertigo associated with changes in head posture, e.g. lying on the pillow at night. Attacks tend to persist for weeks or months before spontaneously resolving, but may recur. Conventional physical examination is normal. Hallpike's manoeuvre is a specific provocation test performed by bringing the patient from a sitting position down onto their back while turning the head briskly in one direction. If positive, there is nystagmus with rotation towards the side of the lesion and the patient's symptoms are replicated. It is caused by debris in the semicircular canals and can be treated by Epley's manoeuvre.
- **Acute vestibular failure** is a common clinical problem where patients complain of the sudden onset of nausea, vomiting and severe vertigo. On examination, there is nystagmus on lateral gaze and unsteadiness. This condition, which has a good prognosis and tends to resolve over days to weeks, has a variety of synonyms such as 'acute labyrinthitis' and 'vestibular neuronitis' which suggest a possible viral, postviral or inflammatory origin, but betray our ignorance of the true pathogenesis. It sometimes occurs after an upper respiratory tract infection.
- **Ménière's disease**: recurrent attacks of vertigo, tinnitus and decreased hearing occur in middle life and ultimately may progress to deafness. The attacks build up over minutes, last for hours and then gradually resolve. The key to the diagnosis is to document fluctuating levels of hearing loss.
- **Chronic vestibular failure**: this has a number of causes and presents with a more insidious form of dizziness, which can be rather non-specific in character. Age-related vestibular degeneration is increasingly being recognized.
- **Drugs**, such as high-dose aminoglycosides and furosemide (frusemide), can cause vestibular failure.

Central causes of vertigo

- **Vertebrobasilar ischaemia** is a rarer cause of isolated dizziness than usually thought. Attacks of dizziness of abrupt onset and lasting for several minutes are typical. Most patients with vertebrobasilar ischaemia have other symptoms of brainstem involvement. Brainstem stroke also usually produces other physical signs.
- **Migraine** can cause transient vertigo. Other symptoms of brainstem involvement are usual. A migrainous headache may or may not follow.
- **Brainstem disease**, including multiple sclerosis.

Mixed causes of vertigo

- **Acoustic neuroma**: a benign Schwann cell tumour arising on the vestibular portion of cranial nerve VIII, either isolated or caused by neurofibromatosis type 2 (see Chapter 208), causing deafness and often vertigo. Brainstem compression may cause ataxia and, if severe, aqueduct compression and hydrocephalus. Sensation to the cornea is lost. Magnetic resonance imaging confirms the diagnosis. Surgery may be curative.

59 Weakness

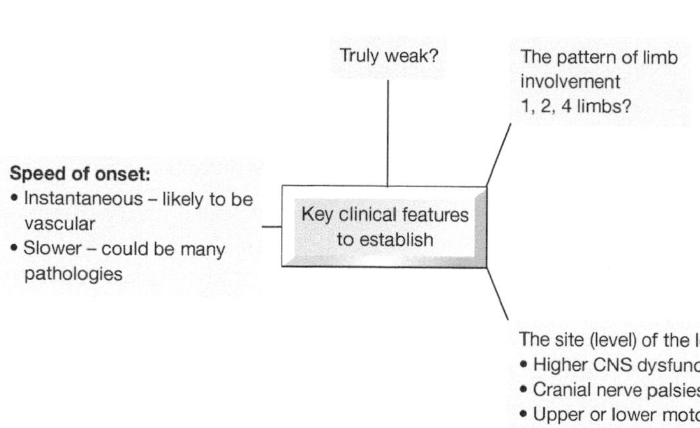

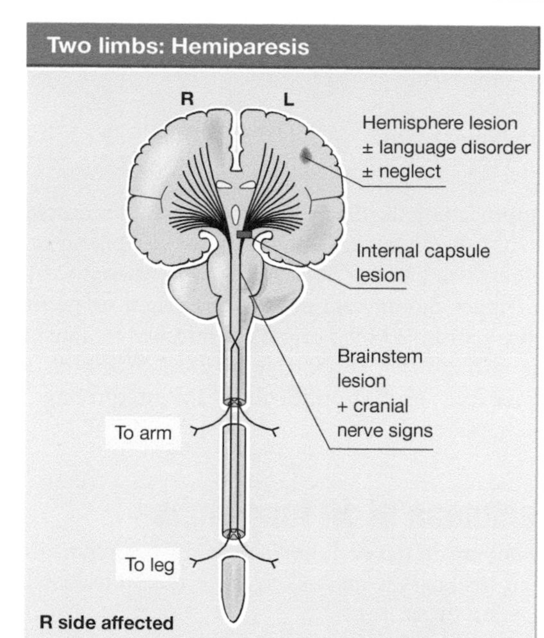

One limb: Monoparesis

R L

Motor cortex lesion

Internal capsule lesion
No sensory loss, e.g. clumsy hand/ dysarthria syndrome

Plexus lesion, e.g. brachial LMN signs

Motor neuron disease – UMN + LMN signs

L limb affected

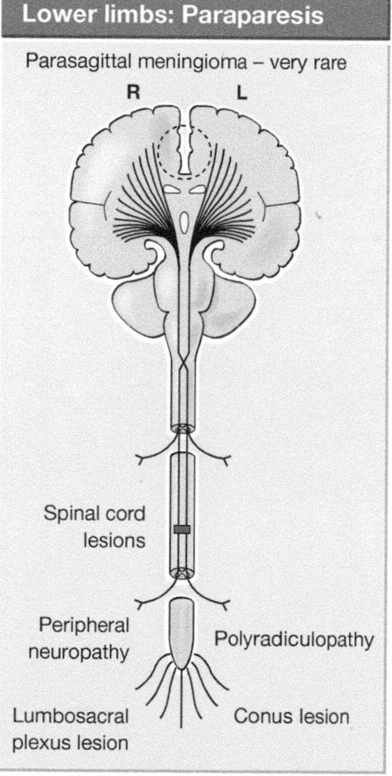

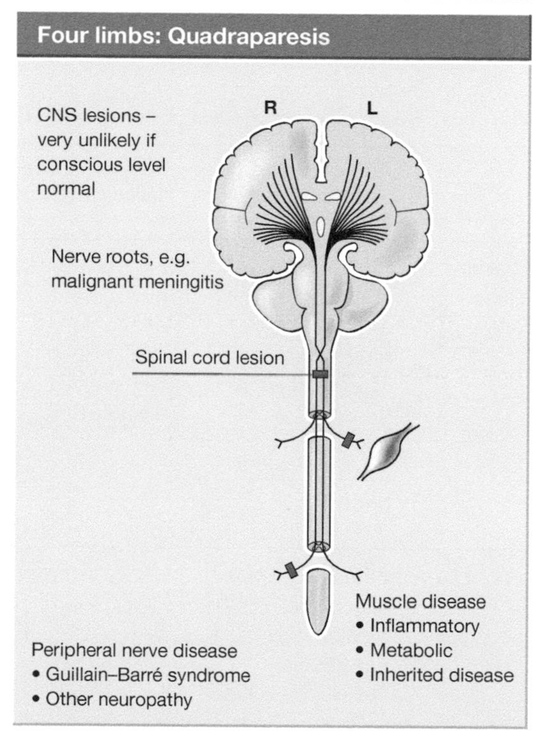

Medicine at a Glance, Fifth Edition. Edited by Patrick Davey and Alex Pitcher.

Companion website: www.wiley.com/go/medicine5e

Weakness may be used loosely by patients to include fatigue or tiredness – it is vital to establish that any weakness is genuine, i.e. has led to loss of function (although loss of function may also relate to sensory loss, dyspraxia or inco-ordination, e.g. as a result of cerebellar disease). It is useful to ask the patient to list the specific activities that cannot be performed (walking, climbing stairs, rising from sitting to standing, reaching above the head, writing, unscrewing lids, etc.). Motor weakness may result from lesions affecting:

- the brain.
- the spinal cord.
- nerves, neuromuscular junctions or muscles.

In approaching the diagnosis of weakness, it is crucial to establish whether the problem is of central or peripheral origin (neuroanatomy, see Chapter 56). Differences between weakness of central (upper motor neuron [UMN]) origin or peripheral (lower motor neuron [LMN]) origin are outlined in Table 59.1. Finally, bear in mind that co-existing medical conditions such as joint disease can lead to difficulties in interpreting neurological weakness.

Weakness of all four limbs

Depending on the evolution and associated physical signs, generalized weakness is most likely to be due to lesions in one of the following structures.

Cerebral hemispheres

It is very unlikely that a patient with a *normal level of consciousness* and generalized weakness has a hemispheric lesion of the brain.

Brainstem

A pontine haemorrhage or other lesion can lead to complete quadriplegia, including the face (locked-in syndrome). Consciousness is usually markedly depressed in the early stages.

Spinal cord

The degree to which weakness is generalized and affects the upper and lower limbs depends on the level of involvement of the spinal cord. Complete weakness affecting all four limbs occurs only if the spinal lesion is above C5. The pathological diagnosis is often suspected from the speed of onset of symptoms.

- Acute: cord compression, anterior spinal artery thrombosis and acute transverse myelitis.
- Subacute: intrinsic spinal cord tumours, vascular malformations of the dura, vitamin B_{12} deficiency and malignant meningeal infiltration.
- Chronic: benign tumours, syringomyelia and inherited conditions – hereditary spastic paraparesis (although this usually affects only the legs), spinocerebellar ataxias (e.g. Friedreich ataxia) and tropical spastic paraparesis caused by human T-lymphocyte virus 1 infection.

Table 59.1 Weakness of central and peripheral origin

	Upper motor neuron (usually pyramidal tract)	Extrapyramidal or basal ganglia disorders	Lower motor neuron	Muscular	Neuromuscular junction
Pattern of weakness	Limb weakness often incomplete, affecting large movements Most marked in the extensors of upper limb and flexors of lower limb	No true loss of muscle power, but failure of integration of agonist and antagonist muscles Generalized throughout a whole limb	Usually marked, affecting specific muscle groups, except in diffuse polyneuropathies Maximal distally in polyneuropathies	Usually generalized, unless one muscle is injured Maximal proximally and usually symmetrical: neck and swallowing and eye muscles may be involved	Variable but fatiguable, ptosis and extraocular muscle weakness common
Tone	Spasticity: velocity-dependent resistance to movement Clasp knife reflex Clonus	Rigidity	Decreased	Normal or decreased	Normal
Reflexes	Brisk	Normal	Reduced or absent	Normal	Normal or depressed (Eaton–Lambert syndrome)
Muscle appearance	Disuse atrophy after prolonged weakness, but no true wasting	Normal	Segmental wasting; fasciculation if lesion at the level of anterior horn cell	Normal or atrophic	Usually normal

Nerve roots

Inflammation, such as that caused by viral infection (cytomegalovirus, varicella zoster virus) of the nerve roots, can cause weakness in all four limbs, as can malignant infiltration spread through the cerebrospinal fluid (malignant meningitis).

Polyneuropathy

Diffuse nerve damage can cause weakness of all four limbs, such as occurs in Guillain–Barré syndrome (see Chapter 211), chronic inflammatory demyelinating polyneuropathy or inherited neuropathies such as hereditary motor and sensory neuropathy. Other causes include critical illness polyneuropathy, diphtheria, sarcoidosis, Lyme disease, borreliosis and amyloid. In general, there is a distal predominant pattern of weakness.

Muscle disease

Inflammatory, metabolic or inherited muscle disease can all produce a diffuse weakness (see Chapter 210).

Weakness of one limb

This is a difficult problem clinically and can arise from lesions almost anywhere in the nervous system.

Cortical lesions

Cortical lesions affecting the motor pathways to the limbs can start as a problem isolated to one limb. UMN signs are found. Lacunar strokes affecting the basis pontis can give rise to clumsiness and weakness of one hand.

Motor neuron disease

Motor neuron disease not infrequently begins in one limb with foot drop or wasting of the intrinsic hand muscles, although subtle signs can often be seen in other limbs.

Spinal cord lesions

Spinal cord lesions at the appropriate level can give rise to weakness of one leg associated with loss of pain and temperature in the contralateral leg.

Plexopathy

A plexopathy (brachial or lumbosacral) can affect an arm or a leg. Inflammatory diseases such as brachial neuritis or diabetic amyotrophy are examples.

Involvement of multiple large motor nerves (mononeuritis multiplex)

Mononeuritis multiplex can present in one limb or asymmetrically involve several limbs. Mononeuritis multiplex is usually a consequence of an underlying systemic disease process (see Table 59.1). Multiple root lesions can produce a similar pattern.

Isolated mononeuropathy

An isolated mononeuropathy, e.g. femoral, can give rise to isolated weakness of one limb.

Weakness of one side of the body

A hemiparesis can arise in a wide variety of locations.

Contralateral cerebral hemisphere

Damage to the contralateral cerebral hemisphere can cause weakness down one side of the body, when it may be associated with other physical signs (e.g. language dysfunction in the dominant hemisphere, neglect in the non-dominant hemisphere).

Brainstem

Vascular occlusion in this area can cause a number of eponymous syndromes.

- In the midbrain there will be hemiplegia with a contralateral third nerve palsy (Weber syndrome).
- In the pons, the weakness will be associated with conjugate gaze deviation towards the weak limbs and there may be a contralateral LMN facial weakness.

Spinal cord

See Chapter 209.

Weakness of both lower limbs (paraparesis)

- Spinal cord lesion.
- Peripheral neuropathy.
- Bilateral involvement of the lumbosacral plexus.
- Motor neuron disease.

Rarely, bilateral parasagittal lesions in the brain, classically a meningioma (although this is very rare), or other bilateral pathologies may also be responsible.

Weakness of both upper limbs

- Spinal cord lesion.
- Unusual forms of motor neuron disease.
- Bilateral brachial neuritis.

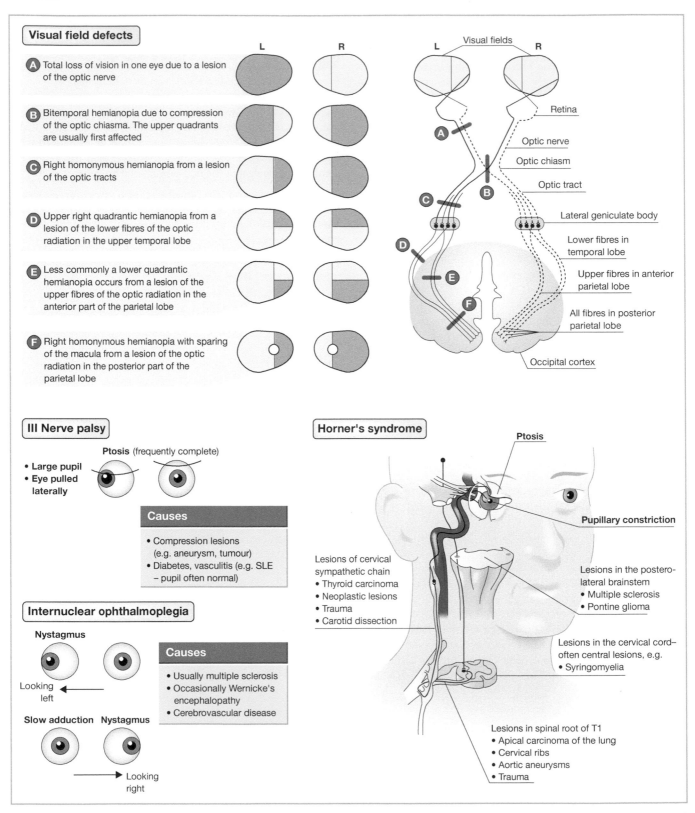

Disturbance of vision: a neurological perspective

Visual field defects

L R

A Total loss of vision in one eye due to a lesion of the optic nerve

B Bitemporal hemianopia due to compression of the optic chiasma. The upper quadrants are usually first affected

C Right homonymous hemianopia from a lesion of the optic tracts

D Upper right quadrantic hemianopia from a lesion of the lower fibres of the optic radiation in the upper temporal lobe

E Less commonly a lower quadrantic hemianopia occurs from a lesion of the upper fibres of the optic radiation in the anterior part of the parietal lobe

F Right homonymous hemianopia with sparing of the macula from a lesion of the optic radiation in the posterior part of the parietal lobe

Visual fields
L
R
Retina
Optic nerve
Optic chiasm
Optic tract
Lateral geniculate body
Lower fibres in temporal lobe
Upper fibres in anterior parietal lobe
All fibres in posterior parietal lobe
Occipital cortex
A
B
C
D
E
F

III Nerve palsy

- **Large pupil**
- **Eye pulled laterally**

Ptosis (frequently complete)

Causes

- Compression lesions (e.g. aneurysm, tumour)
- Diabetes, vasculitis (e.g. SLE – pupil often normal)

Internuclear ophthalmoplegia

Nystagmus

Looking left

Slow adduction **Nystagmus**

Looking right

Causes

- Usually multiple sclerosis
- Occasionally Wernicke's encephalopathy
- Cerebrovascular disease

Horner's syndrome

Ptosis

Pupillary constriction

Lesions of cervical sympathetic chain
- Thyroid carcinoma
- Neoplastic lesions
- Trauma
- Carotid dissection

Lesions in the postero-lateral brainstem
- Multiple sclerosis
- Pontine glioma

Lesions in the cervical cord– often central lesions, e.g.
- Syringomyelia

Lesions in spinal root of T1
- Apical carcinoma of the lung
- Cervical ribs
- Aortic aneurysms
- Trauma

Medicine at a Glance, Fifth Edition. Edited by Patrick Davey and Alex Pitcher.

Companion website: www.wiley.com/go/medicine5e

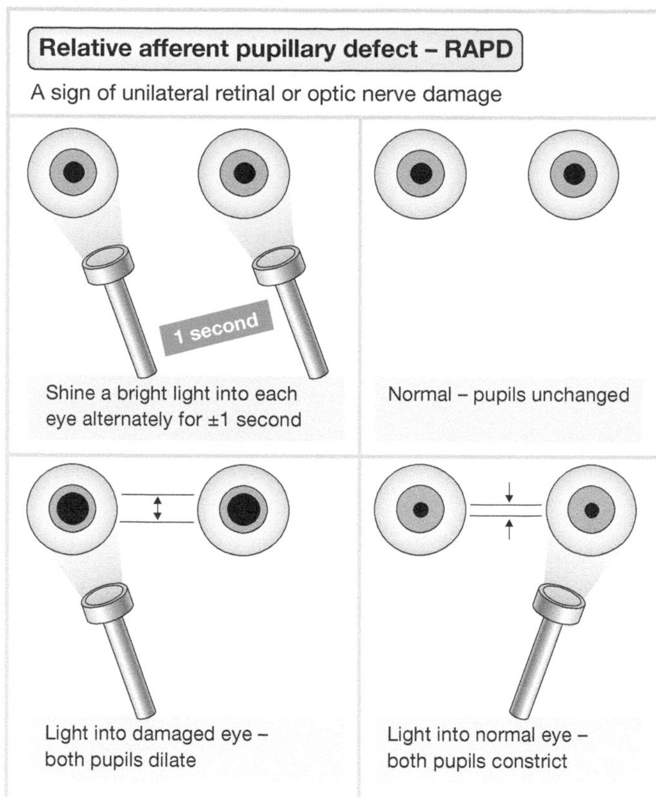

Relative afferent pupillary defect - RAPD
A sign of unilateral retinal or optic nerve damage
1 second
Shine a bright light into each eye alternately for ±1 second
Normal – pupils unchanged
Light into damaged eye – both pupils dilate
Light into normal eye – both pupils constrict

Visual loss

Monocular visual loss

This is a lesion anterior to the optic chiasma.

- The eye: cornea, lens and vitreous, e.g. cataract or vitreous haemorrhage.
- The retina, especially the fovea, e.g. diabetic retinopathy or macular degeneration.
- The optic nerve, e.g. optic neuritis or ischaemic optic neuropathy.

Bilateral involvement of these structures causes bilateral visual loss.

Binocular visual loss

This is a lesion at or behind the chiasma.

- Optic chiasma: classically bitemporal.
- Optic radiation: homonymous – either quadrantanopia (superior: temporal lobe, affecting Meyer's loop; inferior: parietal) or hemianopia.
- Visual cortex: homonymous, often hemianopia.

Typical clinical presentations of 'neurological' causes of visual loss

Brief monocular or binocular visual loss

- Amaurosis fugax: brief unilateral blindness lasting minutes (see Chapter 201).
- Brief transient visual obscurations, caused by idiopathic intracranial hypertension with papilloedema, may occur in one or both eyes. More common in obese young women with headache. The cause is often undefined; some cases are the result of sagittal sinus thrombosis. Acute papilloedema alone has an enlarged blind spot but no visual loss.

Sudden painless loss of vision in one eye

Sudden painless loss of vision in one eye is the result of:

- anterior ischaemic optic neuropathy: profound, irreversible visual loss with a pale swollen optic disc; caused by atheroma emboli or temporal arteritis (see Chapter 222)
- established retinal arterial or venous occlusion: visible with the ophthalmoscope.

Rapid progressive monocular visual loss

Rapid and progressive monocular loss of vision as a result of optic neuritis typically comes on over a few days. Symptoms range from clouding of vision with a vague central scotoma to marked monocular blindness. Pain is variable, but characteristically occurs on looking to one side. Signs comprise loss of colour vision, a relative afferent pupil defect, papilloedema early on and optic atrophy weeks/months later. Eyesight improves over a few weeks, although diminished colour vision may be permanent. If the brain shows evidence of demyelinating lesions on magnetic resonance imaging, there is at least an 80% chance of subsequent multiple sclerosis (MS).

Progressive night blindness

Progressive night blindness occurs in retinitis pigmentosa (RP), and causes peripheral concentric field loss and spicular pigmentation on fundoscopy. Genetically, there are many types, with X-linked or autosomal (dominant or recessive) inheritance. RP is associated with certain neurological syndromes, e.g. Refsum or Usher syndrome.

Bitemporal quadrantic or hemianopia

Bitemporal quadrantic or hemianopia is found in a pituitary lesion that compresses the optic chiasma, usually a macroadenoma. This is often slowly progressive and relatively asymptomatic, unless endocrine features are prominent or pituitary infarction occurs (see Chapters 159 and 164).

Homonymous hemianopia

Homonymous hemianopia may indicate a structural lesion of the hemisphere affecting the optic radiation or visual cortex (rarely the optic tract). Common causes include infarct, haemorrhage and tumour.

Visual neglect and visual hallucinations

Visual neglect suggests a parietal lobe lesion, in the presence of intact visual fields. Visual hallucinations, including macropsia or micropsia, result from disease of the visual cortex.

Migraine

See Chapter 63.

Double vision

Double vision may be the result of lesions of the oculomotor cranial nerves, the brain (usually the brainstem), neuromuscular junction or muscles or other disease of the orbit (e.g. Graves ophthalmopathy,

Table 60.1 Mitochondrial diseases (prevalence is 10–15 per 100 000, i.e. about 6000–9000 in the UK)

Syndrome	Clinical features
MELAS syndrome (*M*itochondrial *e*ncephalomyopathy *l*actic *a*cidosis and *s*troke-like episodes)	Seizures Episodes of unconsciousness with lactic acidosis stroke-like episodes
PEO (*P*rogressive *e*xternal *o*phthalmoplegia)	Ptosis, external ophthalmoplegia, limb myopathy Kearns–Sayre syndrome variant; develops age ≤20 years, + pigmentary retinopathy, ataxia and heart block
MERRF (*M*yoclonic *e*pilepsy with *r*agged *r*ed *f*ibres)	Myoclonic epilepsy Cerebellar ataxia Myopathy
NARP (*N*europathy, *a*taxia and *r*etinitis *p*igmentosa)	Proximal muscle weakness, sensory neuropathy, retinal pigmentary degeneration, developmental delay; dementia Ataxia, seizures
LHON (*L*eber's *h*ereditary *o*ptic *n*europathy)	Painless subacute visual loss Scotomas Abnormal colour vision
Others, including aminoglycoside-induced deafness (AID), maternally inherited Leigh syndrome (MILS), Pearson syndrome (PS)	Variable, usually suggested by the title; cardiomyopathy and deafness common in AID, sideroblastic anaemia and pancreatic failure in PS

head trauma). It is useful to establish the pattern, e.g. worse in one direction, on near or far vision, or at different times of the day.

Cranial nerve palsies

- In **sixth nerve palsy**, horizontal doubling – worse in the distance and on looking laterally – occurs. Looking straight ahead, there is a convergent squint as the affected eye is held adducted (unopposed medial rectus action). Causes include raised intracranial pressure, compression of the sixth nerve and microvascular disease. In children, sixth nerve palsy can follow a viral infection.
- **Fourth nerve palsy** is rare and causes diplopia on looking down, in and near, i.e. reading, eating and walking down stairs. On examination, there is failure to depress the eye when held in adduction (on abduction, the eye is depressed by the inferior rectus).
- In **third nerve palsy**, diplopia is complex and occurs in most directions. Ptosis (often complete) and pupil dilation occur (compare Horner syndrome which has partial ptosis and pupil constriction). The eye is abducted as a result of unopposed lateral rectus action. It is caused by compressive lesions, e.g. posterior communicating artery aneurysms, tumours and microvascular disease (hypertension, diabetes – pupil usually spared).

Internuclear ophthalmoplegia

Internuclear ophthalmoplegia is caused by medial longitudinal fasciculus damage, which connects the third and sixth nerve nuclei to allow fluent rapid lateral gaze. There is failure of prompt ipsilateral adduction on saccadic movement, and contralateral abducting nystagmus may be seen. Usually a sign of MS (especially if bilateral) but can also occur in other inflammatory lesions and vascular events in the brainstem. It is frequently asymptomatic.

Brainstem lesions

Diplopia with other cranial nerve signs suggests brainstem disease (or cavernous sinus/orbital apex, depending on which nerves are involved). Isolated nuclear cranial nerve palsies may be found, but failure of conjugate gaze is more common. The eyes may be held in skew deviation; there may be gaze instability, nystagmus or failure of upgaze/downgaze. Causes include MS, stroke or tumour, or Wernicke encephalopathy.

Cerebellar disease

Cerebellar disease may affect conjugate gaze but instability of vision is the usual symptom, rather than diplopia. Nystagmus is common.

Myasthenia gravis

Myasthenia gravis almost always has eye involvement. Diplopia is a common presentation, usually with ptosis. Any muscles can be affected, but the medial rectus is particularly susceptible. The pattern of doubling and the precise signs found are variable and may include fatigue.

Mitochondrial myopathies

Mitochondrial myopathies can present with chronic progressive external ophthalmoplegia and ptosis. They are rarely associated with diplopia, as malalignment is so gradual. Mitochondrial diseases are rare, though important. They can present in multiple different ways (Table 60.1). Damage to the external eye muscles, retina and/or optic nerve is commonly found in the many different forms of mitochondrial disease, and causes defects in vision appropriate for the location of the damage.

Thyroid disease

See Chapter 161.

Pupils

Large

- Both pupils enlarge in response to dim lighting, fear, intoxication (e.g. cannabis, deadly nightshade) or death.
- One pupil enlarged may be the result of parasympathetic palsy (e.g. third nerve compression), Adie's pupil or iris paralysis (e.g. dilating drops or trauma).

Small

- Both pupils constrict with bright light, near focus, intoxication (e.g. opiates or cholinesterase inhibitors) or pontine haemorrhage.
- One constricted pupil may be the result of a sympathetic palsy (Horner's syndrome), pilocarpine use or iritis.

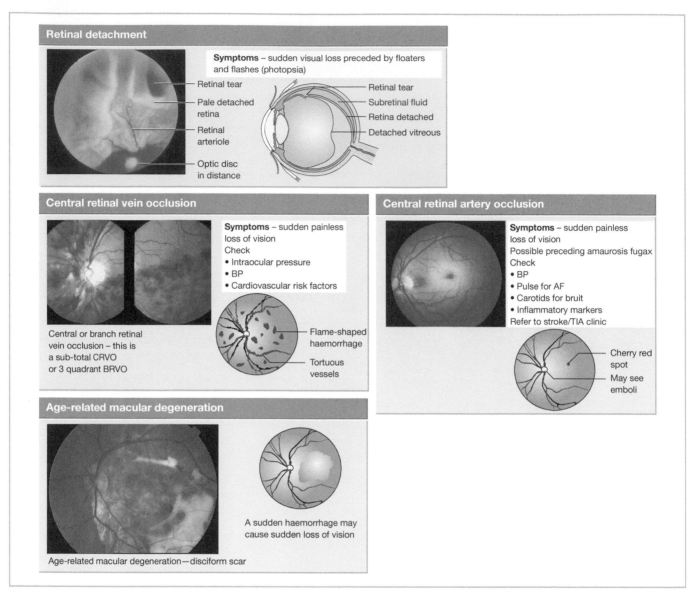

Sudden painless loss of vision

Retinal detachment

Symptoms – sudden visual loss preceded by floaters and flashes (photopsia)

Retinal tear
Pale detached retina
Retinal arteriole
Optic disc in distance

Retinal tear
Subretinal fluid
Retina detached
Detached vitreous

Central retinal vein occlusion

Symptoms – sudden painless loss of vision
Check
- Intraocular pressure
- BP
- Cardiovascular risk factors

Flame-shaped haemorrhage
Tortuous vessels

Central or branch retinal vein occlusion – this is a sub-total CRVO or 3 quadrant BRVO

Central retinal artery occlusion

Symptoms – sudden painless loss of vision
Possible preceding amaurosis fugax
Check
- BP
- Pulse for AF
- Carotids for bruit
- Inflammatory markers

Refer to stroke/TIA clinic

Cherry red spot
May see emboli

Age-related macular degeneration

A sudden haemorrhage may cause sudden loss of vision

Age-related macular degeneration—disciform scar

For sudden painless loss of vision, you will get your clues for the aetiology and be able to make a likely diagnosis from a really good history. Some causes are urgent, needing emergency ophthalmology assessment and possible surgery or systemic treatment. It's important to be able to identify these.

More urgent

Retinal detachment

This is when the retina separates from the underlying layers of the eyeball.

- *History*: usually unilateral loss of vision, often starting as a black 'curtain' coming up or down. When the patch of visual loss crosses the midline, this means the macula has detached, and visual loss will be much more profound.
- *Clues*: the patient may be shortsighted (myopic), or have had recent cataract surgery. There may have been preceding floaters and/or flashing lights.
- *Examination*: loss of part or all of the visual field in one eye. Relative afferent pupillary defect (RAPD) if the detachment is extensive.
- *Management*: urgent referral to ophthalmology – urgent or emergency surgery will be required.

Medicine at a Glance, Fifth Edition. Edited by Patrick Davey and Alex Pitcher.

Companion website: www.wiley.com/go/medicine5e

Central or branch retinal artery occlusion (CRAO/BRAO)

- *History*: usually very sudden profound loss of part or all the vision in one eye.
- *Clues*: very sudden onset, with no preceding symptoms. The patient may be older, with cardiovascular risk factors, or symptoms of giant cell arteritis (GCA). There may be a known source of emboli such as carotid atheroma or atrial fibrillation.
- *Examination*: pale retina with cherry red spot, sometimes a visible embolus. RAPD if the vision loss is severe.
- *Management*: urgent referral: sometimes an embolus can be dislodged with first aid treatment (e.g. reduction of intraocular pressure) if the patient is seen within a few hours. Medical referral for source of emboli and consideration of giant cell arteritis as a cause.

Non-arteritic ischaemic optic neuropathy (NAION)

Ischaemia of the optic nerve caused by occlusion of the small ciliary blood vessels supplying it.

- *History*: non-arteritic means 'not associated with GCA'. If there are symptoms of GCA, such as jaw or head pain or claudication, consider arteritic optic neuropathy as a diagnosis. NAION presents as painless, often altitudinal loss of vision in one eye.
- *Clues*: altitudinal loss is characteristic, may be a stepwise progression. The patient usually has vascular risk factors, including smoking, or the use of drugs such as sildenafil, or they may have had a hypotensive episode.
- *Examination*: there may be segmental or 360° swelling of the optic disc. If the posterior optic nerve is involved, the disc may be normal.
- *Management*: it is essential to immediately exclude GCA with the help of rheumatology if necessary. Manage risk factors for vascular occlusion.

Vitreous haemorrhage

Blood in the vitreous gel. This is an urgent condition as it may herald retinal detachment, aggressive diabetic retinopathy or accidental or non-accidental injury.

- *History*: floaters, droplets or worms in the vision, progressing to blurred vision, which can be profound if the bleed is severe.
- *Clues*: the history may be classic, as above. The patient may be diabetic, have 'wet' macular degeneration or be on anticoagulants.
- *Examination*: there will usually be no view of the retina with the direct ophthalmoscope. Sometimes you can focus on red blood cells on the back of the lens or in the vitreous.
- *Management*: urgent referral to ophthalmology. A B-scan (ultrasound) will help diagnose retinal detachment; sometimes vitrectomy surgery is needed to reveal the cause.

Less urgent

Central or branch retinal vein occlusion (CRVO/BRVO)

- *History*: painless unilateral blurring of part or all of the vision which can develop over a few hours.
- *Clues*: the patient is often older and hypertensive. There is an association with glaucoma/raised intraocular pressure (IOP), diabetes, systemic inflammation and 'sticky blood'.
- *Examination*: multiple haemorrhages throughout the retina.
- *Management*: assessment for medical predisposing factors and systemic disease. Ophthalmological referral for treatment of IOP and management of complications.

Cerebrovascular accident

- *History*: visual loss following an infarct or bleed affecting the optic radiation or visual cortex causes sudden loss of part of the vision in both eyes. Usually there will be other neurology.
- *Clues*: the patient may have other signs of a stroke, or vascular risk factors, and may notice that the visual loss is bilateral.
- *Examination*: confrontation visual fields should reveal a corresponding defect in each eye, although the loss may be worse in one eye.
- *Management*: referral to stroke physicians and ophthalmology.

Migraine

- *History*: slow onset of scintillations or zigzags expanding over the vision of both eyes (although patients often only report it in one eye), resolving over 30–60 minutes, possibly followed by headache.
- *Clues*: a normal eye examination with a history of migraine.
- *Examination*: if you are able to examine the patient while they still have the symptoms, you can demonstrate that the scintillations are in both eyes.
- *Management*: reassurance of normal eye exam. Advice to discuss with GP. The onset of migraine in later life merits imaging.

Age-related macular degeneration (AMD)

- *History*: central visual loss in one eye, with preserved peripheral vision. There is often distortion of the vision as the macula is affected.
- *Clues*: a known history of AMD, distortion or central scotoma, older patient.
- *Examination*: you may see pigment or haemorrhage in the posterior pole with the direct ophthalmoscope.
- *Management*: prompt referral to ophthalmology, as the patient may need urgent intravitreal injection or surgery.

Tremor and other involuntary movements

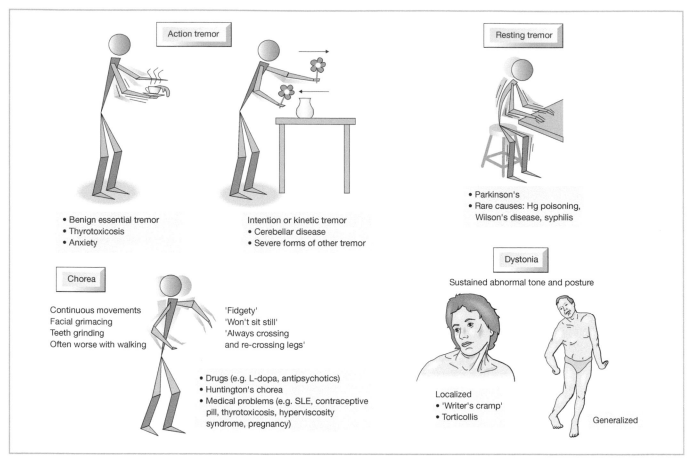

Understanding and interpreting movement disorders depends on having a precise grasp of the terminology used to describe the phenomenology of abnormal movement and posture.

Tremor is the *involuntary, rhythmical oscillation* of a muscle group around a joint. It should be distinguished from other involuntary movements such as dyskinesia, chorea, myoclonus, tics and mannerisms (defined later). Measuring the frequency of the tremor is not often of value in distinguishing the cause. There are, in clinical practice, only three common types of tremor (Table 62.1).

1 Resting tremor: if asymmetrical, this is almost pathognomonic of idiopathic **Parkinson disease**.
2 Postural tremor, which is usually the result of **essential tremor**.
3 Action or kinetic tremor, which is a feature of **cerebellar dysfunction**.

Common causes of tremor

Essential tremor

Essential tremor is usually symmetrical and barely present at rest, becomes pronounced on movement and posture (the rattling of a teacup is suggestive of the diagnosis), and can be relieved by small amounts of alcohol, although this effect wanes with time. It is often associated with a family history and is very rarely disabling.

Cerebellar disease

The characteristic feature of cerebellar tremor is that it is brought out at the end of movement. The head may be involved. Isolated tremor is most unusual and usually there are other signs of cerebellar dysfunction.

Parkinsonism

Parkinson tremor is of asymmetrical onset, is most prominent at rest, and is reduced by voluntary action (see Chapter 212). Head tremor is not characteristic of idiopathic Parkinson disease, but the jaw is frequently involved.

Dystonic tremor

See section on dystonias.

Drugs and toxins

- Alcohol withdrawal: though tremor is extremely common, and indeed almost universal in alcohol withdrawal, the clinical condition is usually dominated by other features, especially neuropsychiatric ones, including difficult behaviour, acute confusional

Medicine at a Glance, Fifth Edition. Edited by Patrick Davey and Alex Pitcher.

Companion website: www.wiley.com/go/medicine5e

Table 62.1 Types of tremor and their features

	Maximal	Distribution	Response to movement	Involvement of head
Essential tremor	Action and postural	Symmetrical	Worse	If severe
Parkinsonian	Rest, abolished by action	Asymmetrical	Abolished	Never (but does involve jaw)
Cerebellar	Kinetic	Symmetrical, frequently head	Accentuated at end of movement	Frequent

state, hallucinations and seizures. Patients are not infrequently jaundiced, with other stigmata of liver disease, such as spider naevi, ascites, etc.

- Sodium valproate.
- Lithium.
- Caffeine.
- Heavy metal poisoning.

Metabolic

- **Thyrotoxicosis**.
- **Phaeochromocytoma**.
- **Hepatic encephalopathy**.
- **Wilson's disease**: rare (one in 33 000–100 000), autosomal recessive disease caused by mutations/deletions of the ATP7B gene. Fifty percent present with movement disorders and neuropsychiatric disturbance (nearly all patients with neurological symptoms have Kayser–Fleischer rings), the remainder with liver disease, anaemia or by proband screening. Screening for Wilson disease, which is a treatable cause of neurodegeneration, should be considered in any patient presenting with new-onset tremor below the age of 50 years.

Other abnormal movements

Myoclonus

This comprises brief, explosive 'electric shock'-like activation of a group of muscles, often involving a whole limb. It is reasonable to think of this as an 'epileptic' phenomenon which can arise from anywhere in the central nervous system, including the brainstem and spinal cord. There are a very large number of causes, ranging from vascular disease, drugs and metabolic derangements to neurodegenerative disease such as spongiform encephalopathies.

Dystonias

These are sustained, abnormal tone and posture of a group of muscles, which can be:

- **focal**, e.g. writer's cramp, torticollis (now known as 'idiopathic cervical dystonia') and hemifacial spasm
- **generalized**, e.g. generalized torsion dystonia, a condition of abnormal writhing movements, which may be genetic (dominantly inherited) or symptomatic of other conditions (drugs, structural lesions of the brain, neurodegenerative disease).

Dystonia frequently presents as a tremor which can be misdiagnosed as either Parkinson disease or essential tremor. Dystonic tremor commonly affects the upper limb, when it is usually unilateral or markedly asymmetrical, or the head, resulting in a 'no-no' side-to-side tremor.

Chorea

These are continuous, random, flowing or dancing movements of the extremities, which in its mildest form may be turned into semipurposeful movements such that the patient just appears fidgety. The definition of the ad hoc Committee on Classification of the World Federation of Neurology is helpful, and states that chorea is 'a state of excessive, spontaneous movements, irregularly timed, non-repetitive, randomly distributed and abrupt in character. These movements may vary in severity from restlessness with mild intermittent exaggeration of gesture and expression, fidgeting movements of the hands, unstable dance-like gait to a continuous flow of disabling, violent movements.'

There are multiple causes.

- **Drug-induced syndromes**: continuous dyskinesia merging into chorea not infrequently complicates long-term Parkinson disease, where long-term treatment with dopamine and its agonists may be contributory. Similarly, the restless movements complicating long-term treatment with dopamine antagonists, such as the neuroleptic drugs used for major psychosis, can appear choreiform.
- **Huntington disease** (HD): abnormal movements are the presenting symptom in 50–75% of HD patients. Indeed, choreiform movements can, occasionally, be so profound as to result in severe weight loss due to the high-energy expenditure resulting from nearly continuous motor activity. Chorea is particularly prevalent in those who present at an older age; HD presenting in childhood is dominated by rigidity and cognitive decline. In the majority of patients presenting in mid-adult life, personality change (e.g. impulsivity) may precede chorea with overt cognitive decline occurring later.
- **Sydenham chorea**: this is a complication of rheumatic fever, which most typically occurs some 1–6 months after an acute attack of rheumatic fever. However, it has been described as occurring up to 30 years after the acute attack. This means that the history is often the vital aspect of the diagnosis, rather than the finding of raised antistreptococcal antibodies. Chorea often occurs in isolation.
- **Systemic lupus erythematosus (SLE)**.
- **Oral contraceptive pill**.
- **Hyperviscosity syndromes**.
- **Pregnancy**.
- **Thyrotoxicosis**: while tremor is almost universal in hyperthyroidism chorea, and well described, it is extraordinarily rare. It usually resolves on successfully treating the overactive thyroid.
- **Antiphospholipid syndrome**: most patients (c. 90%) with this syndrome who develop chorea are female, about 25% develop symptoms either on the pill or when pregnant; it is unilateral in 45%, and 35% have abnormalities on brain magnetic resonance imaging.
- There are many **other causes**, including Wilson disease.

Dyskinesias

These are disorders of movement integration, which may have choreiform or dystonic components. The term is usually used for drug-induced movements caused by neuroleptics or Parkinson disease or its treatment.

Tics

Tics are stereotyped explosive movements, under partial voluntary control, which are recognizably part of the normal movement repertoire (e.g. blinking or winking).

63 Headache and facial pain

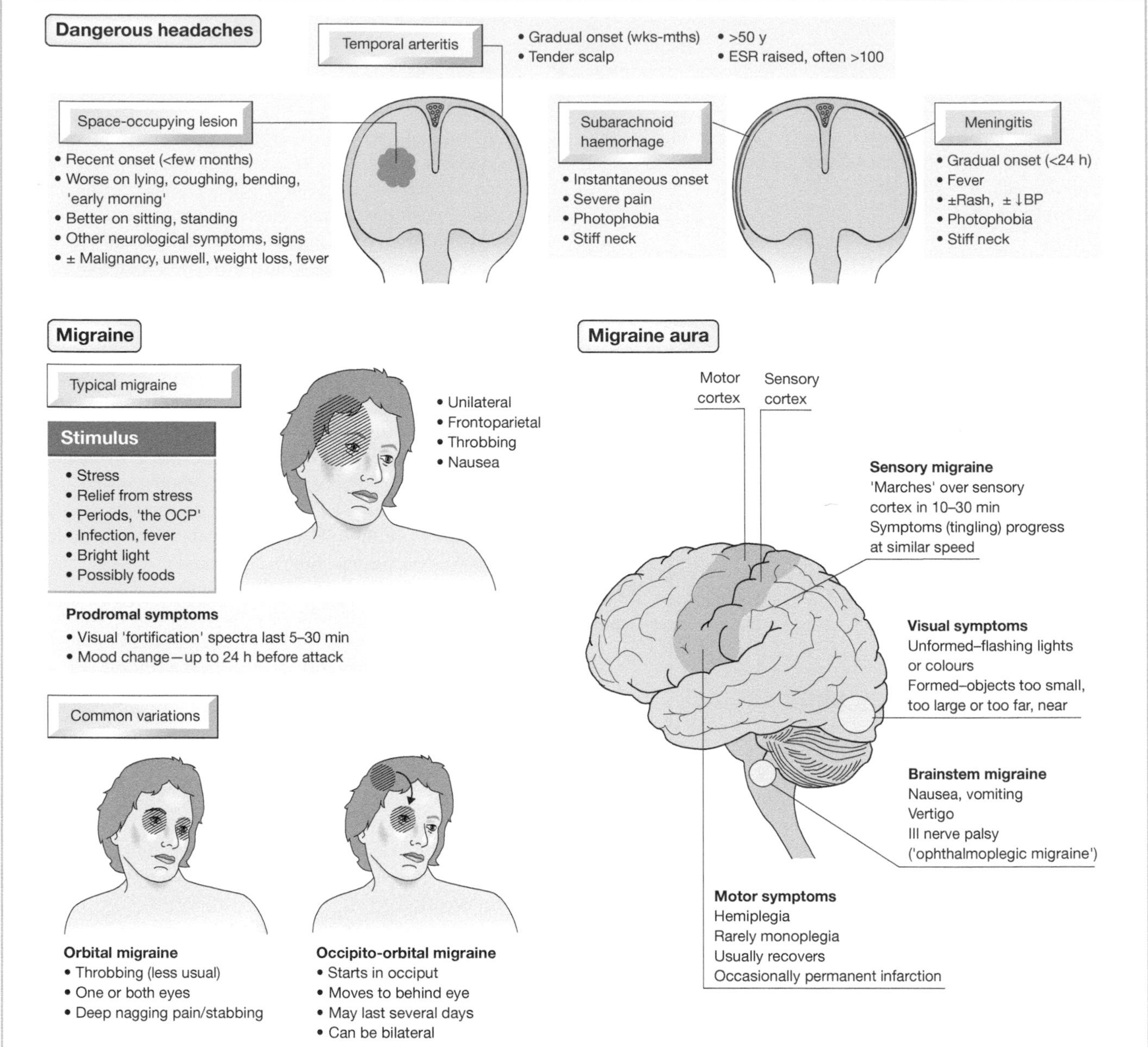
Dangerous headaches
Temporal arteritis
• Gradual onset (wks-mths) • >50 y
• Tender scalp • ESR raised, often >100
Space-occupying lesion
• Recent onset (<few months)
• Worse on lying, coughing, bending, 'early morning'
• Better on sitting, standing
• Other neurological symptoms, signs
• ± Malignancy, unwell, weight loss, fever
Subarachnoid haemorhage
• Instantaneous onset
• Severe pain
• Photophobia
• Stiff neck
Meningitis
• Gradual onset (<24 h)
• Fever
• ±Rash, ± ↓BP
• Photophobia
• Stiff neck
Migraine
Typical migraine
Stimulus
• Stress
• Relief from stress
• Periods, 'the OCP'
• Infection, fever
• Bright light
• Possibly foods
• Unilateral
• Frontoparietal
• Throbbing
• Nausea
Prodromal symptoms
• Visual 'fortification' spectra last 5–30 min
• Mood change—up to 24 h before attack
Common variations
Orbital migraine
• Throbbing (less usual)
• One or both eyes
• Deep nagging pain/stabbing
Occipito-orbital migraine
• Starts in occiput
• Moves to behind eye
• May last several days
• Can be bilateral
Migraine aura
Motor cortex
Sensory cortex
Sensory migraine
'Marches' over sensory cortex in 10–30 min
Symptoms (tingling) progress at similar speed
Visual symptoms
Unformed–flashing lights or colours
Formed–objects too small, too large or too far, near
Brainstem migraine
Nausea, vomiting
Vertigo
III nerve palsy
('ophthalmoplegic migraine')
Motor symptoms
Hemiplegia
Rarely monoplegia
Usually recovers
Occasionally permanent infarction

Headache is a subjective sensation, so the patient and not the doctor has to define its presence or absence. The brain is insensate: pain in the head and face arises from the trigeminovascular system, which supplies the meninges, or from bony or ligamentous structures. As an isolated symptom (i.e. no other symptoms or neurological signs), it is almost never indicative of structural brain disease (and is referred to as 'primary headache'). The following isolated headaches are exceptions and may indicate underlying disease.

- 'Thunderclap' headache: may be the result of subarachnoid or intracerebral haemorrhage.
- Headache gradually increasing in severity over several hours with fever, photophobia and neck stiffness (not all components need be present) suggests acute meningitis, a medical emergency. Immediate intravenous antibiotics are given if definitive diagnosis (usually established by lumbar puncture) is unavoidably delayed. Chronic meningitis may cause isolated headache that is progressive over days to weeks.

Medicine at a Glance, Fifth Edition. Edited by Patrick Davey and Alex Pitcher.

Companion website: www.wiley.com/go/medicine5e

- Exertional headache, or headache occurring exclusively on coughing, sneezing or stooping: occasionally caused by vascular malformations of the brain or lesions of the foramen magnum, e.g. the Arnold–Chiari malformation.
- Postural headache: may indicate abnormalities of cerebrospinal fluid pressure (high or low).
- Headache waking the patient from sleep: although most often the result of benign conditions, e.g. migraine, this should prompt a search for a structural lesion by careful physical examination (e.g. for hemiplegia) and consideration of neuroimaging.
- New and continuous headache in those aged over 50 years raises the possibility of temporal arteritis. The scalp may be tender. A raised erythrocyte sedimentation rate (ESR) supports the diagnosis (see Chapter 222).

Classification of primary headache

Migraine

The core features of migraine are headache, typically but not exclusively unilateral, nausea and vomiting, and variable constitutional upset (fatigue, carbohydrate craving, diuresis), which usually lasts <48 hours. There are two main types.

- **Migraine with aura**: there is a prodrome of neurological symptoms, evolving gradually over a few minutes, unlike stroke or transient ischaemia where symptoms arise instantaneously. These prodromal symptoms comprise the following.
  - Visual phenomena: positive (scintillations, fortification spectra, etc.) or negative (scotomata, hemianopia).
  - Altered sensations of the face or limbs.
  - Occasional rare variants such as 'basilar' migraine with double vision and vertigo, and ophthalmoplegic and hemiplegic migraine.
- **Migraine without aura**: there are no accompanying neurological symptoms or signs but nausea and the other constitutional features are still present.

Acute attacks may respond to simple analgesia if given quickly (paracetamol or high-dose aspirin in soluble form; codeine-based preparations are contraindicated because of nausea and rebound headache). Triptans (e.g. sumatriptan) are usually reserved for severe recurrent attacks and ergotamine is now used rarely. Prophylaxis is indicated for debilitating attacks occurring several times a month; propranolol and topiramate have been shown to work in selected patients.

Tension-type headache

This is an unsatisfactory term because patients believe that they are being criticized as being tense. The relationship to psychosocial stress is uncertain and variable but the symptoms are still disabling. The key features are:

- a dull generalized headache, usually poorly localized (occasionally localized over the eyes), sometimes referred to as a 'fuzzy head'
- poor response to over-the-counter analgesia
- worsening throughout the day
- duration of days to weeks.

Some neurologists consider this to be a variant of migraine and it is not uncommon to find both types of headache in the same patient or to find a cluster of migraines merging into tension headache. They do not usually respond to antimigraine therapy but some respond to low-dose amitriptyline.

Chronic daily headache

This describes patients who have a non-specific, non-disabling headache on most days (4% of the UK population). It is unresponsive to simple analgesia and difficult to treat.

Cluster headache

This is more common in men (9:1) and characterized by episodes of severe unilateral headache of extreme to excruciating intensity, often arising from sleep. Eye watering may occur; duration is 10–60 minutes. Patients prefer to move around. Occurs in clusters, typically daily for 6–8 weeks before disappearing completely. Acute treatment is with triptan antimigraine therapy; some respond to high-flow oxygen. Prophylaxis is with verapamil or lithium. Once started, clusters can sometimes be aborted with a reducing course of prednisolone.

Indomethacin-responsive headaches

These are a group of unusual headache syndromes, defined by the specific response to indomethacin. Paroxysmal hemicrania is a unilateral, lancinating headache of great severity, which continues throughout the day. Patients describe paroxysms of sharp jabbing, lasting for seconds and often localized behind the eye. If it becomes chronic, it is known as 'hemicrania continua'.

Facial pain

- **Trigeminal neuralgia** causes a unilateral, lancinating facial pain in the distribution of the trigeminal nerve (usually maxillary or mandibular), typically arising in middle age. Bilateral symptoms can be the result of multiple sclerosis. Patients usually report that the pain is precipitated by tactile stimulation of the face (shaving, brushing teeth, hot or cold drinks, the wind). The pain can be difficult to control. Most patients respond to carbamazepine but the effect is not always sustained. A minority of patients have vascular compression of the trigeminal nerve shown by magnetic resonance imaging, and may respond to surgical decompression of the artery in the posterior fossa.
- **Postherpetic neuralgia**: this troublesome condition affects 30% of people after an episode of shingles. Risk factors are age and late treatment with aciclovir. The most common location is in the ophthalmic trigeminal division, but it can occur anywhere. Although it is difficult to treat, carbamazepine or amitriptyline are worth trying. In many, symptoms abate after several years.
- **'Atypical facial pain'**, by definition, does not have any of the distinguishing features of the aforementioned conditions. It is most common in young women, and not associated with physical signs. Amitriptyline is the treatment of choice.

Other causes of headache

- Analgesic overuse headache is a major problem.
- Benign paroxysmal headache (triggered by cold, exertion or coughing).
- Temporomandibular joint dysfunction.
- Sinusitis.
- Dental caries.

64 Episodic alterations in awareness and consciousness

Syncope

Miscellaneous causes

These include:
- Alcohol-related
- Pulmonary embolus
- Pulmonary hypertension
- Aortic stenosis
- Sepsis
- GI bleed
- Psychogenic

Neurological causes
- Seizures (40%)
- Cerebrovascular disease (40%)

Vasomotor syncope

Situational syncope = cough, micturition syncope, etc.
Neurocardiogenic syncope including vasovagal syncope
Carotid sinus hypersensitivity
Drug induced
Postural hypotension

'Vasomotor syncope' = syncope due to a 'disorder of the control of the circulation' → inappropriate ↓heart rate and/or vasodilation → ↓blood pressure → syncope

Not diagnosed

Arrhythmias

Ventricular tachycardia (95% mono morphic VT)
Brady–tachy syndromes
Sinus bradycardia
AV block
Pacemaker failure
SVT

- 66% tachyarrhythmias
- 33% bradyarrhythmias

Syncope in the elderly

Carotid sinus hypersensitivity

Defined as ≥ 3 s asystole (cardio-inhibitory) or ≥ 50 mmHg BP drop (vasodepressor), or both (mixed), after 5 s carotid sinus massage
- Vasodepressor 55%
- Cardio-inhibitory 15%
- Mixed 30%

Other
Vestibular disease
Cardiovascular disease, including aortic stenosis
Epilepsy
Arrhythmias
Postural hypotension
Neurocardiogenic syncope

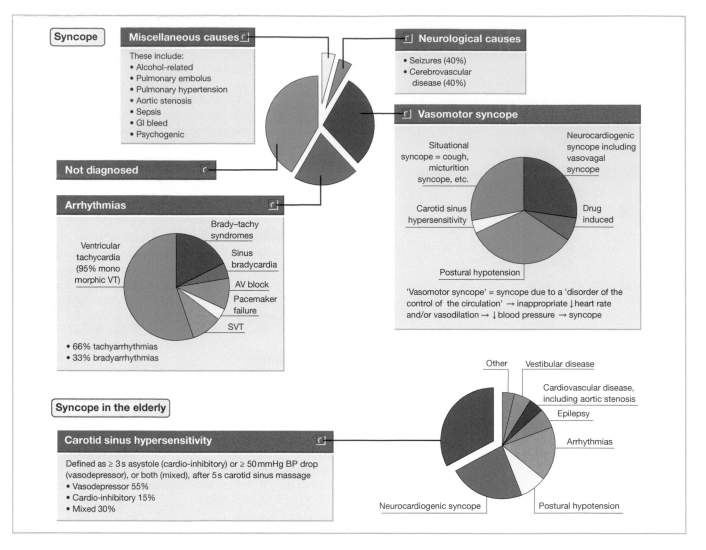

Blackouts and near blackouts are frightening experiences. The most helpful diagnostic approach is to obtain a full history from the patient and an accurate witness, because the examination and special investigations may add little. The features of diagnostic value to focus on are as follows.

- What happens immediately before the attack? A prodrome (warning) suggests a vasovagal cause, whereas no warning is a feature of primary generalized epilepsy or Stokes–Adams attacks. Patients with temporal lobe epilepsy (which is rarer than many other causes of loss of consciousness) can have an unusual prodrome, with any form of hallucination, strange epigastric sensations and *déjà/jamais vu* ('thoughts of having/never having been here before').
- What does the patient look like during the attack? Abnormal movements suggest epilepsy. Pallor or an appearance 'as if dead' suggest a cardiovascular cause. These distinctions are not absolute – for example, some 40% of patients with vasomotor forms of syncope have some minor twitching during the attack, and a few (especially those kept in the upright position) have more generalized hypoxic seizures (termed 'secondary hypoxic seizures').
- What is the memory of the attack itself? Remembrance of events during the attack suggests that consciousness was not fully lost. This is often so in minor cardiovascular events, in partial epilepsy and, especially, in hyperventilation.
- Did injury occur? Major injury suggests an absence of warning, as well as total loss of consciousness. Attacks with injury are strongly associated with significant underlying pathology.
- What happens immediately afterwards? Postevent confusion suggests epilepsy, whereas postevent flushing or sweating suggests a cardiovascular cause.
- What do witnesses say? This can be the key to diagnosis.

Medicine at a Glance, Fifth Edition. Edited by Patrick Davey and Alex Pitcher.

Companion website: www.wiley.com/go/medicine5e

- Are attacks recurrent? If so, are they all similar (stereotyped attacks suggest a single underlying aetiology)? Do they all occur in the standing position (which suggests postural hypotension or neurocardiogenic syncope), on effort (see below) or in the same psychological situation (which suggests vasovagal attacks or hyperventilation)?
- The patient's age alters the probability of disease: ≤30 years – vasovagal syncope and epilepsy are more likely; ≥60 years – cardiac causes and micturition syncope are more likely. However, any cause can occur at any age.

Cardiovascular causes of loss of consciousness

Consciousness is disrupted if there is a decrease in blood supply to the brain, either from a decreased cardiac output or hypotension from inappropriate vasodilation. Such cardiovascular diseases are characterized by faintness (presyncope, which means that patients feel that they are about to black out) or actual loss of consciousness (syncope) of brief duration (always less than a few minutes), with pallor during the attack, to the extent that the patient may 'appear dead'. Sweating afterwards is a good clue to a cardiovascular aetiology. Full consciousness returns rapidly. There are different variants of cardiovascular syncope.

Vasovagal syncope This is a common cause of altered consciousness at any age with the following features.

- A coherent account of the events leading up to the attack is given by the patient. Attacks may be precipitated by emotional stimuli and often recur in the same context.
- Loss of consciousness is preceded by: (i) a feeling of light-headedness or dysequilibrium, which is occasionally prolonged; (ii) ringing in the ears or a progressive alteration in sound quality; (iii) a feeling of warmth or flushing.
- The warning prodrome may be absent in elderly people in whom the picture may be of sudden drop attacks. Younger people often recall slowly falling to the ground before 'blacking out'.
- The patient is fully orientated as he/she comes round, although may feel weak, nauseated and light-headed. Recovery is complete within minutes. Prolonged confusion raises the suspicion that the attack is epileptic.
- Brief, non-sustained jerking of the limbs is common and those who faint with a full bladder may be incontinent. The diagnosis is complicated in those rare patients who faint and have a secondary anoxic convulsive seizure, from maintenance of the upright position.

Postural hypotension Here the autonomic nervous system fails to prevent a fall of blood pressure (BP) on standing. Characterized by symptoms of vasovagal syncope on standing, never when sitting or lying.

- Patients are usually elderly. The condition may be provoked or exacerbated by drugs (diuretics, antihypertensives, antipsychotics) and dehydration (e.g. fluid deprivation, diuretics, gastrointestinal [GI] bleed). Autonomic failure is also a common cause, e.g. diabetic neuropathy, Parkinson disease and related disorders.
- The diagnosis is established by demonstrating a progressive fall in BP on standing over several minutes.

It differs from hypotensive cardioneurogenic syncope in that the BP fall starts immediately, not after a delay, and there is never any

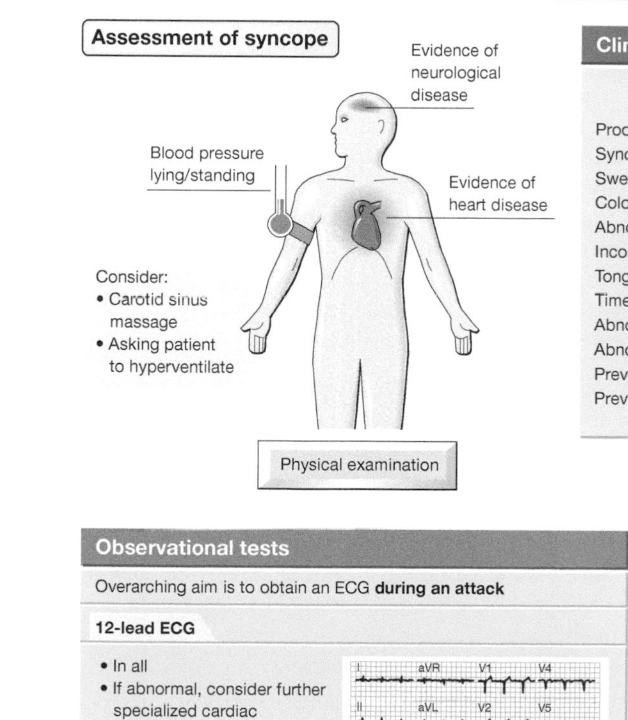

Clinical differences between cardiac and neurogenic syncope

	Cardiac	Neurogenic
Prodrome	0 – +	++
Syncope duration	Secs – mins	Mins – hours
Sweating	++	0
Colour during attack	Pale 'as if dead'	Normal – cyanosed
Abnormal movements	0 (unless 2 fitting)	++
Incontinence	0 – ±	+
Tongue biting	0	+
Time to full recovery	0 – few mins	Hours
Abnormal ECG outside attack	++	0
Abnormal EEG outside attack	0	+
Previous MI	++ (VT likely)	0
Previous CVA	0	+ (epilepsy likely)

Observational tests

Overarching aim is to obtain an ECG **during an attack**

12-lead ECG

- In all
- If abnormal, consider further specialized cardiac investigations

Prolonged ECG monitoring

- 24-hour ECG: 4% chance of diagnosing the cause of syncope. Usually only useful if symptoms occur every 2–7 days
- External loop recorder: useful if symptoms occur every 2–3 weeks
- Implantable ECG recorder – e.g. cardiac reveal device – useful if symptoms occur 2–3 x per year

Provocative tests

Aim to provoke symptoms and monitor ECG, blood pressure, heart rate (occasionally EEG)

Tilt table testing (TTT)

'Circulatory stress test'. Used to diagnose neurocardiogenic syncope. Dark, quiet room. Patient strapped to table and tilted upright (passive TTT), or GTN, isoprenaline given (active TTT). Useful if symptoms atypical, or injury occurs.
Problems with TTT:
- High false-positive, false-negative rates
- Poor reproducibility

Ventricular stimulation study (VSTIM)

Aims to induce the causative ventricular arrhythmia in a controlled manner, by pacing the ventricle, and introducing early extrasystoles. Very useful in ischaemic heart disease (IHD) and syncope with no other cause
- Good predictive accuracy in IHD
- May lead to implantation of implantable defibrillator

absolute bradycardia. Treatment is for the underlying disease (diabetes, dehydration). If this is not possible, fludrocortisone may help.
Micturition syncope Patients usually have prostatic hypertrophy. Prolonged straining to initiate micturition decreases venous return to the heart. Cardiac output falls and syncope results. Syncope prevents straining and thus improves cardiac venous return and output, restoring consciousness. A variant of micturition syncope is cough syncope, which occurs in individuals with chronic lung disease and prolonged paroxysms of coughing. The diagnosis is made from the history alone.
Stokes–Adams Attacks describe a specific pattern of syncope, unheralded, with complete loss of consciousness lasting <2–3 minutes. The absence of warning means that patients often fall heavily and sustain significant facial or limb injuries, in contrast to patients who simply faint and are not usually injured. Witnesses state that patients become pale, cyanotic and then reactively hyperaemic on recovery. Afterwards, there is a rapid (less than a few minutes) restoration of all mental and physical faculties. Attacks are usually the result of the temporary asystole that accompanies the onset of third-degree heart block; if not, then they may be caused by ventricular tachycardia (VT).
Syncopal (presyncopal) tachyarrhythmias To cause syncope, tachyarrhythmias must be either very fast or associated with moderately severe, structural heart disease. VT is the most common underlying rhythm disturbance, although atrial fibrillation is occasionally the culprit. Patients complain of fast palpitations before fainting. Total loss of consciousness is unlikely to last for more than a few minutes, although a depressed conscious level can last much longer. The 12-lead electrocardiogram (ECG), 24-hour ECG taping (Holter monitoring) or specialized cardiac investigation (e.g. ventricular stimulation study) may be diagnostic. If not, and an arrhythmia seems likely, implantation of a solid-state device to continually record the heart rhythm may be appropriate.
GTN syncope Glyceryl trinitrate (GTN) syncope is the result of excess consumption while the patient is standing. Vasodilation occurs, resulting in syncope. Patients may have failed to understand the role of GTN, and are taking it inappropriately. More usually, GTN syncope is associated with severe cardiac disease: either unacceptable angina, such that a coronary intervention is required (see Chapter 85), or impaired left ventricular function or aortic stenosis.
Effort syncope Syncope on effort occurs either because the heart cannot increase the cardiac output as a result of a fixed obstruction (such as in severe aortic stenosis commonly, in hypertrophic obstructive cardiomyopathy less commonly, and in severe pulmonary hypertension rarely) or because exercise provokes an arrhythmia. Cardiac ultrasonography and exercise testing are usually diagnostic.
Cardioneurogenic syncope This is a confusing term applied to an autonomic reflex, activated only in the standing position, whereby either the heart rate or BP or both drop sufficiently to cause syncope. Characteristically, patients are standing still, feel faint for 30 seconds to several minutes, and then faint and fall down. Sitting down early on may terminate the attack. The diagnosis is confirmed by replicating symptoms and heart rate/BP changes on tilt table testing.
Carotid hypersensitivity syndrome Patients have hypersensitive carotid baroreceptors, which are activated inappropriately by neck turning (often when looking upwards). Inappropriate bradycardia, sometimes with reflex vasodilation, occurs and the patient faints. The diagnosis is confirmed by eliciting symptoms and severe bradycardia on carotid sinus massage.

Terminology

Most doctors define syncope as a 'loss of consciousness with loss of postural reflexes'. The definition does not imply any particular mechanism. Thus syncope can occur from a cardiac cause or equally from a neurological one.

Neurological causes of loss of consciousness

The most common neurological disease underlying loss of consciousness is **epilepsy**, although very occasionally brainstem ischaemia is the cause. Epilepsy resulting in loss of consciousness is classified as generalized epilepsy and is caused by abnormal electrical discharges disrupting the function of the major subcortical structures that maintain consciousness.

- If the abnormal electrical discharges originate in these subcortical structures, unconsciousness occurs immediately and the epilepsy is termed **primary generalized**. Patients have no warning and instantaneous collapse occurs. *Beware*: the absence of a warning is also a feature of some localized seizures that progress unusually rapidly to secondary generalized seizures.
- If these subcortical structures are involved by electrical discharges spreading from a more distant focus, it is termed **secondary generalized**. In this situation, patients often experience some symptoms referable to the first structure involved, i.e. there is usually an aura or attenuated seizures.
- Seizures without loss of consciousness are termed **partial seizures** and may be simple (normal awareness) or complex (loss of awareness) (for further discussion, see Chapter 205).

Features that are strongly in favour of epilepsy as a cause of loss of consciousness are:

- a good witness account, although this is often absent
- postictal confusion (ictal = the epileptic attack itself) lasting some time, e.g. often for many hours; postictal headache
- muscular aching and tongue biting
- incontinence, which can also occur in other situations, is suggestive but non-specific
- known cerebrovascular disease, i.e. a previous stroke, or a degenerative brain condition increases the probability that a collapse relates to a seizure disorder.

Examination immediately after a seizure may show sleepiness for the first few hours, and bilateral extensor plantar responses for the first day, as well as signs referable to any underlying pathology (see Chapter 56). Generalized seizures cause skeletal muscle fibre damage, so muscle enzymes (e.g. creatine kinase, aspartate transaminase) are often elevated, as are serum prolactin levels for the first day or so. Electroencephalograph (EEG) recordings show abnormal interictal activity in 50% of patients with epilepsy.

Transient loss of consciousness

Brainstem ischaemia can result in falls, with loss of consciousness. Conscious level is usually only transiently disturbed (<1 min). The diagnosis is one of exclusion in a patient with cerebrovascular disease. There are no abnormal movements, the patient does not change colour and no rhythm disturbances are found. The presence of true vertigo (i.e. the external visual world is perceived to 'spin') may be a helpful clue. This syndrome is very rare and is overdiagnosed.

Prognosis in syncope

Prognosis in syncope varies greatly – in some patients, syncope is due to highly dangerous pathology (e.g. complete heart block) with a very poor natural history (untreated, acquired, complete heart block leads to death within a few weeks or months). At the other extreme, vasomotor syncope is associated with a normal life expectancy. It is crucial to determine how likely it is that dangerous pathology underlies the syncope. The clues to this can often be obtained fairly easily.

- If the heart is structurally abnormal (especially left ventricular damage following a myocardial infarction [MI]) or there is a known cardiomyopathy (or complex congenital heart disease) then a high-grade ventricular arrhythmia could underlie syncope (e.g. VT). Patients with syncopal VT are likely to experience further attacks, and the concern is that if the first episode of VT reduced cardiac output enough to cause syncope, the second may reduce myocardial blood flow enough to provoke ventricular fibrillation. Thus, syncope from a ventricular arrhythmia is a warning that the patient is at high risk of dying. The clue that VT is the cause of syncope is the presence of damage to the heart, diagnosed from the history (e.g. previous MI, known heart muscle disease, high alcohol intake, or the presence of multiple risk factors for ischaemic heart disease [IHD] – e.g. smoking, age, diabetes, etc.), examination and ECG (most patients with structural heart disease have some ECG abnormality). A cardiac ultrasound can be useful.
- Rarely, certain genetic diseases underlie dangerous ventricular arrhythmias; the most common of these is the still rare Brugada syndrome (prevalence one in 1000); another dangerous genetic disease is hereditary long QT syndrome. Most genetic illnesses cause characteristic abnormalities on the resting ECG; the real clue to their presence is the finding of sudden death in young family members.

Other causes of altered consciousness

- **Hyperventilation** occurs in young adults and there is usually a history of perioral and peripheral paraesthesiae, anxiety and specific provocations.
- **Hypoglycaemia** is associated with sweating, anxiety and confusion before loss of consciousness. Drugs for diabetes are the only common cause. Rarely, it may be caused by insulin-secreting pancreatic tumours.
- **Narcolepsy** is not strictly speaking a disorder that leads to loss of consciousness but, because of its curious manifestations, it is often misdiagnosed as epilepsy or patients are labelled as 'functional'. It is fundamentally a disorder of the central nervous system regulation of arousal and the cardinal diagnostic feature is a short rapid eye movement (REM) sleep latency. The four aspects to the full-blown narcolepsy syndrome are: (i) excessive daytime somnolence with an irresistible desire to sleep which cannot be overcome; (ii) cataplexy, a sudden loss of body tone; this may range from full falling to the ground to as mild a feeling as jaw dropping, and is usually precipitated by emotional stimuli such as jokes or arguments; (iii) sleep paralysis; and (iv) hypnagogic hallucinations.
- **Migraine** is often associated with mild, non-specific feelings of dissociation but can very rarely lead to frank coma.
- **Transient global amnesia** is a syndrome of obscure aetiology in which there is complete loss of new memory formation for a period of hours. Patients may appear relatively normal to external observers but are disorientated and ask repetitive and inconsequential questions. It may be a migrainous phenomenon but rarely recurs.
- **Psychogenic disorder** is always a dangerous diagnosis for the non-specialist to make, but psychological illness occasionally underlies blackouts. However, most patients with psychological/psychiatric illness who black out have genuine organic diseases. Occasionally, patients mimic seizures (i.e. have 'pseudoseizures'); this also occurs in psychologically disturbed patients who also have genuine seizures.

Table 64.1 Incidence rates of syncope per 1000 person-years of follow-up increased with age among both men and women

Rate per 1000 person-years				
Age	Men	Women	Average	Average change
20–29 years	2.6	4.7	3.7	–
30–39 years	3.8	3.2	3.5	−0.2
40–49 years	3.2	3.8	3.5	0
50–59 years	5.0	3.9	4.5	+1
60–69 years	5.7	5.4	5.6	+1.1
70–79 years	11.1	11.1	11.1	+5.5
≥80 years	16.1	19.5	17.8	+6.7

Table 64.2 Prognosis of syncope according to cause

Probability of survival (P)						
Follow-up	No syncope	Vasovagal and other causes	Unknown cause	Neurological cause	Cardiac cause	Difference between vasovagal and other causes vs cardiac cause
Year 1	0.99	0.99	0.94	0.92	0.89	−0.1
Year 2	0.92	0.92	0.9	0.88	0.81	−0.11
Year 3	0.91	0.9	0.88	0.81	0.7	−0.2
Year 4	0.88	0.88	0.82	0.79	0.64	−0.24
Year 5	0.85	0.85	0.8	0.7	0.56	−0.29
Year 10	0.7	0.7	0.55	0.48	0.4	−0.3
Year 15	0.51	0.52	0.4	0.25	0.18	−0.34
Year 20	0.38	0.37	0.19	0.14	0	−0.37

Note: The category 'vasovagal and other causes' includes vasovagal, orthostatic, medication-induced and other, infrequent, causes of syncope

Data from: N Engl J Med 2002: 347; 878–85e

65 The red eye

Diagnosis	How common? 1–6	Symptoms	Signs	Treatment
Conjunctivitis Bacterial Viral Allergic	 1 1 1	Sticky Sticky/watery Itchy	Redness all over Pink lids Source: Casey 2016, p.003 / with permission of Elsevier.	Topical antibiotics Topical lubricants Topical antihistamine and mast cell stabilizer
Subconjunctival haemorrhage	1	None	Confluent dense red patch	Nil
Episcleritis	2	Mild discomfort	Sectoral redness	Nil or topical lubricants
Iritis	2	Photophobia and pain	Redness around limbus, small or distorted pupil	Topical steroids and pupil dilation
Scleritis	5	Severe radiating pain	Intense red/ purple colour	Systemic immunosuppression
Marginal keratitis	3	Foreign body sensation	Peripheral white ulcer, locally red	Topical antibiotic and steroid
Corneal abrasion	1	Very painful and watery	No infiltrate, abrasion stains with fluorescein	Topical antibiotics
Keratitis (bacterial)	4	Painful and sticky	White staining ulcer visible	Topical antibiotics after samples taken
Keratitis (viral)	4	Gritty, sticky	Dendritic staining ulcer	Topical antivirals
Angle closure glaucoma	5	Very painful, nausea, unwell	Hazy cornea, dilated pupil	Topical and systemic treatment to reduce pressure

The eye has a limited way of expressing problems, and the conjunctiva (white part of the eye) being red is one of them. With slit lamp examination it is possible to tell which layer of the eye is inflamed, but it is much more difficult with the naked eye or direct ophthalmoscope. This is why a really good history and a sensible examination are important. You will get your clues for aetiology and be able to make a likely diagnosis from the history. Important diagnostic clues come from whether the eye is painful or just uncomfortable, and whether the vision is affected.

No pain/just uncomfortable, with normal vision

Conjunctivitis – common

An inflammation of the conjunctiva of any cause. The eyes are usually uniformly pink, more so towards the fornices. All types may start in one eye and then spread bilaterally. History and examination clues help identify the likely cause.

Bacterial – common

- *History*: a very sticky eye. If it fails to settle quickly with treatment, consider chlamydia (needs referral to sexual health clinic).
- *Treatment*: swabs (including chlamydial), then chloramphenicol drops hourly for 24 h, then qds for five days. Reconsider the diagnosis if not settling.

Viral – common

- *History*: sticky and watery but less so than bacterial, usually bilateral, there may be a known contact. Sometimes a palpable preauricular node.
- *Treatment*: fastidious personal hygiene, avoid spread with towels, etc. Swabs to confirm diagnosis. Artificial tear drops may help comfort. Adenoviral conjunctivitis can progress to keratitis so referral is appropriate if the symptoms progress.

Allergic – common

- *History*: itching is the crucial clue. There may be a watery or stringy discharge with a personal or family history of atopy. NB:

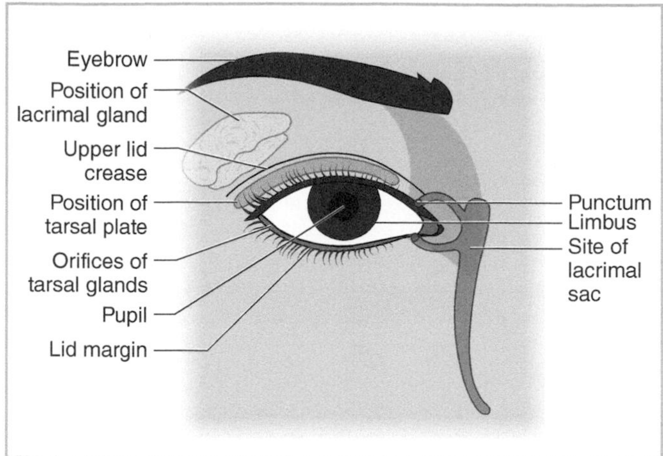

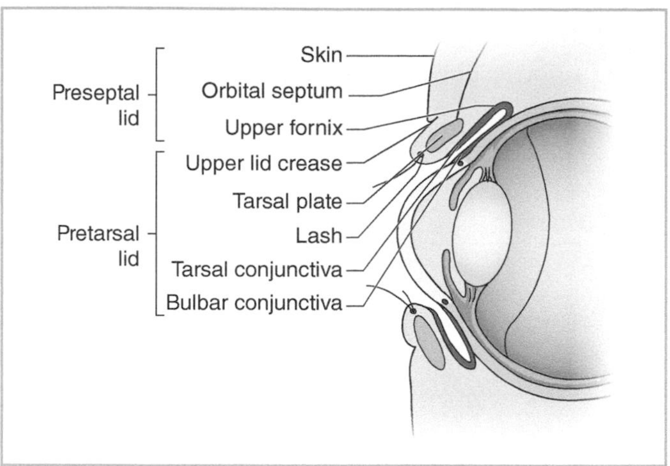

Severity can range from mild (e.g. hayfever eyes) to sight threatening (vernal or atopic keratoconjunctivitis).

- *Treatment*: topical antihistamine or mast cell stabilizing drops as first line. Referral to ophthalmology if persistent or worsening.

Subconjunctival haemorrhage – common

Bleed from the surface of the eye contained underneath the conjunctiva. History: bright, uniform redness (i.e. not injection of the conjunctival vessels). No treatment required. Can be associated with hypertension; can be very dramatic if the patient is on anticoagulants.

Episcleritis – not uncommon

Inflammation of the episclera – the layer immediately underneath the conjunctiva.

- *History*: a slightly uncomfortable eye with sectoral injection (nasally or temporally), without discharge
- *Treatment*: none required, although artificial tears may help. There is no need to investigate for systemic associations as these are very rarely found.

Painful, vision might be affected

Iritis – not uncommon

An inflammation of the iris (which is part of the uveal tract, and so it is also known as anterior uveitis).

- *History*: photophobia, with redness of the conjunctiva around the limbus (not cornea). The vision is usually a bit blurred. The pupil might be small or stuck down to the lens, causing it to be misshapen. Severe cases may have a hypopyon (pus in the anterior chamber, seen as a white level inferiorly). There have often been previous episodes, or a known associated systemic problem such as ankylosing spondylitis.
- *Treatment*: referral to ophthalmology for treatment with topical steroids and dilating drops, and consideration of systemic causes.

Scleritis – very rare

A necrotizing inflammation of the sclera.

- *History*: a deep red/purple discolouration of the eye, with nasty, gnawing radiating pain.
- *Treatment*: urgent referral to ophthalmology. Systemic immunosuppression may be required to prevent complications.

Marginal keratitis – uncommon

This is a corneal ulcer, associated with lid margin disease.

- *History*: a gritty, red eye, with redness localized around a white spot on the peripheral cornea. There may be known associated blepharitis (crusty lids).
- *Treatment*: responds well to a topical steroid/antibiotic mix, but should be assessed on the microscope to be sure of the diagnosis.

Painful, vision affected

Keratitis

It means inflammation of the cornea. Typically, will be very painful, photophobic, watery eyes with redness around the limbus.

Corneal abrasion – uncommon

- *History*: not strictly a keratitis, but a scrape on the cornea. There will be a history of trauma, typically with a fingernail or foliage. The abrasion stains with fluorescein, but there is **no** white infiltrate.
- *Treatment*: these heal quickly, but will be painful while they do. Topical chloramphenicol is used to prevent infection; if there is a history of significant trauma, full assessment is needed.

Bacterial keratitis – rare

- *History*: a painful eye with a white spot on the cornea, staining with fluorescein. If severe, there may be a hypopyon. Contact lens use is a risk factor.
- *Treatment*: these ulcers are usually 'scraped' to get microbiology samples, and started on empirical intensive topical antibiotics while the results are pending.

Viral keratitis (usually herpes simplex keratitis) – rare

- *History*: gritty, watery eye, with possible a history of cold sores. Typically causes branching, dendritic ulcer, staining with fluorescein.
- *Treatment*: don't start topical steroids! Refer to ophthalmology for an accurate diagnosis and prompt treatment with a topical antiviral (ganciclovir or aciclovir).

Acute angle closure glaucoma – very rare

When the normal drainage channels for the aqueous humour become blocked because of natural thickening of the lens in combination with pupil dilation, the pressure in the eye goes up, and the eye becomes ischaemic.

- *History*: an older person, with a very painful red eye, systemically unwell, vomiting, with a visibly cloudy cornea and mid dilated fixed pupil.
- *Treatment*: **urgent!** Treatment is needed to reduce the intraocular pressure, treat the nausea and rehydrate the patient.

Introduction to rheumatological disease

Figure 66.1

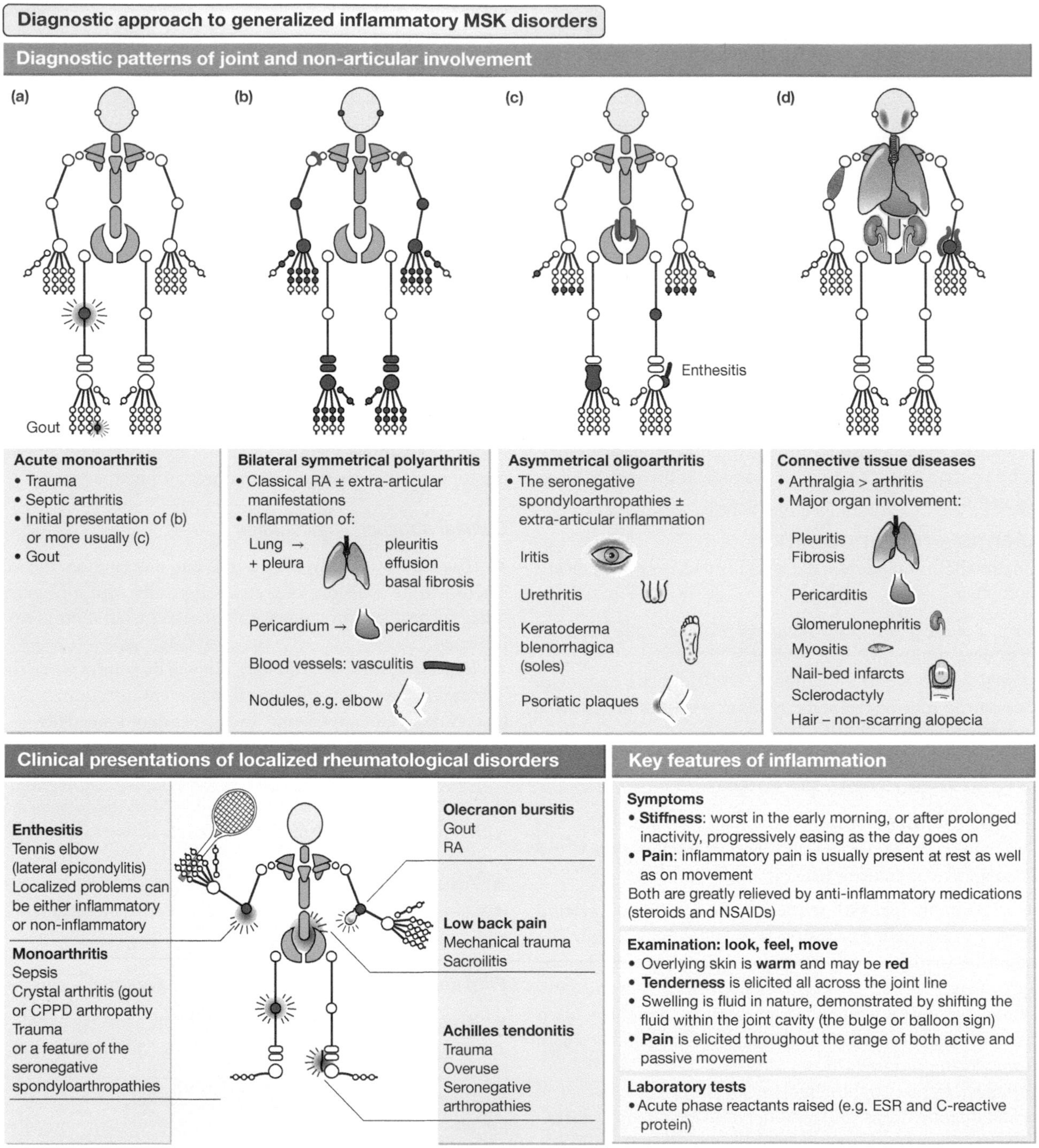

Diagnostic approach to generalized inflammatory MSK disorders

Diagnostic patterns of joint and non-articular involvement

(a) Gout

(b)

(c) Enthesitis

(d)

Acute monoarthritis
- Trauma
- Septic arthritis
- Initial presentation of (b) or more usually (c)
- Gout

Bilateral symmetrical polyarthritis
- Classical RA ± extra-articular manifestations
- Inflammation of:

Lung → + pleura → pleuritis, effusion, basal fibrosis

Pericardium → pericarditis

Blood vessels: vasculitis

Nodules, e.g. elbow

Asymmetrical oligoarthritis
- The seronegative spondyloarthropathies ± extra-articular inflammation

Iritis

Urethritis

Keratoderma blenorrhagica (soles)

Psoriatic plaques

Connective tissue diseases
- Arthralgia > arthritis
- Major organ involvement:

Pleuritis
Fibrosis

Pericarditis

Glomerulonephritis

Myositis

Nail-bed infarcts
Sclerodactyly

Hair – non-scarring alopecia

Clinical presentations of localized rheumatological disorders

Enthesitis
Tennis elbow (lateral epicondylitis)
Localized problems can be either inflammatory or non-inflammatory

Monoarthritis
Sepsis
Crystal arthritis (gout or CPPD arthropathy
Trauma
or a feature of the seronegative spondyloarthropathies

Olecranon bursitis
Gout
RA

Low back pain
Mechanical trauma
Sacroilitis

Achilles tendonitis
Trauma
Overuse
Seronegative arthropathies

Key features of inflammation

Symptoms
- **Stiffness**: worst in the early morning, or after prolonged inactivity, progressively easing as the day goes on
- **Pain**: inflammatory pain is usually present at rest as well as on movement

Both are greatly relieved by anti-inflammatory medications (steroids and NSAIDs)

Examination: look, feel, move
- Overlying skin is **warm** and may be **red**
- **Tenderness** is elicited all across the joint line
- Swelling is fluid in nature, demonstrated by shifting the fluid within the joint cavity (the bulge or balloon sign)
- **Pain** is elicited throughout the range of both active and passive movement

Laboratory tests
- Acute phase reactants raised (e.g. ESR and C-reactive protein)

Rheumatology is a very hands-on clinical specialty in which the history and examination remain the foundations of diagnosis and management. Clinical diagnosis largely depends on the correct elicitation of clinical signs and clinical pattern recognition. Three general patterns are recognized in clinical rheumatology.

1 **Localized musculoskeletal disorders**: involving a single swollen joint/painful area (e.g. 'frozen shoulder', low back pain, 'tennis elbow'). These may be of inflammatory, infectious or mechanical origin, and usually present as regional pain syndromes.

2 **Generalized inflammatory musculoskeletal disorders** causing predominant symptoms in and/or around the joints, e.g. rheumatoid arthritis (RA, synovial joint inflammation) or psoriatic arthritis (PsA, synovitis, enthesitis, dactylitis). Non-articular manifestations occur but joint symptoms tend to predominate.

3 **Generalized inflammatory musculoskeletal disorders with prominent systemic and non-articular manifestations**: e.g. systemic lupus erythematosus (SLE) which affects joints, skin and serosal surfaces as well as major organs such as the kidney or

brain and can present with major systemic upset and symptoms arising from any affected organ.

Key points in clinical assessment

A careful and detailed clinical assessment is integral to both diagnosis and management of rheumatological conditions. See Figure 66.1 above for patterns of presentation.

History

- **Inflammation** is a key feature of the systemic rheumatic diseases and should be sought (features in diagram above).
- **MSK symptoms** may arise in/localize to joint, bone, muscle or periarticular structures.
  - **Joints.**
    - **Acute joint inflammation** (synovitis) causes redness, pain, swelling, tenderness and stiffness which is *characteristically worse in the early morning or after inactivity*. Onset may be sudden/explosive or gradual and progressive.
    - **Distribution** of inflamed joints – large/small/mixed and symmetrical vs asymmetrical. Pattern of involvement is usually characteristic of particular diseases.
    - **Severity of inflammation**: number of inflamed joints, duration of early morning stiffness (hours), functional impact (inability to undertake activities of daily living or work/leisure) and disability/loss of participation.
    - **Osteoarthritis** (OA) causes joint pain and stiffness that is usually worse on movement/activity and at the end of the day (**gelling**). Joint movement may be accompanied by audible joint **crepitus**.
    - **Joint deformity** may occur in both OA and inflammatory arthritis. It is usually a feature of late presentation or chronic disease and is associated with disability.
  - **Bone pain** arises when there is destruction of the integrity of normal bone and is multifactorial. It has the following characteristics.
    - Deep-seated, intense, unrelenting.
    - Unaffected by posture, position or movement.
    - Characteristically disturbs sleep ('wakes me up at night').
    - Unresponsive to anti-inflammatory therapies.
  - Causes of bony pain include:
    - fracture (trauma, osteoporosis, 'stress', myeloma)
    - osteonecrosis (may be secondary to steroids)
    - neoplasia; primary (e.g. osteoid osteoma) or secondary (commonly) from breast, lung, thyroid, renal or prostate
    - metabolic (Paget disease)
    - infection (osteomyelitis, spinal TB).
  - **Muscle pain** is usually experienced as a localized dull ache (myalgia) accompanied by weakness of the affected muscle or group and is extremely common. Patterns of muscle symptoms may be suggestive of the diagnosis.
    - Localised myalgia and tenderness with weakness are usually due to local injury, trauma or overuse. Occasionally may be due to focal myositis (muscle inflammation).
    - Diffuse myalgia with tenderness and weakness is suggestive of myositis (muscle inflammation, often immune mediated, e.g. PMR, PAN, DM, though could be due to viral infection, drugs such as statins, or sarcoidosis).
    - Muscle stiffness, especially of the proximal girdles, is suggestive of polymyalgia rheumatica and may also accompany giant cell arteritis.
    - Muscle weakness in the absence of other symptoms is suggestive of a non-inflammatory myopathy (e.g alcoholism, uraemia, hyperthyroidism, Cushing disease, cancer myopathy) or a neurological cause.
- **Constitutional symptoms** of systemic inflammation include persistent debilitating fatigue or lassitude, malaise, unintended weight loss and occasionally fever.
- **Non-articular symptoms**: a full systems enquiry is required to screen for/determine extent of possible organ involvement and should include eyes, ENT, skin, mucosae and vasculature as well as the major systems.
- Where constitutional and non-articular inflammatory symptoms predominate, systemic inflammatory diseases such as lupus, vasculitis or other connective tissue disease should be considered.
- **Non-inflammatory** rheumatic conditions are usually localized/regional without features of inflammation or constitutional upset.

Examination

Examination of the **locomotor system** is based on the **'look, feel, move'** paradigm. Always enquire about any painful areas in advance to avoid causing pain and distress.

1 **Look** for attitude (how the joint/affected part is held); swelling; deformity; asymmetry; muscle wasting around the joint; redness of the overlying skin. Note the pattern of affected joints, e.g. small vs large, symmetrical vs asymmetrical (see Figure 66.1 above for characteristic patterns of joint disease).
2 **Feel** for heat; character of swelling (bony [nodal OA] vs boggy [synovitis] vs fluid [effusion] vs other, e.g. subcutaneous rheumatoid nodule); tenderness in relation to underlying anatomical structure. Maximum tenderness elicited by mild/moderate direct pressure (sufficient to blanch the examining finger nail) over the joint line is consistent with synovitis/arthritis; over periarticular structures (tendon, enthesis) suggests tendonitis or enthesitis.
3 **Move** (active then passive). Note any restriction in joint movement: restriction throughout the range of active and passive motion suggests inflammatory synovitis of the affected joint; end-of-range pain and restriction (often with crepitus) suggest osteoarthritis. **Crepitus** is a 'creaking' feeling under the examiner's hand on passive movement; audible crepitus usually indicates advanced joint destruction. Pain only in specific planes or on specific movements suggests a localized periarticular or mechanical problem. Active resisted movements that stress the involved structure aggravate pain arising from tendonitis, enthesitis and bursitis. Long-standing disease may produce deformities such as 'fixed flexion' or angular deformities (varus/valgus).

Systems examination

Full systems examination is undertaken to (i) inform diagnosis and (ii) determine the presence/extent of non-articular involvement in systematic disease. Findings may include the following (see also Figure 66.1 above).

- **Systemic/general:** evidence of weight loss, fever, generalized lymphadenopathy.
- **Skin:** psoriasis (characteristic rash may be limited to the scalp, umbilicus, nails or natal cleft); butterfly rash of SLE; palpable purpura or ulceration of systemic vasculitis; skin thickening and tightening (scleroderma) of systemic sclerosis; Gottron's papules (dermatomyositis).
- **Mucosae:** oral dryness (primary Sjogren syndrome) or ulceration (SLE or Behçet vasculitis).
- **Eyes:** conjunctivitis, scleritis (RA); iritis (ankylosing spondylitis or Behçet).
- **Respiratory:** shortness of breath (RA or connective tissue disease-associated interstitial lung disease or pleural effusion).
- **Cardiovascular:** Raynaud (systemic sclerosis, other CTDs), palpitations (SLE), venous thromboembolism (Behçet vasculitis, antiphospholipid syndrome).

- **GI:** heartburn (systemic sclerosis); diarrhea (seronegative spondyloarthropathy).
- **Neurological:** seizures (SLE, vasculitis); chorea (SLE); mononeuritis (vasculitis, SLE).
- **Psychological:** depression is a common co-morbidity. Psychosis may be a feature of CNS inflammation in SLE.

Investigation

On the basis of the history and examination, a presumptive diagnosis can often be made (see Figure 66.1 above). Diagnostic (or classification) criteria for the rheumatic diseases include a combination of clinical, laboratory and/or radiological/pathological criteria. Further investigation should be informed by the clinical findings and include serological tests and appropriate imaging. An overview of immunological tests and imaging in diagnosis and management of the rheumatic diseases is presented in Table 66.1.

Laboratory tests in rheumatological disease

- **Inflammatory markers** (ESR, CRP) are usually raised in inflammatory rheumatological conditions and are useful screening tests.
- **Others**: serum uric acid (gout); ferritin (Still disease, HLH); C3 and C4 complement levels (SLE); CK (myositis).
- **Immunological tests**: see Table 66.1.

Table 66.1 Immunological tests in rheumatology.

Test	Target antigen (if applicable) and method	Clinical indication	Interpretation and comments
Screening tests			
ANA (antinuclear antibody)	Nuclear antigens Test: indirect immunofluorescent antibody (IIF) (gold standard) Others: e.g. ELISA(immunoassay). Higher throughput but lower sensitivity	Clinical features suggestive of connective tissue disease (CTD), including SLE	+ve ANA titre ≥1:160 found in CTD or SLE –ve ANA by IIF (high sensitivity) makes CTD or SLE very unlikely. Pattern of immunofluorescence useful e.g. homogeneous staining of dsDNA ab. +ve ANA –> do follow-up ENA and dsDNA(below). +ANA also found in infection, liver disease, malignancy, older age, 10% of the healthy population (low titre)
Rheumatoid factor (RF)	Antigenic determinants of Fc fragment of IgG RF usually of IgM class Test: Rose–Waaler or Latex test	Clinical features suggestive of inflammatory arthritis, particularly RA	**RF in RA** Moderate sensitivity (50–75%) and specificity (65–70%). High-titre RF predicts poor outcomes in RA. +ve RF also found in: SLE; Sjogren syndrome; systemic sclerosis (SSc), cryoglobulinaemia (type II) Infection (e.g. viral hepatitis, tuberculosis, infective endocarditis), Neoplasia, e.g. lymphoma, 5% of healthy individuals
Anti-CCP/ACPA (anticyclic citrullinated peptide antibody)	Antigenic determinants of proteins containing citrulline residues from post-translational modification. Test: ELISA	Clinical features suggestive of inflammatory arthritis, particularly RA	In RA, ACPA sensitivity (50–75%) similar to RF, but higher specificity (90–95%). Combining RF and ACPA (both positive or both negative) improves diagnostic accuracy. Anti-CCP antibodies/ACPA precede clinical RA, predict poor prognosis and better treatment response
ENA (extractable nuclear antigen) antibody screen	Antigens on nuclear components, e.g. ribosomes, centromere	Positive ANA or clinical suspicion of specific CTD	Specific antibodies have strong or specific disease associations, e.g. anti scl-70 and anti-RNA polymerase III (diffuse cutaneous SSc), anticentromere (limited cutaneous SSc/CREST syndrome), anti-jo1 (antisynthetase syndrome), anti-Ro (SS-A) and anti-La (SS-B) (SLE, Sjogren syndrome), anti-Smith (SLE), anti-RNP and U1RNP (MCTD/SSc)
ANCA (antineutrophil cytoplasmic antibody)	Neutrophil cytoplasmic antigens: myeloperoxidase (MPO) serine proteinase (PR3)	Clinical features suggestive of vasculitis, e.g. constitutional, palpable purpura, end-organ symptoms (e.g. ENT, renal)	Associated with immune-mediated systemic vasculitis. Immunofluorescence staining patterns: perinuclear, p-anca; granular cytoplasmic, c-ANCA. Follow-up tests: specific antibodies to MPO and PR3
Second-level tests			
Anti-dsDNA (double-stranded DNA) antibody	**DNA**	Positive ANA and clinical features suggestive of SLE	Rising titres may indicate active inflammation in those who produce dsDNA antibodies

Table 66.1 (Continued)

Test	Target antigen (if applicable) and method	Clinical indication	Interpretation and comments
Extended myositis panel	Specific nuclear and nucleolar targets	Specialist use in immune-mediated inflammatory myopathies	Used in specialist clinical practice only
Anti-MPO and anti-PR3 antibody	Neutrophil cytoplasmic antigens: myelo-peroxidase serine proteinase	Positive ANCA, clinical features of systemic vasculitis	Overlap may occur but generally MPO Ab associated with EGPA and MPA PR3 Ab associated with GPA
Antiphospholipid antibodies Antibodies to anticardiolipin and β_2-glycoprotein I	Phospholipids present on vascular endothelium IgG and IgM isotypes Test: ELISA	Recurrent miscarriage, 3rd trimester loss Unprovoked VTE Pregnancy planning in those with CTD/SLE	1 or 2 (of 3) laboratory criteria for antiphospholipid syndrome (APS) (the other is +ve lupus anticoagulant) Can be tested even if patient anticoagulated Testing technically difficult; must be positive ×2 >12 weeks apart Positive laboratory criteria *not sufficient* for diagnosis of APS (also requires clinical event). APS may be primary or in association with systemic rheumatic disease
Lupus anticoagulant (AC)	Standard clotting tests: APTT or DRVVT (non-correctable prolongation)	As for anticardiolipin Ab	Prolongs clotting time *in vitro* and does not correct with addition of normal plasma (as would factor deficiencies). Cannot test if anticoagulated

Core principles in rheumatology

Modern-day rheumatology has benefited from the development of targeted treatments arising out of our improved understanding of disease pathogenesis and mechanisms. Patient care has benefited from the development and widespread adoption of international criteria for diagnosis or classification and management of the major rheumatological diseases by the American College of Rheumatology (ACR) and the European Alliance of Associations for Rheumatology (EULAR). In this era, core broad principles apply to management of the inflammatory rheumatic diseases. Disease-specific guidelines are subject to continuous review and can be found in the relevant chapters.

Principles for diagnosis of the rheumatic diseases

- Rheumatological diseases have characteristic clinical, laboratory, radiological and pathological features. Diagnosis requires consideration of all three parameters but is firmly guided by a full, accurate **clinical assessment**. This is an important core competency.
- **Laboratory tests** have less than perfect sensitivity and specificity for rheumatic diseases and test performance may vary from lab to lab. False-positive and false-negative results are thus expected. The utility of a test in clinical practice can be ascertained from its **likelihood ratios** (LR) (positive +LR and negative -LR). These are calculated from its sensitivity and specificity characteristics. Most immunological tests used in the rheumatic diseases have moderate LRs at best (excepting the LR of ANA, which is high), and are most useful when there is a moderate to high clinical (pretest) probability of the condition. They are *not* indicated in the absence of clinical features of rheumatic diseases and should not be used as screens for fatigue, lassitude or non-specific/generalized pain without specific rheumatological features. In such cases, the test adds a healthcare cost and may generate unnecessary worry for the patient. Similarly, screening tests (e.g. ANA) or specific diagnostic tests (e.g. ENA, ANCA) should not be repeated when a diagnosis is established. Some tests, e.g. anti dsDNA, anti-PR3 or -MPO antibody titres, inflammatory markers or complement levels, may be helpful in monitoring disease activity.
- **Radiology: plain radiographs** of joints are useful to determine interval progression (e.g. erosion) or complication (e.g. secondary OA) in established inflammatory disease but are not sensitive indicators of early joint disease. Targeted use of more sensitive techniques such as dynamic power Doppler ultrasound or MRI is preferred where available. Other diagnostic imaging techniques include CT, DEXA (for bone density), bone scintigraphy (for Paget, secondaries, osteomyelitis), and FDG-PET, particularly useful for large vessel vasculitis.
- **Collaborative international classification criteria** have been developed for most rheumatological diseases, e.g. RA, SLE. These are designed for use in clinical trials, mandating that they are highly specific, i.e. only those with the disease will be enrolled (low false-positive rate). Their use in clinical practice for *diagnosis* is limited by the concomitant reduction in sensitivity; their rigid application may miss early disease or disease in evolution and the importance of expert evaluation by a rheumatologist cannot be overstated.

Principles of management

- The overall aim of management of all rheumatic disease is to improve patient quality of life.
- This is achieved by disease modification, which comprises: timely/effective amelioration of symptoms and clinical features/signs, maximization/normalization of physical and social function, minimization of organ or structural damage/deformity.
- Disease modification is augmented by attending to disease **co-morbidities** and to the **adverse or unwanted effects** of medications (by prevention/screening/management thereof).

- **Collaborative international clinical guidelines** have been agreed for the expert management of rheumatological diseases, e.g. RA, SLE, gout, OA. They are tailored to the context and clinical nuance of individual patients. These are:
  1. **Patient centred**: all care decisions are made in partnership and informed by patient preferences, priorities and concerns.
  2. **Multidisciplinary:** A **specialist-led multidisciplinary team holistic approach** to patient care attends to all aspects of disease; physical/biological, psychological and social/participatory.
  3. **Evidence based.**
  4. **Outcome based**: The target outcome for many rheumatological conditions is now that of **disease remission** or **very low disease activity**.
- An algorithmic or stepwise **treat-to-target** approach is adopted in most clinical guidelines. Regular interval patient assessment ± laboratory/imaging updates guide decisions for escalation (remission induction) *or* maintenance *or* de-escalation (inactive disease with low risk of recurrence) of therapy.
- **Co-morbidities,** which may be general (e.g. age-related), disease associated (e.g. increased cardiovascular risk in RA) or medication associated (e.g. increased infection risk with immunosuppressant therapy).
- **Cost**: clinical guidelines have a cost-conscious approach and include lower-cost options (including generic and biosimilars) where there is evidence for these.

Figure 66.2 Approach to bone and muscle pain

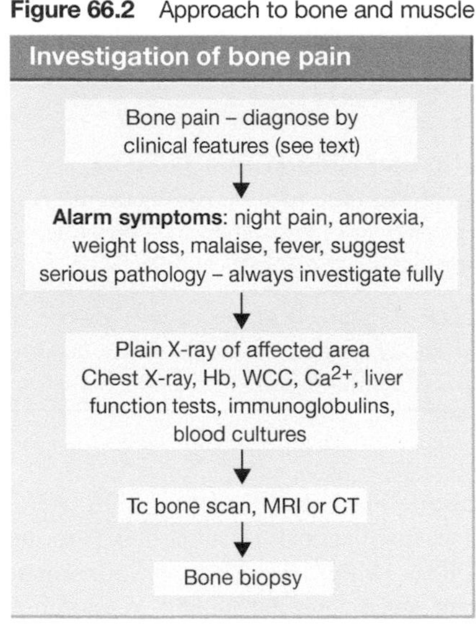

Investigation of bone pain
Bone pain – diagnose by clinical features (see text)
Alarm symptoms: night pain, anorexia, weight loss, malaise, fever, suggest serious pathology – always investigate fully
Plain X-ray of affected area
Chest X-ray, Hb, WCC, Ca2+, liver function tests, immunoglobulins, blood cultures
Tc bone scan, MRI or CT
Bone biopsy

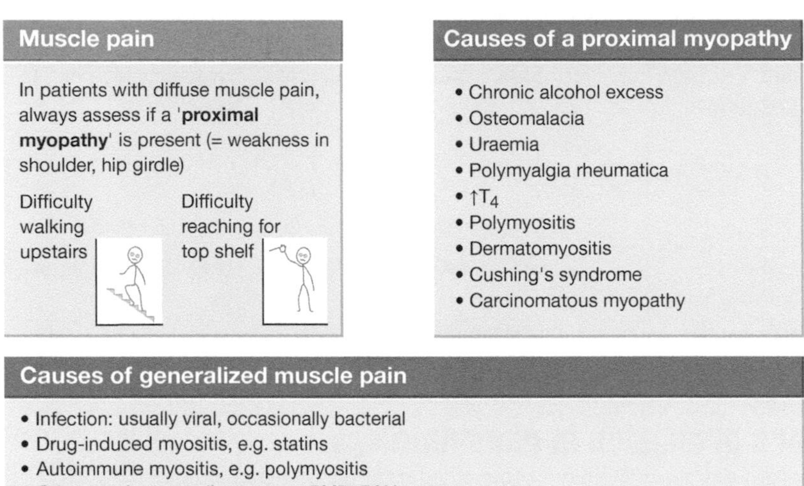

Muscle pain
In patients with diffuse muscle pain, always assess if a 'proximal myopathy' is present (= weakness in shoulder, hip girdle)
Difficulty walking upstairs
Difficulty reaching for top shelf
Causes of a proximal myopathy
• Chronic alcohol excess
• Osteomalacia
• Uraemia
• Polymyalgia rheumatica
• ↑T4
• Polymyositis
• Dermatomyositis
• Cushing's syndrome
• Carcinomatous myopathy

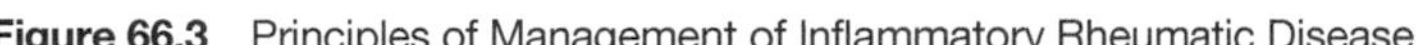

• Infection: usually viral, occasionally bacterial
• Drug-induced myositis, e.g. statins
• Autoimmune myositis, e.g. polymyositis

• Miscellaneous other causes, e.g. sarcoidosis, fibromyalgia

Figure 66.3 Principles of Management of Inflammatory Rheumatic Disease

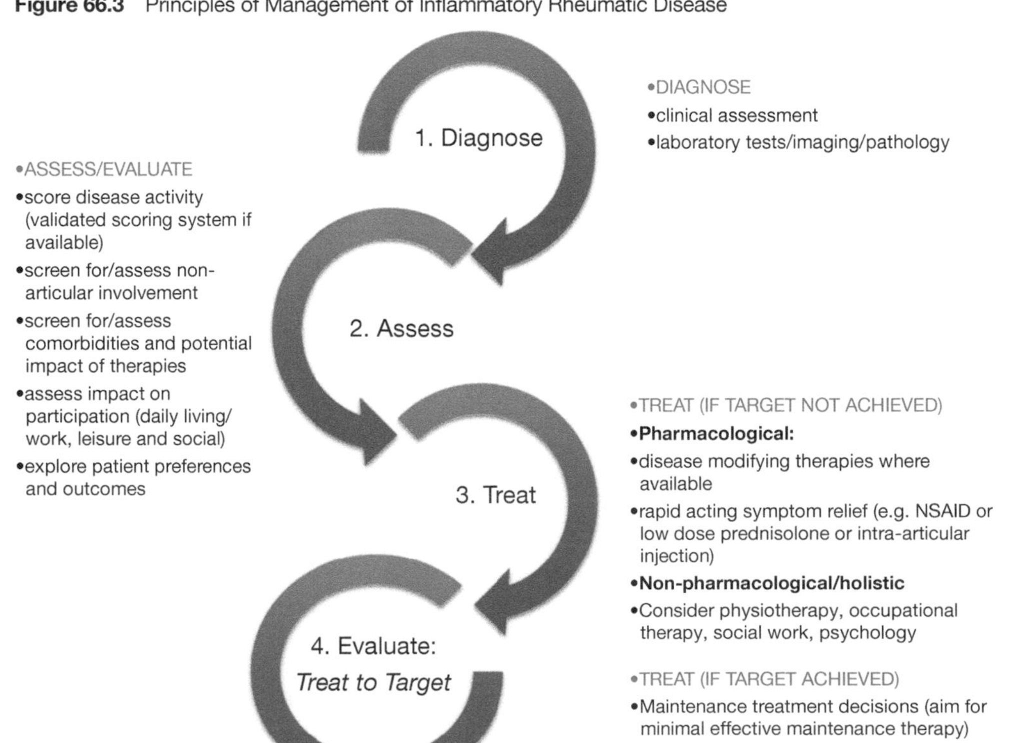

1. Diagnose

•ASSESS/EVALUATE
•score disease activity (validated scoring system if available)

•screen for/assess comorbidities and potential impact of therapies
•assess impact on participation (daily living/ work, leisure and social)

•TREAT (IF TARGET NOT ACHIEVED)

•Consider physiotherapy, occupational therapy, social work, psychology
4. Evaluate:

•TREAT (IF TARGET ACHIEVED)

Table 66.2 Approach to Musculoskeletal Imaging in Rheumatology

Screening Tests		
	Utility: Visualisation of	Comments
Plain Film Radiographs (X-ray)	o Erosions (inflammatory arthritis) o Osteoarthritis (subchondral sclerosis, cartilage loss, osteophytes) o Joint alignment/mal-alignment o Osteoporotic fracture o Pagetic bone change	Widely available, generally inexpensive Limited utility in early disease and non-bone pathology
Ultrasound	o Soft tissue structures, e.g. tendons, rotator cuff o joint inflammation (synovitis) and damage o early erosions in inflammation o clarifies physical exam findings, e.g. shoulder o guides needle placement for intra-articular injection	Point of care utility – may speed up diagnosis No radiation exposure
MRI Magnetic Resonance Imaging	Detailed visualization of all relevant MSK tissues and structures including tendons, joints, cartilage, muscles, nerves and spinal cord	Increasingly available but may be expensive No radiation exposure
CT Computed Tomography	Detailed visualization of all relevant MSK tissues and structures	Consider radiation exposure
DEXA Dual Energy X-Ray Absorptiometry	Measurement of bone density as surrogate for bone strength Measured in g/cm^2 or as T score	Included in FRAX © Score to estimate fracture risk
Bone Scintigraphy	Useful for detecting areas of increased activity in Paget's disease or osteomyelitis (bone infection) or stress fracture	Tc-99m diphosphonate administered intravenously. Three phase uptake scan
FDG PET Fluorodeoxyglucose (*FDG*)-positron emission tomography (*PET*)	Specialist use only for the evaluation of activity in known or suspected large vessel vasculitis	Usually in conjunction with CT Enhanced FDG uptake in the lining of large vessels in active vasculitis

Low back pain and other regional pain syndromes

Structures which may cause back pain

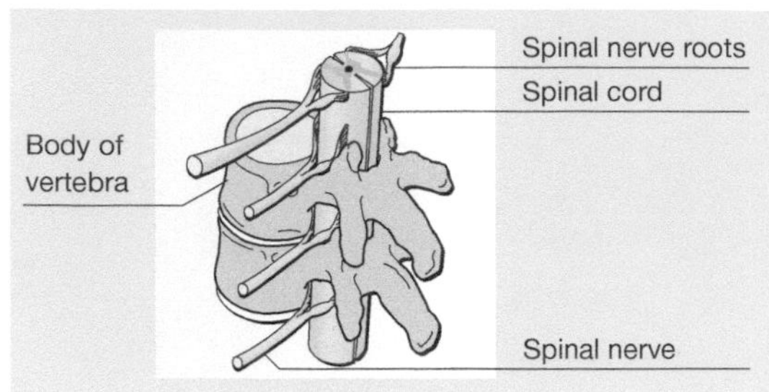

Clinical features of back pain
- Apophyseal joints → pain ↑ on back extension
- Disc prolapse → pain ↑ by flexion ± nerve root signs (e.g. 'sciatica')
- Bone disease → constant, severe pain
- Entheses/ligaments → localized pain, no radiation

- Stress fracture of pars interarticularis = spondylolysis
- Bony slip of vertebra on another = spondylolisthesis

Management of low back pain

Causes
- Prolapsed disc
- Osteoporotic fracture
- Non-inflammatory joint/ ligament disease

History + examination suggests

Mechanical origin

Clinical features
- Sudden onset
- Eased by rest
- Unilateral symptoms
- ↑ by coughing/sneezing
- Previous episodes

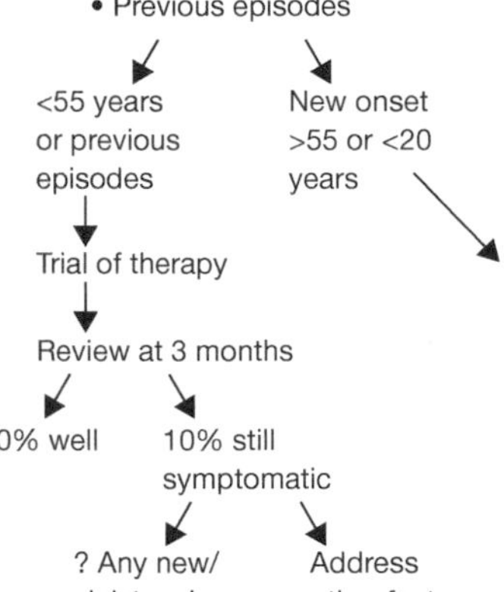

<55 years or previous episodes → Trial of therapy → Review at 3 months
- 90% well
- 10% still symptomatic
  - ? Any new/ sinister signs or symptoms → Investigate and treat appropriately
  - Address other factors (see text)

New onset >55 or <20 years → (Investigations)

Systemic or inflammatory origin

- Predominant stiffness (>30 minutes in a.m.)
- Gradual onset → progressive
- ↑ Pain with rest
- Disturbs sleep
- Stiff/rigid spine on exam
- Symmetrical restriction SIJ tenderness

↓

Investigations
- Inflammatory markers (CRP, ESR)
- WCC, Hb
- Ca, PO_4, alk phos
- Protein electrophoresis
- Blood cultures if appropriate + image: plain X-ray, CT, MRI

↓

Diagnosis
Sacroiliitis
Neoplasia
Epidural abscess
Paget's disease
(Abdominal visceral origin)

↓

Institute appropriate treatment

Cauda equina syndrome

= compression of cauda equina by posterior disc herniation
- Persistent + progressive
- Leg pain on walking
- Normal leg pulses
- Pain eased by leaning forwards
- Stiff spine on exam
- Neurology is **bladder/bowel** dysfunction + **appears late**

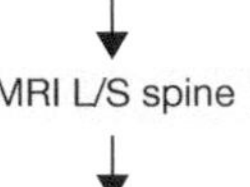

MRI L/S spine
↓
Surgical intervention

Causes of low back pain

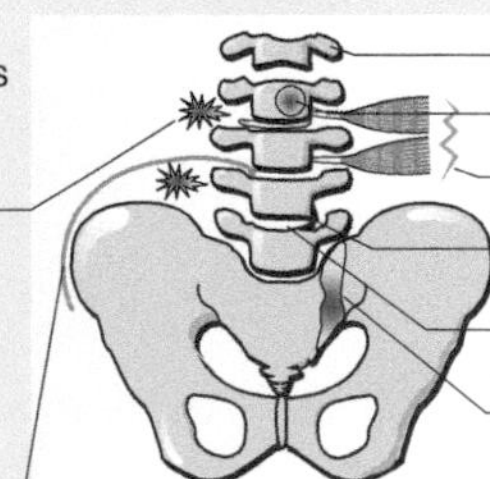

Medicine at a Glance, Fifth Edition. Edited by Patrick Davey and Alex Pitcher.

Companion website: www.wiley.com/go/medicine5e

Low back pain

Low back pain is common and disabling. The lifetime incidence is 65–80%, representing about 10% of rheumatological problems in general practice. The economic cost in 1990 was $24 billion in the USA and it is much more now.

Aetiology and nomenclature

The different causes of low back pain are as follows.

- **Mechanical** low back pain: arising from anatomical structures such as muscle, ligament or intervertebral disc or facet joints due to trauma, deformity or degenerative change.
- **Systemic illness** such as inflammatory spondylitis, infection, malignancy, myeloma or Paget disease.
- **Sciatica**: pain that radiates from the buttock down the back of the leg and into the foot, often accompanied by paraesthesia in the same distribution. It is commonly due to compression of a lumbosacral nerve root by a protruding intervertebral disc or facet joint hypertrophy.

Symptoms

- Mechanical back pain causes localized symptoms, which may be referred to other sites around the pelvic girdle and upper legs. It does not extend below the knee unless there is additional nerve root compression causing sciatica. In this case, symptoms and signs in the anatomical distribution of the sciatic nerve occur (see figure below).
- Central canal narrowing stenosis (large central disc prolapse and/or osteophyte formation) may cause compression of the cauda equina, giving rise to distinct symptoms of bilateral leg claudication. Bladder/bowel dysfunction constitutes a medical emergency.
- Lateral recess stenosis may occur as a result of posterolateral protrusion of the disc, osteophytes around a degenerate zygoapophyseal joint, or a combination of the two. Sciatica is prominent on standing or walking for any extended periods of time; nocturnal pain in the leg (with or without paraesthesia) typically wakes the patient in the early hours and may be eased by walking around. Neurological signs may be minor or absent but can sometimes be provoked by activity.
- Features suggestive of systemic/inflammatory illness (malaise, fevers, weight loss, severe pain) or cauda equina compression (paraparesis, bladder involvement) should prompt complete systemic examination and investigations.

Natural history of low back pain

Most episodes of low back pain are self-limiting and not incapacitating.

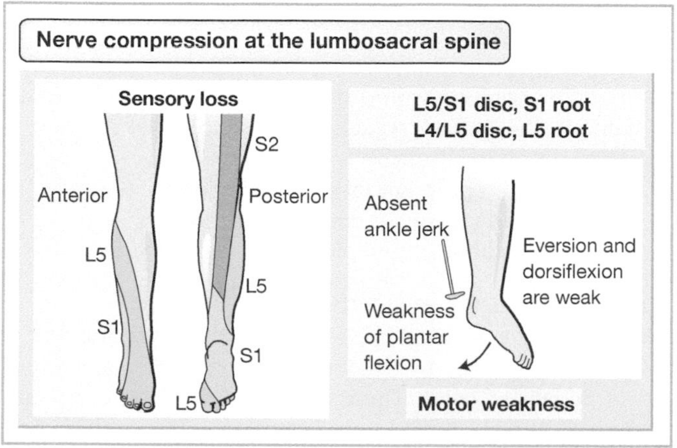

- 90% are due to 'mechanical' back pain.
- 50% are better one week after onset.
- <10% of patients have pain persistent for more than six months. These patients enter a 'chronic pain cycle', are the least likely to return to full employment/activity, and account for 80% of the costs incurred in care.
- 10% are due to underlying systemic or inflammatory illness.

Clinical approach

The aims of the clinical evaluation are:

- to discriminate between mechanical and systemic causes
- to identify features that suggest the need for advanced imaging studies ± early surgical referral.

Examination

Routine back examination is shown on the next page. Pointers towards serious underlying disease include:

- patients with systemic or inflammatory features
- those >55 or <25 years old with new-onset low back pain
- those unresponsive to a 6–8-week trial of conservative therapy for mechanical low back pain.

Management

Initial treatment consists of reassurance and education; simple analgesia ± non-steroidal anti-inflammatory drugs. Bed rest has a limited role in the acute phase (≤48 h) with early mobilization, followed by a graded exercise programme. Ninety percent of cases settle.

For unresponsive patients with no new physical findings, the following should be done.

- Identification of occupational, physical and psychosocial contributions.
- Development of a patient-tailored rehabilitation programme, which may include cognitive behavioural approaches.
- Identification of specific anatomical lesions causing the pain (e.g. facet joints, disc lesions, nerve roots, bones).

Where such lesions can be identified, the following **specific measures** may be useful.

- **Facet joint injection** with local anaesthetic and corticosteroids. This is sometimes therapeutic and is particularly helpful in localizing a painful segment prior to considering spinal fusion.
- **Local anaesthetic injections** around nerve roots to confirm compression at specific levels prior to surgical decompression, particularly when there are lesions at multiple levels.
- **Chemonucleolysis** by intradisc injection of chymopapain to relieve compression symptoms from a bulging disc.
- **Surgery** is performed to relieve nerve compression due to disc herniation using the technique of partial laminectomy/discectomy. It is much more effective at relieving sciatica than back pain. It may be combined with spinal fusion at the corresponding level.

Regional pain syndromes

Regional rheumatic pain syndromes are very common. They may be difficult to diagnose with confidence. In particular, pain arising in a localized area, such as the shoulder or hip, presents a clinical challenge. Pain may arise from numerous articular or

Back examination

Examine patient while standing

- **Gait**: look for any abnormality whilst walking and turning, and note whether walking aids are required. Normal gait involves stance (60%) and swing (40%) phases
- **Back**: look for any abnormality including scoliosis, which is described by the side of the vertebral concavity. Cervical lordosis, thoracic kyphosis and lumbar lordosis are normal, i.e. looking at the patient from the side, with the patient facing to the right, a lordosis is a curve shaped like a closing bracket ')', whereas a kyphosis is shaped like an opening bracket '('
- Check for any localized tenderness in the spine (press, and then 'bang' on each of the vertebral processes in turn) – local tenderness may indicate infection
- Look at the progression of the thoracic kyphosis; a useful measure is the distance from the wall to the tragus (ear lobe) when the patient stands with his/her back to the wall
- Forward bending; measure the increase in length between L5/S1 vertebrae and points 10 cm above and 5 cm below (Schober's test) – it should be ≥ 4 cm. (Incidentally, the finger to floor distance on bending forward is not a good measure of spinal stiffness as it may vary with hip mobility)
- Lateral flexion; ask the patient to reach down laterally to the knee joint. This can normally be achieved, but may be restricted in ankylosing spondylitis
- Hyperextension; which is arching the back backwards. Usually 10 from the vertical can be achieved

Examine patients while sitting

- Cervical spine; examine for flexion (i.e. bending the neck forward), extension (i.e. bending the neck backwards), lateral flexion (i.e. tilting the head to one side), and rotation (i.e. moving the head to the left and right). The angle attained is measured from the face forward position – normal ranges are: flexion and extension 70, lateral flexion 40, rotation 80

Pelvis examination

Examine while standing

- Look for asymmetry of the pelvis, which may suggest unequal leg length
- Trendelenburg's test. Ask the patient to stand on one leg – a dropped pelvis on the side of the raised leg (= +ve Trendelenburg test) suggests muscle weakness or hip pathology

Examine while supine

- Sacroiliac tenderness; press the anterior superior iliac spines gently apart. This will cause sacroiliac pain if they are inflamed. With the patient prone, press on the sacrum – this will cause pain if there is sacroiliac joint inflammation
- True and apparent leg lengths. Measure from the anterior superior iliac spine and umbilicus, respectively, to the medial malleolus; an apparent difference may indicate lateral tilting of the pelvis
- Hip flexion; bring the leg in towards the chest with the knees flexed – the normal limit is 110
- Hip extension; with the patient prone, extend the hip – the normal range is 0–30. This will exacerbate the symptoms if there is nerve root irritation, as the femoral nerve will be stretched
- Internal and external rotation, abduction and adduction of the hip. Rotate each hip internally (normal range 25), and externally (normal range 45) with the hip flexed, then measure the range of abduction (normal range 50) and adduction (normal 30)
- Traction manoeuvres. Assess the sciatic nerve by straight leg raising (and record the angle of elevation). Dorsiflex the foot whilst raised (Lasègue's test). This will exacerbate symptoms of lumbosacral root compression

periarticular structures, or may be referred from a more distant organ or structure site.

Differential diagnosis

The differential diagnosis of regional pain is dependent on a good knowledge of the regional anatomy and a precise history and examination. The differential diagnoses for pain around the hip, shoulder and wrist are shown on the next page.

History

- Details of all factors relevant to pain: nature and severity, radiation, factors that relieve or exacerbate, movements that provoke pain.
- Causative factors such as trauma or overuse related to work or leisure.
- Features suggestive of a more widespread inflammatory or systemic condition.

A complete neuromuscular examination is performed. **Look** for swelling, redness, muscle wasting and posture in which the affected part is held. **Feel** carefully to localize where the tenderness is maximal. **Move** carefully and so determine the range of active, then passive, motion around the appropriate joints. Note which movements provoke pain.

Ask the patient to perform these movements against resistance. Lesions such as tendonitis, enthesitis and bursitis are often more painful on movement against resistance.

Principles of management

- Exclude serious systemic disease and infection by appropriate tests, e.g. synovial fluid microscopy for crystals from gouty bursitis or micro-organisms from septic bursitis.
- Educate the patient regarding avoidance or correction of mechanical triggers. Reassure.
- Advise on an appropriate level of activity/exercises.
- Splinting (particularly for synovitis and tenosynovitis).
- Analgesia, including intralesional steroid/local anaesthetic.

Prognosis and outcome

Many of these conditions are self-limiting and respond well to simple measures, as above. Most will be asymptomatic within 12–18 months of onset. Those who receive prompt advice and therapy usually do better. A small percentage of cases fail to settle, and it may be necessary to alter work or sporting techniques.

Pain in the shoulder

Referred pain

1. Cervical spine
   - Up into neck
   - ± Down into forearm + hand
2. Myocardial infarction
3. Diaphragmatic irritation

Local causes

4. AC joint arthritis
5. Supraspinatus tendonitis (painful mid-arc)
6. Subacromial bursitis
7. Glenohumeral arthritis
8. Bicipital tendonitis

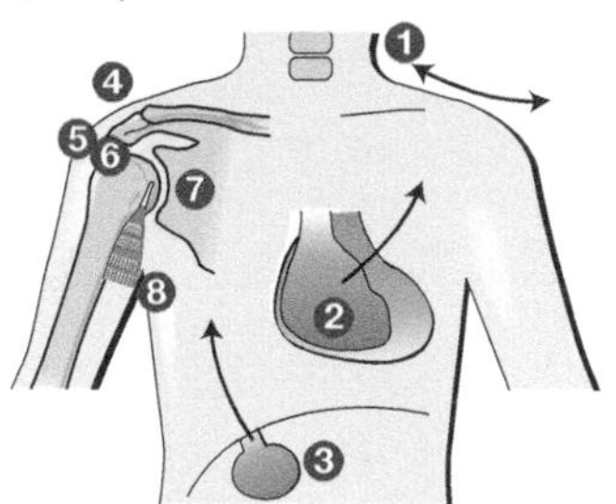

Pain in the hip

Structures giving rise to pain around the hip and buttocks

1. Sacroiliac joint
2. Hip joint (OA, RA, sepsis)
3. Trochanteric bursa (overuse, mechanical imbalance)
4. Ischiogluteal bursa (posterior)
5. Insertion of adductor tendon

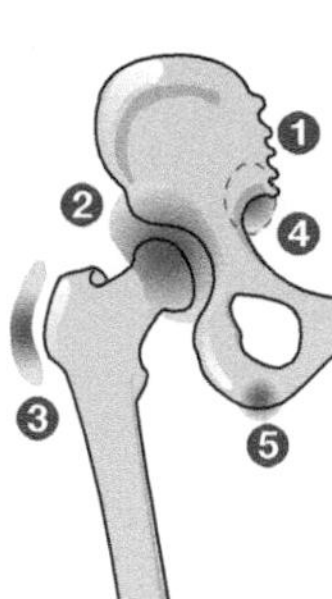

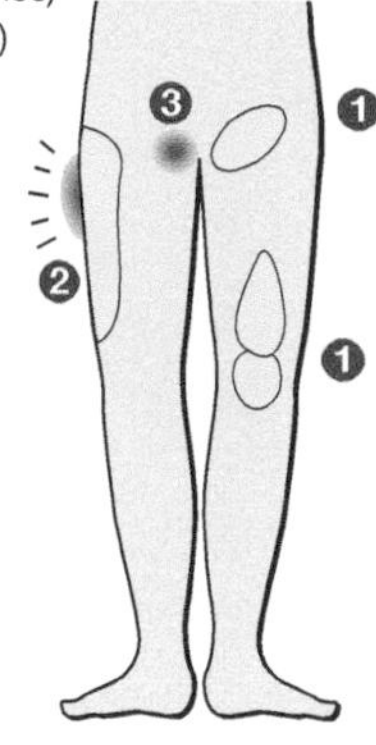

Patterns of pain around the hip

1. Intrinsic hip **or knee** joint pain
2. Trochanteric bursitis
3. Adductor tendonitis

Pain in the wrist/hand

1. 1st carpometacarpal (CMC) OA
2. De Quervain's tenosynovitis (maximal around radial styloid)
3. Dorsal (extensor) tenosynovitis

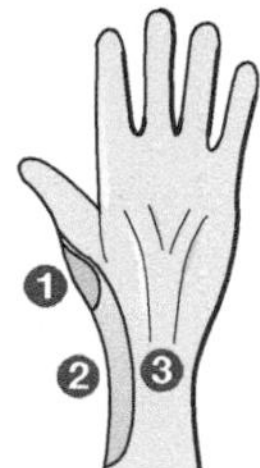

Dorsal view of hand

Origin of pain	Nomenclature and causes	Structures involved in regional pain syndromes 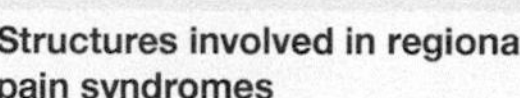	Characteristic features and examples
Synovium (1)	**Synovitis** Inflammatory arthritis Crystal deposition	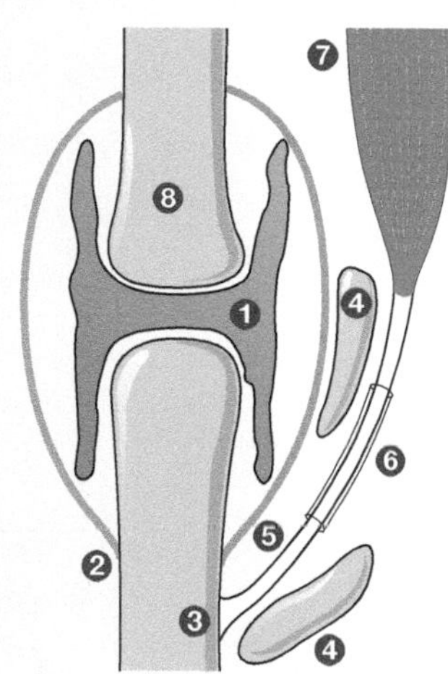	Swelling, heat and tenderness of the joint. Limited passive and active motion at the joint. Pain throughout *all* movements in all planes, e.g. rheumatoid arthritis, gout
Capsule (2) or ligament (enthesis) insertion (3)	**Capsulitis, enthesitis** Trauma Overuse		Localized pain and tenderness Movement restricted in a single plane Pain exacerbated by movement against resistance, e.g. tennis elbow (lateral epicondylitis)
Bursa (4)	**Bursitis** Mechanical Calcific Systemic		Often palpable, with defined limits to swelling Tenderness localized Pressure causes: pre- or infrapatellar bursitis (housemaid's knee) Underlying diseases: olecranon bursitis (gout), sepsis
Tendon (5) / synovial lining of tendon sheaths (6)	**Tendonitis** Overuse **Tenosynovitis** Inflammation		Pain minimal or absent on performing a movement passively which causes pain when performed actively Pain exacerbated by performing the movement against resistance: supraspinatus tendonitis, Achilles tendonitis Tenosynovitis results in swelling and tenderness of the whole tendon sheaths, e.g. extensor tenosynovitis at the wrist in RA
Muscle (7)	**Myositis** Inflammation **Muscle tear** Overuse		See inflammatory muscle diseases
Bone (8)	Fracture/tumour Infection		Persistent pain, wakes at night, unrelated to any specific movement, often not responsive to simple analgesia. See bone pain (Chapter 66)

68 Introduction to dermatology

Dermatological assessmentof a rash

1. Take a history 2. Note the distribution of the rash

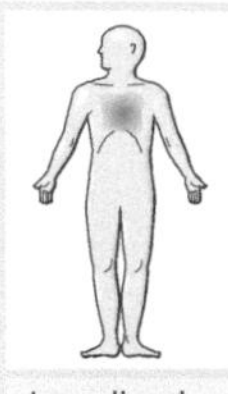
Localized

Generalized

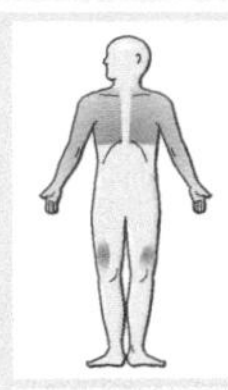
Symmetric

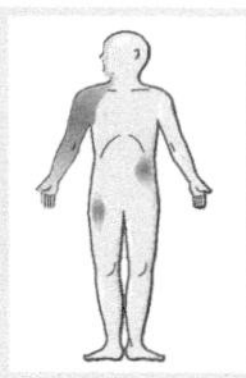
Asymmetric

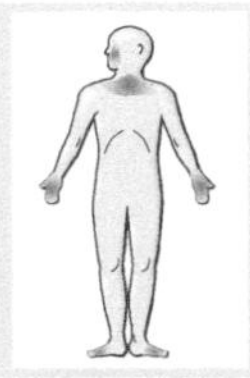
Photosensitive

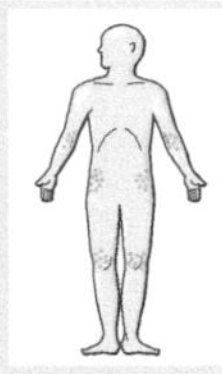
Grouped

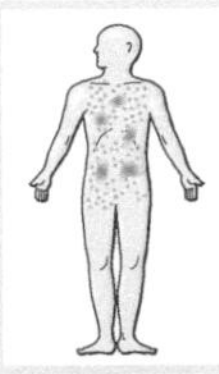
Coalescing

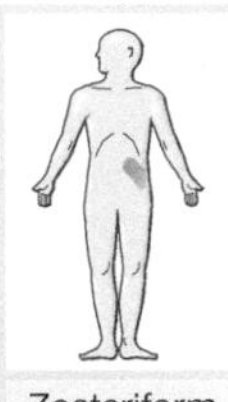
Zosteriform

3. Describe the type of eruption

Erythema

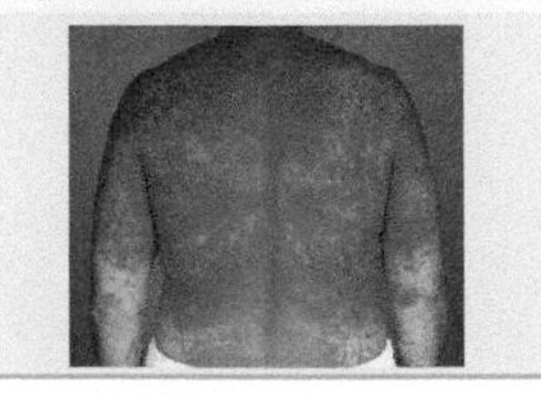

Red and scaly rash

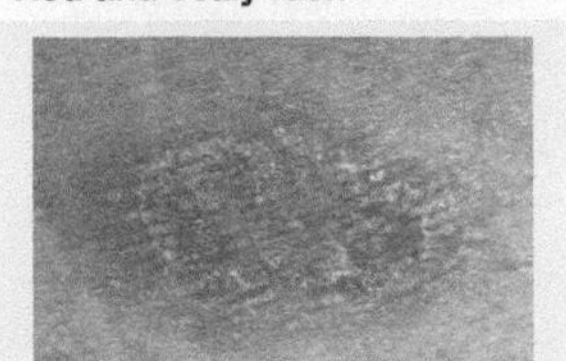

Urticaria

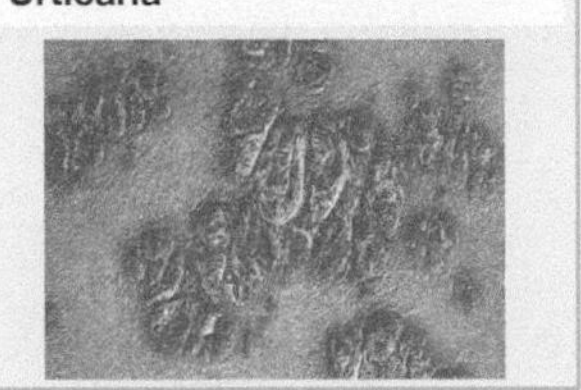

Vesicobullous

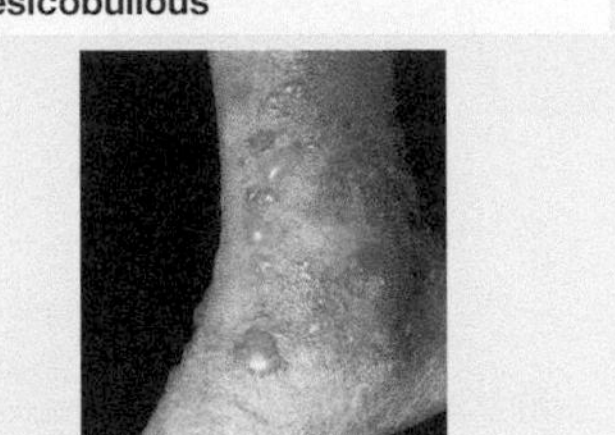

4. Examine individual lesions and determine the principal morphologies

Plaques Large elevated lesions

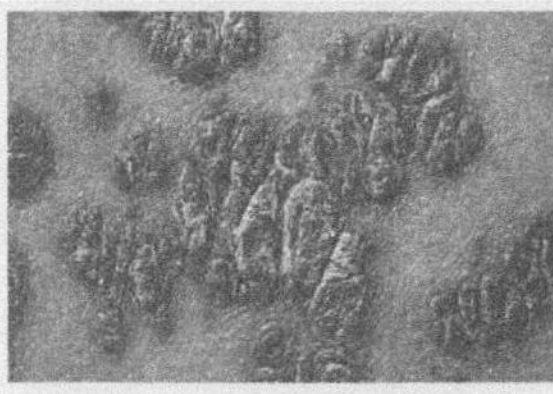

Vesicles Small (<5mm) blisters

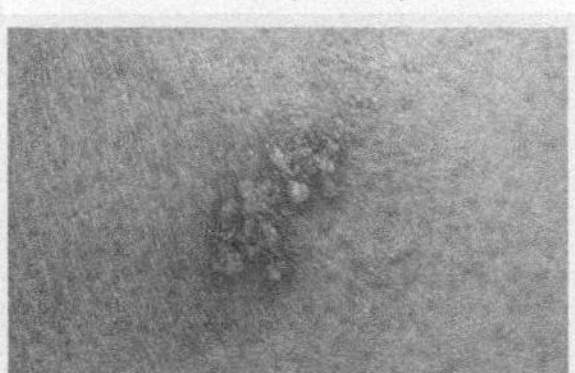

Macules (small) and **patches** (larger) — impalpable lesions

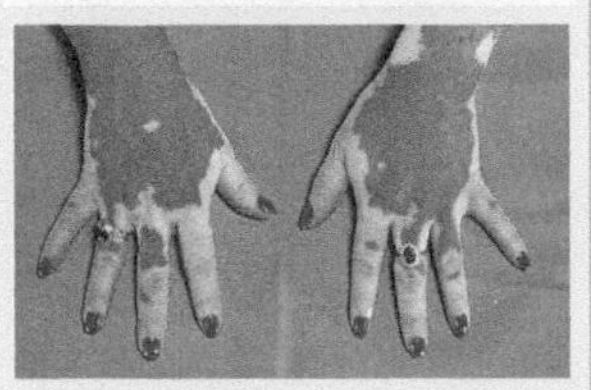

Papules (small) and **nodules** (larger) — palpable lesions

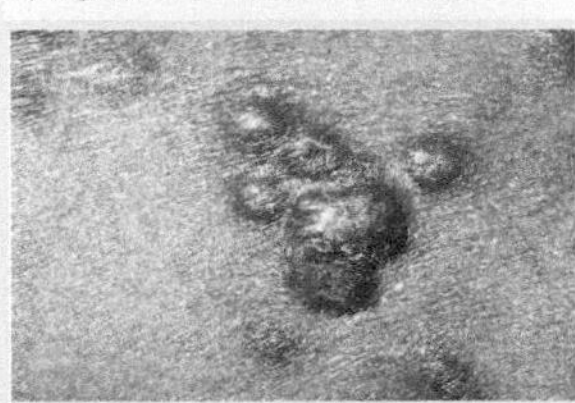

Bullae Large (>5mm) blisters

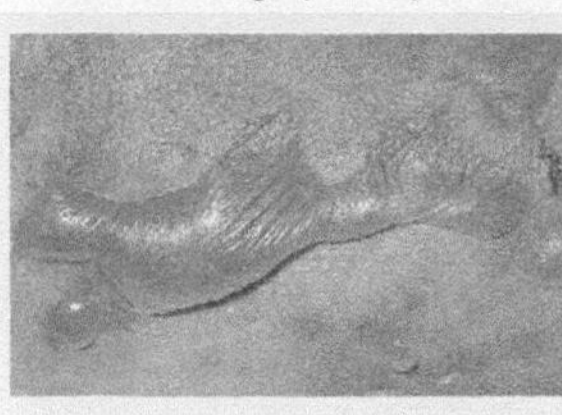

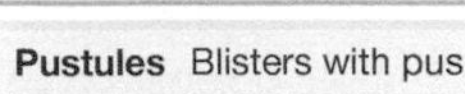
Pustules Blisters with pus

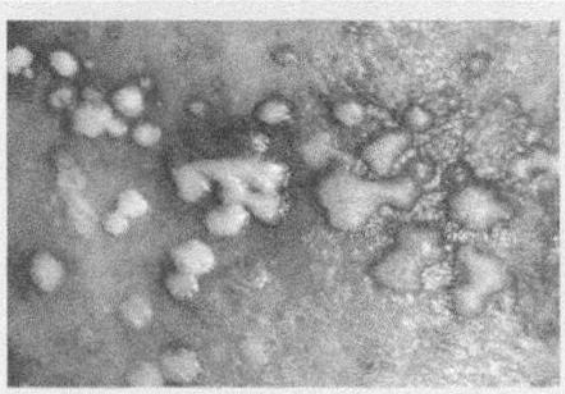

Wheals Cutaneous oedema

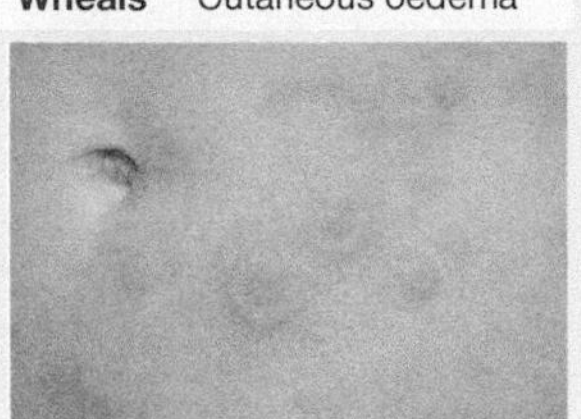

Nodule/tumour Large palpable lesion

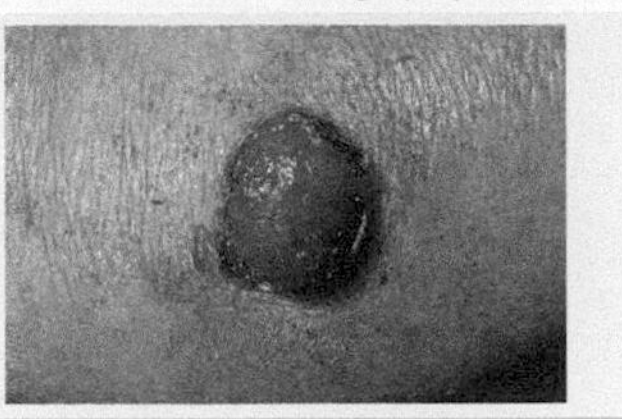

5. Examine other areas (hair, mouth, nails, genitalia) as indicated: carry out a general examination if appropriate

6. Use bedside tests when necessary

Wood's light – in fungal infection and erythrasma (as illustrated)

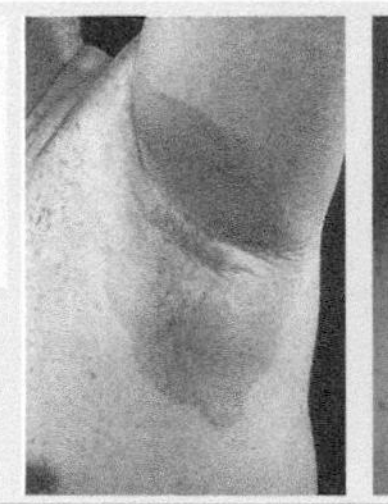

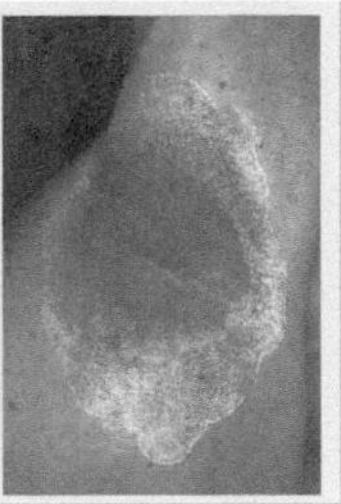

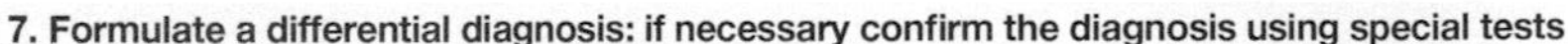
7. Formulate a differential diagnosis: if necessary confirm the diagnosis using special tests

Skin patch tests

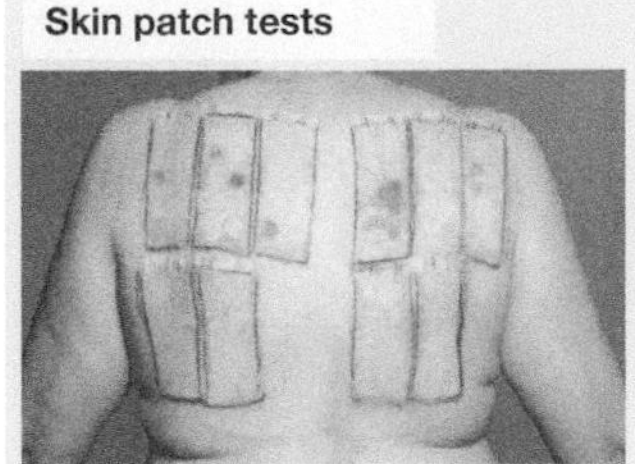

Biopsy
Direct immunofluorescence demonstrating (light green) autoantibodies against intercellular desmosomes in pemphigus vulgaris

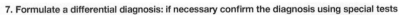

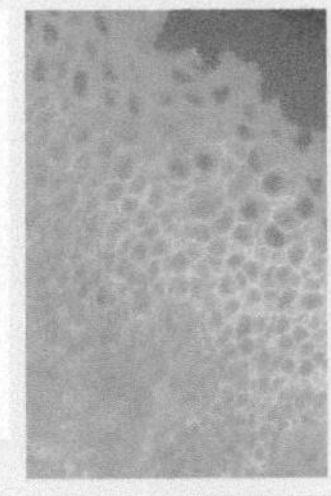

Medicine at a Glance, Fifth Edition. Edited by Patrick Davey and Alex Pitcher.

Companion website: www.wiley.com/go/medicine5e

Dermatologists achieve a clinical diagnosis by taking a history (which itself often establishes the diagnosis) and examining the skin.

History

Most patients present with a rash or a lump/bump. Other symptoms include itch/pruritus (see Chapter 69), flushing (see Chapter 37), pain, hair loss, nail changes (see Chapter 70) and ulceration. It is important to ask about the spatiotemporal characteristics of the presenting symptoms, for example:

- When did the rash or lump appear?
- Where did it spread to?
- When did it ulcerate or bleed?

Determine age, racial background, occupation, sexual orientation, drug history (could a rash represent an adverse drug reaction?), family history (there is a genetic predisposition in eczema, psoriasis and skin cancer), past medical history and current health, associated symptoms (e.g. joints, genitals) and sun history (easy burning or tanning, lifelong sun exposure, sunburn, sun beds) as sunlight may relieve or exacerbate a rash.

Examination

Skin examination is performed in a good light with the patient lying supine on a couch, using the naked eye first, then a magnifying glass. Undertake a general medical examination (see Chapter 10) when relevant.

- For a **rash**, ascertain its distribution: asymmetrical (suggests exogenous cause, e.g. local infection), symmetrical (endogenous cause), localized or widespread. Note the morphology: is it an erythema or urticaria, red and scaly (eczematous, psoriasiform or lichenoid), or vasculitis, vesicobullous or erythroderma? Check other sites that may be affected. Complete by examining the scalp, eyes, mouth, hands and nails, breasts, anogenital area and feet. Assess for lymphadenopathy.
- For a **lump/bump**, note its site and morphology (increasingly, a dermascope is used for morphological assessment of pigmented lesions), and the draining lymph nodes and liver (for distant metastases). Note skin phenotypes that predispose to cancer (fair, freckling, degree and type of moles, iris lentigines). A precise clinical diagnosis is often feasible but the prime objective is to differentiate benign from malignant lesions.

Morphology

Important morphological terms include the following.

- **Macule**: flat, no change in surface markings.
- **Papule**: circumscribed palpable lesion.
- **Nodule**: palpable mass ≥1 cm.
- **Vesicles and bullae** (blisters): visible accumulations of fluid (vesicles are small, bullae are larger).
- Other terms include telangiectasia, erosion, ulcer, plaque, wheal, comedone, pustule, abscess, cyst, scar, atrophy, purpura and sclerosis.

Special investigations

After physical examination (including urinalysis), the differential diagnosis can be further explored using special investigations.

- Wood's light: ultraviolet radiation of wavelength 360 nm, useful in demonstrating pigmentary diseases and fungal infections.
- Microbiology: swab for bacteria, scrapings for fungi.
- Biopsy for histology (± immunofluorescence): useful in diagnosing many conditions and to exclude malignancy.
- Patch testing: putative allergens are applied to the skin and the resulting reaction is read at 48 and 96 hours.
- Blood tests (e.g. for syphilis, HIV, lupus, iron deficiency).

Dermatological treatment

In the skin, a range of pathological processes (inflammation, infection, fibrosis, dysplasia, neoplasia) results in thousands of named diseases, some of which have specific treatments (see individual chapters). Some general principles of management can be outlined.

Supportive treatments

- Moisturizing the skin and avoiding soap.
- Avoiding the sun and wearing a sunscreen.
- Providing reassurance and psychological support.

Specific treatments

These can be dietary or involve drugs, phototherapy or surgery.

- **Diet**: essential fatty acids (e.g. fish and evening primrose oils) may be useful in inflammatory dermatoses; antioxidants in fruit and vegetables may protect against skin cancer.
- **Drugs** may be applied topically or taken orally.
  - Topical treatments include emollients and soap substitutes, shampoos, sunscreens, antibacterials, antifungals, keratolytics, steroids, calcineurin inhibitors, retinoids and cytotoxics.
  - Systemic treatments include antibacterials, antifungals, antihistamines, anti-inflammatory drugs (e.g. dapsone), antimalarials, retinoids, steroids and 'biological immunomodulators'.
- **Phototherapy**: ultraviolet B and PUVA (psoralens and ultraviolet A) photochemotherapy may be useful in severe dermatoses and mycosis fungoides.
- **Surgery** is used for diagnosis by biopsy and may be curative for skin cancer.

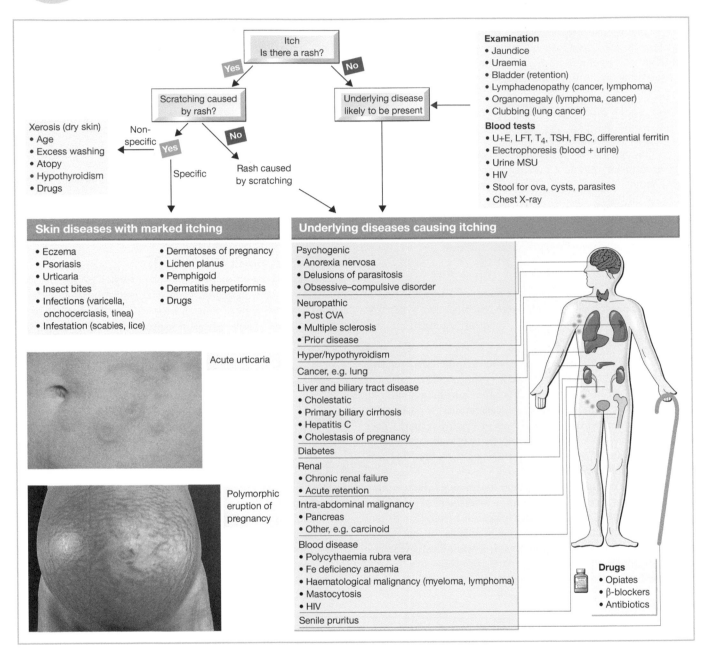

Pruritus and rashes

Itch
Is there a rash?

Yes → Scratching caused by rash?

- Yes, Non-specific → Xerosis (dry skin)
  - Age
  - Excess washing
  - Atopy
  - Hypothyroidism
  - Drugs
- Yes, Specific → Skin diseases with marked itching
- No → Rash caused by scratching → Underlying diseases causing itching

No → Underlying disease likely to be present → Underlying diseases causing itching

Examination
- Jaundice
- Uraemia
- Bladder (retention)
- Lymphadenopathy (cancer, lymphoma)
- Organomegaly (lymphoma, cancer)
- Clubbing (lung cancer)

Blood tests
- U+E, LFT, T_4, TSH, FBC, differential ferritin
- Electrophoresis (blood + urine)
- Urine MSU
- HIV
- Stool for ova, cysts, parasites
- Chest X-ray

Skin diseases with marked itching
- Eczema
- Psoriasis
- Urticaria
- Insect bites
- Infections (varicella, onchocerciasis, tinea)
- Infestation (scabies, lice)
- Dermatoses of pregnancy
- Lichen planus
- Pemphigoid
- Dermatitis herpetiformis
- Drugs

Acute urticaria

Polymorphic eruption of pregnancy

Underlying diseases causing itching

Psychogenic
- Anorexia nervosa
- Delusions of parasitosis
- Obsessive–compulsive disorder

Neuropathic
- Post CVA
- Multiple sclerosis
- Prior disease

Hyper/hypothyroidism

Cancer, e.g. lung

Liver and biliary tract disease
- Cholestatic
- Primary biliary cirrhosis
- Hepatitis C
- Cholestasis of pregnancy

Diabetes

Renal
- Chronic renal failure
- Acute retention

Intra-abdominal malignancy
- Pancreas
- Other, e.g. carcinoid

Blood disease
- Polycythaemia rubra vera
- Fe deficiency anaemia
- Haematological malignancy (myeloma, lymphoma)
- Mastocytosis
- HIV

Senile pruritus

Drugs
- Opiates
- β-blockers
- Antibiotics

Pruritus

Pruritus (itching) may be localized or generalized. Primary skin disease, underlying systemic disease or, rarely, a psychological condition must be considered.

History

Localized pruritus suggests a local cause. Generalized pruritus may relate to dermatological or systemic disease. If a rash is present, determine whether the itching occurred before (suggests underlying systemic disorder, with the signs caused by scratching) or after (suggests underlying skin disease) the rash. Undertake a general assessment including a drug history.

Examination and treatment

Excoriations, eczematization and impetiginization are non-specific secondary signs from scratching and infection. Determine

Medicine at a Glance, Fifth Edition. Edited by Patrick Davey and Alex Pitcher.

Companion website: www.wiley.com/go/medicine5e

whether there are any signs of a primary dermatosis or underlying disease. Treatment is for the underlying cause and includes emollients and antihistamines.

Rashes

Distinguish the distribution, the type of rash and the morphology (see Chapter 68).

Erythemas

The principal causes of erythema in the skin are listed in Table 69.1.

Urticarial lesions

The principal causes are as follows.

- Idiopathic urticaria.
- Drug eruptions.
- Prodromal bullous pemphigoid.
- Henoch–Schönlein purpura.

Red scaly patches

The causes of red scaly patches are listed in Table 69.2.

Erythroderma

Erythroderma is a widespread, confluent, erythematous eruption that may develop acutely or insidiously. Causes, complications and treatment are listed in the figure below.

Blistering

Blistering is common and examples include acute eczema, herpes, impetigo and insect bites. Some drug eruptions are bullous, e.g. toxic epidermal necrolysis (see Chapter 227), as are some systemic diseases, e.g. porphyria cutanea tarda and amyloid. Primary bullous disease is discussed in Chapter 227.

Vasculitis

Vasculitis can be localized to the skin or involve internal organs (see Chapter 220). Vasculitic manifestations range from erythema, livedo reticularis and urticaria, to palpable purpuric papules, nodules, necrosis and infarction, depending on the calibre of the vessel involved, the nature of the inflammatory response and the severity of the vasculitic insult.

Table 69.1 Causes of erythema

- Toxic erythema: drug or viral
- Specific viral exanthems
- Erythema chronicum migrans – Lyme borreliosis
- Erythema multiforme (see Chapter 231)
- Erythema nodosum (see Chapter 229)
- Erythema marginatum – very rare reticular erythema
- Still disease – diurnal angulated macular erythema
- Erythema ab igne – from close contact with heat

Table 69.2 Eruptions that may have red scaly patches

- Eczema/dermatitis
- Psoriasis
- Lichen planus
- Lichen sclerosus
- Pityriasis rosea
- Lupus erythematosus
- Dermatomyositis
- Tinea
- Pityriasis versicolor
- Mycosis fungoides
- Solar keratosis
- Bowen disease
- Paget disease
- Superficial basal cell carcinoma
- Drug eruption

Flushing (see Chapter 37)

Skin diseases to consider are rosacea (see Chapter 225), urticaria (see Chapter 223) and erythromelalgia.

Pustules

Causes of pustules include acne (see Chapter 225), rosacea, impetigo and autoimmune blistering diseases.

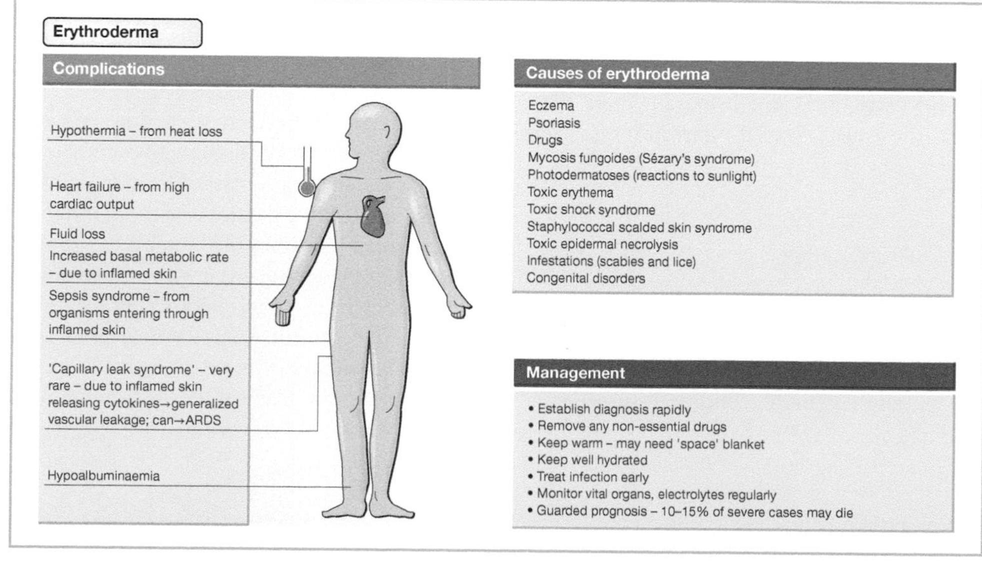

Erythroderma
Complications
Hypothermia – from heat loss
Heart failure – from high cardiac output
Fluid loss
Increased basal metabolic rate – due to inflamed skin
Sepsis syndrome – from organisms entering through inflamed skin
'Capillary leak syndrome' – very rare – due to inflamed skin releasing cytokines→generalized vascular leakage; can→ARDS
Hypoalbuminaemia
Causes of erythroderma
Eczema
Psoriasis
Drugs
Mycosis fungoides (Sézary's syndrome)
Photodermatoses (reactions to sunlight)
Toxic erythema
Toxic shock syndrome
Staphylococcal scalded skin syndrome
Toxic epidermal necrolysis
Infestations (scabies and lice)
Congenital disorders
Management
• Establish diagnosis rapidly
• Remove any non-essential drugs
• Keep warm – may need 'space' blanket
• Keep well hydrated
• Treat infection early
• Monitor vital organs, electrolytes regularly
• Guarded prognosis – 10–15% of severe cases may die

70 Hair and nail disorders

Hair loss

Alopecia areata

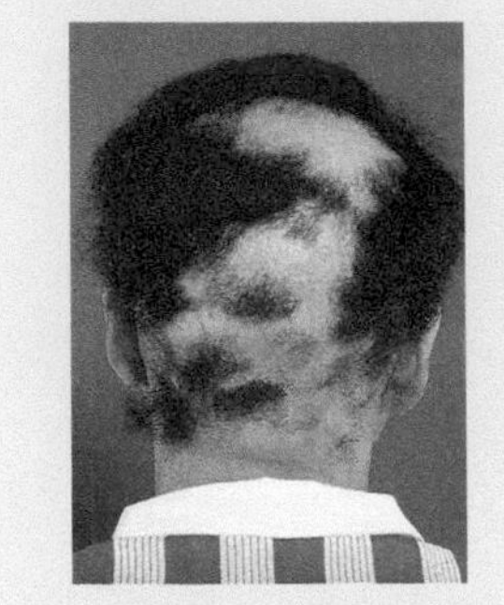

Tinea capitis. Erythema, scale, hair loss and scarring

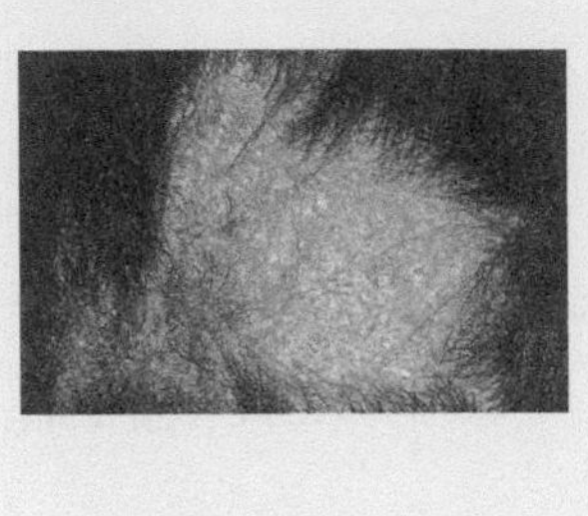

Cicatricial (scarring) Lichen planus

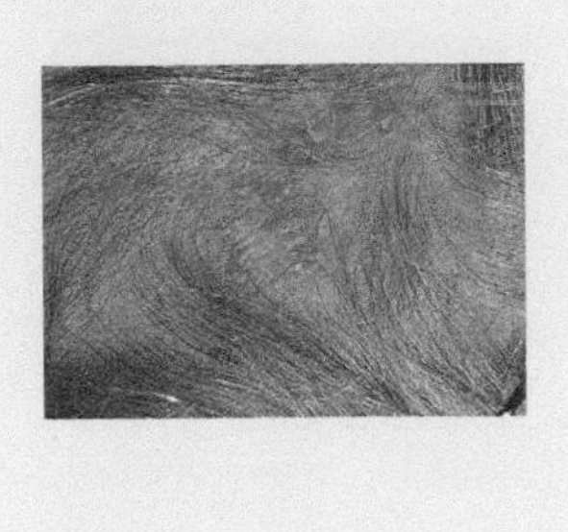

Discoid lupus erythematosus

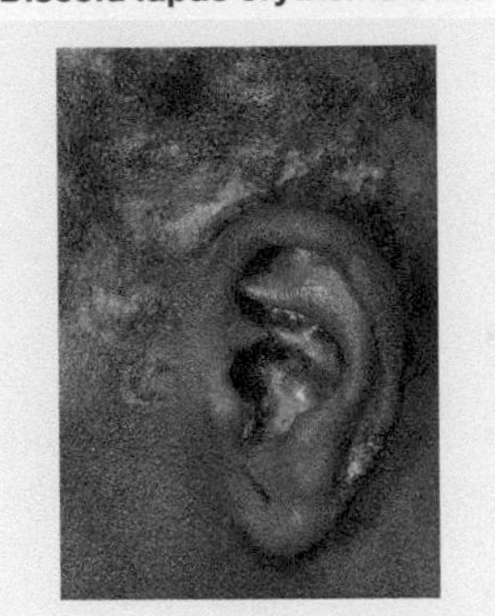

Hirsutes and hypertrichosis

- **Hirsutes** describes coarse terminal hair in women at sites where it would be normal in a postpubertal male (see Chapter 39). Virilizing tumours of adrenal or ovarian origin are rare (but examine for deepening of the voice and clitoromegaly), as are situations of extreme insulin resistance. Idiopathic hirsutes is common, as is the polycystic ovary syndrome, which may present with other features of cutaneous virilization such as acne, and androgenic alopecia (also obesity, oligomenorrhoea and infertility). Late-onset congenital adrenal hyperplasia (CAH) can cause hirsutes alone. CAH is usually due to 21-hydroxylase deficiency (10% due to 11β-hydroxylase or 3β-hydroxysteroid deficiency).
- **Hypertrichosis** is the appearance of excess, usually vellus, hair in non-androgen-dependent sites. Causes include the following.
  - **Localized**: Becker naevus, spina bifida occulta, post inflammatory disorder (trauma, porphyria cutanea tarda, arthritis), occlusion, paraneoplastic hypertrichosis lanuginose (lymphoma).
  - **Generalized**: hypothyroidism, malnutrition, anorexia, drugs (ciclosporine, corticosteroids, phenytoin, psoralens and ultraviolet A [PUVA]).

Tests in hirsutes and hypertrichosis are listed in Table 70.1. Treatment is directed at the cause; topical eflornithine may be helpful.

Table 70.1 Investigations of excess hair growth

- Thyroid function, glucose
- Luteinizing hormome, follicle-stimulating hormone, testosterone, sex hormone-binding globulin, prolactin
- 0900 cortisol, 17α-hydroxyprogesterone
- Dihydroepiandrosterone, androstenedione
- Pelvic ultrasound

Alopecia

Alopecia, or hair loss, is common. It may be subdivided into male pattern, localized or generalized. A *scarring* process must be identified and treated with alacrity. The duration of the process, sites affected and the patient's general condition (pregnancy, nutrition, health) must be ascertained. On examination, elicit local signs (erythema, scarring, pustulosis) and look for signs of a more widespread dermatosis or systemic illness. Helpful investigations include hair microscopy, telogen count, mycology, microbiology, skin biopsy and tests for an underlying systemic illness (full blood count, renal and liver function, iron studies [ferritin], systemic lupus erythematosus [SLE], HIV and syphilis).

- **Diffuse non-scarring alopecia**: the differential diagnosis includes systemic disease, thyroid disorders and other endocrinopathies, iron deficiency anaemia, skin diseases (such as psoriasis, seborrhoeic dermatitis and alopecia areata) and drugs (such as lithium or cytotoxics).
- **Androgenic alopecia**: in men, this is physiological and consists of focal frontal and vertical loss with eventual confluence of baldness and occipital sparing. Finasteride 1 mg daily is licensed for treatment. In women, the picture is of more diffuse thinning. Minoxidil 2–5% solution/foam may help some cases. In women, the antiandrogen cyproterone acetate given with ethinyl oestradiol to regulate the menstrual cycle has some effect. Other drugs used include spironolactone and metformin (in polcystic ovarian syndrome).
- **Alopecia areata**: this refers to focal areas of complete, non-scarring alopecia. Topical or intralesional corticosteroids can

Medicine at a Glance, Fifth Edition. Edited by Patrick Davey and Alex Pitcher.

Companion website: www.wiley.com/go/medicine5e

help, as well as topical immunotherapy and immunosuppressive drugs. The prognosis is unpredictable, although patients with nail pits or widespread hair loss do worse. Occasionally, patients may have or develop another organ-specific autoimmune disease.

- **Scarring alopecia**: the differential diagnosis includes infection and inflammatory dermatoses (see Table 70.2). Skin biopsy is essential. Diagnosis and treatment must be prompt to save the hair. The principal differential diagnoses are tinea capitis (treat with systemic antifungals), lichen planus (topical/systemic corticosteroids) and lupus erythematosus (topical/systemic steroids and systemic antimalarials).

Nail disorders

The key points in diagnosing nail disorders are to establish whether the signs point to an underlying disease or to a treatable cause of nail dystrophy. The common nail disorders are as follows.

- **Clubbing**: there are many causes for clubbing (see figure below); in practice, lung cancer is the most common.
- **Dystrophy** (misshapen, abnormally growing nails): a common cause is fungal infection; exclude by examination of clippings. Peripheral vascular disease or severe Raynaud phenomenon, psoriasis and trauma are other common causes.
- **Onycholysis** (premature seaparation of the nail plate from the nail bed) occurs commonly in psoriasis, tinea and drug eruptions. Aggressive nail manicure may also be responsible.
- **Nail pits** are found in psoriasis, eczema and alopecia areata.
- **Leuconychia** (white nails) occurs most commonly as small white spots where it is of no significance. Pathological leuconychia occurs mainly in long-standing systemic disease such as cirrhosis, diabetes mellitus, cardiac failure and severe anaemia.
- **Koilonychia** (spoon-shaped nails) may be associated with local nail dystrophy or with a dermatosis such as psoriasis or lichen simplex. Rarely, it is a sign of iron deficiency.
- **Splinter haemorrhages** occur with trauma, in autoimmune rheumatic disease and endocarditis.

Table 70.2 Causes of scarring alopecia
Infections
• Tinea capitis and kerion
• Staphylococcal folliculitis/folliculitis decalvans
• Syphilis
• Herpes simplex and zoster
• Lupus vulgaris (tuberculosis)
Other skin diseases
• Lichen planus
• Lupus erythematosus (especially discoid lupus erythematosus)
• Sarcoid
• Scleroderma
• Basal cell carcinoma
• Acne keloidalis nuchae (keloid reaction to acne)

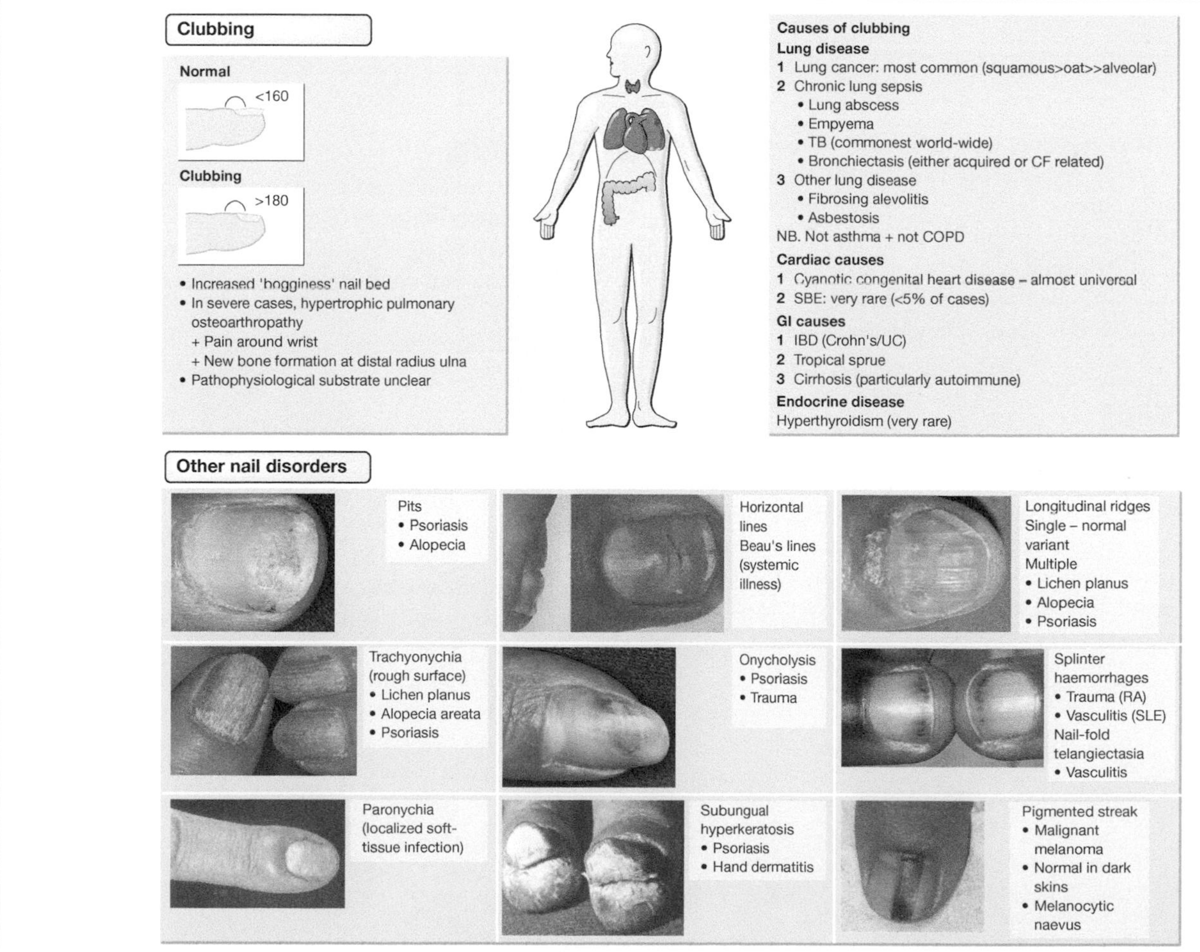

71 Leg ulcers

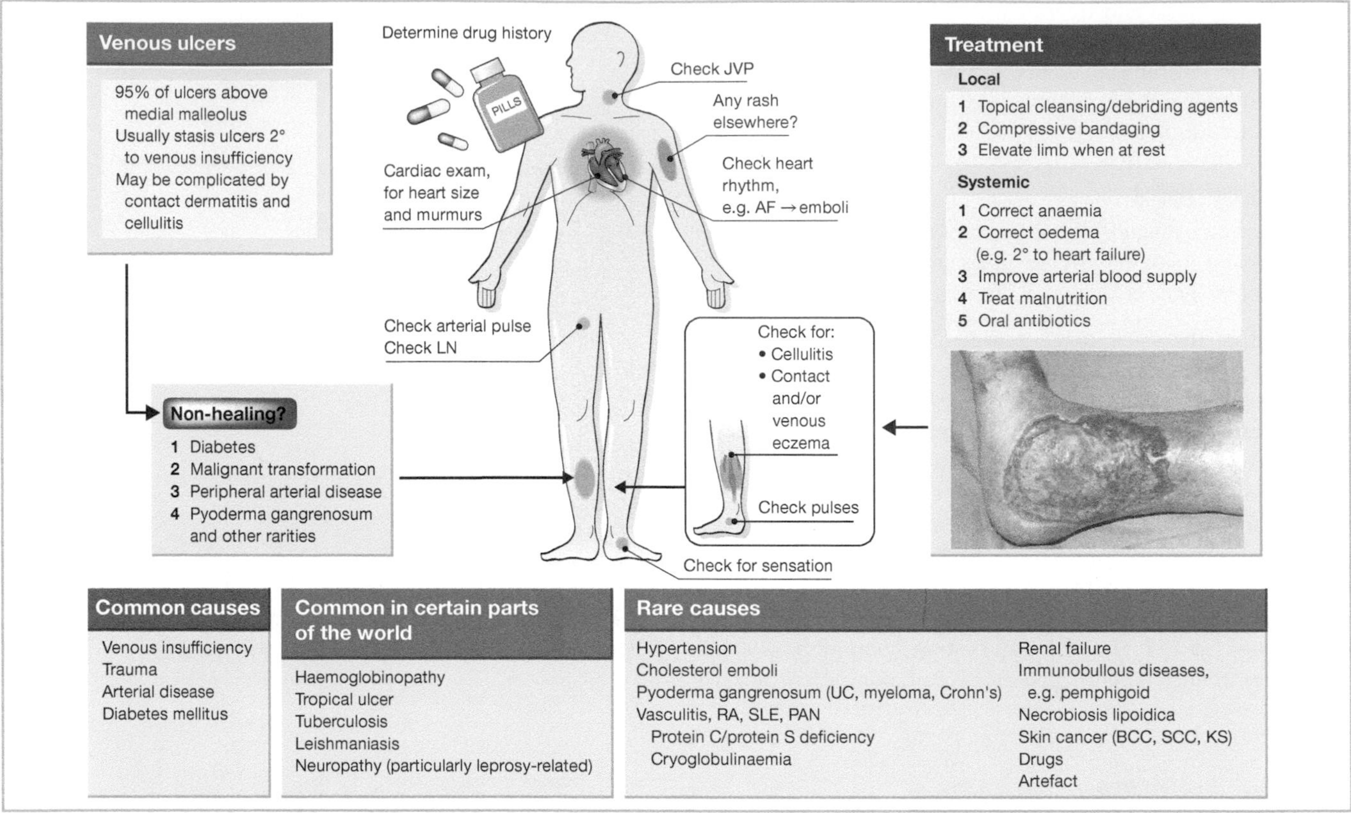

Venous ulcers
95% of ulcers above medial malleolus
Usually stasis ulcers 2° to venous insufficiency
May be complicated by contact dermatitis and cellulitis
Determine drug history
PILLS
Check JVP
Any rash elsewhere?
Cardiac exam, for heart size and murmurs
Check heart rhythm, e.g. AF → emboli
Check arterial pulse
Check LN
Non-healing?
1 Diabetes
2 Malignant transformation
3 Peripheral arterial disease
4 Pyoderma gangrenosum and other rarities
Check for:
• Cellulitis
• Contact and/or venous eczema
Check pulses
Check for sensation
Treatment
Local
1 Topical cleansing/debriding agents
2 Compressive bandaging
3 Elevate limb when at rest
Systemic
1 Correct anaemia
2 Correct oedema (e.g. 2° to heart failure)
3 Improve arterial blood supply
4 Treat malnutrition
5 Oral antibiotics
Common causes
Venous insufficiency
Trauma
Arterial disease
Diabetes mellitus
Common in certain parts of the world
Haemoglobinopathy
Tropical ulcer
Tuberculosis
Leishmaniasis
Neuropathy (particularly leprosy-related)
Rare causes
Hypertension
Cholesterol emboli
Pyoderma gangrenosum (UC, myeloma, Crohn's)
Vasculitis, RA, SLE, PAN
Protein C/protein S deficiency
Cryoglobulinaemia
Renal failure
Immunobullous diseases, e.g. pemphigoid
Necrobiosis lipoidica
Skin cancer (BCC, SCC, KS)
Drugs
Artefact

Most leg ulceration is the result of venous disease, although other causes should always be considered. The common causes for acute deterioration in chronic leg ulcers are infection (cellulitis) and allergic contact dermatitis (resulting from a topical medicament or dressing). All chronic ulcers are at risk of malignant transformation (Marjolin squamous carcinoma), so regular reassessment, especially in elderly people, should occur.

Clinical features

It is important to determine the duration of ulceration, the degree of associated pain (e.g. whether diabetic neuropathy is present), the presence of associated infection and systemic upset (e.g. sepsis), and whether the patient has diabetes, renal failure, arthritis or a connective tissue disease, a haemoglobinopathy or inflammatory bowel disease. Topical agents and dressings may cause contact dermatitis.

Examination

This should be particularly for stasis or contact eczema, venous and arterial insufficiency, inguinal lymphadenopathy and cellulitis.

Investigations

Investigations should be used in selected cases to determine the arterial blood supply to the leg (Doppler studies and/or angiography) and venous drainage (leg and pelvic ultrasonography). Skin biopsy (including immunofluorescence) is necessary when the cause is in doubt.

Treatment

Exclude and treat the different factors (see figure above). Maximize the arterial blood supply (e.g. angioplasty), and treat anaemia and infection (systemic antibiotics continued long term), heart failure and malnutrition (protein, iron, vitamin C or zinc deficiency).

Encourage regular exercise and weight loss. Elevate the limb at rest and apply compressive bandaging (non-adherent or paraffin gauze), after using a topical cleansing and/or debriding agent to encourage granulation tissue formation. Other measures include mild-to-moderate potency steroids to non-ulcerated eczematous skin. Beware of contact sensitization to topical applications. If a clean granulating ulcer base can be achieved, consider 'pinch' skin grafting.

Medicine at a Glance, Fifth Edition. Edited by Patrick Davey and Alex Pitcher.

Companion website: www.wiley.com/go/medicine5e

72 Photodermatoses

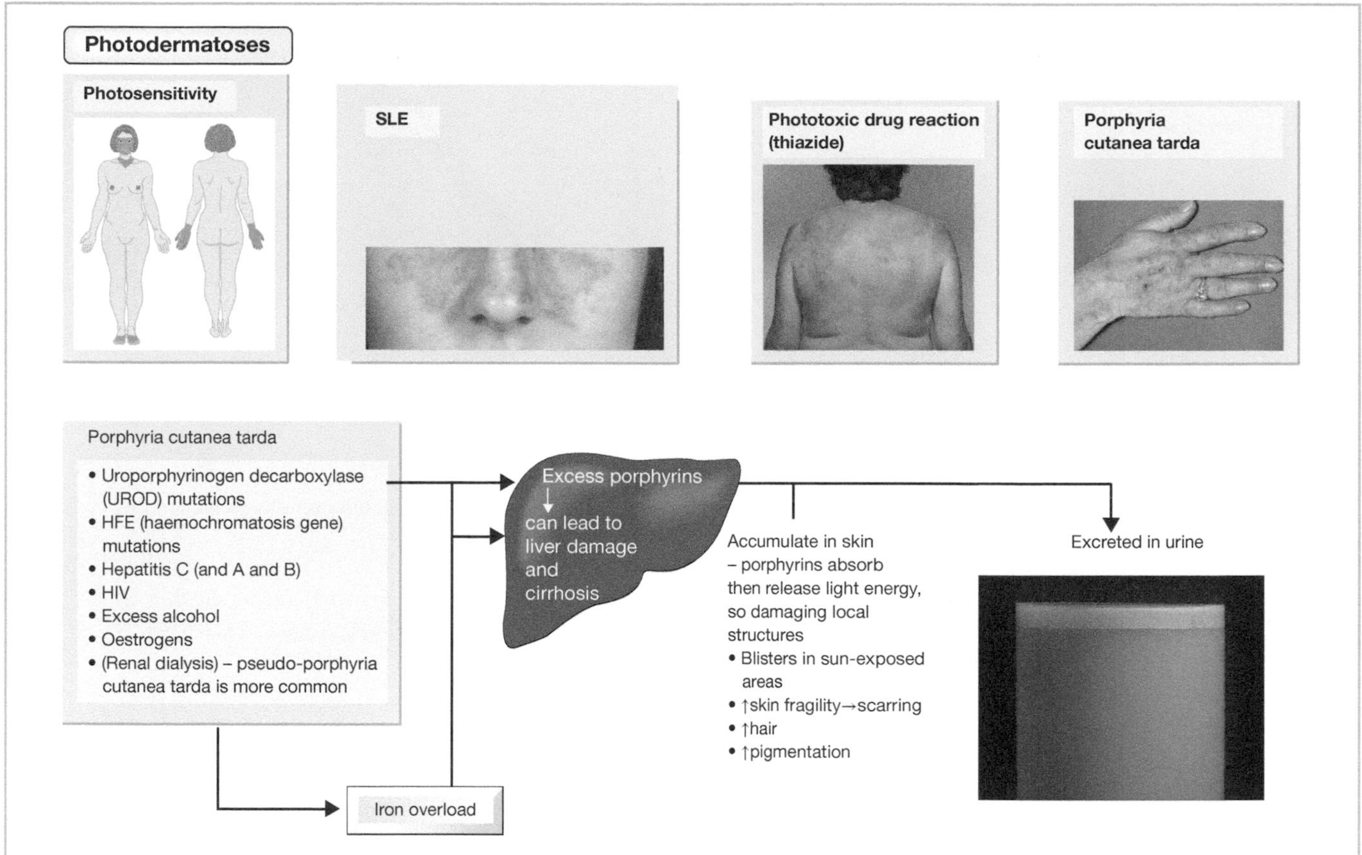
Photodermatoses
Photosensitivity
SLE
Phototoxic drug reaction (thiazide)
Porphyria cutanea tarda
Porphyria cutanea tarda
• Uroporphyrinogen decarboxylase (UROD) mutations
• HFE (haemochromatosis gene) mutations
• Hepatitis C (and A and B)
• HIV
• Excess alcohol
• Oestrogens
• (Renal dialysis) – pseudo-porphyria cutanea tarda is more common
Excess porphyrins
can lead to liver damage and cirrhosis
Accumulate in skin – porphyrins absorb then release light energy, so damaging local structures
• Blisters in sun-exposed areas
• ↑skin fragility→scarring
• ↑hair
• ↑pigmentation
Excreted in urine
Iron overload

A cardinal clue that an eruption is sunlight related (i.e. a photodermatosis) is its distribution in sun-exposed areas (forehead, cheeks, ears, nose, chin, anterior chest in a 'V' distribution, hands) with sparing of areas photo-protected by clothes or natural shadows (around the orbit, behind the ears, under the chin). Some primary dermatoses (e.g. psoriasis, acne) can improve with sunlight. Photo-eruptions occur in the following conditions.

- **Atopic eczema** (this also sometimes improves with sunlight).
- **Systemic lupus erythematosus** (SLE) (see Chapter 221).
- **Lichen planus**.
- **Drug eruptions**.
  - In phototoxic drug eruptions (increased susceptibility to the normal effects of sunlight), sunburn occurs within minutes of sun exposure, e.g. with amiodarone, thiazides or tetracycline. Extracts from many plants can act as topical sun sensitizers.
  - Photoallergic drug reactions are idiosyncratic inflammatory reactions (resembling contact dermatitis) to, for example, phenothiazines and angiotensin-converting enzyme inhibitors.
- **Polymorphic light eruption**: this is the most common photodermatosis. It can cause erythema, papules, urticarial wheals and plaques usually 4–6 hours after (early summer) sun exposure. Topical steroids may help short term. Sun avoidance and sunscreens are essential. Prophylactic psoralens and ultraviolet A (PUVA) or ultraviolet B (before holidays) can be used. Gradual exposure to sunlight results in tolerance, which lasts until the following year.
- **Solar urticaria** is rare, but is characterized by an immediate urticarial response to sun exposure. It fades in the shade.
- **Porphyrias** result from deficiencies in the enzymes synthesizing haem. Haem precursors are deposited in the skin, resulting in disease. Porphyria cutanea tarda may be familial or sporadically affect young women (related to alcohol and the contraceptive pill) or middle-aged men (alcoholism). There is an association with hepatitis B/C, HIV and renal dialysis. Skin fragility and photosensitive blistering with scarring occur on exposed sites, especially the hands. Hypertrichosis occurs on the face. Clinical and/or biochemical liver disease may occur. There is a deficiency of uroporphyrinogen decarboxylase activity and uroporphyrin III is found in the urine and faeces. Treatment is avoidance of alcohol, oestrogen and sunlight, venesection and/or low-dose hydroxychloroquine.
- **Pellagra** (niacin deficiency) may result in a classic tetrad of features (diarrhoea, dementia, dermatitis, death). The classic cutaneous manifestation is an eruption around the neck, 'Casal's necklace'.

Medicine at a Glance, Fifth Edition. Edited by Patrick Davey and Alex Pitcher.

Companion website: www.wiley.com/go/medicine5e

73 Pelvic pain

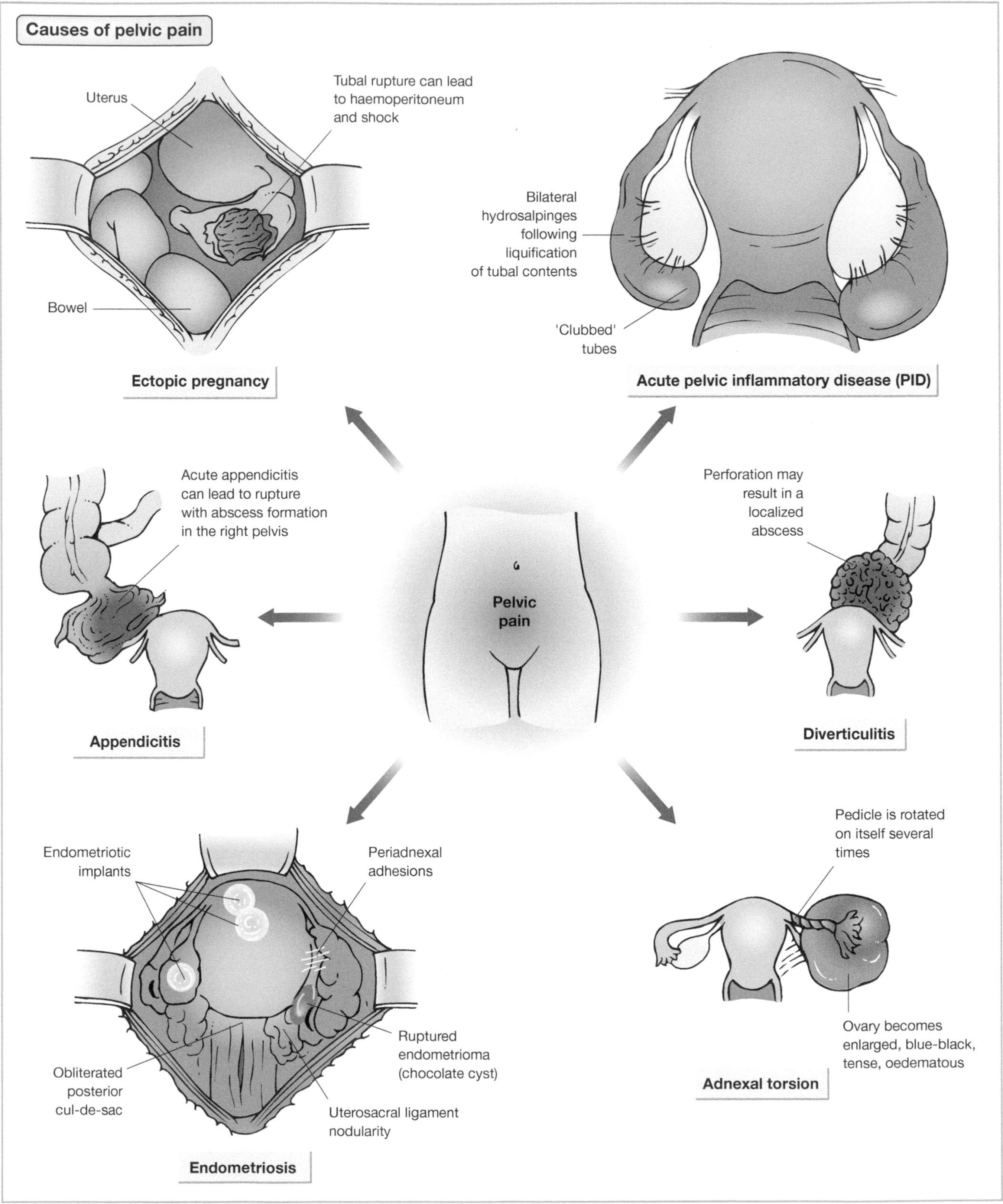

Medicine at a Glance, Fifth Edition. Edited by Patrick Davey and Alex Pitcher.

Companion website: www.wiley.com/go/medicine5e

As pain arising from the pelvis is a subjective perception rather than an objective sensation, accurately determining the aetiology is often difficult. Dysmenorrhoea (uterine pain associated with menses) is the most common gynaecological pain complaint.

Clinical approach

- The history provides a description of the nature, intensity and distribution of the pain, its relationship to periods and sexual intercourse. However, imprecise localization is typical with intra-abdominal processes, and ovarian pain often radiates to the loin.
- Date last menstrual period (LMP) started should be recorded along with method of contraception if sexually active. New partner(s) should be enquired after, if PID is suspected.
- Recent pelvic procedures, including fertility tests and treatments, should be asked about, as should recent pregnancies and their outcomes.
- If the pain is acute, or acute on chronic, examination must include vital signs and temperature.
- Physical examination includes a comprehensive abdominal and gynaecological examination. Specific attention should be paid to trying to reproduce the pain symptoms. Cervical excitation (pain reproduced by sharply lifting the cervix on bimanual examination) is a sign of pelvic peritonitis.
- Pregnancy must be excluded by testing urine for hCG in all premenopausal women and girls if the pain is acute.
- Cervical swab for chlamydia/gonorrhoea PCR or culture, vaginal swab for culture and urinalysis (with microscopy and culture if positive for signs of urinary tract infection) are frequently helpful.
- Pelvic ultrasonography is usually the most helpful initial imaging study for a gynaecological cause; this should be transvaginal, unless the patient is a virgin or declines (having understood that more information is obtained by this route). If a transabdominal approach is needed, the bladder must be full.
- Specialized diagnostic studies based on the presumptive diagnosis may require consultation with other specialists in radiology, general surgery, gastroenterology or urology.

Acute pelvic pain

Potentially catastrophic causes (ectopic pregnancy, ruptured appendix) require timely intervention to quickly diagnose and treat. Ectopic pregnancy can be fatal. Ruptured appendix can lead to pelvic adhesion formation, affecting future fertility.

Gynaecological causes

There are three main categories: pregnancy, infection and ovarian cyst accidents.

- **Ectopic pregnancy**: in all women of reproductive age, the first priority in evaluating acute pelvic pain is to rule out the possibility of a ruptured ectopic pregnancy. There may or may not be vaginal bleeding and an apparent LMP of less than four weeks ago does not rule out pregnancy.
- **Threatened, inevitable or incomplete miscarriages** are generally accompanied by midline pelvic pain, usually of a crampy, intermittent nature, and vaginal bleeding.
- **Acute pelvic inflammatory disease** (PID) is an ascending infection that often presents with high fever, severe pelvic pain (usually bilateral), nausea and evidence of cervical motion tenderness in sexually active women. It may be associated with abnormal vaginal bleeding or discharge, the latter typically purulent. PID can also occur after a pelvic procedure, especially one involving passing an instrument through the cervix, with or without instillation of fluid, e.g. hysteroscopy, hysterosalpingogram, insertion of intrauterine contraceptive device/system. It can also follow pregnancy, especially after miscarriage or termination, prolonged ruptured membranes, manual removal of placenta or caesarean birth.
- **Rupture of an ovarian cyst**: rupture of a follicular/simple cyst or haemorrhagic corpus luteum is a common cause of acute pelvic pain. The pain may be very severe and is often associated with signs or symptoms of peritonism. The condition is usually self-limiting with limited intraperitoneal bleeding, although sometimes a ruptured corpus luteum causes a significant haematoperitoneum. Endometrioma can rupture, although less commonly, and when they do, it is usually a slow leak, which can also be seen with dermoid cysts.
- **Adnexal torsion:** an adnexal mass, but typically an enlarged ovary, may twist on its vascular pedicle, causing severe unilateral pain by suddenly and intermittently compromising its blood supply. Typically, the pain will wax and wane (colicky pain), with associated nausea and vomiting. It will often radiate to the loin and can be mistaken for musculoskeletal causes. Torsion may be associated with a low-grade fever and inflammatory markers can be elevated. If it is not corrected soon enough, the ovary will become necrotic and its function compromised. There is a risk of the necrotic tissue forming an abscess. Torsion is seen most commonly in adolescents or women of reproductive age. Dermoid cysts are a common cause, but endometrioma rarely do, as they often tether the ovary to adjacent structures. It can occur immediately after or within a couple of weeks of egg collection for IVF, when the ovary is still larger than normal. Non-ovarian causes include paraovarian cysts, fibromas, broad ligament fibroids and occasionally an enlarged fallopian tube (hydro/haematosalpinx). Torsion is rarely seen after the menopause, in which case, malignant enlargement of the adnexum should be considered and appropriate work-up performed before surgery.

Non-gynaecological causes

- **Appendicitis** is the most common acute surgical condition of the abdomen, occurring in all age groups. Classically, the pain is initially diffuse and centred in the umbilical area but after several hours, it localizes to the right lower quadrant (McBurney's point). It is often accompanied by low-grade fever, anorexia, diarrhoea and leukocytosis.
- **Diverticulitis** occurs most frequently in older people. It is characterized by left-sided pelvic pain, diarrhoea which may be bloody, fever and leukocytosis.
- **Urinary tract disorders** (cystitis, pyelonephritis, renal calculi) can cause acute or referred suprapubic pain, pressure and/or dysuria.
- **Mesenteric lymphadenitis** most often follows an upper respiratory infection in young people. The pain is usually more diffuse and less severe than in appendicitis.

Chronic pelvic pain

Pelvic pain is common, and when the condition persists for longer than six months, it is considered chronic. It may be constant or intermittent, and usually has a gynaecological cause when significantly related to the menstrual cycle, although the symptoms of some non-gynaecological causes can also show a degree of variation with the cycle, e.g. irritable bowel syndrome. It is often multifactorial. New pelvic pain in postmenopausal women should be considered suspicious of malignancy until proven otherwise.

- Chronic pelvic pain accounts for 10% of all visits to gynaecologists and 20–30% of laparoscopies.
- A third to one half of women who undergo laparoscopy for chronic pelvic pain will have no identifiable cause. In some cases, identified pathology may not be the cause. Painful periods, in the absence of any pathological findings, may be due to excessive prostaglandin production by the uterus.
- Patients and physicians may both become frustrated because the condition is difficult to cure or manage adequately.

Gynaecological causes

- **Endometriosis** has a spectrum of pain that ranges from dysmenorrhoea (painful periods – with pain typically starting a few days before the start of the period) to severe, intractable, continuous pain which may be disabling. It can cause pain on intercourse (dyspareunia) and/or on defaecation (dyschezia), sometimes associated with bowel disturbance. Peritoneal endometriosis may not be detected on imaging, although ovarian endometriosis usually is. The severity of pain often does not correlate with the degree of pelvic pathology seen at laparoscopy/laparotomy.
- **Adenomyosis** is a common condition in older and multiparous women that was previously only confirmed histologically after hysterectomy with the finding of endometrial glands and stroma within the myometrium (uterine muscle). It is a cause of painful and heavy periods, pain on intercourse and abnormal uterine bleeding, and may be associated with infertility. One-third may have no symptoms. Clinically, the uterus is enlarged, boggy and mildly tender to bimanual palpation. The higher resolution and more ubiquitous use of transvaginal ultrasonography are identifying features indicative of ademomyosis in more and younger women, although a consensus on diagnostic criteria is awaited and the significance of it in younger women is unclear. Like endometriosis, it can cause symptoms in adolescents, but regresses after the menopause.
- **Fibroids** are the most frequent (benign) tumours found in the female pelvis. They may cause pain by either putting pressure on adjacent organs or, less frequently, undergoing degeneration, which can also be a cause of acute pain. Fibroids may co-exist with endometriosis and/or adenomyosis.
- **Genital prolapse** may lead to complaints of heaviness, pressure, a dropping sensation or pelvic aching.
- **Chronic PID** is usually a result of persistent hydrosalpinx, tubo-ovarian mass or pelvic adhesions.

Treatments that suppress ovarian function (combined hormonal contraception [CHC], gonadotropin releasing hormone analogues [GnRHa]) or the endometrium (progesterone-only contraception, including long-acting) often benefit chronic pelvic pain of different aetiologies and non-steroidal anti-inflammatory drugs may be helpful. If dysmenorrhoea is associated with heavy menstrual flow, oral tranexamic acid and/or NSAIDs can reduce blood loss and thereby reduce pain.

Non-gynaecological causes

- **Gastrointestinal disorders** such as constipation, irritable bowel syndrome, inflammatory bowel disease, coeliac disease.
- **Interstitial cystitis** (chronic inflammatory condition of the bladder).
- **Adhesions** caused by previous intraperitoneal infection (appendicitis, diverticulitis, PID) or surgeries.
- **Musculoskeletal problems** such as muscle strain of the abdominal wall or pelvic floor may causing trigger points; joint issues or nerve entrapment, including after surgery.
- **Somatoform disorders** are characterized by physical pain and symptoms that mimic disease, but are related to psychological and social factors. There is a complex relationship between physical or sexual abuse (in childhood and ongoing) and chronic pelvic pain. Depression is more common in those with pelvic pain, possibly as a consequence, but treating the depression may improve quality of life/daily functioning. Assessment should include time for the patient to express their concerns and sensitive enquiry to elicit psychological and social issues. Where there is no clear physical cause, possibly after laparoscopy but not always, a treatment plan should be made in partnership with the patient, using a holistic approach which may include analgesia, dietary changes, physiotherapy, complementary therapies such as acupuncture, and psychological therapies. Referral to a pain clinic may be helpful.

74 Urinary incontinence

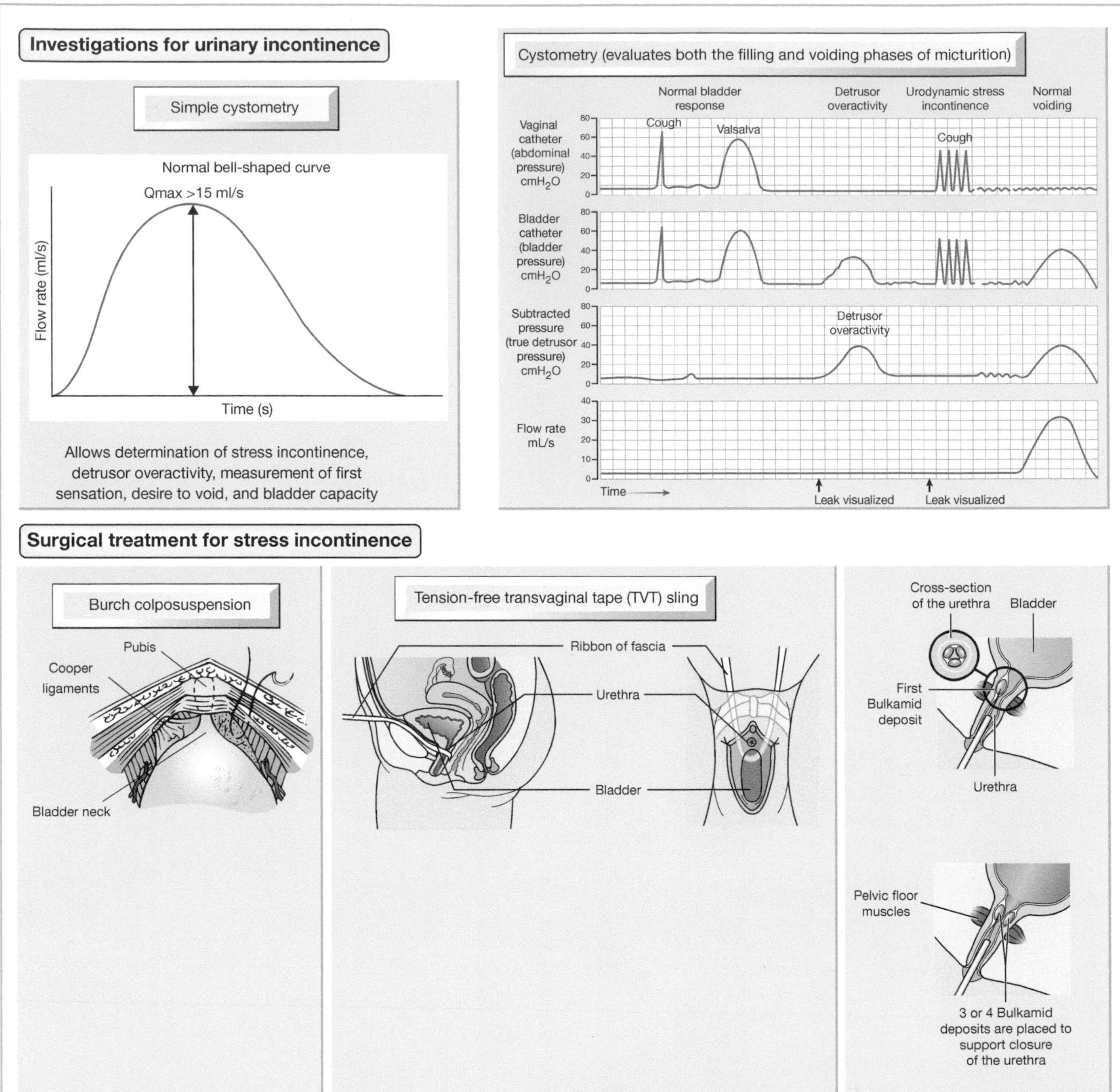

- **Definition**: involuntary leakage of urine that is sufficient in frequency and amount to cause physical and/or emotional distress.
- **Incidence**: highly prevalent in women across their adult lifespan; severity increases linearly with age in women: 4–8% ultimately seek medical attention. Nine to 39% of women aged >60 years report daily urinary incontinence.

Diagnosis

There are six main steps in diagnosis.

1 **History**. A detailed history is important to determine the type, severity, burden and duration of symptoms and rule out medication causes. Emotional distress often does not correlate well with the amount of urine loss that can be demonstrated.

2 **Physical examination**.
- **General examination** to rule out delirium and atrophic urethritis, restricted mobility or stool impaction.
- **Urogynaecological examination** may reveal severe vulvar excoriation from continual dampness. The vaginal tissue should be inspected for signs of atrophy, stenosis, bladder neck mobility (*Q-tip test*) and atrophic urethritis. The patient is asked to cough repeatedly or undergo a Valsalva manoeuvre with a full bladder in the lithotomy or standing position to induce urine leakage. Rectal examination can evaluate rectal sphincter tone or the presence of faecal impaction.

3 **Urinalysis and urine culture**. Many relevant metabolic and urinary tract disorders can be screened by a simple urinalysis.

A culture is essential to rule out infection before proceeding with further evaluation.

4 **Residual urine volume after voiding.** A catheterized postvoid residual (PVR) urine specimen should be obtained to exclude urinary retention (normal PVR ≤100 ml) or infection.

5 **Frequency–volume bladder chart.** More than seven voids per day suggests a problem with frequency, but this is highly dependent on habit and fluid intake. Patients can be notoriously inaccurate in estimating urinary frequency and should be encouraged to keep a 'urinary diary' for several days as part of their initial evaluation.

6 **Urodynamics** is a group of tests designed to aid in determining the aetiology of lower urinary tract dysfunction.

- Uroflowmetry. Simple non-invasive test where the woman is asked to void into flowmeter. A graph of flow rate (ml/s) against time (s) is recorded. In a normal graph, the maximum flow rate (Qmax) should be above 15 ml/s. Qmax, however, is dependent on the volume voided, which should be more than 150 ml for the test to be valid. Qmax is artificially reduced if the voided volume is too small or large. Qmax is of relevance as a reduced value may be a predictor of voiding difficulty.
- Filling and voiding cystometry.
  - The patient has two catheters in the bladder, one for filling the bladder with fluid and the other for measuring bladder pressure. The patient also has a pressure catheter in the rectum that measures intra-abdominal pressure.
  - Cystometry is carried out after uroflowmetry. Insertion of the bladder catheters also provides a postvoid residual measurement.
  - Cystometry carries a small risk of UTI and haematuria.
- Filling cystometry. The bladder is filled slowly with normal saline, usually at a rate of 50–100 ml/min. As it fills, the bladder pressure catheter measures intravesical pressure (Pves) while the rectal pressure catheter measures intra-abdominal pressure (Pabd). The detrusor pressure (Pdet) can be calculated by subtracting Pabd from Pves (Pves − Pabd = Pdet). Pdet and Pabd are necessary in order to diagnose urodynamic stress incontinence (USI) and detrusor overactivity (DOA).
- Voiding cystometry. The patient is asked to void with the pressure lincs *in situ* to assess detrusor pressures needed to void, flow pattern and then postvoid residual is assessed with ultrasound.

Types of urinary incontinence

Stress urinary incontinence

Patients have involuntary loss of small amounts of urine with coughing, laughing, sneezing, exercising or other movements that increase intra-abdominal pressure due to urethral sphincter weakness and/or pelvic floor weakness.

- **Aetiology**: physical changes resulting from pregnancy, childbirth and menopause often result in weaknesses in the pelvic floor and urethral support structures and nerve damage. Young women active in sports may also experience this.
- **Mechanism**: if the fascial support is weakened, the urethra can move downward at times of increased abdominal pressure, causing bladder pressure to exceed urethral sphincter closure pressure (hypermobile urethra). Incomplete urethral closure may be due to scarring or neuromuscular damage, and can cause a more severe form of stress urinary incontinence – intrinsic sphincter deficiency.
- **Diagnosis**: stress urinary incontinence (SUI) is suggested by the history, physical examination and a positive stress test (demonstrable loss of urine while the patient is being examined). Urodynamic stress incontinence is also seen.
- **Non-surgical treatment** includes pelvic muscle (Kegel) exercises, biofeedback (pressure measurement device notifies the patient when correct muscle contraction is performed and reinforces correct technique) and pessaries.
- **Surgical treatment.**
  - *Burch colposuspension* involves suture placement at the Cooper ligament. The Marshall–Marchetti–Krantz variation has sutures going through the periosteum of the pubic symphysis. Either can be laparoscopic or via a Pfanennstiel incision.
  - *Autologous fascial sling*: a strip of fascia is taken from the abdominal wall layers and placed underneath the urethra. This strip is passed on either side to be fixed back to the abdominal wall. This is achieved via a Pfannenstiel incision to harvest the fascia and also to facilitate the exit points of the fascia as it is passed under the urethra vaginally and up either side of the bladder neck so it can be anchored to the abdominal wall. This is an alternative to the synthetic midurethral sling.
  - *Collagen periurethral injections* (e.g. Bulkamid®) are designed as a treatment for SUI resulting from intrinsic sphincter deficiency.

At present in the UK, the use of synthetic midurethral slings (TVT) for the management of stress urinary incontinence is paused due to concerns about mesh erosion and other complications.

Urge urinary incontinence

Patients experience involuntary leakage for no apparent reason while suddenly feeling an urgent need to urinate. This may be accompanied by urinary frequency and nocturia, and patients often describe their bladder as 'overactive'.

- **Aetiology**: involuntary detrusor muscle contractions. Detrusor overactivity can be due to loss of central nervous system inhibitory pathways, local irritants or bladder outlet obstruction.
- **Mechanism**: frequently idiopathic, but results from damage to the nerves of the bladder, the nervous system (spinal cord and brain) or the muscles themselves.
- **Treatment**: behaviour modification (bladder drills, biofeedback) and/or pharmacological therapy (anticholinergics, e.g. oxybutynin chloride, β3 agonists, e.g. mirabegron), injection of the detrusor muscle with botulinum toxin A or neuromodulation.

Overflow urinary incontinence

Patients experience continuous, unstoppable dribbling of urine, or continuing to dribble for some time after they have passed urine.

- **Aetiology**: the bladder is always full and overflows, resulting in frequent or continuous urine leakage.
- **Mechanism**: weak bladder detrusor muscles, resulting in incomplete emptying, or a blocked urethra (outflow obstruction) due to advanced vaginal prolapse, or after an anti-incontinence procedure that has overcorrected the problem.
- **Treatment**: catheter drainage, followed by treatment of the underlying condition.

Other types of incontinence

- **Mixed incontinence** usually refers to the common combination of stress and urge incontinence occurring together.
- **Transient incontinence** is often triggered by medications, urinary tract infections, mental impairment, restricted mobility or stool impaction (severe constipation), which can push against the urinary tract and obstruct outflow.
- **Functional incontinence** occurs when a person does not recognize the need to go to the toilet, recognize where the toilet is or get to the toilet in time due to confusion, dementia, poor eyesight or poor mobility.

75 Attempted suicide by drug poisoning

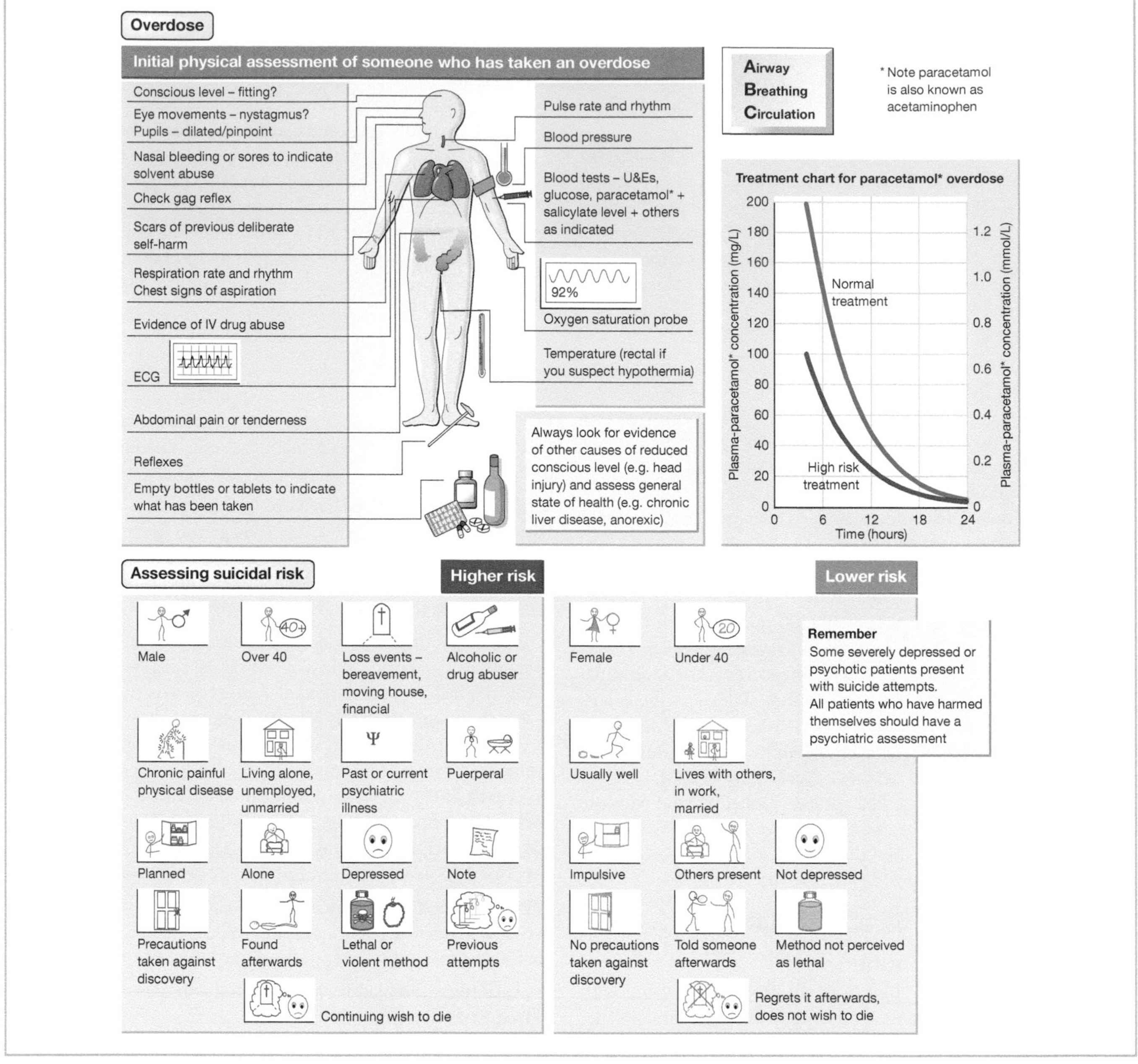

Poisoning is a common reason for hospital admission. Most poisonings are deliberate, although some are accidental. Attempted suicide may be the first presentation of psychiatric illness.

History

The key facts to establish are the circumstances of the attempt, psychiatric history (past and present) and past medical history.

Important points in the history are what was taken, when, how much and in what circumstances. How do they feel about it now? What was their suicide intent and risk? Psychiatric history should include the presence of current or past psychiatric illness and previous attempts; completed suicide rates are higher in patients with previous attempts.

Risk is increased by a history of bipolar disorder, depression, psychotic disorder, personality disorder and substance abuse (particularly alcohol). Anorexia also carries a risk and affects medical treatment. Likewise, medical illness and drug use affect treatment, e.g. liver disease or enzyme-inducing drugs lower the treatment threshold for paracetamol.

Medicine at a Glance, Fifth Edition. Edited by Patrick Davey and Alex Pitcher.

Companion website: www.wiley.com/go/medicine5e

Drug information

The National Poisons Information Service (NPIS) provides expert advice on all aspects of acute and chronic poisoning via its poisons information database TOXBASE® (www.TOXBASE.org or via an app) or for individual advice on more serious or complex cases via the NPIS 24-hour telephone service (www.npis.org).

Examination

Overdose patients may be unconscious, fully alert or anything in between. Assess **a**irway, **b**reathing and **c**irculation (ABC). Look for the following.

- Hypotension, arrhythmias, e.g. with antiarrhythmics and tricyclics.
- Respiratory depression, e.g. with opiates.
- Aspiration if vomiting with reduced conscious level (unprotected airway).
- Hypothermia with barbiturate or phenothiazine. Hyperthermia with CNS stimulants.
- Glucose and electrolyte imbalance should be measured.
- Convulsions and coma: common in severe poisoning with many drugs.

Immediate treatment

- Consider activated charcoal, which binds many poisons in the gastrointestinal tract, reducing absorption. It is most effective if used within one hour, although for drugs that delay gastric emptying or modified-release preparations, it is useful for longer or repeated doses. The only common side-effect is constipation (give a laxative). It is not useful for corrosives, alcohols, lithium, iron or pesticide ingestion.
- Gastric lavage is rarely used nowadays. It is only helpful within 1–2 hours, in conscious patients, with non-corrosive toxins.
- Ipecacuanha, which induces vomiting, is not used because it does not prevent absorption.
- Haemodialysis may be needed for severe salicylate, phenobarbital (phenobarbitone), methanol or ethylene glycol poisoning. Haemoperfusion can be used for theophylline and barbiturate poisoning.

Some specific commonly ingested poisons

Paracetamol

For paracetamol, 12 g (24 tablets) is a potentially fatal dose in most patients, whereas 7.5 g may be lethal in high-risk individuals. Symptoms are delayed up to three days after the overdose, when nausea, vomiting and abdominal pain, and late fulminant hepatic failure, can occur. Paracetamol is metabolized by liver conjugation; when this pathway is saturated, a toxic metabolite is formed, usually inactivated by glutathione. When glutathione stores run out, this metabolite binds to cell proteins, causing cell death. Lower doses are toxic in people on enzyme-inducing drugs (e.g. phenytoin, carbamazepine, rifampicin) and undernourished people (anorexia, alcoholism, starvation).

Management

- Consider activated charcoal if presenting within one hour of ingestion of >150 mg/kg paracetamol.
- Acetylcysteine, according to the NIPS paracetamol normogram, to increase liver glutathione if the paracetamol level is high four hours after ingestion, continued, in high-risk individuals, until paracetamol is no longer detected. Oral acetylcysteine may be used on specialist advice.
- Monitor urea and electrolytes (U&Es), glucose, liver function tests and clotting initially and 24 hours after ingestion.
- In severe overdose, patients may require haemodialysis and/or liver support, including transplantation (liver transplantation criteria available on TOXBASE).

Tricyclic antidepressants

Tricyclic antidepressants are highly toxic and fatal cardiac arrhythmias may occur soon after ingestion. Toxicity causes drowsiness, dilated pupils, dry mouth, tachycardia and urinary retention (anticholinergic effects), and hypothermia with hyperreflexia. In severe toxicity, convulsions, coma, respiratory depression, hypotension, arrhythmias and cardiac arrest may occur.

Management

- Consider activated charcoal.
- Twelve-lead ECG – check cardiac rhythm, QRS duration and QT interval. Perform continuous cardiac monitoring.
- Consider 50–100 mL of 8.4% sodium bicarbonate if QRS >120 msec or hypotension unresponsive to fluids.
- Consider intubation ± ventilation if respiration is inadequate or there are convulsions or arrhythmias (hyperventilation and bicarbonate improve arrhythmias).
- On recovery, delirium, agitation and visual and auditory hallucinations are common and respond to diazepam.

Opioids

Opioids cause respiratory depression, pinpoint pupils and hypotension, vomiting, fits and pulmonary oedema. Naloxone, a specific antidote, is given. The half-life of naloxone is very short (less than opioid), so an intravenous (IV) infusion is often needed.

Salicylates

Salicylates cause restlessness, flushing, sweating and hyperventilation. Nausea, vomiting and tinnitus are common. Confusion, coma, hyperthermia and convulsions are rare but associated with high mortality. Cardiac arrest may occur in severe overdose. Electrolyte abnormalities are common, such as hypokalaemic alkalosis (vomiting), respiratory alkalosis (hyperventilation) or a metabolic acidosis (uncoupling of oxidative phosphorylation). Dehydration and hyperpyrexia occur. Glucose control is impaired, causing hypo- or hyperglycaemia. A bleeding tendency may develop.

Management

- Consider activated charcoal if presenting within one hour of ingestion of 125 mg/kg or more.
- Treat hypokalaemia and give IV fluids.
- Consider correction of metabolic acidosis with sodium bicarbonate once potassium is within normal range.
- Consider urine alkalinization of plasma salicylate concentration >500 mg/L (or 350 mg/L in children). Forced alkaline diuresis is no longer used.
- Consider haemodialysis (or haemodiafiltration) in severe poisoning.
- Monitor vital signs and cardiac rhythm. Hyperthermia requires urgent treatment.
- Check full blood count, U&Es, clotting, glucose and gases; chest X-ray for pulmonary oedema.

Benzodiazepines

In overdose, benzodiazepines cause drowsiness, ataxia, dysarthria, nystagmus and respiratory depression. Flumazenil, a specific antidote, is not routinely used but can be considered in patients poisoned only by benzodiazepine and who would otherwise require intubation and ventilation for reduced respiration or coma. It should not be used in people with a history of seizures or chronic benzodiazepine use or if tricyclics have been taken.

Alcohol

Alcohol may be taken as part of the attempt or before the attempt, acutely or chronically. Alcoholism affects liver function, and thus affects any drugs or poisons that affect the liver, such as paracetamol. Acute alcohol intoxication depresses the conscious level and respiration – even small quantities of alcohol potentiate central nervous system depressants.

76 Anaphylaxis

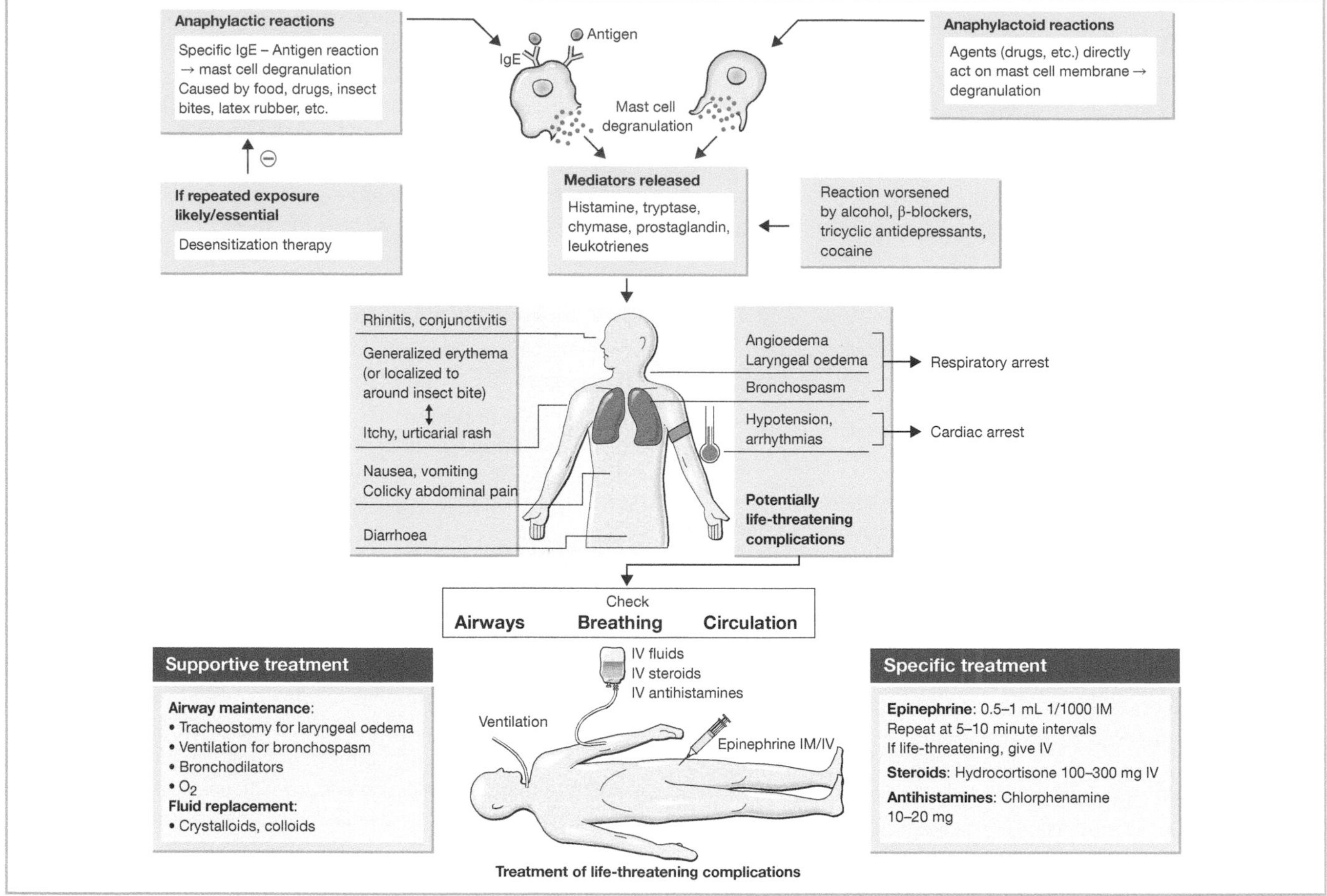

Anaphylaxis is an acute, generalized, life-threatening allergic reaction, affecting one in 10 000 individuals/year, and is the cause of one in every 2700 hospital admissions.

Mechanism

Anaphylaxis results from the rapid systemic release of large quantities of biologically active mediators from mast cells and basophils, triggered by the interaction of the allergen with specific IgE antibodies bound to cell membranes. Cell activation results in the release of preformed mediators stored in granules (including histamine, tryptase and chymase) and of newly formed mediators (including prostaglandins and leukotrienes). These mediators cause capillary leakage, mucosal oedema and smooth muscle contraction.

Anaphylactoid reactions result from the non-specific degranulation of mast cells by drugs, chemicals or other triggers, and do not involve IgE-based sensitivity. These reactions are clinically indistinguishable from anaphylactic reactions. Acutely, discrimination is unnecessary as the management is the same. However, discrimination between IgE-mediated and non-IgE-mediated disease may subsequently be important in identifying the precipitating agent.

Clinical features

Patients present with a range of clinical features.

- Feeling of impending doom.
- Generalized pruritus.
- Erythema and/or urticaria, though some 50% of patients may not experience any rash.
- Angioedema.
- Bronchospasm.
- Laryngeal oedema ± stridor.
- Rhinitis.
- Conjunctivitis.
- Nausea, vomiting, abdominal pain, uterine contractions.
- Palpitations, cardiac arrhythmias.
- Hypotension.
- Cardiorespiratory arrest.

The symptoms are usually of rapid onset, within minutes of exposure, although they may be delayed up to several hours. Route of exposure to the triggering agent, as well as quantity of antigen, rate of administration and co-existent features such as alcohol and

Medicine at a Glance, Fifth Edition. Edited by Patrick Davey and Alex Pitcher.

Companion website: www.wiley.com/go/medicine5e

exercise determine the severity of a reaction. Reactions are not always of the same degree of severity, even on exposure to the same allergen.

The immediate symptoms are caused by the release of stored histamine. Occasionally, the symptoms of anaphylaxis recur after some hours, a *biphasic reaction*, so all individuals should be kept under observation for at least six hours after an anaphylactic episode. Late-phase reactions are caused by synthesis *de novo* by the mast cells of leukotrienes, which have similar biological properties to histamine. The late reaction can be blocked by early administration of corticosteroids.

Source of allergen

The most common causes of anaphylaxis are **foods**. The majority of food reactions are to peanuts (a pea, not a nut!) and to tree nuts (hazelnut, almond, brazil nut, walnut, cashew, etc.). Peanut-allergic patients often also have allergy to tree nuts as well as other legumes. Peanuts and almonds may be present as a hidden allergen in many different foods. Particular care needs to be taken with oriental food. Shellfish and fish are potent causes of severe allergic reactions, and miniscule levels of exposure may cause severe reactions. Any other food is capable of causing reactions.

Other causes include the following.

- **Stinging insects** (bees, bumblebees, wasps, hornets, fire ants) can cause severe reactions.
- Severe reactions to **latex**. Awareness of the problem of latex in healthcare settings has led to a reduction in the use of latex-containing products and thus in the number of new cases. Most patients with latex allergy, however, have type IV delayed hypersensitivity reactions, mainly against the chemicals in the rubber rather than the rubber proteins, leading to contact dermatitis.
- Many **drugs** can cause IgE-mediated reactions, including penicillins, muscle relaxants (which are all highly cross-reactive), other anaesthetic agents and biological products such as vaccines. Opiate drugs such as morphine and codeine cause anaphylactoid reactions due to direct degranulation of mast cells; fentanyl does not seem to have this effect. Non-steroidal anti-inflammatory drugs also cause severe reactions through non-IgE mechanisms. Radiocontrast media, particularly non-ionic media, are potent mast cell degranulating agents.
- **Exercise**, alone or with foods, particularly wheat or shellfish, can trigger anaphylaxis.
- In some cases, **no cause** can be identified despite extensive searching (idiopathic anaphylaxis).

Differential diagnosis

Some clinical features of anaphylaxis are similar to other local or systemic disease. Accurate clinical assessment is essential.

- Shock (see Chapter 18).
- Airway obstruction: status asthmaticus, acute bacterial epiglottitis, acute foreign body upper airway obstruction.
- Mediator release: mastocytosis (excessive collections of mast cells in the gut, skin and bone marrow), carcinoid syndrome.
- Recurrent angioedema: inherited and acquired C1 esterase inhibitor deficiency, drug-induced angioedema; idiopathic angioedema.
- Vasovagal syncope.
- Factitious anaphylaxis (usually occurring in patients with known anaphylaxis).
- Globus hystericus (characterized by a lack of evidence of airway obstruction, despite protestations of swelling in the throat, and no rash or other symptoms).

Management

Acute management

Anaphylaxis is an acute medical emergency, which in the absence of appropriate treatment carries a significant mortality. Resuscitation should follow the normal rules of **a**irway, **b**reathing and **c**irculation (ABC).

- Airway maintenance: look for obstruction (swollen tongue, stridor). Administer high-flow oxygen. Consider a tracheotomy if complete airway obstruction is likely.
- Check breathing: full resuscitation if not breathing.
- Circulation: check pulse and blood pressure. Patients with excess histamine are usually warm and vasodilated with hypotension. Pulse is rapid. Obtain intravenous (IV) access.
- Adrenaline: *early* administration of adrenaline (epinephrine) is essential; 0.5 ml 1/1000 solution intramuscular (0.5 mg IM, Resuscitation Council UK guideline), repeat at five minutes intervals if no response; further doses may be required. Do not administer subcutaneously (poor absorption). In the hospital setting, IV adrenaline may be administered *only* with appropriate electrocardiogram monitoring. It must be given well diluted (10 ml 1/10 000 solution diluted into 100 ml normal saline and administered via an infusion pump).
- Corticosteroids: hydrocortisone 200 mg IV (this prevents late reactions).
- Antihistamines: chlorphenamine 10 mg IV (this is traditional but not of proven value).
- Fluid replacement: use colloid or crystalloid to restore blood pressure.
- Use nebulized salbutamol for bronchospasm.
- Keep under observation for a minimum of six hours before discharge, even if there is rapid recovery.
- Do not discharge without a clear plan for further investigation and follow-up (NICE guidelines).
- If appropriate, discharge with adrenaline (epinephrine) ×2 for self-administration (MHRA guidance).

Subsequent management

All individuals who have experienced anaphylaxis should be referred to a clinical immunologist or allergist for further investigation to identify the trigger factor and to educate the patient in avoidance and management of subsequent episodes. Consideration should be given to supplying adrenaline (epinephrine) for self-administration. Preloaded administration devices are available (Epipen®, Jext®, Emerade®); training must be provided with the chosen device. Patients should be advised to wear a Medic-Alert® bracelet, or equivalent. In the specific event of bee or wasp venom-induced anaphylaxis, immunotherapy with graded concentrations of allergen is effective in reducing the risk of further reactions. For drug allergy, confirmatory skin prick and intradermal testing are appropriate; this may be followed, if negative, by oral drug challenge (antibiotics).

Prognosis

The natural history and prognosis of anaphylaxis are variable. There are no predictors of the severity of further reactions. Avoidance remains the mainstay. Anxiety is extremely common and needs to be addressed. If the trigger factor cannot be identified or cannot be avoided, recurrence may be common and should be anticipated. Many children will grow out of early food-induced reactions such as egg, although peanut sensitivity is often life-long. Food challenges may be required to prove loss of sensitization, especially if a career in the armed forces is being considered.

77 Allergic reactions

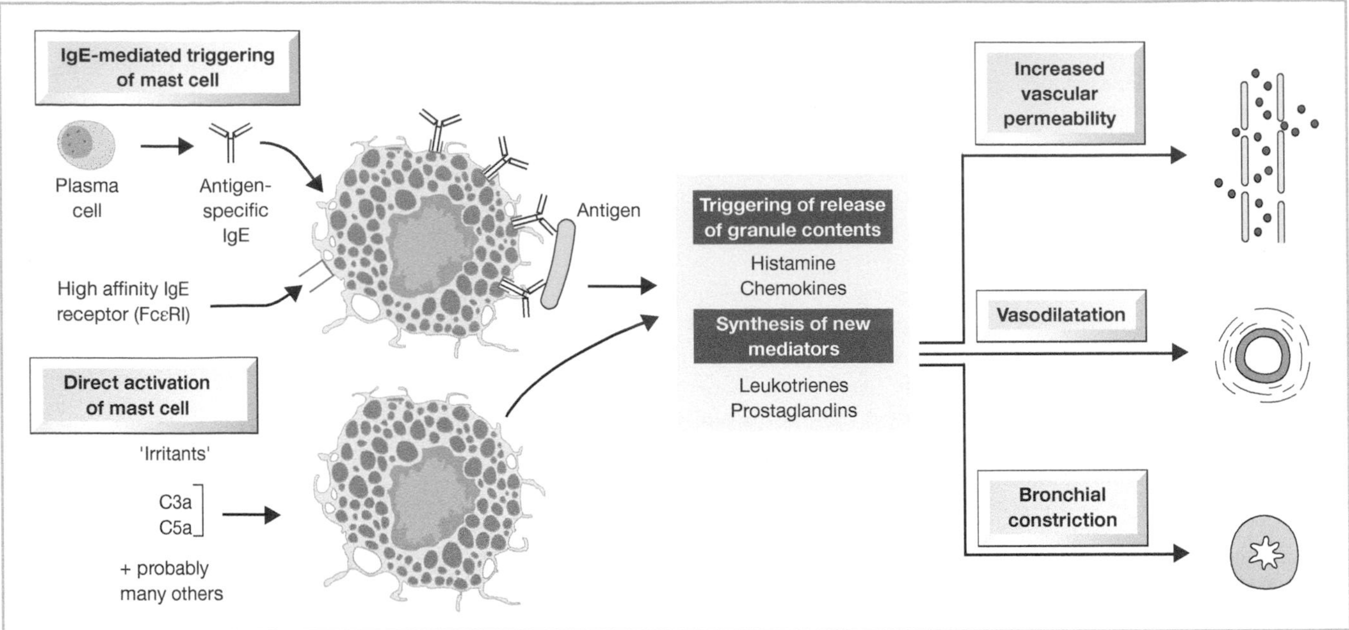

The severity of an allergic reaction depends upon the dose, site of allergen exposure and individual characteristics including medication and previous history. In most cases, the history provides the key to the diagnosis, especially as in non-urgent situations most patients will have few physical signs. Allergic disorders include:

- summer hayfever (pollen-induced allergic rhinoconjunctivitis)
- perennial rhinitis (house dust mites, pets)
- allergic asthma (including occupational asthma)
- allergy to drugs
- food allergy and food intolerance, oral allergy syndrome
- allergy to stinging insects
- allergic skin disorders, e.g. atopic eczema
- anaphylaxis (acute generalized allergic reaction)
- urticaria (see Chapter 223)
- angioedema.

Inhalant allergy

Allergy to inhalant allergens such as house dust mite, animal danders and pollens (grasses, trees, weeds) will trigger allergic rhinoconjunctivitis, sinusitis and asthma. Typical features include sneezing, blocked and running nose, headache and sinus pain, and itchy red eyes often with discharge, with or without asthmatic symptoms. Onset is rapid on exposure, but symptoms may be chronic if exposure cannot be avoided. A good history will usually identify the most likely triggers.

Diagnosis is by the skin prick test or a blood test, the 'RAST' test (radioallergosorbent test). Management is via topical treatments to the eye (sodium cromoglicate, nedocromil sodium), nose (nasal steroid sprays such as beclomethasone, mometasone, triamcinolone, fluticasone) and lung (inhaled bronchodilators such as salbutamol, salmeterol, formeterol and steroids, beclomethasone, budesonide, fluticasone), accompanied by oral antihistamines (potent non-sedating, long-acting antihistamines such as fexofenadine, cetirizine, levocetirizine). For upper airway allergy, desensitization by immunotherapy is possible for patients whose symptoms cannot be controlled on maximal medical therapy, including oral steroids. Injectable steroids (e.g. Kenalog®) are no longer recommended for the management of summer hay fever.

Food allergy

Food 'allergy' is blamed for a plethora of symptoms, not all of which are related to true, IgE-mediated food allergy. There is no evidence that irritable bowel symptoms are related to food allergy, although sufferers often complain of bloating with wheat-based products. Excess nasal catarrh is sometimes associated with milk intolerance. Anaphylaxis represents the severe end of the spectrum of disease, but urticaria and angioedema may represent less severe reactions. Eczema is associated with food allergies in children, often to dairy products and wheat, but adult eczema is less commonly helped by dietary manipulation.

The oral allergy syndrome, also known as the pollen-fruit syndrome, is the association of inhalant allergy to birch pollen in association with lip and tongue swelling when eating soft fruits such as peaches, nectarines, apples, almonds and other closely

Medicine at a Glance, Fifth Edition. Edited by Patrick Davey and Alex Pitcher.

Companion website: www.wiley.com/go/medicine5e

related fruits. This syndrome is rarely associated with anaphylaxis. The allergens are heat labile and destroyed by cooking.

Occasionally, it may be necessary to undertake an elimination diet with sequential reintroduction of foods to identify foods causing the symptoms. Double-blind, placebo-controlled challenge is the gold standard for investigation of food-related symptoms.

Angioedema

Angioedema relates to deep tissue swelling, which is usually non-itchy. It may occur alone or with urticaria. Bradykinin is the main trigger. It often presents acutely to accident and emergency (A&E) and acute medical services. It must be distinguished from systemic allergic reactions.

Hereditary angioedema is extremely rare and is due to deficiency of the complement regulatory protein C1 esterase inhibitor (see Chapter 223). Acquired angioedema caused by autoantibodies against the inhibitor may very rarely be seen in older patients in association with lymphoma and myeloma or in association with other autoimmune disease such as systemic lupus erythematosus. The most common causes of angioedema, however, are stress, infections and allergic reactions to foods and drugs. The most common drugs causing angioedema are angiotensin-converting enzyme (ACE) inhibitors, which cause angioedema by preventing the breakdown of bradykinin, non-steroidal anti-inflammatory drugs and statins (cholesterol-lowering drugs). Many cases, particularly of nocturnal angioedema, do not have an identifiable trigger (idiopathic).

Antihistamines are often ineffective in many cases of angioedema without urticaria, but tranexamic acid, an antifibrinolytic drug, may be valuable in preventing swelling where there is no avoidable trigger identified. Acute attacks usually require treatment with intravenous or oral corticosteroids. Adrenaline (epinephrine) should be reserved for angioedema where there is clear laryngeal involvement.

Urticaria

The typical rash in urticaria is that of wheal and flare (nettle rash), caused by histamine. The rash may be generalized and patients may feel systemically unwell. Presentation to A&E is common. The causes of acute urticaria are stress, infection, allergy and physical causes (sun, pressure, water, vibration, heat, cold), in association with thyroid disease or haematinic deficiency. However, in many cases there is no identifiable cause. Chronic urticaria, lasting beyond six weeks, is rarely associated with allergy (see also Chapter 223).

Acute treatment is with high-dose antihistamine given orally (cetirizine 10–20 mg daily) or intravenously (chlorphenamine 10 mg IV) and 24–48 hours of oral corticosteroid (prednisolone 20 mg/day). Treatment of chronic urticaria is with long-acting non-sedating antihistamines, and it may be necessary to use larger doses than those normally used, up to 4× normal dose. Montelukast may also be helpful. Corticosteroid therapy should be avoided in chronic urticaria apart from emergency management, as the risks of side-effects outweigh the benefits. Chronic spontaneous urticaria may respond to the anti-IgE monoclonal antibody omalizumab, given by monthly injection. Severe cases may require treatment with immunosuppressive drugs such as ciclosporin.

Investigation of allergic disease

Skin prick tests are cheap, quick and used to support the diagnosis. The patient is exposed to standardized solutions of allergen extract through a skin prick to the forearm. Positive (histamine) and negative (saline) controls are included. A wheal >2 mm greater than the negative control is a positive test. Testing should be carried out with great caution in patients who have had anaphylaxis. Skin must be normal so this type of testing is inappropriate in patients with active eczema.

Antihistamines should be discontinued for one week before testing as they abolish the response. Other drugs such as calcium channel blockers (for hypertension) and antidepressant drugs also interfere with the tests.

Intradermal testing is often used to investigate suspected drug allergy, if prick testing is negative. Diluted solutions of the drugs are injected intradermally, alongside appropriate control solutions.

The RAST test measures specific IgE in a blood sample to the putative antigen. This laboratory test is a useful alternative when skin prick tests are not available, or if a patient is on antihistamines. The results are similar to skin prick tests for inhalant allergens and nuts, but are not so useful for drug allergy and certain foods with labile allergens (fruits).

Measurement of the levels of the mast cell tryptase are valuable in identifying severe allergic reactions and in identifying patients with mastocytosis, a condition with excess mast cells, who are prone to severe allergic reactions.

78 Cardiac and respiratory arrest

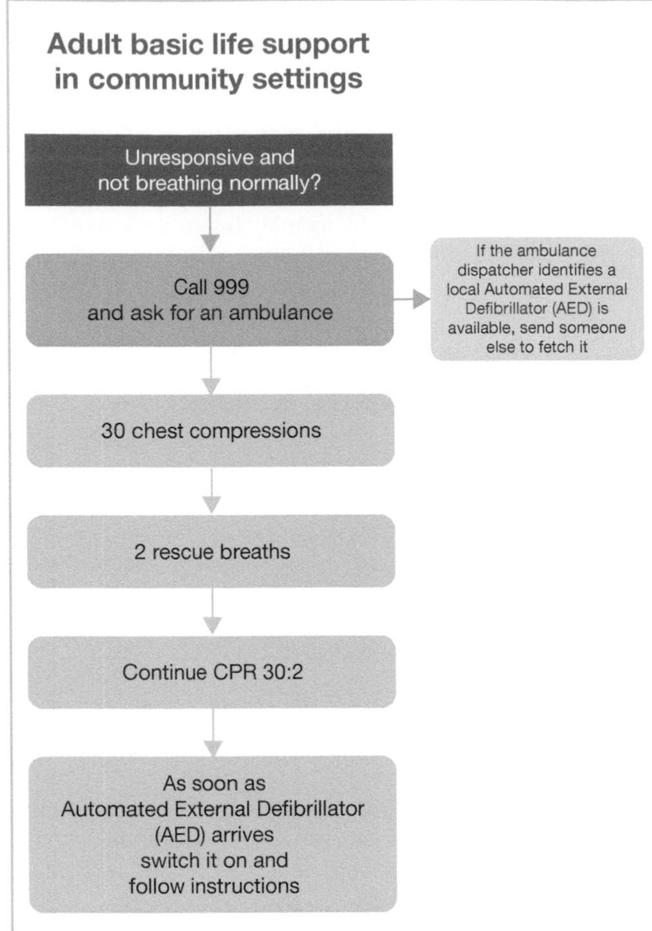

Adult basic life support in community settings
Unresponsive and not breathing normally?
Call 999 and ask for an ambulance
If the ambulance dispatcher identifies a local Automated External Defibrillator (AED) is available, send someone else to fetch it
30 chest compressions
2 rescue breaths
Continue CPR 30:2
As soon as Automated External Defibrillator (AED) arrives switch it on and follow instructions

Cardiac and respiratory arrests are common in the community and in hospital. The common causes of circulatory failure, 'cardiac arrest', are sufficiently severe to cause unconsciousness and compromise life.

Causes of cardiac and respiratory arrest

Cardiac arrest

- **Ventricular arrhythmias**: these can be due to acute coronary occlusions, scar tissue late after a myocardial infarction (MI), heart failure of any aetiology, and metabolic disturbance (e.g. hypo- and hyperkalaemia, hypoxaemia, drugs including tricyclic antidepressants, non-sedating antihistamines, major antipsychotics, macrolide antibiotics, etc.).
- **Bradyarrhythmias**: due to conducting tissue disease, e.g. complete heart block, during MI, following prolonged ventricular arrhythmias or respiratory arrest (see ALS section).
- **Cardiogenic shock**: often caused by large MIs or advanced heart failure.

Medicine at a Glance, Fifth Edition. Edited by Patrick Davey and Alex Pitcher.

Companion website: www.wiley.com/go/medicine5e

Pulseless electrical activity (also known as electromechanical dissociation)

If circulatory failure occurs and QRS complexes are seen on the electrocardiogram (ECG) monitor, pulseless electrical activity is diagnosed.

In all cases, consider reversible causes of cardiac arrest, including the following.

- **Hypovolaemia**: e.g. stab wounds, torrential gastrointestinal or retroperitoneal haemorrhage (e.g. ruptured abdominal aortic aneurysm).
- **Hypo/hyperthermia**.
- **Hypoxia**.
- **Hypo/hyperkalaemia or other metabolic derangement**.
- **Pericardial tamponade**: stab wounds, recent MI (where it indicates cardiac rupture), malignancy or immediately after cardiac surgery.
- **Thrombosis – coronary or pulmonary embolus**.
- **Tension pneumothorax**: in people with asthma, in chronic lung diseases, especially chronic obstructive pulmonary disease (COPD), or after trauma.
- **Toxins**.

Respiratory arrest

There are a number of common causes of failure to breathe sufficiently to maintain life – 'respiratory arrest'.

- **Severe lung disease**: pneumonia, severe airway obstruction (e.g. asthma, exacerbation of COPD, end-stage COPD, etc.).
- **Airway obstruction**: foreign body, or the tongue in a comatose patient.
- **Left ventricular failure**.
- **Brain injury**: stroke, overdose of narcotic drugs (e.g. opiates) or hypnotics (e.g. major tranquillizers, etc.).

Cardiopulmonary resuscitation

Cardiopulmonary resuscitation (CPR) is applied for the immediate treatment of cardiac and/or respiratory arrest. CPR constitutes support for both the circulation and respiration, and is a generic treatment applicable to most cases of cardiac/respiratory arrest. However, it does not remove the need to make an accurate diagnosis so that specific therapy for a potentially reversible cause, when available, can be given early on when it is most likely to be life saving. Always evaluate for reversible causes.

Key principles underlying CPR

- **Appropriateness**: treatment aims to restore the patient to a high quality of life. If this is not possible, consider whether CPR is appropriate. 'Do not attempt cardiopulmonary resuscitation' (DNACPR) orders (always clearly recorded in the notes) are made on the basis of:
  - the chance of immediate CPR success (relates to age and disease)

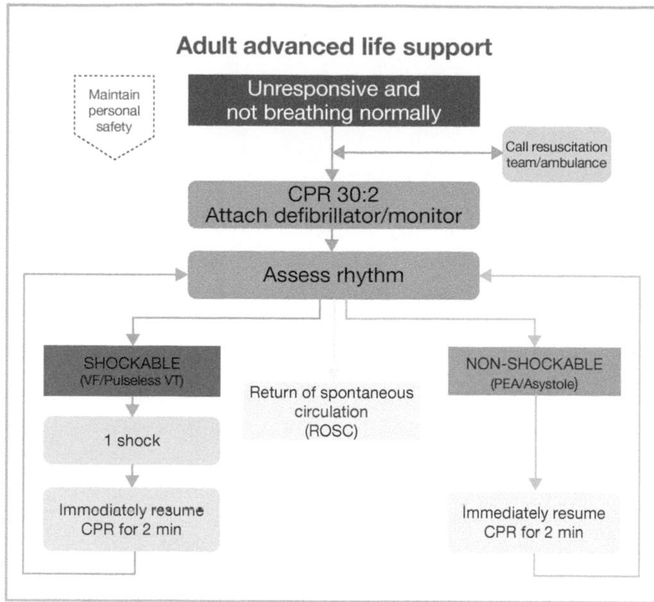

- the chance of restoring long-term high-quality life (relates to pre-existing quality of life)
- patient's wishes, which must be established.

- **Speed**: after total circulatory/respiratory failure, irreversible hypoxic brain injury follows within 3–4 minutes (unless extreme hypothermia is present). Furthermore, cardiac anoxia develops quickly, preventing successful restoration of the circulation. High-quality chest compressions should be started immediately, with access to a defibrillator and assessment of cardiac rhythm as soon as possible.

Basic life support

If someone is unresponsive and not breathing normally in the community, immediately call for help and send someone to fetch a defibrillator if available. Assess the airway and remove any obstruction. Determine within 10 seconds whether breathing is normal.

- Look for chest movement.
- Listen at the victim's mouth for breath sounds.
- Feel for air on your cheek.

Begin chest compressions by pushing the sternum down 4–5 cm each time, at a rate of 100/min, alternating 30 compressions to two slow, effective rescue breaths into the mouth (each of 700–1000 ml), with the nose pinched shut, sufficient to make the chest rise and fall. Chest compressions restore 30% of normal cerebral perfusion. Continue this algorithm until movement or spontaneous breathing occurs, or until an automated external defibrillator (AED) arrives, in which case switch it on and follow instructions. In prolonged arrest and if available, consider applying an external automated mechanical chest compression device, e.g. LUCAS.

Advanced life support

Advanced life support (ALS) (i.e. equipment is available; see ALS algorithm): apply BLS, attach defibrillator and diagnose the heart rhythm as shockable or non-shockable.

- **Shockable rhythms: ventricular fibrillation** (VF) and **pulseless ventricular tachycardia** (VT) are the common survivable causes of cardiac arrest. Success rates decline by 7–10% for every minute that defibrillation is delayed. Give a single shock (unless the cardiac arrest was witnessed, in which case up to three stacked shocks may be given), immediately resuming CPR thereafter. After successful cardioversion, transient (≥10 s) asystole and/or a weak pulse (myocardial stunning) may occur; accordingly chest compressions are continued unless there are signs of return of spontaneous circulation (such as waking or purposeful movement). If VF/VT persists, secure the airway (endotracheal tube, laryngeal mask airway) and ventilate at 10 breaths/min, continuing chest compression uninterrupted. Establish intravenous (IV) access (or intraosseous access if intravenous access cannot be obtained). Give adrenaline (epinephrine) after the third shock and every 3–5 minutes thereafter to improve the efficacy of CPR (α-adrenergic actions cause vasoconstriction, increasing myocardial and cerebral perfusion pressures). Refractory VF/VT may respond to further shocks with alternative pad positions or IV amiodarone (after three shocks). Assess for and treat reversible causes. Continue until the circulation is restored or the decision is made to stop. Consider bicarbonate in tricyclic antidepressant overdose or if hyperkalaemia is present.
- **Non-shockable rhythms**, including **PEA** and **asystole**, have a lower survival rate. Resume CPR and administer adrenaline immediately, with further doses every 3–5 minutes. Complete heart block may respond to pacing (external or transvenous) and/or isoprenaline. Beware spurious asystole: VF with a low voltage trace or incorrectly applied electrodes. Assess for and treat reversible causes.

Discontinue CPR, after consultation with other team members, when the situation is deemed irrecoverable, based on duration of CPR and whether a stable circulation was ever attained. Pupil dilation is an unreliable sign of irreversible brain damage.

Give high-quality chest compressions, and:

- Give oxygen
- Use waveform capnography
- Continuous compressions if advanced airway
- Minimise interruptions to compressions
- Intravenous or intraosseous access
- Give adrenaline every 3–5 min
- Give amiodarone after 3 shocks
- Identify and treat reversible causes

Identify and treat reversible causes

- Hypoxia
- Hypovolaemia
- Hypo-/hyperkalaemia/metabolic
- Hypo/hyperthermia
- Thrombosis – coronary or pulmonary
- Tension pneumothorax
- Tamponade – cardiac
- Toxins

Consider ultrasound imaging to identify reversible causes

Consider

- Coronary angiography/percutaneous coronary intervention
- Mechanical chest compressions to facilitate transfer/treatment
- Extracorporeal CPR

After ROSC

- Use an ABCDE approach
- Aim for SpO_2 of 94–98% and normal $PaCO_2$
- 12-lead ECG
- Identify and treat cause
- Targeted temperature management

79 Delirium

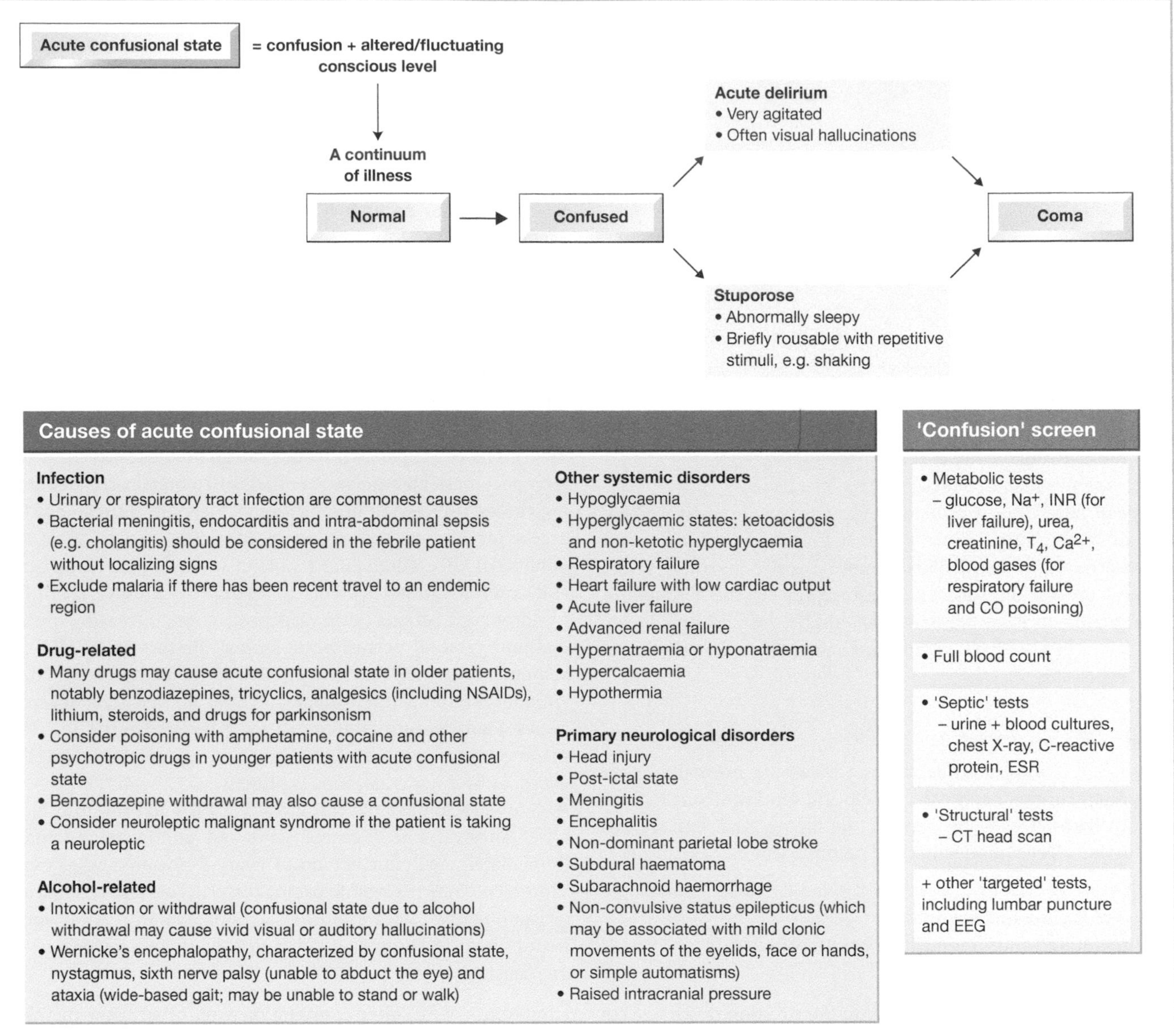

Acute confusional state
= confusion + altered/fluctuating conscious level
A continuum of illness
Normal
Confused
Acute delirium
• Very agitated
• Often visual hallucinations
Stuporose
• Abnormally sleepy
• Briefly rousable with repetitive stimuli, e.g. shaking
Coma
Causes of acute confusional state
Infection
• Urinary or respiratory tract infection are commonest causes
• Bacterial meningitis, endocarditis and intra-abdominal sepsis (e.g. cholangitis) should be considered in the febrile patient without localizing signs
• Exclude malaria if there has been recent travel to an endemic region
Drug-related
• Many drugs may cause acute confusional state in older patients, notably benzodiazepines, tricyclics, analgesics (including NSAIDs), lithium, steroids, and drugs for parkinsonism
• Consider poisoning with amphetamine, cocaine and other psychotropic drugs in younger patients with acute confusional state
• Benzodiazepine withdrawal may also cause a confusional state
• Consider neuroleptic malignant syndrome if the patient is taking a neuroleptic
Alcohol-related
• Intoxication or withdrawal (confusional state due to alcohol withdrawal may cause vivid visual or auditory hallucinations)
• Wernicke's encephalopathy, characterized by confusional state, nystagmus, sixth nerve palsy (unable to abduct the eye) and ataxia (wide-based gait; may be unable to stand or walk)
Other systemic disorders
• Hypoglycaemia
• Hyperglycaemic states: ketoacidosis and non-ketotic hyperglycaemia
• Respiratory failure
• Heart failure with low cardiac output
• Acute liver failure
• Advanced renal failure
• Hypernatraemia or hyponatraemia
• Hypercalcaemia
• Hypothermia
Primary neurological disorders
• Head injury
• Post-ictal state
• Meningitis
• Encephalitis
• Non-dominant parietal lobe stroke
• Subdural haematoma
• Subarachnoid haemorrhage
• Non-convulsive status epilepticus (which may be associated with mild clonic movements of the eyelids, face or hands, or simple automatisms)
• Raised intracranial pressure
'Confusion' screen
• Metabolic tests
– glucose, Na^+, INR (for liver failure), urea, creatinine, T_4, Ca^{2+}, blood gases (for respiratory failure and CO poisoning)
• Full blood count
• 'Septic' tests
– urine + blood cultures, chest X-ray, C-reactive protein, ESR
• 'Structural' tests
– CT head scan
+ other 'targeted' tests, including lumbar puncture and EEG

Delirium is a functional brain disorder characterized by clouding of consciousness and impaired cognitive function, which develops over hours or days, and typically fluctuates over the course of the day. Present on hospital admission in around 15% of patients aged over 65, and developing after admission in a further 20%, delirium is a common manifestation of a wide range of systemic disorders (notably infection) or an adverse effect of medications, especially those with an anticholinergic effect. In patients of all ages, it may reflect a primary neurological disorder. Common causes of delirium by context are shown in Table 79.1.

The term 'acute confusional state' is often used synonymously with delirium, although delirium is preferred, as confusion (an inability to think with usual clarity) is not specific to delirium. Delirium may be associated with increased or decreased psychomotor activity (hyperactive and hypoactive variants), hallucinations and delusions. Pronounced psychomotor and sympathetic hyperactivity are more often seen with delirium due to alcohol/substance intoxication or withdrawal (delirium tremens) in younger patients, but no cause is specific to a clinical subtype.

Medicine at a Glance, Fifth Edition. Edited by Patrick Davey and Alex Pitcher.

Companion website: www.wiley.com/go/medicine5e

Table 79.1 Causes of delirium by context

Patient group	Common causes
Older patient in emergency department	Acute infection (e.g. urinary tract or lower respiratory tract) Adverse effect of medication Electrolyte disorder Stroke
Younger patient in emergency department	Alcohol intoxication Poisoning with psychoactive drug Primary neurological disorder (e.g. encephalitis)
Patient with alcohol use disorder or alcoholic liver disease	Alcohol intoxication or withdrawal Liver failure Acute infection (e.g. spontaneous bacterial peritonitis, pneumonia)
Patient with cancer	Brain or meningeal metastases Electrolyte disorder (e.g. hypercalcaemia or hyponatraemia) Adverse effect of medication (e.g. opioid toxicity) Paraneoplastic effect
Older patient after surgery	Acute infection Pain Adverse effect of medication Urinary retention Faecal impaction

Source: Reproduced with permission from the National Institute for Health and Care Excellence (NICE).

There are two aspects to the diagnosis of delirium: recognition of the syndrome and identification of its cause or causes. Any patient with an abnormal mental state may have a disease which is an immediate threat to life (e.g. respiratory failure), and you should therefore begin with a rapid ABCDE assessment (see Table 10.1, Chapter 10). to ensure that the airway, breathing and circulation are not compromised, and hypoglycaemia excluded, before exploring the diagnosis.

Recognition of delirium

Delirium is a clinical diagnosis, based on examination of the patient's mental state supplemented by a collateral history from family members, carers or hospital staff.

The duration of the abnormal mental state (developing over hours or days) helps distinguish delirium from dementia, with which it may co-exist, as dementia renders the brain vulnerable to delirium. Delirium may be obvious from the patient's behaviour and speech, but you should also suspect the disorder in any older patient labelled as difficult, depressed, unco-operative or a 'poor historian'. Testing for delirium can be done in a few minutes using the 4AT assessment tool (Table 79.2).

Diagnosing the cause of delirium

Having made an ABCDE assessment, you should complete a focused history and examination, and arrange appropriate investigation.

History

Establish current symptoms, context and past history by talking to family members, carers or hospital staff, and reviewing the patient's medical and nursing records. Check prescribed medications. Many drugs may cause delirium, notably benzodiazepines, opioid analgesics, high-dose corticosteroids and medications for parkinsonism. If the patient was admitted with delirium, establish which drugs were prescribed in primary care, and ask relatives to collect all medications in the home.

Examination

Review the physiological observations and make a systematic examination. Check for focal chest signs, abdominal tenderness or guarding, urinary retention, faecal impaction, pressure ulceration and cellulitis. Are there abnormal neurological signs? As a minimum, examine for neck stiffness and lateralized weakness, and check the plantar responses.

Investigation

As a general rule, all patients with delirium should have a full blood count, biochemical profile, measurement of C-reactive protein level, urine stick test and chest X-ray. Additional investigations will be guided by the context and clinical findings.

Neuroimaging (by CT or MRI) is indicated:

- if delirium followed a fall or head injury
- if there are new focal neurological signs
- if there is papilloedema or other evidence of raised intracranial pressure
- if the patient has cancer or HIV-AIDS
- if the patient's behaviour prevents adequate neurological examination
- or if no systemic cause for the delirium is apparent.

Examination of the cerebrospinal fluid should be done (assuming no contraindication to lumbar puncture):

- if meningitis or encephalitis is suspected
- if the patient is febrile and no systemic focus of infection is found
- or if the cause of delirium remains unclear.

Prevention and management of delirium

As well as being highly distressing to patients and their families, delirium is a major threat to health. It predisposes to injury, falls, dehydration, malnutrition, incontinence and pressure ulceration, and may also result in an irreversible worsening of cognitive function. Delirium should therefore be prevented if possible. Multicomponent intervention (Table 79.3) can reduce the incidence of delirium in patients at risk, such as older patients having major surgery, and should be an integral part of the care of these patients.

In a patient with delirium, your aim is promptly to identify and treat the underlying cause, in a setting where safe care can be delivered; this includes anticipation and prevention of potential complications (see Table 79.3). Physical restraint should be avoided if possible. Short-term (one week or less) therapy with haloperidol should only be used if the patient is severely distressed or likely to injure themselves or others.

Table 79.2 The 4AT assessment test for delirium and cognitive impairment

[1] ALERTNESS	
This includes patients who may be markedly drowsy (e.g. difficult to rouse and/or obviously sleepy during assessment) or agitated/hyperactive. Observe the patient. If asleep, attempt to wake with speech or gentle touch on shoulder. Ask the patient to state their name and address to assist rating.	
Normal (fully alert, but not agitated, throughout assessment)	0
Mild sleepiness for <10 seconds after waking, then normal	0
Clearly abnormal	4
[2] AMT4	
Age, date of birth, place (name of the hospital or building), current year.	
No mistakes	0
1 mistake	1
2 or more mistakes/untestable	2
[3] ATTENTION	
Ask the patient: 'Please tell me the months of the year in backwards order, starting at December'. To assist initial understanding, one prompt of 'what is the month before December?' is permitted.	
Achieves 7 months or more correctly	0
Starts but scores <7 months/refuses to start	1
Untestable (cannot start because unwell, drowsy, inattentive)	2
[4] ACUTE CHANGE OR FLUCTUATING COURSE	
Evidence of significant change or fluctuation in: alertness, cognition, other mental function (e.g. paranoia, hallucinations) arising over the last 2 weeks and still evident in last 24h.	
No	0
Yes	4

4AT score:
4 or above: possible delirium +/- cognitive impairment
1-3: possible cognitive impairment
0: delirium or severe cognitive impairment unlikely (but delirium still possible if information incomplete)

Source: Further information and guidance notes available at www.the4at.com

Table 79.3 Prevention and management of delirium

Clinical factors that can contribute to delirium	Preventive interventions and actions
Disorientation	Provide clear signage, soft lighting, a 24-hour clock and a calendar, all easily visible to the patient Introduce cognitively stimulating activities Facilitate regular visits from family and friends
Dehydration and/or constipation	Ensure an adequate fluid intake Take advice where necessary when managing fluid balance in patients with co-morbidities such as heart failure or chronic kidney disease Look for and treat constipation
Infection	Look for and treat infection Avoid unnecessary bladder catheterization Implement good infection control procedures
Pain	Find out whether the patient has pain Look out for non-verbal signs of pain, particularly in those with communication difficulties If patients have been prescribed pain relief, ensure they receive it
Polypharmacy effects	Review the medications the patient is taking and stop those which may be contributing to delirium
Poor nutrition	Assess nutritional status using a validated tool Measure the height and weight and calculate the body mass index If the patient is malnourished, obtain the advice of a dietician on an appropriate diet If patients have dentures, ensure they are well-fitting
Restricted or limited mobility or immobility	Encourage patients to carry out active range-of-motion exercises, to walk about if they can, and mobilize early after surgery
Sensory impairment	Ensure hearing and visual aids (in good working order) are available to and used by patients who need them
Sleep disturbance	Promote good sleep patterns and sleep hygiene by scheduling medication rounds to avoid disturbing sleep, and reducing noise to a minimum during sleep periods

Source: Adapted from NICE clinical guideline 103 (2010).

80 Coma

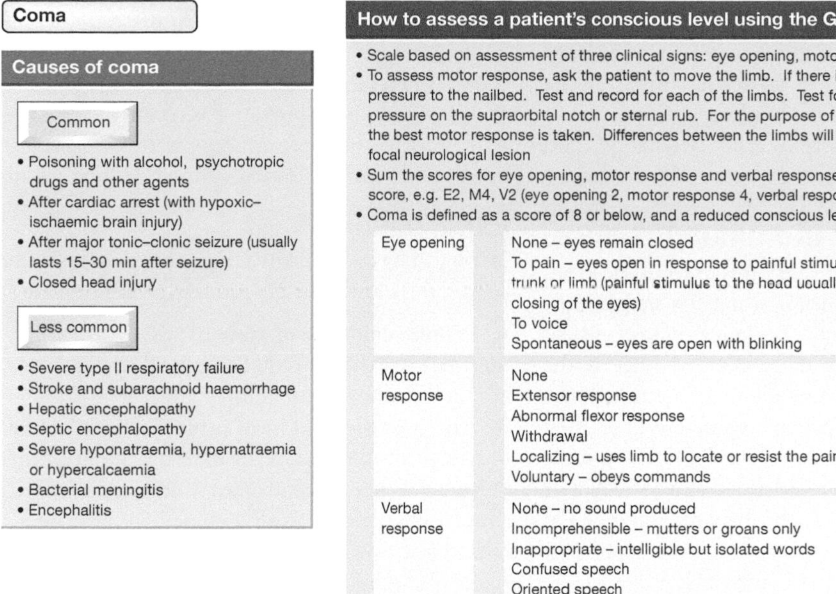

Coma

Causes of coma

Common

- Poisoning with alcohol, psychotropic drugs and other agents
- After cardiac arrest (with hypoxic–ischaemic brain injury)
- After major tonic–clonic seizure (usually lasts 15–30 min after seizure)
- Closed head injury

Less common

- Severe type II respiratory failure
- Stroke and subarachnoid haemorrhage
- Hepatic encephalopathy
- Septic encephalopathy
- Severe hyponatraemia, hypernatraemia or hypercalcaemia
- Bacterial meningitis
- Encephalitis

How to assess a patient's conscious level using the Glasgow Coma Scale

- Scale based on assessment of three clinical signs: eye opening, motor response and verbal response
- To assess motor response, ask the patient to move the limb. If there is no response, apply firm pressure to the nailbed. Test and record for each of the limbs. Test for a localizing response by pressure on the supraorbital notch or sternal rub. For the purpose of assessment of conscious level, the best motor response is taken. Differences between the limbs will be important in identifying any focal neurological lesion
- Sum the scores for eye opening, motor response and verbal response; also record the elements of the score, e.g. E2, M4, V2 (eye opening 2, motor response 4, verbal response 2)
- Coma is defined as a score of 8 or below, and a reduced conscious level as a score of 9–14

Eye opening	None – eyes remain closed	1
	To pain – eyes open in response to painful stimulus applied to trunk or limb (painful stimulus to the head usually provokes closing of the eyes)	2
	To voice	3
	Spontaneous – eyes are open with blinking	4
Motor response	None	1
	Extensor response	2
	Abnormal flexor response	3
	Withdrawal	4
	Localizing – uses limb to locate or resist the painful stimulus	5
	Voluntary – obeys commands	6
Verbal response	None – no sound produced	1
	Incomprehensible – mutters or groans only	2
	Inappropriate – intelligible but isolated words	3
	Confused speech	4
	Oriented speech	5
	Total	**3–15**

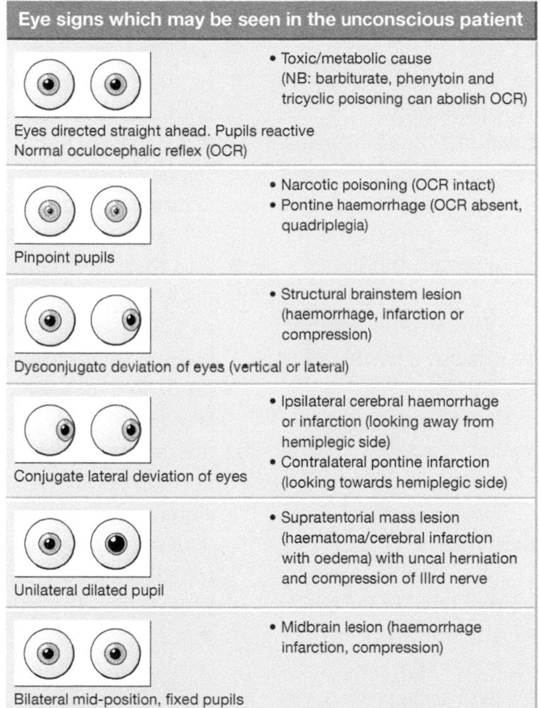

Coma is a pathological state of unconsciousness from which the patient cannot be roused to wakefulness by stimuli. It reflects dysfunction of the brainstem reticular system and its thalamic projections, or diffuse injury of both cerebral hemispheres. A unilateral lesion of a cerebral hemisphere (such as a haemorrhagic stroke) will not cause coma unless there is secondary compression of the contralateral hemisphere or brainstem.

Causes of coma you are likely to see in the emergency department include head trauma, poisoning, stroke, hypoxic-ischaemic brain injury following cardiac arrest, seizures

Medicine at a Glance, Fifth Edition. Edited by Patrick Davey and Alex Pitcher.

Companion website: www.wiley.com/go/medicine5e

or postictal state, intracranial infection and metabolic disorders. Poisoning, due to ingestion of sedative drugs, often with alcohol, is the cause of non-traumatic coma in 80% of patients under 40, but only 10% of those over 60, in whom stroke is the most common diagnosis. Be aware that several diseases may be contributing to coma (e.g. opioid poisoning complicated by respiratory arrest with resultant hypoxic-ischaemic brain injury; alcohol intoxication complicated by head injury).

Coma is a medical emergency, because the comatose patient is at high risk of permanent brain injury or death, caused by the underlying disease or its secondary effects. Immediate action is needed to stabilize the airway, breathing and circulation, and correct hypoglycaemia if present, before exploring the diagnosis.

Assessment of the level of consciousness

Consciousness is a continuum from full alertness to complete unresponsiveness, and can be graded clinically using the simple four-point AVPU scale (A, alert; V, responds to voice; P, responds to painful stimuli; U, unresponsive). A more detailed scale is the Glasgow Coma Scale (GCS), based on eye opening, motor response and verbal response. How to assess a patient's conscious level using the GCS is summarized in the figure above. The GCS gives a score of 15 (alert) to 3 (unresponsive). Coma is defined as a score of 8 or below, and a reduced conscious level as a score between 9 and 14. On the AVPU scale, A corresponds with a GCS of 15, V with a GCS of around 13, P with a GCS of around 8 and U with a GCS of 3.

Priorities in the management of the comatose patient

- Immediately assess the patient using the ABCDE (airway, breathing, circulation, disability, exposure) approach.
- Stabilize the airway, breathing and circulation. One of the major risks of impaired consciousness is the loss of the ability to protect the airway. As a general rule, patients with a GCS score of 8 or below (P, responds to painful stimuli, or U, unresponsive, on the AVPU scale) need endotracheal intubation to protect the airway.
- Exclude/treat hypoglycaemia.
- If Wernicke encephalopathy is possible (because of coma in the setting of alcohol use disorder or malnutrition), give thiamine intravenously, before the administration of glucose.
- Give naloxone if opioid poisoning is possible (respiratory rate <12/min, pinpoint pupils, or the circumstances suggest it), and flumazenil if the patient has received benzodiazepine in hospital (e.g. for procedural sedation).
- Treat generalized seizures along standard lines.
- Diagnose and treat the underlying cause. This is done by clinical assessment and computed tomography (CT) of the brain, together with other investigations. The age of the patient, their long-term health conditions, the setting in which coma occurred, and the findings on examination and CT will usually limit the differential diagnosis to a handful of diseases.

Clinical assessment of the comatose patient

History

Obtain the history from all available sources: ambulance personnel, family and friends, GP and hospital records, and the patient's belongings. Establish the following.

- The setting and time course of the loss of consciousness. Was loss of consciousness abrupt (e.g. subarachnoid haemorrhage [SAH], seizure), gradual (e.g. poisoning, bacterial meningitis) or fluctuating (e.g. recurring seizures, subdural haematoma, metabolic encephalopathy)?
- If loss of consciousness was preceded by neurological or other symptoms.
- The long-term health conditions of the patient: systemic (e.g. chronic obstructive pulmonary disease, chronic liver disease), neurological (e.g. epilepsy) and psychiatric.
- A complete list of current medications. If the patient was admitted with coma, find out exactly what medications were being taken prior to admission (if necessary, contact the patient's GP to check prescribed medications, and ask a family member to collect all medications in the home).
- If there has been previous or recent alcohol or substance use.
- If there has been recent foreign travel (raising the possibility of infectious diseases acquired abroad, such as falciparum malaria).

Examination

Having addressed the ABCDE priorities, complete your examination (see figure below). Key questions to be answered are as follows.

- **Is there evidence of systemic disease?** Is there fever or hypothermia? Are there signs of chronic liver disease (e.g. spider naevi, ascites) or other organ failure?
- **Are there signs of head injury?** Check for scalp laceration or bruising, bleeding from the external auditory meatus or nose. If there are signs of head injury, additional cervical spine injury should be suspected until excluded, and the neck must be immobilized in a collar and X-rayed before testing for neck stiffness and the oculocephalic response.
- **Is there neck stiffness?** Neck stiffness is a sign of meningeal irritation, and may be seen in meningitis, subarachnoid haemorrhage and cerebral or cerebellar haemorrhage with extension into the subarachoid space.
- **Is intracranial infection possible?** If bacterial meningitis or viral encephalitis is possible (e.g. consistent history, fever, neck stiffness), take blood for culture and start antimicrobial treatment immediately, with cefotaxime or ceftriaxone (plus amoxycillin in patients over 60, or with immunocompromise or alcohol use disorder) and aciclovir.
- **Are there focal neurological signs?** Examine the eyes and limbs carefully.
  - Check the position of the eyes, the size and symmetry of the pupils and their response to bright light, and examine the fundi. Eye signs which may be seen in the unconscious patient are illustrated in the figure above. With the exception of coma due to opioid poisoning (characterized by pinpoint pupils), normal pupils usually indicate a toxic/metabolic cause of coma.
  - Examine the fundi: if you see spontaneous pulsation of the retinal veins, the intracranial pressure is normal. Subhyaloid haemorrhages may be seen in SAH.
  - Check the corneal reflex: a normal response bilaterally (eyelid closure and upward deviation of the eyes) indicates normal function of the midbrain and pons. The corneal reflex may be lost in deep coma due to a toxic/metabolic cause.
  - Provided the cervical spine is stable, check the oculocephalic response: this is a simple test of an intact brainstem. Rotate the head to the left and right. In an unconscious patient with an intact brainstem, both eyes rotate counter to movement of the head.
  - Check limb tone, limb response to a painful stimulus (nail-bed pressure), the tendon reflexes and plantar responses. Consistent asymmetry between right- and left-sided findings usually indicates a structural neurological cause.

The absence of neck stiffness or focal neurological signs usually indicates a toxic/metabolic cause of coma, but some brain disorders (e.g. hypoxic-ischaemic injury) may not give focal signs.

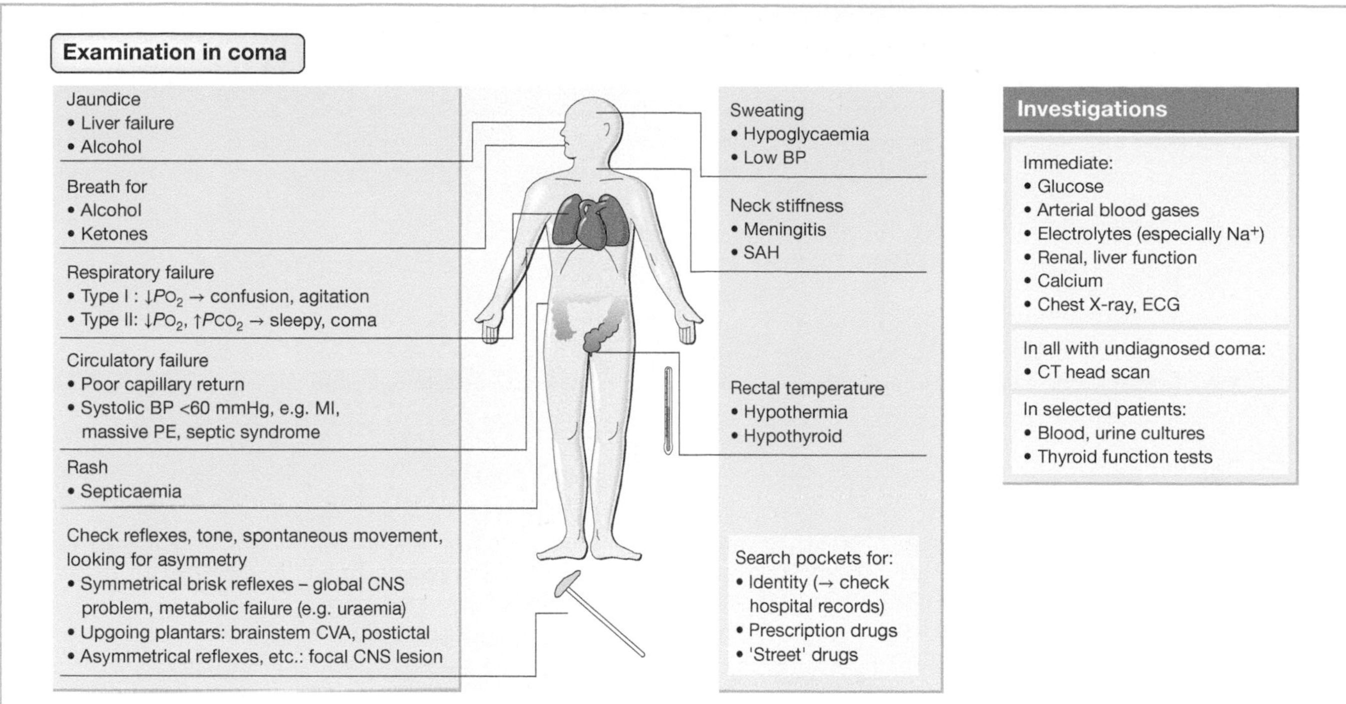

Abnormal eye signs are typically found in structural disorders affecting the brainstem, either a primary event (e.g. haemorrhage) or due to compression or distortion from an expanding supratentorial or posterior fossa mass lesion.

Urgent investigation

- **Computed tomography (CT)** should be done in all patients, unless there is a clear toxic cause of coma in a young patient, with no features to suggest additional pathology. CT is very sensitive for intracranial haemorrhage (>95% positive in SAH and intracerebral haemorrhage) and can identify mass lessions, hydrocephalus, marked cerebral oedema and large cerebral hemisphere ischaemic strokes. If CT shows haemorrhage or other structural pathology, an urgent neurosurgical opinion is needed. Non-contrast CT may be normal in early ischaemic stroke, especially of the brainstem or cerebellum, hypoxic-ischaemic brain injury and white matter disorders (e.g. central pontine myelinolyis).
- **A chest X-ray** should be taken to exclude pneumonia.
- **An ECG** should be recorded in all patients over 50 and in younger patients if there is hypotension, co-existent heart disease or suspected ingestion of cardiotoxic drugs.
- **Arterial blood gases and pH** should be checked. Respiratory failure may result in coma or complicate coma from other disorders.
- **Key blood tests** are **full blood count**, **coagulation screen** and **biochemical profile**. A **toxicology screen** and **measurement of plasma paracetamol and salicylate levels** should be done if poisoining is possible. **Blood culture** should be taken if there is fever or hypothermia.

Additional investigation

- **Examination of the cerebrospinal fluid** (assuming no contraindication to lumbar puncture [LP]), if the cause of coma is unexplained by CT and other tests above, to rule out meningitis and encephalitis.
- **Magnetic resonance imaging (MRI)** of the brain, if the diagnosis remains unclear or you suspect a cause to which CT is insensitive (see above).
- **Electroencephalography (EEG)** if the clinical findings suggest non-convulsive status epilepticus. EEG can be diagnostically useful if the cause of coma is still unclear after neuro-imaging and other tests.
- Other tests which may be helpful in specific circumstances include measurement of **plasma osmolality** (raised in poisoning with ethanol, ethylene glycol, isopropyl alcohol or methanol), **plasma ammonia** (raised in hepatic encephalopathy) and **red cell transketolase** (low in Wernicke encephalopathy due to thiamine deficiency).

Further management

- Nurse the patient in a high-dependency or intensive care unit.
- Monitor physiological observations and the level of consciousness initially every 15–30 min.
- Maintain airway patency, breathing and circulation.
- Maintain blood glucose between 8 and 10 mmol/L. Avoid hypoglycaemia.
- Treat the underlying cause or causes. Neurosurgical advice should be sought urgently for patients with coma due to head injury or structural brain diseases.
- Anticipate, prevent or treat the complications of coma (e.g. pressure necrosis of skin or muscle, corneal abrasions, inhalation pneumonia).
- Induced hypothermia (target 36 °C, for 24 h) should be instituted if coma has followed cardiac arrest, as this improves the neurological prognosis.

Prognosis

Patients with coma may make a complete recovery (for example, after poisoning with psychoactive drugs), survive with varying degrees of brain injury, or die from brain death or systemic disease. The prognosis largely depends on the cause of coma, and is poor when there is major structural brain disease. For a given cause, the depth of coma and the status of brainstem reflexes influence prognosis (better with normal brainstem function).

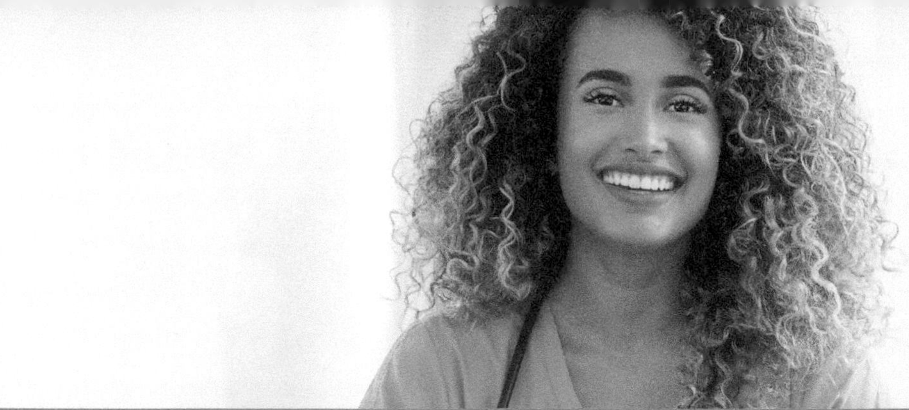

Chapters

Cardiovascular disease

Respiratory disease

Gastroenterology

Renal medicine

Endocrinology

Diseases and treatments at a glance

81 Hypertension

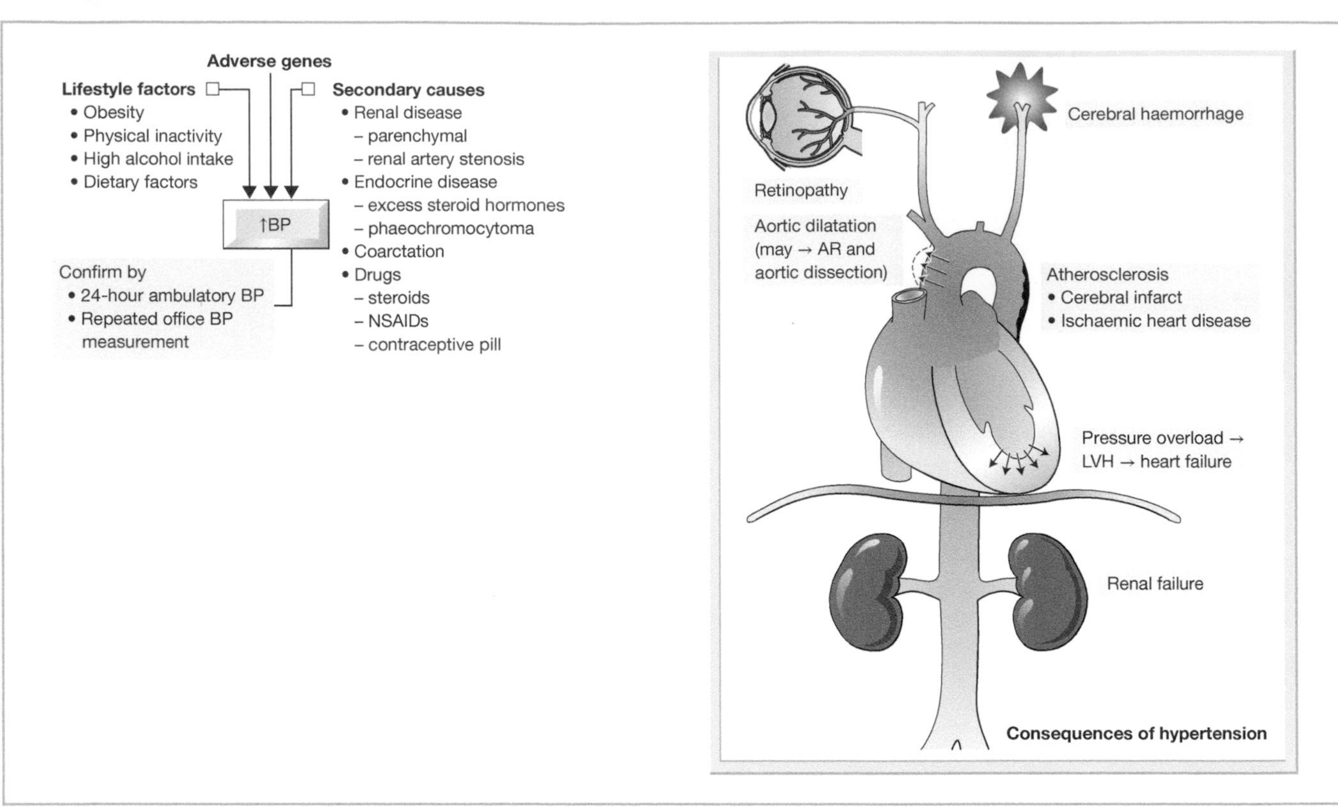

Definition

Blood pressure (BP) is distributed continuously. The incidence of complications is proportional to BP, so there is no absolute definition of hypertension. Treatment is often beneficial with sustained BP >140/90 mmHg.

Incidence

Increases with age. Prevalence of mild hypertension is 2% in those aged 25 years or less, rising to 25% in those in their 50s and 50% in those in their 70s.

Pathophysiology

Most (95%) hypertension is **essential hypertension**, a combination of numerous genetic and environmental factors that results in a hypertensive phenotype. **Secondary hypertension**, caused by an identifiable cause, is uncommon, and suggested by:

- renal dysfunction (look for a raised creatinine and/or dipstick haematuria or proteinurea). If there is ischaemic heart disease (IHD)/peripheral vascular disease (PVD), consider renal artery stenosis
- young age (especially 30 years or less); consider coarctation or rare genetic causes of hypertension (Liddle syndrome, Gordon syndrome, Geller syndrome and others)
- severe treatment-resistant hypertension
- hypokalaemia (in the absence of diuretics), which suggests mineralocorticoid excess (Cushing or Conn syndrome).

Clinical features

Hypertension is usually asymptomatic, until end-organ damage occurs. Most headaches in hypertension are *not* related to BP. Arrange urgent assessment/treatment for patients with severe hypertension (>180/120 mmHg) who have retinal haemorrhage/papilloedema or new confusion, chest pain, heart failure or acute kidney injury.

Effects of hypertension

The long-term risk of hypertension is end-organ damage.

- **Cerebrovascular disease**: especially thrombotic and haemorrhagic stroke.
- **Vascular disease**: coronary and peripheral artery disease.
- **Left ventricular hypertrophy** (LVH) is a compensatory response to a chronically elevated BP. It is an independent predictor of early death (sudden cardiac death from ventricular arrhythmias, heart failure, myocardial infarction (MI) or cerebrovascular accident). Heart failure in hypertension may relate to the abnormalities in hypertrophied myocyte function (long-standing hypertrophied muscle develops first diastolic and later systolic

Medicine at a Glance, Fifth Edition. Edited by Patrick Davey and Alex Pitcher.

Companion website: www.wiley.com/go/medicine5e

Table 81.1 Classification of hypertension

Category	Systolic blood pressure (mmHg)	Diastolic blood pressure (mmHg)
Optimal blood pressure	<120	<80
Normal blood pressure	<140	<90
Stage 1 hypertension	140–159	90–99
Stage 2 hypertension	160–179	100–119
Stage 3 hypertension	≥180	≥120

contractile failure) or to coronary disease, which is more likely in long-standing hypertension.

- **Chronic kidney disease**: hypertension leads to renovascular damage and glomerular loss.

Severity

Hypertension is classed according to the presence of end-organ damage and the BP level (Table 81.1).

Investigations

- **Confirm hypertension**: arrange ambulatory blood pressure monitoring to confirm a diagnosis in patients with a clinic blood pressure of between 140/90 mmHg and 180/120 mmHg.
- **Assess for secondary causes**: renal disease (dipstick urine, check creatinine, renal size, non-invasive renal artery imaging by magnetic resonance imaging). Exclude coarctation (clinical examination demonstrating decreased femoral pulse strength, and often 'radiofemoral' delay or 'rib notching' on chest X-ray), hypokalaemia (Cushing and Conn syndromes) and phaeochromocytoma (see Chapter 163).
- **Assess end-organ damage**: electrocardiogram, echocardiography (for LVH), renal function.

Treatment

Treatment essentially abolishes the excess stroke and coronary risk.

Overall approach

Other cardiovascular risk factors must also be addressed, e.g. smoking, diabetes control, cholesterol (statin therapy is often indicated).

Non-pharmacological measures

Lifestyle modification (weight loss, lower salt and alcohol intake, regular exercise) may be sufficient in mild hypertension. Pharmacological therapy is used if the BP is too high on several recordings or on 24-hour BP monitoring.

Pharmacological treatments

Large long-term clinical trials have shown a clear mortality reduction from treating hypertension, principally from fewer strokes, but also from less sudden cardiac death, heart failure and MI. The benefit of treatment relates to the degree of hypertension, i.e. the more severe the hypertension, the greater the impact of treatment. However, even mild hypertension benefits from treatment when the risk of end-organ damage is high or already present (e.g. people who are older, people with diabetes, previous MI, etc.). The risk reduction is related to the lowering of BP. Except for β-blockers, there is *little good evidence that any drug is better than any other*, although individual drugs are particularly suited to some patients.

- **Angiotensin-converting enzyme (ACE) inhibitors** (e.g. ramipril, lisinopril, enalapril) exert their antihypertensive effects by blocking the formation of angiotensin II. Mortality data are strong for patients with heart failure, impaired LV function or known coronary artery disease. May cause profound hypotension or acute renal failure in those with renovascular hypertension, i.e. bilateral renal artery stenosis. Side-effects include dry cough (common) and angioedema.
- **Angiotensin II receptor antagonists** (e.g. losartan, valsartan) antagonize the angiotensin II–renin axis. They have comparable efficacy to ACE inhibitors, although trial data supporting their use are less comprehensive. They are indicated in heart failure or impaired LV function if a cough from ACE inhibitor is troublesome. Effects on renal function in renovascular hypertension are similar.
- **β-blockers** (e.g. atenolol and metoprolol) reduce heart rate and BP by antagonizing adrenergic signalling. β-blockers are not first-line treatments for hypertension, though there is good evidence for long-term benefit for some drugs (bisoprolol, carvedilol, nebivolol, metoprolol) in left ventricular (LV) dysfunction. Side-effects can include lethargy, impotence, cold peripheries, exacerbation of diabetes and hyperlipidaemia. They are contraindicated in people with asthma; use with caution in PVD.
- **Diuretics** (e.g. bendrofluazide) are safe and effective.
- **Spironolactone and related drugs** are also, often, very effective, with few symptomatic side-effects (gynaecomastia can occur) although they do require close monitoring of renal function and potassium.
- **Calcium channel antagonists** are vasodilators that lower BP. Nifedipine (and possibly amlodipine) causes a reflex tachycardia unless a β-blocker is co-prescribed. Diltiazem and verapamil cause a bradycardia. Side-effects include flushing, ankle oedema and worsening heart failure (not with amlodipine).
- **α-antagonists** (e.g. doxazosin) are vasodilators that lower BP by antagonism of the α-adrenergic receptors in the peripheral vasculature.
- **SGLT-2 inhibitors,** while not usually indicated for BP control, may be considered if there are additional indications (diabetes, heart failure), and do reduce BP significantly.
- **Other drugs** include centrally acting agents (e.g. methyldopa, moxonidine).

Guidelines in treating hypertension

The choice of antihypertensive therapy is influenced by other diseases/risk factors, e.g. patients with heart failure with reduced ejection fraction or coronary disease benefit from a β-blocker and ACE inhibitor. β-blockers should generally be avoided in asthma. Those with prostatic symptoms find α-blockers relieve these as well as their hypertension.

In general, the first-line therapies are ACE inhibitors (preferred in those with type 2 diabetes and those aged under 55 and not of black African or African-Caribbean family origin) or calcium channel blockers (in those aged over 55 or over or those of black African or African-Caribbean family origin without type 2 diabetes). Angiotension receptor antagonists are used in those intolerant to ACE inhibitors, e.g. due to cough.

If hypertension remains uncontrolled, the next step is to add another agent (either an ACE inhibitor or calcium channel blocker, or a thiazide diuretic). Step 3 is a combination of an ACE inhibitor, calcium channel blocker and a thiazide diuretic.

If hypertension is not controlled with the above approach, remember to assess for adherence to therapy, lifestyle factors and reversible causes. Consider adding in higher dose/alternative diuretics (e.g. spironolactone, α-blockers, β-blockers or others).

Hypertension urgencies and emergencies

Rarely, patients present with severe, uncontrolled hypertension and severe resulting end-organ damage, which requires urgent treatment. It is important to distinguish a hypertension emergency from hypertension resulting from pain or distress related to a different condition, which does not usually require specific treatment.

Symptoms of a hypertension emergency may include headache, confusion ('hypertensive encephalopathy') or other acute end-organ damage (aortic dissection or heart failure). However, hypertension in the context of an ischaemic stroke is not usually treated immediately. Patients with hypertension emergencies are admitted to hospital because the risks of end-organ damage and life-threatening complications are high. Oral agents are given, unless the patient is critically unwell (repeated hypertensive seizures, severe LV failure, aortic dissection) when cautious intravenous therapy may be given; however, BP lowering must be gradual because sudden falls in BP can precipitate a stroke. Intravenous agents include intravenous nitrates and labetolol, a β-blocker that also has α-adrenergic antagonist effects.

82 Hyperlipidaemia

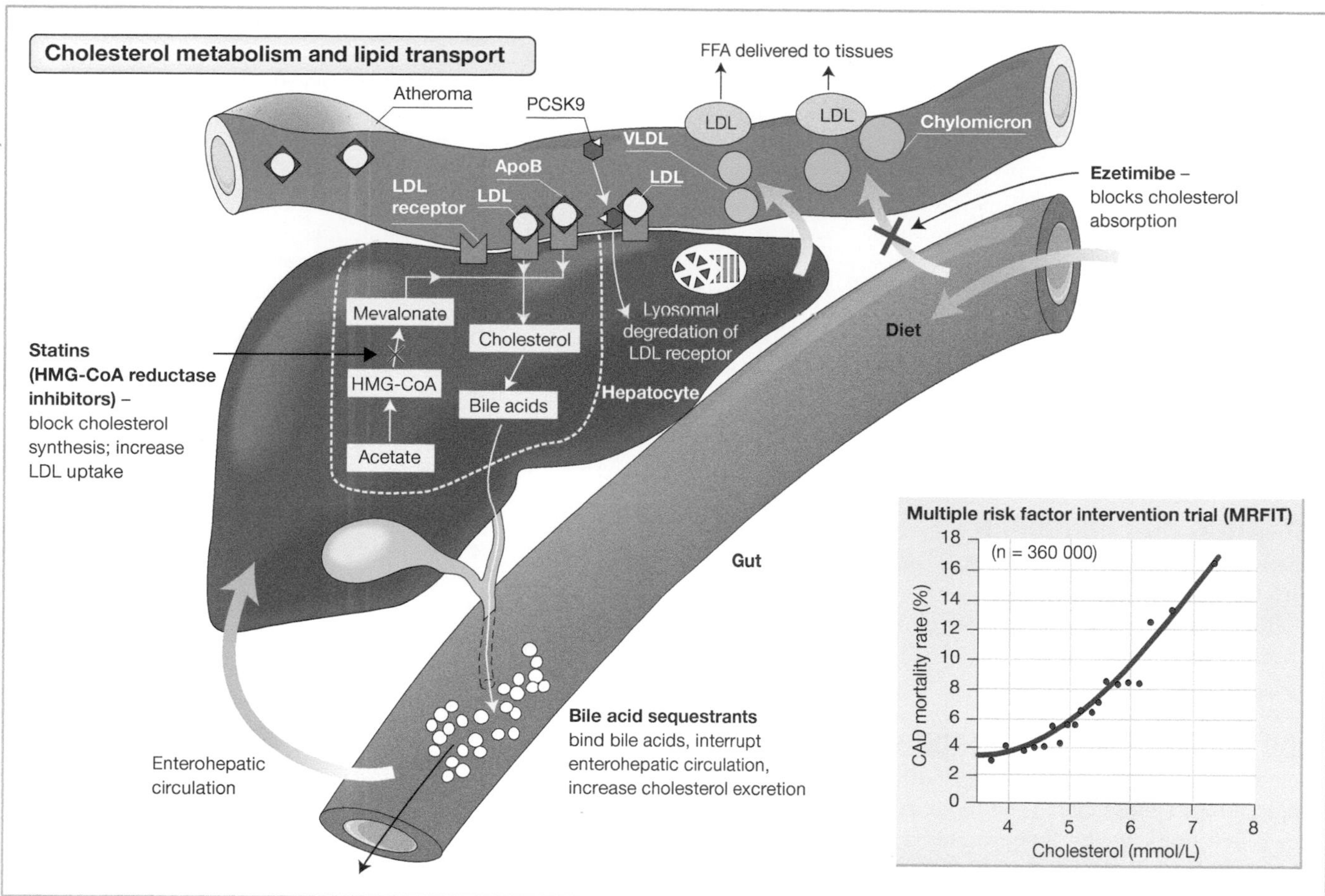

Medicine at a Glance, Fifth Edition. Edited by Patrick Davey and Alex Pitcher.

Companion website: www.wiley.com/go/medicine5e

Table 82.1 Composition and function of lipoproteins and apoproteins

	Composition	Function	Major apoproteins
Chylomicrons	Rich in triglyceride (85%) Very large particle (200–500 nm) with low density Very little protein (2%)	Transports lipid from the gut to the liver in the postprandial state	**ApoCII**: activator of lipoprotein lipase enzyme that breaks down triglycerides for delivery to tissues **ApoE** (see below)
VLDL	Rich in triglyceride Size 50–80 nm	Transports lipid from the liver to the tissues	**ApoCII** (see above) **ApoB$_{100}$** **ApoE**: binds to ApoE receptors on hepatocytes, mediates uptake of lipoprotein remnants after catabolism
LDL	Rich in cholesterol Size 20 nm	Produced by catabolism of VLDL, via intermediate-density lipoprotein. Taken up by liver	**ApoB$_{100}$**: the ligand for the LDL receptor on hepatocytes; mediates uptake of LDL **ApoE** (see above)
HDL	Smallest (8 nm) and most dense lipoprotein >50% protein	Carries cholesterol esters back to the liver from tissues and other lipoproteins ('reverse cholesterol transport')	**ApoAI**: activates LCAT enzyme that esterifies cholesterol

Definition and incidence

Hyperlipidaemia is defined as elevated levels of cholesterol and/or triglycerides. Hypercholesterolaemia is common: ≥60% of the UK population have a total cholesterol >5.2 mmol/L and 3% >7.5 mmol/L.

Lipid metabolism and lipoproteins

Cholesterol and triglycerides are transported in the bloodstream complexed with phospholipid and proteins (**apoproteins**) in particles called **lipoproteins. Apoproteins** act as signalling molecules or enzymes and play very important roles in controlling lipid transport. The different classes of lipoproteins transport lipids between different tissues and are defined by characteristic compositions of lipids and apoproteins (see Table 82.1). Cholesterol is principally metabolized in the liver. Blood levels are controlled by the balance between blood uptake, cholesterol production (activity of cholesterol biosynthetic pathway) and gastrointestinal (GI) excretion (bile acids).

Secondary hyperlipidaemias

Before deciding whether a hyperlipidaemia is primary, diseases producing secondary hyperlipidaemias should be excluded.

- Diabetes.
- Hypothyroidism.
- Chronic renal failure or nephrotic syndrome.
- Chronic liver disease, especially alcoholic.
- Chronic biliary obstruction.
- Drugs: steroids, oestrogens.

Genetic hyperlipidaemias

Single gene defects in lipid metabolism causing extreme hyperlipidaemias are rare. However, common genetic variability or heterozygote status is a very important determinant of cholesterol levels in the general population.

- **Familial hypercholesterolaemia**: a group of single gene disorders affecting the low-density lipoprotein (LDL) receptor and causing deficient or absent uptake of LDL particles, which therefore accumulate in the bloodstream. Homozygotes (1/1 000 000) have extremely high cholesterol levels (10–25 mmol/L) and coronary artery disease (CAD) in their teens or twenties. Heterozygotes (1/500) have moderately high cholesterol (7–12 mmol/L) and are at risk of premature CAD. Patients may have corneal arcus, xanthelasmas and tendon xanthomas.
- **Polygenetic hypercholesterolaemia and familial combined hyperlipidaemia**: inherited conditions (1/300–600) characterized by moderately elevated cholesterol (7–12 mmol/L) with or without high triglycerides, not caused by a single gene disorder, although in some inheritance is apparently autosomal dominant. Very important cause of increased atherosclerosis risk in the population. Very high triglycerides may cause pancreatitis.
- **Apoprotein E genotype**: genetic variation in the *ApoE* gene results in different isoforms of the ApoE protein. The *ApoE2* isoform binds less avidly to hepatic receptors, resulting in hyperlipidaemia. *ApoE2* homozygotes are uncommon (1/100) but *ApoE2* heterozygotes (15% of the population) appear to have a significantly increased risk of CAD.
- **Lipoprotein lipase deficiency and ApoCII deficiency**: extremely rare. There are very elevated chylomicrons, eruptive xanthomas, hepatomegaly and pancreatitis.
- Conversely, mutations in genes including *PCSK9* and *ANGPTL3* have been identified and result in *low* levels of cholesterol and hypolipidaemia and can therefore be targeted with new therapies.

Lipids in atherosclerosis

Studies have identified elevated plasma cholesterol as an important risk factor for the development of CAD.

- Total cholesterol >6.5 mmol/L doubles the risk of lethal CAD; >7.8 mmol/L increases the risk four-fold.
- Reducing total cholesterol by 20% reduces the coronary risk by 10%.

● The strongest association is with LDL cholesterol, whereas high-density lipoprotein (HDL) cholesterol is protective. The Total Cholesterol:HDL cholesterol ratio is a useful indicator, a ratio of >4 indicating high risk. The greater the LDL reduction, the greater the reduction in cardiovascular risk.

Elevated cholesterol (especially oxidized LDL) damages the endothelium early in atherosclerosis and is taken up into the lipid core of established plaques by macrophages (foam cells). Lowering LDL cholesterol reduces cholesterol deposition into atherosclerotic plaques and may reverse this process. Crucially, cholesterol lowering stabilizes plaques, reducing the risk of acute plaque rupture.

Lipid lowering and risk factor modification

● **Lipid lowering by diet**: reducing fat intake, especially high cholesterol foods (red meat, eggs, high-fat diet, dairy products), lowers cholesterol by 1 mmol/L and reduces body weight. However, diet alone is *insufficient* in patients with elevated cholesterol and CAD.

● **Lipid-lowering drugs**: should be strongly recommended to essentially all patients who have established cardiovascular disease such as a myocardial infarction, ischaemic stroke/TIA or peripheral vascular disease (*secondary* prevention). High-dose, high-intensity statins are used to target an LDL-C goal of <1.4 mmol/L. For *primary* prevention, lipid-lowering therapy is generally recommended to those with a 10% or greater risk of developing cardiovascular disease over the next 10 years (which can be estimated using a scoring system such as QRISK3).

1 **HMG-CoA reductase inhibitors ('statins', e.g. atorvastatin, rosuvastatin, simvastatin)**: these are potent agents that inhibit hydroxymethylglutaryl coenzyme (HMG-CoA) reductase, the rate-limiting enzyme in cholesterol biosynthesis. This increases hepatic cholesterol uptake because reduced intracellular cholesterol biosynthesis increases expression of cell surface LDL receptors. For this reason, they may be less effective in patients with familial hypercholesterolaemia. Statins typically lower LDL cholesterol by 30% or more, and may modestly increase HDL cholesterol. They have relatively little effect on plasma triglycerides.

2 Large intervention trials (e.g. 4S, WOSCOPS, CARE, LIPID, Heart Protection Study) show that cholesterol lowering with statins significantly reduces the subsequent incidence of coronary events. The benefits are apparent within months, implying that changes in the composition of atherosclerotic plaques occur rapidly. Angiographic and intravascular imaging studies also show that statins can result in regression of established atheroma.

3 **Cholesterol absorption inhibitors**: ezetimibe inhibits intestinal uptake of dietary and biliary cholesterol. As a result, the liver increases clearance of LDL from the blood.

4 **Fibric acid derivatives ('fibrates', e.g. bezafibrate, fenofibrate)**: these agents reduce cholesterol moderately, but also reduce triglycerides and increase HDL cholesterol. The mechanism of action is complex but involves stimulation of lipoprotein lipase activity (increases chylomicrons and very low-density lipoprotein [VLDL] catabolism) and increased cholesterol excretion via bile acids. They are more useful in patients with mixed hyperlipidaemia and/or low HDL.

5 **PCSK9 inhibitors (alirocumab; evolocumab)** are administered subcutaneously and are an option for treating primary non-familial hypercholesterolaemia or mixed dyslipidaemia where there is either high or very high cardiovascular risk *and* LDL-C greater than 4.0 mmol/L or 3.5 mmol/L respectively. Longer acting agents targeting PCSK9 production using RNA silencing technology (e.g. inclisiran), are now available, and can lower LDL by about half, for over 6 months after a single subcutaneous injection.

6 **Bile acid sequestrants, e.g. cholestyramine**: these lower cholesterol by binding cholesterol in the GI tract, interrupting the enterohepatic circulation and so increasing cholesterol excretion. They have an unpleasant taste and may have intolerable GI side-effects. They can be effective and remain useful in familial hypercholesterolaemia.

Multiple risk factor modification

Lipid lowering represents only one aspect of reducing coronary risk and needs to be considered in the context of the whole coronary risk factor profile for that individual patient. Aggressive lipid lowering is more important in patients who already have an adverse risk factor profile (diabetes, hypertension, smoking) because *multiple risk factors are synergistic in increasing coronary risk*. In contrast, isolated mild hypercholesterolaemia in a patient without other risk factors could be managed by dietary intervention.

83 Acute coronary syndromes

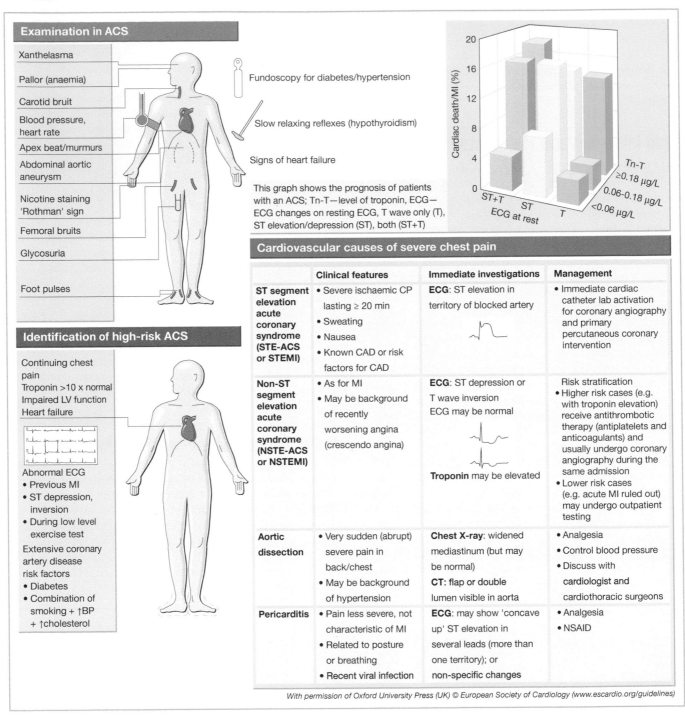

Examination in ACS

Xanthelasma
Pallor (anaemia)
Carotid bruit
Blood pressure, heart rate
Apex beat/murmurs
Abdominal aortic aneurysm
Nicotine staining 'Rothman' sign
Femoral bruits
Glycosuria
Foot pulses
Fundoscopy for diabetes/hypertension
Slow relaxing reflexes (hypothyroidism)
Signs of heart failure

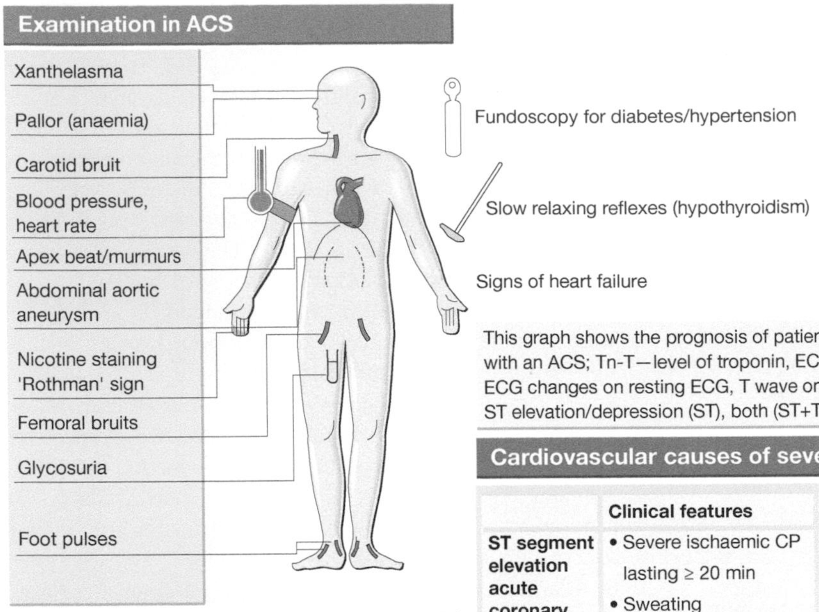

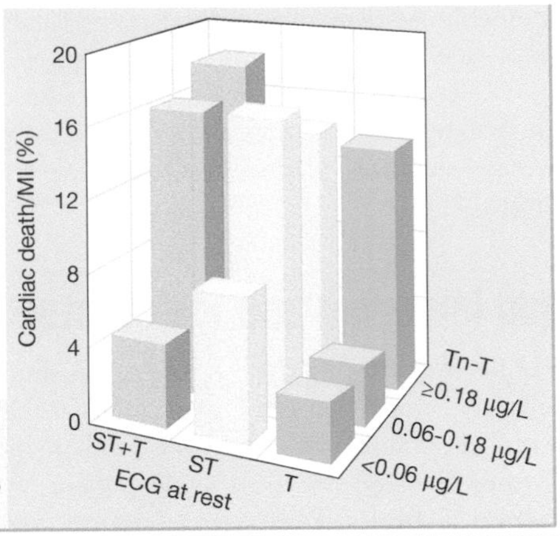

This graph shows the prognosis of patients with an ACS; Tn-T—level of troponin, ECG—ECG changes on resting ECG, T wave only (T), ST elevation/depression (ST), both (ST+T)

Cardiac death/MI (%)
0
4
8
12
16
20
ST+T
ST
T
ECG at rest
Tn-T
≥0.18 μg/L
0.06-0.18 μg/L
<0.06 μg/L

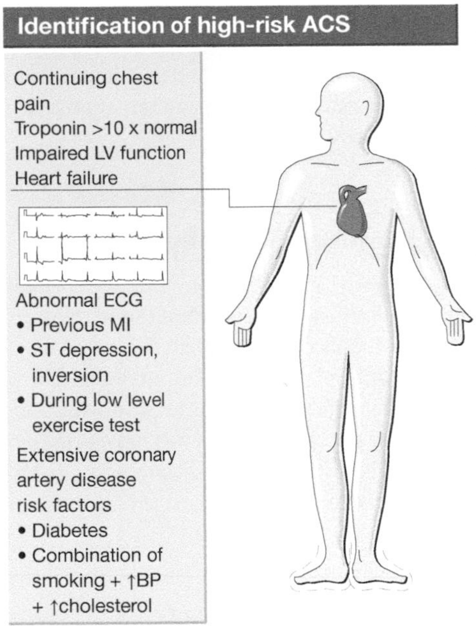

Identification of high-risk ACS

Continuing chest pain
Troponin >10 x normal
Impaired LV function
Heart failure
Abnormal ECG
• Previous MI
• ST depression, inversion
• During low level exercise test
Extensive coronary artery disease
risk factors
• Diabetes
• Combination of smoking + ↑BP + ↑cholesterol

Cardiovascular causes of severe chest pain

	Clinical features	Immediate investigations	Management
ST segment elevation acute coronary syndrome (STE-ACS or STEMI)	• Severe ischaemic CP lasting ≥ 20 min • Sweating • Nausea • Known CAD or risk factors for CAD	**ECG**: ST elevation in territory of blocked artery	• Immediate cardiac catheter lab activation for coronary angiography and primary percutaneous coronary intervention
Non-ST segment elevation acute coronary syndrome (NSTE-ACS or NSTEMI)	• As for MI • May be background of recently worsening angina (crescendo angina)	**ECG**: ST depression or T wave inversion ECG may be normal **Troponin** may be elevated	Risk stratification • Higher risk cases (e.g. with troponin elevation) receive antithrombotic therapy (antiplatelets and anticoagulants) and usually undergo coronary angiography during the same admission • Lower risk cases (e.g. acute MI ruled out) may undergo outpatient testing
Aortic dissection	• Very sudden (abrupt) severe pain in back/chest • May be background of hypertension	**Chest X-ray**: widened mediastinum (but may be normal) **CT:** flap or double lumen visible in aorta	• Analgesia • Control blood pressure • Discuss with cardiologist and cardiothoracic surgeons
Pericarditis	• Pain less severe, not characteristic of MI • Related to posture or breathing • Recent viral infection	**ECG**: may show 'concave up' ST elevation in several leads (more than one territory); or non-specific changes	• Analgesia • NSAID

With permission of Oxford University Press (UK) © European Society of Cardiology (www.escardio.org/guidelines)

Medicine at a Glance, Fifth Edition. Edited by Patrick Davey and Alex Pitcher.

Companion website: www.wiley.com/go/medicine5e

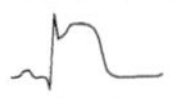

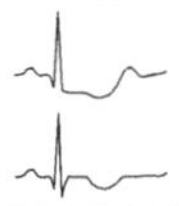

Figure 83.1 Central illustration. ACS, acute coronary syndrome; CABG, coronary artery bypass grafting; ECG, electrocardiogram; LMWH, low molecularweight heparin; NSTE-ACS, non-ST-elevation acute coronary syndrome; PCI, percutaneous coronary intervention; PPCI, primary percutaneous coronary intervention; STEMI, ST-elevation myocardial infarction; UFH, unfractionated heparin. Patients with acute coronary syndrome (ACS) can initially present with a wide variety of clinical signs and symptoms and it is important that there is a high degree of awareness of this amongst both the general public and healthcare providers. If ACS is suspected, think 'A.C.S.' for the initial triage and assessment. This involves performing an electrocardiogram (ECG) to assess for **A**bnormalities or evidence of ischaemia, taking a targeted clinical history to assess the clinical **C**ontext of the presentation, and carrying out a targeted clinical examination to assess for clinical and haemodynamic **S**tability. Based on the initial assessment, the healthcare provider can decide whether immediate invasive management is required. Patients with ST-elevation myocardial infarction (STEMI) require primary percutaneous coronary intervention (PPCI) (or fibrinolysis if PPCI within 120 min is not feasible); patients with non-ST-elevation ACS (NSTE-ACS) with very high-risk features require immediate angiography ± PCI if indicated; patients with NSTE-ACS and high-risk features should undergo inpatient angiography (angiography within 24 h should be considered). A combination of antiplatelet and anticoagulant therapy is indicated acutely for patients with ACS. The majority of patients with ACS will eventually undergo revascularization, most commonly with PCI. Once the final diagnosis of ACS has been established, it is important to implement measures to prevent recurrent events and to optimize cardiovascular risk. This consists of medical therapy, lifestyle changes and cardiac rehabilitation, as well as consideration of psychosocial factors.

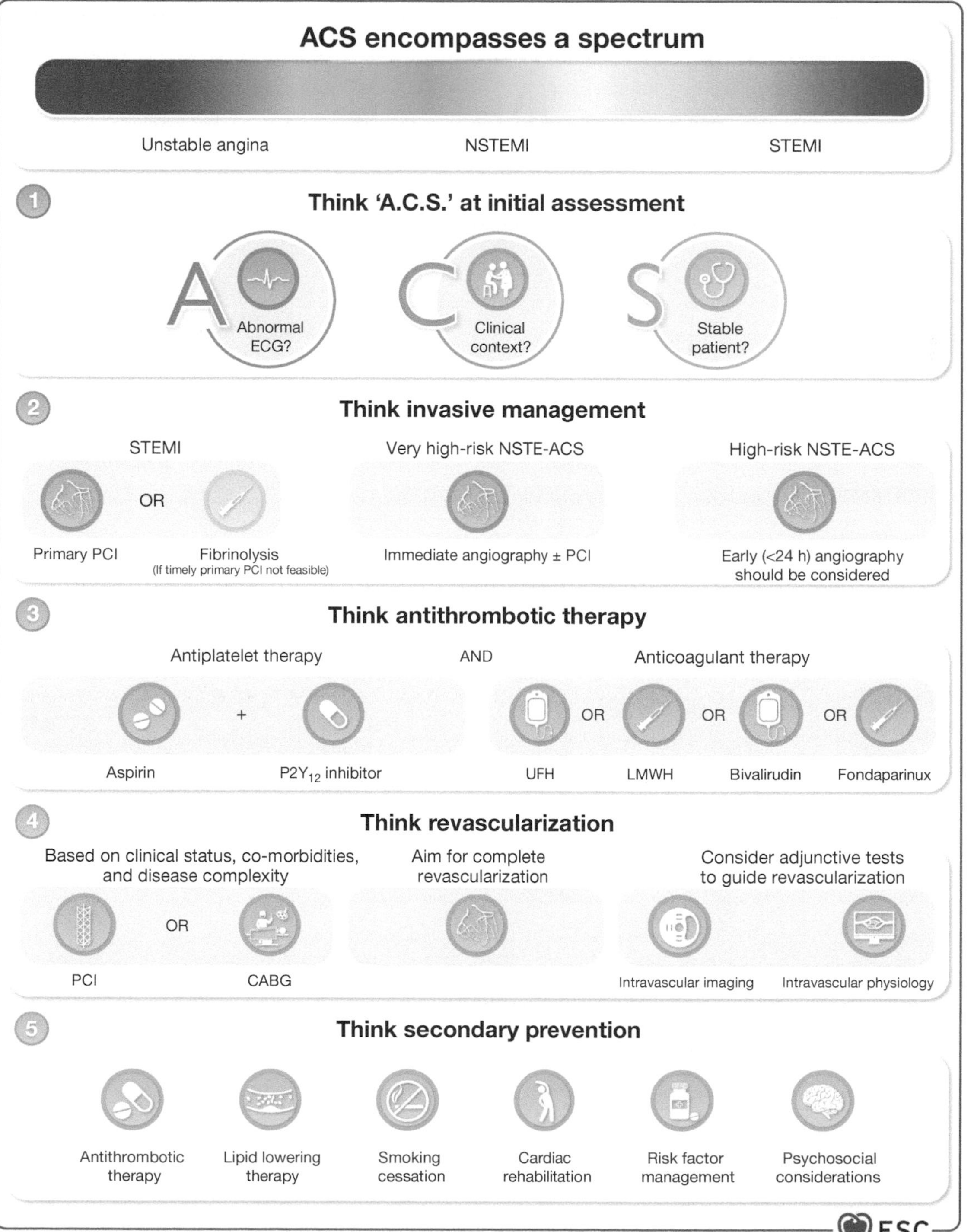

Figure 83.2 The spectrum of clinical presentations, electrocardiographic findings, and high-sensitivity cardiac troponin levels in patients with acute coronary syndrome. ACS, acute coronary syndrome; ECG, electrocardiogram; hs-cTn, high-sensitivity cardiac troponin; NSTE-ACS, non-ST-elevation acute coronary syndrome; NSTEMI, non-ST-elevation myocardial infarction; STEMI, ST-elevation myocardial infarction.

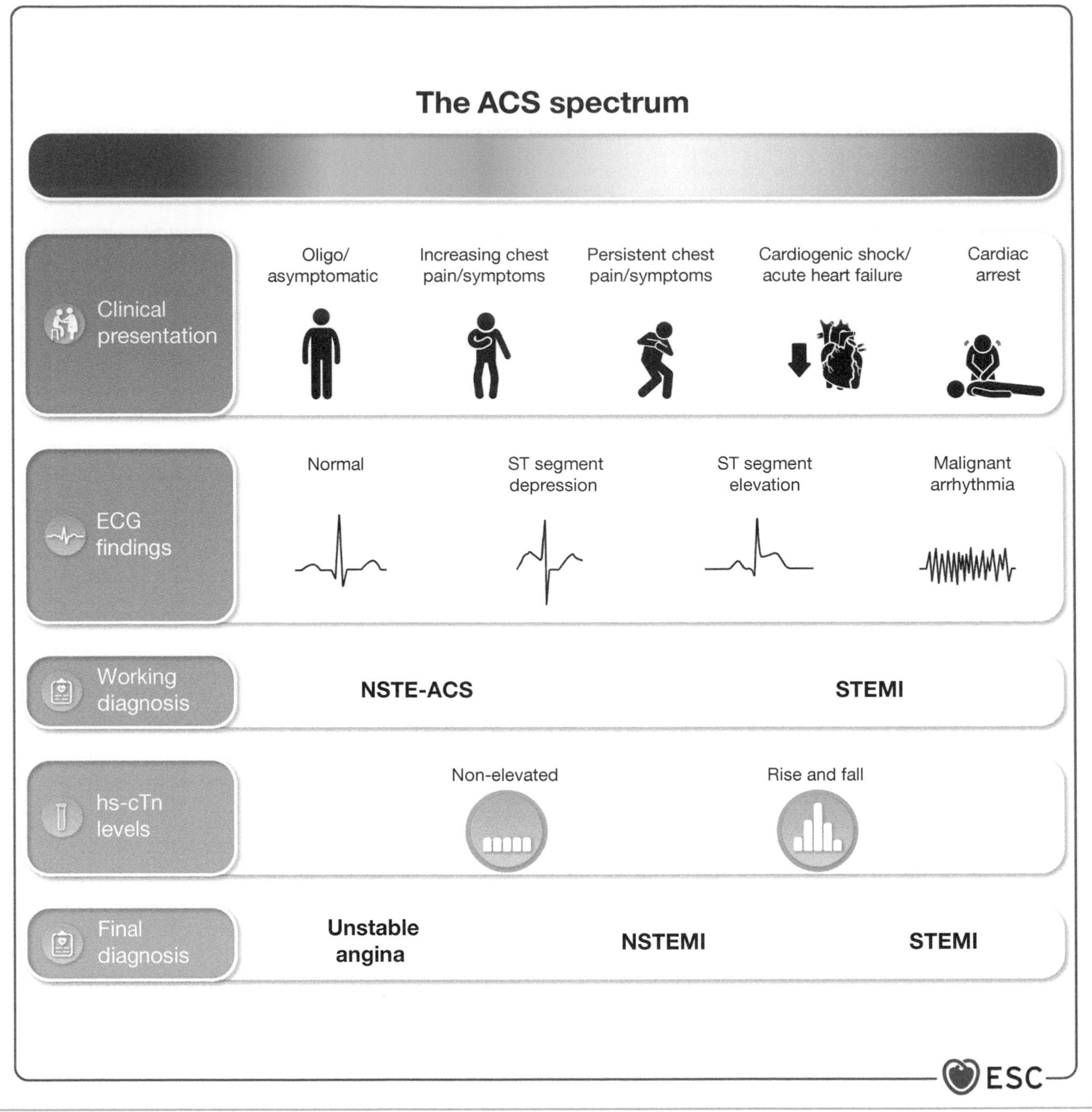

Acute chest pain is a common presentation in the emergency department and accounts for 10% of medical patients. Management aims to separate out, and treat early, patients with high-risk acute coronary syndromes (ACSs) including acute myocardial infarction (MI), be it ST segment elevation myocardial infarction (STEMI) (see Chapter 84) or non-ST segment elevation myocardial infarction (non-STEMI) from other life-threatening diagnoses such as aortic dissection and from less life-threatening causes of pain such as pericarditis or gastro-oesophageal pain.

General approach

The initial assessment of the patient should enable a diagnosis or differential diagnosis that guides immediate management and enables administration of emergency treatment with as little delay as possible. Rapid clinical assessment by history and examination is combined with simple investigations such as electrocardiogram (ECG) and chest X-ray.

Diagnosis of myocardial ischaemia

Myocardial ischaemia is presumptively diagnosed when a patient at risk of coronary disease experiences:

- tight retrosternal chest pain, especially if it is severe. Radiation into the neck, or down the left arm, increases the probability of MI
- pains occurring for >4 weeks with a strong relationship to exercise. However, if pains are present for <2 weeks, often (surprisingly) there is no/little relationship with effort
- pains felt during a previous *unambiguous* episode of MI being similar to the current pains.

If multiple episodes of pain are present over several weeks, they should each be of short duration (i.e. <20–30 min). If they are of longer duration, then almost always if they are due to myocardial ischaemia, infarction will have occurred, and leave easily picked up diagnostic clues such as abnormalities on the resting ECG and/or a raised troponin. Put another way, if a patient presents with multiple recent episodes of prolonged chest pain and the ECG is normal and the troponin is not raised, then myocardial ischaemia becomes less likely.

Differential diagnosis of myocardial ischaemia

The differential diagnosis is broad, and must always be fully considered quickly (see Chapter 13). In essence, all possible causes of chest pain must be evaluated; if you do not, you may miss important disease processes and so fail to treat them. If you assume all chest pain with ST elevation is due to acute thrombotic occlusion of a coronary artery leading to MI, you will miss the cases where coronary occlusion is due to an aortic dissection (and if you miss this diagnosis, you will order the wrong tests at the wrong time and also give potent antiplatelet therapy inappropriately). You will also miss the cases where chest pain is due to perimyocarditis, and cases where chest pain relates to cocaine. All of these have specific treatments, which differ radically from the other.

With chest pain, always ask what is going on, and what pathology is driving the process. Do not assume that only ACSs can produce ECG changes, or that the only cause of an elevated troponin level is an ACS (see Chapter 13), and always consider a broad differential diagnosis. Always test your possible diagnosis against the data you have available on the patient, be it the demographics, the exact symptoms or the easily obtainable investigatory data.

If at the end of this process you are still in doubt about the diagnosis, first ask yourself the question whether greater clarity would change your approach to management. If it would not (e.g. very frail patient with advanced dementia), then stop investigating. If greater clarity would change management, do the one test that provides you with the answer; in suspected ACS, this will often be a coronary angiogram.

Physical examination

This is often unrevealing, but may show evidence of risk factors (nicotine-stained hands, cholesterol deposits around the eyes, hypertension, vascular disease elsewhere) or complications (arrhythmias, heart failure), or suggest other diagnoses. On top of the routine cardiovascular examination, always feel for all pulses (occasionally absent pulses may point to the rare diagnosis of aortic dissection) and measure oxygen saturations (low Po_2 is most commonly due to heart failure, but may reflect chronic obstructive pulmonary disease or be the only sign that a pulmonary embolism [PE] is present).

Investigations

The important investigations early on in suspected MI are as follows.

- **ECGs** repeated whenever there is chest pain, and in any case frequently whilst in hospital. An ECG should be repeated whenever there is chest pain, as an ACS may at any time evolve into a STEMI, requiring immediate reperfusion therapy (using percutaneous coronary intervention [PCI]). Make sure that you know how to read an ECG.
- **Biomarkers** of myocardial necrosis. A variety of troponin assays exist; modern assays are highly sensitive and can even detect low circulating levels of troponin in many healthy people. Be aware that there are many causes of a rise in troponin, only one of which is an ACS (see Table 83.1). It is often helpful to repeat a

Table 83.1 Possible non-acute coronary syndrome causes of troponin elevation. Bold indicates important differential diagnoses

- **Chronic or acute renal dysfunction**
- Severe congestive **heart failure** – acute and chronic
- **Hypertensive crisis**
- **Tachy- or bradyarrhythmias**
- **Pulmonary embolism**, severe pulmonary hypertension
- Inflammatory diseases, e.g. **myocarditis**
- Acute neurological disease, including **stroke** or subarachnoid haemorrhage
- Aortic dissection, aortic valve disease or hypertrophic cardiomyopathy
- Cardiac contusion, ablation, pacing, cardioversion or endomyocardial biopsy
- Hypothyroidism
- Apical ballooning syndrome (Takotsubo cardiomyopathy)
- Infiltrative diseases, e.g. amyloidosis, haemochromatosis, sarcoidosis, scleroderma
- Drug toxicity, e.g. Adriamycin, 5-fluorouracil, herceptin, snake venoms
- Burns, if affecting >30% of body surface area
- Rhabdomyolysis
- Critically ill patients, especially with respiratory failure or sepsis

Source: Hamm et al. 2011. With permission of Oxford University Press (UK) © European Society of Cardiology (www.escardio.org/guidelines).

negative or borderline troponin test in order to establish whether there has been a rise or fall to suggest a recent ACS.

- **Chest X-ray** (CXR) to evaluate for alternative pathologies and complicating heart failure. This should be done in most patients at presentation but should not delay emergency angiography in STEMI. In these patients, the CXR should be done immediately following the PCI procedure.
- **Haemoglobin**: anaemia is a common provocotant of myocardial ischaemia, and if the patient is anaemic, ask why (cancer, gastrointestinal [GI] bleeding, haematinic deficiency, primary bone marrow problem, etc.) and in particular, might antiplatelet therapy exacerbate the anaemia (e.g. if it is due to GI bleeding from peptic ulceration)?
- **Lipid profile** (on admission, because acute MI artefactually lowers cholesterol from days to months afterwards), triglycerides and glucose.
- **Renal function** as many patients will require CT or invasive angiography.

Acute coronary syndromes including acute STEMI

The common pathology underlying acute coronary events is the rupture or erosion of a coronary artery plaque, leading to intracoronary thrombosis. The resulting clinical syndrome depends on whether the coronary artery has occluded (usually but not always producing an ECG showing STEMI), or whether it is only partially or transiently (<20 min at a time) occluded (non-STEMI).

Damage to the heart can result from the occlusion itself. However, even if the occlusion is not complete, myocardial necrosis can still result from thrombus embolizing down the coronary artery, infarcting distal tissue. So, there are several forms of ACS defined by the ECG and troponin (see Table 83.2).

- **ST elevation MI (STEMI)**: here the ECG shows ST segment elevation, and the troponin is elevated. Therapy to reopen the occluded artery is time-critical and aims to minimize loss of myocytes and reduce the risk of arrhythmia and heart failure, and is discussed further in Chapter 84. STEMI is diagnosed from the history, and ECG and troponin testing should not delay treatment.
- **Non-ST elevation MI (non-STEMI)**: by definition, there must be a troponin rise. Almost any ECG change can occur, the most common being ST depression/T wave inversion, though transient self-terminating ST elevation can also occur. True troponin-negative ACS is rare in the era of highly sensitive troponin assays.

Table 83.2 Quick guide to acute coronary syndromes

ECG	Troponin	ACS diagnosis[a]
ST elevation	+ to +++	STEMI
No ST elevation (other repolarization changes may occur)	+	Non-STEMI
No ST elevation (other repolarization changes may occur)	No rise or trivial rise	Unstable angina/ troponin –ve ACS

[a] There is a differential diagnosis for all these ECG/troponin combinations, and only the ACS component is given here.

Immediate treatment of ACS

Patients with STEMI are at high risk of early adverse events (see Chapter 84 for MI complications, which are the same for STEMI and non-STEMI), and so constitute a medical emergency requiring immediate treatment followed by close monitoring on a cardiology unit. Many health systems will divert STEMI patients directly to cardiac catheter laboratories. In contrast, NSTEMI patients do not generally require immediate angiography and PCI unless there is ongoing chest pain, dynamic ECG change or other very high-risk features. Most NSTEMI patients benefit from:

- dual antiplatelet therapy: aspirin (chewed), and one of clopidogrel, prasugrel or ticagrelor according to local protocols
- subcutaneous low molecular weight (LMW) heparin or fondaparinux
- high-dose statin therapy (such as atorvastatin 80 mg od)
- ACE inhibitors and β-blockers are also often begun in hospital, depending upon LV function.

Patients with lower risk chest pain in whom MI has been excluded are sometimes evaluated with non-invasive testing (CT coronary angiography or functional tests) on an outpatient basis.

Immediate treatment of suspected ACS

This is a common problem – you think your patient may have an ACS, but for various reasons you are not sure. What should you do? As in all diagnostic dilemmas – and these are very common in acute medicine – first, do no harm; second, try and clarify the situation as soon as possible using the highest yield tests; third, always consider the differential diagnosis. Once you have done so, treat the most likely diagnosis in the standard fashion, and if possible the most likely dangerous cause, always bearing in mind that treatment for one condition may exacerbate another.

In patients with suspected but not confirmed ACS who are at low bleeding risk, the balance of risks and benefits usually favours early administration of antiplatelets whilst additional biomarker testing is performed. In patients with higher bleeding risk, it may be preferable to await biomarker/imaging results before beginning treatment and individualizing the choice of second antiplatelet agent if ACS is confirmed (bleeding risk with clopidogrel is probably lower than for prasugrel/ticagrelor). Some patients with acute aortic dissection are misdiagnosed with ACS and inappropriately receive antiplatelets and anticoagulants, further increasing the risk of fatal haemorrhage and intraoperative complication. Ultrasound and CT may be helpful complementary investigations where available quickly.

There is an almost endless combination of actual and possible diagnoses in chest pain, particularly in the ageing population, and you will have to tailor your approach to the individual. However, the basic principle always remains the same: if more data would change your approach, get the data.

Risk stratification of ACSs

After immediate medical management, further investigation and treatment are determined by the risk of further cardiac events. Factors associated with higher risk include:

- ST segment depression on the presentation ECG or dynamic ST changes later

- elevated troponin levels
- recurrent episodes of chest pain
- diabetes, previous MI, impaired left ventricular (LV) function, heart failure.

Higher risk patients undergo early **cardiac catheterization**, as many have unstable coronary lesions which benefit from PCI, or severe multivessel coronary artery disease needing coronary artery bypass graft (CABG) surgery. Acute coronary syndromes differ from stable angina in that treatment of culprit coronary lesions improves clinical outcomes, principally by reducing the risk of myocardial infarction.

In addition to medical therapy and revascularization, ACS patients should have aggressive antiatherogenic risk factor management.

- Lifestyle changes: no smoking, regular exercise, ideal weight, modest alcohol intake. None of these are easy to do. Doctors must, sympathetically, emphasize the harm that cigarettes do, and should offer nicotine replacement therapy. Exercise should be for a minimum of 20 minutes cardiovascular exercise sufficiently intense to induce some breathlessness at least three times a week. There are no easy approaches to weight reduction; however, if patients have class III obesity (body mass index >40 kg/m^2) after recovery from the MI, bariatric surgery may have a role. In most overweight patients, a sympathetic approach, with an understanding that these patients will need considerable support (e.g. as provided by weight loss organizations), is appropriate. Alcohol should be in the 14–21 units per week range for men, and 7–14 for women.
- Cholesterol reduction is with high-intensity statins at high dose. Additional therapies (ezetimibe, PCSK9 inhibitors and other emerging options) may be required in patients not reaching target lipid levels at the best tolerated dose of statins.
- Blood pressure (BP) reduced to a target <140/80 mmHg (<130/80 in diabetes or heart failure), using non-pharmacological approaches and drugs as necessary.
- Long-term antiplatelet agents: in troponin-positive ACS, the risk of reinfarction (sometimes leading to death) is greatly increased in the months following an ACS, so a second antiplatelet is added to aspirin for a period of time after an ACS. This is also essential when PCI with drug-eluting stents has been performed.
- Most benefit from angiotensin-converting enzyme inhibitors, even when LV function is not impaired.
- In those with very severely impaired LV function following revascularization and medical therapy, there is a role for device therapy (either implantable cardioverter defibrillators [ICDs] or cardiac resynchronization therapy [CRT] – see Chapter 87).

Coronary angiography

Coronary angiography is the definitive investigation to evaluate and often treat coronary disease. It is not the only possible coronary investigation (see Chapter 85), though it is by far the most commonly used one in ACS, where a complete assessment of coronary anatomy is needed, along with the option to treat using PCI in appropriate cases.

How coronary angiography is performed

Coronary angiography involves passing a catheter (a small-calibre, long, flexible plastic tube, about 90–120 cm or so long) through a peripheral artery (preferably the radial or sometimes the femoral artery) into the ascending aorta, and then manipulating the catheter so its end sits just in the mouth of the coronary artery. Radio-opaque contrast is injected into the artery (about 2–8 ml over 3–4 s) and an X-ray is taken. These X-rays pass through all the thoracic structures to a greater or lesser extent, but not through any of the contrast contained within the artery. The pictures obtained are therefore a negative image of the lumen of the artery, and any obstruction or occlusion can be seen, as can the general state of the coronary arteries.

The procedure takes about 20 minutes, and takes place in a specially constructed and sterile X-ray room, usually one whose sole purpose is the study of coronary arteries. Patients lie flat on the X-ray table, and may be given intravenous sedation (usually a diazepam-type drug, though if the patient is very anxious, sick or in pain, an opiate is used). They are covered in sterile drapes, local anaesthetic is injected over the artery to be entered, and an arterial sheath placed within the artery using a standard Seldinger technique. A small guidewire (a 'J' wire) is passed through the sheath to the ascending aorta, and over this the diagnostic catheter is passed, to the coronaries, as above.

Indications

The major indication for coronary angiography is the diagnosis and treatment of acute coronary syndromes. Non-invasive testing is usually performed initially in chronic coronary syndromes, with coronary angiography reserved for patients with high-risk features (e.g. significant disease of the left main coronary artery) or symptoms refractory to antianginal therapy.

Benefits

Benefits of coronary angiography include a better understanding of the coronary anatomy, which may lead to interventions that reduce the risk of MI and prolong life (in ACS and in those with some forms of very severe coronary disease) and that may also relieve symptoms. Some interventions relieve symptoms but do not reduce the risk of death or MI (e.g. PCI in most cases of chronic stable angina).

Risks

Risks of coronary angiography include heart attack, stroke, renal failure (usually from the contrast in those with pre-existing impaired renal function) and bleeding, usually but not exclusively around the access site (there is a higher risk of a major bleed with the femoral approach and the radial approach is preferred where possible). Any of these severe complications can lead to death. The overall chance of a severe complication is around 1 in 1000, higher in the elderly, those with diabetes or those with renal failure.

Invasive cardiac assessment beyond coronary angiography

Invasive coronary angiography generally provides an excellent assessment of coronary anatomy and disease. Sometimes, additional invasive diagnostic techniques provide additional information and optimize therapy.

- **Fractional flow reserve** is a technique in which a small pressure probe, attached to a tiny wire, is passed down the coronary artery beyond the narrowing to be investigated. The pressure drop over the narrowing is measured, first at rest, then when coronary arterial dilation (and so increased coronary blood flow) is provoked using the coronary vasodilator adenosine. The pressure before (from the catheter tip) and after the narrowing is measured – more haemodynamically significant stenoses result in a greater pressure drop during stress. Treating lesions with a greater degree of haemodynamic significance is probably more likely to lead to greater improvement in symptoms following PCI.

- **Intracoronary imaging (intravascular ultrasound/optical coherence tomography** [OCT]) refers to a range of techniques where very small imaging probes (ultrasound or OCT) are placed on a guidewire into the coronary artery, allowing three-dimensional imaging of the lumen of the artery. It can be very useful to define lesion characteristics, evaluate for other pathology such as coronary dissection and optimize stent deployment.

Percutaneous coronary intervention

Percutaneous coronary intervention involves passing an angioplasty balloon over a fine guidewire previously steered down the artery and across a coronary lesion. Inflating the balloon opens the artery up. **Stents** are inserted to help maintain short- and long-term patency (i.e. to lessen restenosis). The large majority of unstable coronary lesions can be treated with PCI, with CABG generally reserved for complex coronary disease, often in the context of diabetes.

Restenosis of the stented artery can occur from six weeks onwards to about one year following PCI. Intimal hyperplasia (a process switched on by balloon injury to the vessel wall, and going on for up to a year) impinges on the lumen of the artery sufficient to produce recurrent angina in 10–20% of patients, and is termed 'restenosis'. Further PCI (especially with drug-eluting stents) may establish long-term patency. Essentially, all modern PCI is performed using **drug-eluting stents** which greatly reduce the problem of in-stent restenosis by inhibiting vascular smooth muscle cell growth.

Benefits

Percutaneous coronary intervention in STEMI is termed primary PCI (primary indicating the first therapy, as opposed to PCI following thrombolysis, where it could be termed secondary, or for those who do not respond to thrombolysis, termed bail-out PCI). Primary PCI is modestly more effective than thrombolysis in improving prognosis in STEMIs but has a markedly lower risk of intracranial hemorrhage and allows definitive treatment. It is therefore the preferred treatment for most patients with STEMI. PCI in NSTEMI also reduces the risk of myocardial infarction and improves outcomes.

In chronic stable angina, there is unlikely to be any reduction in the subsequent MI rate, and so prognosis is usually unaffected by PCI in this setting, with possible exceptions for those very few patients who have a tight narrowing in a very large artery (such as the left main stem) proximally, with a lot of still viable tissue beyond the narrowing. The primary indication is therefore for the relief of angina that cannot be adequately controlled with medical therapy. However, the situation changes in unstable coronary syndromes, where PCI does improve prognosis. Those who have the greatest increase in prognosis are those with the most severe expressions of coronary disease, those in cardiogenic shock (early on), those with STEMIs and those with high-risk non-STEMIs.

Risks

The risks of PCI are the same complications as for diagnostic angiography, but the overall rate of a major complication, including causing an MI, is higher. Overall, about 0.5–1% of patients suffer a major complication.

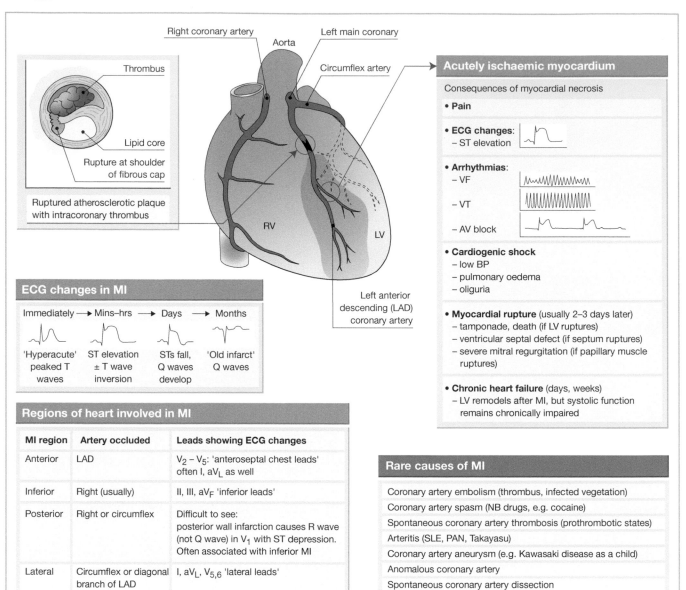

ST segment elevation myocardial infarction

Right coronary artery
Aorta
Left main coronary
Circumflex artery
Thrombus
Lipid core
Rupture at shoulder of fibrous cap
Ruptured atherosclerotic plaque with intracoronary thrombus
RV
LV
Left anterior descending (LAD) coronary artery

Acutely ischaemic myocardium

Consequences of myocardial necrosis

- **Pain**
- **ECG changes**:
  - ST elevation
- **Arrhythmias**:
  - VF
  - VT
  - AV block
- **Cardiogenic shock**
  - low BP
  - pulmonary oedema
  - oliguria
- **Myocardial rupture** (usually 2–3 days later)
  - tamponade, death (if LV ruptures)
  - ventricular septal defect (if septum ruptures)
  - severe mitral regurgitation (if papillary muscle ruptures)
- **Chronic heart failure** (days, weeks)
  - LV remodels after MI, but systolic function remains chronically impaired

ECG changes in MI

Immediately →	Mins–hrs →	Days →	Months
'Hyperacute' peaked T waves	ST elevation ± T wave inversion	STs fall, Q waves develop	'Old infarct' Q waves

Regions of heart involved in MI

MI region	Artery occluded	Leads showing ECG changes
Anterior	LAD	$V_2 - V_5$: 'anteroseptal chest leads' often I, aV_L as well
Inferior	Right (usually)	II, III, aV_F 'inferior leads'
Posterior	Right or circumflex	Difficult to see: posterior wall infarction causes R wave (not Q wave) in V_1 with ST depression. Often associated with inferior MI
Lateral	Circumflex or diagonal branch of LAD	I, aV_L, $V_{5,6}$ 'lateral leads'

Rare causes of MI

- Coronary artery embolism (thrombus, infected vegetation)
- Coronary artery spasm (NB drugs, e.g. cocaine)
- Spontaneous coronary artery thrombosis (prothrombotic states)
- Arteritis (SLE, PAN, Takayasu)
- Coronary artery aneurysm (e.g. Kawasaki disease as a child)
- Anomalous coronary artery
- Spontaneous coronary artery dissection

Medicine at a Glance, Fifth Edition. Edited by Patrick Davey and Alex Pitcher.

Companion website: www.wiley.com/go/medicine5e

Demographics

- **Definition**: ischaemic injury of the myocardium as a result of acute occlusion of a coronary artery. This results in a typical electrocardiogram (ECG), that showing an ST segment elevation myocardial infarction (STEMI). The relevance of separating out STEMI from other forms of myocardial infarction (MI) is that STEMIs benefit from immediate therapy to open the occluded coronary artery (using primary percutaneous coronary intervention [PPCI] or, rarely, fibrinolysis); treatment is time critical. Other forms of MI need immediate *medical* therapy and early but not necessarily immediate angiography (± PCI or coronary artery bypass graft [CABG]).
- **Incidence**: very common; 250 000 MIs per year in the UK (one every 2 min), with 100 000 deaths.
- **Pathogenesis**: an MI occurs when a coronary artery occludes, the myocardium supplied by that artery becomes ischaemic and necrosis occurs over several hours; early restoration of blood flow may abort the infarction and limit necrosis. The overwhelmingly common cause is **atheromatous coronary artery disease** (CAD), when an existing coronary atheromatous plaque (not necessarily one severely narrowing the artery) becomes eroded or ruptures, causing a sudden expansion of the plaque and thrombosis of the coronary artery lumen. Other causes of MI occur very occasionally (see figure).

Clinical features

- **Classic presentation**: severe, crushing central chest pain ≥20 minutes, unrelieved by nitrates, associated with sweating, pallor and nausea. However, as STEMI is common, atypical manifestations are also common; the intensity of the chest pain may be surprisingly mild (or even absent), the location may be atypical (jaw/arm only, unusual place on the chest, such as left shoulder only, etc.). Sometimes patients present only with the autonomic features (sweating, vomiting), or just feeling unwell. As acute coronary syndrome (ACS) accounts for a large proportion of acute medical admissions, if you see a patient in this context and the diagnosis is not immediately apparent, always do an ECG to help rule out a STEMI.
- **Other presentations** include arrhythmia, cardiac arrest or acute heart failure.
- May be atypical in **elderly people** (collapse or confusion) and in those with **diabetes**, who may have no chest pain, and develop worsening of metabolic status or heart failure. Up to one-third of patients with MI are 'silent', that is to say, patients do not recognize their symptoms as being due to something serious and do not present to hospital. Such infarcts only come to light later, either when patients have cardiac imaging carried out for other purposes, or when patients present with late complications of MI, such as heart failure or arrhythmias.
- Most patients have risk factors or known CAD; 50% have no preceding angina (and so 50% do!).

Investigations

Initial investigations (especially the ECG) should quickly establish the diagnosis.

- The diagnostic hallmark of acute MI is ST segment elevation. However, not all ST segment elevation is due to acute STEMI – some is due to old infarction, some to pericarditis, some is physiological, some the consequences of bundle branch block (BBB), hyperkalaemia and rarely Brugada syndrome. The usual clues to ST elevation reflecting STEMI are: (i) the exact nature of the ST elevation (convex upwards); (ii) the regional distribution (reflecting the coronary arteries) and presence of reciprocal ST depression; and (iii) the clinical context. You should become very familiar with the ECG signs of STEMI, and how to exclude other causes. Experienced ECG readers can frequently detect patterns diagnostic of acute coronary occlusion before classic STEMI criteria are met.
- With right BBB, it is usually fairly easy to see if there is an underlying STEMI. STEMI can be more challenging to diagnose with left BBB or in paced rhythms and should therefore be considered whenever there is an appropriate clinical context.
- Eighty percent of patients are subsequently shown to have had an MI present with other ECG changes such as ST depression and T-wave inversion (or no localizing ECG features). These patients are treated with medical therapy initially, but are monitored closely and may still require expedited angiography if high-risk features such as persistent chest pain occur.

Important differential diagnoses to exclude are **acute aortic syndromes** (a wide mediastinum on chest X-ray is regarded as being a classic sign but is of low specificity and sensitivity, loss of pulses, aortic regurgitation) and **pericarditis** (widespread non-specific changes on ECG). **Acute pulmonary embolism** is a common and serious cause of acute chest pain, and is probably the most common condition to be inappropriately diagnosed as an acute MI. Always consider acute pulmonary embolism (PE) in the differential of all chest pain.

Management

Patients with STEMI are usually diagnosed by the emergency first responders (ambulance service) and such patients should be immediately transferred to the primary PCI facility. If the diagnosis is made in the emergency department, likewise, immediate transfer to the catheter laboratory with primary PCI facilities should occur. Patients with non-STEMI or other actual or potential serious cardiac illness should be moved to a coronary care unit (CCU) for monitoring and further assessment.

- Once STEMI is diagnosed, or considered likely, immediate treatment during transfer for emergency angiography includes: (i) antiplatelet drugs (aspirin 300 mg and a second antiplatelet drug according to local procotols, usually ticagrelor or clopidogrel) and (ii) pain relief with opiate analgesia. Supplemental oxygen is no longer routinely recommended unless there is hypoxia (SaO_2 <90%).
- Immediate coronary angioplasty/stenting (**primary PCI**) is the treatment of choice and is time critical.
- Thrombolysis, usually with tissue plasminogen activator (tPA) or related thrombolytics, is an alternative only where rapid primary PCI is not rapidly available.
- Diuretic for pulmonary oedema.
- Angiotensin-converting enzyme (ACE) inhibitor (day 2 or 3), especially if there is clinical heart failure, or significantly impaired left ventricular (LV) function (anterior MI, large enzyme release, impaired left ventricle on echocardiography).

Complications

Rapid reperfusion using primary PCI substantially reduces the risk of major complication from STEMI.

Immediate/hours

- **Ventricular arrhythmias** (ventricular tachycardia [VT] or ventricular fibrillation [VF]) occurring within 24 hours or less are the principal cause of prehospital death. Patients should be monitored close to a defibrillator. Early VT/VF (provided the patient survives) is not associated with a worse long-term outlook.

- **Heart block** most commonly complicates inferior MI, and can usually be reversed by reopening the infarct vessel but may require temporary pacing.
- **Atrial arrhythmias**, especially atrial fibrillation (AF), may compromise cardiac output and need immediate cardioversion or, at the very least, heart rate slowing and heparin. AF is more likely in those with more severe and extensive coronary disease, and so is a marker for a worse prognosis.
- **Failed or delayed reperfusion** is the failure of treatment to re-establish adequate blood flow in the occluded artery. It is diagnosed in the catheter laboratory and may lead to persisting ST elevation. The mechanisms are likely to involve microvascular obstruction, perhaps due to embolizing thrombus, or distal spread of vasoactive substances, and remain a target for therapeutic investigation.

Hours/days

Cardiac rupture into the pericardium is uncommon, but typically occurs on days 2–5 and is commonly fatal. **Heart failure** with pulmonary oedema results from acute impairment of LV function. **Cardiogenic shock** occurs when cardiac output is inadequate to maintain arterial blood pressure (BP), resulting from the following.

- **Severe impairment of LV function**: some heart muscle is irreparably damaged, but some is reversibly stunned and may improve its contractile function, provided the patient can be carried over the acute period. If patients develop cardiogenic shock early on during an MI, immediate angiography is often indicated to reperfuse occluded arteries and in time hopefully improve contractile function and outcome. Mechanical cardiac support may be needed.
- **Infarction of the right ventricle** (usually in inferior MI): in this situation the right heart needs a high (not normal) filling pressure (i.e. right atrial pressure) to operate anywhere like normally. If the filling pressure is normal or low (dehydration from sweating and inadequate fluid intake is common in acute MI), then right heart output falls, causing inadequate left heart filling. Treatment of right ventricular infarction is by diagnosing it (inferior infarct and cardiac ultrasound showing a dilated, poorly functioning right heart with reasonable LV function) and then giving intravenous fluids.
- **Mechanical catastrophe** such as: (i) **ventricular septal rupture**, with a new loud pansystolic murmur at the lower left sternal edge; or (ii) **papillary muscle rupture**, with severe mitral regurgitation; murmur may not be loud, but severe pulmonary oedema is out of proportion to apparent LV damage. Both require *immediate* cardiological assessment with a view to surgical repair.

Days/weeks

- **Chronic heart failure**: LV remodelling after MI may worsen rather than improve LV function. Treat with ACE inhibitors, diuretics, cautious β-blockade and mineralocorticoid receptor antagonists.
- **Ventricular tachycardia**: occurring after 48 hours implies that the myocardial scar is a substrate for re-entrant circuits. β-blockers and amiodarone help but if there is impaired LV function or collapse, the risk of future sudden cardiac death is significant and justifies automatic defibrillator implantation.
- **Dressler syndrome**: usually self-limiting autoimmune pericarditis occurring several weeks after a full-thickness MI. Occasionally requires steroids, more commonly responds to non-steroidal anti-inflammatory drugs.

Prognosis and rehabilitation

The long-term outlook after MI is governed largely by the extent of **LV damage**, and the severity of the underlying **coronary artery disease**. Most post-MI deaths are caused by heart failure, sudden cardiac death or further MI. Secondary prophylaxis to prevent further MI and other vascular events comprises the following aspects.

- **Aspirin** (or another antiplatelet agent such as clopidogrel or ticagrelor), β-blockers and ACE inhibitors.
- **Risk factor modification**: stop smoking, reduce cholesterol (diet and statins and other drugs for lipid management) and treat hypertension and diabetes.
- **Rehabilitation programme** to increase physical exercise, encourage lifestyle changes and provide psychological support.

Risk stratification

Risk stratification requires a full knowledge of cardiac risk factors, cardiac anatomy and functional capacity. Not all data are relevant in everyone, as much risk factor modification is relevant to all – for example, cholesterol reduction with statins improves outlook regardless of whether the starting cholesterol is very high, high or 'average'. Likewise, exercise is good for all, and this must be emphasized. The important aspects of risk stratification and modification are listed below.

- **Lifestyle measures**: smoking must cease, though there is rarely an easy means to achieve this. Likewise, alcohol consumption should be moderate. Regular exercise is vital both to maximize good health and improve prognosis. Achievement of ideal weight is important, both to lessen the atherogenic impact of obesity, which is particularly powerful in the diabetic patient, and to minimize the long-term risk of cancer.
- **Left ventricular function** is a crucial determinant of long-term prognosis, and should be assessed in all patients echocardiographically; this can be done during the MI or, in many, several weeks following the heart attack. Prognosis is worst in those who not only have poor left ventricles but who also have symptoms and signs of heart failure, especially if they have a broad QRS complex on the resting ECG, and ambient complex ventricular arrhythmias on 24-hour ECG recording. Aggressive treatment is with medical therapy, including spironolactone (or the modern equivalent eplerenone), revascularization where appropriate and device therapy, including cardiac resynchronization therapy/implantable cardiovertor defibrillators.
- **Extent of coronary disease**: those with the most extensive coronary disease have the worst outlook, and gain the most from successful revascularization. Most patients with acute STEMI have had angiography performed during the infarct as part of the primary PCI procedure, and so there is knowledge of the extent of bystander coronary disease (that is, coronary narrowings in the non-infarct-related artery). Plans can be made for the most appropriate form of revascularization, be it by further PCI or CABG. All elective revascularization must be discussed beforehand by appropriately constituted multidisciplinary teams including

cardiac surgeons (the 'heart team'). If angiography has not been undertaken acutely, many patients will have this electively, though its benefit must be titrated against risk (highest in the very elderly and those with extensive vascular co-morbidity) and benefit (which is limited in those with other disease processes shortening length and quality of life). However, there is a small cohort of patients who are considered low risk and may not benefit, and this includes: (i) younger patients (increasing age is a powerful adverse risk factor in MI outlook); (ii) completed Q-wave infarct (no further heart muscle to save); (iii) no ongoing symptoms of angina (angina suggests there is a significant volume of heart muscle supplied by a stenosed coronary artery); symptomatology can be tested by an exercise stress test, and evidence of silent myocardial ischaemia can also be sought (silent ischaemia may have the same prognostic significance as symptomatic ischaemia); (iv) no preceding angina (which suggests a plaque event rather than fixed high-grade coronary stenosis); and (v) good left ventricular function.

85 Chronic coronary syndromes

Exercise testing

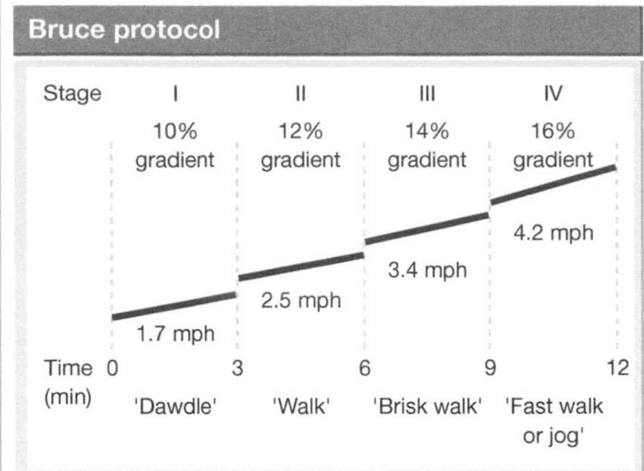

Percutaneous coronary intervention (PCI)

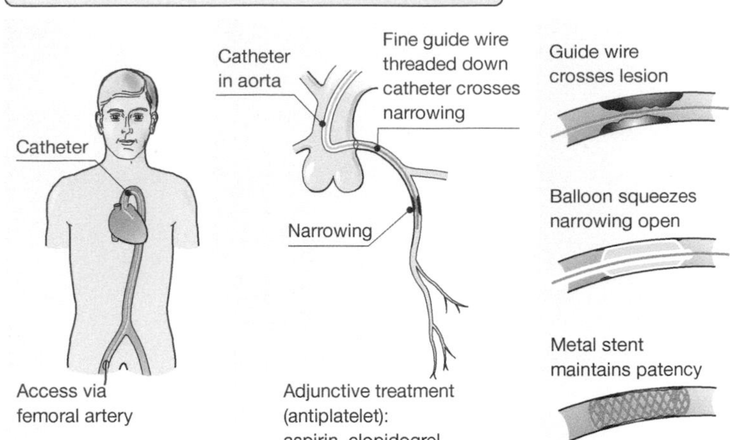

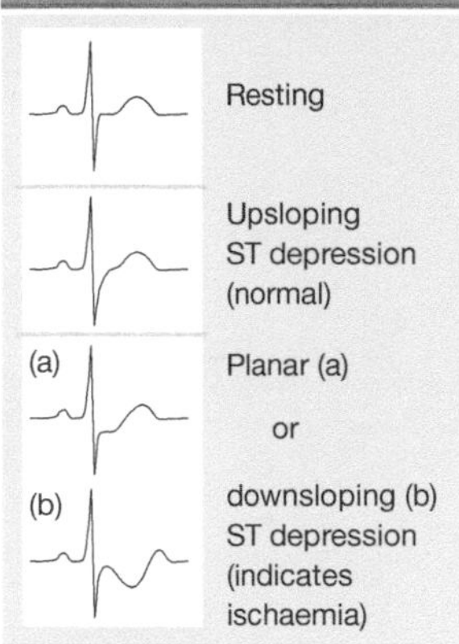

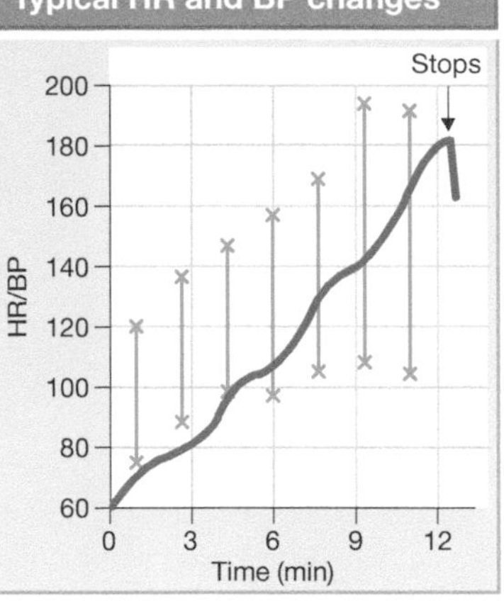

Coronary artery bypass graft (CABG) surgery

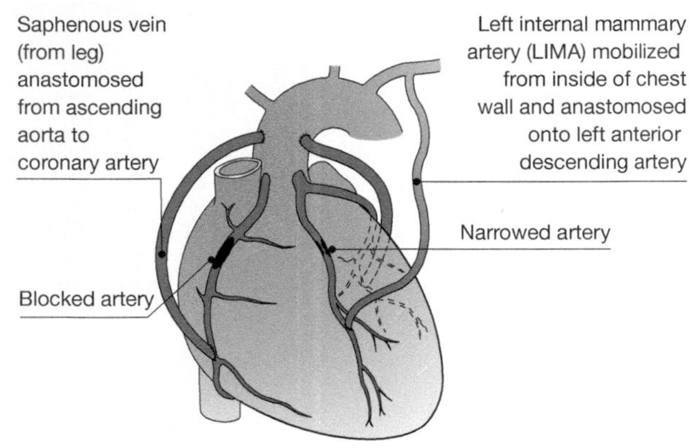

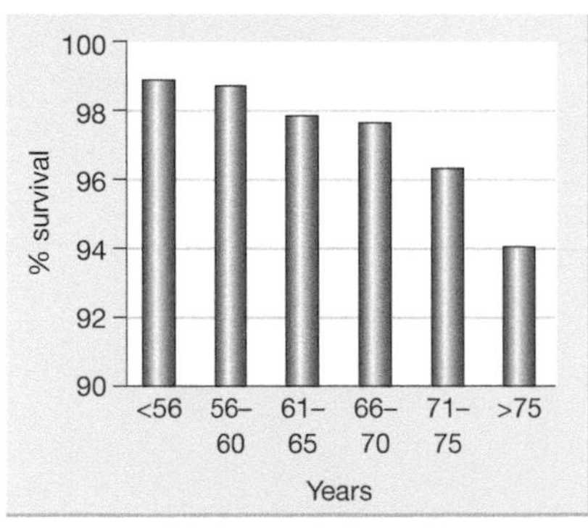

Survival following first time CABG

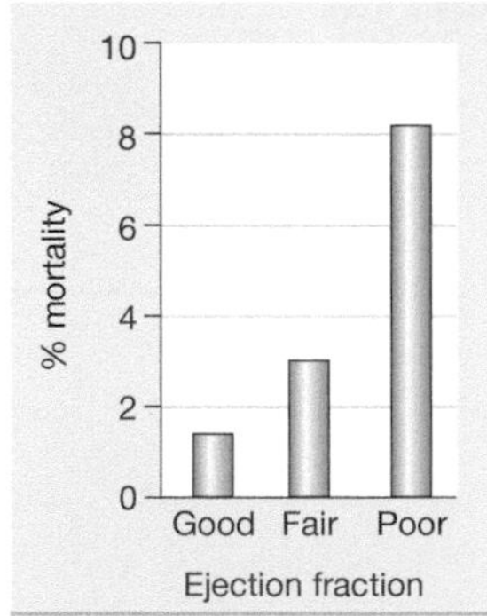

Mortality rate following first time CABG

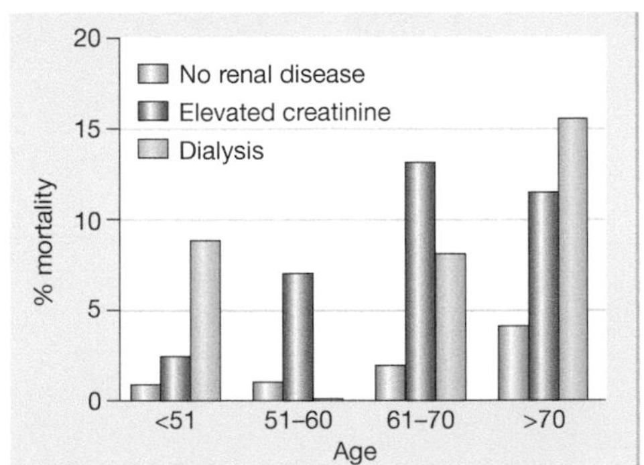

Mortality in first time CABG and renal function

Medicine at a Glance, Fifth Edition. Edited by Patrick Davey and Alex Pitcher.

Companion website: www.wiley.com/go/medicine5e

Chronic chest pain is common, as is coronary artery disease (CAD). The key to managing chronic chest pain is to establish whether symptoms relate to coronary disease and, if they do, estimate the risk of an adverse event occurring.

Diagnosis

Stable angina usually relates to CAD, although other pathologies may be responsible (see Chapter 13). It is a common condition, and while the symptoms often are classic, given how common it is, it not infrequently presents with atypical symptomatology.

The clinical history is the first cornerstone of the diagnosis of angina. Classic symptoms of stable angina include:

- constricting chest discomfort, which may radiate to the jaw, arm, neck or chest
- precipitated by physical exertion
- relieved by rest or nitrates within five minutes.

Typical angina is defined as symptoms meeting all three of these characteristics; atypical angina meets two and non-anginal chest pain meets one or none.

In angina, effort capacity may be decreased by the cold, the wind, on hills or after eating. Symptoms may be atypical – the diagnostic clue is the clear provocation with effort and rapid relief by rest, in the presence of appropriate coronary risk factors (age, sex, etc.). Breathlessness, rather than chest pain, may be an 'anginal equivalent' in people with diabetes.

The diagnosis is usually clear from the history alone. If not, non-invasive investigations confirm the diagnosis and provide risk stratification. Occasionally, coronary angiography is needed for diagnostic purposes.

In terms of diagnosing whether chest pain relates to coronary disease, most cardiologists look for two things: firstly, in the history, a strong relationship between effort provoking symptoms and rest relieving symptoms (Table 85.1). This relationship is almost always present if symptoms have been present long enough (>1–2 months), though for unknown reasons may not be present in the first few weeks of new-onset angina. Beware that inactive people may not show this relationship with effort. Symptoms most typically are retrosternal pain, though some people with angina feel pain symptoms elsewhere, and some feel breathlessness rather than pain. Secondly, cardiologists examining the patient will use the resting electrocardiogram (ECG) to look for clues of aortic stenosis, hypertrophic cardiomyopathy and pulmonary hypertension.

Diagnostic testing in chronic chest pain syndromes

The aims of undertaking diagnostic testing in chronic chest pain syndromes are, firstly, to increase confidence as to whether the symptoms are linked to a diagnosis of obstructive coronary disease or not and, secondly, to provide risk stratification to guide the need for further treatment. A range of non-invasive tests are available and the selection of the optimal test depends upon factors including the pretest probability of coronary disease, local test availability and expertise, and additional factors including patient preference and co-morbidities. Broadly, diagnostic tests can be divided into the following.

1 **Anatomical tests**, which directly visualize the coronary arteries and assess for atherosclerotic plaques.
2 **Functional tests** which assess for deficits in myocardial perfusion or function during stress which might suggest ischaemia resulting from atherosclerotic plaques.

Table 85.1 Percentage of people estimated to have coronary artery disease (CAD) according to typicality of symptoms, age, sex and risk factors.

	Non-anginal chest pain				Atypical angina				Typical angina			
	Men		Women		Men		Women		Men		Women	
Age (years)	Lo	Hi	Lo	Hi	Lo	Hi	Lo	Hi	Lo	Hi	Lo	Hi
35	3	35	1	19	8	59	2	39	39	88	10	78
45	9	47	2	22	21	70	5	43	51	92	20	79
55	23	59	4	25	45	79	10	47	80	95	38	82
65	49	69	9	29	71	86	20	51	93	97	56	84

For men older than 70 with atypical or typical symptoms, assume an estimate >90%. For women older than 70, assume an estimate of 61–90%, EXCEPT women at high risk AND with typical symptoms where a risk of >90% should be assumed.

Values are per cent of people at each mid-decade age with significant CAD.

Hi, high risk = diabetes, smoking and hyperlipidaemia (total cholesterol >6.47 mmol/l).

Lo, low risk = none of these three.

Note: These results are likely to overestimate CAD in primary care populations. If there are resting ECG ST-T changes or Q waves, the likelihood of CAD is higher in each cell of the table.

Source: National Clinical Guideline Centre for Acute and Chronic Conditions, 2010, www.ncbi.nlm.nih.gov/pmc/articles/PMC2913741/

Anatomical tests for coronary artery disease

- **CT coronary angiography**: a bolus of contrast is injected intravenously and after an appropriate delay, this passes through the coronary arteries, at which time its presence is detected and outlined by the CT scan. This allows an anatomical assessment of the arteries to be obtained along with determining the presence of atherosclerotic plaques. Modern multidetector CT platforms provide high anatomical resolution with low radiation dose. CT coronary has the further potential advantage of identifying non-flow limiting plaques which might allow additional treatment for risk factor modification (e.g. with statins).
- **Invasive coronary angiography**: catheters are passed through peripheral arteries to the coronary arteries, and contrast is injected to delineate the lumen using X-rays. Non-invasive testing is generally performed first but using invasive angiography may be reasonable in patients with highly typical symptoms refractory to medical treatment at low workload as it offers the potential for intervention using PCI (see below).

Functional tests for coronary artery disease

- **Stress echocardiography**: this test involves acquiring ultrasound images of the heart whilst increasing the heart rate with either exercise or catecholamines, usually dobutamine. All segments of a normal left ventricle will increase contractile performance with such stimulation. However, regions of the heart subtended by arteries stenosed to a sufficient degree are unable to augment function due to inadequate perfusion. The accuracy of the test is operator dependent. The main advantage of the test is that it is radiation free.
- **Myocardial perfusion scintigraphy**, otherwise known as myocardial single photon emission CT (SPECT). This is an accurate and well-validated test. A radioactive isotope, usually containing technetium 99, is injected intravenously; the isotope is taken up by the heart's tissues proportional to blood flow and can be detected by photomultiplier tubes arranged round the body (the imager is called a gamma camera). The data are then reconstructed into a three-dimensional model of the heart, allowing one to see how much tracer has been taken up in the different coronary artery territories. Injections are made at rest and with stress (either by physical exercise, e.g. treadmill – the preferred modality, or pharmacological, often using a coronary vasodilator such as adenosine or its analogues). Narrowed arteries rarely reduce resting blood flow, so the rest injection allows viable heart to be differentiated from areas of dead heart, i.e. previous myocardial infarction (MI). Narrowed arteries reduce peak blood flow compared to healthy arteries, so leading to less tracer uptake in the supplied territory, which can be imaged using the gamma camera, thus allowing the areas of the heart supplied with narrowed arteries to be determined. This is a good test for assessing the presence of coronary disease, and its severity. A perfusion scan with no or few perfusion abnormalities corresponds to a good prognosis.
- **Cardiac magnetic resonance imaging (CMR)**: CMR provides excellent structural and functional assessment of the myocardium and detects previous myocardial infarctions as well as alternative diagnoses such as cardiomyopathy. For coronary disease, CMR is generally used as a functional test, assessing differences in gadolinium perfusion during vasodilator administration as a surrogate for blood flow. CMR is free from ionizing radiation and provides excellent information, but is less available and more expensive than some other techniques.
- **Exercise stress ECG**: has historically been central to the assessment of stable angina, but imaging tests are now usually preferred on account of increased diagnostic accuracy. Exercise ECG provides excellent assessment of the relationship between exercise and symptoms, and also good data on prognosis – exercise capacity itself is powerfully related to outcome.

Risk stratification

Risk stratification is a key component in the assessment of angina. There are several factors associated with a worse outlook in chronic angina.

- Extensive and severe coronary disease, such as left main coronary artery disease.
- Impaired left ventricular (LV) function (e.g. previous MI, hypertensive heart disease) or overt heart failure.
- Exercise-induced hypotension or arrhythmia.
- Diabetes.
- Vascular disease elsewhere, e.g. peripheral vascular disease.

Treatment

Medical therapy is the cornerstone of treatment for stable CAD and can improve symptoms and prognosis. Many patients are managed on medical therapy alone.

- **Hypercholesterolaemia** (see Chapter 82): all patients should be on statin therapy. If statins cannot be tolerated, try ezetimibe or other agent. Cholesterol reduction by lifestyle measures is important, but is never a substitute for statin therapy.
- **Angiotensin-converting enzyme inhibitors** have antiatherogenic actions in those at high risk of vascular events. This is probably through their BP-lowering action.
- **Antiplatelet agents**: aspirin has prognostic benefit. In aspirin allergy/intolerance, clopidogrel is used (and is marginally superior, a valid difference in higher risk patients). In anyone with a recent (<1 year) ACS, dual antiplatelet therapy with aspirin and clopidogrel (or ticagrelor or prasugrel) for a year from the time of the ACS improves outcome.
- Action should be taken to improve diet (omega-3 fish oils, fruit, decrease animal fats, low cholesterol), lose weight and increase exercise (which lessens blood pressure [BP] by ±10 mmHg and cholesterol by 1.0–1.5 mmol/l).
- Stop smoking – this is vital.
- Treat diabetes and hypertension aggressively (target BP <140/80, unless diabetes is also present, in which case aim for <130/80).

Antianginal medical therapy

- **β-blockers** are commonly used as antianginal therapy. They reduce cardiac work, lessen angina and improve prognosis after an MI and in heart failure.
- **Ivabradine**, a drug acting on the sinus node, has heart rate-slowing properties in patients in sinus rhythm, and can be used as an antianginal, though its main use is in the treatment of patients in heart failure who are in sinus rhythm but who cannot take a β-blocker.
- **Nitrates** are effective in relieving angina. Nitrate tolerance develops if they are given throughout the 24 hours and a 'nitrate-free' period of 12–14 h/day is needed.
- **Nicorandil** is a potassium channel activator, resulting in vasodilation and a reduction in angina.

- **Calcium channel blockers**: second-line therapies are used only when β-blockers are contraindicated. They are contraindicated in heart failure. Only those with heart rate-slowing properties (e.g. diltiazem or verapamil, not nifedipine) can be given as monotherapy in angina.
- **Ranolazine**: this is a newer class of drug, a cardiac potassium channel opener, which is an effective antianginal, and may have other useful mechanisms of action. It is currently used in those with symptoms refractory to other treatments.

Revascularization in CAD

Revascularization in coronary disease can be performed using either percutaneous techniques (PCI) or surgery with coronary artery bypass grafting. The most common aim of revascularization in CAD is to improve symptoms which are not adequately controlled with medication. In a subgroup of patients with high-risk CAD (for example, disease of the left main stem), revascularization may improve prognosis by reducing the risk of MI or death. Historical data support a prognostic benefit from CABG in those with stenoses (>70% luminal narrowing) affecting: (i) all three coronary arteries; or (ii) the left main coronary artery; or (iii) the proximal portion of the left anterior descending artery (though these studies were conducted before contemporary medical therapy was available). Because of the complexity, the choice of revascularization strategy, if any, is individualized according to patient wishes, co-morbidity and coronary anatomy with multidisciplinary decision making by 'heart teams' incorporating cardiac surgeons and cardiologists.

Percutaneous coronary intervention (PCI)

Along with medical therapy, PCI is an option for relieving symptoms in patients with chronic stable angina. With rare exceptions, PCI is not thought to improve survival beyond medical therapy for unstable angina. PCI is, however, associated with improved clinical outcomes in *unstable* coronary syndromes. For further details on PCI, see Chapter 83.

Coronary artery bypass surgery

Coronary surgery is effective at relieving anginal symptoms and in some cases is associated with an improved prognosis.

In CABG, bypass grafts are connected from the aorta to the coronary artery distal to the stenosis. Usually, this requires stopping the heart and supporting the patient by a cardiopulmonary bypass machine (that is to say, a machine that takes deoxygenated blood out of the patient, gives it oxygen and also pressurizes it, so acting like the heart and lungs combined). In many patients it is possible to apply grafts without stopping the heart – so-called 'off-pump surgery'. The claimed advantage of off-pump surgery is a lessened 'systemic inflammatory response syndrome' – this is where the membrane in the heart–lung machine activates components of the blood to turn on an inflammatory response throughout the body, which can result in lung damage, kidney failure and a variety of brain syndromes.

There are two forms of bypass graft.

- **Vein grafts** (from leg saphenous veins) are easy to use and quick to apply, but have an annual failure rate of ±8%. Many patients are therefore informed that these grafts should be expected to last no longer than 10 years. When saphenous grafts fail, patients can have any of the following symptoms: none (surprisingly common, the explanation being that the heart has developed internal bypasses), stable angina, an ACS including acute MI, and sudden cardiac death. Most graft failure can be managed medically (with pills), some requires PCI, and for a very few, redo CABG (which is much higher risk than first-time CABG) can be undertaken.
- **Arterial grafts** are technically more difficult to apply but have a much better long-term survival rate, and therefore a better medium-term patient survival. The most commonly used arterial graft is the internal mammary artery, usually applied to the left anterior descending (LAD) artery. The application of this graft to the LAD artery is powerfully associated with a prolongation of life. This is by far the most important reason for carrying out CABG.

Elective surgery has, in good hands and in low-risk patients, a ±1% mortality rate. However, in those with damaged left ventricles, renal impairment and other co-morbidities, the risk of surgery goes up, as does the benefit from successful surgery. Deciding which of these high-risk patients should have surgery can be a difficult decision, and most units would routinely pass all these decisions to a multidisciplinary team (MDT) meeting where cardiologists, cardiac surgeons and cardiac anaesthetists can together decide what approach is in the best interests of the patient. After surgery, antiatherogenic and antiplatelet measures must continue.

86 Acute aortic dissection

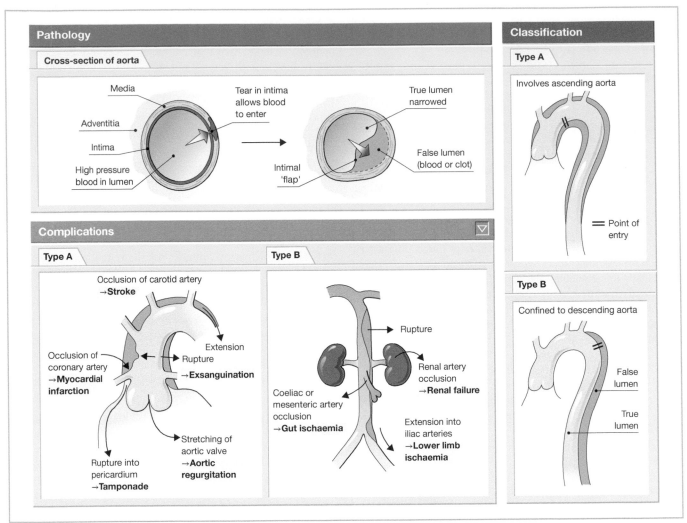

Aortic dissection affects 1/40 000 of the population per year and consists of a tear in the intima of the thoracic aorta, causing bleeding into the aortic wall, and raising a flap. This then propagates distal to the original tear, interrupting vital organ blood supply. Aortic rupture may occur. Aortic dissection is the most common form of acute aortic syndrome, which also includes penetrating ulcer and intramural thrombus.

Risk factors

- Marfan syndrome, Loeys-Dietz syndrome and Vascular Ehlers Danlos syndrome strongly predispose to aortic aneurysm formation, dissection and rupture (see figure below). Exclude acute aortic syndrome in any patient with one of these conditions and new chest pain.
- Hypertension.
- Atherosclerosis.

Pathology

High blood pressure (BP), stretched connective tissues and the presence of diseased intima (atherosclerosis) result in sudden tearing of the intima. Blood enters the layer between the intima and media, and high pressure causes the blood to track longitudinally along the aorta, forwards and backwards from the point of entry, forming a false lumen. Blood in the false lumen may clot or remain liquid with some flow. Dissections are classified into one of two types, depending on whether the ascending aorta is involved.

- **Type A**: the point of intimal tearing is in the ascending aorta. The dissection usually tracks distally to involve the descending aorta and proximally to disrupt the aortic valve apparatus and into the pericardium.
- **Type B**: the point of intimal tearing is in the descending aorta, typically just beyond the origin of the left subclavian artery. It is rare for the tear to propagate proximally.

Medicine at a Glance, Fifth Edition. Edited by Patrick Davey and Alex Pitcher.

Companion website: www.wiley.com/go/medicine5e

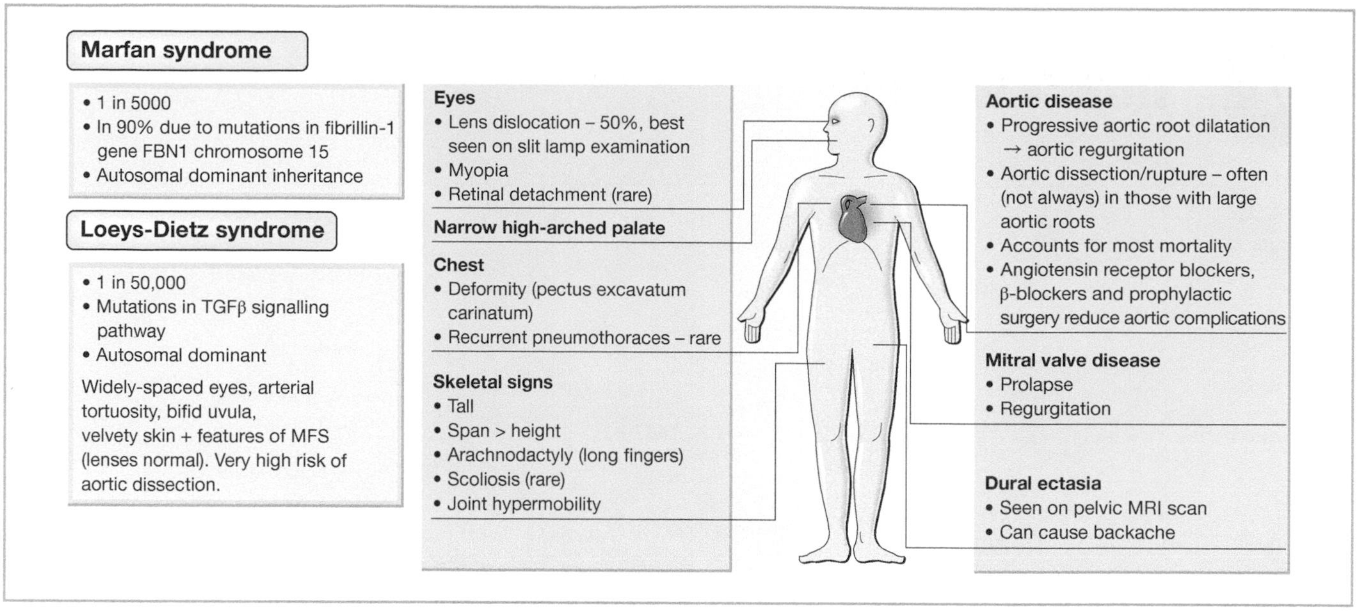

Marfan syndrome

- 1 in 5000
- In 90% due to mutations in fibrillin-1 gene FBN1 chromosome 15
- Autosomal dominant inheritance

Loeys-Dietz syndrome

- 1 in 50,000
- Mutations in TGFβ signalling pathway
- Autosomal dominant

Widely-spaced eyes, arterial tortuosity, bifid uvula, velvety skin + features of MFS (lenses normal). Very high risk of aortic dissection.

Eyes
- Lens dislocation – 50%, best seen on slit lamp examination
- Myopia
- Retinal detachment (rare)

Narrow high-arched palate

Chest
- Deformity (pectus excavatum carinatum)
- Recurrent pneumothoraces – rare

Skeletal signs
- Tall
- Span > height
- Arachnodactyly (long fingers)
- Scoliosis (rare)
- Joint hypermobility

Aortic disease
- Progressive aortic root dilatation → aortic regurgitation
- Aortic dissection/rupture – often (not always) in those with large aortic roots
- Accounts for most mortality
- Angiotensin receptor blockers, β-blockers and prophylactic surgery reduce aortic complications

Mitral valve disease
- Prolapse
- Regurgitation

Dural ectasia
- Seen on pelvic MRI scan
- Can cause backache

Clinical features

The clinical presentation is extremely variable because of the diverse consequences and complications of aortic dissection. Symptoms arise from the stripping of the intima away from the aortic wall (presentation symptoms) and from either the interruption of blood supply to vital organs or rupture. The most common presentation is with abrupt onset of extremely severe pain felt in the chest or back (interscapular), particularly in a middle-aged hypertensive man. The complications of dissection are listed below.

- **Rupture**: catastrophic pain, hypotension and collapse. Often fatal, but may be contained as BP falls. Occurs retroperitoneally, in the mediastinum or into the left (although never the right) pleural space.
- **Pericardial tamponade**: rupture of a type A dissection backwards into the pericardium results in haemopericardium and pericardial tamponade, the clinical features of which are hypotension (pulsus paradoxus) and a raised jugular venous pressure (Kussmaul sign).
- **Aortic regurgitation**: involvement of the aortic root disrupts the aortic valve ring, causing the valve to leak. Early diastolic murmur.
- **Aortic side branch occlusion**: the false lumen compresses the origin of arterial branches as they arise from the aorta. Any branch, at any point along the ascending, descending and abdominal aorta, can be involved. This can lead to a myocardial infarction (MI) (only patients with inferior infarction are seen, because left main coronary dissection is lethal), stroke, upper or lower limb ischaemia, paraparesis caused by spinal artery occlusion, renal failure or gut ischaemia.
- **Extension**: initial dissection may extend along the aorta, typically causing further pain in the direction of the extension.

Investigations

- **ECG**: principally to exclude MI. May show left ventricular hypertrophy from long-standing hypertension.
- **Chest X-ray**: may show widened mediastinum as a result of haemomediastinum, or a pleural effusion, caused by aortic rupture into the (usually left) pleural space.
- **Computed tomography scan**: this is usually the test of choice and should not be delayed. Cross-sectional images of the aorta show flap and true and false lumina when contrast is given.
- **Transthoracic echocardiography** rarely shows the dissection flap but may show complications such as haemopericardium and aortic regurgitation. Transthoracic echocardiography cannot exclude acute aortic syndrome.
- **Transoesophageal echocardiography** is very sensitive in imaging both the ascending and descending aorta. A specialized echo probe is passed down the oesophagus and positioned behind the heart, allowing imaging of the great vessels and heart, unimpeded by ribs or lungs. Images of a high quality are obtained. The procedure requires a highly skilled operator and is invasive, and patients require sedation. Because it may transiently increase the BP, thus provoking extension of the dissection, *it should only be carried out in cardiothoracic centres with access to immediate surgery.*

Management

Aortic dissection is a medical emergency and should be treated with the very highest priority. In both types A and B, the immediate concern is to lower the BP to less than 100 mmHg systolic to prevent further dissection or rupture, using opiate analgesia and intravenous β-blockers. Those with hypotension due to bleeding should be resuscitated to maintain a modest BP only. Specific treatment depends on the site of origination of the flap.

- **Type A dissection**: the risk of catastrophic complications, particularly rupture into the pericardium, is extremely high, with an *hourly* mortality rate of about 2%. Patients should be transferred by blue light/air ambulance to a cardiothoracic centre immediately, whatever the time of day, for immediate surgery to replace the aortic root, with or without a concomitant aortic valve procedure.
- **Type B dissection**: surgery is high risk and therefore not indicated as first-line treatment. Aggressive BP control is indicated, aiming for a systolic BP of <100 mmHg. Surgery is reserved for life-threatening complications, such as threatened rupture. A false lumen may clot and stabilize.

Prognosis

Type A dissection has a very high immediate mortality, but if the patient does not have life-threatening complications (e.g. stroke, paraplegia), the outlook after successful surgery is good. The immediate outlook for type B dissection is better, although there are late complications, including aneurysm formation and rupture.

87 Heart failure

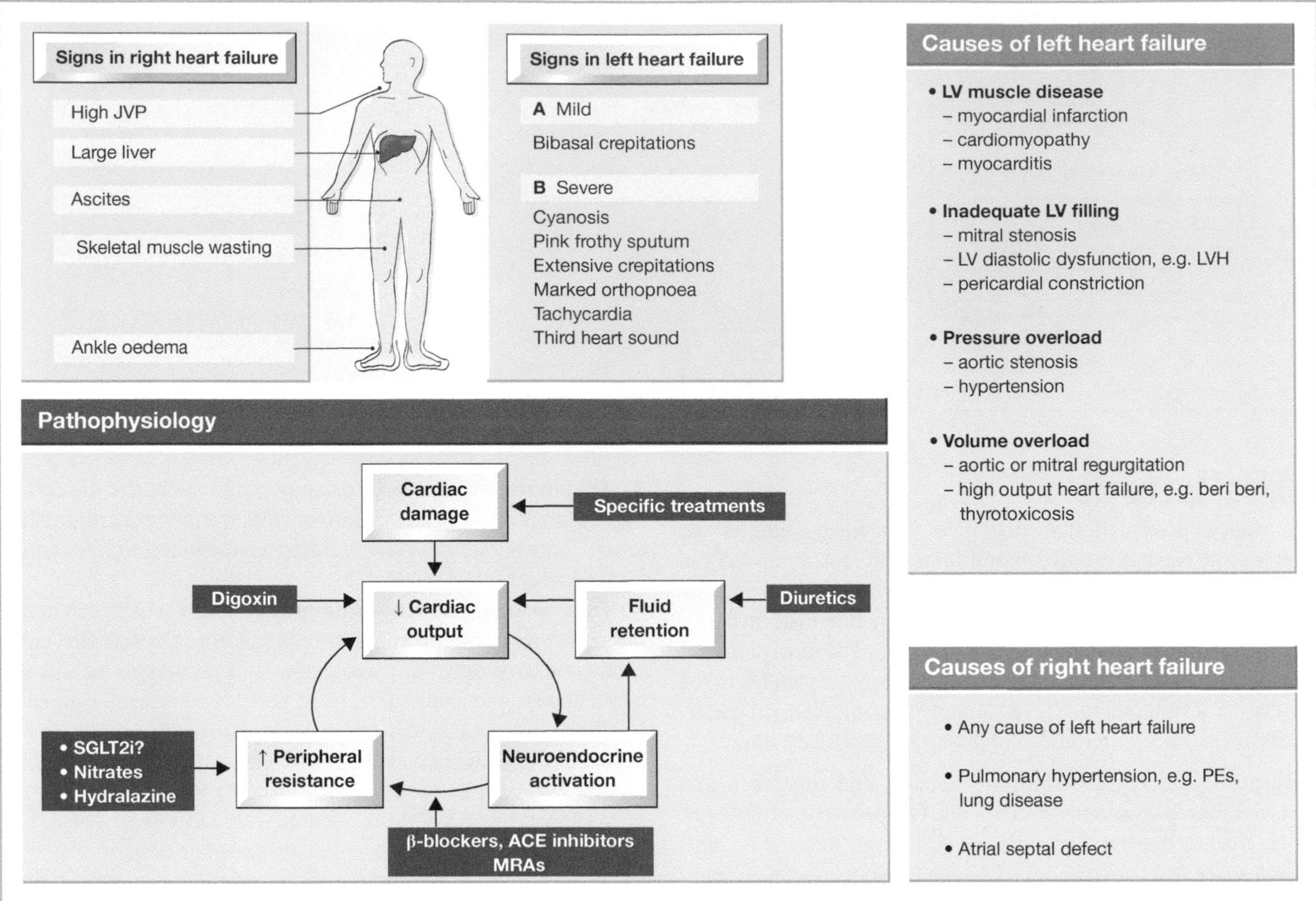

The term *heart failure* is used in several different ways and can be unhelpful to use with patients in some situations, but the term is widely used, usually to mean the clinical syndrome that arises when the function of the heart is seriously impaired. Most doctors need to be able to recognize it, to understand why it might occur, and to be able to initiate treatment. Obvious cases are easy to diagnose, but subtle cases, in which only a few features are present, can be more difficult for the inexperienced or unwary clinician. Sometimes, only subtle features are present despite severe impairment of heart function.

Symptoms and signs

- **Left heart failure**: breathlessness, which is worse when lying down (orthopnoea), especially in the middle of the night (paroxysmal nocturnal dyspnoea, PND). Classically, when PND occurs, patients feel the need to get up and fling open the window to get air. Typically, symptoms improve within minutes of getting up. Signs comprise tachypnoea, tachycardia, third heart sound ('gallop rhythm') and bibasal inspiratory pulmonary crepitations.
- **Right heart failure**: fluid retention in the legs, and in severe cases ascites. Signs comprise raised JVP and peripheral oedema. If ascites is more prominent than leg oedema *and the venous pressure is up* (indicating a high probability of a cardiac problem) then consider the very rare diagnosis of pericardial constriction.

Very commonly, both left and right heart failure commonly co-exist, usually because chronic left heart failure results in secondary pulmonary hypertension and right heart failure. Chronic biventricular failure is termed 'congestive cardiac failure'.

- **Chronic heart failure**: in long-standing heart failure the heart may enlarge (cardiomegaly) and secondary mitral/tricuspid regurgitation occurs. Skeletal muscle loss ('cardiac cachexia') may be substantial and responsible for fatigue, tiredness and weakness. The New York Heart Association classification grades severity (Table 87.1). Prognosis relates to many factors, but symptom severity is an important predictor (Box 87.1; see also Table 87.1).

Medicine at a Glance, Fifth Edition. Edited by Patrick Davey and Alex Pitcher.

Companion website: www.wiley.com/go/medicine5e

Table 87.1 New York Heart Association (NYHA) classification.

NYHA class	Breathlessness	Estimated annual mortality
I	None	<5%
II	On strenuous exercise	5–10%
III	On moderate effort	10–15%
IV	At rest	30–40%

Box 87.1 General predictors of worse prognosis.

The following indicators have been independently associated with a limited prognosis in heart failure.

- Recent cardiac hospitalization (triples one-year mortality)
- Elevated blood urea nitrogen (defined by upper limit of normal) and/or creatinine ≥1.4 mg/d (120 µmol/l)
- Systolic blood pressure <100 mmHg and/or pulse >100 bpm (each doubles one-year mortality)
- Decreased left ventricular ejection fraction (linearly correlated with survival at LVEF ≤45%)
- Ventricular dysrhythmias, treatment resistant
- Anaemia (each 1 g/dl reduction in haemoglobin is associated with a 16% increase in mortality)
- Hyponatremia (serum sodium ≤135 mEq/l)
- Cachexia
- Reduced functional capacity
- Co-morbidities: diabetes, depression, chronic obstructive pulmonary disease, cirrhosis, cerebrovascular disease, cancer and HIV-associated cardiomyopathy

Pathophysiology

Heart failure is a **syndrome** because, despite many different causes, once present the symptoms, signs and pathophysiology are similar. An inadequate cardiac output stimulates compensatory mechanisms resembling the response to hypovolaemia. Initially beneficial, these in turn become maladaptive.

- **Neurohormonal activation** occurs with increases in vasoconstrictors (renin, angiotensin II and catecholamines amongst others, and there are many others) provoking salt and water retention and increasing cardiac afterload. These decrease left ventricular (LV) emptying and depress cardiac output further, producing greater neuroendocrine activation, so increasing afterload, etc., resulting in a vicious downward spiral. Some neurohormones are used to help diagnose the syndrome of heart failure, particularly B-type natriuretic peptide (BNP). A normal level effectively excludes most heart failure; a very raised level is strongly associated with heart failure; a mildly or moderately raised level could indicate heart failure, but equally is associated with many other disease processes.
- **Ventricular dilation**: impaired systolic function (reduced ejection fraction) and fluid retention increase ventricular volume (dilation). A dilated heart is mechanically inefficient (law of Laplace). If energy supply is limited (e.g. coronary disease), this may lead to further contractile failure and neuroendocrine activation.

Classification

The most common classification of heart failure is performed according to the left ventricular ejection fraction (LVEF), a measure of the change in left ventricular volume from diastole to systole, which can be estimated using cardiac imaging (usually echocardiography). A normal LVEF is usually >55%.

- **Heart failure with reduced ejection fraction** (HFrEF) occurs where the primary problem is a failure of the left ventricle to contract adequately. This form of heart failure is fairly easy to understand: the heart does not expel enough blood to meet systemic requirements, resulting in a reduced ejection fraction and increasingly large intracardiac dimensions. HFrEF is diagnosed when there are symptoms or signs of heart failure, and the LVEF is reduced. This may result from loss of cardiomyocytes, for instance due to a large myocardial infarction, or from abnormal function of myocytes due to a cardiomyopathy.
- **Heart failure with preserved ejection fraction** (HFpEF) where the main problem is impaired relaxation of the ventricle with increased ventricular wall stiffness. HFpEF probably accounts for around half of hospital admissions with heart failure. HFpEF is more difficult to conceptualize, diagnose and treat than HFrEF. Despite preserved systolic function, ventricular relaxation is impaired, which results in high intracardiac and pulmonary venous pressures, especially during exercise which is when symptoms tend to occur. HFpEF is common in the elderly, those with hypertension, high body mass index and atrial fibrillation. Clinical diagnosis depends on accurately determining consistent symptoms and signs, assessing risk factors for HFpEF, measuring natriuretic peptides and assessing additional echocardiographic parameters of diastolic function beyond LVEF. Scoring systems integrating these parameters may help.

Alternative classification systems for heart failure exist, though none are ideal. Another system groups heart failure syndromes according to the clinical signs.

- **Acute heart failure** is largely synonymous with left heart failure and results from a sudden failure to maintain cardiac output. There is insufficient time for compensatory mechanisms to develop and the clinical picture is dominated by acute pulmonary oedema. Such patients are usually quite unwell and require immediate hospital admission.
- **Chronic heart failure (CHF)**: cardiac output declines gradually, symptoms and signs are less florid, and features relating to compensatory mechanisms dominate. Patients, while unwell, can often be managed on an outpatient basis.

Demographics and prognosis

Heart failure affects 1–2% of those aged ≥65 years and 10% of those aged ≥75 years. The natural history of untreated heart failure is poor; in severe heart failure, ≥50% die within three years though this risk can be mitigated with contemporary treatments. Sudden death due to arrhythmia is a common mode of death in heart failure.

Aetiology

Any disease that damages or overloads the pumping ability of the heart can result in cardiac failure. Common conditions include coronary disease, hypertension, age, obesity and alcohol-related disease. Valvular heart disease can be either age-related (aortic stenosis) or rheumatic. In some countries, infections are relevant (e.g. South American trypanosomiasis in Brazil).

Provoking/exacerbating factors

It is vital to consider whether there are contributory factors in any patient presenting with new-onset or decompensated heart failure.

- **Arrhythmias** (e.g. atrial fibrillation [AF]), which can often provoke symptoms of heart failure in someone with a previously asymptomatic damaged heart. For example, patients with hypertensive heart disease not infrequently present out of the blue with heart failure provoked by tachycardia resulting from new-onset AF.
- **Drug issues** (non-compliance, fluid-retaining drugs, e.g. non-steroidal anti-inflammatory drugs): these are all common.
- **Anaemia**: anaemia and iron deficiency are common in severe heart failure.
- **Infection**, e.g. pneumonia, urinary tract infection.
- **Thyroid disease**.

Investigations

The aims of investigations are to confirm the diagnosis of the heart failure syndrome, to ascertain the underlying cause, to assess severity and guide and monitor treatment.

- **Echocardiography**: essential, simple, non-invasive tool for diagnosing aetiology and severity and ruling out important valvular heart disease. However, you should be aware that there are limitations to the technique.
  - In obese subjects, and in some other patients, it may not be possible to obtain good views of the heart and the study therefore may not be of diagnostic quality (after checking the name of the patient, the next most important aspect to check is the echocardiographer's assessment of the adequacy of the views, and you will find this information on the echo report).
  - An apparently normal echo does not rule out heart failure – an incomplete study may miss evidence of HFpEF and rare causes such as pericardial constriction (a rare but important cause of heart failure).
  - An abnormal cardiac ultrasound does not mean that a patient inevitably has heart failure! Heart failure is the syndrome that results from a cardiac abnormality – just having a cardiac abnormality does not necessarily mean that symptoms inevitably have accrued from this. Put another way, always be clear in your own mind as to whether the symptoms you are exploring are heart failure, and use the test to evaluate causation, rather than use the test to explore directly whether symptoms are heart-related. If you don't follow this rule, you will find a heart abnormality, label this as the cause of the patient's symptoms and so miss the serious pathology that is causing the symptoms, such as severe chronic obstructive pulmonary disease (COPD), pulmonary emboli, interstitial lung disease, anaemia, etc.
- **Electrocardiogram (ECG)**: look for old myocardial infarction, LVH (e.g. hypertension, aortic stenosis), T-wave changes that are associated with critical coronary disease (e.g. symmetrical pan-anterior T-wave inversion) or cardiomyopathy (asymmetrical widespread T-wave inversion). Look for arrhythmias (e.g. AF).
- **Chest X-ray**: large heart, pulmonary congestion (Kerley B lines) or pulmonary oedema. Be aware that some reports labelling obese patients as having cardiomegaly are wrong – the cardiac silhoutte is increased by pericardial fat, rather than by the heart being genuinely enlarged.
- **Biochemistry**: electrolytes must be measured, as a common mode of death in heart failure is sudden cardiac death due to ventricular fibrillation, the probability of which is increased by hypokalaemia, which itself occurs readily with loop diuretic therapy. Potassium-sparing diuretics lessen mortality in heart failure. Monitor renal function and haematology (anaemia). Check thyroid function.
- **Cardiac MRI**: useful for accurate measurement of the ejection fraction. Patterns of fibrosis (late gadolinium enhancement) may help to determine the cause of heart failure (e.g. previous myocardial infarctions, non-ischemic dilated cardiomyopathy, amyloidosis).
- **Coronary CT or cardiac catheterization**: to exclude critical coronary artery disease (CAD), or to assess CAD severity and treatment options in those with known ischaemic heart disease.
- **Ambulatory ECG** recording to investigate arrhythmias.

Treatment

- **General measures**: treat the underlying cause and any arrhythmias. Reduce salt and water intake, and monitor treatment by measuring body weights. Treat hypertension and CAD risk factors vigorously – aim for a blood pressure (BP) not above 130/80.
- **Specific measures**: if possible, treat the cause of the heart failure – valve surgery for valve disease, meticulous heart rate control for any rate-related cardiomyopathies (this is where heart failure has resulted from an uncontrolled arrhythmia driving the heart too fast for too long, e.g. an atrial tachycardia for 2–3 months with a heart rate of >140 bpm), teetotal status in those with alcohol-related heart disease, etc. Revascularization is a complex issue in HFrEF due to coronary disease, but if large areas of the heart either with reversible ischaemia or hibernation are found, revascularization may be appropriate and may improve LV function and outlook.
- **Diuretics** are the mainstay of symptomatic treatment. The dose should be sufficiently large to remove pulmonary and/or peripheral oedema. The principal side-effect is hypokalaemia (give potassium supplements or sparing diuretic, e.g. amiloride).

There are currently no evidence-based therapies to improve prognosis in HFpEF, although HFpEF may be the result of an underlying condition (such as cardiac amyloidosis) which may have specific treatment options. However, a number of therapies are under evaluation at present which may emerge as treatment options in the near future.

In contrast, medical therapy in HFrEF improves both symptoms and prognosis and is essential.

- **Angiotensin-converting enzyme (ACE) inhibitors** block conversion of angiotensin I to II, interrupting the maladaptive neuroendocrine response, vasodilating and lowering BP. Several large, randomized, controlled trials show they improve symptoms, quality of life and prognosis in overt heart failure or impaired LV function. They may provoke renal failure in bilateral renal artery stenosis (check urea and electrolytes). The most common other side-effect is a persistent dry cough in 5%.

- **Angiotensin II receptor antagonists (ARB)** (e.g. losartan) block angiotensin II by direct antagonism of its receptor. They have similar effects and benefits to ACE inhibitors and are an alternative to ACE inhibitors, but are not used in conjunction with them.
- **Angiotensin/neprilysin inhibition (ARNI):** sacubitril/valsartan is a combination of the angiotensin II receptor antagonist valsartan and sacubitril, which is an inhibitor of natriuretic peptide breakdown. A large trial has demonstrated superiority for sacubitril/valsartan compared to enalapril, in reducing the risk of death and hospitalization in heart failure and it is now increasingly widely used instead of ACE inhibitors or angiotensin receptor blockers in selected patients with HFrEF.
- **β-Blockers** (e.g. bisoprolol, metoprolol, carvedilol) were historically felt to be contraindicated in heart failure, and still should not be initiated in patients in acute decompensated pulmonary oedema. However, high circulating catecholamines and down-regulation of adrenergic receptors are detrimental in heart failure. β-Blockers (started at low doses and increased slowly) reverse these abnormalities and improve functional status and prognosis. They reduce both pump failure and arrhythmic sudden deaths. Ivabradine may be used when the heart rate remains elevated despite β-blockers, or when β-blockers cannot be tolerated or are contraindicated (e.g. asthma).
- **Mineralocorticoid receptor antagonists** (e.g. spironolactone and eplerenone) are potassium-sparing diuretics and improve prognosis in HFrEF.
- **Sodium glucose co-transporter 2 (SGLT2) inhibitors** (e.g. dapagliflozin) promote renal excretion of glucose and reduce mortality and heart failure hospitalizations in HFrEF, including in those without diabetes.
- **Digoxin** has a positive inotropic effect in sinus rhythm and results in symptomatic improvement and a reduction in hospital admissions, although it has no mortality benefit. It is used mainly to control the ventricular rate resulting from atrial arrhythmia.
- **Device therapy**: patients with HFrEF have an increased risk of death due to ventricular arrhythmia. In selected patients, this risk can be reduced with an **implantable cardioverter defibrillator** (ICD), which can monitor for ventricular arrhythmias and deliver either rapid pacing or a high-energy shock to defibrillate VT or VF. Patients with HFrEF also commonly have left bundle branch block (LBBB) which leads to inefficient, dyssynchronous ventricular activation. This means that different parts of the ventricle contract at different times. This leads to a loss of cardiac output, as blood can move around the ventricle, as one segment contracts against a segment yet to contract, rather than contributing to cardiac output. Patients with HFrEF and LBBB contraction may benefit from **cardiac resynchronization therapy (CRT)**, in which pacemaker leads are placed in the right ventricle and the lateral wall of the left ventricle (via the coronary sinus). These two ventricular leads allow simultaneous activation of two widely separated parts of the ventricle, so minimizing inco-ordinated contraction and maximizing cardiac output. When CRT is combined with an ICD, it is referred to as CRT-D.

Complications

- **Ventricular arrhythmias** are common and may cause syncope or **sudden cardiac death** (25–50% of deaths in CHF). In those successfully resuscitated, ICDs are usually offered.
- **Atrial fibrillation** commonly complicates CHF, when it can provoke a dramatic deterioration. Treatment of the AF is indicated using rate or rhythm control strategies as appropriate, and anticoagulation (because the combination of heart failure and atrial fibrillation is associated with elevated thromboembolic risks).
- **Progressive pump failure** may respond to increasing doses of diuretics. Mechanical circulatory support and heart transplantation are options in selected patients.

Aortic valve disease

Aortic stenosis (AS)

Causes of valvar AS
- Calcific stenosis of a tricuspid aortic valve
- Bicuspid aortic valve

Other causes of left ventricular outflow tract (LVOT) obstruction
- Hypertrophic cardiomyopathy
- Membrane (very rare)
- Supravalvar AS (very rare)

Impaired systolic flow of blood from left ventricle to aorta by narrowed aortic valve

Pressure (mmHg)
160
100
0
70 mmHg gradient
Ao pressure
LV pressure

Aortic regurgitation

Causes of AR
- Stretched aortic root
  - hypertension
  - Marfan
  - other cause of aortopathy
- Abnormal aortic valve
  - bicuspid
  - degenerative
  - endocarditis

Pressure (mmHg)
140
100
60
50
0
Ao
LV
Ao pressure 'collapses' rapidly during diastole
Wide pulse pressure
LV pressure rises during diastole due to additional volume load
Ao-LV pressure difference gradually falls as diastole progresses, so murmur is decrescendo

Pathology

Intra-valve membrane
- Presents in infancy

Calcification in a bicuspid valve
- Presents 40–60 yrs

Calcification in a tricuspid valve
- Presents 60–100 yrs
- Very common

Beware:
Hypertrophic cardiomyopathy can be mistaken clinically for aortic stenosis

Clinical features

Pulse	Precordium	Auscultation
Aortic stenosis Slow rising (low pulse pressure)	Apex is forceful (hypertrophy)	Ejection click if valve mobile Soft or absent A_2 if valve immobile EC S_1 A_2 P_2 S_1 Harsh, ejection systolic murmur, radiates to carotids
Aortic regurgitation Collapsing (high pulse pressure)	Apex diffuse and displaced (volume overload)	Early diastolic decrescendo murmur at left sternal edge (right sternal edge if due to aortic aneursym) S_1 A_2 P_2 S_1 Ejection systolic murmur due to increased stroke volume

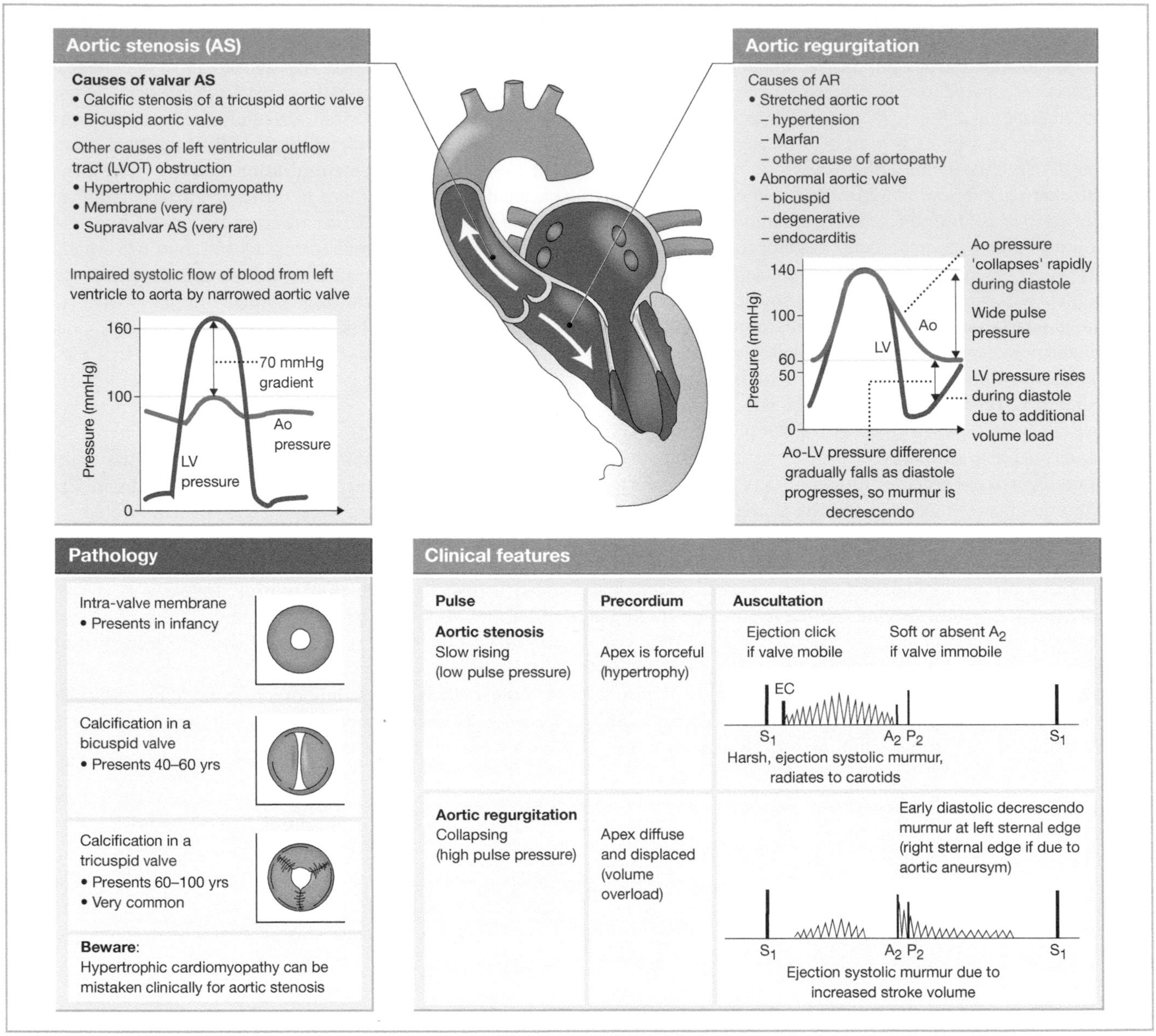

Aortic stenosis

There are three major causes of aortic stenosis.

1 Calcific/degenerative aortic stenosis of a normal valve: the most common aortic valve lesion, occurring from age 65 onwards. At age 80, about 10% of the population have it. Calcification may occur earlier in those with renal failure or hypercholesterolaemia.
2 Premature calcification of a congenitally **bicuspid aortic valve**: patients typically develop symptoms from age 40 years onwards.
3 Congenital aortic stenosis: this is very rare, and may be the result of a bicuspid valve, or a subaortic membrane, constricting the left ventricular (LV) outflow tract.

Symptoms

There is a classic triad of symptoms associated with aortic stenosis. All are exertional and progressive.

- **Effort dyspnoea.**
- **Effort angina.**
- **Effort dizziness or syncope.**
- **Sudden cardiac death** is rare in those without any of the above symptoms, but becomes increasingly likely as other symptoms develop. For this reason asymptomatic patients are followed up, whereas symptomatic patients undergo valve intervention.

Medicine at a Glance, Fifth Edition. Edited by Patrick Davey and Alex Pitcher.

Companion website: www.wiley.com/go/medicine5e

Angina at rest is usually caused by concomitant coronary disease rather than aortic stenosis. Syncope at rest is usually the result of atrioventricular (AV) block (e.g. complete heart block) because concomitant conducting tissue disease is common.

Signs

Ejection systolic murmur is often harsh and loud. The area where the murmur is heard loudest varies – usually it is the middle of the left sternal edge, sometimes in the 'aortic' area (second right intercostal space) and occasionally in the 'mitral' area, i.e. at the apex (fifth intercostal space, midclavicular line). The murmur often radiates into the carotids. A slow rising pulse, absent second heart sound and signs of LV hypertrophy (LVH) indicate severity. Signs of complicating heart failure may also be present.

Investigations

Echocardiography is the key investigation and allows assessment of LV function and valve structure (e.g. bicuspid or tricuspid, calcified or not) and severity of stenosis. Stenosis severity is usually quoted as the peak velocity of blood (determined from the Doppler ultrasonic probe) through the valve (a value of >3.5 m/s generally indicates that the aortic stenosis may be sufficiently severe to cause symptoms).

Other parameters including valve area can also be estimated from echocardiography and are helpful when LV function is reduced. Cardiac computed tomography (CT) and magnetic resonance (CMR) provide direct estimates of valve area via planimetry, and are helpful in planning intervention. Invasive cardiac catheterisation may be used before surgery to determine whether there is coronary disease that may need intervention at the same time as the valve (bypass grafting or PCI). A chest X-ray is useful if complicating heart failure is suspected. An electrocardiogram (ECG) may show LVH, and occasionally conducting tissue disease (calcium from the valve 'burrows' down into the interventricular septum, interfering with electrical impulse propagation).

- **Creatinine**: impaired renal function is an important predictor of increased operative risk.
- **Cholesterol and glucose**: aortic valve disease may be a marker for other atherosclerotic vascular disease.
- **Full blood count**: there is an association between angiodysplasia and aortic stenosis. As aortic stenosis can induce functional von Willebrand disease, iron deficiency may occur.

Treatment

In the absence of symptoms, most patients can be followed with periodic echocardiography to monitor LV function and the severity of the aortic stenosis. When symptoms occur, or the left ventricular function deteriorates, or the degree of stenosis becomes very severe, there is a higher risk of clinical deterioration. Valve intervention using surgical or transcatheter valve replacement is therefore usually recommended at this point.

- **Surgical aortic valve replacement (SAVR)**: usually used for patients at low/intermediate operative risk. Under general anaesthesia, via a midline sternotomy, the heart–lung machine is connected, the aorta is clamped and cut open, and under direct vision the old damaged aortic valve is cut out and an artificial one sewn in (either metallic or bioprosthetic or, rarely, a homograft). Operative mortality is usually 1–5%.
- **Transcatheter valve implantation/replacement (TAVI/TAVR)**: has become a mainstream alternative to surgical aortic valve replacement, especially in patients with moderate or greater surgical risk. A new aortic valve is delivered via a peripheral artery (usually femoral) via a wire and deployed across the existing valve using a balloon.

The choice of surgical or transcatheter intervention is individualized according to the patient's anatomy, co-morbidities and views, with decision making by a multidisciplinary heart team.

Aortic regurgitation

There are two pathologies that give rise to aortic regurgitation (AR). They can usually be distinguished echocardiographically.

- **Disease processes affecting the aortic valve** (including rheumatic heart disease, endocarditis, systemic lupus erythematosus). Calcific aortic stenosis is also often associated with significant AR.
- **Diseases resulting in dilation of the aortic root** and thus the aortic valve ring (including aortic aneurysm caused by hypertension, Marfan syndrome, ankylosing spondylitis or syphilis, or the rarer annuloectasia, which is idiopathic dilation of the aortic root). Aortic dissection disrupts the aortic root, causing acute AR.

Symptoms

With gradual-onset AR, even if the leak is severe, symptoms are often mild or absent. If the leak worsens, or if LV decompensation occurs, dyspnoea develops, on effort or at rest.

Signs

Collapsing pulse with a volume-overloaded left ventricle (hyperdynamic apex beat). The diastolic blood pressure (BP), which relates directly to how much blood has leaked back from the aorta into the left ventricle, is a good guide to the severity of chronic AR (low diastolic BP = severe AR). Wide pulse pressure may cause:

- Corrigan sign (visible carotid pulsations)
- De Musset sign (head bobbing)
- Quinke sign (nail-bed pulsations)
- pistol shot femorals (also known as Traube phenomenon): femoral artery auscultation reveals a loud sound during systole, likened to a pistol shot, due to the large forward stroke volume.
- Duroziez murmur, a to-and-fro murmur heard when the femoral artery is auscultated and slight pressure is placed on the stethoscope, relates to the large forward and backward flow in the aorta from the AR.

An early diastolic murmur is heard along the left sternal edge (with the patient leaning forward in end-expiration), unless the AR is caused by an aortic root aneurysm, when the murmur is loudest along the right sternal edge. The murmur may be surprisingly loud in mild AR, and is often quiet in very severe AR, or if the lesion is acute, e.g. endocarditis.

Investigations

Echocardiography is useful for monitoring LV function, determining whether the regurgitation is the result of a valve or aortic root problem, and determining its severity. Although the aortic root diameter can be measured, if there is substantial enlargement, computed tomography or magnetic resonance imaging of the thoracic aorta is needed to determine how much of the aortic arch (and descending aorta) is enlarged. A chest X-ray may show an enlarged heart or aortic aneurysm; an ECG usually shows LVH. Coronary angiography is useful to assess for concomitant coronary disease once surgery has been decided on.

Treatment

Angiotensin-converting enzyme (ACE) inhibitors (and possibly other vasodilators such as calcium channel blockers) may reduce the decline in LV function with significant AR. Increasing LV dimensions and symptoms are indications for AV intervention. If AR is the result of dilation of the aortic root, valve and root replacements are necessary. Surgical aortic valve replacement is commonly the intervention of choice for AR, but some patients at higher risk may have a transcatheter option.

89 Mitral valve disease

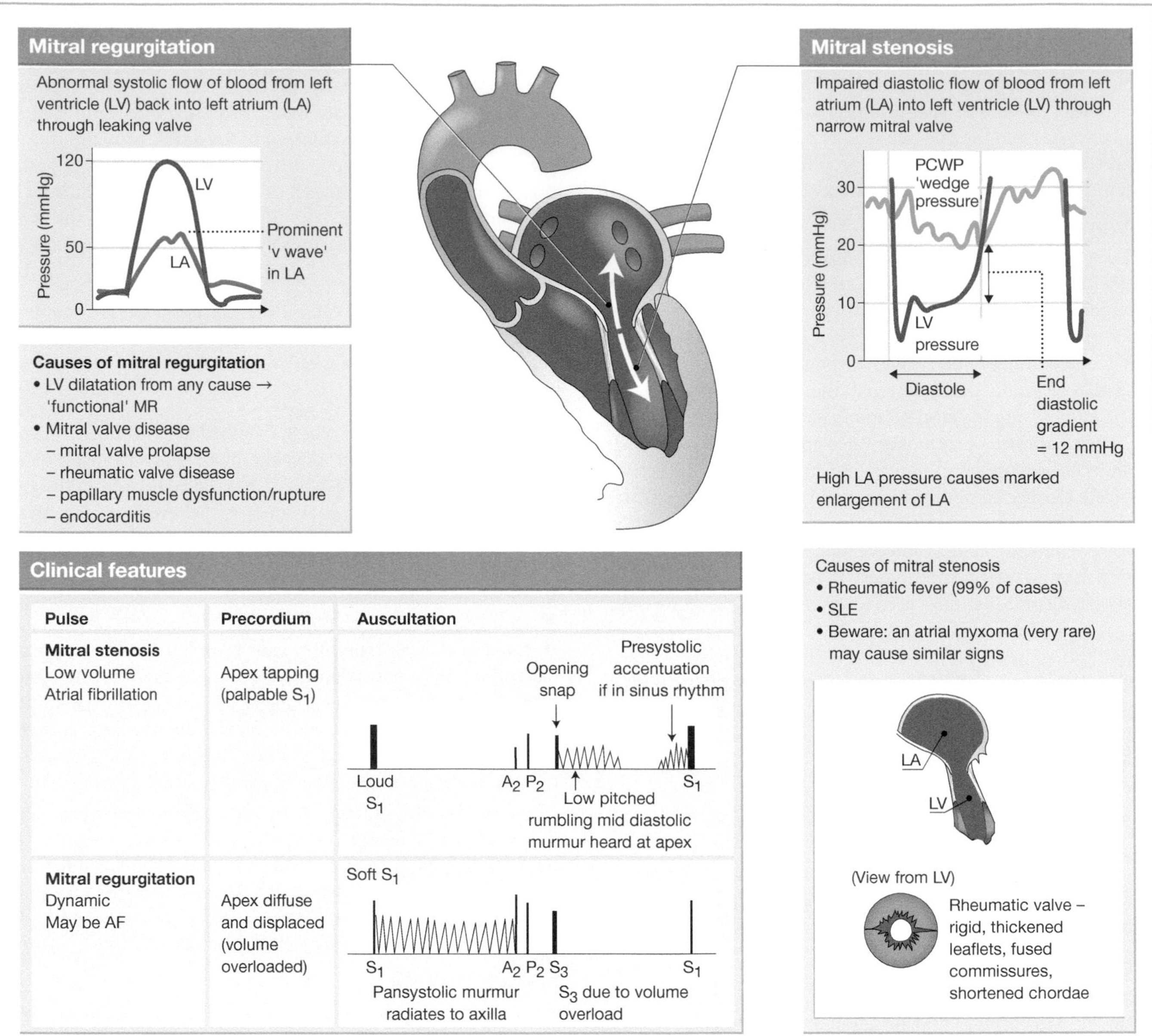

Mitral stenosis

Although, on a worldwide basis, mitral stenosis is still very common, this is now a rare lesion in the developed world, because of the decline in the incidence of rheumatic valve disease. In practice, all mitral stenosis relates to previous rheumatic fever.

Symptoms

Half of those diagnosed have documented/remembered childhood rheumatic fever. Symptomatic mitral stenosis develops within a few years in deprived communities, but may take decades in the West. Typically there is the gradual onset of progressive exertional dyspnoea, as a result of chronic heart failure, in those aged 40–50 years. Sudden and severe symptoms occur with the onset of atrial fibrillation (AF). Mitral stenosis with AF is a very potent substrate for systemic thromboemboli (e.g. a stroke) that are sometimes the first manifestation of the lesion.

Signs

- Female > male.
- Mitral facies (malar flush).

Medicine at a Glance, Fifth Edition. Edited by Patrick Davey and Alex Pitcher.

Companion website: www.wiley.com/go/medicine5e

- May be signs of chronic heart failure: elevated jugular venous pressure, oedema.
- Usually AF.
- Right ventricular 'heave' if there is secondary pulmonary hypertension.
- 'Tapping' apex beat (palpable S_1), which is undisplaced in the absence of significant mitral regurgitation.
- Low-pitched, rumbling, mid-diastolic murmur, best heard with the bell in a left lateral position.
- Opening snap (rigid valve opening) precedes murmur.

Investigations
Echocardiography confirms the diagnosis and follows disease progression. The valve may be 'rheumatic' (thickened and distorted). The velocity of the blood flow during diastole through the mitral valve can be measured using Doppler. In normal individuals, this starts high and then declines rapidly as diastole proceeds. A much slower velocity decline is found in mitral stenosis, and the severity can be deduced from the rate of velocity decline ('pressure half-time'). Pulmonary hypertension can also often be diagnosed from Doppler measurements of regurgitant blood through the tricuspid valve. Concomitant mitral regurgitation (MR) and aortic valve disease likewise can be diagnosed and followed up. An electrocardiogram (ECG) may show left atrial enlargement (when in sinus rhythm) or AF. In pulmonary hypertension, a dominant R wave may appear in chest lead V_1. A chest X-ray may show left atrial enlargement (cardiomegaly, 'splayed' tracheal bifurcation).

Treatment
- **Medical therapy** (with diuretics, digoxin and warfarin) maintains good functional status for decades. The only indication for surgery is when symptoms are not controlled by drugs.
- **Intervention**: there are two approaches.
  - *Mitral valvotomy*: this can be carried out percutaneously in some, using a balloon. Historically, valvotomy was performed via thoracotomy (often made over the left lung, so as to gain easy access to the valve through the left atrium).
  - *Mitral valve replacement*: this is a common operation. Usually, a mechanical valve (rather than a biological one) is used because warfarin is already indicated in patients with AF which is common.

Differential diagnosis
Very rarely, similar symptoms and signs are caused by an atrial myxoma, a benign tumour, usually found in the left atrium attached to the interatrial septum, which grows sufficiently to impede mitral diastolic blood flow. It causes episodic or progressive breathlessness, and occasionally fever and weight loss with an elevated erythrocyte sedimentation rate. Cardiac ultrasonography is diagnostic. Immediate surgery is usually curative.

Mitral prolapse
In mitral valve prolapse (MVP, Barlow syndrome), the mitral valve is larger than usual and/or the chordae attached to the mitral valve are too long. As a consequence, a component of the mitral valve 'prolapses' back into the left atrium during ventricular systole. There may or may not be MR (see next section). In MVP without MR, the usual sign is a 'click', heard in early mid-systole. The 'click' of MVP can be a rather intermittent phenomenon. MVP with MR predisposes to bacterial endocarditis (see Chapter 93). Some patients with apparently isolated mitral prolapse appear to be at increased risk of ventricular arrhythmia.

Mitral regurgitation
Mitral regurgitation is an extremely common valve lesion. Like aortic regurgitation, there are two underlying pathologies.

- Those caused by **intrinsic valve disease** (e.g. myxomatous degeneration, rheumatic heart disease, infective endocarditis) or disease of the valve-related apparatus (e.g. chordal rupture, as in some cases of floppy mitral valve) or of the papillary muscles (e.g. dysfunction/rupture resulting from ischaemia/infarction, usually of the circumflex artery).
- **Secondary** (also termed 'functional') caused by stretching of the valve ring when the left ventricle is dilated, as in many cases of left heart failure. The MR murmur may become dramatically quieter as the heart failure responds to treatment.

Symptoms
Patients are often asymptomatic for many years, unless the lesion has occurred/progressed over a very short time span. Unfortunately, during this asymptomatic period, left ventricular (LV) function may be permanently damaged. Symptoms when they occur are those of heart failure, such as breathlessness, effort intolerance and fatigue.

Signs
- Displaced, diffuse apex resulting from volume overload.
- Loud pansystolic murmur at apex.
- Functional MR may not be pansystolic.
- The murmur radiates up the LV outflow tract (i.e. is heard along the left sternal edge/aortic area) in posterior leaflet mitral valve prolapse, and is heard in the back in anterior mitral valve leaflet prolapse.

Investigations
Echocardiography can be helpful in establishing both the presence of MR and its mechanism. Often, transthoracic echocardiography provides a good estimate of the severity of the MR, but this is not always true, and sometimes transoesophageal echocardiography is needed to determine severity more accurately. This is particularly true if an artificial mitral valve is present (i.e. previous mitral valve replacement). Cardiac ultrasonography is also useful in monitoring LV function, although this can easily be overestimated. Chest X-ray is useful for diagnosing heart failure. An ECG often shows LV hypertrophy, and may show AF.

Treatment
Initially, medical therapy with diuretics and angiotensin-converting enzyme inhibitors is used; they can control symptoms and maintain the systolic function of the left ventricle for years in the face of severe MR. In intrinsic valve disease, when symptoms are intrusive or if the left ventricle enlarges progressively, surgery is indicated. Prognosis after mitral valve repair is better than after mitral valve replacement. Less invasive treatment options, including percutaneous edge-to-edge repair using clips and percutaneous valve replacement, are becoming increasingly available for patients with suitable anatomy.

90 Cardiomyopathies

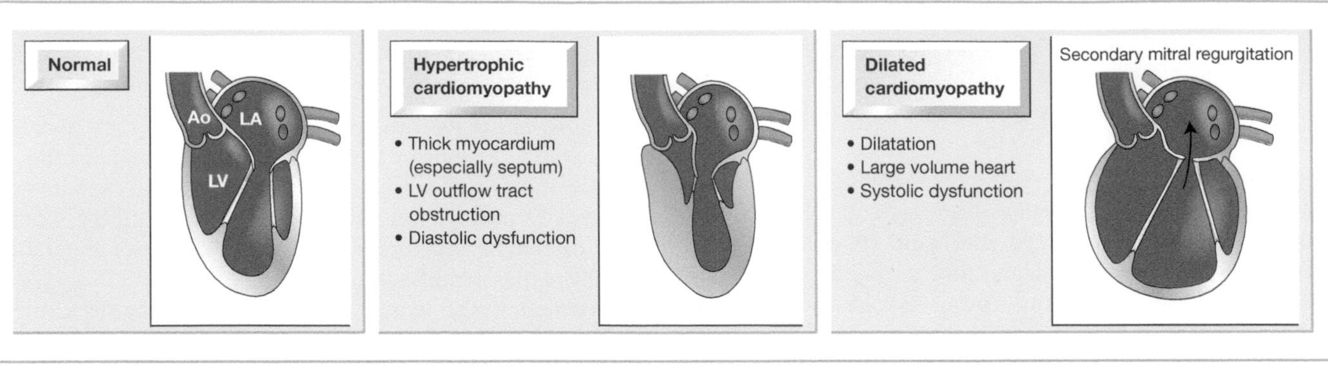

Causes of dilated cardiomyopathy (DCM)	
Genetic	Familial DCM, muscle dystrophies (Duchenne, myotonia, mitochondrial)
Toxins	Alcohol, drugs (anthracyclines)
Endocrine	Hypothyroidism, thyrotoxicosis, phaeochromocytoma
Infection	Viruses (Coxsackie), Trypanosoma species (Chagas' disease)
Dietary	Beri-beri (thiamine)
Infiltrative	Sarcoid, iron overload (haemochromatosis, excess blood transfusions)

Cardiomyopathies are **primary heart muscle diseases**. They are uncommon but not rare, e.g. dilated cardiomyopathy (DCM) underlies 5–10% of heart failure. Cardiomyopathies are currently classified primarily according to the imaging findings, usually by echocardiography or cardiovascular magnetic resonance (CMR).

Dilated cardiomyopathy

Dilated cardiomyopathy (DCM) is defined as the presence of left or biventricular dilation and systolic dysfunction in the absence of abnormal loading conditions (such as hypertension or valve disease) or coronary artery disease sufficient to account for the LV impairment. Clinically, LV or congestive cardiac failure occurs, often severe and progressive, with displacement of the apex beat and prominent S_3. Functional mitral regurgitation (MR) and atrial fibrillation are common. There is an increased risk of thromboembolism.

Several illnesses can cause **secondary DCM**, the most common of which is **excess alcohol**. **'Idiopathic'** or **'primary' DCM** is a diagnosis of exclusion though around one-third of cases have a family history, suggesting a significant genetic contribution for which some genes are defined with potentially causative mutations identified in around 25% of sporadic cases, and a high rate in patients with a family history.

Treatment is standard heart failure therapy including renin-angiotensin-aldosterone antagonists and diuretics (see Chapter 87). **Cardiac transplantation** is an important option for younger patients with severe refractory heart failure.

Hypertrophic cardiomyopathy

Hypertrophic cardiomyopathy is common (prevalence of 1:500) and is characterized by abnormal myocardial hypertrophy in the absence of a clear cause. A family history is positive in around 60% of cases and numerous genetic variants (>500) have been identified. The myocardial structure is abnormal (**myocyte disarray** and **interstitial fibrosis**). Hypertrophy results in a small LV cavity, diastolic dysfunction and secondary MR. When the septum is hypertrophied, this can result in dynamic LV outflow tract obstruction. Whilst this is often asymptomatic, severe hypertrophy and outflow tract obstruction may cause exertion breathlessness, chest pain or dizziness. The greatest risk is of collapse or sudden death as a result of ventricular arrhythmias, which may be unheralded and occur in otherwise fit patients.

The aims of treatment are to improve symptoms and reduce the risk of sudden cardiac death. Treatment is with the following.

- **β-blockers, calcium channel antagonists, disopyramide, myosin ATPase inhibitors**: these are used to treat exertional symptoms.
- **Devices**: used in those at high risk of ventricular tachycardia. Implantable cardiovertor defibrillators (ICDs) may be justified in patients with high risk (estimated using scoring systems) and/or a strong family history of sudden death.
- **Genetic counselling** and **screening** of asymptomatic family members are important to identify asymptomatic family members who might benefit from treatment.

Arrhythmogenic cardiomyopathy

Arrhythmogenic cardiomyopathy, previously known as arrhythmogenic right ventricular cardiomyopathy (ARVC) is characterized by the replacement of RV myocardium with fatty and fibrous tissue. Diagnosis is according to diagnostic criteria which incorporate cardiac imaging studies, family history, the presence of arrhythmia and resting ECG abnormalities. ICDs may be offered to reduce the risk of sudden cardiac death in patients at high risk. Naxos disease is a recessive form of arrhythmogenic cardiomyopathy which incorporates characteristic keratoderma and hair changes.

Restrictive cardiomyopathy

Restrictive cardiomyopathies include a wide range of pathologies and result in a rigid, stiff and thickened myocardium, usually arising from myocardial infiltration by abnormal materials or from fibrosis. It is probably the least common cause of cardiomyopathy and may cause congestive cardiac failure resulting from diastolic dysfunction. The most common form is amyloid (light chain amyloid AL resulting from multiple myeloma/paraproteinaemia or transthyretin [ATTR] amyloidosis which may be hereditary or wild type). Other causes include metabolic storage diseases, scleroderma, endomyocardial fibrosis and hypereosinophilic syndromes.

New treatments are emerging for specific forms of restrictive cardiomyopathies (e.g. enzyme replacement therapy in Fabry disease, tafamidis for ATTR amyloid, chemotherapy for plasma cell dyscrasia resulting in AL amyloid and others) and so an accurate diagnosis is important.

91 Pericardial disease

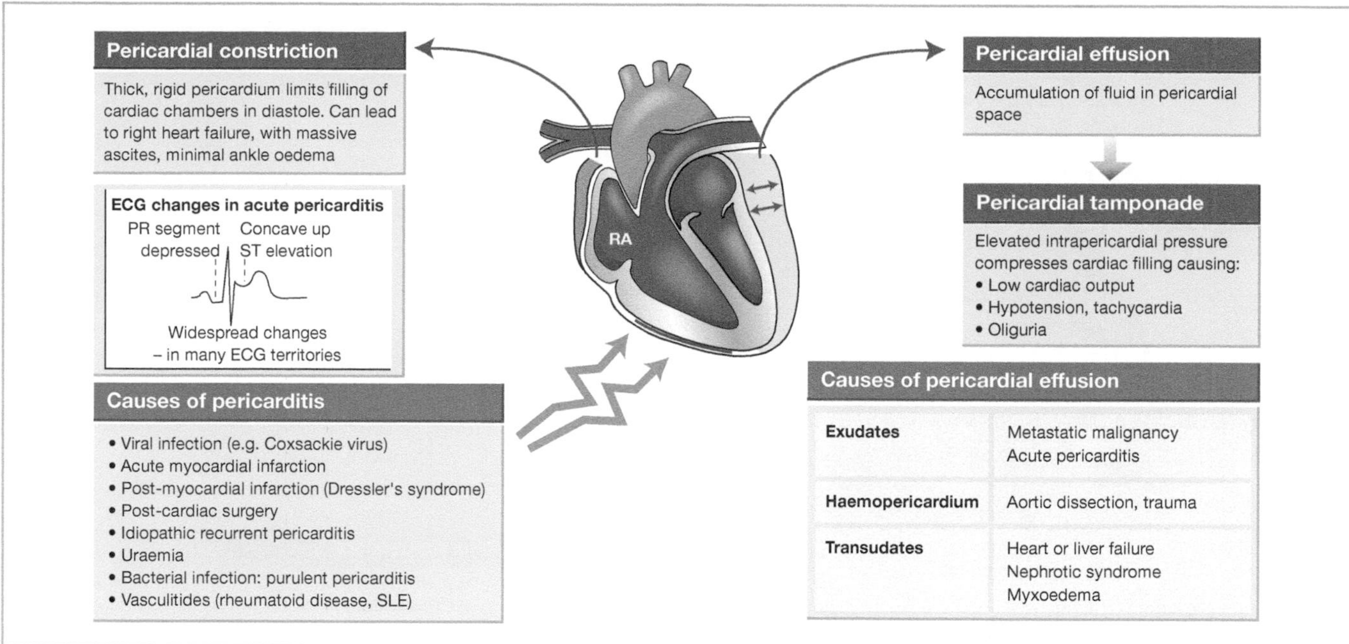

Pericardial constriction
Thick, rigid pericardium limits filling of cardiac chambers in diastole. Can lead to right heart failure, with massive ascites, minimal ankle oedema
ECG changes in acute pericarditis
PR segment depressed
Concave up ST elevation
Widespread changes – in many ECG territories
Causes of pericarditis
• Viral infection (e.g. Coxsackie virus)
• Acute myocardial infarction
• Post-myocardial infarction (Dressler's syndrome)
• Post-cardiac surgery
• Idiopathic recurrent pericarditis
• Uraemia
• Bacterial infection: purulent pericarditis
• Vasculitides (rheumatoid disease, SLE)
RA
Pericardial effusion
Accumulation of fluid in pericardial space
Pericardial tamponade
Elevated intrapericardial pressure compresses cardiac filling causing:
• Low cardiac output
• Hypotension, tachycardia
• Oliguria
Causes of pericardial effusion
Exudates
Metastatic malignancy
Acute pericarditis
Haemopericardium
Aortic dissection, trauma
Transudates
Heart or liver failure
Nephrotic syndrome
Myxoedema

Pericardial disease presents as one of four syndromes. **Pericarditis** describes inflammation of the pericardium, either acute or chronic. The accumulation of fluid within the pericardial space, **pericardial effusion**, can result in **pericardial tamponade**. Chronic or recurrent pericarditis may result in fibrosis of the pericardium, adherence of the visceral and parietal layers and **pericardial constriction**.

Acute pericarditis

Pleuritic chest pain, often positional, is classically relieved by sitting forwards. Many patients experience only a dull central ache without any specific features. A **pericardial rub** may be heard, often only in one position or on inspiration. There may be fever or systemic features. An electrocardiogram (ECG) shows **ST segment elevation** which is concave upwards, typically *affecting leads in multiple territories*, not just one territory as in myocardial infarction. Echocardiography may demonstrate a small pericardial effusion. Specific tests may demonstrate the cause. Non-steroidal anti-inflammatory drugs reduce the pain and inflammation. Colchicine reduces risk of recurrence.

Pericardial effusion

Pericardial effusion refers to the accumulation of fluid within the pericardial space. The effusion is categorized according to the protein content of the fluid into **transudates** which have low protein and **exudates** which have high protein or are bloody (**haemopericardium**). Occasionally, the effusion is **purulent** as a result of bacterial infection. **Cardiac tamponade** is caused by the accumulation of a pericardial effusion to the point where elevated intrapericardial pressures compromise cardiac filling. Slowly enlarging pericardial effusions allow the pericardium to stretch to accommodate the fluid; they may be very large (>1 l) before tamponade occurs. Rapidly growing effusions cause tamponade early on (the pericardium does not comply). A pericardial rub does not exclude tamponade.

Clinical features and treatment of cardiac tamponade

- Low output state (tachycardia, low blood pressure [BP], cold peripheries, oliguria – sometimes the most prominent sign of tamponade is progresive renal failure).
- Greatly elevated jugular venous pressure (JVP) (Kussmaul sign: JVP increases further rather than falls with inspiration).
- Pulsus paradoxus: BP falls with inspiration. The radial pulse may disappear in severe tamponade. Quiet heart sounds, no gallop.
- Large 'globular' heart on chest X-ray, but no pulmonary congestion.

Echocardiography confirms the presence of large pericardial effusions and evidence of tamponade (diastolic collapse of the atrium early on, and of the right ventricle in advanced cases). A simple pericardial effusion without haemodynamic compromise does not need drainage. In contrast, pericardial tamponade is a medical emergency requiring immediate percutaneous or surgical drainage.

Constrictive pericarditis

Acute, chronic or relapsing pericarditis (often caused by tuberculosis or radiotherapy) may cause pericardial fibrosis sufficient to constrict the heart, impede cardiac filling and decrease cardiac output. Progressive **exertional dyspnoea**, peripheral **oedema** and **ascites** occur.

A greatly elevated JVP and pericardial knock (loud diastolic heart sound) are seen. Computed tomography/magnetic resonance imaging, echocardiography and cardiac catheterization can all be used to establish the diagnosis. Diuretics relieve symptoms. Surgery may help.

Medicine at a Glance, Fifth Edition. Edited by Patrick Davey and Alex Pitcher.

Companion website: www.wiley.com/go/medicine5e

92 Pulmonary embolism

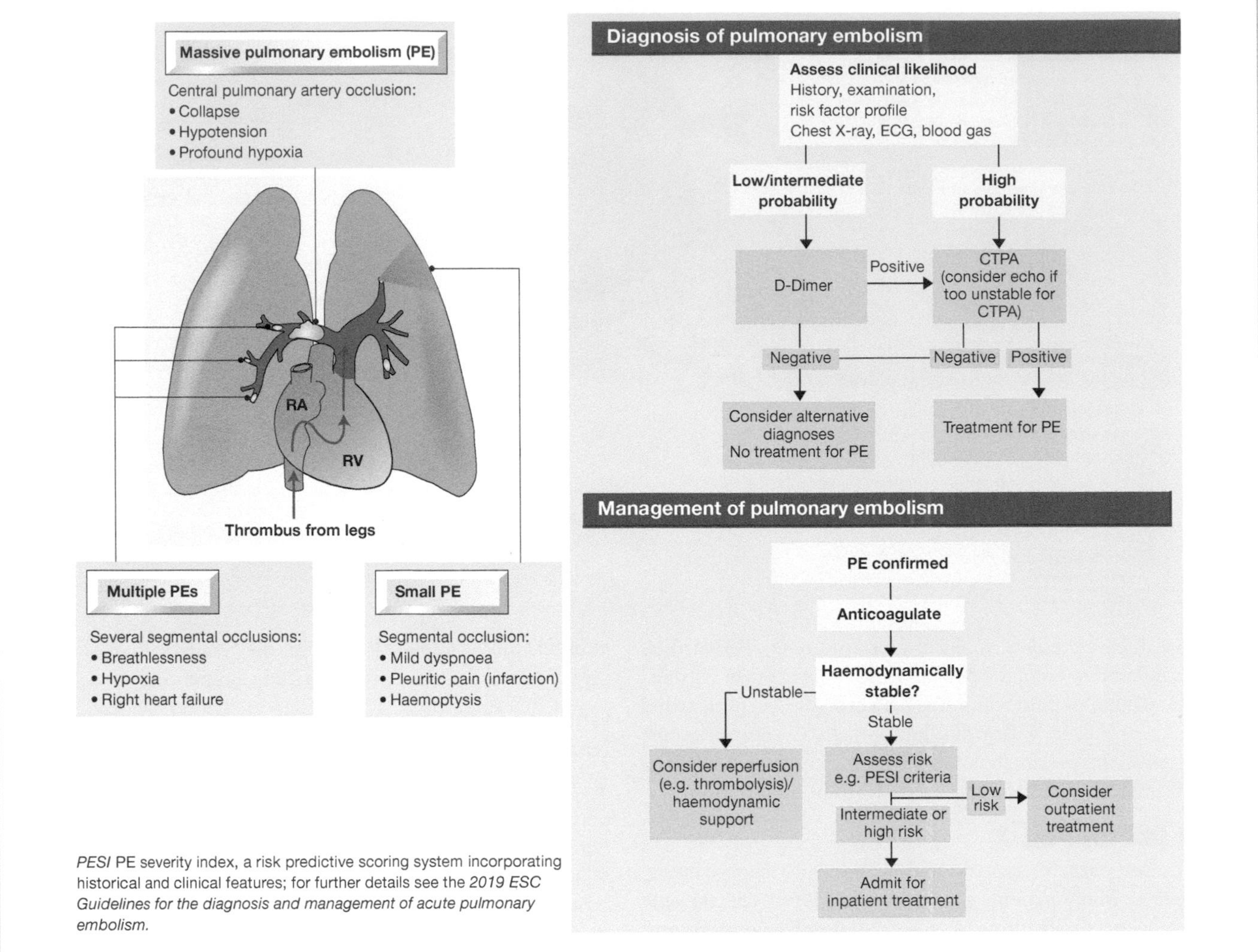

PESI PE severity index, a risk predictive scoring system incorporating historical and clinical features; for further details see the *2019 ESC Guidelines for the diagnosis and management of acute pulmonary embolism.*

Definition

Pulmonary embolisms (PEs) result when thrombi (often from the deep veins of the thigh or pelvis) embolize via the right heart into the pulmonary arteries.

Risk factors

Predisposing factors are found in the majority of patients and are an important clue to diagnosis. PEs are classified as either provoked or unprovoked, which guides the duration for which anticoagulation is required. Factors suggesting a 'provoked' PE include the following.

- Surgery less than 12 weeks ago.
- Immobilization for more than three days in the last four weeks.
- Previous deep venous thrombosis (DVT)/PE or family history.
- Lower limb fracture.
- Malignancy.
- Postpartum.
- Long-distance travel, especially in cramped conditions.

Medicine at a Glance, Fifth Edition. Edited by Patrick Davey and Alex Pitcher.

Companion website: www.wiley.com/go/medicine5e

Clinical features

The clinical presentation of PE can be varied, so a high degree of clinical suspicion is required. PEs cause hypoxia from ventilation/perfusion ($\dot{V}/\dot{Q}$) mismatch and interrupt pulmonary blood flow, causing pulmonary infarcts (so inflaming the pleura) and lowering cardiac output. These features are responsible for the three distinct clinical syndromes with which pulmonary thromboembolic disease presents.

1 Pleurisy and/or haemoptysis: small or moderate-sized PEs cause pulmonary infarction. Dyspnoea is absent or minor.
2 Dyspnoea with hypoxia in the absence of other causes: this suggests a moderate or large PE or repeated PEs over a period of time. There may be signs of cardiopulmonary disturbance (tachycardia, tachypnoea, elevated jugular venous pressure [JVP], left parasternal lift from acute right heart strain). Pleurisy/haemoptysis is often absent.
3 Circulatory collapse: large or massive PE. Typically a high-risk patient (e.g. post surgery) with unheralded collapse or unexplained clinical deterioration, and with hypotension, tachycardia and hypoxia.

Investigations

An assessment of the likelihood of PE, based on clinical, blood gas and chest X-ray (CXR) parameters, remains central to the diagnosis of PE, and directs early therapy. Later therapy is guided by more specific tests, e.g. CT pulmonary angiography or $\dot{V}/\dot{Q}$ scans.

- **Chest X-ray**: evaluates for other conditions, e.g. pneumonia, pneumothorax, pulmonary oedema. In PE, the CXR abnormalities are minimal/minor in relation to the degree of cardiorespiratory compromise.
- **Arterial blood gases**: haemodynamically significant PE causes $\dot{V}/\dot{Q}$ mismatching and hypoxia. Compensatory hyperventilation results in a reduced $PaCO_2$. The alveolar–arterial gradient is increased (see Chapter 100). *In hypoxaemia with a normal/near normal CXR, always consider the diagnosis of PE.*
- **Electrocardiogram (ECG)**: abnormalities are common, but are usually non-specific and not diagnostically useful, e.g. sinus tachycardia, minor ST and T-wave abnormalities (especially in V_{1-3}). In large or massive PE, the more classic ECG features of acute right ventricular strain (S_1, Q_3, T_3 which is rare), right bundle branch block or atrial fibrillation may occur.
- **D-dimers** are cross-linked fibrin degradation products. A normal D-dimer level implies a very low probability of PE. High D-dimers are found in many conditions (e.g. recent surgery, malignancy and inflammatory states), including PE.
- **Computed tomography (CT)**: spiral CT (CT pulmonary angiography) allows imaging of the pulmonary arteries to detect thrombi with high sensitivity and specificity. It has essentially replaced $\dot{V}/\dot{Q}$ scanning and invasive pulmonary angiography, and is especially useful when the CXR is abnormal, for any reason. Another reason why it is taking over from conventional $\dot{V}/\dot{Q}$ scanning is that it may well allow the cause of symptoms to be diagnosed even if they are not due to pulmonary emboli – for example, interstitial lung disease, heart failure and even coronary disease (whose probability can be partly estimated from the degree of coronary calcification seen).
- **$\dot{V}/\dot{Q}$ scanning**: isotope $\dot{V}/\dot{Q}$ scanning relies on the fact that a significant PE results in regional hypoperfusion of a segment or lobe of the lung without a corresponding defect in ventilation. To simplify the procedure, a normal CXR is sometimes used as a surrogate to imply normal ventilation. It is widely used, but with significant diagnostic limitations.
  - Strengths: a high probability scan or a normal scan is diagnostically powerful (>95%), especially in the setting of high or low clinical suspicion.
  - Limitations: 75% of scans are in the low or intermediate categories, which are less useful in confirming or excluding the diagnosis. Even a high probability $\dot{V}/\dot{Q}$ scan fails to detect >50% of PEs.
- **Echocardiography**: occasionally detects large thrombi in the pulmonary artery, or the right atrium or ventricle. More commonly, echocardiography shows right heart dilation and strain (i.e. poor systolic contractile function).
- **Pulmonary angiography**: historically the 'gold standard' investigation for the diagnosis of PE but now rarely used unless interventional treatment such as catheter-directed thrombolysis or mechanical thrombectomy is performed.

Treatment (Table 92.1)

- **Oxygen**: should be given to treat hypoxia in patients with suspected PE.
- **Anticoagulation**: should be administered when there is clinical suspicion of PE, while investigations are completed. Subcutaneous low molecular weight heparin (LMWH) or direct oral anticoagulants (DOAC) are commonly used, according to local protocols. Intravenous (IV) heparin is less commonly used and is generally reserved for large or massive PE.
- **Thrombolysis**: streptokinase or tissue plasminogen activator (tPA) promotes dissolution of thrombi. It is indicated for confirmed PE with haemodynamic instability.
- **Anticoagulants**: DOACs, warfarin and LMWH can all be used to provide anticoagulation. DOACs offer predictable anticoagulation without the need for monitoring, whilst LMWH is more commonly used for cancer-associated VTE. The duration of anticoagulation depends on whether the PE was provoked or unprovoked. The duration is usually at least three months for a provoked PE, but may be given long term for an unprovoked or recurrent PE or where risk factors persist.

Table 92.1 Management of pulmonary embolism (PE).

Low-risk PE	Confirm diagnosis using imaging (e.g. CT pulmonary angiogram or $\dot{V}/\dot{Q}$ scan) and anticoagulated with DOAC, warfarin or LMWH
Intermediate- or high-risk PE	Supplemental oxygen if hypoxic, anticoagulation and consider intravenous fluids if chest X-ray and ECG exclude myocardial infarction/pulmonary oedema. Imaging with CT pulmonary angiography if clinical conditions and local availability allow. If haemodynamic collapse, thrombolysis with tPA, then continued IV heparin. In some centres catheter-directed thrombolysis, catheter or surgical embolectomy is used in high-risk cases on a case-by-case basis
Multiple chronic PE	Anticoagulation. Refer for cardiological assessment

Chronic thromboembolic disease

Although the usual mode of presentation of PE is with an acute illness, occasionally patients present with a more chronic picture. The typical history is of several months' progressive breathlessness, markedly limiting the time of presentation. The physical signs are of cyanosis with marked pulmonary hypertension (left parasternal lift, raised JVP, sometimes peripheral oedema). Investigations show marked hypoxaemia; $\dot{V}/\dot{Q}$ scanning is usually floridly abnormal and CT often shows large thrombi in the central pulmonary arteries. Echocardiography allows determination of the pulmonary artery pressure, often 70–80 mmHg.

Treatment is problematic. Much thrombus is endothelialized and only rarely regresses on standard anticoagulant therapy. In a few selected patients, surgical pulmonary thromboembolectomy has a role.

Thrombophilia

Rare disorders of blood coagulation predispose to thromboembolism, and should be considered in the following.

- Patients aged <40 years with no other risk factors.
- Those with a first-degree relative with a history of venous thromboembolism.
- Patients with previous episodes of venous thromboembolism.

Deficiencies of proteins S, protein C or antithrombin III are the most common of these rare disorders (see Chapter 190). Other procoagulant states include lupus anticoagulant (anticardiolipin antibodies) and homocystinuria. More common are genetic polymorphisms in genes encoding clotting proteins – these increase thromboembolic risk, e.g. factor V Leiden.

93 Cardiac infections

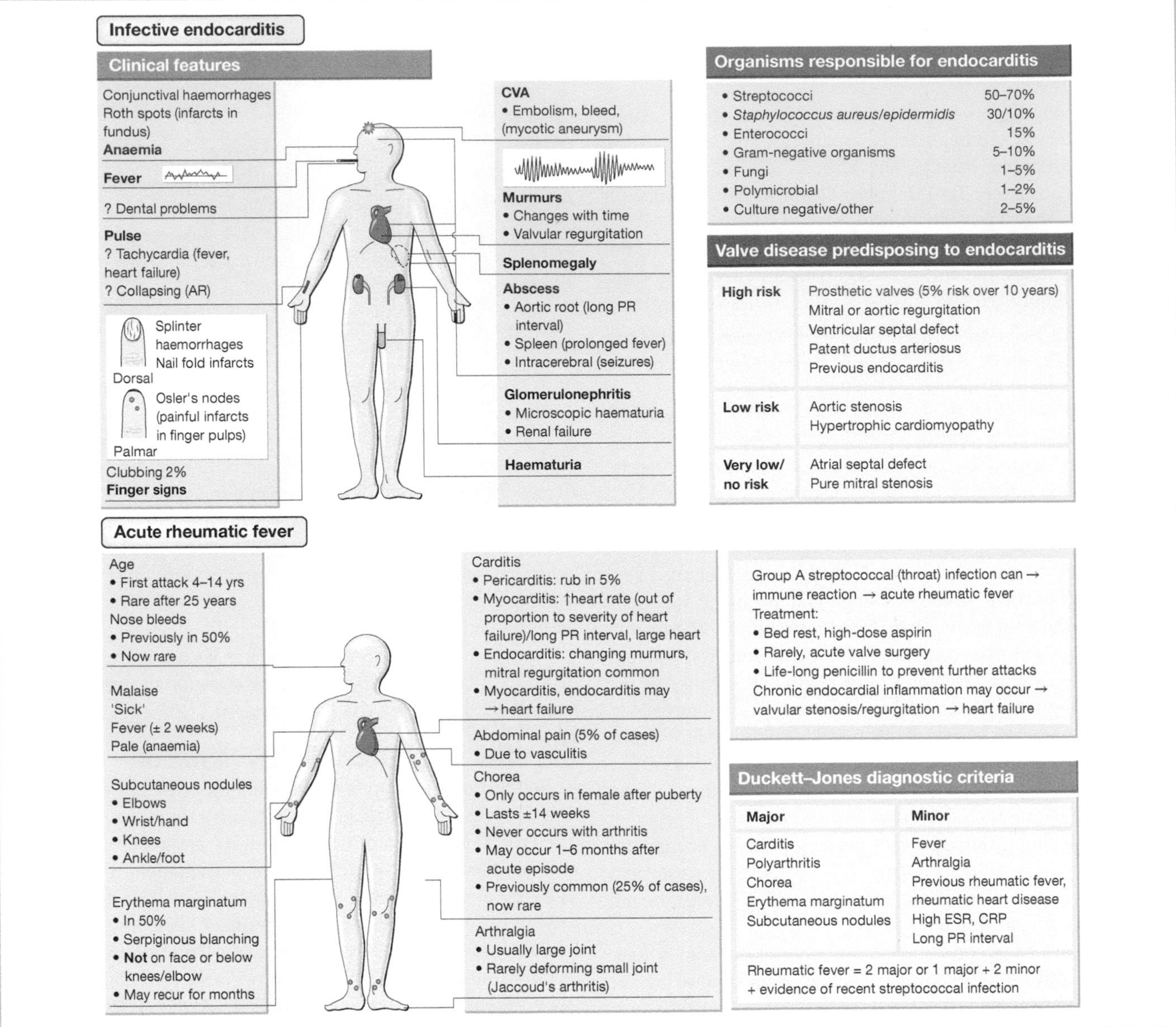

Infective endocarditis

This is infection of the heart, usually the heart valves, which are commonly diseased or prosthetic. There are about 3000 cases/year in the UK.

Aetiology and pathogenesis

Blood-borne organisms settle on a heart valve. Fibrin deposits together with micro-organisms form **vegetations** on a valve leaflet or cusp. The clinical manifestations are from valve damage (heart failure), embolization of infected material from the heart (abscesses, infarction of vital organs) or the immune response to chronic infection (renal failure).

The most common source of infection is the mouth after dental procedures or a tooth abscess. Skin infections (*Staphylococcus aureus*) and the gastrointestinal tract are also common sources. Intravenous drug abusers are at risk of tricuspid valve endocarditis and infection with unusual organisms (coliforms, fungi, etc.). Prosthetic valves are at high risk of infection <3 months after surgery from skin-related organisms (e.g. *S. epidermidis*, *S. aureus*), and later from the same organisms as native valves.

Clinical features

Presentation is typically non-specific, so a high clinical suspicion is required. The duration of symptoms before diagnosis is often weeks or months.

Medicine at a Glance, Fifth Edition. Edited by Patrick Davey and Alex Pitcher.

Companion website: www.wiley.com/go/medicine5e

- **Systemic features**: these are common, especially with low virulence organisms, e.g. *Streptococcus viridans*. There is fatigue, fever, anaemia or weight loss. A common and surprising symptom is back pain of obscure origin.
- **Valve destruction** by infection causes valvular regurgitation, not stenosis, leading to heart failure, and new or changing heart murmurs. Murmurs are common in endocarditis.
- **Systemic complications** result from 'seeding' of infection caused by bacteraemia or embolism of infected vegetation fragments, leading to new infection or abscess formation at distant sites, and/or manifestations of thromboembolism.
  - Cerebrovascular accident (CVA) from embolism, or haemorrhage resulting from ruptured mycotic aneurysm.
  - Finger/toe gangrene caused by embolism ± vasculitis.
  - Renal or splenic abscess or infarction.
  - Mesenteric embolism (ischaemic bowel and an acute abdomen).
  - Joint infection.
  - Bone infection: this is quite a common occurrence in infective endocarditis, and often affects the vertebrae. The most common symptom is back pain, though sometimes persistent sepsis is the diagnostic clue. The investigation of choice is bone magnetic resonance imaging; treatment is usually medical, though rarely surgical debridement is needed.
- **Acute renal failure**: this may occur from immune complex disease, haemodynamic upset (acute heart failure), damage during cardiac surgery and nephrotoxic antibiotics. Close monitoring of renal function throughout the illness is mandatory.

The physical examination often only reveals evidence of fever (temperature), mild weight loss, murmurs and sometimes complicating heart failure. The classic signs of clubbing, splinter haemorrhages and more substantial hand infarcts (Osler nodes) are rare in the current era. Splenomegaly is common. Dipstick haematuria is common.

Investigations

- **Blood tests**: the most important investigation is blood culture, three sets of which detect an organism in 97% of cases.
  - Systemic inflammatory markers: erythrocyte sedimentation rate (ESR) and C-reactive protein (CRP) are usually elevated.
  - Anaemia of chronic disease and elevated white cell count.
  - Urine dipstick and microscopy (haematuria).
- **Transthoracic echocardiography**: in patients with a low probability of endocarditis and sterile blood cultures, the diagnostic yield of transthoracic echocardiography is low. In patients with moderate or greater probability and a typical organism in blood cultures, a transthoracic echocardiogram becomes extremely valuable in making the diagnosis, assessing the degree and consequences of valvular damage and guiding subsequent management. It is increasingly accepted that a high-quality transthoracic echocardiogram (which will not be possible in all patients) showing no endocarditis has useful negative predictive value with a moderate or lower pretest probability.
- **Transoesophageal echocardiography**: useful when transthoracic images are suboptimal or for assessing prosthetic valves, because better acoustic windows allow more detailed imaging. It is also useful in assessing complications of endocarditis (abscess formation or acute valvular destruction) before surgery.

Treatment and prognosis

Antibiotic therapy is the mainstay of treatment, based on blood culture findings and organism sensitivities. This requires close collaboration with microbiologists. Antibiotics are usually intravenous, often in drug combinations in order to attain the best antibacterial killing and tissue penetration. Treatment commonly continues for four or six weeks, though some data suggest that shorter courses may be equivalent in some cases. **Endocarditis surgery** to remove and replace the infected valve is sometimes indicated for:

- severe valvular destruction causing heart failure
- abscess formation
- failure to eradicate infection despite prolonged antibiotic therapy
- prosthetic valve endocarditis.

Prognosis is variable, but overall mortality rate is 10–20%. Optimal endocarditis care is delivered by an 'endocarditis team' involving cardiologists, imaging specialists, microbiologists and cardiac surgeons.

Antibiotic prophylaxis to prevent infective endocarditis

Patients with significant risk factors for endocarditis, including congenital heart disease or prosthetic valves, should have antibiotics before undergoing procedures that provoke bacteraemia (dental procedures involving the gums and other invasive procedures, e.g. lower gastrointestinal endoscopy). Follow local protocols.

Myocarditis

Myocarditis is inflammation of the heart muscle caused by the following.

- **Viral infections**, e.g. Coxsackie, mumps and influenza. Subclinical infection is common in HIV infection. SARS-CoV-2 infection.
- **Autoimmune disease**: the most common myocarditis on a worldwide basis is rheumatic fever.
- **Toxin damage** such as from diphtheria infection.
- **Bacterial infection**: may occur in severe septicaemia, although other features dominate the clinical picture.
- **Radiation exposure**: much more common before targeted beam therapy.

The clinical features depend on the severity and duration of the inflammation. Many patients with myocarditis will remain systemically well and recover without specific treatment. The diagnosis may be clear clinically, but if uncertainty exists, cardiac MRI may reveal lesions in a characteristic pattern and help to exclude an acute coronary syndrome. A small proportion of patients will develop **fulminant myocarditis** where the dominant feature is acute heart failure. The patient may be critically unwell, breathless and in a low output state. Mortality is high and an endomyocardial biopsy and mechanical support may be needed.

A particularly distressing manifestation of acute myocarditis is **sudden cardiac death**, which may be more prevalent in athletic sufferers. In **chronic myocarditis**, e.g. South American trypanosomiasis (*Trypanosoma cruzii*) infection, patients may present with chronic heart failure. Investigations include the following.

- **Echocardiography**: shows impaired systolic contractile function, and in chronic processes dilation of the left ventricle and atrium.
- **Cardiac enzymes**: elevated and, unlike myocardial infarction, often stay high for many days or weeks before declining.
- **Inflammatory markers**: CRP and ESR are usually high.
- **Serological tests**: may reveal the responsible organism.

Treatment and prognosis

There is rarely any specific treatment. Immunosuppression may be used in fulminant myocarditis depending upon biopsy findings. If LV dysfunction is present following an episode of myocarditis, standard heart failure therapy is given (see Chapter 87).

Pericarditis

See Chapter 91.

Rheumatic fever

See figure.

94 Tachyarrhythmias

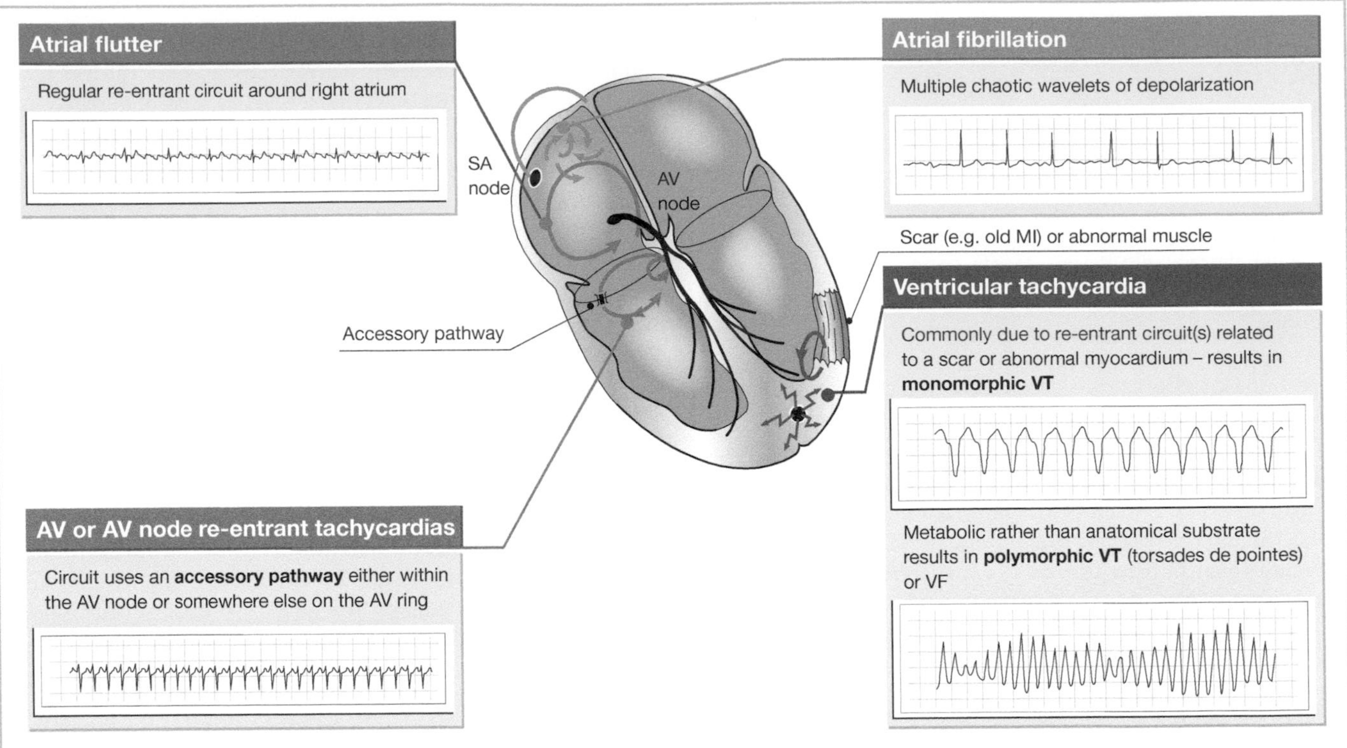

Arrhythmias are abnormal heart rhythms, either fast (tachyarrhythmias) or slow (bradyarrhythmias). The most common sustained arrhythmia, atrial fibrillation (AF), occurs in 1% of those aged 50 years or more, and 10% of the over-80s. Sudden cardiac death is often the result of arrhythmias (usually ventricular tachycardia [VT] and ventricular fibrillation [VF]) and causes 15–40% of deaths in coronary artery disease or heart failure.

Clinical features

Arrhythmias may be asymptomatic, cause intermittent minor palpitations, or be the cause of blackouts, severe cardiovascular compromise or cardiac arrest. **Palpitation** is an abnormal awareness of the heart beat; however, it does not necessarily mean that the heart rhythm is abnormal.

Key facts for understanding arrhythmias

The heart beat is initiated by the fastest pacemaker focus. During a tachyarrhythmia, the normal sinus node depolarizations are 'suppressed' by the faster depolarizations of the abnormal focus. The surface electrocardiogram (ECG) is a 'superimposed' graph of both atrial and ventricular activity. Atrial and ventricular activity are not necessarily linked during arrhythmias, so they need to be considered separately. Arrhythmias can be categorized according to where the initial depolarization originates.

- **Supraventricular arrhythmias** originate in the atria or around the atrioventricular (AV) node.
- **Ventricular arrhythmias** originate in the ventricles.

In the normal heart, the only communication between the atria and ventricles is the AV node, so the ventricular rate during arrhythmias arising in the atria is governed not just by the arrhythmia itself but by conduction through the AV node. The normal AV node acts as a 'turnstile', because it conducts depolarizations slowly and is refractory for a relatively long period after each depolarization. Abnormal additional conducting pathways between the atria and ventricles ('accessory pathways') are fairly common, and in some people may allow depolarizations to spread from the atria to ventricles, or from the ventricles to the atria, without necessarily passing fully through the AV node. This allows re-entry circuits to be set up, and in some circumstances bypasses the normal 'safety valve' of the AV node.

Medicine at a Glance, Fifth Edition. Edited by Patrick Davey and Alex Pitcher.

Companion website: www.wiley.com/go/medicine5e

Supraventricular arrhythmias

Atrial fibrillation

Pathophysiology

The atria depolarize spontaneously in a rapid (frequently >300 bpm), unco-ordinated fashion, bombarding the AV node continuously with electrical impulses. Conduction to the ventricles is limited by AV node refractoriness (often to <200 bpm) and occurs unpredictably, causing an *irregularly irregular* ventricular response. Heart rates in AF can vary widely, but in untreated AF are typically around 100–150 bpm. AF is very common, with a lifetime risk of around 30%.

Classification

There are several different forms of AF.

- **Paroxysmal AF**, where AF terminates either spontaneously or with intervention within seven days of onset.
- **Persistent AF**, where AF is sustained beyond seven days.
- **Permanent AF**, where AF is accepted to be permanent, and the patient and physician accept that no further attempts to restore sinus rhythm will be undertaken.

ECG diagnosis

The QRS rate is usually fast and irregularly irregular. No P-waves are visible; the baseline may be flat or show fast, small depolarizations. The key diagnostic feature is that no other cardiac rhythm is truly irregularly irregular.

Clinical features

There are many possible different symptoms in AF.

- Most patients present with **fast irregular palpitations** that are typically cardiac (i.e. sudden onset, defined duration, sudden offset).
- Some patients present with additional symptoms of **breathlessness**. In many patients who are breathless with AF, there is a cardiac pathology beyond AF, most commonly impaired left ventricular (LV) function, occasionally cardiomyopathy or coronary disease.
- Many patients present with vague and **ill-defined symptoms of loss of good health** – only recognized as being due to AF once the AF is terminated and they feel better – or effort intolerance, due to the marked tachycardia during exercise in AF impairing cardiac efficiency and so limiting exercise capacity.
- In some patients, distressingly, the first sign of AF is a **stroke** (see Treatment section). These are most commonly patients who have not felt palpitations or have not recognized palpitations as being a possible sign of a cardiac illness.
- In a very few patients, **syncope** occurs. This is very rare, and the only situation is where there is underlying sinus node disease. The sinus node disease itself can predispose to AF. During an

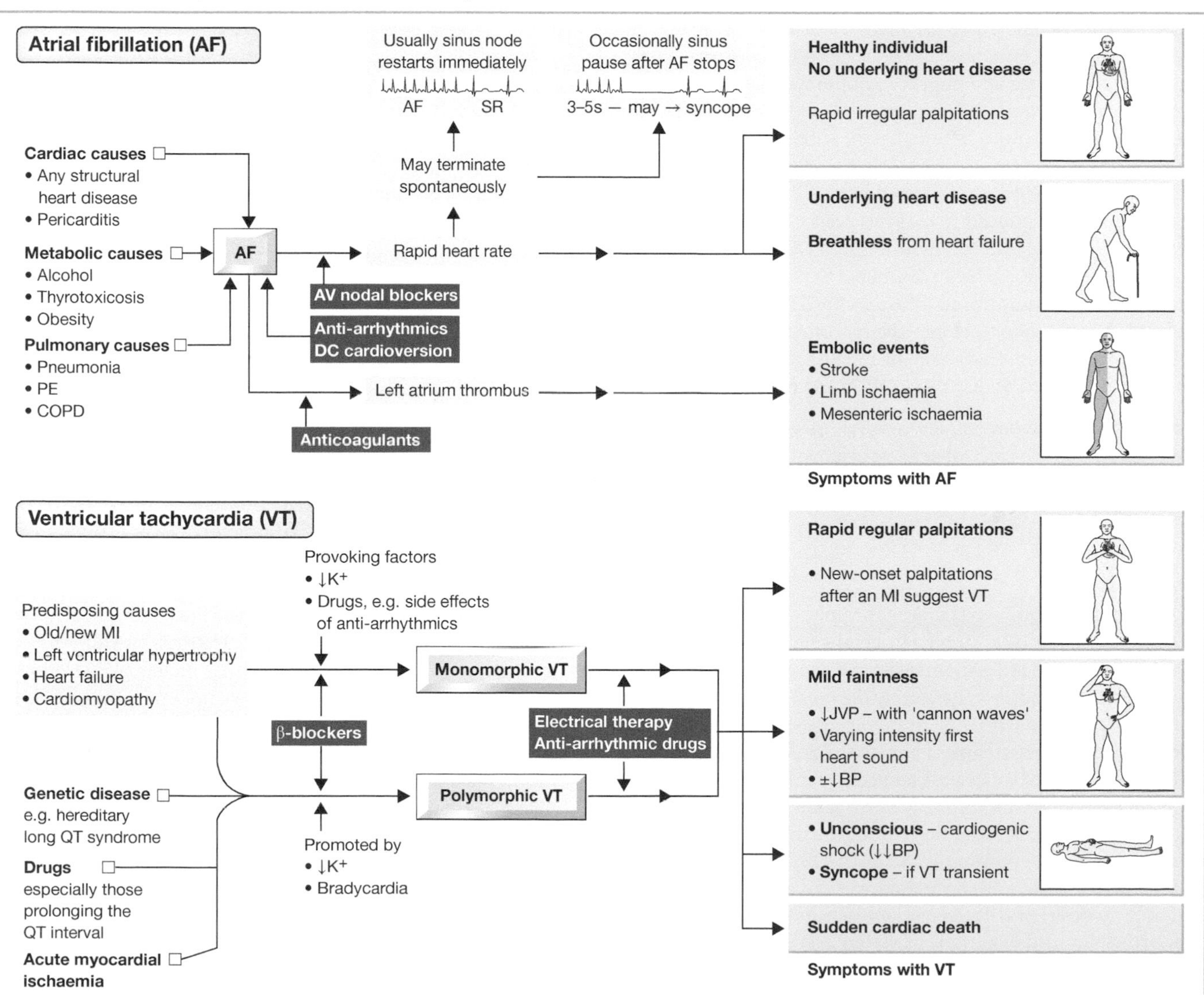

episode of AF, sinus node function is suppressed, and when the AF terminates, due to the sinus node disease it takes unusually long for sinus node function to restart, and a period of asystole can occur, occasionally lasting tens of seconds, sufficient to cause syncope. It must be emphasized that this is rare, and for the vast majority of patients who come to hospital with a blackout and are found to be in AF, the AF is not relevant to their blackout.

- In some patients, the AF itself does not give rise to symptoms of palpitations, or, initially, any other symptoms. The heart rate can then be 140–180 bpm for several months, and the patient can develop a **'rate-related cardiomyopathy or tachycardiomyopathy'**, a condition where after several months of rapid heart rate LV function falls dramatically. Patients then present with symptoms and signs of congestive heart failure (see Chapter 87). With meticulous heart rate control, LV function almost always returns to normal.
- In many patients with AF, **no symptoms** are present, and the condition is only picked up during a medical examination for another condition. These patients must have formal thromboembolic risk evaluation carried out to minimize the long-term risk of stroke.

Aetiology

Frequently, no cause of AF is found in otherwise well outpatients. AF incidence increases with age, and at any age is more common in men than women. There are many associations with AF, and treatment of certain medical and lifestyle risk factors may reduce the risk of recurrence and improve symptom control.

- **Cardiac**: hypertension, ischaemic heart disease, mitral valve disease (especially mitral stenosis), pericarditis and cardiomyopathy or heart failure (any cause).
- **Metabolic**: obesity is associated with AF and weight loss is associated with a reduced risk of recurrence and improved outcomes from AF treatment. Thyrotoxicosis is also associated with AF and may require separate treatment.
- **Alcohol:** is commonly associated with AF and alcohol abstinence has been shown to reduce the risk of AF recurrence.
- **Pulmonary**: pulmonary embolism (PE), pneumonia, chronic obstructive pulmonary disease (COPD) and cor pulmonale.

In acute hospital inpatient settings, AF may be precipitated by infection, anaemia, electrolyte derangement and other causes. Spontaneous reversion of the AF following treatment of these factors is common. Whether long-term anticoagulation improves outcomes in this setting is less clear.

Treatment

- **Anticoagulation**: systemic thromboembolism (stroke, embolic occlusion of a limb or visceral artery) is the most significant risk in AF. All patients with AF should be evaluated for their stroke risk and *this is probably the most important aspect of caring for patients with AF*. Systemic emboli may arise from thrombus in the left atrium. The risk is especially high in those with structural cardiac disease (especially mitral stenosis), large left atria (≥40 mm) and those aged 65 years or over. The risk of systemic emboli in AF can be estimated using scoring systems, of which the most common is the CHA_2DS_2-VASc score. Those with a score ≥2 are anticoagulated with an anticoagulant (now preferably a novel oral anticoagulant such as apixaban, rivaroxaban, edoxaban or dabigatran) or warfarin (this remains the preferred option for patients with prosthetic mechanical heart valves and/or moderate or severe mitral stenosis). The benefit from anticoagulants is balanced against the risk of bleeding. A score (HASBLED) summarizes some of these risk factors (**H**ypertension, **A**bnormal renal/liver function, **S**troke, **B**leeding history or predisposition, **L**abile INR, **E**lderly, **D**rugs/alcohol concomitantly), though there is no clear cut-off score and, unhelpfully, there is significant overlap between stroke and bleeding risk factors. If there is an absolute contraindication to anticoagulation, occluding the left atrial appendage with a closure device may be an alternative to reduce stroke risk. The thromboembolic risk is essentially the same in paroxysmal, persistent or permanent AF, and remains high regardless of the frequency of symptoms, and so a return to sinus rhythm does not mean that anticoagulants can be stopped. If a patient with documented AF has a high CHA_2DS_2-VASc score, they should remain on anticoagulants indefinitely regardless of whether they revert to sinus rhythm.
- **Rhythm control**: having assessed and, if appropriate, modified stroke risk, the next step is to assess the heart rate. The optimal ventricular rate target is unclear, but a resting rate of <110 bpm is probably acceptable in the first instance though many cardiologists prefer <90 bpm. The ventricular rate may be decreased by reducing conduction through the AV node using β-blockers, digoxin and/or certain calcium channel antagonists. Some patients will require a combination of these drugs. The intention of rate control is to reduce symptoms arising from AF and prevent tachycardia-mediated cardiomyopathy rather than terminating the AF, though reversion to sinus rhythm may occur spontaneously during rate control treatment.
- Approaches to rhythm control include the following.
  - *Drugs* (amiodarone, flecainide, sotalol and others) can cardiovert AF back to sinus rhythm and/or prevent further episodes of AF. *The primary goal of rhythm control in AF is to reduce symptoms*, and in general, rhythm control is not thought to improve outcomes compared to rate control (though there are rare exceptions). DC cardioversion under anaesthesia/deep sedation is very effective in restoring sinus rhythm provided that AF has been present for <1 year, and the heart is not structurally abnormal.
  - *Ablation*: if ongoing episodes of AF are troublesome despite antiarrhythmic drugs, or there is actual or possible concern over drug side-effects, ablation of certain electrical structures in the left atrium can reduce AF burden. There are several different techniques; all use ablating catheters inserted into the left atrium via the femoral vein, right heart and across the interatrial septum. The ablation circuits can isolate the pulmonary veins, often the initial source of the abnormal electrical impulses in AF, or channel the electricity within the left atrium, preventing self re-entering AF circuits. AF ablation is frequently performed to reduce symptoms arising despite medical treatment in AF, and the risk is low (though up to 1–2% of patients may have a major complication and around half of patients may require additional ablation procedures to obtain a satisfactory result).

Supraventricular tachycardias

The terminology can get confusing as many arrhythmias, including AF, are supraventricular in origin. However, the term 'supraventricular tachycardia' (SVT) is most commonly used to refer only to regular narrow complex tachycardias, which have a range of causes. It is commonly not possible to reliably separate these without an invasive electrophysiology study, though the principles of acute management are similar.

Pathogenesis

The potential for a re-entrant circuit is established by the presence of an additional electrical pathway. This can be either:

- an extension arising from the AV node and forming a potential circuit (termed dual AV nodal physiology with 'fast' and 'slow' pathways): this is the most common additional pathway and is the cause of AV nodal re-entrant tachycardia (AVNRT), or
- between the atria and ventricles, which can cause AV re-entrant tachycardia (AVRT). Evidence of this additional pathway may be seen in the ECG during normal sinus rhythm (see next section).

ECG diagnosis

A regular, narrow QRS complex tachycardia, usually at a rate of 150–200 bpm, is found. Regular P-waves may be visible interspersed between the QRS complexes. Often the P-waves are of an abnormal shape, as they are activated retrogradely, either by impulses passing up an accessory pathway from the ventricle, as in orthodromic tachycardia complicating Wolf–Parkinson–White (WPW) syndrome, or more commonly by impulses passing up from the AV node, as during an episode of AVNRT. In the latter, the P-wave is upside down and follows closely just after the QRS complex.

Clinical features

They usually present as recurrent attacks of rapid palpitations, lasting from a few minutes to hours or even days.

Treatment

Temporarily blocking conduction through the AV node will stop SVTs in which the re-entrant circuit involves the AV node (including AVNRT and AVRT). It may also unmask crucial clues to diagnosis in SVTs with a circuit that does not involve the AV node (e.g. by revealing flutter waves in atrial flutter), but will not terminate these arrhythmias.

- **Vagotonic manoeuvres** that increase vagal tone (e.g. Valsalva manoeuvre, swallowing cold drinks or carotid sinus massage); patients may discover these themselves.
- **Drug treatment**: slows or blocks conduction in the AV node.
  - Intravenous (IV) adenosine transiently blocks AV node conduction, terminating any tachycardia using the AV node as part of the circuit (i.e. both AVRT and AVNRT), so restoring sinus rhythm.
  - β-blockers (or verapamil, flecainide as alternatives) are useful as long-term oral prophylaxis or intermittent therapy.
- **Radiofrequency ablation**: increasingly the treatment of choice, especially if the SVT is recurrent. During an electrophysiological study, attempts are made to induce the arrhythmia in order to diagnose, and it may then be possible to destroy the culprit pathway by applying radiofrequency energy. Successful ablation is commonly curative in AVNRT, AVRT and atrial flutter.

Accessory pathways, pre-excitation and WPW syndrome

An accessory pathway, which conducts atrial depolarizations directly into the ventricular myocardium, bypassing the AV node, characterizes the WPW syndrome; pre-excitation, AV reciprocating tachycardias and pre-excited AF may occur.

- **Pre-excitation**: atrial impulses are propagated more quickly to the ventricle by the accessory pathway than by the normal AV node. The part of the myocardium into which the accessory pathway is inserted depolarizes earlier (i.e. is pre-excited) than the part of the ventricle depolarized by the normally conducted beat. This shortens the PR interval on the ECG. Electrical activity propagates slowly from the pre-excited ventricular myocardium by myocyte-to-myocyte transmission, not through specialized conducting tissue, so slurring the first part of the QRS complex (δ wave).
- **Atrial fibrillation in WPW syndrome**: normally the AV node acts as a 'safety valve' preventing an over-rapid ventricular response in AF. Some (about 5–10%) accessory pathways conduct impulses more frequently than the normal AV node, allowing AF to be conducted to the ventricles very rapidly, shortening diastole, impairing ventricular filling and lessening cardiac output, so that haemodynamic collapse or VF ('sudden cardiac death') occurs. Risk assessment and prevention of sudden cardiac death are therefore crucial in WPW syndrome. The ECG in 'pre-excited' AF has very abnormal, wide QRS complexes, because ventricular depolarization is largely from the impulse conducted down the accessory pathway. Pre-excited AF is usually treated with immediate direct current (DC) cardioversion as there is a risk of degeneration to VF. All patients with pre-excitation should have formal electrophysiological studies to assess the risk of the accessory pathway, and if it is high then the pathway is ablated, which is usually curative.

Atrial flutter

Pathophysiology

In its most common form ('typical' atrial flutter), the atria depolarize in a rapid co-ordinated fashion, as a result of a macro re-entry circuit moving anticlockwise around the right atrium. Atrial depolarizations occur at a rate of 300/min; conduction to the ventricles is limited to every second, third or fourth depolarization, because of AV node refractoriness.

ECG diagnosis

The QRS rate is exactly 150/min if alternate flutter waves are conducted ('atrial flutter with 2:1 AV block') or can be other divisibles of the flutter rate, e.g. 100 (3:1), 75 (4:1), sometimes varying every few beats. Continuous sawtooth 'flutter waves' are usually visible instead of P-waves, most obviously in leads II, III, aVf and V1. *If a regular tachycardia has a constant rate of exactly 150/min, always think of atrial flutter* even if flutter waves are not obvious – they may be obscured by the QRS/T waves.

Clinical features

The pulse rate is usually 150 and regular. The patient may be asymptomatic, experience rapid palpitation or breathlessness, or be in heart failure. The incidence and causes of atrial flutter are similar to those of AF; these two arrhythmias commonly occur in the same patient.

Treatment

In typical atrial flutter, radiofrequency ablation is safe and has excellent success rates and may be considered in all patients.

Ventricular tachycardias

Pathogenesis

Rapid depolarizations arise in the ventricular myocardium, as a result of:

- re-entrant circuit(s) in an anatomically abnormal substrate such as myocardial infarction (MI) scar tissue. The ECG shows monomorphic VT.
- abnormal triggered activity in ventricular myocardium, resulting from electrophysiological/metabolic disturbances that often prolong the QT interval, such as acute ischaemia and drugs. The ECG shows polymorphic VT.

The most powerful stimulus to VT is myocardial damage, e.g. in heart failure VT is common. For each 10% decrease in ejection fraction, the chance of an arrhythmic death occurring increases by 65%. If patients with impaired LV function develop syncope, unless there is clear evidence for an alternative diagnosis, VT should be strongly suspected.

ECG diagnosis

The QRS complexes are broad with an abnormal shape. VT should *always be suspected* when patients known to have heart disease (especially recent or remote MI) present with a regular tachycardia with broad QRS complexes.

- In monomorphic VT, the QRS morphology is uniform; typically the rate is 120–190 bpm. There may be evidence of independent atrial activity, i.e. dissociated P-waves, or fusion and capture beats of narrower QRS complex.
- Polymorphic VT (Table 94.1) is less regular, more chaotic and sometimes with a characteristic phasic variation in the QRS morphology – 'torsades de pointes' is the combination of polymorphic VT with prolonged QT interval. Polymorphic VT is inherently unstable and often degenerates early on into VF.

Table 94.1 Causes of polymorphic ventricular tachycardia

- Acute ischaemia
- Drugs (cause prolongation of the QT interval): quinidine, sotalol, amiodarone, tricyclic antidepressants, antihistamines
- Hypokalaemia
- Hypomagnesaemia
- Hypocalcaemia
- Bradycardias (any cause)
- Congenital QT prolongation syndromes (ion channel mutations)

Source: Eur Heart J. 2010. Reproduced with permission of Oxford University Press.

Clinical features

The pulse rate is fast or may be weak, or there may be no pulse palpable. The patient may be in acute cardiac failure, be severely compromised, suffer cardiac arrest (pulseless VT) or be relatively well, except for rapid palpitation or breathlessness. A good clinical state in a patient does not exclude VT, and the risk of haemodynamic deterioration remains.

Treatment

- **Pulseless VT or impending cardiovascular collapse**: DC cardioversion, either immediate or after urgent anaesthesia/sedation.
- **Haemodynamically stable VT**: Drug treatment with antiarrhythmics (e.g. IV lidocaine [lignocaine] or amiodarone or others). If drugs are unsuccessful, DC cardioversion may be required.

Condition	Points
C – Congestive heart failure (or left ventricular systolic dysfunction)	1
H – **Hypertension**: blood pressure consistently above 140/90 mmHg (or treated hypertension on medication)	1
A_2 – Age ≥75 years	2
D – Diabetes mellitus	1
S_2 – Prior **stroke** or **TIA** or **thromboembolism**	2
V – Vascular disease (e.g. peripheral artery disease, myocardial infarction, aortic plaque)	1
A – Age 65–74 years	1
Sc – Sex category (i.e. female gender)	1

Annual stroke risk	
CHA_2DS_2-VASc score	**Stroke risk %**
0	0
1	1.3
2	2.2
3	3.2
4	4.0
5	6.7
6	9.8
7	9.6
8	6.7
9	15.2

Causes of sudden death

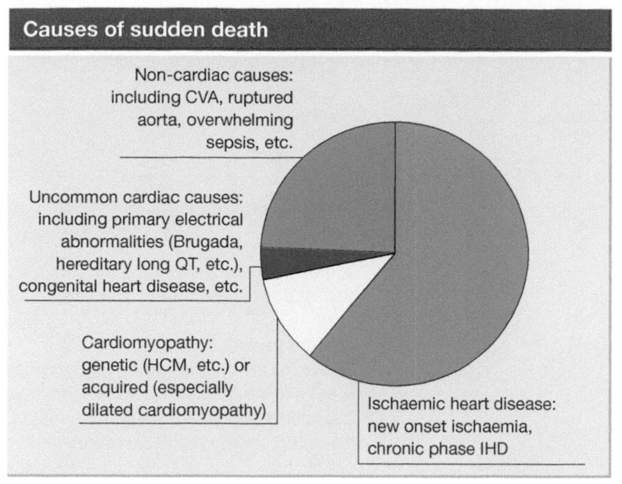

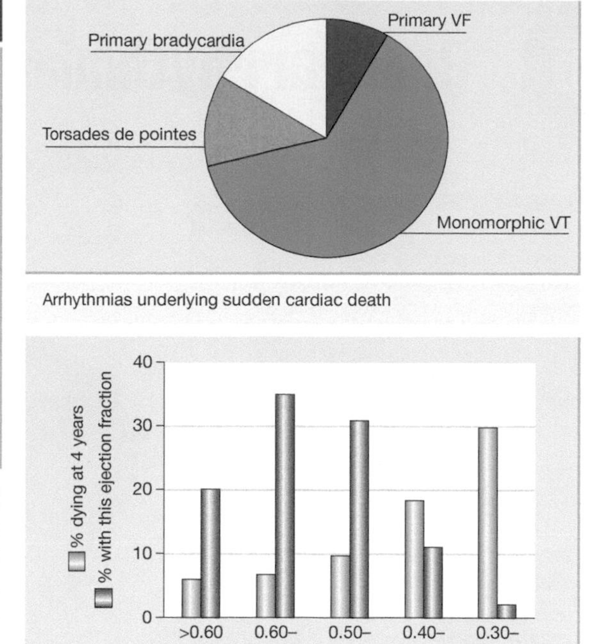

Arrhythmias underlying sudden cardiac death

The role of ejection fraction in predicting death at 4 years following an acute MI. Ejection fraction is the proportion of blood ejected from the heart with each cardiac cycle, i.e. the (end-diastolic – end-systolic volume) /end-diastolic volume. Ejection fraction is plotted against % dying; the highest risk of death is in those with the lowest ejection fraction (affects a rather small proportion of the post MI population)

Polymorphic VT: patients with sustained polymorphic VT and haemodynamic compromise require immediate DC cardioversion. Intravenous magnesium (e.g. 8 mM over 10–15 minutes) may be used not only to break the arrhythmia but also to reduce recurrence risk. Avoidance of any QT prolonging drugs and correction of underlying metabolic or ischaemic issues are crucial. Slow heart rates prolong the QT interval and may increase the risk of polymorphic VT; increasing the heart rate by pacing often prevents or dramatically reduces the incidence of polymorphic VT.

Prevention of future episodes

- **Long-term drug therapy**: β-blockers, amiodarone, angiotensin-converting enzyme inhibitors and spironolactone to improve LV function and maintain K^+.
- **Revascularization** (coronary artery bypass graft or percutaneous coronary intervention): for severe coronary disease.
- **Implantable cardioverter defibrillators** (ICDs): monitor the cardiac rhythm and deliver antitachycardia therapy (overdrive pacing and/or intracardiac shocks) if VT or VF is detected. They are indicated for survivors of cardiac arrest, and in VT with impaired LV function.

Ventricular fibrillation

Ventricular fibrillation (VF) is often lethal, especially out of hospital, but provided patients can be resuscitated (see Chapter 78) without major neurological damage, it is important to determine the underlying cause, and this usually needs full cardiac and coronary imaging.

- **Ischaemic heart disease (IHD)**: either acute MI, which is then treated in the standard fashion, or critical coronary stenosis, treated with complete revascularization. If there is no new ischaemia, and the problem relates to an old MI-related scar, the treatment is an ICD.
- **Other structural heart disease**: especially cardiomyopathies. Many patients in these categories need an ICD.
- **Channelopathies**: these are usually genetically mediated proarrhythmic conditions, and include hereditary long QT syndrome and Brugada syndrome, among others.

95 Bradyarrhythmias

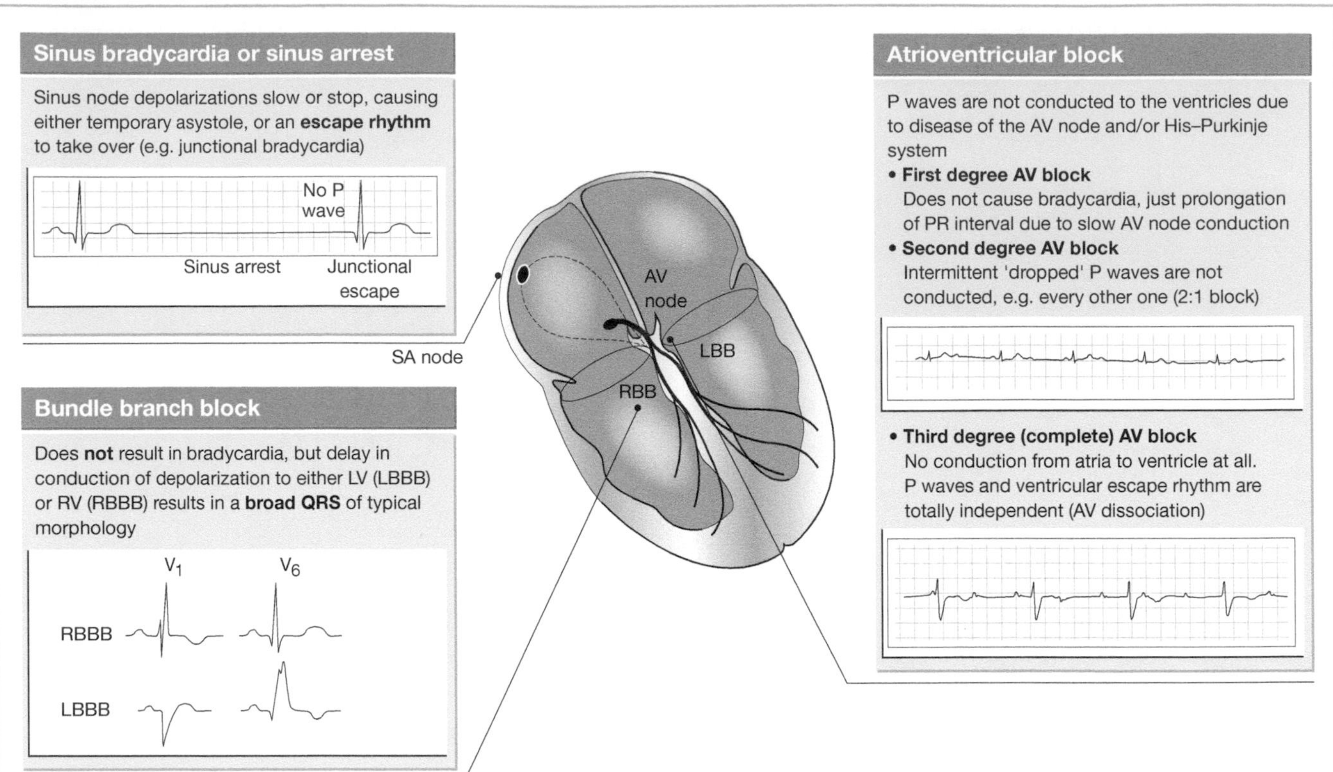
Sinus bradycardia or sinus arrest
Sinus node depolarizations slow or stop, causing either temporary asystole, or an escape rhythm to take over (e.g. junctional bradycardia)
No P wave
Sinus arrest
Junctional escape
SA node
Bundle branch block
Does not result in bradycardia, but delay in conduction of depolarization to either LV (LBBB) or RV (RBBB) results in a broad QRS of typical morphology
V1
V6
RBBB
LBBB
AV node
LBB
RBB
Atrioventricular block
P waves are not conducted to the ventricles due to disease of the AV node and/or His–Purkinje system
• First degree AV block
Does not cause bradycardia, just prolongation of PR interval due to slow AV node conduction
• Second degree AV block
Intermittent 'dropped' P waves are not conducted, e.g. every other one (2:1 block)
• Third degree (complete) AV block
No conduction from atria to ventricle at all.
P waves and ventricular escape rhythm are totally independent (AV dissociation)

Type of AV block	ECG features	Site/cause of impaired conduction	Natural history/treatment
First degree	Prolonged PR interval only	AV node May be functional, due to drugs or high vagal tone	If functional – progression unusual If due to AV node disease, progression common Usual treatment is observation only
Second degree	Some P waves are not conducted		
Mobitz I (Wenckebach)	Progressive PR interval prolongation leads to 'dropped' beat	AV node. May be functional, due to drugs or high vagal tone	May be benign, BUT often needs a pacemaker
Mobitz II	Only every second or third P wave is conducted	Usually structural AV node/His bundle disease	Always progresses to CHB Early permanent pacemaker
Third degree (complete) **Complete heart block (CHB)**	No P waves are conducted P waves and ventricular escape rhythm are completely independent (AV dissociation)	Structural disease of AV node and/or conducting system	Urgent pacemaker Immediate pacemaker if any history of syncope, or heart rate <35 bpm

Definition and clinical features

Bradyarrhythmias are abnormally slow heart beats (<60/min). Mild or transient bradyarrhythmias may be asymptomatic or even physiological, e.g. sinus bradycardia during sleep or in a healthy athlete. Symptomatic bradycardias commonly cause dizziness or syncope, or less commonly fatigue or heart failure. Palpitations are not a feature of bradyarrhythmias. The classic syncopal episode caused by a bradyarrhythmia is a **Stokes–Adams attack**. The characteristics are as follows.

Medicine at a Glance, Fifth Edition. Edited by Patrick Davey and Alex Pitcher.

Companion website: www.wiley.com/go/medicine5e

- Sudden onset without warning (within a few seconds). A warning, typically lasting up to a minute, is not typical for Stokes–Adams attacks, and rather suggests that the diagnosis is a form of fainting (vasomotor syncope), or just possibly an epileptiform seizure.
- Immediate collapse with loss of consciousness.
- Pale and still 'as if dead'.
- Duration a few seconds to 1–2 minutes.
- Rapid recovery back to normal, only transient disorientation at most for a few minutes, and no focal neurological symptoms or

signs. Prolonged time to full recovery suggests some form of epilepsy, or that a secondary anoxic seizure has complicated the attack.

Aetiology

Bradyarrhythmias arise either from failure of the sinoatrial (SA) node to provide regular depolarizations (**sinoatrial disease**), or by failure of the conducting system to convey the depolarizations into the ventricles (**atrioventricular [AV] block** or **complete heart block**). The total absence of any depolarizations (**asystole**) is usually prevented for more than a few seconds by the emergence of an **escape rhythm**, arising from the next most active intrinsic cardiac pacemaker. When the sinus node stops, this is usually the AV node (**junctional escape rhythm**); when AV conduction is blocked, a **ventricular escape rhythm** arises either from the conducting tissues or from the ventricular myocardium itself. The 'lower' (i.e. further away from the SA node) the escape rhythm, the slower it is. Both sinoatrial node disease and atrioventricular block are much more common in elderly than young patients.

Sinoatrial node disease

This is a dysfunction of the sinus node that manifests either as inappropriate **sinus bradycardia** or by periods of **sinus arrest**. It may be one aspect of the **sick sinus syndrome**, where patients experience both episodes of bradyarrhythmias (also known as sinus node dysfunction) and episodes of atrial tachyarrhythmias such as atrial fibrillation (AF). The bradycardias in SA node disease may be exacerbated by drugs used to control tachyarrhythmias, such as β-blockers or digoxin. Another manifestation of SA node disease is 'fainting' (syncope) or feeling faint (presyncope), occurring at the moment that an episode of AF stops. The usual mechanism for this is a prolonged sinus pause before the intrinsic SA node pacemaker starts up (see Chapter 94).

Sinoatrial node disease often has no particular cause, though it can relate to coronary disease, drugs (particularly long-term amiodarone) and occasionally hypothyroidism. It can also complicate many forms of heart disease, especially congenital. The prognosis of SA node disease not associated with any heart disease is good.

Atrioventricular block

Disease of either the AV node and/or the conducting system results in failure of transmission of the P-waves to the ventricles. AV block is classified according to the extent of the failure of transmission, seen on the electrocardiogram (ECG), and this is broadly related to the site and extent of the disease in the AV node/His–Purkinje system.

The clinical signs depend on the type of AV block. First-degree block is difficult to detect clinically as the first heart sound may be quiet. Second-degree block usually has a heart rate of <50 bpm. In third-degree block, the atria, which beat independently of the ventricles, occasionally contract on a closed tricuspid valve. Blood cannot leave the atria for the ventricle and instead will be propelled into the neck veins, seen as a prominent jugular venous pressure (JVP) pulsation – 'cannon' waves.

Investigations

Distinguishing arrhythmic syncope from other causes of dizziness or syncope (e.g. vasovagal episode, seizure, postural hypotension, transient ischaemic attack [TIA]) can be challenging. The clinical history and additional information from a witness are extremely important and may be the only information on which to base management decisions. The diagnostic investigation is an ECG during an episode, which will of course usually not be available initially. It is therefore essential to perform risk stratification in all patients with syncope and, where there is concern for arrhythmia, additional monitoring on an inpatient or outpatient may be required depending upon the outcome of risk stratification.

- **Twelve-lead ECG**: provides essential risk stratification in all forms of syncope. For suspected bradycardia, it may show evidence of conducting system disease, e.g. first-degree AV block or bundle branch block (BBB). The likelihood of intermittent high-grade AV block is higher in those with a greater degree of conducting tissue disease, e.g. bifascicular block with first-degree AV block.
- **Ambulatory ECG recording (Holter monitor)**: this is commonly used to detect the occurrence of both tachyarrhythmias and bradyarrhythmias but is often not useful as the duration of recording is usually 24–48 hours and so episodes occurring less frequently than this are unlikely to be documented. It may provide useful information on heart rate variability.
- **Wearables:** a new range of wearable devices can provide ambulatory ECG monitoring. These now include watches, home ECG monitors, adhesive patches and many others. If used correctly, these can provide high-quality traces of cardiac rhythm and are especially helpful if used whilst symptomatic.
- **Implantable loop recorder**: loop recorders are very small, implantable ECG recorders, about 1 × 4 × 0.5 cm, implanted under the skin on the left side of the chest, which continually record the ECG. They are primarily used to document cardiac rhythm when there is concern for significant arrhythmia and when symptoms are infrequent, i.e. separated by months.

Treatment

Minor bradyarrhythmias that do not cause symptoms do not require specific treatment. SA node disease requires treatment only if symptomatic or if a potentially exacerbating medication cannot be stopped. Asymptomatic first-degree AV block, BBB and Wenckebach block also do not require pacemaker implantation. However, patients with higher degrees of AV block (Mobitz II and complete heart block) are usually offered pacemaker implantation even if not symptomatic, because there is a higher risk of future syncope or even of sudden death.

- **Pacemaker implantation** is the preferred treatment for symptomatic bradyarrhythmias and AV block. A permanent pacemaker is a small electronic device that generates regular pulses to depolarize the heart through an electrode inserted into the right side of the heart through the venous system. A **single-chamber pacemaker** has an electrode in the right ventricle. A **dual-chamber pacemaker** paces both the atrium and the ventricle through two electrodes, and can pace the ventricle synchronously after each P-wave that is sensed in the atrium. This helps to restore normal AV synchrony, and allows the heart beat to change rate in track with the sinus node.
- **Pacemaker nomenclature** is as follows.
  - First letter: chamber paced (V, ventricle; A, atrium; D, dual).
  - Second letter: chamber sensed (V, A, D or O for none).
  - Third letter: pacemaker response to the detection of cardiac electrical activity (I, inhibited; T, triggered; D, both).
  - Fourth letter: relates to whether the pacemaker delivers quicker pacing on physical activity (R, rate responsive, e.g. VVIR).

So, using this system, single-chamber pacemakers are usually programmed VVI, which means that the ventricle is paced and sensed, and if electricity is detected (i.e. the ventricle has fired normally) then the system is inhibited (i.e. is silent).

The most common dual-chamber programming mode is DDD, where D stands for both atrial (A) and ventricular (V) leads. So, A and V can be paced, A and V are sensed, and the response can either be inhibited (I, as above) or triggered (T).

A dual-chamber pacemaker is preferred in most patients. The exception is when there is permanent atrial fibrillation (an atrial lead would be unable to pace a fibrillating atrium), and so a single-chamber pacemaker is used.

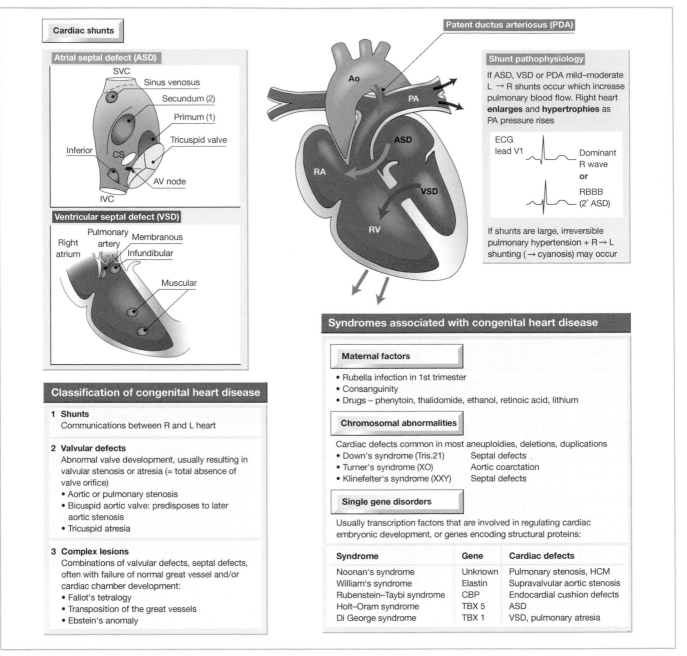

Congenital heart disease

Cardiac shunts

Atrial septal defect (ASD)

SVC
Sinus venosus
Secundum (2)
Primum (1)
Tricuspid valve
Inferior
CS
AV node
IVC

Ventricular septal defect (VSD)

Right atrium
Pulmonary artery
Membranous
Infundibular
Muscular

Patent ductus arteriosus (PDA)

Ao
PA
ASD
RA
VSD
RV

Shunt pathophysiology

If ASD, VSD or PDA mild–moderate L → R shunts occur which increase pulmonary blood flow. Right heart **enlarges** and **hypertrophies** as PA pressure rises

ECG lead V1
Dominant R wave
or
RBBB (2° ASD)

If shunts are large, irreversible pulmonary hypertension + R → L shunting (→ cyanosis) may occur

Classification of congenital heart disease

1 Shunts
Communications between R and L heart

2 Valvular defects
Abnormal valve development, usually resulting in valvular stenosis or atresia (= total absence of valve orifice)
- Aortic or pulmonary stenosis
- Bicuspid aortic valve: predisposes to later aortic stenosis
- Tricuspid atresia

3 Complex lesions
Combinations of valvular defects, septal defects, often with failure of normal great vessel and/or cardiac chamber development:
- Fallot's tetralogy
- Transposition of the great vessels
- Ebstein's anomaly

Syndromes associated with congenital heart disease

Maternal factors
- Rubella infection in 1st trimester
- Consanguinity
- Drugs – phenytoin, thalidomide, ethanol, retinoic acid, lithium

Chromosomal abnormalities

Cardiac defects common in most aneuploidies, deletions, duplications

• Down's syndrome (Tris.21)	Septal defects
• Turner's syndrome (XO)	Aortic coarctation
• Klinefelter's syndrome (XXY)	Septal defects

Single gene disorders

Usually transcription factors that are involved in regulating cardiac embryonic development, or genes encoding structural proteins:

Syndrome	Gene	Cardiac defects
Noonan's syndrome	Unknown	Pulmonary stenosis, HCM
William's syndrome	Elastin	Supravalvular aortic stenosis
Rubenstein–Taybi syndrome	CBP	Endocardial cushion defects
Holt–Oram syndrome	TBX 5	ASD
Di George syndrome	TBX 1	VSD, pulmonary atresia

Definition and incidence

Congenital heart disease (CHD) is an abnormal embryological cardiac development, or persistence of some parts of the fetal circulation after birth resulting in structural cardiac defects. The conditions discussed here (along with congenital aortic and pulmonary stenosis) account for 80% of CHD. The incidence of complex defects is 8/1000 live births. Non-complex defects are more common, e.g. bicuspid aortic valve affects 2%.

Medicine at a Glance, Fifth Edition. Edited by Patrick Davey and Alex Pitcher.

Companion website: www.wiley.com/go/medicine5e

Classification

See figure above.

Ventricular septal defect

Ventricular septal defect (VSD) is the most common example of CHD. A defect in the interventricular septum allows systolic blood flow from the left to right ventricle.

- **Small defects** produce high-velocity jets and a loud murmur (maladie de Roger) that is not of haemodynamic significance.
- **Large defects** may have a quiet murmur and a large left-to-right shunt. Untreated, this may cause pulmonary hypertension and Eisenmenger syndrome. Treatment is closure (usually surgical) before pulmonary hypertension develops.

There is a high risk of endocarditis (especially in small defects), so antibiotic prophylaxis is essential.

Atrial septal defect

Atrial septal defect (ASD) comprises 10% of CHD. A defect in the interatrial septum allows shunting of blood from the left to right atrium.

- Secundum ASD: 70%.
- Primum ASD: 30%; often involves the atrioventricular (AV) valves with mitral or tricuspid regurgitation. May be associated with other defects including VSD.

Left-to-right shunting increases pulmonary blood flow, producing a systolic pulmonary flow murmur, wide fixed splitting of the second heart sound and right ventricular hypertrophy (RVH). An electrocardiogram (ECG) shows right bundle branch block (RBBB) with right axis deviation and RVH (secundum) or left axis deviation with RVH (primum). Supraventricular tachycardias, e.g. atrial fibrillation, are common. ASDs may be undetected until adult life when they present with exertional dyspnoea and fatigue. The diagnosis is confirmed by transoesophageal cardiac ultrasonography. Treatment is closure of the defect, either by surgery or by a percutaneous closure device.

Patent ductus arteriosus

Patent ductus arteriosus (PDA) comprises 15% of CHD. The ductus arteriosus fails to close after birth, resulting in left-to-right shunting from the aorta to the pulmonary artery and a continuous (machinery) murmur. A large duct with a significant shunt leads to left ventricular hypertrophy (LVH) and heart failure, or pulmonary hypertension and Eisenmenger syndrome. Duct endocarditis is a significant long-term risk.

Treatment in neonates involves indomethacin blockade of prostaglandin production, which may provoke duct closure. Ducts remaining open require surgical ligation or percutaneous closure (coil or umbrella devices).

Eisenmenger syndrome

This describes irreversible pulmonary hypertension (from the high pulmonary blood flow of large left-to-right shunts) with shunt reversal (from left to right to right to left) resulting from the high right-sided heart pressures. Patients experience worsening symptoms with breathlessness; there is cyanosis, clubbing and signs of severe pulmonary hypertension. Surgical closure of left-to-right shunts must be undertaken before Eisenmenger syndrome develops; the only surgical treatment for established Eisenmenger syndrome is heart–lung transplantation.

Coarctation of the aorta

This comprises 5% of CHD. A developmentally hypoplastic segment of the aorta causes narrowing of the aorta and a significant pressure gradient, usually (98%), immediately distal to the origin of the left subclavian artery. Sixty percent also have a bicuspid aortic valve. Blood flow to the lower body is maintained by an increase in collateral flow (which may be huge) via the mammary arteries and intercostal arteries. Usually presents as (upper limb) hypertension with absent or weak femoral pulses and radial–femoral delay. There are features of LVH and palpable collaterals around the scapulae. There may be signs of bicuspid aortic valve and systolic murmur from the coarctation. The diagnosis is by echocardiography, computed tomography or magnetic resonance imaging. Treatment is surgical correction of the narrowing, preferably in older childhood (allows a sufficient increase in aortic calibre). Percutaneous dilation using a balloon is sometimes a viable alternative.

Complex congenital heart disease

In complex CHD, there are abnormal relationships of the arteries, ventricles and great vessels, abnormalities of chamber development, often with septal defects, and/or valvular lesions.

Tetralogy of Fallot

This is the most common 'complex' CHD (10% of CHD), involving a combination of VSD with right-to-left shunting, due to:

- **pulmonary stenosis**, either infundibular or valvar
- **right ventricular overload** and hypertrophy
- **dextro position** of the aorta so that it over-rides the VSD.

There is cyanosis, clubbing, signs of RVH and a pulmonary systolic murmur (the large VSD does not generate a murmur). Children with Fallot tetralogy experience exertional breathlessness, dizziness and growth retardation. Squatting kinks the femoral arteries, increases systemic resistance and reduces the right-to-left shunt.

Surgery aims to either:

- totally **correct the defects**, if the pulmonary arteries are large enough; or
- **increase pulmonary blood flow** using systemic to pulmonary artery shunts.
  - *Blalock–Taussig shunt*: subclavian artery to pulmonary artery.
  - *Waterston shunt*: ascending aorta to right pulmonary artery.
  - *Potts shunt*: descending aorta to left pulmonary artery.

Ebstein's anomaly

The tricuspid valve is displaced downwards into the right ventricle, resulting in a very small right ventricular cavity and a very large right atrium. There is tricuspid regurgitation and usually an ASD; 20% have accessory pathways (Wolff–Parkinson–White syndrome).

Transposition of the great arteries

There is ventriculo-arterial discordance: the aorta arises from the right ventricle and the pulmonary artery from the left ventricle. In isolation, this is incompatible with life (totally separate pulmonary and systemic circulations); an associated ASD usually allows shunting. Surgical treatments include the following.

- **Balloon septostomy** (Rashkind): increases shunting and reduces cyanosis.
- **Interatrial shunt** (Mustard or Senning operation): directs systemic venous return from the right atrium across the ASD into the morphological left ventricle; pulmonary venous return passes in the opposite direction and into the aorta.
- **Arterial 'switch' operation** totally corrects the defect by reconnecting the aorta to the left ventricle and the pulmonary artery to the right ventricle and has replaced interatrial shunt procedures.
- **Congenitally corrected transposition**: the right and left ventricles and AV valves are interchanged (venous return drains via the right atrium into a morphological left ventricle, which ejects blood into the pulmonary artery). Usually well tolerated in childhood but heart failure may occur in adult life (the morphological right ventricle may be unable to sustain systemic pressures long term).

Adult congenital heart disease

Advances in surgical and percutaneous treatment of congenital heart diseases have transformed the outlook for affected children, many of whom now survive into adulthood and may have normal or near-normal life expectancy. Adult congenital heart disease specialists work in multidisciplinary teams to provide care to this population, who have unique health needs.

97 Lung function tests

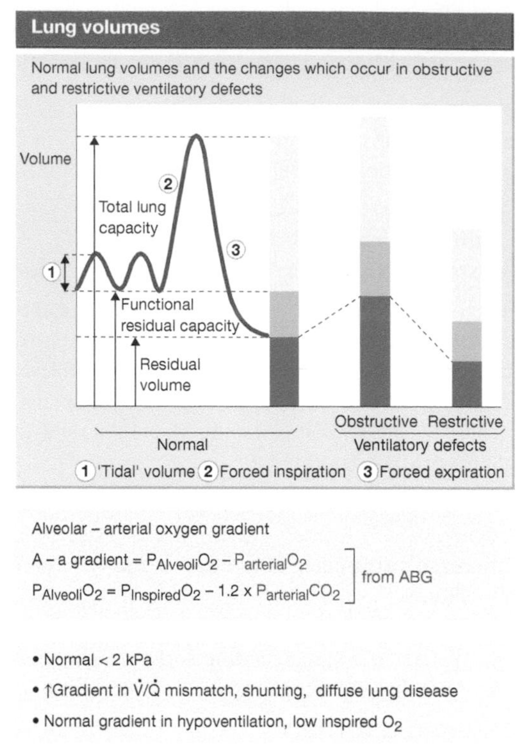

Lung volumes
Normal lung volumes and the changes which occur in obstructive and restrictive ventilatory defects
Volume
Total lung capacity
Functional residual capacity
Residual volume
Normal
Obstructive Restrictive
Ventilatory defects
1 'Tidal' volume 2 Forced inspiration 3 Forced expiration
Alveolar – arterial oxygen gradient
A – a gradient = $P_{Alveoli}O_2 - P_{arterial}O_2$
$P_{Alveoli}O_2 = P_{Inspired}O_2 - 1.2 \times P_{arterial}CO_2$
from ABG
• Normal < 2 kPa
• ↑Gradient in $\dot{V}/\dot{Q}$ mismatch, shunting, diffuse lung disease
• Normal gradient in hypoventilation, low inspired O_2

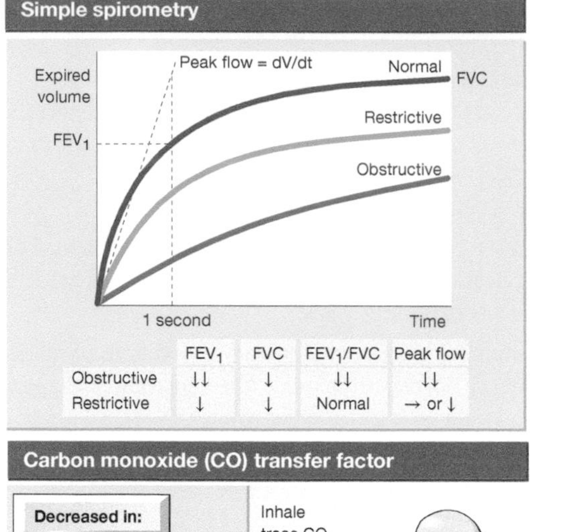

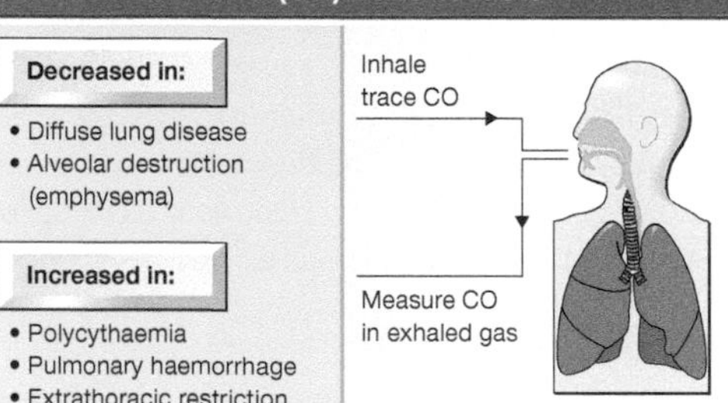

Carbon monoxide (CO) transfer factor
Decreased in:
• Diffuse lung disease
• Alveolar destruction (emphysema)
Increased in:
• Polycythaemia
• Pulmonary haemorrhage
• Extrathoracic restriction
Inhale trace CO
Measure CO in exhaled gas

Spirometric tests of airway function

These are simple, cheap and reproducible.

- **Forced expiratory volume in one second** (FEV_1).
- **Forced vital capacity** (FVC): the total volume of air expelled by a forced expiration after maximal inspiration.
- **FEV_1/FVC ratio** (%): the percentage of FVC exhaled in one second during forced expiration. These measures allow for the classification of lung diseases into restrictive or obstructive. In obstructive disease, the ratio is less than 70% and in restrictive disease, there is reduction of both FEV_1 and FVC with a normal or high ratio.
- **Peak expiratory flow rate (PEFR)**: fastest flow rate attained at the start of a forced expiration after maximal inspiration. Useful for monitoring changes in airflow obstruction. This is effort dependent and can be reduced in restrictive disease so it is not useful in isolation as a diagnostic test.
- **Reversibility testing**: measurement of airway function before and after an inhaled bronchodilator. An improvement of ≥20% and 300 mL represents a positive test.

Lung volumes

Total lung capacity (TLC) is measured by dilution of an inert gas such as helium or in an enclosed box (total body plethysmograph).

- **TLC**: the total amount of gas in the lungs at maximal inspiration. Residual volume is the amount of gas left in the lung after maximal expiration and is derived from the TLC and vital capacity (VC).
- **Functional residual capacity (FRC)**: the amount of gas left in the lung at end expiration during tidal breathing, derived by helium dilution during tidal breathing.

Tests of gas exchange

- **Carbon monoxide transfer factor (*K*co)**: measured by inhalation of a trace of CO, which is avidly taken up by haemoglobin. Assesses the size and efficiency of the gas-exchanging area.
- **Pulse oximetry**: measured by the absorbance of light by haemoglobin; used to assess hypoxaemia and in particular the response to oxygen therapy. CO_2 is not measured.
- **Blood gas analysis** (see Chapters 97 and 98).

Other investigations

- **Fractional exhaled nitric oxide levels** (FeNO): this gas is produced by inflamed airways. The test can be used to diagnose asthma and to decide if increased anti-inflammatory treatment with inhaled steroids is likely to work. Levels above 40 parts per billion are abnormal.
- **Flow–volume loops** are useful for diagnosing large airway obstruction of both intra- and extrathoracic airways.
- **Tests of respiratory muscles**: muscle power is measured by breathing against a closed orifice or by a sniff. Maximal inspiratory pressure is measured at FRC and expiratory pressure at TLC. Values <60 cmH_2O are abnormal.

Medicine at a Glance, Fifth Edition. Edited by Patrick Davey and Alex Pitcher.

Companion website: www.wiley.com/go/medicine5e

98 Overnight oximetry and sleep apnoea

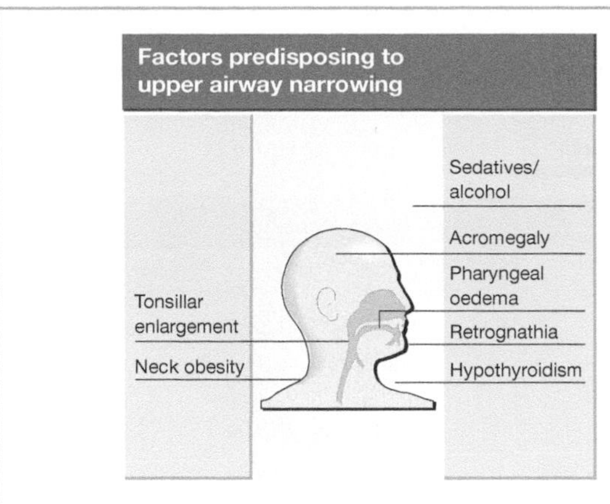

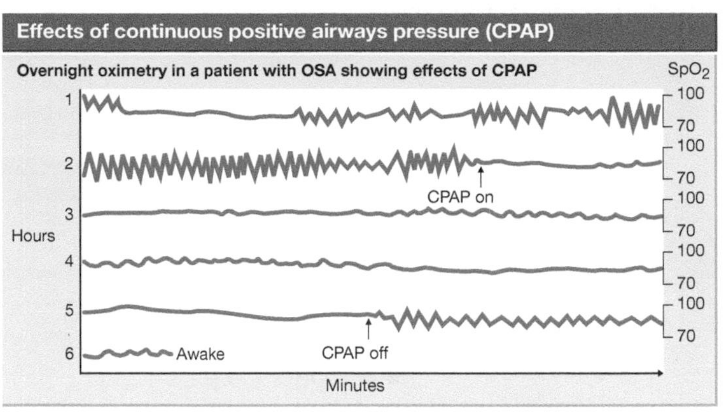

Sleep apnoea is mostly caused by obstruction to the upper airway – obstructive sleep apnoea (OSA). Less commonly, it relates to disturbed control of breathing in conditions such as heart failure and stroke. Pathological episodes of nocturnal apnoea or desaturation due to hypoventilation often occur during rapid eye movement (REM) sleep in:

- brainstem disease, either as a result of hypnotics or as a preterminal event in many conditions
- motor weakness, most commonly motor neuron disease, occasionally from previous poliomyelitis
- OSA (see below)
- chronic obstructive pulmonary disease (COPD).

Apnoea leads to hypoxaemia, sometimes profound, arousal and waking. Frequent episodes disturb sleep, resulting in daytime sleepiness. Severe sleep apnoea may lead to nocturnal arrhythmias or right-sided heart failure.

Obstructive sleep apnoea

A syndrome of upper airway collapse leading to sleep disruption which results in symptoms, usually of daytime sleepiness. It is very common: 5% of middle-aged adult men are affected. It is more common in men but increasingly recognized in women.

Aetiology

Obstructive sleep apnoea is caused by upper airway narrowing and obstruction due to reduction in muscle tone during sleep. Arousal from sleep results. Sleep fragmentation causes the predominant symptom of excessive daytime sleepiness. Factors leading to upper airway narrowing predispose to OSA.

- Neck obesity, retrognathia and tonsillar enlargement.
- Endocrine abnormalities, including acromegaly, amyloidosis and hypothyroidism predispose to upper airway obstruction by enlarged tissues around the oropharynx.
- Neuromuscular disease or myopathy.
- Alcohol, sedatives and sleep deprivation worsen the effects of an anatomically narrow airway.

Clinical features

Classic symptoms are snoring in association with excessive daytime sleepiness. A partner may describe the episodes of obstruction with apnoea, terminating with a sudden loud gasp. Sleepiness may impair performance at work and there is a seven-fold increased risk of motor accidents. Potential symptoms are morning headache, poor concentration and impotence. Examination reveals factors predisposing to upper airway narrowing (see above). Hypertension is a common finding.

Investigations

Occasional obstructions are common in snorers and do not require investigation unless associated with sleepiness. Overnight sleep studies including video and pulse oximetry confirm the diagnosis. Apnoea typically decreases oxygen saturation by ≥4%; such episodes may occur many times each hour (see figure). Full polysomnography studies include measurement of electroencephalograph, airflow, ribcage and abdominal movement, as well as recordings of snoring and continuous oximetry. Endocrine or neurophysiology studies are occasionally appropriate. The degree of patient-reported sleepiness can be assessed using the Epworth sleepiness questionnaire.

Treatment and prognosis

Avoid alcohol and sedatives. Treat any underlying illness.

- **Severe cases**: continuous positive airway pressure (CPAP) delivered overnight by a tight-fitting nasal mask splints the upper airway open, prevents obstruction and arousal, and results in rapid improvement in symptoms. NICE guidance recommends CPAP for severe OSA and moderate OSA when associated with significant sleepiness. Treatment of severe OSA with CPAP improves 24 h mean blood pressure significantly.
- **Milder cases**: weight loss and/or mandibular advancement devices may be sufficient. CPAP is used if symptoms have a significant impact on quality of life.
- **Surgery**: tonsillectomy may be curative, particularly in young patients with significant tonsillar enlargement. Palatal surgery may help but the benefit is not permanent and can make future application of CPAP difficult.

Effective treatment results in rapid improvement of symptoms.

Medicine at a Glance, Fifth Edition. Edited by Patrick Davey and Alex Pitcher.

Companion website: www.wiley.com/go/medicine5e

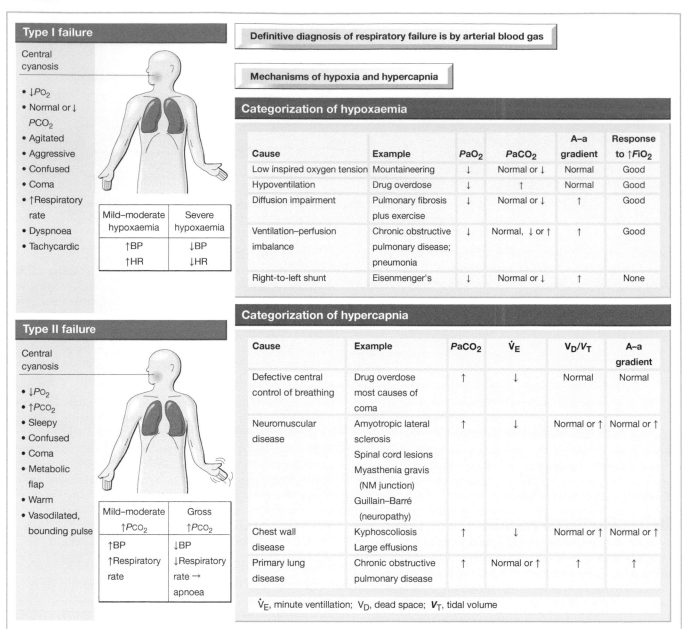

99 Respiratory failure

Type I failure

Central cyanosis

- ↓Po_2
- Normal or ↓ PCO_2
- Agitated
- Aggressive
- Confused
- Coma
- ↑Respiratory rate
- Dyspnoea
- Tachycardic

Mild–moderate hypoxaemia	Severe hypoxaemia
↑BP ↑HR	↓BP ↓HR

Type II failure

Central cyanosis

- ↓Po_2
- ↑Pco_2
- Sleepy
- Confused
- Coma
- Metabolic flap
- Warm
- Vasodilated, bounding pulse

Mild–moderate ↑Pco_2	Gross ↑Pco_2
↑BP ↑Respiratory rate	↓BP ↓Respiratory rate → apnoea

Definitive diagnosis of respiratory failure is by arterial blood gas

Mechanisms of hypoxia and hypercapnia

Categorization of hypoxaemia

Cause	Example	PaO_2	$PaCO_2$	A–a gradient	Response to ↑FiO_2
Low inspired oxygen tension	Mountaineering	↓	Normal or ↓	Normal	Good
Hypoventilation	Drug overdose	↓	↑	Normal	Good
Diffusion impairment	Pulmonary fibrosis plus exercise	↓	Normal or ↓	↑	Good
Ventilation–perfusion imbalance	Chronic obstructive pulmonary disease; pneumonia	↓	Normal, ↓ or ↑	↑	Good
Right-to-left shunt	Eisenmenger's	↓	Normal or ↓	↑	None

Categorization of hypercapnia

Cause	Example	$PaCO_2$	$\dot{V}_E$	V_D/V_T	A–a gradient
Defective central control of breathing	Drug overdose most causes of coma	↑	↓	Normal	Normal
Neuromuscular disease	Amyotropic lateral sclerosis Spinal cord lesions Myasthenia gravis (NM junction) Guillain–Barré (neuropathy)	↑	↓	Normal or ↑	Normal or ↑
Chest wall disease	Kyphoscoliosis Large effusions	↑	↓	Normal or ↑	Normal or ↑
Primary lung disease	Chronic obstructive pulmonary disease	↑	Normal or ↑	↑	↑

$\dot{V}_E$, minute ventillation; V_D, dead space; V_T, tidal volume

Respiratory failure may be acute, chronic or acute-on-chronic (e.g. a patient with an exacerbation of chronic obstructive pulmonary disease [COPD] and pre-existing hypoxia). Abnormal levels of arterial oxygen (PaO_2 <8 kPa) or carbon dioxide ($PaCO_2$ >6.0 kPa) are used to define the presence of respiratory failure, which is thus divided into:

- hypoxaemic (type I): failure of oxygenation
- hypercapnic (type II): failure of ventilation to remove CO_2.

Generally, hypercapnic failure is the result of a disorder with respiratory muscles ('pump failure'), whereas hypoxaemic failure is due to pulmonary pathology. However, type II respiratory failure often supersedes type I failure as the patient becomes exhausted.

What is the A–a gradient?

Alveolar O_2 and CO_2 levels are interdependent and a high alveolar partial pressure of carbon dioxide results in a lower partial pressure of oxygen. The alveolar–arterial oxygen gradient (A–a gradient) is calculated from the alveolar gas equation and is a measure of ventilation and perfusion mismatch (reflecting the severity of lung disease).

Medicine at a Glance, Fifth Edition. Edited by Patrick Davey and Alex Pitcher.

Companion website: www.wiley.com/go/medicine5e

$$A-a \text{ gradient} = FiO_2 \text{ (atmospheric pressure} - \text{water pressure)} - PaO_2 - 1.25\,(Pco_2)$$
$$= 0.21(101\text{kPa} - 6.3\text{ kPa}) - PaO_2 - 1.25(Pco_2)$$
$$= 19.9\text{ kPa} - PaO_2 - 1.25(Pco_2)(\text{on air} - 21\%\text{ oxygen})$$

A normal A–a gradient is 2–4 kPa; it increases with age and at FiO_2 >0.28 (FiO_2 = fraction of O_2 in inspired air). Certain disease processes also increase the A–a gradient; measuring the A–a gradient is thus helpful in ruling in or out these diseases in patients with respiratory failure.

Causes of hypoxaemia

- **Shunt**: the lung is perfused but not ventilated (the opposite of dead space). A right-to-left shunt leads to hypoxaemia that does not respond to 100% oxygen.
- **Ventilation/perfusion mismatch** ($\dot{V}/\dot{Q}$ mismatch): *this is by far the most common form*, even in diseases like pulmonary fibrosis where one might expect diffusion block. Poorly ventilated alveoli contribute to hypoxaemia, which is overcome by an increase in FiO_2.
- **Diffusion block**: a thickened interstitium between alveolus and capillary (uncommon). Only important during exercise when erythrocytes have insufficient time to equilibrate for gas exchange.
- **Low FiO_2 at altitude.**
- **Hypoventilation**: ventilation is inversely proportional to $PaCO_2$. The interdependence of PaO_2 and $PaCO_2$ thus leads to hypoxaemia in hypoventilation.

All causes of hypoxaemia other than true shunts improve with an increase in FiO_2.

Causes of hypercapnia

This is a failure of ventilation, which may be caused by central nervous system, neuromuscular, chest wall or primary lung diseases. There is either insufficient respiratory drive or ineffective (increased dead space) ventilation.

Symptoms and signs of respiratory failure

See figure above.

Treatment of respiratory failure

It is important to establish whether the onset of respiratory failure is acute, chronic or acute-on-chronic, and the underlying aetiology. Patients need to be appropriately monitored in a critical care area. Ideally, monitoring should include respiratory rate, continuous electrocardiogram (ECG), oximetry, arterial line (blood pressure [BP], arterial blood gas [ABG] analysis) and Glasgow Coma Score (GCS). Although, as discussed below, one can treat the consequences of respiratory failure (hypoxaemia and hypercapnia), the *cornerstone of management is treating the underlying disease process*. This is considered in the following chapters on specific respiratory diseases.

Hypoxaemia

Oxygen may be delivered by variable or fixed performance devices.

Variable performance devices: air is entrained during breathing while oxygen is delivered from a reservoir. The latter may be the nasopharynx, mask or reservoir bag. The FiO_2 delivered to the lungs therefore depends on the oxygen flow rate, the patient's inspiratory flow, respiratory rate and the amount of air entrained. Examples include the following.

- **Nasal cannulae**: oxygen flow rates up to 4 l/min (higher rates dry the nasal mucosa). The nasopharynx acts as a reservoir. FiO_2 varies between breaths for a given flow rate depending on the patient's respiration; delivers between 24% and 34%.
- **Facemask**: flow rates must exceed 5 l/min to stop rebreathing of CO_2. Mask provides additional reservoir to oro/nasopharynx. FiO_2 can be 50–60% at 15 l/min.
- **Non-rebreathing masks**: these have a reservoir bag, which should be full before placing on the patient. A one-way valve stops exhaled air entering the oxygen reservoir. High flow rates of 10–15 l/min provide FiO_2 >60% (often approaching 100%).

Fixed performance devices: these are independent of the patient's pattern of breathing and use the Venturi device to entrain air into the mask, exceeding inspiratory flow and thus delivering a fixed oxygen concentration. Typically, they are colour-coded and deliver 24% (blue), 28% (white), 35% (yellow), 40% (red) or 60% (green) FiO_2 for a prescribed flow rate.

High-flow nasal oxygen (HFNO): this is a relatively new technology which provides heated and humidified gas at flow rates up to 60 l/minute via nasal cannulae at FiO_2 of 0.21–1.0. It has a number of physiological effects including a reduction in dead space and increased CO_2 clearance, provision of CPAP in the range 3–7 cmH_2O with the mouth closed, and improved secretion clearance through provided humidified gases.

Continuous positive airway pressure (CPAP): uses a tight-fitting mask and a flow generator to deliver a positive pressure throughout the respiratory cycle (5–15 cmH_2O). This increases functional residual capacity, thereby recruiting more alveoli and improving oxygenation.

Intubation and mechanical ventilation: may be required if hypoxia does not respond to treating the underlying disease, oxygen therapy and/or CPAP.

What is adequate oxygenation?

Generally, one should aim for oxygen saturations exceeding 90% as this puts the patient on the flat part of the oxygen dissociation curve. Further increases in PaO_2 will have only small effects on oxygen delivery (as almost all oxygen in blood is bound to haemoglobin). The British Thoracic Society guidelines for emergency oxygen use in adults recommend saturations of 94–98% for most acutely ill patients or 88–92% for those at risk of hypercapnia. However, caution should be exercised about relying too much on oxygen saturation alone as it can overestimate haemoglobin oxygen saturation, particularly in some ethnic groups. Despite adequate oxygen, the patient may continue to deteriorate and require invasive ventilation. Furthermore, oximetry gives no information on the patient's CO_2 or pH. Some patients (e.g. many with COPD) with chronic hypoxia depend on hypoxaemic pulmonary vasoconstriction to improve V/Q relationships. Oxygen therapy may remove this hypoxic pulmonary vasoconstriction, leading to oxygen-induced hypercapnia, which may be avoided by titrating oxygen to saturations of 88–92%.

It is essential to continue to monitor patients when supplemental oxygen is prescribed and ideally an ABG should be performed.

Hypercapnia

Any sedative drugs should be reversed or avoided (opiates, benzodiazepines). If hypercapnia and respiratory acidosis persist despite treating the underlying condition, artificial ventilation should be considered. Non-invasive ventilation is now widely available and can be delivered via nasal, face, full face or helmet interfaces. It is not a substitute for invasive ventilation, which should be adopted if this method fails.

Indications for intubation and mechanical ventilation in respiratory failure

- Apnoea.
- ↑ Acidosis, $PaCO_2$.
- PaO_2 <8 kPa despite FiO_2 >0.5 (± CPAP).
- GCS <8.
- Unable to clear pulmonary secretions by conventional methods.
- Tiring; ↑ respiratory rate, tachycardia, dyskinetic respiratory pattern.

Arterial blood gas analysis

Arterial blood gas analysis

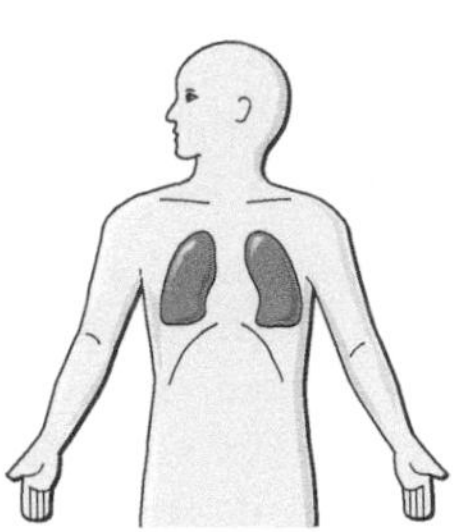

An arterial blood gas from a patient having taken an overdose of opiate shows a pH of 7.29, PaO_2 8 kPa and $PaCO_2$ 8 kPa on room air. The patient has a respiratory acidosis and is hypoxaemic because of hypoventilation, but has a normal A-a gradient as the lungs are normal

$PAO_2 = FiO_2$ (atmospheric pressure – water vapour pressure) – (1.25 x $PaCO_2$)
PAO_2 = 0.21 (101–6.3) – (1.25 x 8)
PAO_2 = 19.9 – 10 = 9.9kPa
A-a gradient ($P_AO_2 - PaO_2$) = 9.9 – 8 = 1.9 kPa (normal 2–4 kPa)

Henderson–Hasselbalch equation

The bicarbonate buffer system

$$CO_2 + H_2O \overset{\text{Carbonic anhydrase}}{\leftrightarrow} H_2CO_3 \leftrightarrow HCO_3^- + H^+$$

The Henderson–Hasselbalch equation

→ $K = [HCO_3^-] \times [H^+] / [H_2CO_3]$
From the law of mass action
K = dissociation constant

→ $K_A = [HCO_3^-] \times [H^+] / [H_2CO_3]$
At equilibrium $[CO_2] \propto [H_2CO_3]$
K_A = corrected dissociation constant

→ $\log K_A = \log [H^+] + \log ([HCO_3^-] / [CO_2])$

→ $-\log [H^+] = -\log K_A + \log ([HCO_3^-] / [CO_2])$

→ $pH = pK_A + \log ([HCO_3^-] / [CO_2])$
(Henderson–Hasselbalch equation)

Respiratory acidosis

$PaCO_2$ increases, pH falls: compensation kidneys retain HCO_3^-
- Central nervous system depression: sedatives, CNS disease
- Lung disease: COPD, pneumonia, asthma, pulmonary oedema, ARDS
- Musculoskelatal disorders: kyphoscoliosis, chest trauma, Guillain–Barré, myasthenia gravis

Respiratory alkalosis

$PaCO_2$ falls, pH increases: compensation kidneys excrete HCO_3^-
- Catastrophic CNS event
- Altitude
- Drugs: salicylates
- Anxiety

Metabolic acidosis

HCO_3^- falls, pH falls: compensation $PaCO_2$ falls

Increased anion gap
- Ketoacidosis: diabetic ketoacidosis, alcohol, starvation
- Poisons: methanol, ethylene glycol, salicylates
- Renal failure
- Lactic acidosis: sepsis, cardiac failure, metformin

Normal anion gap
- GI loss of HCO_3^-: diarrhoea, ileostomy
- Renal loss of HCO_3^-: proximal renal tubular acidosis, carbonic anhydrase inhibitor

Metabolic alkalosis

HCO_3^- increases, pH increases: compensation minute volume falls and $PaCO_2$ rises (this is the least complete form of compensation because of the effect of hypercapnia and hypoxia on respiratory drive)
- H^+ ion loss: vomiting, diuretics, hypokalaemia
- Bicarbonate administration
- Cushing's and Conn's syndrome

The ability to correctly interpret arterial blood gas (ABG) samples is essential for the management of critically ill patients. Blood gas analysers have three electrodes which measure pH, PaO_2 and $PaCO_2$ at 37 °C. Values for bicarbonate (HCO_3^-), base excess (BE) and oxygen saturations (SaO_2) are then *calculated* from these variables. Some blood gas analysers used in critical care or the emergency department have a co-oximeter and also *measure* SaO_2, carboxyhaemoglobin, methaemoglobin and haemoglobin content. They also measure lactate. An ABG provides information about the patient's oxygenation (PaO_2 and SaO_2), ventilation ($PaCO_2$) and acid–base balance (pH, $PaCO_2$, bicarbonate, BE). It is only possible to interpret whether the patient is oxygenating normally if the inspired oxygen fraction is recorded; it is therefore essential that the concentration of oxygen the patient receives is written down.

Although the vast majority of blood gas samples are arterial, occasionally these samples are venous or capillary. Venous samples should generally not be used; however, in critical care, a central venous oxygen saturation ($ScvO_2$) may be obtained in shock states to assess if global oxygen delivery has been adequate (see Chapter 18). In respiratory clinics, the application of a topical vasodilator to the earlobe allows a capillary sample to be drawn, which approximates closely to an arterial sample. To avoid spurious measurements of PaO_2 and $PaCO_2$, once the sample is drawn any air should be expelled, and if the measurement is not performed immediately, the sample should be transported on ice.

Medicine at a Glance, Fifth Edition. Edited by Patrick Davey and Alex Pitcher.

Companion website: www.wiley.com/go/medicine5e

Blood gas values

Normal values for an ABG are as follows.

- pH 7.35–7.45.
- $PaCO_2$ 4.5–6 kPa.
- PaO_2 10–13 kPa.
- HCO_3^- 22–26 mmol/L.
- BE −2 to +2.

The arterial partial pressure of oxygen (PaO_2) is lower than the alveolar partial pressure (P_AO_2) because of imperfections in ventilation/perfusion ($\dot{V}/\dot{Q}$) matching, even in normal lungs. This alveolar–arterial (A–a) gradient is approximately 2–4 kPa in normal lungs (at the higher end of the range with increased age). Gas in the alveolus differs from inspired air in that the partial pressure of carbon dioxide is much higher and therefore within the alveolus, the partial pressures of oxygen and carbon dioxide are interdependent. This relationship is defined by the alveolar gas equation:

$$P_AO_2 = FiO_2(\text{atmospheric pressure} - \text{water vapour pressure}) - (1.25 \times PaCO_2)$$

The alveolar gas equation enables one to deduce the P_AO_2 and hence the A–a gradient (see Chapter 99). Any significant cardiopulmonary disease can increase the A–a gradient and in effect this represents increased $\dot{V}/\dot{Q}$ mismatch. Simple hypoventilation (with normal lungs) will result in hypercapnia and hypoxia but the A–a gradient remains normal.

The $PaCO_2$ is inversely proportional to effective minute volume. Acute changes in $PaCO_2$ lead to predictable changes in pH. Thus, pH falls by 0.1 for a 2.6 kPa rise, and rises by 0.1 for a 1.3 kPa fall in $PaCO_2$ with respect to normal. Changes in pH outside this range have a metabolic contribution.

pH is the negative log of the hydrogen ion concentration and homeostatic mechanisms generally keep this value within a narrow range. Since this is a logarithmic scale, a change in pH of one unit represents a ten-fold change in hydrogen ion concentration. Bicarbonate (actual and standard) (and BE) are calculated from the pH and $PaCO_2$ using the Henderson–Hasselbalch equation. The actual bicarbonate is the calculated bicarbonate using the $PaCO_2$ measured in the sample, whilst the standard bicarbonate is the calculated value using a 'normal' $PaCO_2$ (usually 5.3 kPa). The purpose of the two values is to help differentiate the components of acid–base disturbance. For example, in a pure respiratory acidosis (low pH and high $PaCO_2$) actual bicarbonate will be low, but standard bicarbonate will be normal. BE is a measure of the amount of acid or alkali that must be added under standard conditions (37 °C and $PaCO_2$ 5.3 kPa) to return the pH to 7.4 and is thus a measure of the metabolic component of acid–base abnormalities.

Acid–base homeostasis

The body tightly regulates pH within a narrow range by the use of buffers and the excretion of acid by the kidneys and lungs. Buffers bind or release hydrogen ions and limit sudden changes in pH. The principal buffers in blood are haemoglobin, plasma proteins and bicarbonate but it is the latter which is the most important. Carbon dioxide combines with water to form carbonic acid, which then dissociates into a hydrogen ion and bicarbonate.

The Henderson–Hasselbalch equation describes the relationship between pH, $PaCO_2$ and bicarbonate. Since $PaCO_2$ and bicarbonate can be controlled independently by the lungs and kidneys, respectively, these organs regulate changes in pH. Thus when a metabolic acidosis develops, minute ventilation increases to reduce $PaCO_2$ and to return pH towards normal. Similarly, during hypoventilation (reduced minute volume), $PaCO_2$ rises and an acute respiratory acidosis develops. If this situation persists over several days, the kidneys retain bicarbonate and pH returns towards normal. Compensation by the lungs can occur quickly as minute volume is regulated instantaneously, whereas renal compensation occurs over days. In any case where compensation occurs it is rarely complete; in other words, the pH returns towards normal but not quite to the previous level. Disorders of acid–base homeostasis can therefore be defined as respiratory acidosis, metabolic acidosis, respiratory alkalosis and metabolic alkalosis (see figure and Chapter 142).

The **anion gap** is used in the differential diagnosis of metabolic acidosis; it is:

$$([Na^+]+[K^+])-([Cl^-]+[HCO_3^-])=8-16\ \text{mmol/L}$$

Since electrical neutrality always exists, the gap represents unmeasured cations (Ca^{2+}, Mg^{2+}) and anions (PO_4^{2-}, sulfates, albumin, organic acids). In some diseases the gap is increased because of other unmeasured anions, e.g. ketones in diabetic ketoacidosis, ethylene glycol or salicylate in poisoning.

A practical approach to blood gas interpretation

- Note the inspired fraction of oxygen; is the patient hypoxaemic? In other words, is the PaO_2 low? Does the patient have an oxygenation problem? The PaO_2 may be normal (say 12 kPa), but if this is taken on 60% oxygen, there is an oxygenation problem. This will be manifested by an increase in the A–a gradient (see Chapter 99 for what represents adequate oxygenation).
- Is the pH normal or is the patient acidotic (<7.35) or alkalotic (>7.45)?
- Examine the $PaCO_2$ and standard bicarbonate to see if the problem is respiratory or metabolic.
- Check to see if there is compensation.
- In a metabolic acidosis, calculate the anion gap.

101 Chest X-ray anatomy

Normal adult male chest X-ray

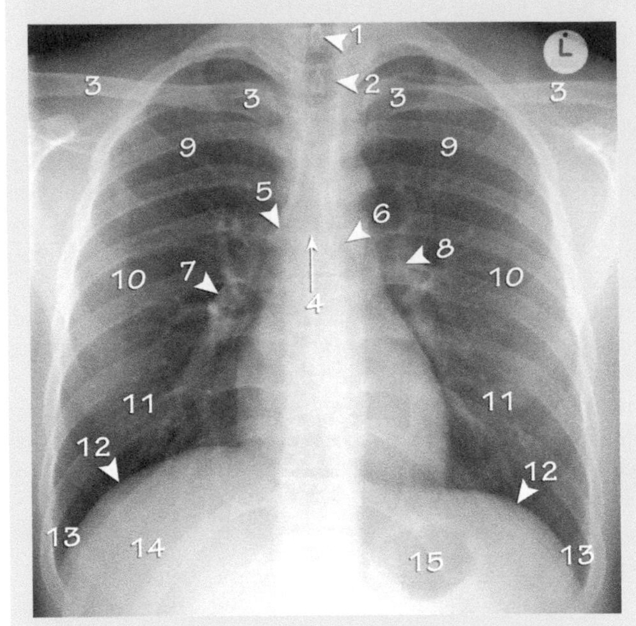

Normal adult female chest X-ray

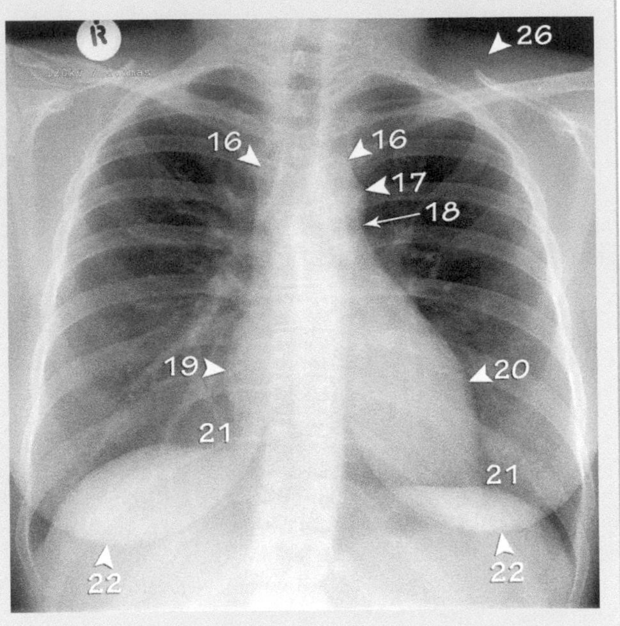

Normal adult male chest X-ray

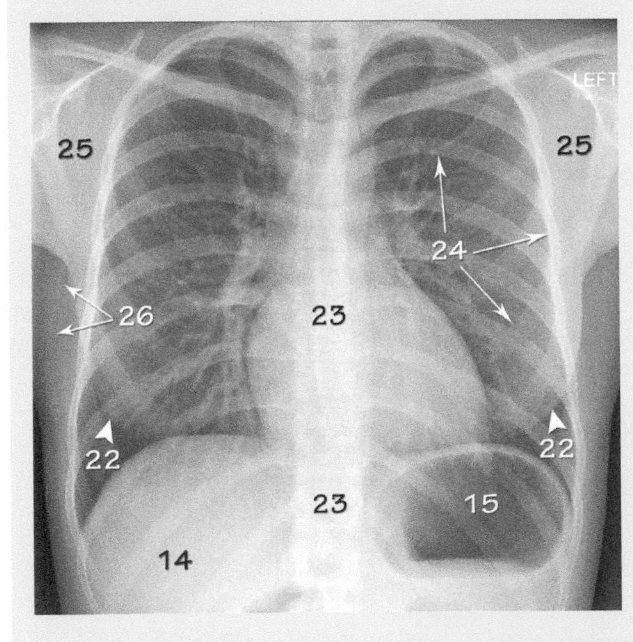

Key

- **1** Spinous process
- **2** Trachea
- **3** Clavicle
- **4** Carina
- **5** Right main bronchus
- **6** Left main bronchus
- **7** Right pulmonary artery
- **8** Left pulmonary artery
- **9** Upper lung zone
- **10** Middle lung zone
- **11** Lower lung zone
- **12** Diaphragm
- **13** Costophrenic angle
- **14** Liver
- **15** Stomach bubble
- **16** Sternum
- **17** Aortic knuckle
- **18** Aorto-pulmonary window
- **19** Right atrial edge
- **20** Left ventricular edge
- **21** Cardiophrenic angles
- **22** Breast
- **23** Spine
- **24** 5th rib (left)
- **25** Scapula
- **26** Fat in soft tissue

Medicine at a Glance, Fifth Edition. Edited by Patrick Davey and Alex Pitcher.

Companion website: www.wiley.com/go/medicine5e

Chest anatomy seen on posteroanterior view

The five principal densities seen on plain imaging should be used as reference points to identify anatomical and pathological structures.

- **Black** – air/gas
- **Dark grey** – fat
- **Light grey** – soft tissue/fluid
- **White** – bone and calcified structures
- **Bright white** – metal

It is important to remember that adjacent structures of different densities form defined edges.

Important anatomical landmarks and structures on a normal chest X-ray

Airways and lungs

These are dark areas due to their high air content.

- **Trachea**: seen as a central vertical lucent tubular structure overlying the vertebral column. The right edge of the trachea, otherwise known as the right paratracheal stripe, is usually thin and well defined because it lies adjacent to the air-dense lung. The left edge, however, lies adjacent to the oesophagus (posterior to the trachea) and great vessels (left of the trachea) and therefore blends in due to their soft tissue density.
- **Carina**: the bifurcation of the trachea.
- **Right main bronchus**: shorter, wider and more vertical than the left main bronchus. This increases the chance of aspiration affecting the right lung.
- **Left main bronchus**: more horizontal due to its passage over the left atrium of the heart.
- **Left lung**: the upper, lingula and lower lobes are not clearly demarcated on a posteroanterior (PA) chest X-ray (CXR). It is therefore best to describe the location of a lesion in terms of upper, middle and lower lung 'zones'. Each zone can then be compared with its counterpart in the contralateral lung.
- **Right lung**: the upper and middle lobes are delineated by the horizontal fissure, which is often visible. The lower lobe cannot be clearly demarcated from the other lobes. Displacement of the horizontal fissure may help determine the location of a disease process.

Mediastinum

The mediastinum is the middle part of the chest and includes all the organs *except the lungs*, i.e. the heart, great vessels, trachea, oesophagus, thymus, lymph nodes, phrenic and vagus nerves. Due to the similar soft tissue densities of these adjacent structures, it may be difficult to clearly identify individual structures. The contours of the heart, aorta and trachea are, however, usually identifiable.

Heart

The heart appears as a large soft tissue density structure. The heart borders are made up of the following.

- **Left border** (superior to inferior): aortic knuckle/arch, aortopulmonary window, left atrial appendage, left ventricle.
- **Right border** (superior to inferior): superior vena cava, right atrium.
- **Inferior border** (in contact with diaphragm): right ventricle.

Hila

The hila are seen as concave structures formed by the configuration of the divergent pulmonary vessels and bronchi. The *left hilum is usually slightly higher* than the right.

Hemidiaphragms

The highest point of the *right hemidiaphragm is slightly higher* than that of the left to accommodate the liver. A dark rounded area is usually seen under the left hemidiaphragm, which is the *gastric air bubble*. This should not be confused with free intra-abdominal gas, which forms a dark crescent under the diaphragm (pneumoperitoneum).

Costophrenic and cardiophrenic angles

Each hemidiaphragm forms a sharp angle at the point of contact with the thoracic wall, known as the costophrenic angle. Loss or blunting of this angle may be due to lung pathology or fluid accumulation in the pleural space (pleural effusion). Each hemidiaphragm also forms an angle at the point of contact with the pericardium, known as the cardiophrenic angle.

Bones and soft tissues

The bones visible on a CXR include the following.

- **Spine**: lower cervical spine to upper lumbar spine.
- **Sternum**.
- **Ribs**.
- **Clavicles**.
- **Scapulae**.
- **Upper left and right humerus**.

The soft tissues visible on a CXR include:

- **breasts**: may mimic lung shadowing, particularly if large or asymmetrical
- **normal soft tissues of the neck and thoracic wall**: may be separated by layers of well-defined fat tissue, which appear darker.

102 Basic chest X-ray interpretation

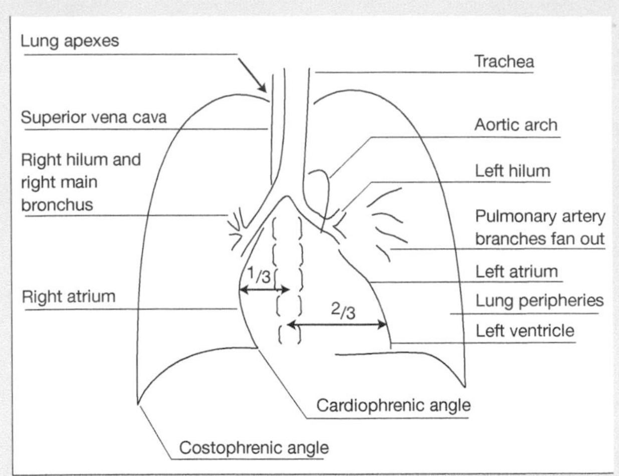

Structures seen in the normal chest X-ray. An abnormality may be obvious but if not, check the apices (lung cancer or tuberculosis is commonly restricted to this area), the bases (small pleural effusions can easily be missed), behind the mediastinal contents for, amongst others, signs of left lower lobe collapse (the sail sign). If the patient is genuinely in respiratory failure (confirmed by blood gases) and the chest X-ray is normal, think of: (1) pulmonary emboli (common) – a cardiac ultrasound may help early management (expect some right heart dilation and decrease in function); (2) *Pneumocystis jirovecii* pneumonia (rare in the UK) – reviewing the history may help; (3) early pneumonia; (4) early ARDS. For (3) and (4), repeating the chest X-ray after a few hours may help (treat empirically in the meantime)

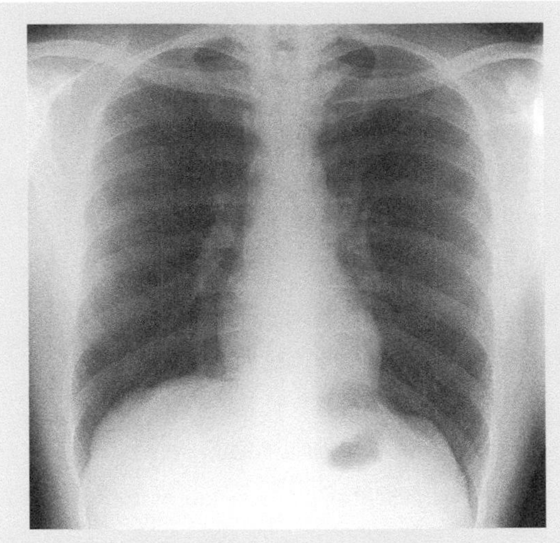

This is a normal chest X-ray. How do we recognize normality here? Largely by experience; always look at the X-rays of your patients, and interpret them before you have seen the official report. You should check the X-ray systematically; check name, date of birth, date of X-ray, then look at the lungs – are they normal, the hilar regions, then the cardiac silhouette for shape and size. Next look at the mediastinum for masses and tracheal shift, then the diaphragms (are they too high, too flat?) and also ensure that the costophrenic angles are clear, sharp and deep. Finally check the bones for abnormalities, such as rib fractures, malignant deposits, etc., and the soft tissues (has there been a mastectomy, etc.?)

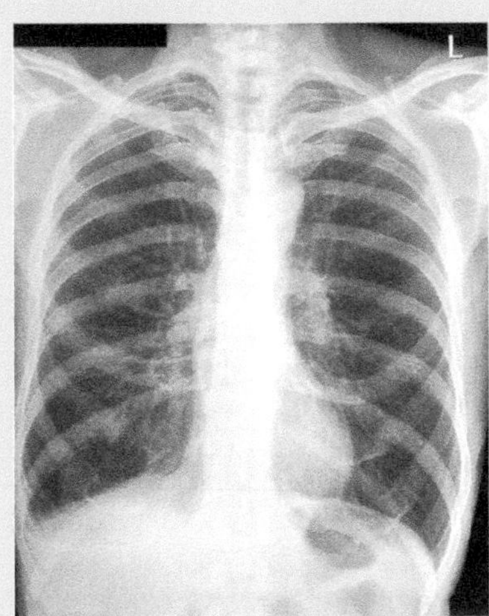

Typical chest X-ray in COPD; the lungs are hyperinflated. There are several radiological signs for this; counting the posterior ribs (i.e. the ribs just as they leave the spinal column) – normal is 8–9, so ≥10 is abnormal. Alternatively, count the number of the last rib that can be seen crossing the diaphragm. The 8th rib can be seen here, ≥7 is abnormal. The diaphragms are flat and the heart shadow is 'thin'. BEWARE that though COPD can be strongly suggested from the chest X-ray, it cannot really be diagnosed from it. Always confirm the presence of COPD by lung function tests, and its functional impact by, among other tests, blood gases. As pneumothoraces are common in COPD, these should always be looked for (they can 'hide' in the lung apexes); as cigarette smoking is almost universal, always look for radiological evidence of lung cancer in these patients

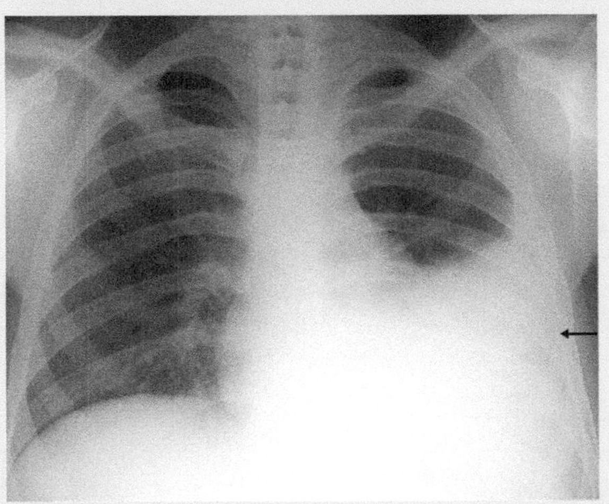

This chest X-ray shows a large left pleural effusion. Instead of the normal appearance, with the lung clearly visible to the diaphragm, only the top half of the lung is visible. It is not possible to see the left border of the heart, nor the left diaphragm, unlike normal. This is because both these structures have pleural fluid abutting against them; clearly defined edges in X-rays rely on there being differences in composition between adjacent structures, e.g. air (lungs) and fluid (heart). These edges disappear when the composition becomes identical, as with a pleural effusion

Medicine at a Glance, Fifth Edition. Edited by Patrick Davey and Alex Pitcher.

Companion website: www.wiley.com/go/medicine5e

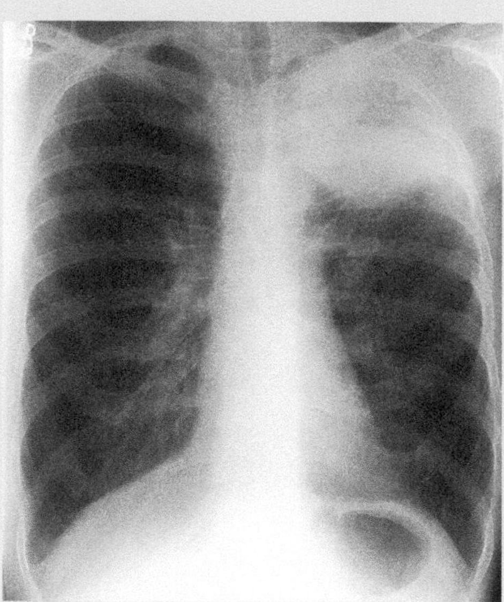

This chest X-ray shows an obvious abnormality at the top (apex) of the left lung. There is a roughly circular structure, quite large, white (so fluid-filled) for which there is a differential diagnosis, including consolidation and even tumour. It has a 'fluid level' within it; in other words, about halfway up, there is a line, above which one can see an air-filled space (darker area); this is a typical appearance of an area of consolidation, with abscess formation, in this case, due to tuberculosis (the clue to this diagnosis being the apical position)

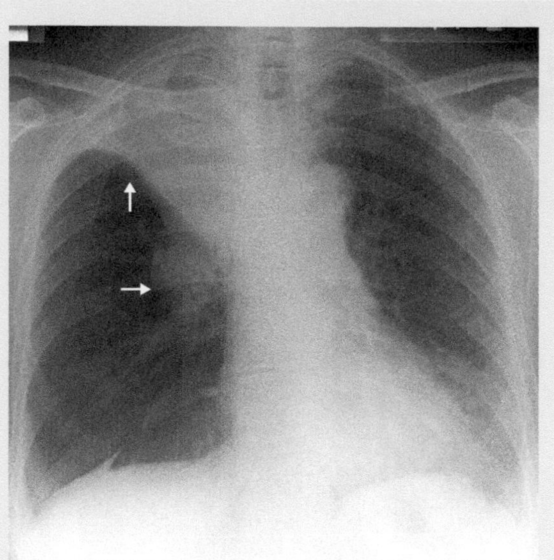

Right upper lobe collapse. There is a wedge-shaped opacification radiating out from the hilum. The horizontal fissure has been pulled up, implying that whatever is going on has led to loss of upper lobe lung volume, and hence the compensatory fissure movement. Inspection of the right hilum reveals a mass, hence the diagnosis here is a tumour (almost certainly malignant) in the right hilum obstructing the bronchus leading to the right upper lobes, resulting in collapse of this lobe

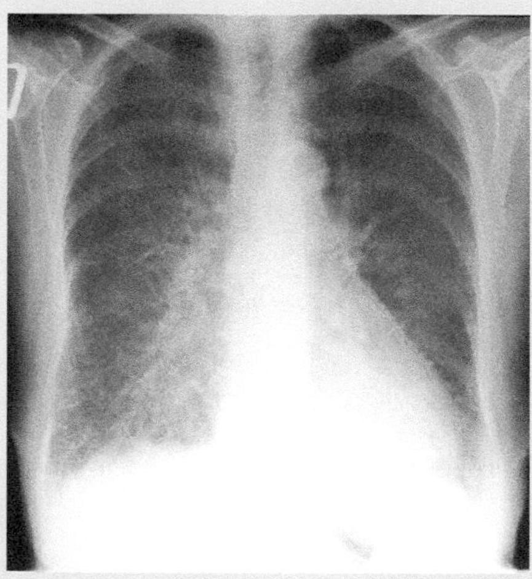

A chest X-ray from a patient with left heart failure (= pulmonary oedema). There are a number of characteristic findings: (1) the heart is enlarged (the normal cardiothoracic ratio is ≤50%; (2) there is interstitial pulmonary oedema ('fuzzy' shadows), especially in the mid and lower zones (where the pulmonary venous pressure is highest – provided the patient has been upright!); (3) the upper lobe veins, which are usually smaller than the lower lobe ones, have become enlarged (upper lobe venous diversion, otherwise known as pulmonary venous imbalance). There is fluid in the lymphatics, seen as Kerley B lines (short horizontal lines 1–2 cm in length, extending horizontally from the lower outer lung fields; heart failure is the most common cause, though malignancy and infection rarely can underlie them; (4) there are small bilateral pleural effusions (shadowing at both lung bases). The shape of the heart usually gives no clues as to the cause of the heart failure; occasionally, enlargement of the left atrium, seen as: (1) great splaying of the left and right bronchi to ≥90°, (2) a large 3rd bulge down the left heart border – the aorta is the 1st, the pulmonary artery the 2nd and the ventricle the 4th – leads one to suspect mitral valve disease

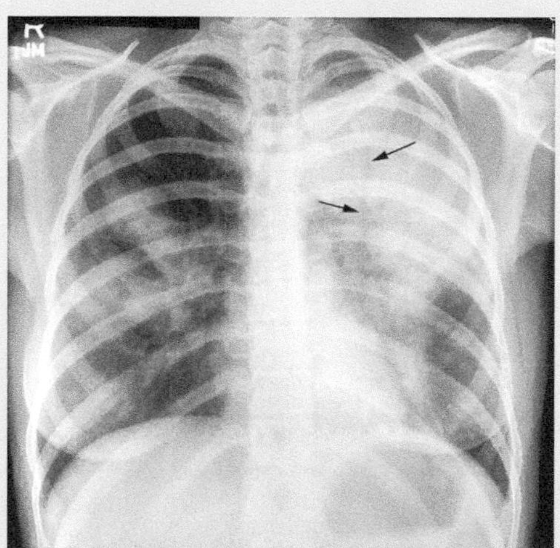

A chest X-ray from a patient with pneumococcal pneumonia. There is extensive shadowing of the left upper zone, within which an air bronchogram (arrows) is seen. An air bronchogram is a pathognomonic sign of consolidation – and by far the most common cause of consolidation is an infective process. There is also some patchy shadowing in the right midzone. Respiratory failure is unusual in otherwise well patients who develop pneumonia, but can occur if the infection is severe, or if there is underlying lung disease, such as COPD (which the chest X-ray may underestimate). BEWARE also that patients immobile from septic processes can develop pulmonary emboli, which can contribute to hypoxaemia. Clinical deterioration in a patient known to have pneumonia may relate to worsening of the infective process, but also may be due to PEs

103 Chest X-ray cases 1

(a) Cardiomegaly

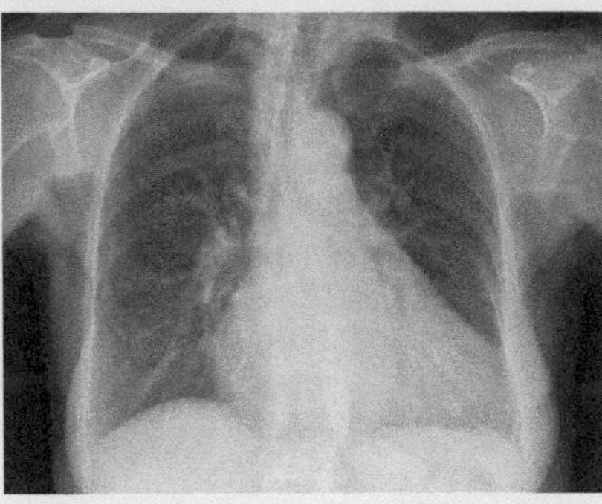

The heart is abnormally large. It takes up greater than 50% of the internal width of the thorax. The patient was known to have left ventricular failure

(b) Pulmonary oedema

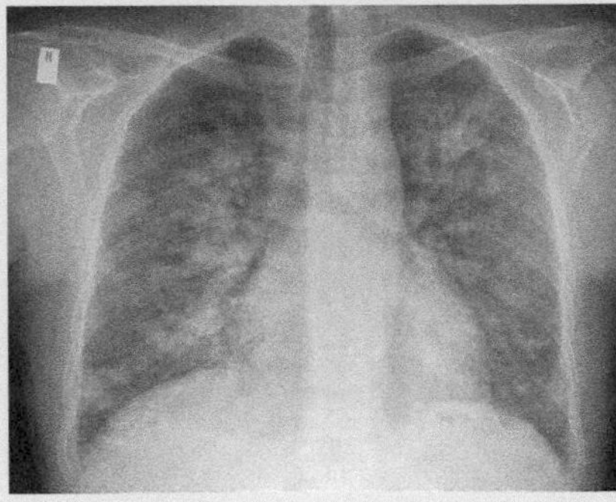

The heart is not enlarged but there are signs of pulmonary oedema with shadowing spreading from the hila. The patient was diabetic and presented with acute myocardial infarction and left ventricular failure

(c) Kerley B lines

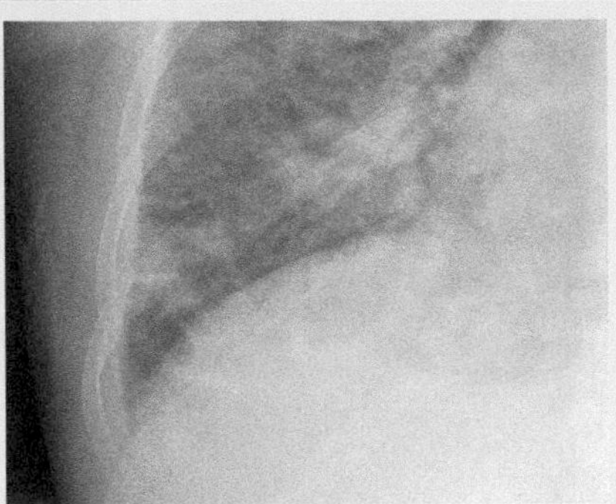

Close-up of costophrenic angle of pulmonary oedema (b). Here septal 'Kerley B' lines are seen. These are horizontal lines that reach the pleural surface. They are caused by fluid between the interlobular septa and are a specific sign of pulmonary oedema

(d) Pleural effusions

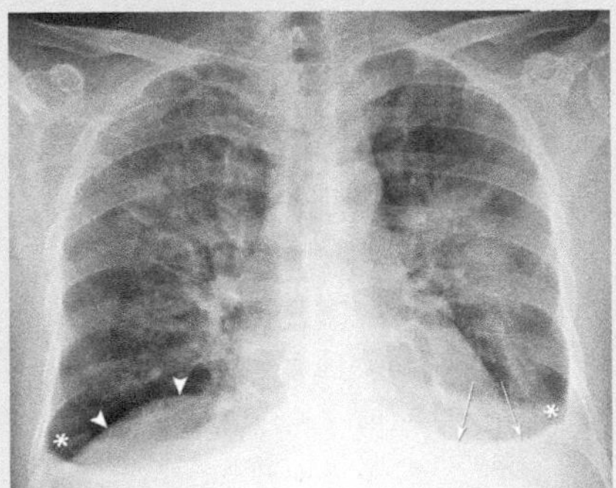

This patient with heart failure has pulmonary oedema and fluid is filling the pleural cavities forming pleural effusions (arrows). The costophrenic angles (*) are blunted. The dome of the diaphragm is still visible (arrowheads)

(e) Prosthetic heart valves

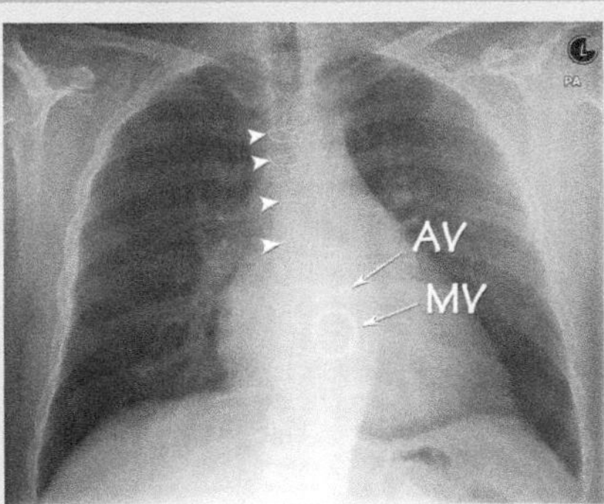

The heart is enlarged due to left ventricular failure. There is evidence of previous cardiac surgery with midline sternotomy wires (arrowheads) and metallic replacements of both the aortic valve (AV) and the mitral valve (MV)

(f) Asbestos plaques

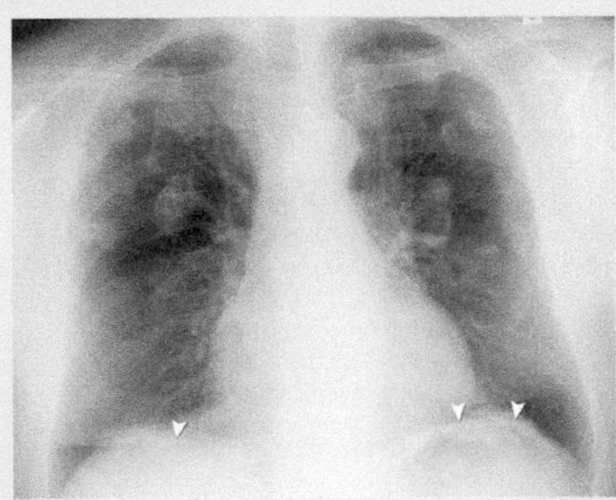

There are multiple dense irregular-shaped opacities over both lungs. These are typical appearances of asbestos plaques. The give-away sign is the layering of dense material over the diaphragm (arrowheads)

Medicine at a Glance, Fifth Edition. Edited by Patrick Davey and Alex Pitcher.

Companion website: www.wiley.com/go/medicine5e

Cardiomegaly

Cardiomegaly is an abnormal enlargement of the heart where the *maximum width of the heart shadow is greater than 50% of the maximum internal width of the thorax*. Causes include the following.

- **Hypertrophy**: caused by an increase in afterload of a particular chamber (e.g. aortic stenosis, hypertension).
- **Dilation**: secondary to toxic, metabolic or infectious agents causing myocardial damage.

Hypertrophy of either ventricle does not usually enlarge the heart shadow unless there is synchronous dilation. Cardiomegaly is usually abnormal, except in athletes, and is associated with other cardiovascular pathology. The shape of an enlarged heart on a chest X-ray (CXR) will depend upon the chamber affected and it may point to the cause.

- A 'globular' shape occurs with pericardial effusion or generalized cardiomyopathy.
- Left ventricular (LV) dilation causes lengthening and rounding of the left heart border and a downward extension of the apex.
- Right ventricular dilation lifts the apex off the hemidiaphragm.
- Left atrial enlargement causes a double density along the right heart border, comprising the left and right atrial edges. Other signs include left atrial appendage prominence and bronchial splaying of the bronchi at the carina.

Pulmonary oedema

Pulmonary oedema occurs when fluid leaks into the lung interstitium from the pulmonary vasculature, leading to impairment of gaseous exchange. It is caused by an *increase in vascular hydrostatic pressure* (e.g. cardiogenic causes – LV dysfunction, mitral stenosis), a *decrease in plasma oncotic pressure* (e.g. liver failure, renal failure) or an *increase in pulmonary capillary membrane permeability* (e.g. adult respiratory distress syndrome, aspiration, inhalation injury, neurogenic pulmonary oedema, multiple blood transfusions).

The CXR features of pulmonary oedema include the following.

- **Absence/presence of cardiomegaly**: cardiomegaly is often seen with cardiogenic causes although it may be normal in size in the early stages. The heart is usually normal in size with non-cardiogenic causes.
- **Upper lobe blood diversion**: the upper lobe blood vessels are normally narrower than the lower lobe vessels. In cardiogenic pulmonary oedema, lower zone alveolar hypoxia causes arteriolar vasoconstriction, diverting blood to the upper lobes to optimize gaseous exchange.
- **Alveolar shadowing**: this represents oedema in the alveoli. It predominates in the lower zones if the cause is cardiogenic, and more diffusely if non-cardiogenic. In acute cardiogenic cases, alveolar shadowing spreads out from the hila in the shape of bats' wings.
- **Kerley lines**: these represent interstitial oedema. They are thin linear shadows caused by interstitial fluid or cellular infiltration.
  - *Kerley A lines*: these represent distension of channels between peripheral and central lung lymphatics. They are unbranching lines (over 2 cm long) extending from the periphery towards the hilum.
  - *Kerley B/septal lines*: these represent oedema of the interlobular septa and are characteristic of pulmonary oedema. They are 1 cm long, thin, horizontal and parallel and seen peripherally above the costophrenic angles.
- **Pleural effusions**: pleural fluid causes blunting of the costophrenic angles.

Pleural effusion

Pleural effusion is excess fluid in the pleural space. Aspiration allows biochemical division into transudates (<30 g/l of protein) and exudates (>30 g/l of protein). Transudates are caused by LV failure, pulmonary embolism and cirrhosis. Exudates are caused by infection, neoplasia and inflammatory conditions, e.g. rheumatoid arthritis or systemic lupus erythematosus. CXR is the primary diagnostic tool for detecting pleural effusions and may point to the cause, e.g. an enlarged heart shadow, lung mass, parenchymal disease, apical fibrosis or bone metastases. Effusions collect in gravity-dependent areas (lung bases when positioned upright). The CXR appearances of pleural effusions include:

- small effusions, which *blunt the costophrenic angles with a meniscus*
- large effusions, which can cause *complete 'white-out'* of the lungs and lung collapse, and push the mediastinum away from the side of the effusion.

Prosthetic heart valves

Normal heart valves may become dysfunctional due to acute and chronic disease, e.g. bacterial endocarditis, aortic stenosis or rheumatic fever. Replacement valves are designed to restore normal function and may be mechanical or biological tissue grafts. *Mechanical valves are radio-opaque*, appearing as white artefacts within the heart shadow on CXR. The major classes of mechanical valves include 'caged ball', 'tilting disc' and 'bileaflet'. A prosthetic mitral valve is larger and aligned more anteroposteriorly than a prosthetic aortic valve, which is smaller and aligned more obliquely on a posteroanterior (PA) CXR.

Pleural plaques

Pleural plaques are focal areas of pleural fibrosis caused by *previous exposure to asbestos*. Pleural calcification is a late sign, occurring in approximately half of those with asbestos-related disease. It is most easily seen along the diaphragmatic pleura. The CXR features include the following.

- **Widespread distribution**: commonly midlung, paravertebral, diaphragmatic, peripheral and bilateral.
- **Peripheral pleural thickening**: appears as a thickened white line, often non-uniform around the edge of the lung.
- **Calcified plaques**: mimic the appearance of a 'holly leaf' with dense, irregular, rolled edges and relatively lucent centres. Plaques evolve slowly and previous CXRs should be reviewed for comparison.

Table 103.1 Classic chest X-ray features 1.

• **Cardiomegaly**	Heart shadow greater than 50% of thoracic cage width
• **Pulmonary oedema**	
Cardiogenic	Bilateral alveolar shadowing, bats' wings, upper lobe blood diversion, Kerley A lines, Kerley B lines, cardiomegaly, effusion, cardiac pathology signs (sternotomy wires, prosthetic valve, pacemaker/defibrillator)
Non-cardiogenic	Normal heart size, diffuse alveolar shadowing
• **Pleural effusion**	Costophrenic angle blunting, meniscus, 'white-out'
• **Pleural plaques**	Peripheral pleural thickening, pleural calcific deposits

104 Chest X-ray cases 2

(a) Simple pneumothorax

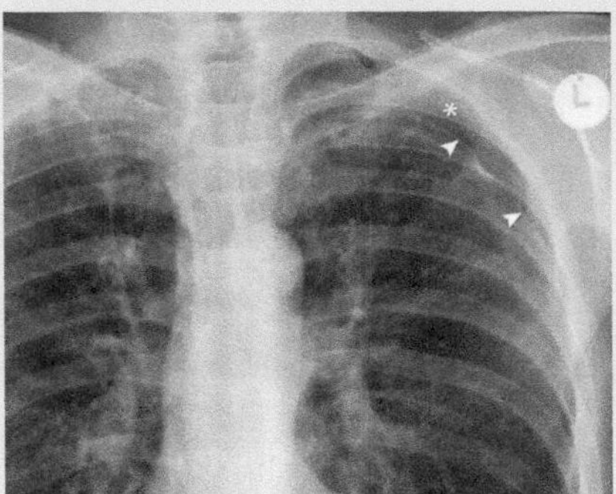

The edge of the left lung can be seen as a thin well-defined line (arrowheads). Beyond this line there are no further lung markings because air is collecting in the pleural cavity (*)

(b) Chest drain

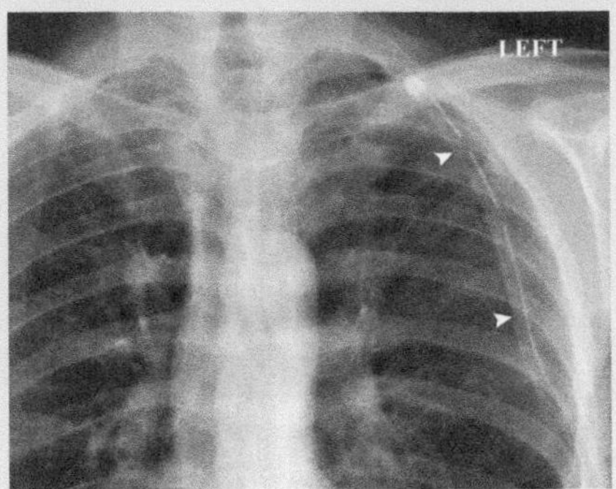

A tube has been inserted to drain air from the pleural cavity. It has been placed appropriately with its tip pointing high up towards the apex of the hemithorax. (Same patient as in (a).)

(c) Tension pneumothorax

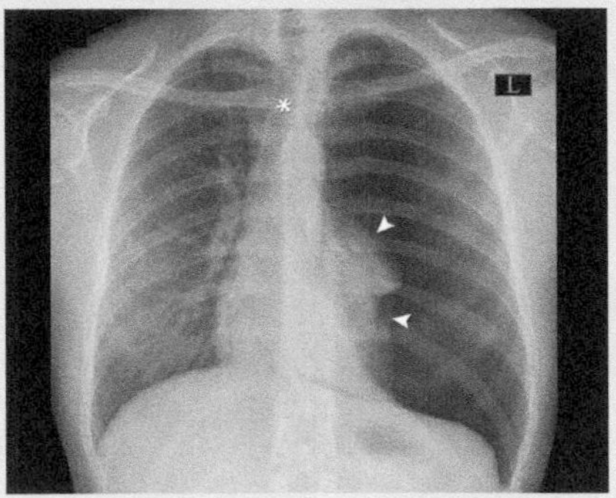

The left lung (arrowheads) is being compressed, the left hemidiaphragm is depressed, and the trachea (*) is pushed towards the right. Immediate aspiration is required

(d) Hydropneumothorax

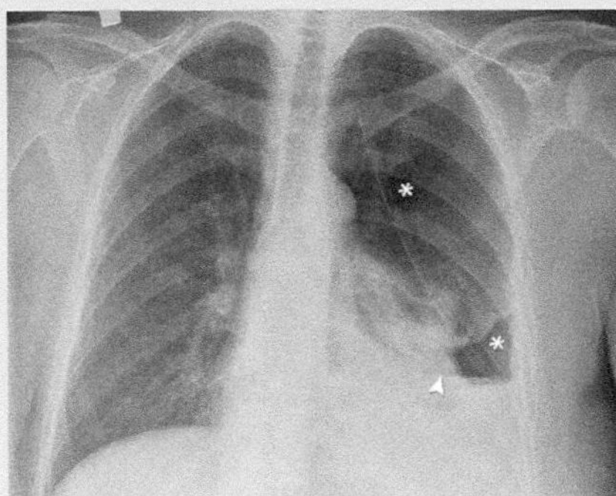

This patient has both a pneumothorax (*) and a pleural effusion (arrowhead) due to an oesophageal rupture. The fluid level does not have the curved meniscus sign of a simple effusion. Note the presence of a chest drain. Haemopneumothorax has identical appearances and is often associated with rib fractures

(e) Lower left lobe collapse

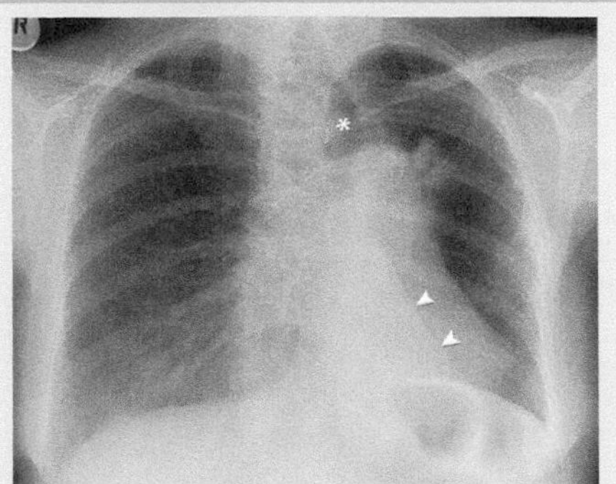

The left lower lobe bronchus is occluded with collapse of this lobe. The edge of the collapsed lobe forms the 'sail sign' (arrowheads). The trachea (*) is pulled towards the side of volume loss

(f) Right upper lobe collapse

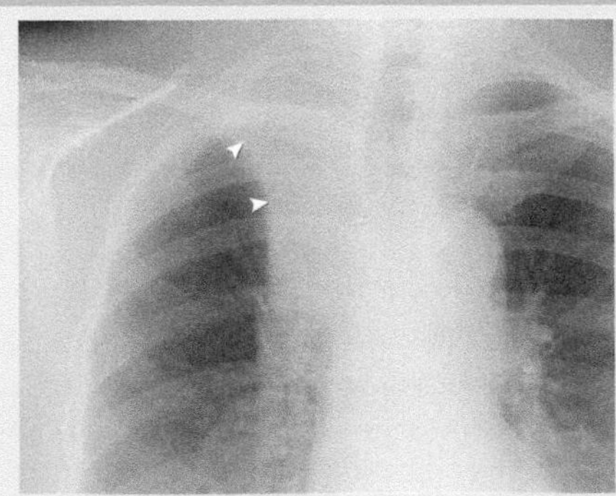

The horizontal fissure (arrowheads) has been pulled upwards due to volume loss of the right upper lobe. The patients in both (e) and (f) had an occluding bronchial carcinoma

Medicine at a Glance, Fifth Edition. Edited by Patrick Davey and Alex Pitcher.

Companion website: www.wiley.com/go/medicine5e

Pneumothorax

Pneumothorax is the presence of air in the pleural cavity. During normal ventilation, the thoracic volume increases to create relative negative intrathoracic pressure for lung inflation. However, in the presence of a pleural defect, air enters the potential pleural space and breaks this pressure potential, thereby compromising lung inflation. This impairs gaseous exchange and may cause breathlessness.

- **Simple pneumothorax** is common and occurs in healthy chests, especially in tall, slim, young males. Secondary pneumothoraces can arise in individuals with underlying disease, e.g. chronic obstructive pulmonary disease, asthma, barotrauma, penetrating chest trauma and pneumonia.
- **Tension pneumothorax** is a medical emergency where air accumulates under pressure in the pleural space due to the formation of a one-way valve at the point of injury, permitting air to enter but not to escape. It can develop from a simple pneumothorax, often following traumatic injury, and requires emergency decompression.

Chest X-ray (CXR) features include the following.

- **Linear pleural shadow, with absence of lung markings** beyond this linear shadow in the peripheral thorax.
- **Air in the pleural cavity will rise to the apices** in an upright CXR. It is therefore vital to review the apical areas.

Haemothorax

A haemothorax is a pleural effusion due to the accumulation of blood within the pleural cavity. It most commonly arises from blunt or penetrating chest trauma. Non-traumatic haemothorax is less common and can result from malignancy, blood dyscrasias, pulmonary infarction and tuberculosis. CXR is the primary diagnostic investigation and the typical appearances on *upright* imaging are *identical to a pleural effusion* (meniscus, blunting of the costophrenic angle, 'white-out' and/or mediastinal shift with a large haemothorax).

Approximately 200–300 ml of blood is required to obliterate the costophrenic angle on an upright CXR. In the acute trauma setting, however, a portable supine CXR is often the first and only view available upon which management decisions are based. Unfortunately, the presence and size of haemothoraces are extremely difficult to evaluate on supine images. In blunt trauma cases, there may be other associated injuries, e.g. rib fractures, pneumothorax or damage to the great vessels. These should be excluded on the CXR.

In the context of a traumatic pneumothorax, the presence of a pleural effusion is almost always due to the accumulation of blood in the pleural cavity (haemopneumothorax). There is no meniscal sign due to a direct interface between the pleural air and blood.

Lobar collapse

Collapse of a single lobe causes characteristic patterns on CXR.

- **Right upper lobe collapse**: the horizontal fissure is pulled up and there is a soft tissue shadow in the right upper zone. The remainder of the lung expands to fill the void.
- **(Right) middle lobe collapse** (there is no left middle lobe): the horizontal and oblique fissures are pulled closer and there is loss of interface between the right heart border and the lung (*silhouette sign*). The lateral CXR demonstrates a wedge-shaped opacity stretching from the hilum anteroinferiorly.
- **Right lower lobe collapse**: there is a soft tissue shadow in the right lower zone and loss of interface between the right hemidiaphragm and lung (*silhouette sign*). The collapsed lobe appears as a triangular opacity behind the right heart border without obscuring it. The lateral CXR demonstrates increased density over the lower thoracic spine caused by the shadow of the collapsed lobe.
- **Left upper lobe collapse**: there is a 'veil-like' shadow cast over the entire left lung due to the anteriorly lying collapsed lobe. Interposition of the lower lobe between the collapsed lobe and aortic arch may be seen as a crescent of air, known as the *Luftsichel sign*.
- **Lingula lobe collapse**: there is loss of interface between the left heart border and the lung (*silhouette sign*).
- **Left lower lobe collapse**: the collapsed lobe is displaced medially and lies behind the heart. A triangular opacity is seen through the heart shadow with a straight left lateral border (*sail sign*). There is also loss of interface between the medial part of the left hemidiaphragm and lung (*silhouette sign*).

Tubes, lines and prostheses

Chest X-ray is the usual method for confirming correct positioning of tubes and lines in the chest.

- *The tip of an endotracheal tube should be midtracheal, 2–3 cm above its bifurcation* at the level of the fourth to fifth thoracic vertebrae. The tip has a radio-opaque marker to enhance its visibility on CXR. If inserted too far, it may enter a bronchus and inflate only one lung, causing contralateral collapse.
- *The tip of a central venous catheter should be in the superior vena cava (SVC), just above the right atrium.* If it is inserted too far, it may cause arrhythmias through direct contact with the heart. It may also erode through the SVC or right atrium, causing haemorrhage and tamponade.
- *The nasogastric tube should follow the central vertical descent of the oesophagus and continue below the left hemidiaphragm into the stomach.* If incorrectly placed, it may enter the trachea or bronchi, perforate the oesophagus or penetrate into the brain through the ethmoid bone.
- *Chest drain*: this tube passes through the chest wall via an intercostal space and its tip lies in the pleural space.
- *Pacemakers and implantable cardioverter defibrillators (ICDs)*: these are usually sited below the lateral left clavicle. Pacing wires connect the pacemaker and/or ICD to the heart muscle. Pacemakers may pace one or more heart chambers. ICDs are used in patients at risk of sudden death from arrhythmia.

Table 104.1 Classic chest X-ray features 2.

• **Haemothorax**	Costophrenic angle blunting, meniscus, 'white-out'
• **Pneumothorax**	Linear pleural shadow with absent lung markings in the periphery beyond
• **Collapse of:**	
Right upper lobe (RUL)	Superiorly displaced horizontal fissure, upper zone shadowing
(Right) middle lobe (R)ML	Right heart silhouette sign, wedge-shaped opacity on lateral CXR
Right lower lobe (RLL)	Right hemidiaphragm silhouette sign, lower zone shadowing, increased lower thoracic spine density on lateral CXR
Left upper lobe (LUL)	Veil-like' shadow, Luftsichel sign
Lingula	Left heart silhouette sign
Left lower lobe (LLL)	Left hemidiaphragm silhouette sign, sail sign

105 Non-invasive ventilation

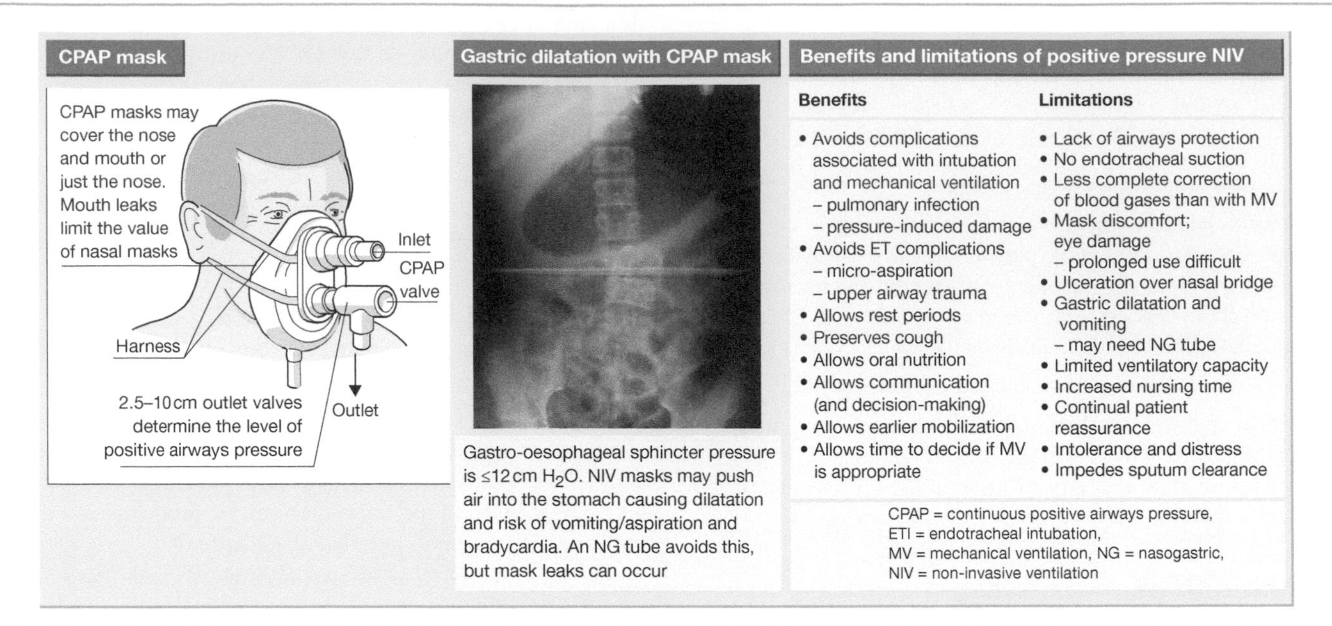

CPAP mask
CPAP masks may cover the nose and mouth or just the nose. Mouth leaks limit the value of nasal masks
Inlet
CPAP valve
Harness
Outlet
2.5–10 cm outlet valves determine the level of positive airways pressure
Gastric dilatation with CPAP mask
Gastro-oesophageal sphincter pressure is ≤12 cm H_2O. NIV masks may push air into the stomach causing dilatation and risk of vomiting/aspiration and bradycardia. An NG tube avoids this, but mask leaks can occur
Benefits and limitations of positive pressure NIV
Benefits
• Avoids complications associated with intubation and mechanical ventilation
– pulmonary infection
– pressure-induced damage
• Avoids ET complications
– micro-aspiration
– upper airway trauma
• Allows rest periods
• Preserves cough
• Allows oral nutrition
• Allows communication (and decision-making)
• Allows earlier mobilization
• Allows time to decide if MV is appropriate
Limitations
• Lack of airways protection
• No endotracheal suction
• Less complete correction of blood gases than with MV
• Mask discomfort; eye damage
– prolonged use difficult
• Ulceration over nasal bridge
• Gastric dilatation and vomiting
– may need NG tube
• Limited ventilatory capacity
• Increased nursing time
• Continual patient reassurance
• Intolerance and distress
• Impedes sputum clearance
CPAP = continuous positive airways pressure,
ETI = endotracheal intubation,
MV = mechanical ventilation, NG = nasogastric,
NIV = non-invasive ventilation

Non-invasive ventilation (NIV) is provided by machines that support ventilation and assist gas exchange through the patient's upper airway by means of a mask or similar interface. Continuous positive airway pressure (CPAP) is applied in the same way but is not a mode of ventilation. It is most successful in alert, co-operative, self-ventilating, haemodynamically stable patients who are able to protect and clear their airways.

Indications

One of the most common uses of NIV is in acute exacerbations of chronic obstructive pulmonary disease (COPD) where a respiratory acidosis (pH <7.35) persists despite optimal medical therapy. It is also used in respiratory failure due to chest wall or neuromuscular disease and cardiogenic pulmonary oedema. It has a role, on occasion, in pneumonia, asthma and as an aid to weaning from mechanical ventilation in the intensive care unit. Prior to initiating NIV, it is important to make a decision whether, if this modality fails, escalation to invasive mechanical ventilation is indicated. Ideally, this should be discussed between the patient, the patient's consultant and the consultant intensivist. There should also be a clear plan of what to do if NIV fails and the patient is not to be intubated.

Non-invasive ventilation should be avoided in refractory hypoxaemia, copious pulmonary secretions, undrained pneumothorax, reduced Glasgow Coma Score, facial trauma, recent upper gastrointestinal surgery and vomiting. A nasogastric tube prevents gastric distension and reduces the risk of aspiration.

Continuous positive airways pressure

CPAP is maintained throughout inspiration and expiration (typically *c.* 5–10 cmH_2O) by a flow generator, although many non-invasive ventilators have a CPAP mode. All the work of breathing (WoB) is provided by the patient; however, the addition of CPAP reduces the WoB by increasing lung compliance. CPAP recruits collapsed lung units and keeps them open during expiration. Consequently, ventilation/perfusion ($\dot{V}/\dot{Q}$) relationships improve and oxygenation increases. Functional residual capacity increases as a result of alveolar recruitment and inflation occurs on the more compliant steep part of the pressure–volume curve; this reduces the WoB.

CPAP is used in cardiogenic pulmonary oedema, pneumonia and obstructive sleep apnoea where it helps prevent upper airways collapse.

Negative and positive pressure ventilation

Non-invasive ventilation can be divided into negative-pressure and positive-pressure types.

- **Negative pressure ventilation** (NPV) was originally developed to support victims of poliomyelitis-induced respiratory paralysis. Patients were placed in *tank ventilators* sealed at the neck. Lowering tank pressures expanded the chest, causing inspiration. Expiration was passive. However, these 'iron lungs' were limited by difficulties with nursing access, poor CO_2 clearance and secretion retention, which caused airways obstruction or pneumonia. NPV has largely been superseded by the development of positive-pressure ventilators and is now rarely used except in

Medicine at a Glance, Fifth Edition. Edited by Patrick Davey and Alex Pitcher.

Companion website: www.wiley.com/go/medicine5e

patients with chronic hypoventilation (e.g. kyphoscoliosis) or as part of rehabilitation programmes (e.g. spinal injury). Current NPV techniques include: (i) *jacket (cuirass) ventilators*, which only produce a negative pressure around the chest but leaks often limit effectiveness; and (ii) *rocking beds*, which utilize gravity to enhance diaphragmatic movement.

- **Positive-pressure NIV** is delivered through tight-fitting interfaces which may be nasal, face mask, full face mask or a helmet. Interfaces come in a variety of sizes and should be carefully matched to individuals to ensure comfort and compliance. The figure lists the potential benefits and disadvantages.

Numerous ventilators are available for NIV, ranging from ventilators used in intensive care with sophisticated monitoring to small, cheap, lightweight ventilators designed for home ventilation. However, it is more important for staff to be familiar with a single type rather than a specific ventilator. Ventilators may be volume or pressure (more common) preset and operate in: (i) triggered mode (also called spontaneous or assist); (ii) assist/control mode (spontaneous or timed) where breaths are triggered by the patient but there is a back-up controlled rate if the patient fails to trigger a breath; and (iii) control mode (mandatory breaths). Bilevel pressure support ventilators are in most frequent use because they are cheap and simple to use. Successful use requires well-trained staff, gradual introduction to a co-operative patient and careful synchronization of breathing with the ventilator.

Several modes of ventilation exist and terminology varies between manufacturers; the most common are listed below.

- **Pressure support ventilation**: delivers an inspiratory pressure (*c.* 10–30 cmH_2O) triggered by the patient and adjusted according to the patient's requirements. It augments tidal volume, clears CO_2 and reduces WoB. Modern NIV ventilators also provide adjustable expiratory positive airway pressure which has the same effects as CPAP.
- **Bilevel positive-pressure ventilation**: alternates between two levels of CPAP while allowing spontaneous respiration. The difference in the two pressures augments alveolar ventilation and CO_2 clearance; the lower pressure maintains alveolar recruitment.

106 Mechanical ventilation

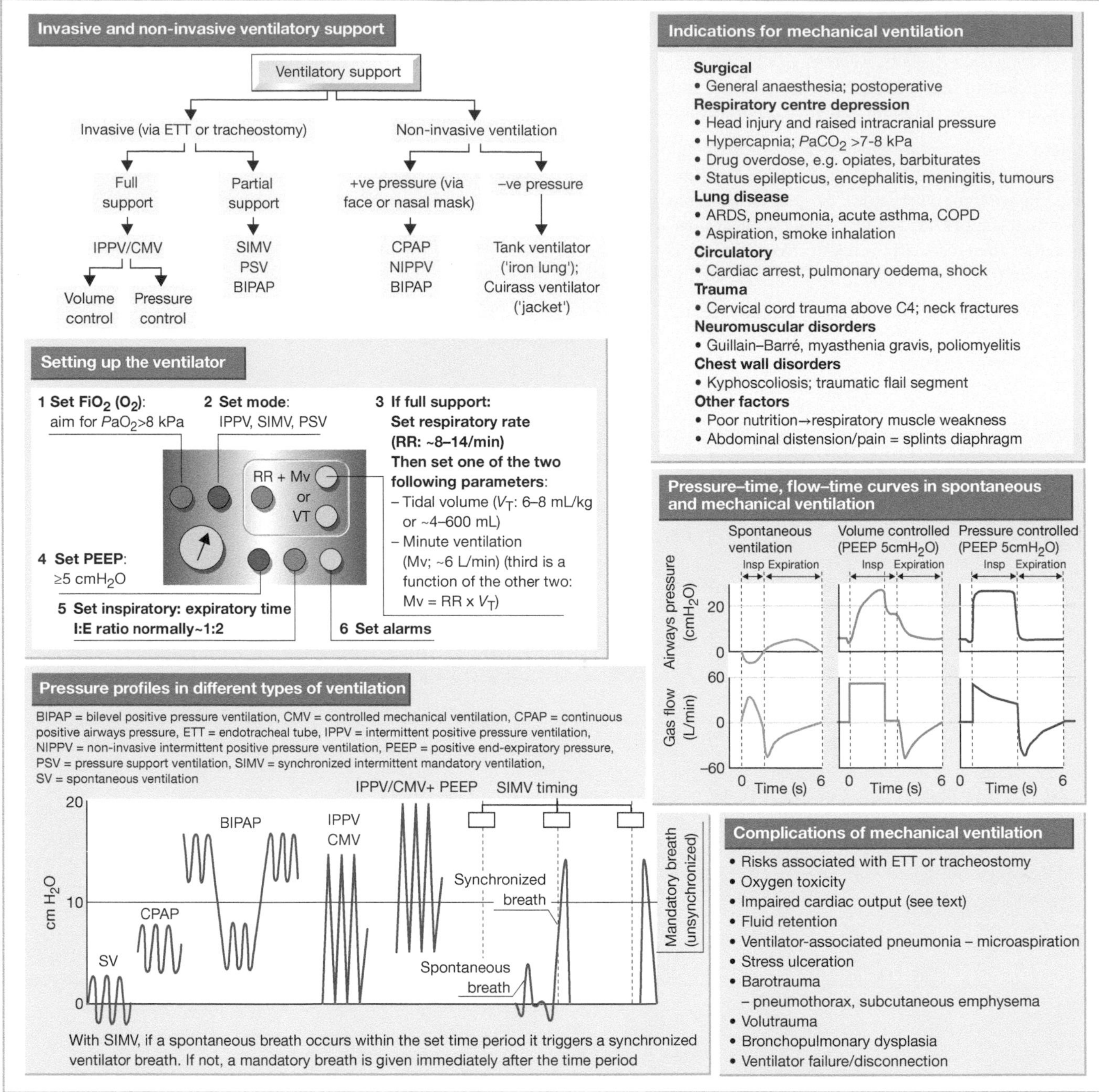

Invasive mechanical ventilation (MV) is frequently required during critical illness to maintain gas exchange and reduce the work of breathing (WoB). This is delivered through an endotracheal tube or tracheostomy (if prolonged ventilation is required) and provides complete or partial respiratory support. Non-invasive ventilation is discussed in Chapter 105.

Indications

Outside the operating theatre, one of the main indications for MV is respiratory failure. However, it is also used in circulatory failure, neurological disease, trauma, poisoning and following prolonged major surgery. MV may also be required to facilitate investigations (such as a computed tomography scan in a head-injured patient who is unable to co-operate) or bronchial toilet.

The decision to intubate and mechanically ventilate a patient requires careful thought as this modality only provides organ support. There needs to be some treatable or reversible cause for why MV is indicated. Generally, such decisions need to be made between the patient's consultant, the consultant intensivist and either the patient (if possible) or family members. It is often difficult to decide exactly when to ventilate a progressively deteriorating patient. There are no simple guidelines. However, hypoxaemia (PO_2 <8 kPa on FiO_2 >0.4), hypercapnia (PCO_2 >7.5 kPa), respiratory/metabolic acidosis (pH <7.2) and other factors such as confusion, exhaustion, poor cough and sputum retention usually indicate the need for MV. *Trends in these variables and any response or failure to treatment are often more helpful than absolute values.*

Ventilator set-up

Typical initial adult intermittent positive-pressure ventilation (IPPV) settings would be: tidal volume (V_T) *c.* 6–8 ml/kg; respiratory frequency (*f*) *c.* 8–14 bpm; and minute ventilation ($M_V = V_T \times f$) *c.* 6 l/min. FiO_2 and M_V are adjusted to maintain PaO_2 >8 kPa and $PaCO_2$ <7 kPa, respectively, but acceptable values depend on individual disease processes. Mechanical ventilation, although life-saving, can itself also cause lung injury. Limiting plateau pressures (Pplat to <30 cmH_2O and V_T to 6–8 ml/kg ideal body weight [IBW]) is often described as lung protective ventilation. More recent concepts of lung-protective ventilation include limiting driving pressure (Pplat – PEEP) or the mechanical power of ventilation (energy delivered from the ventilator to the lung per unit of time). Initially, positive end-expiratory pressure (PEEP) is set at 5 cmH_2O and the inspiratory:expiratory time (I:E ratio) at *c.* 1:2.

Inappropriate ventilation can itself contribute to lung injury or other mechanical complications and generally the ventilator needs to be set by an experienced critical care practitioner.

Mode of ventilation

Modes of ventilation terms are often confusing; they describe whether a breath is: (i) fully or partially supported; (ii) volume or pressure controlled; (iii) mandatory (delivered by the ventilator regardless of patient respiratory effort); or (iv) spontaneously triggered. Modern ventilators with microprocessor controls are sophisticated and provide considerable flexibility, allowing a change from mandatory (all the WoB performed by the ventilator) to partial support modes that minimize sedation requirements and allow patients to be conscious/comfortable. PEEP is generally applied to all modes of invasive mechanical ventilation.

- **Full (mandatory) support modes** (e.g. IPPV or controlled mechanical ventilation): the ventilator initiates, delivers and terminates the breath. The breaths themselves, which are time triggered, may be targeted to a set pressure or volume. In a pressure-controlled mode, inspiratory pressure does not exceed the set value, but V_T may vary according to airway resistance and lung compliance. In volume control, the delivered V_T does not exceed the set value but inspiratory pressures may vary for the same reasons. Controlled mechanical ventilation is uncomfortable if the patient makes any respiratory effort and requires heavy sedation or even neuromuscular blockade. It is used in severe respiratory disease, in circulatory instability or when respiratory drive is absent.
- **Partial support modes** reinforce spontaneous ventilation and are preferred when possible, to allow a reduction in sedation. Breaths are initiated by the patient and detected by sensitive flow/pressure triggers in the ventilator, which then provides inspiratory support.
  - *Synchronized intermittent mandatory ventilation* delivers a set number of mechanically imposed breaths (pressure or volume controlled) which are triggered by the patient. In between mandatory breaths, spontaneous breathing can occur and these may be pressure-supported breaths. The mandatory rate is reduced as the patient becomes ventilator independent during weaning.
  - *Pressure support*: a preset pressure supports every spontaneous breath. The triggering, respiratory rate, V_T and length of inspiration are all determined by the patient. Gradual pressure reductions make it a comfortable and effective mode of weaning.
- **PEEP** describes a positive pressure, maintained throughout expiration, that increases functional residual capacity (i.e. alveolar recruitment), prevents alveolar collapse at end-expiration, reduces $\dot{V}/\dot{Q}$ mismatch and decreases alveolar oedema by increasing lymphatic drainage. PEEP improves oxygenation and oxygen delivery for any ventilation mode if the cardiac output is not reduced by the associated increase in intrathoracic pressure (IP).

Physiological responses to mechanical ventilation

- **Cardiovascular effects** are due to increased IP and alveolar overdistension. Increased IP has two effects on the heart.
  - *Right ventricular (RV) preload reduction* is due to increased right atrial pressure, which reduces venous return and RV cardiac output. However, fluid infusion rapidly restores venous return and cardiac output.
  - *Left ventricular (LV) afterload reduction* is due to reduced LV transmural pressure, which decreases LV work. In the normal heart, any beneficial effect of LV afterload reduction is offset by reduced venous return. However, in the failing heart, cardiac output is relatively insensitive to preload changes but very sensitive to afterload reduction. Consequently, MV may increase cardiac output in heart failure, a useful therapeutic effect.

The overall response to raised IP depends on the state of the heart, vasomotor tone and fluid status (e.g. hypovolaemia). MV also increases lung volumes. Overinflated alveoli compress alveolar blood vessels, increasing pulmonary vascular resistance and causing pulmonary hypertension. Subsequent RV distention displaces the septum into the LV cavity, reducing LV filling and cardiac output, an effect known as interventricular dependence.

- **Respiratory effects**: MV reduces WoB, which increases the proportion of cardiac output going to other potentially ischaemic organs. Re-expansion of collapsed lung segments also improves oxygenation. Unfortunately, supine position, reduced surfactant production and ventilation of poorly perfused lung increase $\dot{V}/\dot{Q}$ mismatch.
- **Fluid retention** is due to antidiuretic hormone secretion.

Complications

Mechanical ventilation may cause or exacerbate lung injury. (ventilator induced lung injury) due to barotrauma (high airway pressures), volutrauma (overdistention of alveoli) and alectotrauma (repeated opening and closing of lung units). Air leaks may develop, causing a pneumothorax or pneumomediastinum; these complications are more frequent when the lungs are stiff (poor compliance), e.g. adult respiratory distress syndrome (ARDS). This has led to the concept of a lung protective strategy where $V_T \leq 6$ ml/kg of IBW and Pplat is < 30 cmH_2O. This strategy frequently leads to respiratory acidosis and is referred to as permissive hypercapnia. PEEP should also be optimized and inspired oxygen kept to the minimal amount to achieve adequate oxygenation. Limiting driving pressure or mechanical power may be a more important lung-protective strategy but there have been no large randomized control trials evaluating these concepts.

The presence of an endotracheal tube circumvents many of the airway's host defence mechanisms and also provides an artificial surface which can be colonized by bacteria, so predisposing individuals to ventilator-associated pneumonia – the most common nosocomial infection in intensive care and greatly increasing length of stay/cost.

Rescue therapies

In severe hypoxaemia, strategies that include prone ventilation, early paralysis or pulmonary vasodilators (e.g. nitric oxide or prostacyclin) may be used. Even then, in some patients with severe respiratory failure, conventional modes of ventilation are insufficient and other rescue therapies may be used including high-frequency oscillatory ventilation (HFOV), airway pressure release ventilation (APRV) and extracorporeal membrane oxygenation (ECMO).

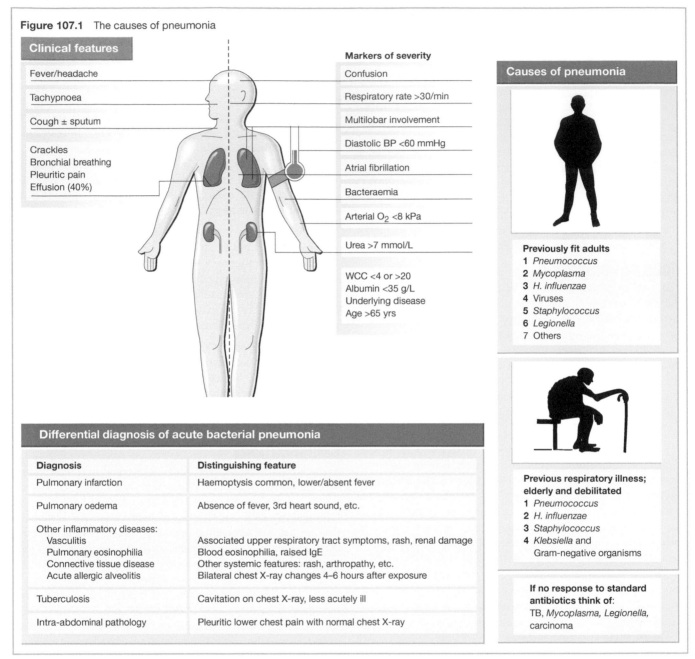

107 Lower respiratory tract infection: pneumonia

Figure 107.1 The causes of pneumonia

Differential diagnosis of acute bacterial pneumonia

Diagnosis	Distinguishing feature
Pulmonary infarction	Haemoptysis common, lower/absent fever
Pulmonary oedema	Absence of fever, 3rd heart sound, etc.
Other inflammatory diseases:	
Vasculitis	Associated upper respiratory tract symptoms, rash, renal damage
Pulmonary eosinophilia	Blood eosinophilia, raised IgE
Connective tissue disease	Other systemic features: rash, arthropathy, etc.
Acute allergic alveolitis	Bilateral chest X-ray changes 4–6 hours after exposure
Tuberculosis	Cavitation on chest X-ray, less acutely ill
Intra-abdominal pathology	Pleuritic lower chest pain with normal chest X-ray

Pneumonia is an acute infective respiratory illness causing radiological shadowing. It is classified according to the setting in which it is acquired, because this influences the likely microbial pathogens and therefore the best empirical treatment.

- Community acquired.
- Hospital acquired (nosocomial).
- Aspiration pneumonia.
- Pneumonia in immunocompromised individuals.

Community-acquired pneumonia

Epidemiology and pathophysiology

Very common. Community incidence is 1–3/1000 in adults. A quarter of cases require hospital admission. M = F, although Legionnaires disease is more common in males. Pneumonia tends to occur at the extremes of age, but it remains an important cause of morbidity and even mortality in young adults.

Infection occurs by droplet spread. Organisms multiply in the lung and, if local defence mechanisms are overcome, pneumonia develops. Tobacco smoke impairs local defences by depressing ciliary function. The causes of pneumonia are listed in Figures 107.1 and 107.2 above.

Clinical features

Fever and cough (initially non-productive) are common symptoms. Chest pain and breathlessness may also occur. Systemic features (more common but not specific to atypical pneumonia) include headache, confusion, myalgia and malaise. A prolonged prodrome is more specific to the atypical organisms. Examination may reveal local signs of consolidation and crackles over the affected lobe.

Figure 107.2 Causes and specific features

Causes and specific features of community-acquired pneumonia

Pathogen	% cases	Specific features
Streptococcus pneumoniae	60–75	Commonest in winter months Lobar involvement >> bronchopneumonic pattern Rapid onset, high fever, herpes labialis, vomiting. Mortality 5–10%
Mycoplasma pneumoniae	5–18	Mainly in autumn. Epidemics every 3–4 years Complications (20%): myocarditis, meningo-encephalitis, rash, haemolytic anaemia (cold haemagglutinin)
Haemophilus influenzae	4–5	Bronchopneumonia. Usually underlying lung disease
Legionella	2–5	Commonest in autumn in previously healthy individuals, from contaminated air conditioning. Key features: confusion, hepatitis, renal impairment, ↓Na^+
Chlamydia psittaci	2	From infected birds. Protracted illness. 50% hepato-splenomegaly
Staphylococcus aureus	1–5	During influenza A epidemics. Rapid progression and high mortality (30%) Cavitation in 50%, pleural effusion/empyema in 15%, pneumothorax
Gram-negative pneumonia	10	Underlying illness, often chronic. Increased chance in nosocomial infections. Often severe pneumonia, with septic shock. *Klebsiella, Pseudomonas, E. coli*
Influenza	5–8	Preceding myalgia + severe prostration. Epidemic
COVID-19	variable	See Chapter 244 on COVID. Usually no symptoms, or mild URTI symptoms, occasionally pneumonia and/or multiorgan failure
Other	2–8	

CURB-65 criteria for severity of pneumonia

1 point for each of the following:

- **C**onfusion
- **U**rea (>7 mmol/L)
- **R**espiratory rate (>30/min)
- **B**lood pressure (systolic BP <90 or diastolic BP <60 mmHg)
- **65** age ≥ 65 years

Risk of ITU admission or death:

0 : 0.7%
1 : 3.2%
2 : 13.0%
3 : 17.0%
4 : 41.5%
5 : 57.0%

Tachypnoea, hypotension, confusion and cyanosis all suggest severe disease. For the differential diagnosis of pneumonia see Figure 107.1.

Investigations

- **Confirm diagnosis**: this is usually done radiologically using a plain chest X-ray (CXR).
- **Define cause**: microbiological diagnosis is achieved by a diagnostic Gram stain, by growing the organism, by demonstrating a characteristic antigen from the organism or serologically (or other diagnostic blood test). Swabs from the upper respiratory tract are used to confirm viral pneumonia. All these tests have advantages and disadvantages and a combined approach may be necessary.
- **Assess severity**: see markers of severity in Figure 107.1. In severe COVID-19 pneumonia, normal markers of severity may be absent. Pulse oximetry can identify patients with hypoxaemia due to severe disease.
- **Identify complications**: complications can be detected by CXR, computed tomography (CT) and bronchoscopy, and include pleural effusion and empyema, lobar collapse (sputum retention), pneumothorax (in cavitating pneumonia and COVID-19) and organizing pneumonia.
- **Exclude cancer**: bronchoscopy should be considered in all people aged ≥50 years who smoke presenting with pneumonia, to exclude underlying lung cancer.

Management and prognosis

- **General supportive measures**: intravenous (IV) fluid, oxygen and physiotherapy.
- **Antibiotic therapy**: according to local guidelines. In severe pneumonia – IV broad-spectrum β-lactam and macrolide (clarithromycin). In less severe cases, ampicillin can be used as the β-lactam and in mild cases, amoxicillin alone is adequate.

The outcome is generally good. Mortality is higher in the elderly. Overall mortality is 5% but increases to 20% if hospital admission is required and 50% if intensive care is needed. Following improvement, particularly in smokers, radiological resolution should be confirmed to exclude underlying pulmonary abnormality, including lung cancer.

Hospital-acquired pneumonia

This is pneumonia occurring ≥2 days after admission to hospital. Infection before this is classified as community acquired.

- Causative organisms are predominantly Gram negative.
- Broad-spectrum antibiotics are necessary.
- High mortality associated with co-morbid factors.

Epidemiology and aetiopathogenesis

This is more common in elderly people, complicates 2–5% of all hospital admissions and accounts for 10–15% of hospital-acquired infections. Several factors predispose patients to the development of pneumonia in hospital – principally increased aspiration risk, reduced host defences and lung/skin instrumentation breaching the normal defences. Although the organisms that cause community-acquired pneumonia also cause infections in hospital, Gram-negative bacteria, *Staphylococcus aureus* and anaerobic organisms are far more likely to be found. Patients with underlying lung disease who develop postoperative pneumonia are still most likely to have pneumococcal or *Haemophilus* infection.

Clinical features and investigations

These are as for community-acquired pneumonia. The severity of illness is often greater as a result of the presence of underlying disease.

Management

- **General supportive treatment**: oxygen, fluids and physiotherapy.
- **Specific antibiotic treatment** needs to cover Gram-negative organisms that are resistant to the antibiotics given in community-acquired pneumonia. Antibiotics for nosocomial pneumonia include the following.

- Third-generation cephalosporin (e.g. cefotaxime) + aminoglycoside.
- Thienamycin (imipenem, meropenem).
- Antipseudomonal penicillin (piperacillin/tazobactam).
- Consider antistaphylococcal ± methicillin-resistant *Staphylococcus aureus* (MRSA) cover (flucloxacillin/vancomycin).

The prognosis depends on the causative organism and underlying disease severity. Pneumonia is often the cause of death in elderly hospital patients. In ventilated patients in intensive care, *Pseudomonas* pneumonia has a 50% mortality rate.

Lung abscess

A lung abscess is localized infection of the lung parenchyma with associated cavitation caused by necrosis. It is an uncommon problem occurring mainly in elderly people.

- Certain specific pneumonic agents are more likely to cavitate: *S. aureus*, *Klebsiella* spp. and anaerobic infection.
- Aspirated gastric contents, typically in those who have lost consciousness, who have bulbar palsy or who have problems with alcohol. Infected sinuses also predispose to anaerobic infection.
- IV drug abusers with right-sided endocarditis can develop multiple lung abscesses.
- Tuberculosis (TB) also causes cavitation, although the presentation is generally less acute.

Clinical features

These are of severe infection with fever and systemic upset. Large amounts of purulent and offensive sputum are produced if an abscess drains into an airway. Rapid weight loss and finger clubbing occur, and make the distinction from cavitating bronchial carcinoma important. Localized clinical signs in the chest may be minimal or there may be signs of consolidation and a pleural rub if there is pleural inflammation.

Investigations

These are as for pneumonia to confirm the diagnosis and the cause, and to assess the severity of the illness. By definition, the CXR will show signs of cavitation, although this must be distinguished from the cavitation found in cancer, TB, vasculitis (GPA) and other rarer causes.

Management and prognosis

Prolonged (six weeks) antibiotics are usually adequate – e.g. amoxicillin, or co-amoxiclav if unwell, and metronidazole to cover *Klebsiella* spp. and anaerobes. Drainage of the abscess usually occurs via the airway and this may be encouraged at bronchoscopy, which will also exclude an underlying obstructing lesion. Percutaneous drainage is not employed because there is a risk of introducing infection into an otherwise sterile pleural cavity.

With adequate drainage and appropriate antibiotics, the prognosis is generally very good.

Pneumonia in the immunocompromised

Definition and epidemiology

This is pneumonia occurring in patients with a deficiency of cellular or humoral immune mechanisms. The incidence is increasing as a result of the use of immunosuppressive drugs (transplantation, vasculitis), chemotherapy (malignancy) and HIV infection. Effective antiretroviral treatment and prophylaxis against *Pneumocystis jirovecii (carinii)* have significantly reduced the incidence of pulmonary infections complicating HIV (see Chapter 168).

Pathophysiology

Pulmonary infection is normally prevented by a combination of mechanical elements (epiglottis, cough and gag reflexes, the mucociliary escalator) and specific immunological mechanisms (macrophage/neutrophils, antibodies produced by B lymphocytes, cellular immunity effected by T lymphocytes). Defects in any of these mechanisms lead to increased risk of infection. Infection with multiple organisms is common. Infections associated with immunosuppression are as follows.

- **Neutropenia**: Gram-negative bacteria, *S. aureus*, fungi (*Candida*, *Aspergillus* spp.).
- **Reduced immunoglobulins**: bacteria (pneumococci, *Haemophilus influenzae*).
- **T-cell defects**: bacteria (pneumococci, *H. influenzae*, *S. aureus*), fungi (*Candida*, *Pneumocystis* spp.), viruses (herpes group, cytomegalovirus, adenovirus) and mycobacteria.

Clinical features and investigations

The diagnosis may be clear with fever, cough and breathlessness with focal clinical signs – symptoms that suggest bacterial infection. Symptoms are often more vague when infection is with opportunistic organisms. Onset may be over several weeks and fever may be absent. A high index of suspicion is necessary in patients known to be immunosuppressed.

- Investigation of the underlying immunological defect may be necessary. Full blood count, immunoglobulin levels and other tests, including for HIV.
- Plain CXR may reveal focal changes. CT may reveal alternative pathology but cannot provide a microbiological diagnosis.
- Standard microbiological investigation includes culture of sputum, blood and pleural fluid. If doubt exists, bronchoalveolar lavage may be necessary, but this has risks and should be reserved for those in whom initial investigation does not achieve a diagnosis. In those who fail to improve or where diagnostic doubt remains, lung biopsy may be necessary.
- At all stages in investigation, close liaison with microbiologists is necessary because specific culture techniques are necessary to identify likely organisms, particularly mycobacteria, viruses and fungi. DNA amplification techniques are used increasingly, particularly for diagnosis of viral infection. Detection of β-glucan in the blood supports a diagnosis of invasive fungal infection.

Management and prognosis

A microbial diagnosis is often not known before treatment is started. In general, broad-spectrum antibacterial agents are necessary while the results of cultures are awaited. Combinations should cover Gram-negative bacteria, including *Pseudomonas* spp., and staphylococci. A combination of antipseudomonal penicillin or third-generation cephalosporin with an aminoglycoside is often used as empirical treatment. Treatment can subsequently be changed according to the results of microbiological investigation. Treatment for viral and fungal infections will include specific antiviral and antifungal agents such as ganciclovir and amphotericin.

Infections often progress rapidly in immunocompromised patients. Achieving an accurate diagnosis to guide treatment is therefore important. Despite full supportive treatment and antibiotics, pulmonary infection in these patients accounts for up to 50–60% of the mortality.

108 Upper respiratory tract infection

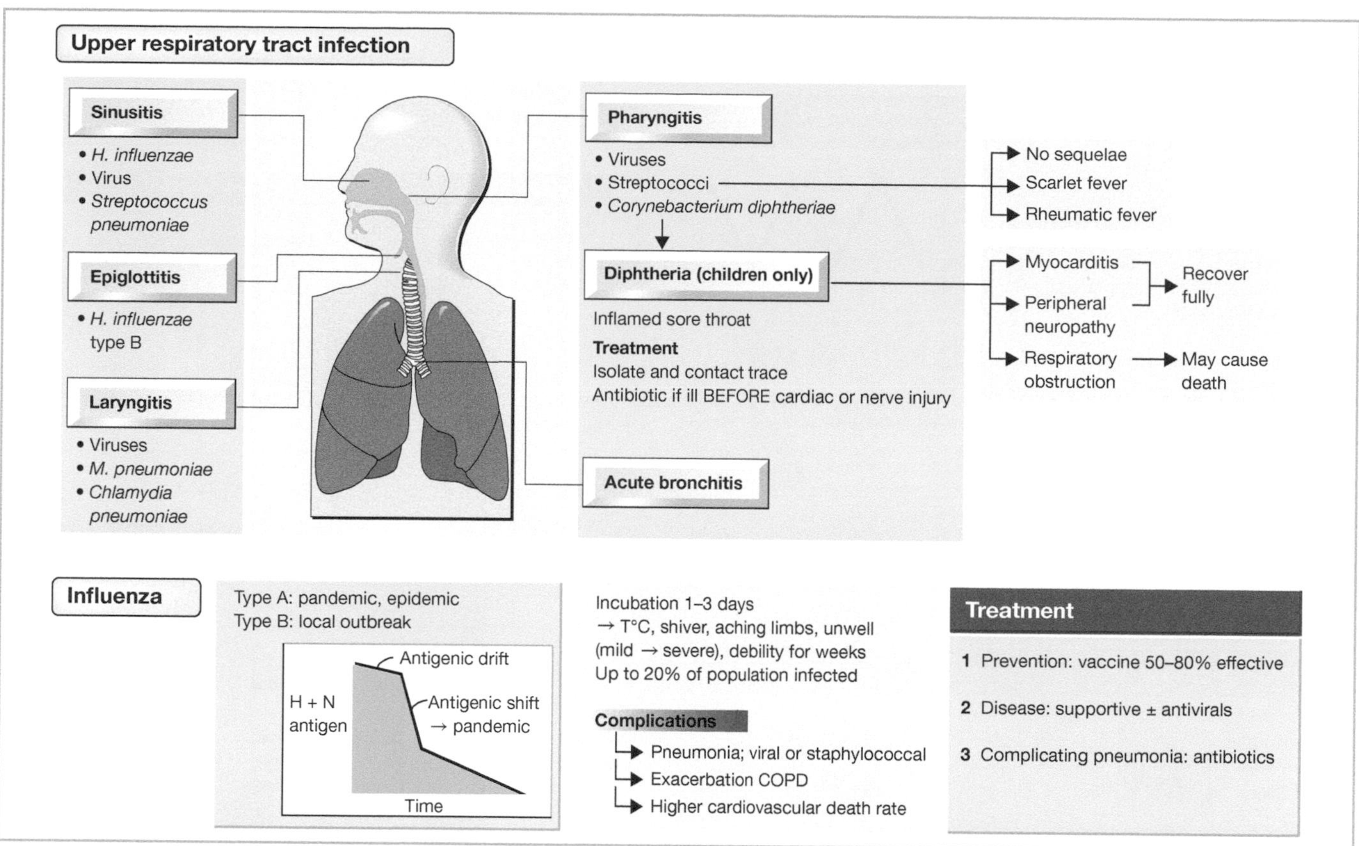

Table 108.1 The common causes of upper respiratory tract infection, their features and management.

	Cause	Features	Investigation	Management	Prognosis
Common cold (coryza)	Viruses	Sneezing, nasal blockage and discharge	None	Symptomatic	Remits in days
Pharyngitis (all ages)	Viral; occasionally streptococcal	Fever, sore throat	Throat swab, ASO titre	Antibiotics if bacterial; surgery if abscess develops	Remits in 1 week if viral
Laryngitis (adults)	Viral; occasionally pneumococci or *Haemophilus* spp.	Fever, hoarse voice	Throat swab	Antibiotics, humidification	Remits in about 1 week
Epiglottitis (children)	*Haemophilus influenzae* (occasional pneumococci)	Fever, sore throat, stridor, upper airway obstruction	Throat swab, blood cultures, lateral neck X-ray	Intravenous antibiotics, humidification, facilities for intubation. Prevention by HiB vaccination	Slow improvement with treatment, risk of death from airway obstruction
Bronchitis (all ages)	Viral; occasional pneumococci or *Haemophilus* spp.	Dry cough, retrosternal soreness, wheeze; sputum if bacterial	Sputum culture	Usually resolves but antibiotics often given	Improves over a week
Sinusitis (all ages)	Various bacteria 15% viral	Headache, facial pain, nasal congestion	None; sinus X ray if severe	Antibiotics; decongestants may help; sinus washout or surgery if persistent	Remits if acute; chronic problems are common

ASO, antistreptolysin O; HiB, *Haemophilus influenzae* B.

Medicine at a Glance, Fifth Edition. Edited by Patrick Davey and Alex Pitcher.

Companion website: www.wiley.com/go/medicine5e

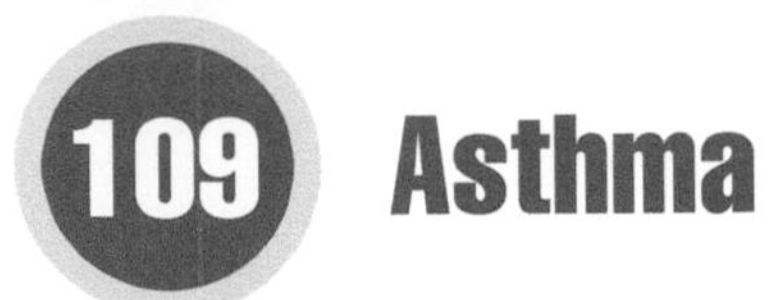

109 Asthma

Asthma

Asthma is an inflammatory condition causing reversible airway obstruction and symptoms of:

- Cough
- Wheeze
- Chest tightness
- Breathlessness

All, or any one

Symptoms respond to β_2 agonists

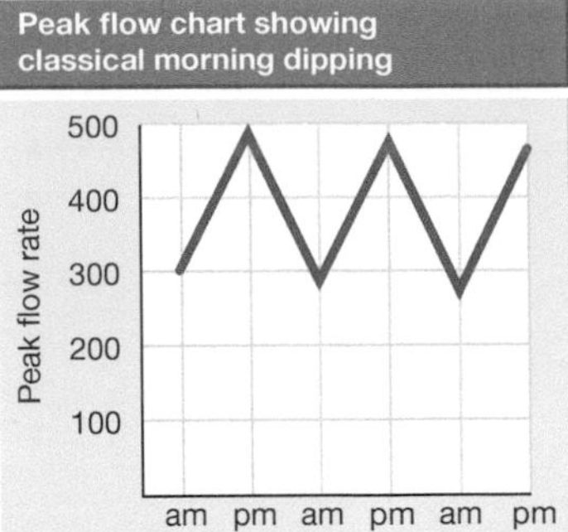

Consider underlying disease when asthma bad, adult onset, abnormal laboratory tests or chest X-ray

1 Allergic bronchopulmonary aspergillosis
2 Churg–Strauss
3 Bronchiectasis

I. Intrinsic	II. Extrinsic
• Adults • Fewer have ↑IgE or +ve skin tests	• Children • Atopic ↑IgE or eosinophils • +ve skin tests

Triggers (may be multifactorial)

Drugs
- Aspirin
- β-blockers

Allergens
- Dust mite
- Cat/dog dander
- Pollens

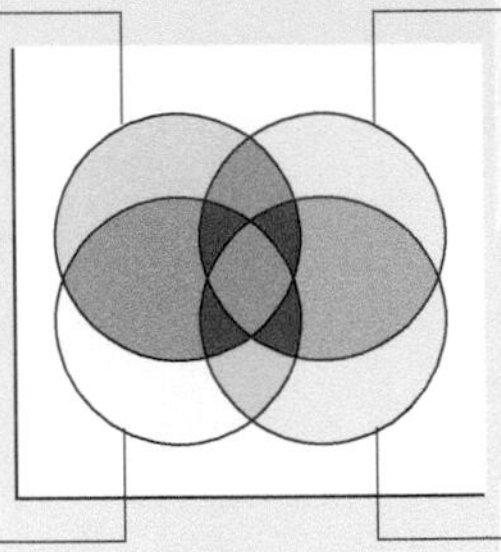

Occupational
- Isocyanates
- Drugs/enzymes
- Wood resin
- Dyes

Environment
- Cold air
- Exercise
- Emotion

Clinical features

1. Air entry
   - Normal
   - Wheezy
   - Silent

   ↑Severe attack
2. ↑Respiratory rate
   Use of accessory muscles of respiration
   - Sternocleidomastoid
   - Pectorals

   Intercostal recession
3. ↑Heart rate
4. ↓Ability to talk
5. Deviated trachea if tension pneumothorax
6. Cyanosis
7. Clammy, sweating
8. Confused

(5–8) In life-threatening attacks

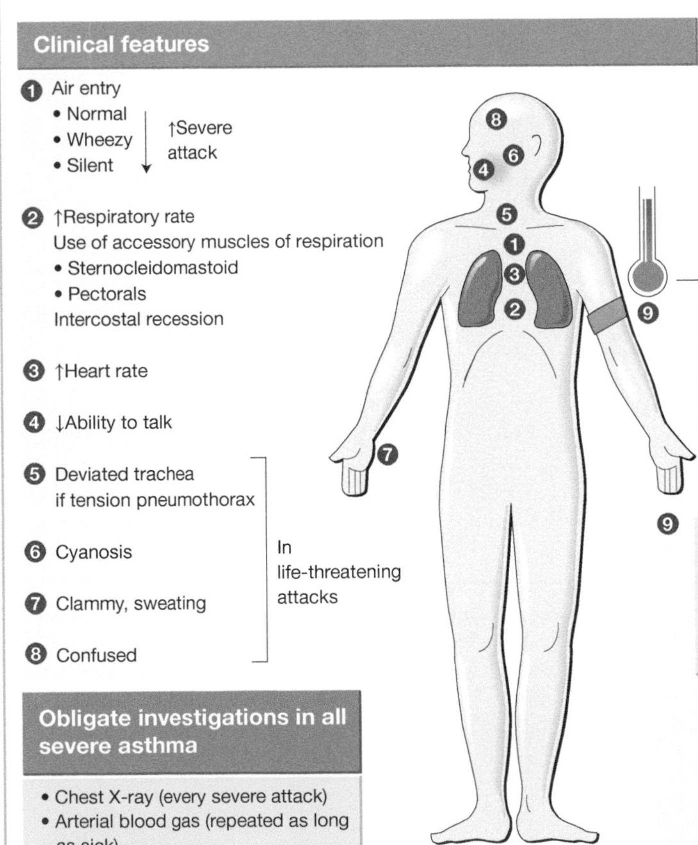

Obligate investigations in all severe asthma

- Chest X-ray (every severe attack)
- Arterial blood gas (repeated as long as sick)

In between attacks	Moderate	Severe	Life-threatening
Normal exam Normal lung function tests	PEFR <65% predicted ↓ Admit to hospital	PEFR <50% Pulse rate >110 Respiratory rate >25 Can't complete sentences Wheezy chest Alert → mild confusion	PEFR <33% Bradycardia Exhaustion Can't talk at all Silent chest Confusion → coma

	Moderate	Severe	Life-threatening
Po_2	↓	↓↓	↓↓↓
Pco_2	↓	→	↑
pH	Ⓝ or ↑	Ⓝ	↓
			Alert ITU

9 **Pulsus paradoxus**

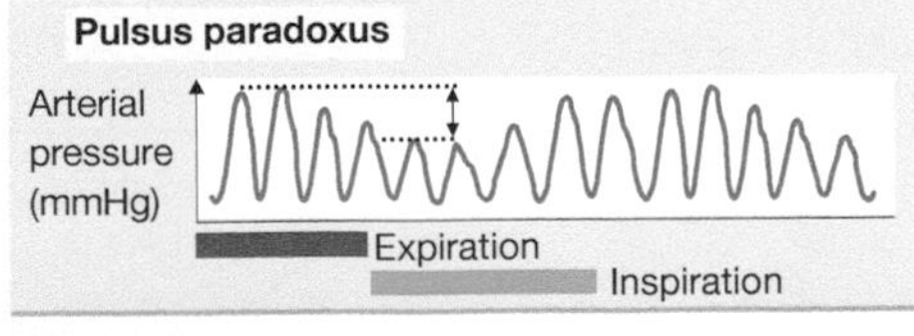

- Normal <5 mmHg
- Moderate 5–10 mmHg
- Severe 10–20 mmHg
- Life-threatening >20 mmHg

NB Large paradox may also arise from tension pneumothorax or from pericardial tamponade

Medicine at a Glance, Fifth Edition. Edited by Patrick Davey and Alex Pitcher.

Companion website: www.wiley.com/go/medicine5e

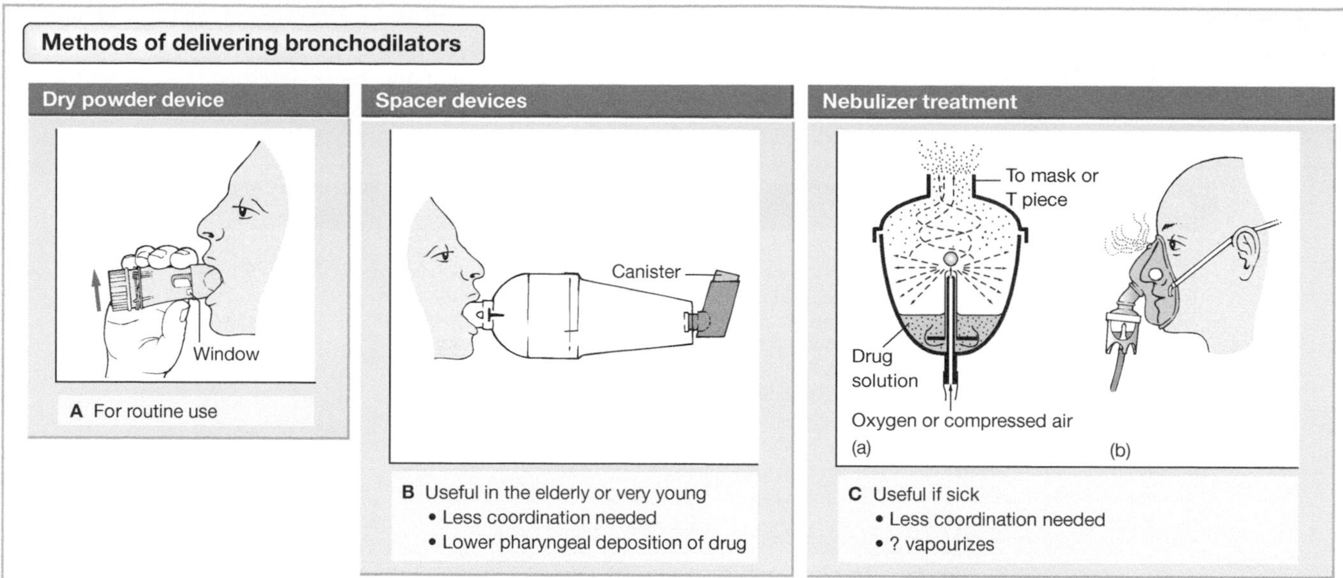

Definition

There is no universally accepted definition. Asthma is present if a combination of cough, wheeze or breathlessness with *variable* airflow obstruction is present.

Epidemiology

Asthma is the single most important cause of respiratory disease morbidity and causes 1500 deaths/year in the UK. The prevalence, currently 10–15%, is increasing in western societies. The incidence of wheeze is highest in childhood (one in three children wheeze and one in seven schoolchildren have a diagnosis of asthma). Asthma is classified as into three categories.

- **Extrinsic**: childhood asthma, associated with atopy (atopy = familial allergic diathesis, manifest as childhood eczema and hay fever). Often remits by teenage years, although it may recur during adult life.
- **Intrinsic**: develops in later life, is less likely to be caused by allergy, may be more progressive and does not respond as well to treatment.
- **Occupational**: relates to industrial/workplace allergens (e.g. photocopier material, baking, soldering, welding, paint spraying, etc.).

Aetiology

Genetics

Asthma runs in families in association with atopy. Genetic studies show linkage to the high-affinity IgE receptor and the T-helper (Th2) cytokine genes (chromosome 5).

Environmental factors

Specific bronchial stimuli include house-dust mite, pollen and cat dander; 3% of people with asthma are sensitive to aspirin.

- **Occupational exposure** to irritants or sensitizers is an important cause of work-related asthma.
- **Non-specific stimuli**: viral infections, cold air, exercise or emotional stress may also precipitate wheeze. High atmospheric levels of ozone (e.g. as found during a thunder storm) or particulate matter predispose to exacerbations of pre-existing asthma.
- **Other environmental factors**, including dietary ones (high Na^+, low Mg^{2+}), reduced incidence of childhood infections (partly as a result of immunization) and increased environmental load of allergens (dust mite) are responsible for increasing prevalence.

Pathology

Airway remodelling occurs with smooth muscle hypertrophy and fibrosis. Histology shows inflammatory cell infiltrate (particularly eosinophils) in airway walls.

Clinical features

Asthma presents with symptoms of cough, wheeze and breathlessness, which vary over time. An obvious trigger such as exercise or allergen exposure may be present. Examination may be normal or may reveal expiratory wheeze.

Investigations

Lung function tests may show airflow obstruction or may be normal. Serial peak flow measurements can be useful in making the diagnosis, and often show a classic pattern of morning dipping. Measurement of exhaled nitric oxide levels which increase due to airway inflammation can support a diagnosis of asthma. In people with known asthma, peak flow measurements are useful markers of severity. Allergy testing, serum IgE and eosinophil count are useful in some patients, in particular those with severe asthma.

Management

The objective of treatment is to keep patients free of symptoms on the minimum therapy.

- **Patient education**: vital for successful management, particularly explanation of the triggers, use and role of medication, and how to detect and react to a deterioration. All patients should be given a written self-management plan.
- **Avoidance of environmental triggers or allergens** is important, especially of cigarette smoke.
- **Chronic asthma**: a stepped care approach is recommended. For severe persistent allergic asthma, biologic treatments targeting raised IgE or eosinophil levels can be useful.
- **Acute asthma**: oxygen, systemic corticosteroids, inhaled β-agonists, anticholinergics and intravenous magnesium or theophyllines if necessary.

Prognosis

Asthma is a chronic disease requiring maintenance treatment. With appropriate treatment, many individuals are symptom free. If asthma is not adequately treated with inhaled corticosteroids, lung function is liable to deteriorate over time and airflow obstruction may become irreversible. Risk factors for death from asthma include poor treatment adherence, intensive therapy unit (ITU) admissions and hospital admission despite steroid treatment.

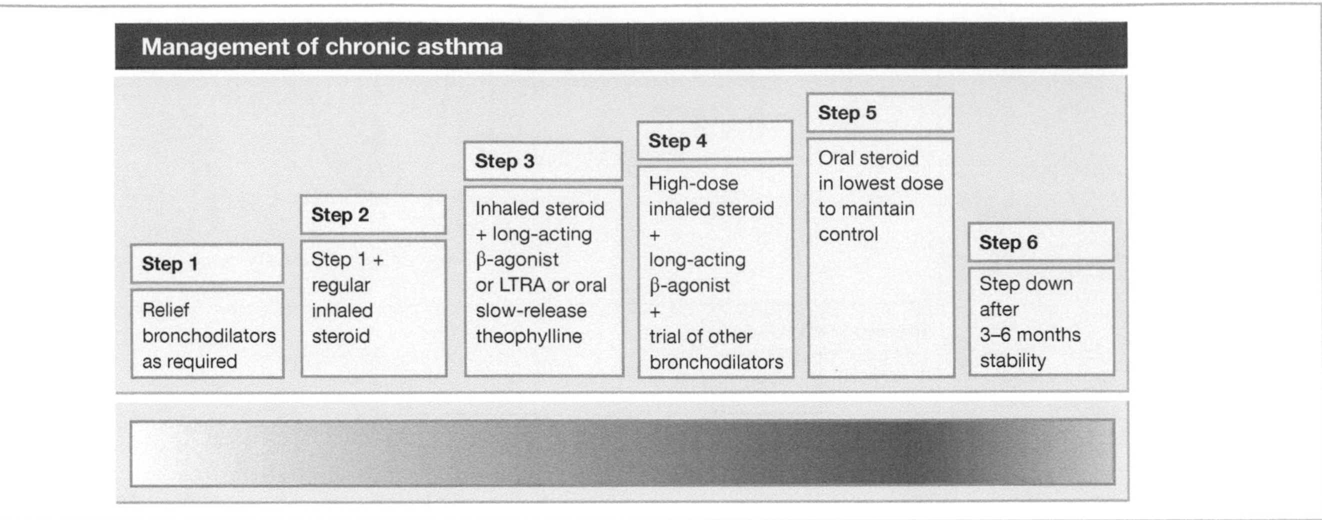

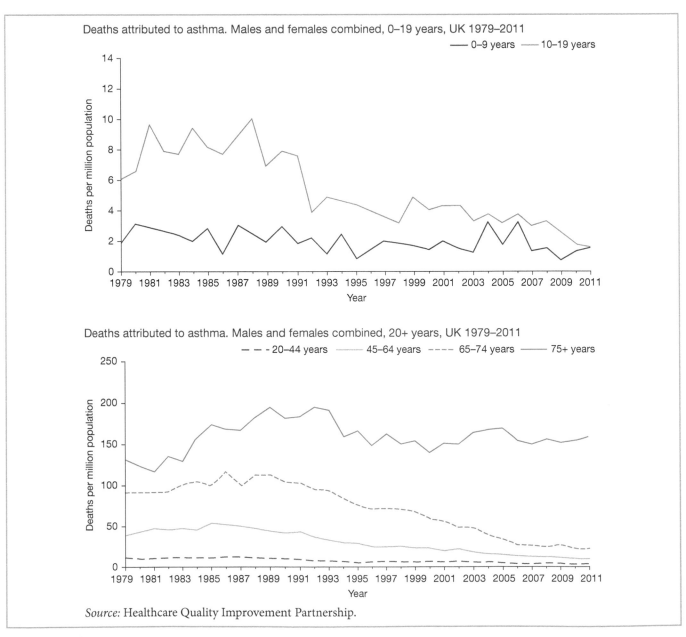

Deaths attributed to asthma. Males and females combined, 0–19 years, UK 1979–2011

0–9 years, 10–19 years; y-axis: Deaths per million population; x-axis: Year

Deaths attributed to asthma. Males and females combined, 20+ years, UK 1979–2011

20–44 years, 45–64 years, 65–74 years, 75+ years; y-axis: Deaths per million population; x-axis: Year

Source: Healthcare Quality Improvement Partnership.

Chronic obstructive pulmonary disease

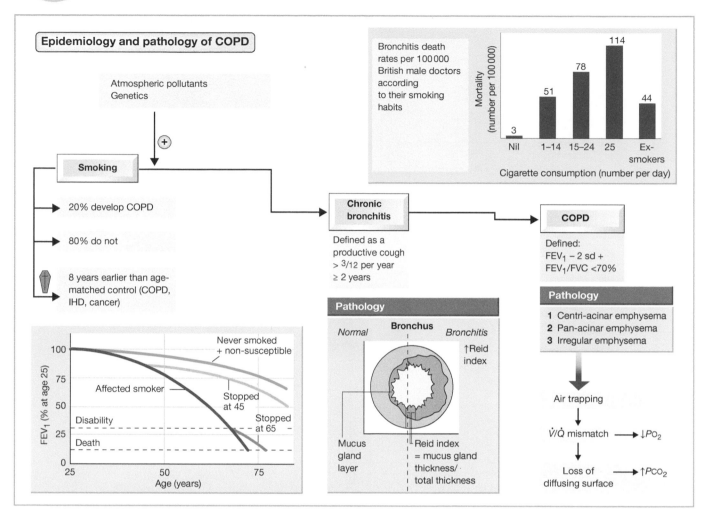

Epidemiology and pathology of COPD

Atmospheric pollutants
Genetics

(+)

Smoking

20% develop COPD
80% do not
8 years earlier than age-matched control (COPD, IHD, cancer)

Bronchitis death rates per 100 000 British male doctors according to their smoking habits

Mortality (number per 100 000)

3, 51, 78, 114, 44

Nil, 1–14, 15–24, 25, Ex-smokers

Cigarette consumption (number per day)

Chronic bronchitis

Defined as a productive cough > 3/12 per year ≥ 2 years

COPD

Defined:
FEV_1 − 2 sd +
FEV_1/FVC <70%

Pathology
1 Centri-acinar emphysema
2 Pan-acinar emphysema
3 Irregular emphysema

Air trapping
$\dot{V}/\dot{Q}$ mismatch → ↓PO_2
Loss of diffusing surface → ↑PCO_2

FEV_1 (% at age 25)
100, 75, 50, 25, 0
Never smoked + non-susceptible
Affected smoker
Stopped at 45
Stopped at 65
Disability
Death
25, 50, 75
Age (years)

Pathology
Bronchus
Normal
Bronchitis
↑Reid index
Mucus gland layer
Reid index = mucus gland thickness/ total thickness

Definition

Chronic obstructive pulmonary disease (COPD) and chronic obstructive airways disease are interchangeable terms. It is a chronic, slowly progressive disorder characterized by fixed or partially reversible airway obstruction, unlike the reversible airway obstruction seen in asthma (see Chapter 109).

Epidemiology

Chronic obstructive pulmonary disease is a major public health problem from which 25 000 people die per year in the UK (5% of all deaths). The UK prevalence is about 3 000 000. Rates are higher in industrialized countries, in inner-city areas, among lower income groups and in elderly people. Rates have plateaued in men but are still rising in women.

Aetiology

- **Environmental factors**: cigarette smoking is the major cause, with additional risk from atmospheric pollutants in the workplace or in the inner city. Some patients have chronic, undiagnosed and untreated asthma.
- **Genetics**: α_1-antitrypsin deficiency predisposes to early development of COPD.

Pathology

Smoking causes bronchial mucus gland hypertrophy and increased mucus production, leading to a productive cough. In chronic bronchitis ('productive cough' >3 months/year for >2 years) the early changes are in the small airways. In addition, destruction of lung tissue with dilation of the distal airspaces

Medicine at a Glance, Fifth Edition. Edited by Patrick Davey and Alex Pitcher.

Companion website: www.wiley.com/go/medicine5e

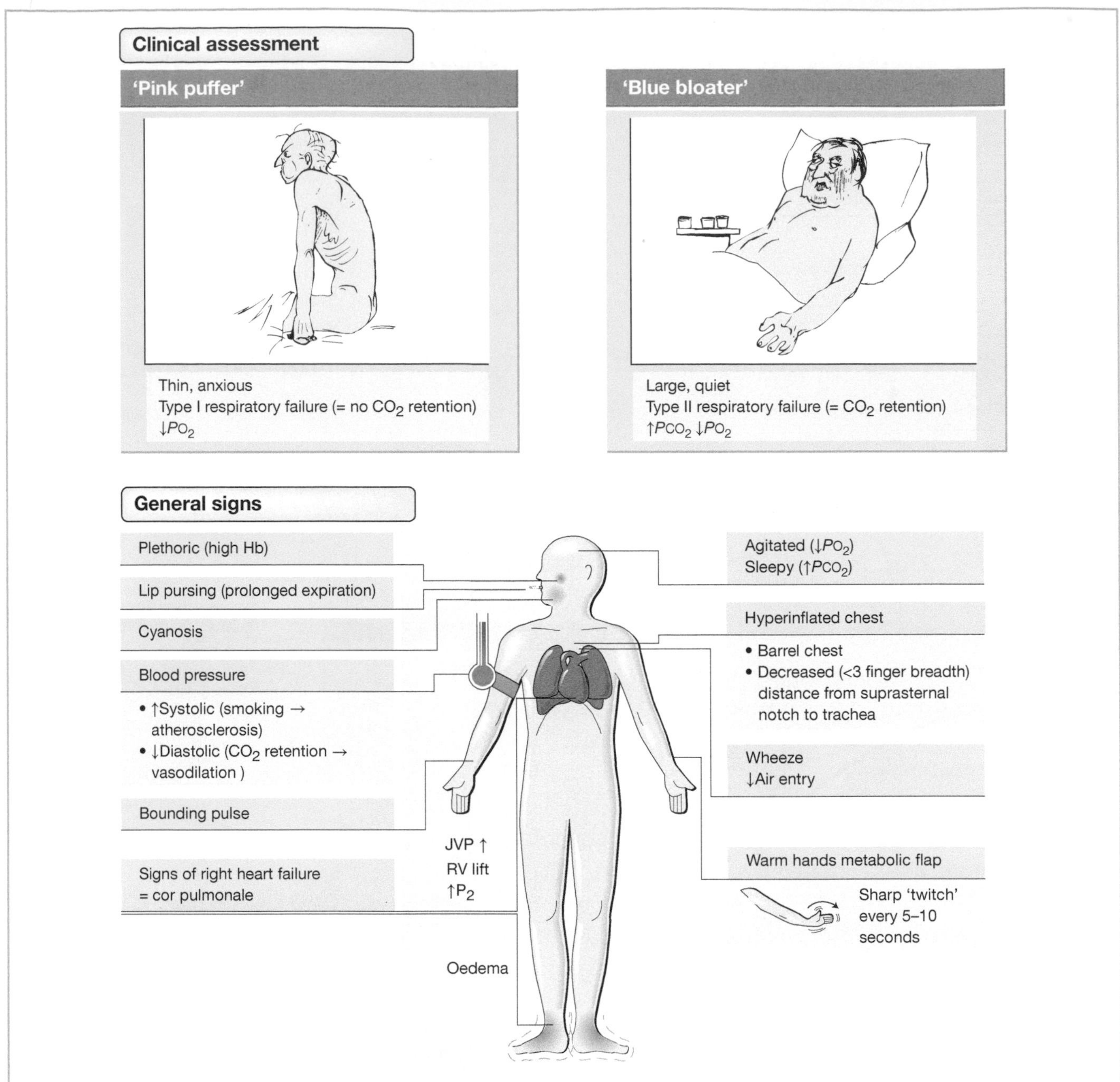

(emphysema) occurs, leading to loss of elastic recoil, hyperinflation, gas trapping and an increase in the work of breathing, causing breathlessness. As the disease progresses, CO_2 levels rise and the drive to respiration switches from CO_2 to hypoxaemia. Supplementary oxygen to correct hypoxaemia can reduce the drive to respiration, provoking respiratory failure.

Clinical features

Slowly progressing symptoms of cough and shortness of breath over several years in a smoker or ex-smoker suggests the diagnosis. Severity of disease is defined by the degree of airflow obstruction (forced expiratory volume in one second [FEV_1]; see Chapter 97).

- **Mild**: FEV_1 80% or higher of age/sex predicted – cough, minimal dyspnoea and normal examination.
- **Moderate**: FEV_1 50–79% – cough, breathless on moderate exertion, wheeze, hyperinflation and reduced air entry.
- **Severe**: FEV_1 30–49% – cough, breathless on minimal exertion, signs of moderate COPD and possibly of cor pulmonale.
- **Very severe**: FEV_1 <30% or <50% with respiratory failure.

Investigations

- **Pulmonary function tests** show airflow obstruction and reduced gas transfer as a result of destruction of lung tissue. Total lung capacity may be normal, or increased as a result of gas trapping. Twenty percent of patients derive benefit from bronchodilators. Response to bronchodilator treatment is not predicted by reversibility testing, which is therefore not recommended.
- **Chest X-ray** (CXR) may be normal but, in emphysema, will reveal hyperinflation with loss of lung markings and a small heart.

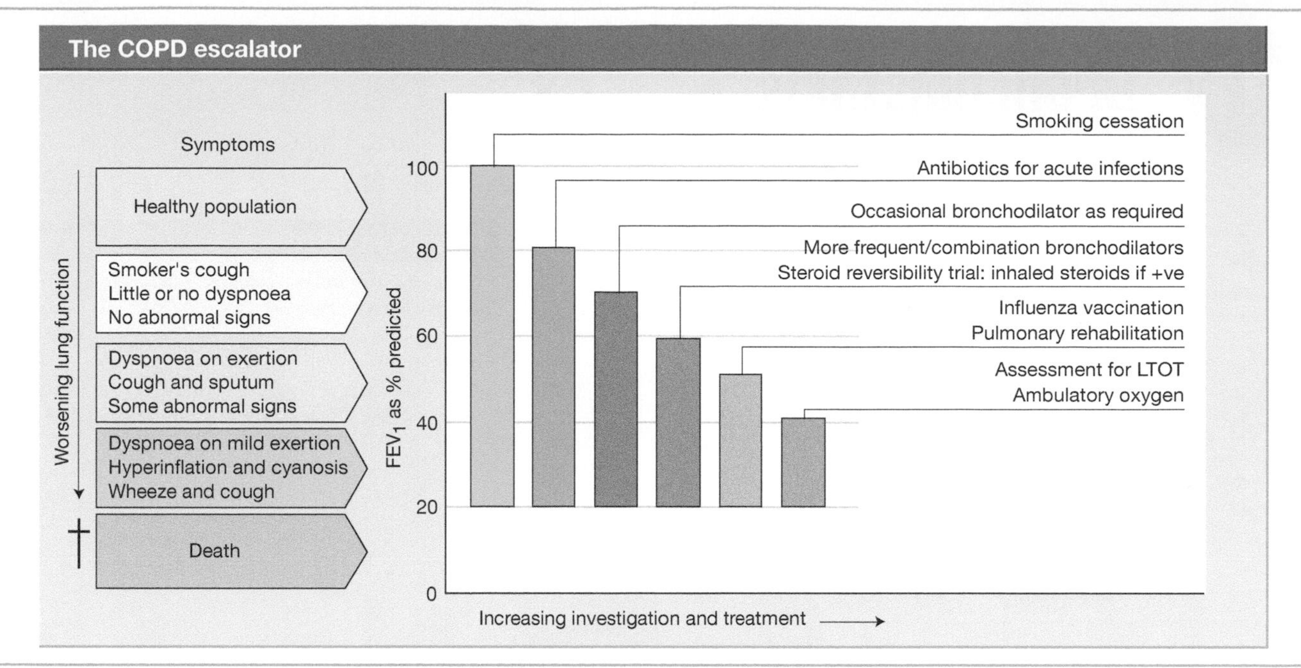

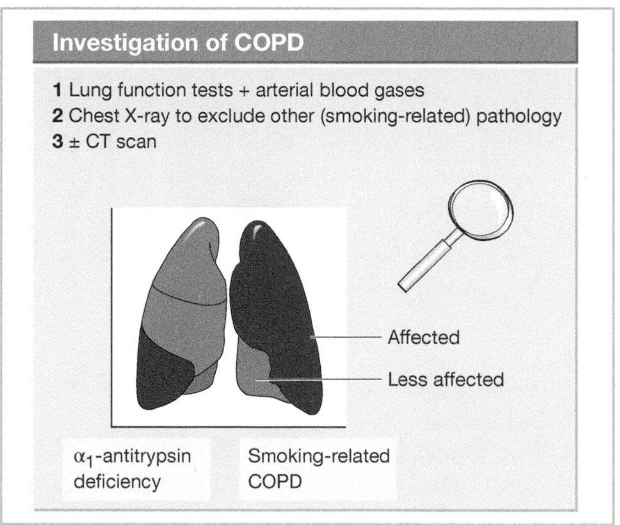

- **Computed tomography** (CT) may confirm emphysematous bullae.
- **Blood gases** should be analysed if there is any suspicion of respiratory failure. In chronic hypoxaemia, the haemoglobin may be increased.

Management

- **Smoking cessation** is a priority.
- **Bronchodilators** (β-agonists or anticholinergics) are used in the 20–40% who benefit. In severe disease, up to 10% of patients derive more benefit if high doses are delivered by nebulizer rather than metered-dose inhaler. A 10-day trial of oral steroids should be considered to determine reversibility (from serial peak flow or spirometry) of airway obstruction if a diagnosis of untreated asthma is suspected. Long-acting bronchodilators are recommended in patients who are still symptomatic on short-acting drugs and in patients with two or more exacerbations per year.
- Long-term **oxygen therapy** (LTOT) for >16 hours daily prolongs life in patients with chronic respiratory failure (i.e. those with a PaO_2 of <7.3 kPa and FEV_1 of <1.5 l).
- In an acute exacerbation, treatment may need to be increased. **Antibiotics** have not been shown to improve outcome, although short-course antibiotics shorten symptom duration of purulent sputum and respiratory deterioration. **Oral steroids** improve recovery from acute exacerbations. Long-term **inhaled steroids** reduce the frequency of exacerbations in those with moderate disease and should be used in those with an FEV_1 of <50% and at least one exacerbation per year.
- **Pulmonary rehabilitation** (especially exercise training) produces significant symptomatic benefit in patients with moderate to severe disease.
- **Resection of large bullae** enables adjacent areas of the lung to reinflate. **Lung volume reduction approaches** (surgery or endobronchial valve insertion) may also produce improvement by improving elastic recoil, maintaining airway patency. Careful selection of patients is important. **Lung transplantation** is used rarely.

Prognosis

This is variable. With continued smoking, decline in lung function will be more rapid than after smoking cessation. LTOT is the only treatment shown to improve life expectancy.

111 Bronchiectasis

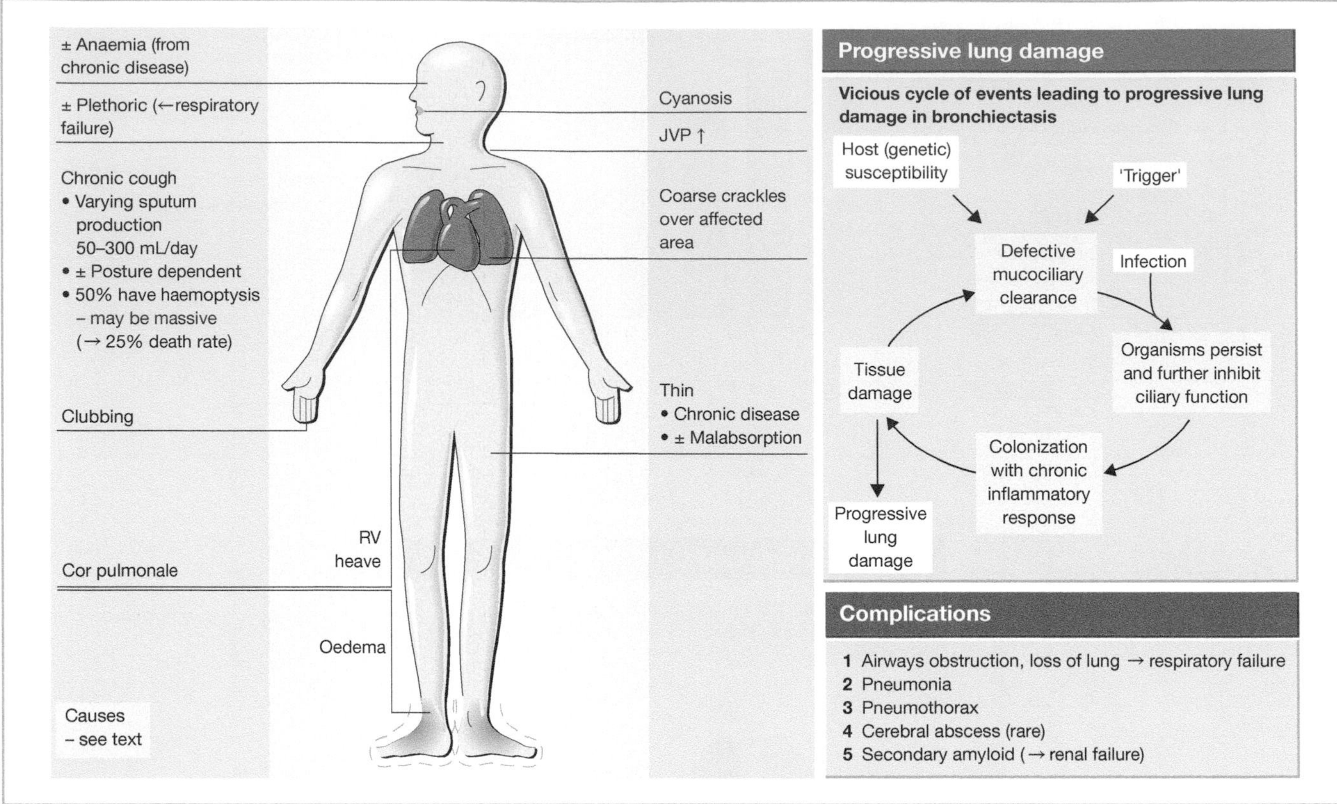

Definition and epidemiology

This is a disease characterized by bronchial wall dilation, often with superadded pulmonary infection. The incidence is unknown. Prevalence is 1/1000 and falling (less childhood whooping cough and tuberculosis). The disease has generally been less severe since the introduction of antibiotic therapy.

Aetiology

This depends on the distribution.

- **Localized bronchiectasis** follows severe pneumonia, or occurs distal to endobronchial (foreign body, tumour) or extrabronchial (tuberculous hilar nodes – Brock syndrome) obstruction.
- **Generalized bronchiectasis**: cystic fibrosis (see Chapter 112), ciliary dyskinesia (Kartagener syndrome), mucus abnormality (Young syndrome) and immune defects (immunoglobulin or complement deficiency, chronic granulomatous disease) cause persistent infection and bronchial wall damage, as do immune complexes (allergic bronchopulmonary aspergillosis, rheumatoid arthritis, inflammatory bowel disease). Underlying pulmonary fibrosis can lead to traction on bronchial walls, causing traction bronchiectasis. Rare disease associations are yellow nail syndrome, α_1-antitrypsin deficiency and Marfan syndrome (Table 111.1).

Pathophysiology

Retention of bronchial secretions occurs and lung infection results. If this is not cleared, the lungs become colonized. In addition, certain bacteria further reduce sputum clearance (e.g. *Pseudomonas aeruginosa*). A vicious cycle is set up and the chronic inflammatory response in the airways leads to tissue damage and bronchial wall dilation.

Clinical features

These are extremely variable. Minor bronchiectasis can be found on computed tomography (CT) scanning during investigation of patients with cough as the only symptom. Some patients have no symptoms or signs. The classic symptoms are of chronic cough and production of large volumes of mucopurulent sputum. Unpleasant breath ('foetor') is common. Haemoptysis occurs in 50% of patients at some stage; 30–40% of patients have associated chronic sinusitis.

- Anaemia, from chronic illness (see Chapter 186), or polycythaemia, from respiratory failure in late disease, may occur.
- Clubbing is found in severe disease.
- Cyanosis and signs of cor pulmonale are present at a late stage in generalized disease.
- Crackles are present in affected areas, particularly during exacerbations, and a significant number of patients have airflow obstruction with wheeze.

Other symptoms and signs relate to the underlying cause (e.g. sinusitis, infertility and dextrocardia in Kartagener syndrome; bronchial carcinoma, etc.).

Complications

The complications are all uncommon.

- Respiratory failure.
- Brain abscess from haematogenous spread of infection.
- Amyloid, with renal failure in long-standing severe disease (see Chapter 147).

Table 111.1 Diseases associated with bronchiectasis.

	General clinical features	Frequency
Cystic fibrosis (CF)	Due to malfunction of the gene coding for the CF transmembrane conductance regulator (CFTR) protein. Usually diagnosed at a young age; lung disease often dominates the clinical pictures. Malabsorption very common; cirrhosis, azoospermia, etc.	1 in 400 (Scotland) 1 in 2000–4000 (most white populations) 1 in 15 000–20 000 (African Americans) 1 in 30 000–100 000 (Asians)
Kartagener syndrome	Due to mutation in gene coding for dynein protein, causes ciliary dysmotility, resulting in sinusitis, situs inversus and infertility in men	1 in 30 000–70 000
Young syndrome	Triad of bronchiectasis, rhinosinusitis and decreased fertility (obstructive azoospermia) due to abnormally viscous mucus	Rare; 15–40% of men with obstructive azoospermia
Immune defects	IgA deficiency: repeated respiratory tract infections, 25% develop autoimmune conditions (e.g. RA, SLE, coeliac disease); IgM deficiency: recurrent infancy/childhood infections with encapsulated organisms. Later on, autoimmune illnesses and malignancy	1 in 600 (Europe) 1 in 250 (Nigeria) 1 in 4000 (China)
Allergic bronchopulmonary aspergillosis (ABPA)	Usually complicates long-standing asthma, leading to worsening of asthma symptoms and transient pulmonary infiltrates on CXR often with eosinophilia	ABPA occurs in 10% of those with long-standing asthma
Rheumatoid arthritis (RA)	Bronchiectasis can occur before overt arthritis, though more common during overt RA	Clinically relevant bronchiectasis in 1–3% of RA sufferers; occult occurrence in 30%
α_1-Antitrypsin deficiency	Chest disease, especially in smokers, at a young age. Symptomatic liver disease (cirrhosis) occurs at a young age	1 in 3000–5000
Marfan syndrome	Family history of premature sudden cardiac death, due to aortic dissection; aortic root enlargement ± dissection; tall, joint hypermobility, lens dislocation	1 in 5000–10 000. Bronchiectasis is a rare complication

Investigations

- The **chest X-ray** usually shows ring shadows or 'tram lines', representing thickened bronchial walls, although it is normal in 10%.
- **High-resolution CT chest scan** will confirm the diagnosis. The typical finding is the 'signet ring' sign – a thick-walled bronchus larger than the adjacent blood vessel.
- **Investigation of the cause**: immunoglobulin estimation, *Aspergillus* precipitins and IgE and relevant tests for cystic fibrosis. CT and/or bronchoscopy can demonstrate localized bronchial obstruction.
- **Saccharin test**: if ciliary abnormalities are suspected, the time taken for saccharin placed in the nose to reach the taste buds is measured. If prolonged, electron microscopy of cilia confirms the diagnosis.
- **Lung function testing**: may reveal airflow obstruction, which is often reversible.
- **Blood gases**: in severe disease if respiratory failure is suspected.
- **Sputum microscopy and culture**: common bacterial pathogens include *Haemophilus* spp., pneumococci and *Pseudomonas* spp. Atypical organisms, including mycobacteria and fungi, may also cause infection and these should be specifically sought.

Management

- **Physiotherapy**: patients should receive physiotherapy advice on twice-daily secretion clearance (active cycle of breathing technique, postural drainage). Supervised physiotherapy is useful during exacerbations.
- **Bronchodilators**: β-agonists, anticholinergics and inhaled steroids are used if reversibility has been demonstrated by formal testing.

Specific treatments

- **Immunoglobulin** replacement in hypogammaglobulinaemia reduces infections.
- Inhaled α_1-antitrypsin has not been shown to benefit deficient patients.
- **Antibiotics**: in high doses and for longer duration than standard courses (10–14 days) are used for infective exacerbations, guided by sensitivity from sputum cultures. Some patients with frequent exacerbations benefit from continuous/rotating antibiotic courses. *Pseudomonas* infection may require the simultaneous use of two antibiotics from different generic groups for a prolonged course (≥14 days).
- **Oxygen**: for symptom relief in hypoxic patients. Patients with chronic hypoxia and cor pulmonale should be prescribed long-term oxygen therapy.
- **Surgery**: resection of localized disease is sometimes effective in single lobar involvement and to control bleeding in massive haemoptysis, but is not useful in widespread disease. Lung transplantation should be considered in young patients with severely impaired lung function (FEV_1 <30% predicted).

Prognosis

Depends on severity. Some patients have few symptoms and lead a normal life with normal life expectancy. Patients with cystic fibrosis or the ciliary dyskinesias that lead to generalized disease tend to progress into respiratory failure.

112 Cystic fibrosis

Clinical features

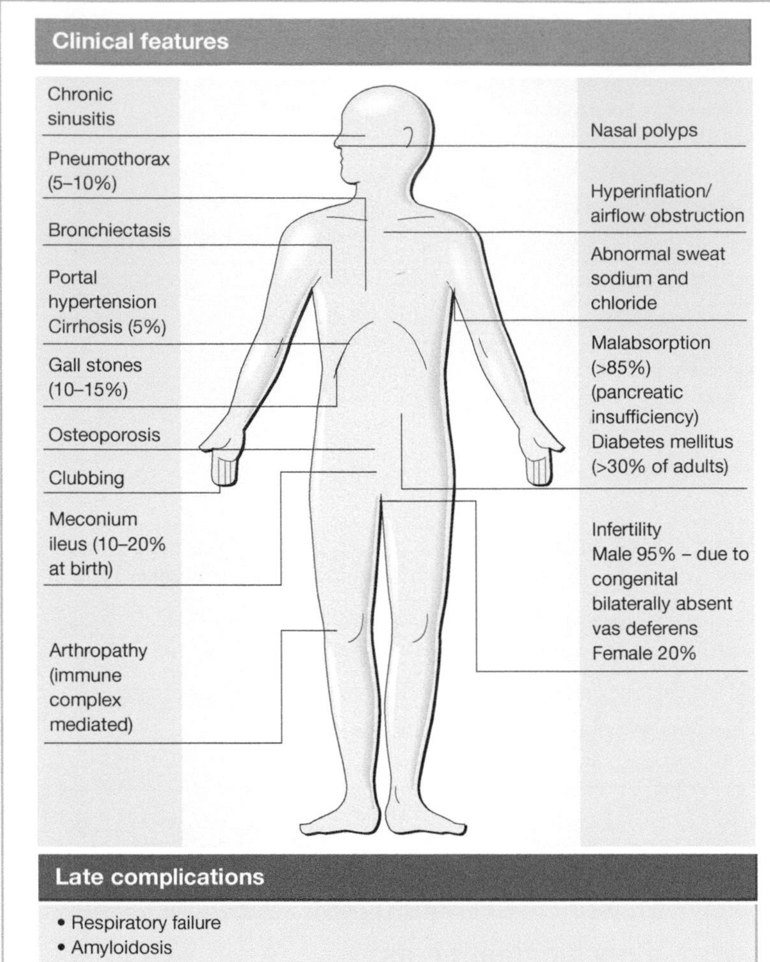

Late complications

- Respiratory failure
- Amyloidosis
- Osteoporosis

SURVIVAL

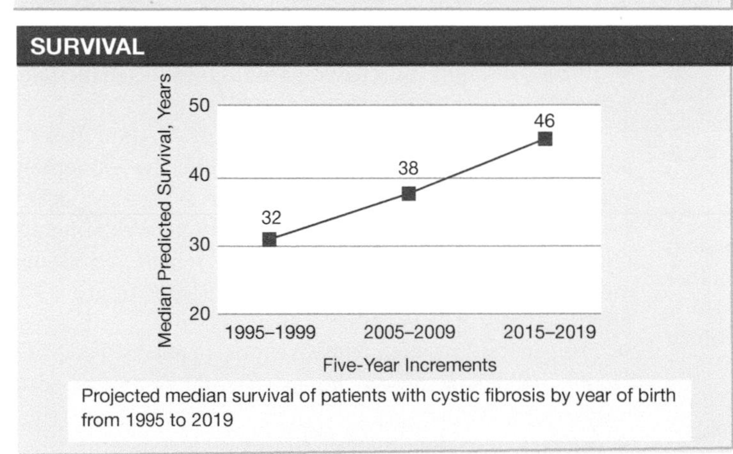

Projected median survival of patients with cystic fibrosis by year of birth from 1995 to 2019

Pathogenesis of cystic fibrosis

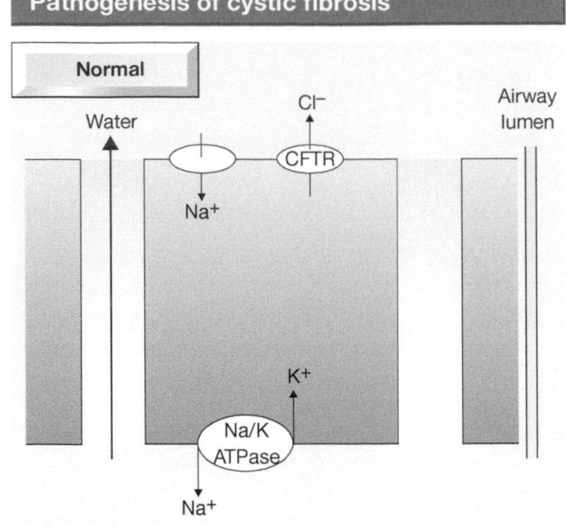

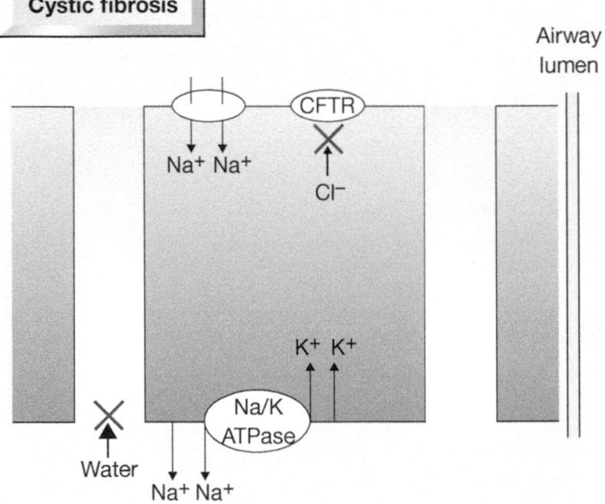

The cystic fibrosis transmembrane conductance regulator (CFTR), in health, acts as a channel allowing chloride ions out of the cell. This in turn keeps sodium in the mucus, which then by osmotic forces drags water into the mucus. In cystic fibrosis, the CFTR fails to allow the passage of chloride ions out of the cell. Sodium is retained intracellularly; this minimizes the osmotic forces that previously dragged water into the airway mucus. The mucus then becomes short of water, and accordingly very viscous

Medicine at a Glance, Fifth Edition. Edited by Patrick Davey and Alex Pitcher.

Companion website: www.wiley.com/go/medicine5e

Definition

Cystic fibrosis is a multisystem genetic disease leading to recurrent respiratory infections, pancreatic insufficiency and abnormal sweat sodium and chloride concentrations.

Epidemiology

Cystic fibrosis is the most common autosomal recessive condition in white people, with a carrier frequency of one in 25–30 and incidence of one in 3000 live births. The incidence is one in 20 000 in Africans/Caribbeans and one in 100 000 in Asians.

Aetiology

The abnormal gene is found on the long arm of chromosome 7 and encodes the cystic fibrosis transmembrane conductance regulator (CFTR), a cellular chloride channel that regulates the movement of salt and water across membranes. Though there are more than 800 known mutations of the gene, the DF508 mutation accounts for 70% of cases in Europeans and causes more severe disease with pancreatic insufficiency. Generally, the genetic mutation correlates only weakly with disease severity. Genetic screening is available for several of the common mutations. Functionally, the defective channel excretes less chloride into the airway lumen and has a three-fold increase in sodium absorption. Water follows sodium uptake, making airway secretions more 'sticky'.

Pathophysiology

The abnormal CFTR results in high concentrations of sodium chloride in sweat and in other secretions, which leads to an increase in the viscosity of bronchial mucus and secretions from the pancreas, liver and reproductive tract. In the lung, mucus clearance is reduced and this predisposes to infection. DNA released from infecting bacteria increases viscosity and exacerbates the problem. Recurrent infection eventually leads to generalized bronchiectasis. Pancreatic secretions are water depleted and therefore more viscid. This leads to reduced secretion of pancreatic enzymes and also local damage to pancreatic tissue, including islet cells. This further worsens secretory function and also results in diabetes mellitus.

Clinical features

- **Pulmonary features**: the lungs are normal at birth but recurrent infections in childhood lead to early-onset bronchiectasis, initially in the upper lobes, and a progressive decline in lung function with airflow obstruction, hyperinflation and breathlessness. In the later stages, clubbing, cor pulmonale and respiratory failure are common. Less severe mutations may result in bronchiectasis presenting in adulthood.
- **Pancreatic features**: pancreatic dysfunction leads to steatorrhoea, malnutrition and deficiency of fat-soluble vitamins. Diabetes is common with increasing age, occurring in more than one-third of patients by their late teens.

Investigations

- **Sweat test**: this is the routine diagnostic test of choice. Sweat sodium and chloride levels are both elevated above 60 mmol/l.
- **Genetic testing**: polymerase chain reaction (PCR) on blood is useful if the genetic mutation is known. Screening using PCR looking for the most common mutations will identify over 90% of cases.
- **Radiology**: early on, the chest X-ray reveals upper lobe bronchiectasis, although later this becomes more diffuse. If there is doubt, computed tomography will confirm this.
- **Lung function tests**: these reveal airflow obstruction with increased residual volume. There is often significant reversibility and this should be assessed. On average, lung function deteriorates by about 3% per year. Lung function impairment correlates well with mortality in late disease.
- **Sputum microbiology**: infection with common respiratory pathogens occurs with increased frequency. Most patients eventually become colonized with *Pseudomonas aeruginosa* which requires more intensive treatment. *Burkholderia cepacia* has also been found with increasing frequency and is important because transmission between patients occurs and it can lead to rapid decline in lung function. Segregation of affected individuals may be necessary. Other important respiratory pathogens include atypical mycobacteria, methicillin-resistant *Staphylococcus aureus* (MRSA) and *Stenotrophomonas maltophilia*.
- **Other routine tests**: full blood count, urea and electrolytes, liver function test, glucose, glycosylated haemoglobin (HbA1c) and glucose tolerance test for diabetes. Abdominal ultrasonography for portal hypertension. Tests for malabsorption (see Chapter 129).

Management

Patients require regular review in specialist units.

- **Lung disease**: this is managed as for bronchiectasis, with regular physiotherapy, bronchodilators and aggressive treatment of infection with antibiotics. Resistant organisms such as *Pseudomonas* spp. require prolonged treatment with at least two antibiotics. Indwelling central venous lines may be required if regular courses of antibiotics are required, and patients or relatives can be trained to administer these at home.
- **Recombinant DNase** is used to improve sputum viscosity and aid clearance by breaking down bacterial DNA in the sputum. One-third to a half of patients demonstrate improved lung function with this treatment.
- **CFTR correctors** have recently been introduced. These drugs bind to elements of the CFTR, improving its function and therefore reducing the impact of the disease in those with the DF508 mutation. Three of these have been combined in the medication Kaftrio®.
- **Influenza immunization** as for all patients with severe lung disease.
- **Nutrition**: nutritional supplements to provide high calorific intake are often required and may require feeding enterostomy for overnight supplements in severe disease. Pancreatic enzymes are taken by mouth to improve digestion and reduce malabsorption. Fat-soluble vitamin supplements are also given, and insulin for diabetes.
- **Lung transplantation**: patients with an FEV_1 ≤30% predicted should be considered for lung or heart–lung transplantation. Survival after transplantation is approximately 55% at five years and 35% at 10 years.
- **Gene therapy**: so far, this has not proved a clinically effective treatment. CFTR can be transfected into respiratory epithelium, but currently only at low levels insufficient to reverse the abnormality in airway secretions. In the future, it is hoped that gene therapy may provide a cure for the disease.

Prognosis

Early diagnosis, improved nutrition and effective treatment of respiratory infections have all led to an improved prognosis. Currently about half of patients with cystic fibrosis will live past the age of 40. Newly diagnosed patients currently have a better prognosis, with 85% anticipated to survive to age 50 years.

113 Sarcoidosis and other granulomatous lung diseases

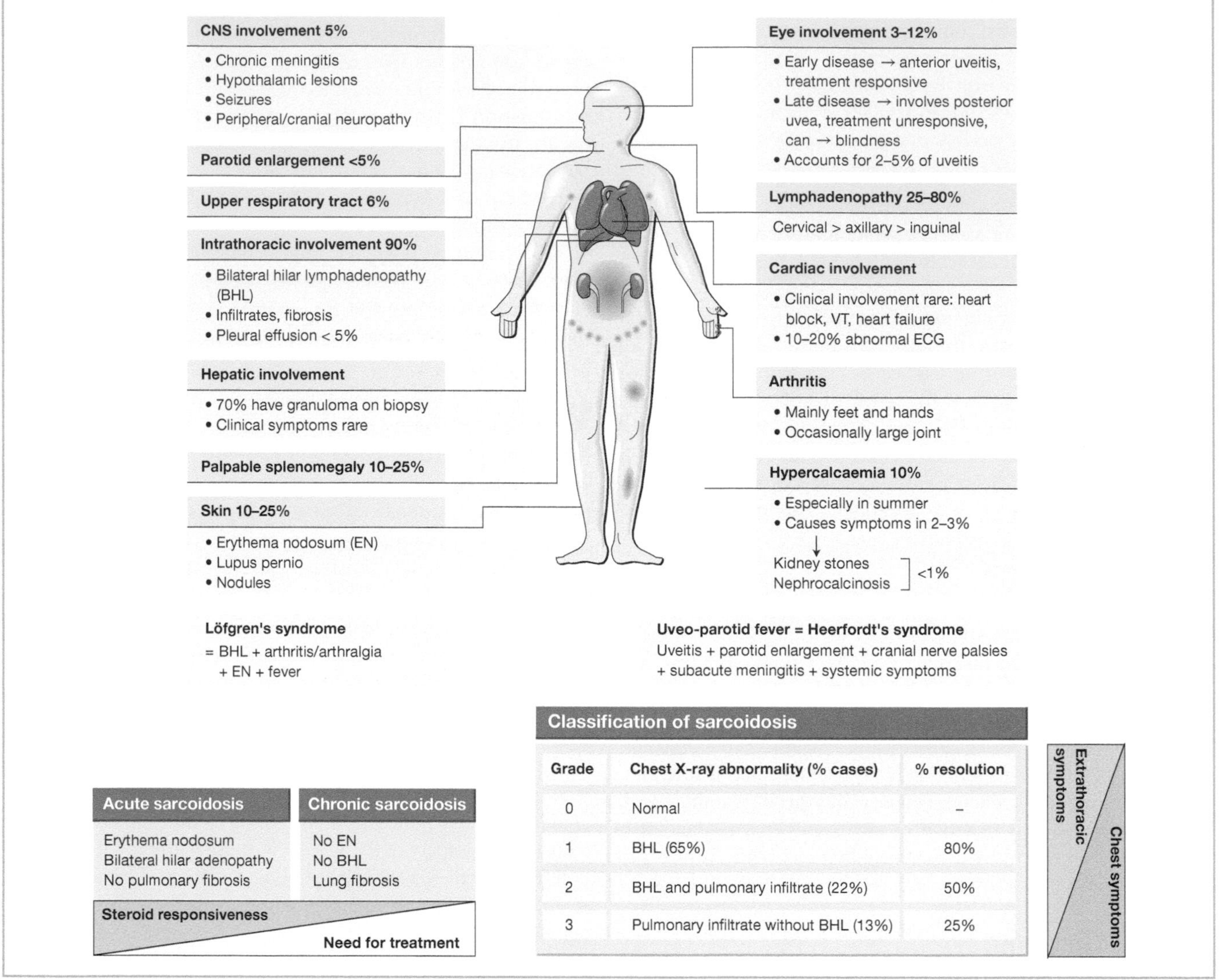

Grade	Chest X-ray abnormality (% cases)	% resolution
0	Normal	–
1	BHL (65%)	80%
2	BHL and pulmonary infiltrate (22%)	50%
3	Pulmonary infiltrate without BHL (13%)	25%

Sarcoidosis

Definition

This is a multisystem disease of unknown aetiology characterized by the presence of non-caseating granulomas in the affected organs. Frequent involvement of the lungs suggests that dust inhalation plays a part in causation. A significant genetic contribution is suggested by an increased incidence in monozygotic twins. Association with the human leukocyte antigen HLA-B8 has been demonstrated, particularly with the combination of arthritis and erythema nodosum. There is no evidence that the disease is the result of tuberculosis although the histology can be similar.

Epidemiology

Females > males. Usually presents in early adult life. Incidence in the UK is 5/100 000. The clinical pattern of sarcoidosis is racially determined, in part caused by the ethnic variation in HLA-B8 incidence (Table 113.1). Sarcoid is 15 times more common in Africans/Caribbeans.

Pathophysiology

The organs most commonly involved are the skin, eyes (see Chapter 65) and respiratory tract. The cause is unknown but the pathological lesion is the non-caseating granuloma. In the lung, a lymphocytic alveolitis is present initially. Subsequent T-lymphocyte-stimulated recruitment of macrophages occurs and these organize into granulomas, which mediate inflammation and long-term damage. A syndrome clinically and histologically indistinguishable from sarcoidosis is found occasionally in patients with underlying malignancy. This should be considered when sarcoidosis presents in older patients.

Medicine at a Glance, Fifth Edition. Edited by Patrick Davey and Alex Pitcher.

Companion website: www.wiley.com/go/medicine5e

Table 113.1 Clinical features (%) of sarcoidosis in different ethnic groups.

Clinical feature	White	Black	Asian
Abnormal chest X-ray	34	7	10
Respiratory symptoms	25	57	55
Systemic symptoms	5	57	55
Erythema nodosum	20	8.5	17
Eye symptoms	7	12	3
Superficial lymphadenopathy	3	34	17

Clinical features

This is a multisystem disease and features depend on the organs involved. Intrathoracic involvement is most common. There are two typical patterns.

1 **Acute presentation** with erythema nodosum, arthralgia and bilateral hilar lymphadenopathy is most common and carries a good prognosis (80% resolution in one year).
2 **Chronic presentation** with slowly progressive breathlessness has a worse prognosis and is associated with progressive pulmonary fibrosis.

Investigations

- **Laboratory tests**: a full blood count may show lymphopenia in active disease. Thrombocytopenia is described. The erythrocyte sedimentation rate is raised in active disease. Serum and urinary calcium are raised in 10%, more commonly so in the summer months, as a result of abnormal vitamin D metabolism. Hypercalcaemia can progress to nephrocalcinosis. Immunoglobulins are diffusely raised in active disease. Serum angiotensin-converting enzyme levels are raised in two-thirds of cases, although this is not specific for sarcoidosis.
- **Chest X-ray** findings are traditionally divided into stages that influence prognosis.
- **High-resolution computed tomography** (HRCT) reveals typical findings of mediastinal nodal disease. Pulmonary parenchymal changes include nodules in a bronchovascular, subpleural and fissural distribution.
- **Pulmonary function tests** are often normal. In fibrotic disease, reduced lung volumes and gas transfer are typical. Obstructive pulmonary function with gas trapping may be found.
- **The Kveim test** involved intradermal injection of a preparation of splenic tissue from a patient with sarcoidosis and subsequent skin biopsy. **It is no longer used** because of concerns over the risk of transmitting infection. Tuberculin tests are negative in two-thirds of patients.
- **Histology** is the best diagnostic test and a tissue diagnosis should always be sought if there is diagnostic doubt or if immunosuppressive treatment is to be used. Transbronchial biopsy is positive in 80%.

Management

- **Observation**: sarcoidosis with a good prognosis (erythema nodosum and bilateral hilar lymphadenopathy) requires no treatment. Non-steroidal anti-inflammatory drugs are used for pain. The chest X-ray is repeated at an interval to document resolution.
- **Oral steroids** are used in symptomatic pulmonary disease, cardiac and neurological sarcoid. Patients with pulmonary disease and radiological changes that persist for longer than six months have a better long-term outcome if given oral steroids (prednisolone 30–40 mg daily, discontinued after a month if no improvement) for three months. Other immunosuppressive drugs (most commonly methotrexate) have been used with some reported benefit.
- **Topical steroids**: for uveitis. Sometimes oral prednisolone is needed.
- **Chloroquine** can be useful in cutaneous and progressive pulmonary disease.

Prognosis

This is worse with older age of onset, more widespread disease and in Africans/Caribbeans. Two-thirds of white and one-third of black patients recover with no treatment. Fewer than 3% of patients die from sarcoidosis.

Beryllium disease

Beryllium is a heavy metal used in the manufacture of fluorescent lighting tubes. Lung disease resulting from exposure is rare.

- **Acute exposure** to fumes leads to an alveolitis, but industry precautions should prevent this occurring.
- **Chronic low-level exposure** can lead to a systemic disease similar to sarcoidosis. Non-caseating granulomas appear in the skin or lungs. Radiologically, there may be nodularity in the lung fields and bilateral hilar lymphadenopathy. The pulmonary abnormality progresses to fibrosis with small lung volumes, impaired gas transfer and respiratory failure. Early treatment with corticosteroids can result in improved lung function. Workers who have been exposed to beryllium undergo regular screening with chest X-rays to detect development of asymptomatic pulmonary disease. They should of course report the development of respiratory symptoms.

Histiocytosis X (Langerhans cell histiocytosis)

Epidemiology

This is a rare multisystem disorder of unknown aetiology occurring more often in males and usually presenting in early adult life. The vast majority of patients are smokers.

Pathophysiology and investigation

Initially, there is infiltration of lung tissue with eosinophils and Langerhans cells. This progresses to granuloma formation, which breaks down to form cystic areas, particularly in the upper zones. Ultimately, pulmonary fibrosis develops. Pneumothorax is common. The diagnosis can be made radiologically. Plain X-rays and HRCT show diffuse nodularity with cyst formation in the characteristic distribution. Lung volume is often well preserved. Pulmonary function tests often reveal a restrictive defect with high residual volume and normal total lung capacity as a result of gas trapping.

Clinical features

Most patients are breathless but 25% are asymptomatic with an abnormal X-ray. Spontaneous pneumothorax is the presenting feature in 10%.

Management

Smoking cessation is essential and complete resolution with no additional treatment is possible. A variety of immunosuppressive regimens have been used. Oral corticosteroids remain the mainstay of treatment in patients with symptomatic disease. Long-term survival is commonly reported.

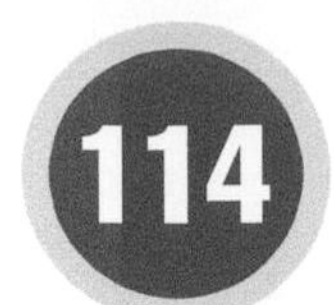

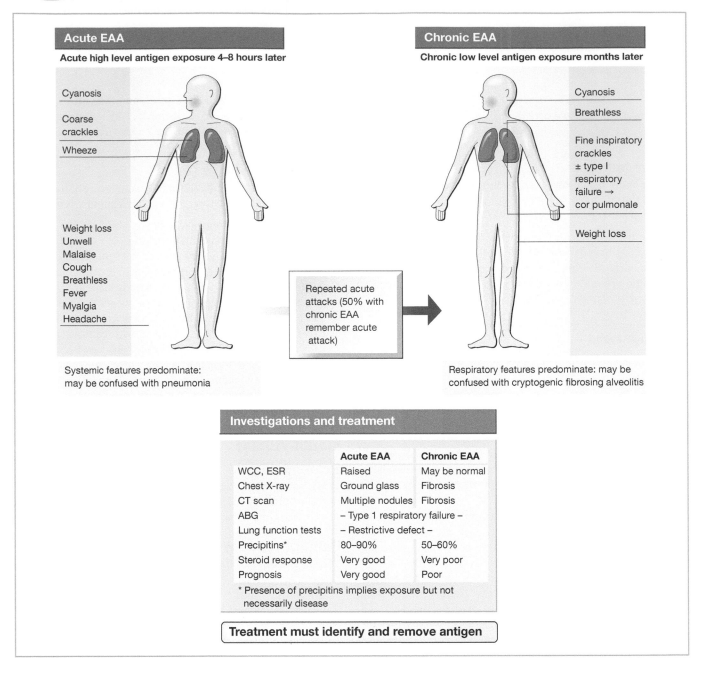

114 Hypersensitivity pneumonitis (extrinsic allergic alveolitis)

Acute EAA

Acute high level antigen exposure 4–8 hours later

Cyanosis
Coarse crackles
Wheeze
Weight loss
Unwell
Malaise
Cough
Breathless
Fever
Myalgia
Headache

Systemic features predominate: may be confused with pneumonia

Repeated acute attacks (50% with chronic EAA remember acute attack)

Chronic EAA

Chronic low level antigen exposure months later

Cyanosis
Breathless
Fine inspiratory crackles ± type I respiratory failure → cor pulmonale
Weight loss

Respiratory features predominate: may be confused with cryptogenic fibrosing alveolitis

Investigations and treatment

	Acute EAA	Chronic EAA
WCC, ESR	Raised	May be normal
Chest X-ray	Ground glass	Fibrosis
CT scan	Multiple nodules	Fibrosis
ABG	– Type 1 respiratory failure –	
Lung function tests	– Restrictive defect –	
Precipitins*	80–90%	50–60%
Steroid response	Very good	Very poor
Prognosis	Very good	Poor

* Presence of precipitins implies exposure but not necessarily disease

Treatment must identify and remove antigen

Definition

This is a condition caused by hypersensitivity to inhaled organic dusts, leading to an inflammatory reaction in the distal airspaces.

Epidemiology

Uncommon: 1–2 per 100 000 in the UK. Mainly in middle-aged people.

Aetiology

Inhalation of a number of antigens may result in a pulmonary inflammatory response. For some causes, see Table 114.1.

Pathophysiology

Extrinsic allergic alveolitis (EAA) is a granulomatous reaction to a variety of organic dusts, including animal proteins (particularly from birds) and microbial spores.

Medicine at a Glance, Fifth Edition. Edited by Patrick Davey and Alex Pitcher.

Companion website: www.wiley.com/go/medicine5e

Table 114.1 Some causes of extrinsic allergic alveolitis – there are many other reported causes.

Disease	Cause	Agent
Farmer's lung	Mouldy hay	Thermophilic actinomycetes
Bird fancier's lung	Pigeon, budgerigar, poultry	Bloom/excreta
Woodworker's lung	Wood	Wood dust
Byssinosis	Cotton dust	? Agent
Suberosis	Cork dust	*Penicillium frequentens*
Humidifier fever	Air humidification units	Variety of agents
Malt worker's lung	Whisky maltings	*Aspergillus clavatus*
Coffee worker's lung	Coffee bean dust	Coffee
Hot tub lung	Aerosols from hot tubs	Non-tuberculous mycobacteria

- Occupational or environmental exposure to these dusts results in an immunological response, with inflammatory cell (neutrophil and lymphocyte) activation in the bronchioles extending distally into the alveoli. Accumulation of giant cells leads to granuloma formation in a bronchocentric distribution.
- Progressive fibrosis results if there is persistent inflammatory cell activation. The formation of granulomas implies that T-cell activation is involved in the pathogenesis of EAA. The presence of IgG serum precipitins implies exposure to an antigenic dust with the formation of immune complexes, but does not relate to the pathology in the lung.

Clinical features

Extrinsic allergic alveolitis may present as acute or chronic alveolitis.

- **Acute allergic alveolitis**: 4–8 hours after exposure to high doses of antigen, systemic features of fever, myalgia and headache develop, with cough and breathlessness. Persistent exposure over weeks can produce considerable weight loss. Examination reveals inspiratory crackles and squeaks.
- **Chronic allergic alveolitis**: presents with progressive exertional breathlessness as a result of pulmonary fibrosis. Prolonged low-level antigen exposure is the cause and there may be a history of acute episodes. Examination reveals inspiratory crackles typical of pulmonary fibrosis.

Investigations

- **Laboratory tests**: in acute alveolitis, a neutrophil leukocytosis may be present. The presence of circulating precipitating antibodies implies antigen exposure but not necessarily disease.
- **Chest X-ray** reveals subtle diffuse ground-glass change with small nodules, which can be confirmed by **high-resolution computed tomography** (HRCT). In chronic alveolitis, fibrosis, typically in the mid and upper zones, is present on the chest X-ray and HRCT.
- **Pulmonary function testing**: shows a restrictive pattern in both acute and chronic disease with impaired gas transfer. Respiratory failure with hypoxaemia may be present in severe acute or chronic fibrotic disease.

The combination of symptoms, radiology, pulmonary function abnormality and the relevant exposure (presence of precipitins) is usually sufficient for a diagnosis. If doubt remains, lung biopsy may be necessary.

Management

This is aimed at optimizing lung function and preventing the development of pulmonary fibrosis. The key is antigen avoidance or reduction of exposure by the use of respiratory protection equipment. Oral corticosteroids (prednisolone 40–60 mg daily for 3–6 months) accelerate the rate of recovery, but do not improve long-term outcome. They should be reserved for patients with acute alveolitis or significant respiratory compromise.

Prognosis

- **Acute disease**: usually full recovery after cessation of exposure.
- **Chronic disease**: progressive and permanent lung damage may occur but long-term survival common.

115 Pulmonary fibrosis

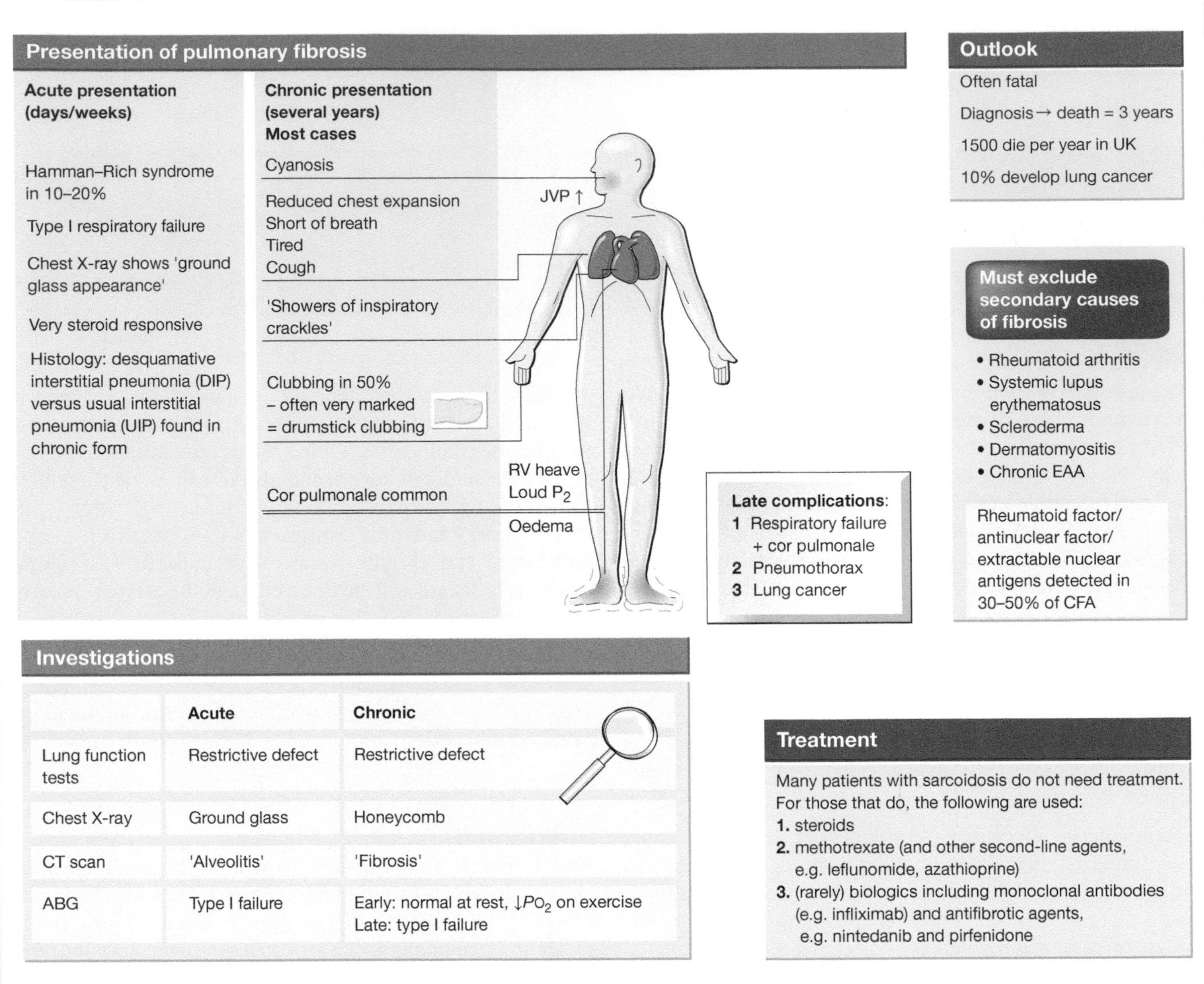

	Acute	Chronic
Lung function tests	Restrictive defect	Restrictive defect
Chest X-ray	Ground glass	Honeycomb
CT scan	'Alveolitis'	'Fibrosis'
ABG	Type I failure	Early: normal at rest, ↓$P\text{O}_2$ on exercise Late: type I failure

Definition

This is a condition involving inflammation and fibrosis of the distal airspaces, defined histologically. The combination of clinical features, restrictive pulmonary function and typical radiological changes suggests the diagnosis, often making a tissue diagnosis redundant.

Aetiology

Unknown, but an identical disease can be caused by several agents, including asbestos, hard metals, drugs and radiation. This suggests that an inhaled or environmental agent is responsible. A number of autoimmune diseases are also associated with pulmonary fibrosis. A few cases are familial, suggesting genetic influence. Some patients with sarcoidosis or hypersensitivity pneumonitis can develop pulmonary fibrosis.

Epidemiology

More frequent with increasing age. Prevalence is increasing and is currently 30/100 000. Idiopathic pulmonary fibrosis (IPF) is more common in males. The median survival from diagnosis is only three years despite intervention. In some individuals, lung function may remain stable for many months.

Medicine at a Glance, Fifth Edition. Edited by Patrick Davey and Alex Pitcher.

Companion website: www.wiley.com/go/medicine5e

Pathology

Histologically, alveolar walls become progressively thickened as a result of organizing inflammatory cell infiltrate with fibroblast proliferation. The main types recognized are as follows.

- **Usual interstitial pneumonia** (UIP) where inflammatory cells are present in the airspaces and fibrosis leads to the contraction of lung tissue and honeycombing.
- **Desquamative interstitial pneumonia** (DIP) in which the predominant infiltrate is the mononuclear cell and fibrosis is less prominent.
- **Non-specific interstitial pneumonia** (NSIP) where there are features that overlap between the above categories.

Lung volume is reduced, diffusion impaired and respiratory failure eventually develops. There is an increased risk of lung cancer (occurs in 10% of patients).

Clinical features

Gradual onset of breathlessness is typical. Cough is very common and is usually non-productive. In 5%, pulmonary fibrosis is an incidental finding and no symptoms are present. Examination reveals clubbing in 50% of those with advanced disease. Showers of fine, late, inspiratory crackles are present on auscultation. Respiratory distress, cyanosis and signs of cor pulmonale may develop. The Hamman–Rich syndrome is a predominantly inflammatory alveolitis of acute onset and more frequently shows a better response to treatment.

Investigations

- **Laboratory tests**: routine blood tests are normal. Blood gases may show hypoxaemia. Weakly positive titres of antinuclear antibodies and rheumatoid factor are present in a quarter. Positive extractable nuclear antigens may reveal a previously unsuspected autoimmune disease.
- **Pulmonary function tests** show reduction in all lung volumes with impaired gas transfer. Gas transfer, total lung capacity and alveolar volume are used as markers of disease progression. The change in forced vital capacity (FVC) in the six months following diagnosis is useful in predicting prognosis. A $<10\%$ change predicts more stable disease with a better prognosis and a $>10\%$ fall in FVC suggests deteriorating disease with a poor prognosis.
- **Chest X-ray** may show diffuse, predominantly basal and peripheral ground-glass change with loss of definition of the heart borders and hemidiaphragms. This may progress to reticulonodular changes and honeycombing.
- **High-resolution computed tomography** (HRCT) reveals subpleural reticulation (usual interstitial pneumonia) and ground-glass change (desquamative interstitial pneumonia), with progression to honeycombing and traction bronchiectasis (usual interstitial pneumonia).
- **Histological** examination may show typical cellular infiltrate or fibrosis. The changes are patchy and transbronchial biopsy may therefore be inadequate.

Frequently, the combination of clinical features and radiological changes is sufficient for the diagnosis to be made.

Management

There is no treatment that improves lung function in usual interstitial pneumonia. Antifibrotic treatment (pirfenidone or nintedinib) can slow the decline in FEV_1 in those with initial values between 50% and 80% of predicted. These drugs have also recently been approved for use in other forms of fibrosis with documented progression on lung function testing or CT.

For those with desquamative interstitial pneumonia, oral corticosteroids are used to treat the inflammatory component. High doses (40–60 mg prednisolone) are often used in patients with severe disease and an acute presentation. In less acutely unwell patients, a lower dose (2 mg prednisolone on alternate days) may be used to reduce treatment side-effects. Additional immunosuppressive drugs such as azathioprine or mycophenolate can be used to reduce the required steroid dose.

For advanced disease, supportive treatment is required. Long-term oxygen for the relief of breathlessness, diuretics for fluid retention in cor pulmonale and antibiotics for infection may all be useful. In young patients with advanced unresponsive disease, lung transplantation should be considered.

Prognosis

In the UK, 1500 people die annually from fibrosing alveolitis. The overall five-year survival rate is only 50%. Current treatment has not influenced this figure. UIP pulmonary fibrosis has a worse overall prognosis than DIP or NSIP. Patients with fibrosis associated with autoimmune disease, sarcoidosis or hypersensitivity pneumonitis also have a much better prognosis, with a life expectancy that can run into decades.

Pulmonary eosinophilia and vasculitis

Causes of pulmonary eosinophilia

Common	Rare	Löffler's syndrome
• Asthma • ABPA • Drugs • Parasites	• Eosinophilic granulomatosis with polyangiitis (Churg-Strauss syndrome) • Chronic eosinophilic pneumonia • Polyarteritis nodosa • Hodgkin's disease	= eosinophilia + transient chest X-ray infiltrate lasting 4–6 weeks Often related to • Drugs • Parasitic worms

Pulmonary eosinophilia

Disease	Features	Investigations	Treatment
Acute eosinophilic pneumonia	Fever, dry cough, dyspnoea, myalgia, chest pain Crackles or wheeze	Eosinophilia Segmental infiltrates; peripheral ground glass on CT Restrictive lung function	Prednisolone 30–40 mg/day Reduce rapidly following improvement
Chronic eosinophilic pneumonia	Cough, fever, dyspnoea, weight loss	Eosinophilia Bilateral peripheral infiltrates Restrictive lung function	Prednisolone 30–40 mg/day Reduce slowly over 6 months
Hypereosinophilic syndrome	Cough, malaise Cardiac failure (myocardial infiltration)	Eosinophilia $<20 \times 10^9$/L Chest X-ray; pulmonary infiltrates and effusions	Prednisolone 30–60 mg/day May require long-term treatment Anticoagulants
Eosinophilic granulomatosis with polyangiitis (Churg-Strauss syndrome)	Asthma, sinusitis, multisystem involvement	Eosinophilia, raised IgE ↑pANCA in 50% Pulmonary infiltrates Pleural effusion in up to 30% Vasculitis on biopsy	Prednisolone 40–60 mg/day reducing over a year Other immunosuppressives in severe disease

Immunologically mediated lung disease

Disease	Features	Investigations	Treatment
Goodpasture's syndrome	Pulmonary haemorrhage (breathless, haemoptysis) Renal failure	Anti-GBM antibody positive ↑ANCA (in some) Pulmonary infiltrates Renal failure – diagnostic renal biopsy	Plasma exchange Prednisolone Other immunosuppressives in severe disease Renal replacement if necessary
Granulomatosis with polyangiitis (formerly Wegener's granulomatosis)	Nose bleeds, sinusitis, cough, haemoptysis, dyspnoea, malaise, weight loss Multisystem involvement	Anaemia, leucocytosis, renal failure Active urine sediment Pulmonary nodules (may cavitate) ↑cANCA in almost all cases Biopsy shows necrotizing granulomatous vasculitis	Prednisolone 40–60 mg/day Cyclophosphamide Renal replacement if necessary

Pulmonary eosinophilia

This is a group of rare diseases, mainly of unknown aetiology, which cause chest X-ray (CXR) abnormalities associated with a raised eosinophil count in peripheral blood. Diseases included in this category include: (i) acute eosinophilic pneumonia; (ii) chronic eosinophilic pneumonia; (iii) hypereosinophilic syndrome; and (iv) eosinophilic granulomatosis with polyangiitis (Churg–Strauss syndrome).

Other diseases that cause pulmonary disease in association with eosinophilia are: (i) asthma; (ii) fungal diseases (including allergic bronchopulmonary aspergillosis [ABPA]); (iii) parasitic infection (e.g. of the filarial parasite *Wuchereria bancrofti*); (iv) drug reactions (see Chapter 119); (v) polyarteritis nodosa; and (vi) Hodgkin disease.

Epidemiology and prognosis

- **Acute and chronic eosinophilic pneumonia** are more common in women; peak incidence is 40–50 years. Fifty percent of patients have asthma. Eosinophilic pneumonia responds well to treatment and recurrence is uncommon. Chronic disease responds less well to treatment and recurrence may require long-term steroid treatment.

Medicine at a Glance, Fifth Edition. Edited by Patrick Davey and Alex Pitcher.

Companion website: www.wiley.com/go/medicine5e

- **Hypereosinophilic syndrome** is very rare, is usually of unknown cause (although it occurs more often in the tropics where it may relate to parasitic infection) and often responds poorly to treatment. Complicating cardiac failure can occur and carries a poor prognosis.
- **Eosinophilic granulomatosis with polyangiitis** (Churg–Strauss syndrome) is a rare form of pulmonary vasculitis (incidence about one per million) affecting small and medium-sized vessels. It occurs in patients with asthma. Antineutrophil cytoplasmic antibody (ANCA) is commonly positive. Untreated vasculitis has a poor prognosis (renal involvement). Vasculitis often responds well to treatment and relapse is unusual.

Vasculitis without eosinophilia

Several vasculitides affect the lung without provoking eosinophilia.

- **Rheumatoid arthritis**: pleural disease (thickening, effusion) is the most common manifestation. Localized nodules or more diffuse fibrosing alveolitis can occur. Extensive nodular fibrosis, called Caplan syndrome, occurs in those with pneumoconiosis (now rarely seen).
- **Systemic lupus erythematosus**: pleural inflammation ('pleurisy') is very common. Pulmonary fibrosis occurs but is rare.
- **Granulomatosis with polyangiitis.**

Granulomatosis with polyangiitis (GPA)

General features

- **Granulomatosis with polyangiitis** is a multisystem vasculitis (see Table 116.1), involving small and medium-sized vessels, associated with ANCA.
- Aetiology is unknown, but may involve an infectious agent.
- Prevalence is about one per 100 000. Men and women are equally affected (i.e. 600 in the UK).
- >90% of GPA patients first seek attention due to symptoms arising from the upper or lower respiratory tract.

Upper airways

- Nasal/sinus disease → congestion and nose bleed. Nasal septum perforation → saddle nose; occurs in up to 30%.
- Subglottic stenosis occurs in 20% → breathlessness (which may be severe), voice change and cough. The diagnosis of subglottic stenosis is suggested by flow–volume loops; this responds very poorly to systemic therapy but may respond to mechanical dilation and local injection of corticosteroids.

Table 116.1 Profile of organ involvement at presentation and during the course of the disease in granulomatosis with polyangiitis.

	Involvement at presentation (%)	Involvement during the disease course (%)
Upper airways	73	92
Lower airways	48	85
Kidneys	20	80
Joint	32	67
Eye	15	52
Skin	13	46
Nerve	1	20

Source: Langford 1999. Reproduced with permission of BMJ Publishing.

Lower airways

- Parenchymal disease: two-thirds of those with parenchymal involvement have symptoms, one-third only have asymptomatic CXR abnormalities.
- Variable changes: bilateral nodular infiltrates, cavitatary disease and pulmonary haemorrhage.
- 15% have inflammation/stenosis of endobronchial airways → cough, wheezing, breathlessness, haemoptysis or lung collapse.
- Major cause of morbidity, but rare cause of mortality.

Renal disease

Glomerulonephritis may rapidly progress to renal failure with no or few symptoms. Renal failure is common (affecting up to 40–50%), and end-stage renal failure requiring dialysis occurs in some 10%. It is detected by dipstick testing of urine (red cells, casts, ↑ creatinine). Common cause of death.

Other features

- Eye disease: many possible manifestations, including (epi)scleritis, conjunctivitis, anterior or posterior uveitis and optic neuritis. Some 8% of patients develop permanent visual loss.
- 15% have mononeuritis multiplex; 8% have central nervous system involvement.

Diagnosis

The diagnosis is made from a biopsy showing a necrotizing vasculitis, with granuloma formation in a clinically relevant setting. Antibodies against neutrophil cytoplasm are found, in two staining patterns.

- **Cytoplasmic ANCA** (cANCA): the antigen is proteinase-3 (PR3), a 2 kDa serine proteinase found in the azurophilic granules of neutrophils. cANCA is found in 70–90% of GPA. Though cANCA has high specificity and sensitivity for GPA, it should not be relied upon in isolation from the clinical situation and appropriate histology, as many patients with GPA do not have cANCA. In some patients, cANCA titre relates to disease activity, though in many it does not.
- **Perinuclear ANCA** (pANCA): the antigen is usually myeloperoxidase. Found in 5–10% of GPA but also many other conditions, so it has a low sensitivity and specificity for the diagnosis of GPA.

Treatment and prognosis

Untreated GPA has a very high mortality. Treatment with cyclophosphamide and prednisolone dramatically reduces morbidity and mortality: 75% achieve complete disease remission, and the two-year survival rate is 80%. The monoclonal antibody rituximab has been shown to be effective for both induction and maintenance treatment of ANCA-positive vasculitis. It has a lower frequency of side-effects and may therefore be preferable to cyclophosphamide.

Drug-related side-effects (sepsis from immunosuppression, late malignancy) are common. *Pneumocystis jirovecii (carinii)* pneumonia is so common as to justify septrin prophylaxis.

Other immunologically mediated disease of the lung

- **Goodpasture syndrome**: results from immune attack by an antibody against the lung and renal glomerular basement membrane (GBM). Pulmonary haemorrhage (causing anaemia, haemoptysis and respiratory failure) occurs usually some days to months before acute renal failure. Anti-GBM antibodies are found, and less frequently a positive ANCA. Treatment is with immunosuppression and plasma exchange.
- **Idiopathic pulmonary haemosiderosis**: a similar disease to Goodpasture's (though renal involvement is uncommon) occurring in young children (>7 years).

117 Fungi and the lung

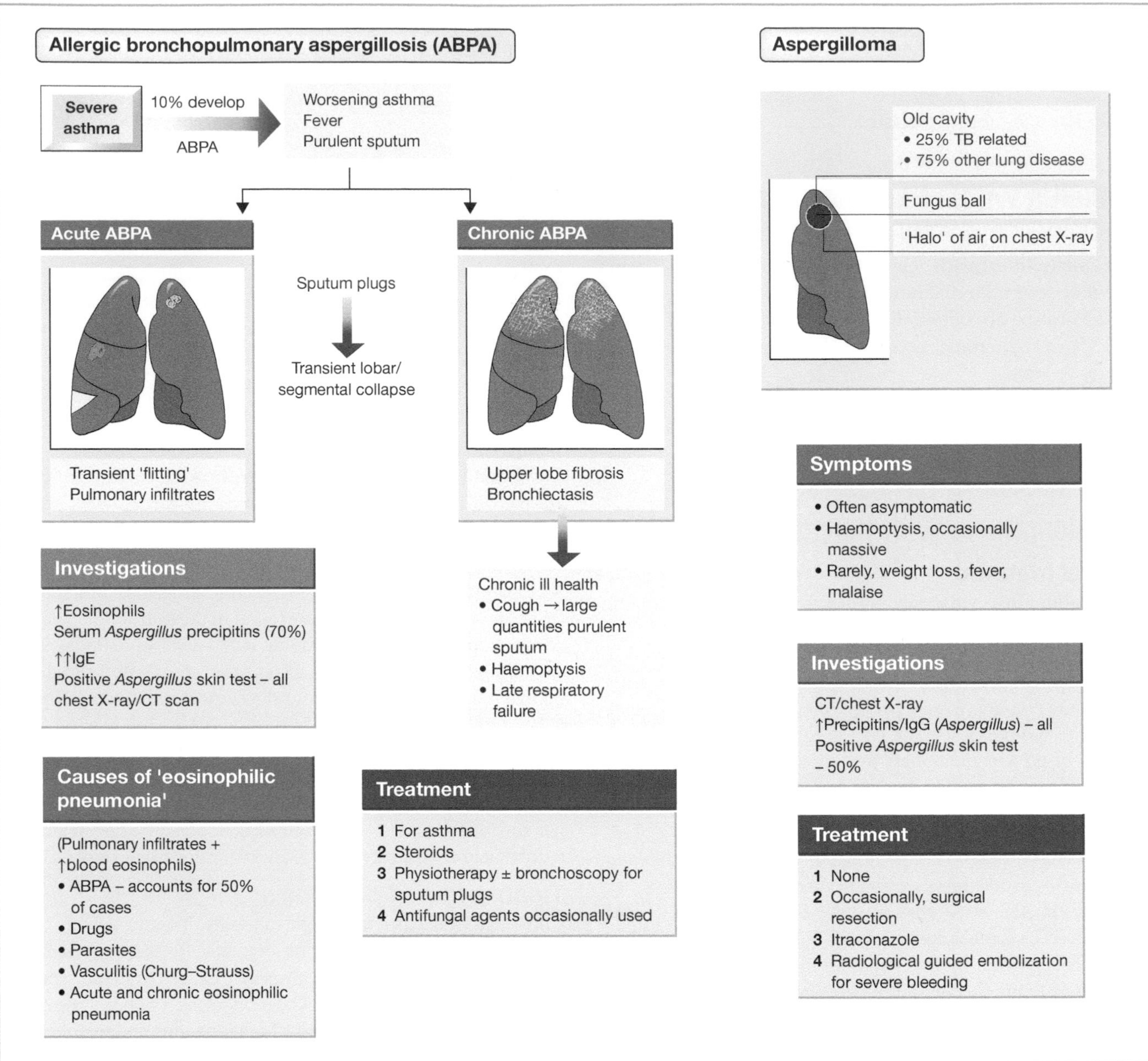

Allergic bronchopulmonary aspergillosis (ABPA)
Severe asthma
10% develop ABPA
Worsening asthma
Fever
Purulent sputum
Acute ABPA
Transient 'flitting'
Pulmonary infiltrates
Sputum plugs
Transient lobar/
segmental collapse
Chronic ABPA
Upper lobe fibrosis
Bronchiectasis
Chronic ill health
• Cough → large quantities purulent sputum
• Haemoptysis
• Late respiratory failure
Investigations
↑Eosinophils
Serum Aspergillus precipitins (70%)
↑↑IgE
Positive Aspergillus skin test – all
chest X-ray/CT scan
Causes of 'eosinophilic pneumonia'
(Pulmonary infiltrates + ↑blood eosinophils)
• ABPA – accounts for 50% of cases
• Drugs
• Parasites
• Vasculitis (Churg–Strauss)
• Acute and chronic eosinophilic pneumonia
Treatment
1 For asthma
2 Steroids
3 Physiotherapy ± bronchoscopy for sputum plugs
4 Antifungal agents occasionally used
Aspergilloma
Old cavity
• 25% TB related
• 75% other lung disease
Fungus ball
'Halo' of air on chest X-ray
Symptoms
• Often asymptomatic
• Haemoptysis, occasionally massive
• Rarely, weight loss, fever, malaise
Investigations
CT/chest X-ray
↑Precipitins/IgG (Aspergillus) – all
Positive Aspergillus skin test – 50%
Treatment
1 None
2 Occasionally, surgical resection
3 Itraconazole
4 Radiological guided embolization for severe bleeding

Common fungal lung infections

Fungal lung infection develops in the immunologically incompetent and in those with chronic lung disease. Infection is usually localized in the immune competent, but those with immune deficiencies develop invasive fungal pneumonia, which has a very high mortality, caused by *Pneumocystis* spp. (see Chapter 168), *Aspergillus* spp., *Candida* spp. and cryptococcosis (see Chapter 169).

Aspergillosis

Aspergillus fumigatus is the most important human pathogen, and disease occurs in immunosuppressed individuals and in those with underlying lung disease. There are three pathologies in lung disease: allergy, colonization and invasion (Table 117.1).

Asthma

Some patients with asthma are allergic to *Aspergillus* spp. Asthma attacks occur when fungal spores are inhaled. They have positive

Medicine at a Glance, Fifth Edition. Edited by Patrick Davey and Alex Pitcher.

Companion website: www.wiley.com/go/medicine5e

Table 117.1 Pathologies of aspergillus lung disease.

Allergic	Asthma
	Allergic bronchopulmonary aspergillosis (ABPA)
	Allergic *Aspergillus* sinusitis
	Allergic alveolitis
	(Bronchocentric granulomatosis)
Colonizing	Aspergilloma
Invasive	Invasive *Aspergillus* pneumonia

skin tests, but such positive reactions are not associated with worse disease, unless allergic bronchopulmonary aspergillosis (ABPA) is also present.

Allergic bronchopulmonary aspergillosis

Epidemiology, aetiology and pathophysiology

This uncommon complication of asthma is found in 10% of difficult asthma cases and underlies some 50% of UK pulmonary eosinophilia. Inhalation of *Aspergillus* spores leads to an IgG- and IgE-mediated hypersensitivity immune reaction, which in turn leads to dense eosinophilic infiltration of lung tissue, mucus plugging and distal collapse. A chronic inflammatory response in the airway wall causes tissue destruction and bronchiectasis. It is not clear why only some patients with asthma develop ABPA, but a genetic predisposition has been suggested.

Clinical features

ABPA patients are usually people with known asthma. Symptoms are of deteriorating asthma with purulent sputum, fever and breathlessness. Transient infiltrates on the chest X-ray (CXR) occur. In chronic bronchiectatic disease, copious purulent sputum production and haemoptysis are present.

Investigations

ABPA should be considered in people with asthma who have an abnormal CXR and high blood eosinophil count.

- **Skin tests**: a positive skin test to *Aspergillus* spp. (or raised serum-specific IgE) is required for diagnosis.
- **Blood tests**: the eosinophil count is raised, particularly in acute episodes. Total serum IgE is markedly elevated. Precipitating antibodies (IgG) are present in 70%.
- **Sputum examination**: fungal hyphae may be present in the sputum.
- **Chest X-ray**: transient ('flitting') perihilar infiltrates are present during acute attacks. Lobar or segmental collapse may occur as a result of bronchial occlusion. In chronic disease, upper lobe contraction, fibrosis and bronchiectasis may occur.

Management and prognosis

Oral corticosteroids (prednisolone) are the mainstay of treatment. They improve asthma control and reduce the growth of *Aspergillus* spp. Inhaled steroids do not affect *Aspergillus* spp. but are used, along with bronchodilators, as part of the overall treatment of asthma. Physiotherapy and sometimes bronchoscopy are necessary for removal of mucus plugs. The antifungal agent itraconazole may reduce the dose of steroids required. ABPA usually progresses to bronchiectasis.

Aspergillus sinusitis

Sinusitis unresponsive to medical treatment in patients with nasal polyps has been found occasionally to be caused by *Aspergillus* spp., and may co-exist with ABPA. The histology and immunology are identical to ABPA.

Allergic alveolitis caused by *Aspergillus* spp.

This rare disease found in malt workers is caused by *A. clavatus* from mouldy barley. The pathology, clinical features and management are as for extrinsic allergic alveolitis of any cause (see Chapter 114).

Aspergilloma

A mycetoma or fungus ball is a collection of fungus.

Aetiology and pathogenesis

The causative organism is *A. fumigatus* in the UK and *A. niger* in the USA. Spores seed a pre-existing lung cavity, often (25%) as a result of previous tuberculosis (TB), and thus in the apex of the lung. Twenty percent of cases are multiple. Spores germinate and a ball of fungus grows to fill the cavity. An immunological reaction to this process occurs. Precipitating antibodies (IgG) are universally present and a positive skin test to *Aspergillus* spp. is found in 50%.

Clinical features

Often asymptomatic and found incidentally on a CXR. The most common symptom is haemoptysis, occurring in 75%, occasionally massive, requiring embolization or surgery. Rarely, systemic features of weight loss, fever and malaise occur. Symptoms of the underlying lung disease are often present.

Investigations

The combination of radiological features (a dense opacity with surrounding halo or crescent) and the presence of precipitating antibodies suggests the diagnosis. In patients with severe underlying lung disease, a computed tomography (CT) scan will define the mycetoma more clearly.

Management and prognosis

Antifungal therapy is often ineffective. Corticosteroids have been used for systemic symptoms but increase the risk of invasion (see Chapter 169). In fit patients with systemic symptoms or significant haemoptysis, surgical resection of the mycetoma or a whole lobe is used. Ten percent cause no problems and resolve. Death occasionally occurs as a result of massive haemoptysis. Invasive disease worsens outcome.

Aspergillus pneumonia

See Chapter 169.

Other fungal lung infections

Histoplasmosis

Histoplasma capsulatum is found worldwide and particularly in the USA, in soil contaminated by bird and bat droppings. Histoplasmosis is not found in the UK. Infection usually causes no symptoms but may lead to a febrile illness with cough, chest pain and dyspnoea, followed by resolution. Ten percent of cases become chronic. In the acute illness, there are bilateral CXR infiltrates with enlarged mediastinal lymph nodes. Calcification of multiple pulmonary nodules can occur, sometimes with cavitation. Diagnosis is made by culture of blood or biopsy specimens or by serological tests, which usually become positive within three weeks of acute infection. Treatment is with amphotericin in severe disease. Itraconazole has been used for chronic disease.

Candida spp.

See Chapter 169.

Cryptococcosis

See Chapter 169.

118 Industrial lung disease

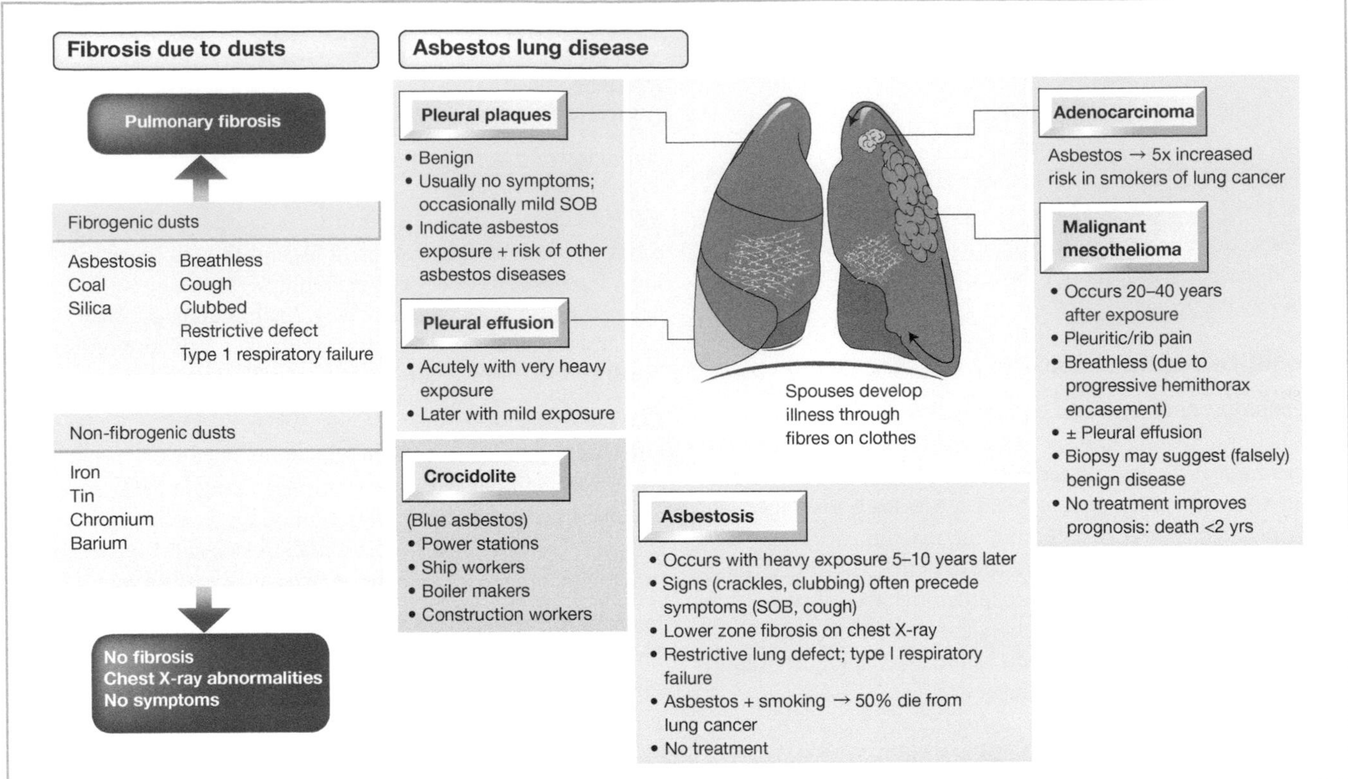

Inhalation of dusts may lead to pulmonary fibrosis or asthma (see Chapter 109).

Dust inhalation diseases

- **Fibrogenic dusts** (asbestos, coal, silica) can impair pulmonary function.
- **Non-fibrogenic dusts** (iron, tin, chromium, barium) lead to a nodular appearance on a chest X-ray (CXR) but do not impair lung function.
- **Organic dusts** can cause extrinsic allergic alveolitis (see Chapter 114).

Asbestosis

Asbestosis is lung fibrosis resulting from asbestos exposure.

Epidemiology

Asbestos-related diseases are industrial diseases (men > women), found in those exposed to blue asbestos (crocidolite). The greater the asbestos exposure, the higher the asbestosis and mesothelioma rates. Symptoms occur decades after exposure. Rates for asbestos-related diseases will increase for some years because effective legal regulation occurred relatively recently and there is often a long delay between exposure and development of disease.

Pathology

Asbestos fibres are small and penetrate distally into the lung. Fibres are engulfed by macrophages that release cytokines, so producing an inflammatory reaction, which leads to progressive fibrosis, mainly in the lower lobes. Pleural plaques are also usually present. Cigarette smoke acts synergistically with asbestos to increase pulmonary fibrosis and lung cancer rates.

Clinical features

Occupational exposure is usually present. Typical symptoms are:

- progressive breathlessness.
- cough.

Clinical signs are of bibasal end-inspiratory crackles, and finger clubbing in 50%. Haemoptysis suggests the development of lung cancer.

Investigations

- **Chest X-ray** reveals symmetrical basal parenchymal changes, and 75% have pleural plaques.
- **High-resolution computed tomography** (HRCT) may be abnormal when the CXR is normal and reveals subpleural changes progressing to honeycombing. Beneath areas of pleural fibrosis, nodular areas of collapse may develop (rounded atelectasis,

Medicine at a Glance, Fifth Edition. Edited by Patrick Davey and Alex Pitcher.

Companion website: www.wiley.com/go/medicine5e

Blesovsky syndrome) which on CXR appear as a mass. HRCT distinguishes these appearances from those of carcinoma.

- **Pulmonary function tests** reveal a restrictive defect with reduced lung volumes and gas transfer. Blood gases show respiratory failure in end-stage disease.

Management

- **Prevention**: risk of progression increases with cumulative dose. Prevention by reduction of exposure has reduced the incidence and severity of disease.
- **Treatment** is ineffective.
- **Prognosis**: 20% of patients with asbestosis die from the disease and 50% from an associated malignancy (lung cancer or mesothelioma).
- **Medicolegal advice**: all patients with asbestosis (and any asbestos injury caused as a result of employment) should be advised to take legal advice on whether they should make a claim for damages against the employer responsible for the asbestos exposure.

Other asbestos-related diseases: mesothelioma

This is a malignant growth arising in the pleura or occasionally in the peritoneum or pericardium; more common in males. Incidence is likely to have peaked (predicted peak 2010–2020). Develops 20–40 years after exposure as a local mass often associated with pleural effusion (>80%), which progressively encases the lung and hemithorax. Histological distinction from benign pleural disease can be difficult even with large biopsies and special staining techniques.

Clinical features

Breathlessness caused by pleural effusion is usual at presentation. Local tumour effects include severe pain due to chest wall invasion, and worsening breathlessness as a result of encasement of the lung.

Investigations

- **Chest X-ray** may reveal pleural nodularity or effusion, and pleural plaques.
- **CT** appearances suggestive of malignancy include pleural nodularity, thickening >1 cm and extension of pleural thickening over the mediastinal pleural surfaces.
- **Pleural aspiration** shows blood-stained fluid (30%). Cytology is often negative. Closed pleural biopsy is positive in 50%. Thoracoscopic biopsy is positive in 90%.

Management

For patients who are fit for chemotherapy, the most commonly used drug combination is pemetrexed and cisplatin. Surgery has been used in early disease and is mainly aimed at disease control rather than cure. Surgery can be combined with chemo-radiotherapy. Treatment is often symptomatic: pleural aspiration for effusion causing breathlessness, often combined with pleurodesis (see Chapter 21). Alternatively, indwelling pleural catheters allowing regular drainage at home can provide symptom relief. Tumour invasion at drainage sites is common and is prevented by local radiotherapy.

Prognosis

Relentless progression occurs with increasing symptoms. Median survival is 12–18 months. Prognosis is better for epithelioid than sarcomatous mesothelioma.

Pleural plaques, pleural thickening and pleural effusion

- **Pleural plaques** are an incidental finding on CXR, implying asbestos exposure and therefore increased risk of other asbestos-related diseases. In themselves, they are a benign problem and of no clinical consequence. They occur in 50% of asbestos-exposed people. Compensation is no longer available for pleural plaques.
- **Diffuse pleural thickening** occurs in 5% of asbestos workers exposed to high doses, and may cause symptoms as a result of restriction of chest wall movement. Lung function tests reveal reduced lung volumes. Such high-level exposure increases the risk of other asbestos-related diseases.
- **Pleural effusion** occurs either at the time of high-level exposure or early after exposure. A blood-stained exudative effusion is typical. Resolution is normal but some patients are left with pleural thickening.

Coal worker's pneumoconiosis

Definition, epidemiology and aetiopathogenesis

This is now a rare lung disease, presenting in elderly men, and caused by inhalation of coal dust. Inhalation of small particles (0.5–7 μm) that are toxic to macrophages initiates the process. Total dose of exposure correlates with disease severity. There are three forms.

- **Simple coal worker's pneumoconiosis** (CWP): inhaled dust is enveloped by inflammatory cells, resulting in small nodules. Simple CWP produces no symptoms.
- **Complicated CWP**: aggregates of small nodules lead to larger nodules >1 cm in diameter. Surrounding emphysema develops. Cavitation of nodules may occur (termed 'progressive massive fibrosis'). Complicated CWP causes progressive breathlessness; cough with black sputum (melanoptysis) may occur, as may cor pulmonale.
- **Caplan syndrome**: large nodules may develop in coal workers with positive rheumatoid factor.

Management

- **Diagnosis** is by CXR (small or large nodules) and pulmonary function tests in complicated CWP (reduced lung volumes with airflow obstruction).
- There is no specific **treatment**. Avoidance of exposure has reduced the incidence. Disability from CWP is compensatable.
- **Prognosis**: as a result of control of dust levels, severe disease is rare. Respiratory failure develops in patients with progressive massive fibrosis.

Silicosis

This is a rare, restrictive, fibrotic lung disease caused by inhalation of silicon dioxide (quartz) particles (mining, sand blasting, pneumatic drilling). Inflammation and damage to local and hilar lymph node structures occur. There are two forms.

- **Acute silicosis** results from high-level exposure and causes rapidly progressive breathlessness, with death within months.
- **Lower level exposure** causes more slowly progressive symptoms and **predisposes to tuberculosis** (TB).

Chest X-ray shows small (1–3 mm) nodules mainly in the upper zones and larger nodules later in the disease. 'Eggshell' calcification of the hilar lymph nodes is pathognomonic.

Management involves reducing dust levels, the use of respiratory protection and regular screening for TB. With avoidance of exposure, prognosis is usually good. Progressive disease or acute silicosis results in death from respiratory failure.

119 Lung disease caused by drugs

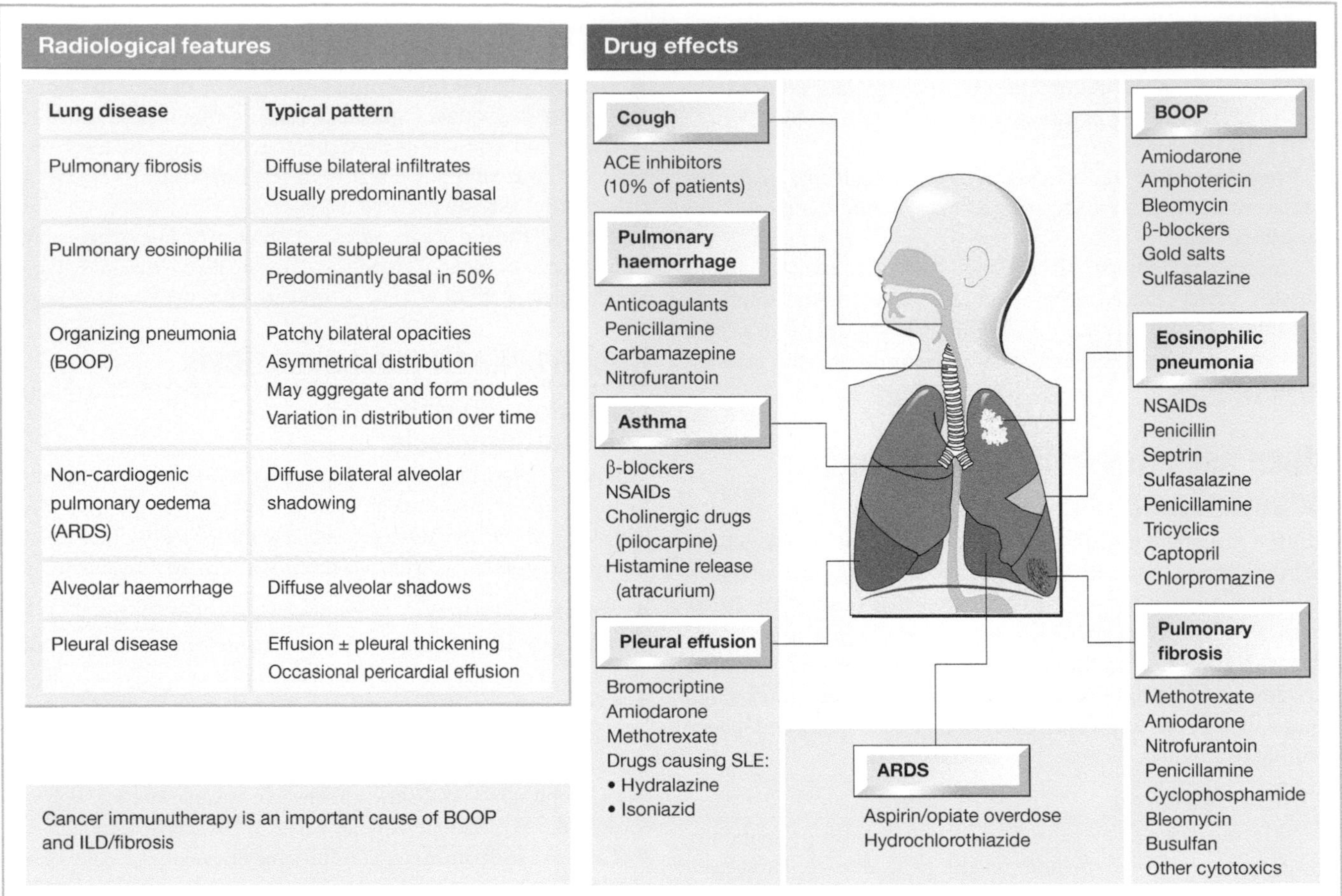

Lung disease	Typical pattern
Pulmonary fibrosis	Diffuse bilateral infiltrates Usually predominantly basal
Pulmonary eosinophilia	Bilateral subpleural opacities Predominantly basal in 50%
Organizing pneumonia (BOOP)	Patchy bilateral opacities Asymmetrical distribution May aggregate and form nodules Variation in distribution over time
Non-cardiogenic pulmonary oedema (ARDS)	Diffuse bilateral alveolar shadowing
Alveolar haemorrhage	Diffuse alveolar shadows
Pleural disease	Effusion ± pleural thickening Occasional pericardial effusion

The effects of drugs on the lung are extremely variable. The figure shows common drug effects on the lung and their major causes. It is by no means exhaustive: virtually any lung disease may be drug-related and thus the differential diagnosis should always include drugs as the cause.

Clinical features

These depend on the nature of the resulting lung disease. Some symptoms relate to a predictable pharmacological effect (e.g. asthma exacerbated by β-blockers). Others may be dose-related (e.g. amiodarone) or idiosyncratic. For patients on drugs commonly associated with pulmonary side-effects (amiodarone, cytotoxic chemotherapeutic agents), baseline pulmonary function tests are helpful to determine whether new symptoms relate to new lung abnormalities.

Radiological features

See figure.

Investigations

These are driven by the nature of the respiratory symptoms. A detailed drug history, including current and previous treatment, should always be sought in any patient with respiratory symptoms. In patients with suspected pulmonary drug toxicity, diagnosis should be based on the following aspects.

- The likelihood of a drug reaction to the drug(s) being taken and exclusion of alternative pathology; this may involve bronchial lavage or biopsy techniques to look for infection or confirm lung pathology.
- Consideration of which drug is responsible. If a drug reaction is confirmed, this will usually result in withdrawal of the agent concerned. Often, no specific treatment is necessary. The consequences of stopping treatment need to be weighed against the likely adverse effects of continuation. Alternative treatment may need to be given to replace the effects of the drug being withdrawn.
- **Reporting to the Medicines & Healthcare products Regulatory Agency (MHRA)**: all patients with drug-induced lung disease should be reported to the committee using the yellow card reporting system (https://yellowcard.mhra.gov.uk).

Medicine at a Glance, Fifth Edition. Edited by Patrick Davey and Alex Pitcher.

Companion website: www.wiley.com/go/medicine5e

120 BOOP and ARDS

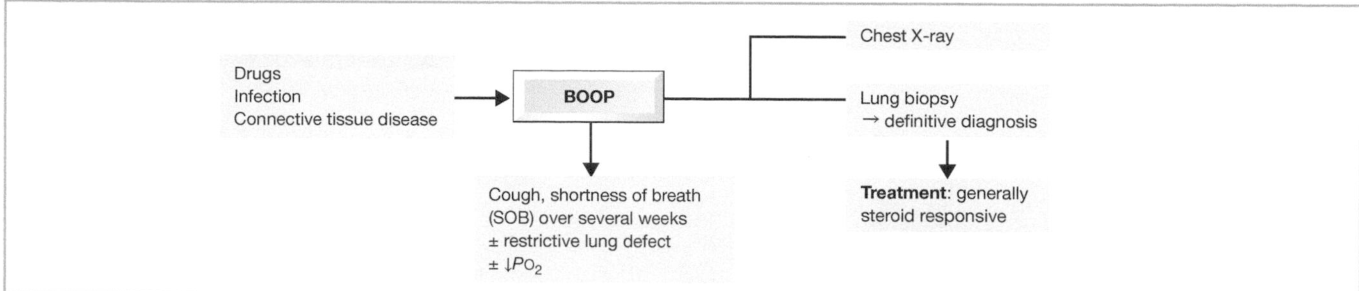

Bronchiolitis obliterans organizing pneumonia

Epidemiology

This rare disease, also known as cryptogenic organizing pneumonia, is of unknown aetiology but may present after infection or drug treatment, or as part of a connective tissue disease. Preponderance in the spring suggests an inhaled agent in some instances. There is no sex difference and no obvious geographical variation; the incidence is 6–7 per 100 000.

Pathophysiology

This is a histological diagnosis. Bronchiolitis obliterans organizing pneumonia (BOOP) is a specific way in which the lung may respond to an inflammatory stimulus. The histology reveals the changes of a pneumonitis with organization of inflammatory cells into granulation tissue. The disease originates in the alveoli with a variable amount of extension into the airways.

Clinical features

BOOP presents with systemic upset, usually over a period of a few weeks. Cough and breathlessness are present in the majority. Fever and weight loss are common. Crackles are often present.

Investigations

Chest X-ray (CXR) and computed tomography (CT) scanning show infiltrates which are often multifocal. The erythrocyte sedimentation rate is almost invariably raised and the eosinophil count is normal. Pulmonary function tests may be normal or show a restrictive defect with impaired gas transfer. In severe disease, blood gases may reveal hypoxaemia. Transbronchial biopsy may help establish the diagnosis but samples are often inadequate. Open lung biopsy is diagnostic.

Management

If a causative drug can be identified, this should be discontinued. Oral corticosteroids (prednisolone 30–40 mg daily) will achieve a rapid improvement in symptoms over days in most patients. Radiological changes can take months to resolve and the steroid course should be reduced over an extended period (several months), as relapse is common (up to a third of cases). Relapse is likely to respond well to further steroid courses.

Acute respiratory distress syndrome

Acute respiratory distress syndrome (ARDS) is a relatively common complication of conditions that activate inflammatory mediators (Table 120.1), resulting in diffuse lung injury, damaged pulmonary vasculature and non-cardiogenic pulmonary oedema. After several days, the inflamed lungs may fibrose, which can interfere with long-term lung function. Key points are as follows.

Table 120.1 Causes of ARDS.

- Sepsis, especially if shock present
- Pneumonia, including influenza
- Chemical lung injury, e.g. toxic gas inhalation, gastric aspiration
- Hypotension, especially if prolonged, or with trauma
- Blood transfusion, especially if massive
- Pancreatitis
- Systemic inflammatory response syndrome (SIRS)
- Disseminated intravascular coagulation
- Obstetric causes; amniotic fluid embolism, pre-eclampsia
- Adverse drug reaction (both prescribed and 'street' drugs, e.g. heroin)
- High-altitude-related lung injury

- ARDS usually occurs in patients already 'sick' for other reasons. Often multiple pathologies underlie ARDS, e.g. sepsis with hypotension.
- Impaired gas exchange occurs, causing breathlessness and central cyanosis. The first indication of ARDS is usually unexplained breathlessness in an already sick patient. Signs include tachycardia, cyanosis (often with confusion and/or agitation) and inspiratory crackles throughout the lung fields.
- CXR may initially be fairly unremarkable, but later shows diffuse 'patchy' infiltrates, which can progress to a 'white-out'. The differential diagnosis includes pneumonia, heart failure and interstitial lung diseases. CT scanning may help differentiate these if doubt exists.
- Intravascular capillary obstruction occurs, causing pulmonary hypertension.
- Treatment involves removing the cause (e.g. sepsis), supporting gas exchange (ventilation, which may be difficult, as the lungs are 'stiff') and other failing organs, and minimizing pulmonary oedema (keeping the patient 'dry' without provoking renal failure).
- Mortality is high at around 30–60%.

Medicine at a Glance, Fifth Edition. Edited by Patrick Davey and Alex Pitcher.

Companion website: www.wiley.com/go/medicine5e

Primary tumours of the lung

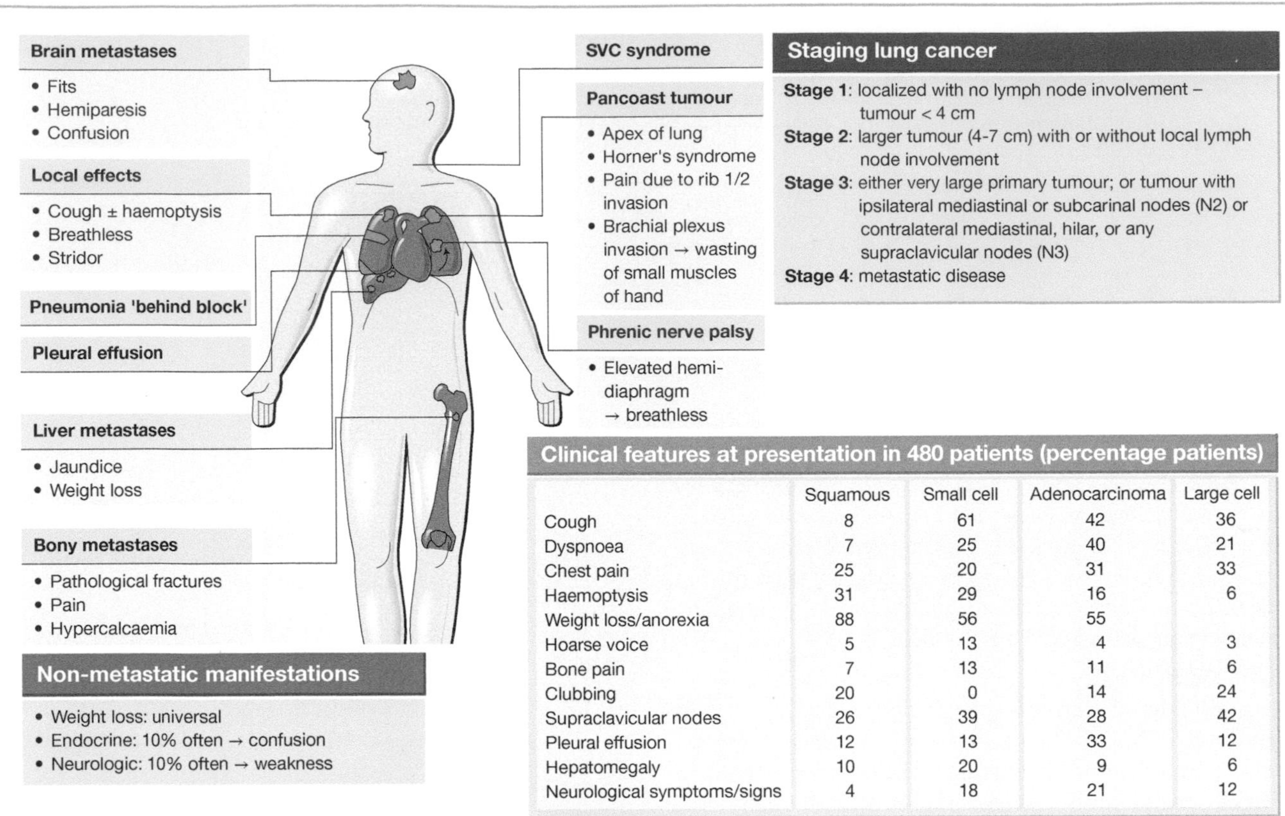

Staging lung cancer

Stage 1: localized with no lymph node involvement – tumour < 4 cm

Stage 2: larger tumour (4-7 cm) with or without local lymph node involvement

Stage 3: either very large primary tumour; or tumour with ipsilateral mediastinal or subcarinal nodes (N2) or contralateral mediastinal, hilar, or any supraclavicular nodes (N3)

Stage 4: metastatic disease

Clinical features at presentation in 480 patients (percentage patients)

	Squamous	Small cell	Adenocarcinoma	Large cell
Cough	8	61	42	36
Dyspnoea	7	25	40	21
Chest pain	25	20	31	33
Haemoptysis	31	29	16	6
Weight loss/anorexia	88	56	55	
Hoarse voice	5	13	4	3
Bone pain	7	13	11	6
Clubbing	20	0	14	24
Supraclavicular nodes	26	39	28	42
Pleural effusion	12	13	33	12
Hepatomegaly	10	20	9	6
Neurological symptoms/signs	4	18	21	12

Non-metastatic manifestations

- Weight loss: universal
- Endocrine: 10% often → confusion
- Neurologic: 10% often → weakness

Cellular types of lung cancer

Cell type	% cases	Features
Adenocarcinoma	45	More often found in the periphery of lung Commonest type seen in non-smokers Can be fast or slow growing Metastases often established early Adenocarcinoma in situ (AIS) arises in distal bronchioles and alveoli Associated with variants in cancer-related genes such as EGFR, ALK, ROS1 for which there are now biological therapies available Associated with mutations of the KRAS proto-oncogene
Squamous	30	Large airways Often fast growing Almost always occurs in current or former heavy smokers Associated with high tumour mutational burden Cavitation occurs Associated with high expression of PD-L1
Small cell	15	Usually centrally located at lung hilum or mediastinum Very fast growing if untreated Metastasizes very early Associated with paraneoplastic syndromes Usually treated with systemic therapy rather than surgery
Large cell	10	Usually highly anaplastic and aggressive Almost always in heavy smokers Poor prognosis

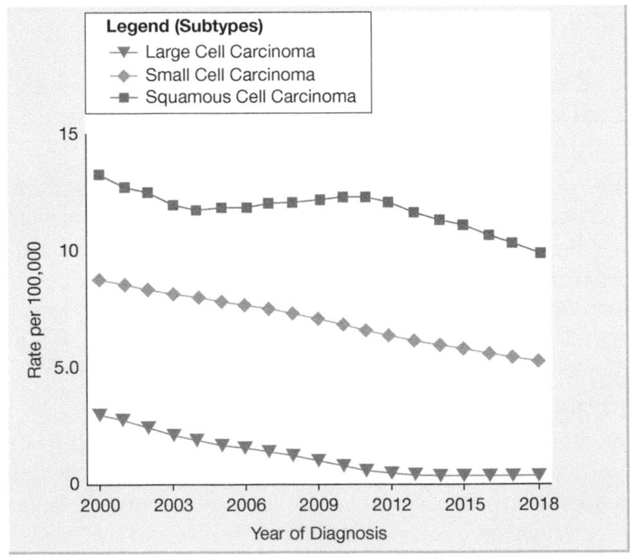

Medicine at a Glance, Fifth Edition. Edited by Patrick Davey and Alex Pitcher.

Companion website: www.wiley.com/go/medicine5e

Epidemiology

Nearly all primary lung tumours are malignant. Lung cancer is the most common malignancy in the western world, with 48 000 cases/year in the UK. Fifty-two percent of cases occur in men and most are the result of cigarette smoking. Women now smoke more and accordingly their lung cancer rates are rising. Rates are falling slowly in men.

Aetiology

- **Tobacco** causes 85% of lung cancers. Cancer is rare in never-smokers but when they do develop lung cancer, it is almost always adenocarcinoma. The more cigarettes smoked, the higher the cancer rates. Low-tar cigarettes are the most common type currently smoked but offer little protection from lung cancer risk. Smoking marijuana with tobacco entails a substantial risk of lung cancer. After smoking cessation, lung cancer risk falls back to that of never-smokers over the next 40 years.
- **Other risk factors**: passive smoking, exposure to asbestos either occupationally or in domestic settings, silica and nickel, and pulmonary fibrosis. Genetic factors play a part.

Clinical features

New or persistent respiratory symptoms in a current or ex-smoker should always raise the suspicion of lung cancer. Symptoms may be absent or non-specific (40%, lack of energy, anorexia, weight loss), as a result of the primary cancer or caused by local spread, distant metastases or non-metastatic manifestations.

- **Effects of the primary cancer**: cough (≥50%); breathlessness resulting from bronchial obstruction, lobar collapse or pleural effusion; haemoptysis (≥35%). Fixed wheeze or stridor suggests large airway narrowing.
- **Effects of local spread**: local pain from chest wall involvement. Apical (Pancoast) tumours may invade the brachial plexus (pain radiating down the arm) and cause Horner syndrome (see Chapter 60). Mediastinal invasion causes recurrent laryngeal nerve palsy (hoarseness), superior vena cava (SVC) obstruction (plethora, facial swelling), phrenic nerve palsy (breathlessness) and oesophageal compression (dysphagia).
- **Effects of distant metastases**: metastases occur in the bone (pain or hypercalcaemia), liver (asymptomatic, capsular pain) or brain (headache, confusion, seizures).
- **Non-metastatic manifestations**: endocrine – syndrome of inappropriate release of antidiuretic hormone (SIADH) (hyponatraemia especially with small cell lung cancer; see Chapter 142) or hypercalcaemia (parathyroid hormone-related peptide in 6% of squamous carcinoma). There is ectopic adrenocorticotrophic hormone (ACTH) secretion in 30% of small cell tumours, although Cushing syndrome rarely has time to develop; gynaecomastia occurs in ≤1% of squamous carcinoma.
- **Neurological symptoms**: usually relate to metastases; non-metastatic manifestations include the Lambert–Eaton myasthenic syndrome with small cell lung cancer (SCLC) (see Chapter 197). Cerebellar degeneration, peripheral neuropathy, encephalopathy, and mixed and sensory neuropathies all occur relatively infrequently.
- **Finger clubbing**: mainly in squamous carcinoma. Advanced clubbing is associated with hypertrophic pulmonary osteoarthropathy, which presents with pain and swelling in the long bones.
- **Other symptoms**: dermatomyositis and the nephrotic syndrome rarely occur.

Investigations

These should confirm the diagnosis and cell type, and stage the disease to determine treatment.

- **Chest X-ray**: usually abnormal by the time symptoms develop.
- **Paraneoplastic syndromes**: diagnosed from the full blood count, urea and electrolytes, and calcium. Additional investigations (such as auto antibodies) might be required.
- **Lung function tests**: low FEV_1 (forced expiratory volume in one second) or gas transfer preclude surgery, radical radiotherapy and percutaneous biopsy.
- **Bronchoscopy, endobronchial ultrasound biopsy (EBUS), percutaneous biopsy**: bronchoscopy produces diagnostic histology in 70% of central lung cancers. Endobronchial ultrasound biopsy (EBUS) is now the investigation of choice in many patients as it yields cells for diagnosis and provides mediastinal staging information. For peripheral tumours, a computed tomography (CT)/ultrasound-guided percutaneous approach is used. If the radiological features are highly suggestive of early-stage carcinoma, excision biopsy is preferable. If lymph node or liver metastases are present, biopsy of these is preferable.
- **Sputum cytology**: only used when invasive procedures are inappropriate (poor pulmonary function, co-morbid factors) and is now rarely performed.

Staging investigations

For **non-SCLC**.

- **Thoracic and abdominal CT**: to include the common sites for metastases – liver and adrenal glands (4%). Small mediastinal nodes <1 cm are not malignant in 25% and, unless 'on-table' mediastinoscopic staging is positive, should not preclude surgery.
- **Isotope bone scanning** for bony metastases (bone pain or hypercalcaemia), although PET scanning (see below) provides information on bone metastases.
- **Brain CT or MRI**: to exclude metatsases.
- **Positron emission tomography (PET) scanning**: can reveal nodal or distant metastases not revealed by other staging methods. Should be used to confirm localized disease in all patients prior to radical treatment (surgery or radical chemo-radiotherapy). Will not reveal brain metastases.

Staging investigations for **SCLC** are broadly similar though PET scanning is not required if CT reveals extensive metastatic disease.

Management

- **Surgery** offers the best chance of cure, but <30% are operable and around 50–60% of these are alive at five years. Surgery usually consists of lobectomy or wedge resection. Pneumonectomy is rarely performed because of poor survival data. Recent surgical advances include the routine use of thoracoscopic and robotic 'keyhole' operations. Perioperative mortality rate is less than 3% for lobectomy and over 6% for pneumonectomy.

- **Radical radiotherapy** is used for inoperable non-SCLC. Radical treatment is suitable for anatomically localized disease, and cures some patients.
- **Palliative radiotherapy** for haemoptysis, cough, breathlessness or local pain. Brain metastases are treated with metastasectomy or stereotactic or wide field radiotherapy. Stereotactic radiotherapy is under investigation for the treatment of oligometastatic disease (i.e. metastases in a limited number of sites)
- **Chemotherapy** is used for SCLC, because surgery is rarely appropriate with this histology. Response occurs in 60–85%; survival gain is approximately 4–6 months. In early-stage SCLC, radiotherapy with chemotherapy reduces local recurrence rates from 75% to 30% and achieves long-term cure in around 15% of patients. Chemotherapy often with immunotherapy (see below) is recommended in non-SCLC for fit patients with metastatic or locally advanced disease. Chemotherapy can be used preoperatively to downstage tumours and improve postoperative survival.
- **Immunotherapy** is now a standard treatment for advanced non-SCLC and SCLC. The most common agents target the immune checkpoint proteins PD-1 and PD-L1. Treatment is given in combination with chemotherapy or as a single agent. Antiangiogenesis antibodies are also used.
- **Biological or targeted therapies** are widely used in non-SCLC for patients with tumours exhibiting single gene variants including EGFR, ALK, ROS1, KRAS, BRAF and MET. Most are available as tablets or capsules and treatment continues until tumour progression.
- **Endobronchial treatments** such as cryotherapy, laser treatment, radiofrequency ablation (RFA) and bronchial or vascular stents can provide relief of symptoms in patients with significant symptomatic disease.
- **Palliative care**: opiates are helpful for pain and dyspnoea. Steroids help non-specific symptoms and improve appetite. Support from carers, family and palliative care specialists is extremely important.

Prognosis

Overall five-year survival for patients with early-stage lung cancer (stage 1) is around 50–60%. For loco-regional stage (stage 2 and some stage 3), survival is 15–30% and for advanced lung cancer (most stages 3 and 4), survival is around 5–7%. Median survival in small cell disease without treatment is 2–4 months and, with extensive disease at presentation, survival is 4–6 weeks without treatment. With treatment, 25% of patients with limited disease at presentation survive two years. In extensive disease, two-year survival falls to less than 5%.

122 Gastrointestinal infections

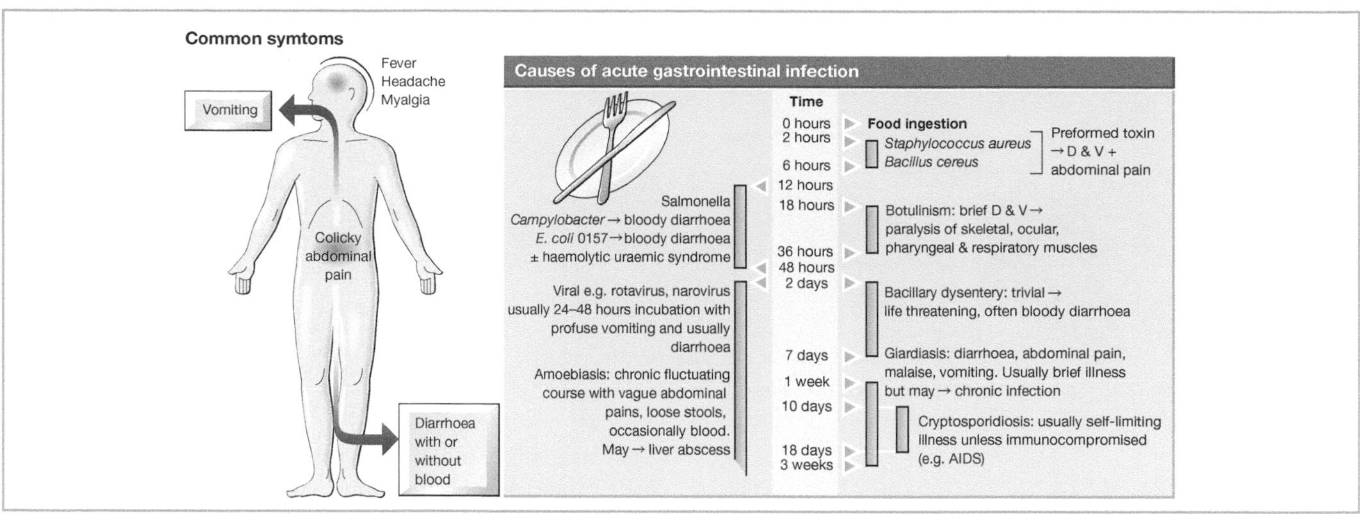

Acute gastroenteritis

Acute and short-lived diarrhoea (with vomiting [D&V] or without) is now a very common complaint. In many cases, the management is empirical and based on history rather than positive cultures. Important causes include the following.

- **Common**: culture negative (viral), *Campylobacter* spp., *Salmonella* spp., cholera (developing countries).
- **Uncommon**: *Shigella* spp.
- **Rare** but important: *Escherichia coli* O157, *Staphylococcus aureus*, *Vibrio parahaemolyticus*, *Clostridium botulinum*.

'Food poisoning' refers to bacterial or viral infection derived from diet and is typically used to denote self-limiting bacterial illnesses.

Clinical features

Symptoms are usually of sudden onset: diarrhoea with or without vomiting, abdominal pain and fever, headache or myalgia. There may be a history of travel or suspect food, and other individuals may also be affected.

Investigations

Most cases settle spontaneously and do not require investigation. In patients sufficiently ill to warrant admission to hospital, investigations should be considered, including stool and blood cultures, full blood count, electrolytes and plain abdominal radiology.

Management and prognosis

Mild cases require no more than an encouragement for oral rehydration. More severe cases may require intravenous fluids. Antibiotics are indicated in septicaemia (i.e. fever, positive blood cultures). Ciprofloxacin is a common first-line agent, active against the common bacterial pathogens (*Salmonella*, *Shigella* and *Campylobacter* spp.) although resistance is becoming more frequent.

If diarrhoea persists for more than three weeks, the patient will need further investigation (e.g. colonoscopy) and should be referred to a gastroenterologist. Common causes of persistent diarrhoea include hypolactasia, postinfective irritable bowel and giardiasis, but consideration should be given to the presence of an unrelated underlying pathology (colitis, coeliac disease).

Chronic infections

Giardiasis

Infection with *Giardia lamblia* may cause a persistent infection. Making a positive diagnosis on culture may prove difficult (even with culture of duodenal aspirates). Empirical treatment with tinidazole or metronidazole is effective.

Tuberculosis

Gastrointestinal tuberculosis (TB) is an important diagnosis that is relatively uncommon in developed nations but very common elsewhere. The diagnosis should be considered in patients from developing countries who have chronic abdominal symptoms. There are a number of possible clinical presentations.

- **Ileocaecal TB**, which mimics Crohn's disease (fever, abdominal pain, weight loss, diarrhoea). The chest X-ray is usually normal and TB is not found elsewhere in the body.
- **Tuberculous peritonitis**: exudative ascites. May require peritoneal biopsy to make the diagnosis.
- **Mesenteric lymphadenopathy**, which may cause right iliac fossa pain and subacute obstructive symptoms. Lymph nodes elsewhere (cervical, mediastinal, peritoneal) are also usually affected.

Treatment is the same as for pulmonary TB.

Amoebiasis

Infection with *Entamoeba histolytica* may cause a variety of clinical presentations; asymptomatic excretion of cysts is the most common finding, amoebic dysentery, non-dysenteric colonic disease and invasive disease/hepatic abscess also can occur. The diagnosis may be made by microscopy of 'hot' stool, looking for ova cysts and parasites, or by histology of colonic biopsies and/or serology. Treatment is with metronidazole followed by diloxanide furoate.

Medicine at a Glance, Fifth Edition. Edited by Patrick Davey and Alex Pitcher.

Companion website: www.wiley.com/go/medicine5e

123 Reflux

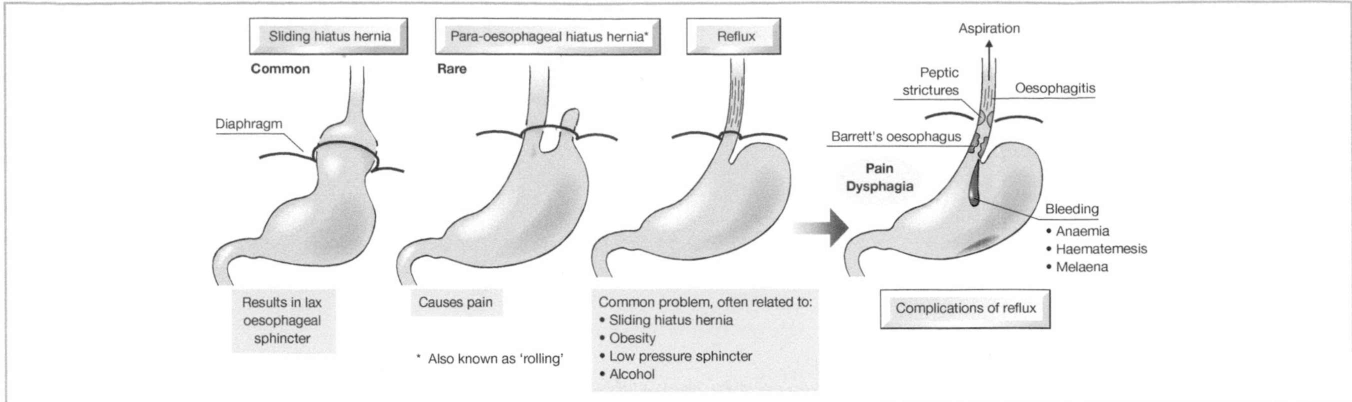

Incidence

Symptoms of gastro-oesophageal reflux are very common in the western world (20–40% of the population).

Pathophysiology

- Laxity of the lower oesophageal sphincter predisposes to episodic reflux of acid and other gastric contents back into the oesophagus.
- Symptoms of reflux will be exacerbated by **lifestyle factors**. Obesity increases intra-abdominal pressure. Smoking, stress and dietary factors (e.g. fatty foods, pastry, alcohol, chocolate) all reduce the pressure in the lower oesophageal sphincter and promote reflux. Symptoms might also be provoked by postural factors, e.g. eating late at night.
- Some patients with symptomatic reflux might be shown to have a hiatal hernia but the two are not synonomous.

Clinical features

Symptomatic reflux is diagnosed on the basis of a good clinical history and many patients will have unremarkable investigations.

- **Heartburn**: reflux most commonly presents with heartburn and occasionally nausea (see Chapter 30). Effortless regurgitation (to be distinguished from vomiting) and belching ('northerly wind') will often be present and the symptoms may have a marked postural element.
- **Chest pain** may be the presenting symptom and results from reflux-precipitated oesophageal spasm. This may be indistinguishable from angina. Cardiac pain should be excluded (often by exercise testing) before the upper gastrointestinal tract is investigated.
- **Transient dysphagia** may be experienced in severe oesophagitis. More predictable dysphagia with food bolus impaction or vomiting suggests the development of a secondary complication such as a peptic oesophageal stricture or even carcinoma.

Investigations

- **Upper gastrointestinal endoscopy** may be useful in reflux. In many, this is normal or it may demonstrate oesophagitis; it should be considered when there are any features suggestive of potential malignancy or ulcer disease.
- **24-hour oesophageal manometry and pH recording**: patients with persistent and troublesome symptoms may benefit from manometry and pH recording, which is used to select those patients who might benefit from antireflux surgery.

Management and prognosis

- **Lifestyle changes**: most patients with reflux symptoms will experience a significant improvement by: 1) limiting chocolate, coffee and alcohol intake 2) maintaining a reasonable body mass index 3) eating regular meals (especially breakfast) and avoiding late-night eating.
- **Antacids**: over-the-counter antacids (often with an alginate) are used intermittently by many reflux sufferers.
- **Proton pump inhibitors** (e.g. omeprazole, lansoprazole) are the most potent treatment for reflux symptoms. Clinical response to a therapeutic trial of acid suppression often proves informative – if not diagnostic.
- **Prokinetics**: patients with more regurgitation than heartburn may be better treated with a prokinetic agent (e.g. domperidone) to aid gastric emptying.
- **Surgery**: antireflux surgery (laparoscopic Nissen fundoplication) is beneficial in those whose symptoms are resistant to medical therapy, who have unacceptable side-effects on proton pump inhibitors (usually diarrhoea) or those with a rolling hiatal hernia and a high risk of incarceration/volvulus. Endoscopic antireflux procedures may become an alternative option for some patients.

Barrett's oesophagus

Barrett's oesophagus is a condition in which the normal stratified squamous epithelium of the lower oesophagus has undergone metaplastic change to show columnar epithelium with goblet cells. It is present in up to 15% of patients with reflux symptoms. This is potentially a premalignant condition, predisposing to lower third oesophageal adenocarcinoma. The incidence of cancer in patients with Barrett's oesophagus is now recognized to be lower than initially feared (0.5%) and although regular surveillance endoscopy and oesophageal biopsies to identify dysplasia have been widely advocated, the benefit of such strategies remains unproved.

- British Society of Gastroenterology guidelines on the diagnosis and management of Barrett's oesophagus. www.bsg.org.uk/clinical-resource/bsg-guidelines-on-the-diagnosis-and-management-of-barretts-oesophagus/.

Medicine at a Glance, Fifth Edition. Edited by Patrick Davey and Alex Pitcher.

Companion website: www.wiley.com/go/medicine5e

124 Peptic ulcer disease

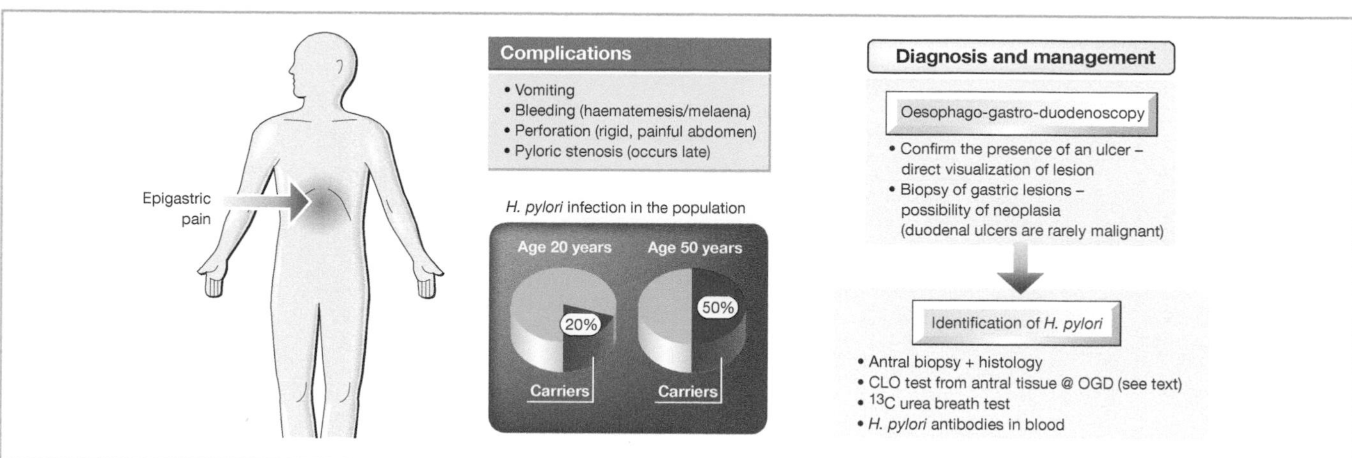

Peptic ulceration of the upper gastrointestinal (GI) tract may occur in either the duodenum or the stomach.

Duodenal ulcer

Duodenal ulcers occur predominantly when gastric acid production exceeds the buffering capacity of the alkali secreted from Brunner's glands and the pancreas. There is a very strong association with the presence of *Helicobacter pylori* and the use of non-steroidal anti-inflammatory drugs (NSAIDs).

Clinical features

- **Gastrointestinal haemorrhage**: now the most common presentation of peptic ulceration (see Chapter 27).
- **Dyspepsia**: abdominal pain has historically been considered to be the classic symptom of a duodenal ulcer but many patients presenting with acute GI bleeding deny indigestion symptoms.
- **Vomiting**: may be the presenting feature if long-standing duodenal ulceration results in pyloric stenosis.
- **Perforation** with peritonitis is occasionally a presenting or complicating feature.

Investigations

- **Endoscopy** is the first-line investigation for patients with dyspepsia and for upper GI bleeding (for diagnosis and endoscopic therapy in bleeding).
- **Testing for *H. pylori***: various tests allow the identification of this organism, which is characteristically very difficult to culture.
  - **Serology**: measurement of *H. pylori*-specific IgG antibodies in blood.
  - **Urease breath test**: ^{13}C radiolabelled urea is ingested, which is split by bacterial urease to produce $^{13}CO_2$, which is then exhaled and detected in the breath.
  - **CLO test** (*Campylobacter*-like organism test), from endoscopically obtained gastric antral biopsy: this test also detects the presence of bacterial (i.e. *H. pylori*) urease causing a colour change in a pH-sensitive gel indicator (changing from yellow to red).
  - **Faecal antigen testing**: possibly more specific and sensitive than serology.

Detection of *H. pylori* alone is not sufficient for a diagnosis of duodenal ulceration, because 20% (aged 20 years) to 50% (aged 50 years) of the population are carriers.

Gastric ulcer

Although there is considerable overlap in the pathophysiology of duodenal and gastric ulcers, the latter commonly occur in circumstances of impaired mucosal defence (e.g. NSAID use). Distinguishing between benign and malignant gastric ulcers can be extremely difficult endoscopically. Biopsies should always be taken and endoscopic follow-up arranged to ensure healing.

Clinical features and investigations

The clinical presentation is similar to duodenal ulcers and GI bleeding is now as common a presentation as indigestion. As newly identified gastric ulcers may represent early gastric cancer, biopsy of the ulcer edge and interval re-endoscopy after six weeks of medical therapy are mandatory.

Management and prognosis

- **Medical therapy** with proton pump inhibitors with or without *H. pylori* eradication results in ulcer healing after 4–6 weeks. Wherever possible, NSAIDs should be stopped.
- ***H. pylori* eradication**: ulcer recurrence is common without eradication of *H. pylori*. Eradication regimens consisting of high doses of a proton pump inhibitor in combination with two different antibiotics are 70–80% successful. Success should be documented using the urease breath test. In failed eradication, re-endoscopy with culture of organisms for antibiotic sensitivity is occasionally indicated.
- **Surgery**: required in those with perforation and recurrent or persistent bleeding. Elective surgery is an infrequent option for persistent ulceration and/or intolerance of medical therapy.

Medicine at a Glance, Fifth Edition. Edited by Patrick Davey and Alex Pitcher.

Companion website: www.wiley.com/go/medicine5e

125 Iron deficiency

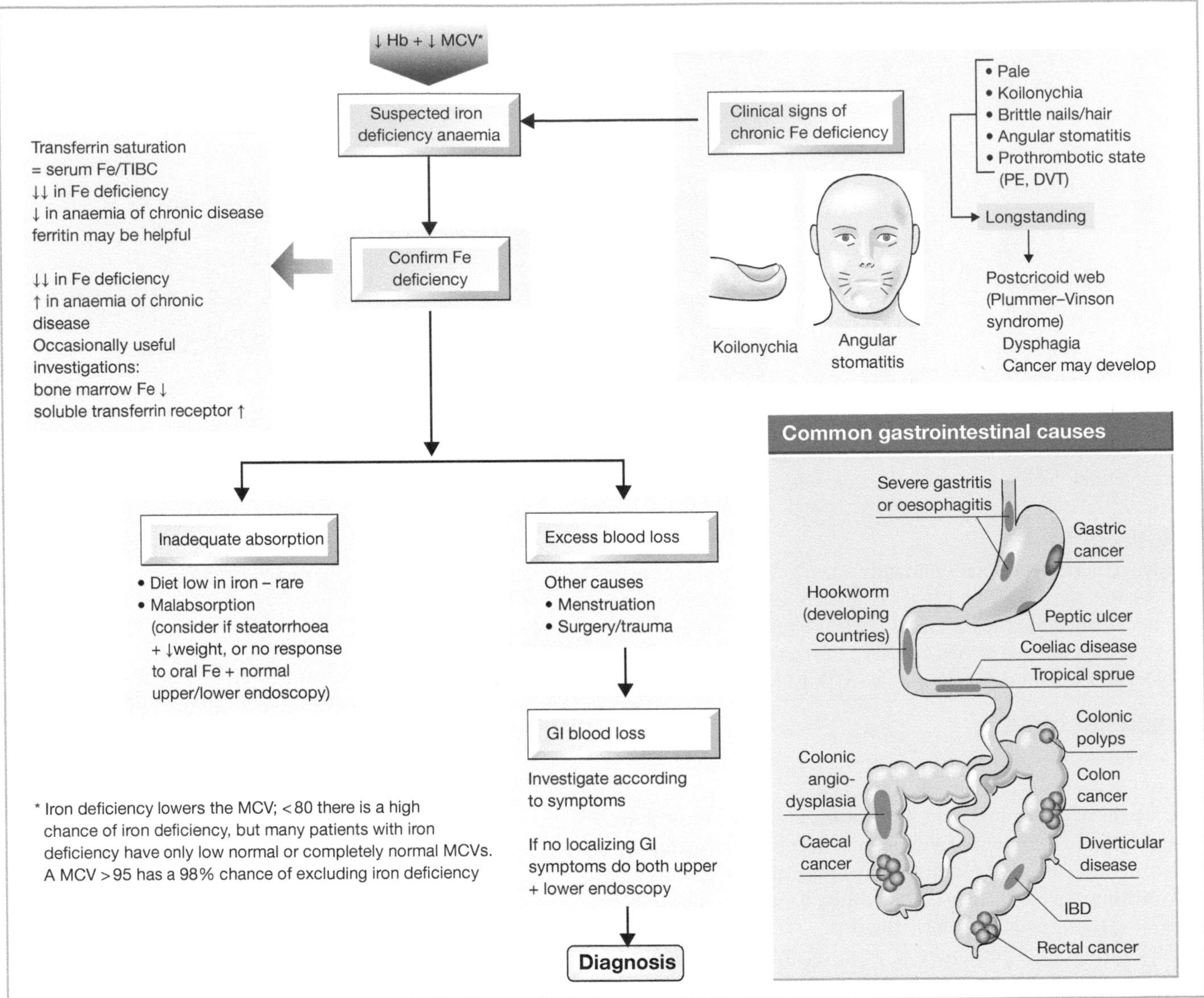

Iron is absorbed in the proximal small intestine. There is no physiological route of iron excretion in humans. Hence there are two potential reasons for iron deficiency.

1 **Reduced iron absorption** from the gastrointestinal (GI) tract, as a result of mucosal disease (coeliac disease) or gastroduodenal surgery (e.g. gastric bypass for weight loss).

2 **Chronic blood loss**, the most common cause, resulting from: (i) menstrual bleeding (premenopausal women); (ii) GI neoplasia (colonic adenomatous polyps, caecal/gastric carcinoma); or (iii) intestinal angiodysplasia. Occasionally, renal causes lead to iron deficiency anaemia, though more commonly these patients present with overt haematuria.

Medicine at a Glance, Fifth Edition. Edited by Patrick Davey and Alex Pitcher.

Companion website: www.wiley.com/go/medicine5e

Clinical features

Many patients do not have GI symptoms, although any symptoms found may prioritize the subsequent investigation.

History

In premenopausal women, a menstrual history should be taken. Previous gastric surgery may predispose to iron deficiency through duodenal bypass (i.e. gastroenterostomy) or gastric cancer.

Examination

In elderly people, an underdiagnosed cause of iron deficiency is intestinal angiodysplasia – small angiodysplastic lesions may be

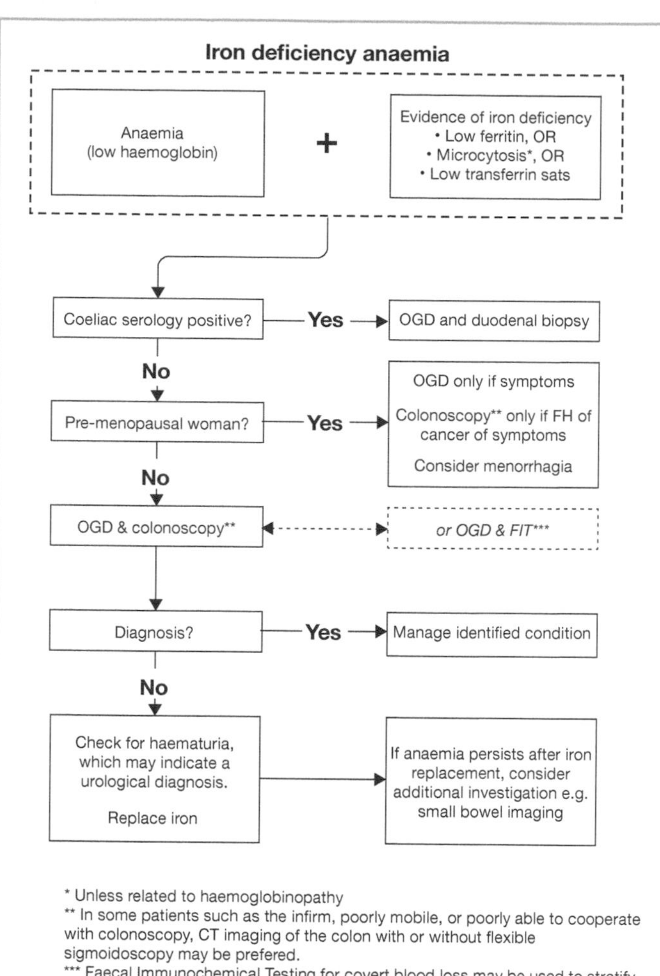

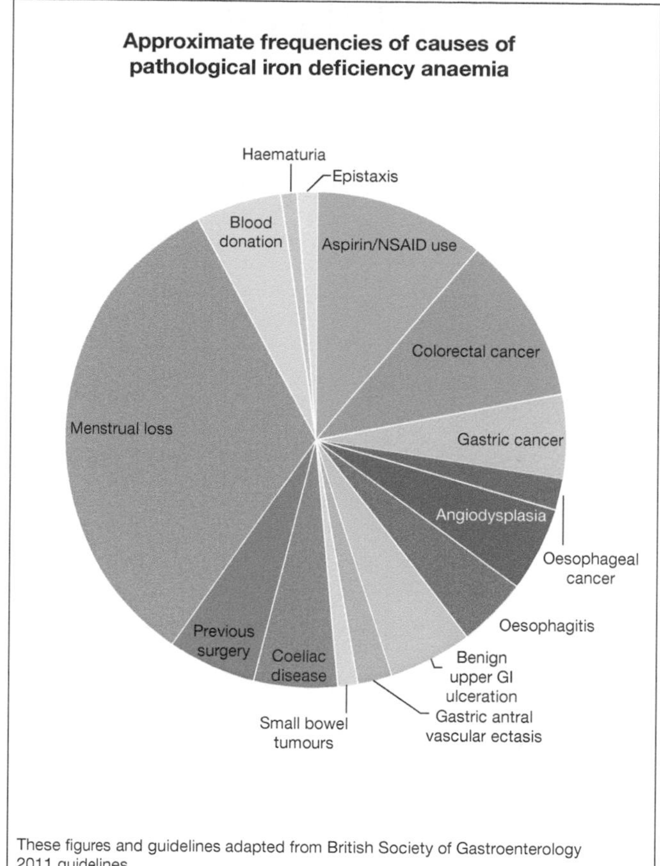

These figures and guidelines adapted from British Society of Gastroenterology 2011 guidelines

seen on the lips or buccal mucosa. Lymphadenopathy should be sought (including Virchow's node). An abdominal mass may be present and each iliac fossa should be carefully palpated. Even without altered bowel habit or rectal bleeding, a rectal examination and sigmoidoscopy are mandatory.

Investigations

- **Blood tests**: a full blood count shows a microcytic anaemia.
- **Ferritin and transferrin saturation** (serum iron divided by total iron-binding capacity [TIBC]) are low. Ferritin is an acute phase reactant and may be raised (or inappropriately 'normal') in the presence of any coexisting inflammation. A microcytic anaemia should always be confirmed as being caused by iron deficiency before treatment/GI investigation.
- **Tissue transglutaminase** antibodies: persistent or recurrent iron deficiency in the absence of obvious loss requires investigation for malabsorption and tissue transglutaminase antibody to exclude coeliac disease.
- **Faecal occult blood**: chemical tests for haem oxygenase (haemoccult) are relatively sensitive – persistently strongly positive results suggest significant GI blood loss (see Chapter 193).
- **Faecal immunchemical test:** antibody-based test that is very sensitive for blood loss and has a high negative predictive value for bowel cancer; used in the UK National Bowel Cancer Screening Programme for example.
- **Colonoscopy and endoscopy**: most patients with iron deficiency require examination of both upper and lower GI tracts. At upper endoscopy, duodenal biopsies should be taken to exclude coeliac disease. Polyps identified at colonoscopy are snared and removed.
- **Computed tomography colonography**: may be considered a suitable alternative to colonoscopy in elderly and frail patients.
- **Small bowel imaging**: if no source is identified, consideration should be given to small bowel imaging, preferably with wireless capsule endoscopy.

Management

- **Treat underlying cause**: GI angiodysplasia can be managed by continuous oral iron replacement (for gastric and colorectal cancer, see Chapters 136 and 137).
- If **no source of GI blood loss is identified**, consideration should be given to either continuous oral iron replacement or a course of replacement, and repeat investigation should the problem recur.
- Intravenous iron in the significant minority who are unable to tolerate, or are refractory to, oral iron.

126 Abnormal liver chemistry

Causes

Common
- Fatty liver
- Alcohol
- Hepatitis C virus infection
- Drug reactions

Uncommon
- Haemochromatosis
- Chronic hepatitis B infection
- Primary biliary cholangitis
- Autoimmune hepatitis

Rare
- α1 Antitrypsin deficiency
- Primary sclerosing cholangitis
- Wilson disease

Approach to abnormal liver chemistry

Liver screen / Liver imaging → Clear diagnosis → Treatment/monitoring

Liver screen / Liver imaging → No clear diagnosis → Liver biopsy

Liver blood tests

	Tests	Causes of abnormality	
Synthetic function	Albumin INR/PT	Synthetic dysfunction, e.g. cirrhosis but also acutely	
Hepatic enzymes	AST ALT	Hepatitis: viral, autoimmune	
Cholestatic enzymes	Alkaline phosphatase γGT	Cholestasis: intra- or extrahepatic obstruction	Hepatic metastasis
Inducible enzymes	γGT	Drugs: alcohol, anticonvulsants, etc.	
Bilirubin		↑in many liver diseases Isolated↑ : – haemolysis (unconjugated) – Gilbert syndrome (unconjugated)	

Chronic liver screen blood tests

Viral serology	Hepatitis B virus serology HBsAg + HBcAb + HBsAb Hepatitis C virus Ab ± HCV PCR
Iron studies	Ferritin Fe, TIBC, TSats
Autoantibodies	ANA, AMA, SMA Liver, kidney, microsomal AA Immunoglobulins
Other	Thyroid function, lipid screen, fasting glucose, α1-AT Tests of copper status in younger patients

CAGE questionnaire for alcohol abuse

Felt the need to:
- **C** ut down
- **A** nger, when told to cut down
- **G** uilt over drinking
- **E** ye opener

Consider: random ethanol, asialotransferrin

Overall approach

Abnormalities in liver chemistry (known as liver function tests or LFTs by some but not actually directly reflective of liver function) accompanied by symptoms are described in the relevant chapters. Abnormalities of liver chemistry in asymptomatic individuals are a frequent reason for outpatient hospital referral. Although these individuals are often not ill at the time of the consultation, the abnormal test may herald an underlying disease and an attempt is made to reach a diagnosis to make prognostic and therapeutic decisions.

Often there is little in the clinical history, although there are many features that should be specifically sought.

- **Alcohol intake is commonly understated/underreported by the patient.** Many patients quote the national recommendations of 14 units/week; one UK unit is 10ml of ethyl alcohol. It is more informative to know whether or not the patient takes alcohol daily and what the patient drinks. Remember that the alcohol concentration of beers varies considerably. The CAGE questionnaire may be useful; a positive answer to two or more questions has a 90% correlation with alcohol dependence.
- Features suggesting hepatitis B or C, including foreign travel (Eastern Europe, Far East and Africa), sexual behaviour and intravenous drug use (past or present).
- Full current and recent medication history, including antibiotics, over-the-counter drugs, herbal and alternative medicines.
- Family history of liver disease or multiorgan pathology such as alcohol, diabetes (e.g. haemochromatosis) or emphysema (e.g. α_1-antitrypsin (α_1-AT) deficiency).
- Other illnesses.

Medicine at a Glance, Fifth Edition. Edited by Patrick Davey and Alex Pitcher.

Companion website: www.wiley.com/go/medicine5e

Table 126.1 Non-alcoholic fatty liver disease: common cause of abnormal liver chemistry.

	Non-alcoholic fatty liver disease (NAFLD)	Non-alcoholic steatohepatitis (NASH) – NAFLD with inflammation	Cirrhosis due to NASH
Epidemiology	• Also known as simple steatosis • Affects 10–25% of the population • Found in 70% of obese subjects • Increasing rates in older subjects	• May affect 2–3% of US population • Found in 25% of those undergoing antiobesity surgery • 40% overweight/obese • 20% diabetic • 20% dyslipidaemic • 50% men	• Occurs in a variable number with NASH; ±3% at 10 years with simple steatosis or non-specific inflammation on biopsy • Occurs in 25–30% at 8–10 years in those with NASH and hepatocyte necrosis on biopsy • 80% of those developing cirrhosis have fibrosis on preceding biopsy for NASH
Clinical features	• Usually asymptomatic • Small proportion 'tired', upper abdominal discomfort	50% have persistent fatigue and/or upper abdominal discomfort	Features of chronic liver disease: • Tired • Other features (see figure in Chapter 134)
Cause	Relates to the 'metabolic syndrome' (insulin resistance)	Primary NASH: • Obesity; especially central pattern Secondary NASH: • Drugs, including amiodarone, methotrexate • Sudden weight loss (e.g. jejunoileal bypass surgery) or weight cycling • Wilson disease, lipodystrophy	• Genetic factors may promote progression from NASH to cirrhosis • Cytokines and reactive oxygen species may also promote cirrhosis
Laboratory data	Biochemistry may be normal or ALT, gGT or ALP elevations with ALT typically > AST	• ALT and AST may be raised • TNF-α may promote progression from simple steatosis to NASH • 20–50% have ↑ ferritin levels	• Features in common with other cirrhosis patients • Liver enzymes may be normal ↔ abnormal • ± ↓ albumin; ± ↑ INR
Imaging	Ultrasound, elastography, CT and MRI can diagnose moderate–severe steatosis	Imaging cannot distinguish NAFLD from NASH	Liver often small, spleen may enlarge with portal hypertension
Histology	Normal liver architecture + lipid accumulation in hepatocytes (lipids comprise 5–10% by weight)	• Steatosis + some inflammation ± fibrosis • BMI >28; ALT >2× normal; age >50 years; triglycerides >1.8; hypertension and diabetes predict fibrosis (confirmatory biopsy needed) • Biopsy shows liver inflammation + variable fibrosis	• Frank cirrhosis • Varying residual steatohepatitis
Treatment	• Weight loss • Exercise	• Control hyperglycaemia • Remove any contributor drugs • Possibly probiotics to reduce gut-derived cytokines, LPS. Possibly vitamin E, etc.	• Standard care for chronic liver disease • Accounts for increasing proportion of liver transplants
Prognosis	Excellent; probably the same as for age-matched controls	Reasonable, though some increase in mortality; cardiovascular death more frequent than liver	• Poor; 15% of hepatocellular carcinomas may relate to NASH or NASH-related cirrhosis

ALP, alkaline phosphatase; ALT, alanine transaminase; AST, aspartate transaminase; BMI, body mass index; CT, computed tomography; gGT, γ-glutamyl transferase; INR, international normalised ratio; LPS, lipopolysaccharide; MRI, magnetic resonance imaging; TNF-α, tumour necrosis factor α.

Examination

Look for signs of chronic liver disease, although these may be sparse. Record the patient's weight and body mass index.

Investigations

Blood tests

A predominant rise in alanine transaminase (ALT) represents a hepatocellular injury, whereas a predominant rise in alkaline phosphatase indicates a 'cholestatic' or biliary pattern. Random ethanol levels may help diagnose occult alcoholic liver disease (and this may also be suggested by increased γ-glutamyl transferase [γ-GT] levels and erythrocyte mean red cell volume). Other routine tests include the following.

- **Viral serology**: hepatitis A does not cause persistently abnormal liver chemistry, although hepatitis B and C can. Hepatitis E may cause chronic hepatitis in the immunosuppressed.
- **Soluble markers of liver fibrosis**: a number of blood tests have been identified as indicators of liver fibrosis (procollagen III peptide, hyaluronidase, TIMP-1 [tissue inhibitor of metalloproteinase 1]). These are probably best employed in combinations.
- **Autoantibodies and immunoglobulins**: primary biliary cirrhosis may present with non-specific malaise and pruritus. Antimitochondrial antibodies will be present in 95% and will often be accompanied by an elevated IgM. Autoimmune hepatitis is usually accompanied by autoantibodies to double-stranded DNA, smooth muscle, soluble liver antigen, liver cytosol and liver–kidney microsomes. The IgG and IgA are usually elevated. Primary sclerosing cholangitis is associated with atypical antineutrophil cytoplasmic antibody (ANCA).
- **Iron studies ± genetic studies** to detect haemochromatosis: the early identification of this common inborn error of metabolism is very important.
- **α_1-AT levels**: the relationship between α_1-AT deficiency and liver disease is very complex but patients should not smoke.
- **Fasting glucose**: diabetes can cause abnormal liver chemistry, as can obesity and, paradoxically, starvation. HbA1c and fasting lipid profile should also be considered.
- **Depressed albumin or prolonged prothrombin time** indicates impaired liver synthetic function.
- The **lipid profile** is often deranged in significant chronic liver disease and should be measured.
- **Liver ultrasonography**: this is mandatory to exclude focal liver abnormality, such as malignancy, and may occasionally identify features suggesting chronic liver disease (e.g. splenomegaly, ascites, intra-abdominal varices). Doppler examination of the portal vein may indicate portal hypertension. Steatosis can be assessed visually.
- **Liver elastography** (e.g. FibroScan®): measurement of liver elasticity (or 'stiffness') with low-amplitude ultrasound has been demonstrated in many liver conditions to correlate with fibrosis and cirrhosis. The controlled attenuation parameter gives an indication of steatosis.
- **Liver biopsy** remains the definitive way of determining prognosis (i.e. the presence of fibrosis), even if a formal diagnosis is not possible.

Management

Management depends on the underlying pathology. Often, the need is for qualified reassurance and an opinion about prognosis. For NASH, only patients with advanced fibrosis are most likely to die from liver disease; otherwise, the typical concurrent cardiovascular risk and malignancy risk are of more pressing concern.

127 Diverticular disease

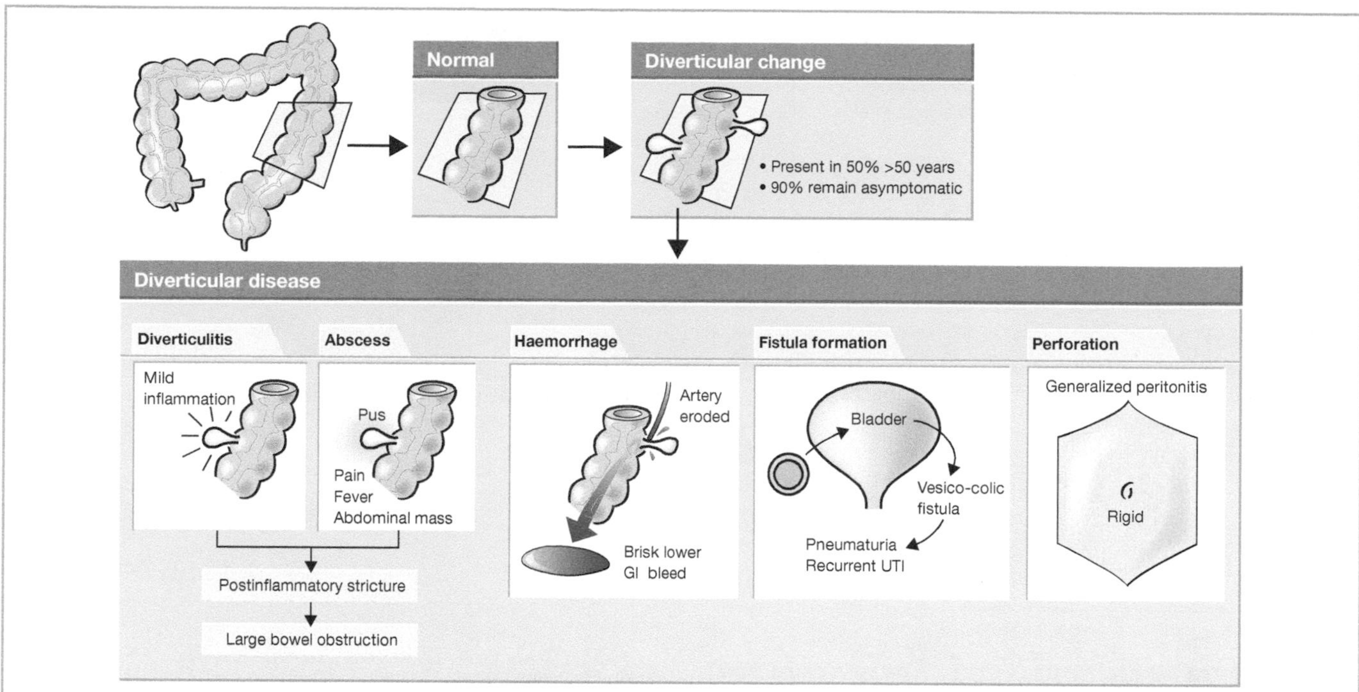

Diverticulosis represents a degenerative change in the colon, resulting in the formation of outpouches or pockets of colonic mucosa extruding through the muscular wall of the bowel. In many elderly people, this may be asymptomatic and the terms 'diverticular change' or 'diverticulosis' may be more appropriate than the more commonly used term 'diverticulitis'.

Incidence

The prevalence increases with age and is 5% at 40 years, rising to 50% at 80 years.

Pathophysiology

There may be an underlying genetic predisposition to diverticular disease but it is best considered as an acquired condition.

Clinical features

Diverticular change itself is asymptomatic and it is the common complications that lead to symptomatic presentation.

- **Diverticulitis**: an associated inflammation of the colon – considered to be precipitated by impaction of faeces within a diverticulum. This may evolve into a diverticular abscess with abdominal pain, fever and a left-sided abdominal mass.
- **Colonic bleeding**: this is a frequent presentation of diverticular disease, possibly because diverticula form at the point of maximal weakness in the colon, i.e. at the point where blood vessels penetrate the muscle coat.
- **Repeated infective episodes** may result in the formation of either a diverticular stricture, presenting with symptoms of colonic obstruction, or a colovesical fistula, presenting with recurrent urinary tract infections (UTIs) or the characteristic symptom of pneumaturia.

Investigations

- **Colonoscopy** or computed tomography (CT) colonography: asymptomatic diverticular change may be demonstrated as an incidental finding at colonoscopy or on other colonic imaging.
- **Abdominal CT**: the best way to demonstrate abscesses. Colovesical fistulae require a high index of suspicion (recurrent UTIs, pneumaturia, etc.), and may need to be sought specifically (i.e. using rectal contrast).

Management and prognosis

The management of diverticular disease is conservative, though surgery is occasionally required.

- **Avoidance of symptomatic constipation**: may reduce the risk of complications.
- **Treatment of complications**: acute diverticulitis requires intravenous fluids, antibiotics and analgesics. Diverticular abscess may require drainage in addition to the above. Bleeding usually settles with supportive treatment.
- **Surgery**: this is usually reserved for complicated diverticular disease (i.e. bleeding, abscess, stricture).

Medicine at a Glance, Fifth Edition. Edited by Patrick Davey and Alex Pitcher.

Companion website: www.wiley.com/go/medicine5e

128 Inflammatory bowel disease

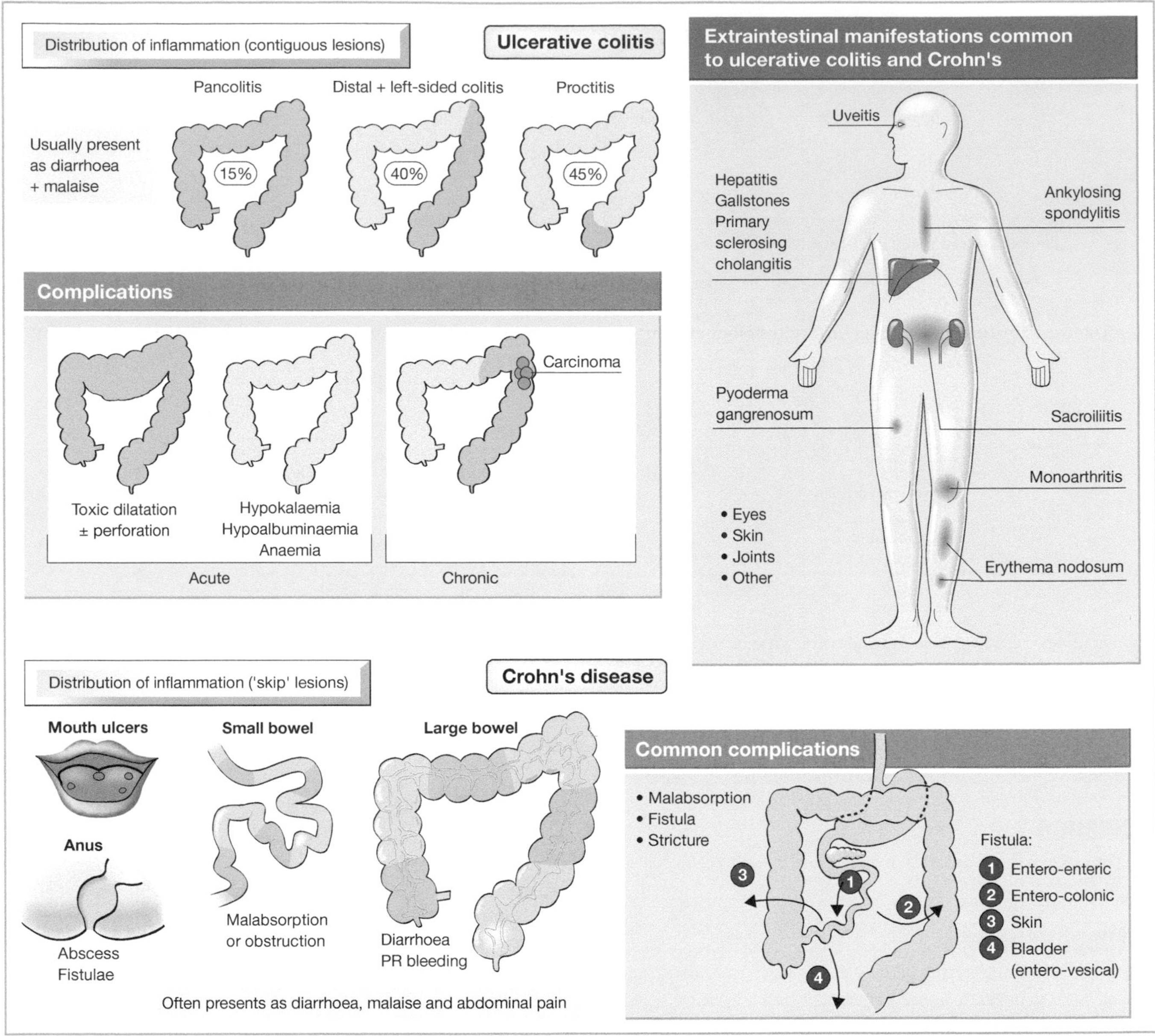

Idiopathic inflammatory bowel disease (IBD) comprises ulcerative colitis (UC), Crohn's disease and the microscopic colitides (lymphocytic and collagenous colitis). In some patients, the distinction between these conditions may prove difficult and the term IBD-U (IBD unclassified) may be used.

Ulcerative colitis

This is the most common form of IBD, affecting up to 500 per 100 000 of the population. It commonly presents in young adults. No unifying cause has been identified, although genetic factors play a major role, with 15% of cases having a clear family history. Smoking appears to protect against UC for unknown reasons, as does prior appendicectomy.

The majority of UC patients present with a chronic illness, but around 15% present acutely with severe colitis. Overall, around 10% need colectomy by five years and 15% by 10 years. There was previously thought to be a markedly elevated risk of colon cancer, but more recent evidence suggests that an elevated risk is largely confined to those with long duration of disease, those with primary sclerosing cholangitis, and those with uncontrolled inflammation.

Medicine at a Glance, Fifth Edition. Edited by Patrick Davey and Alex Pitcher.

Companion website: www.wiley.com/go/medicine5e

Pathophysiology and clinical features

The pathological hallmarks of UC are as follows: inflammation is always present in the rectum, it extends a variable distance proximally in the colon, is continuous and is limited to the mucosa of the bowel (i.e. it is superficial).

- '**Total**' **colitis** (pancolitis) presents with chronic diarrhoea, sometimes with constitutional upset and objective biochemical markers of inflammation.
- '**Distal**' **UC** (left-sided colitis, proctosigmoiditis, proctitis) more often presents with rectal bleeding associated with urge and a sense of incomplete rectal emptying (tenesmus). Constitutional disturbance is less frequent.

With either presentation, there may be extraintestinal manifestations of disease (arthralgia, iritis, skin lesions). Pain is an infrequent feature.

Investigations

The diagnosis is made on the basis of history, histology and imaging. It is crucial to recognize severe colitis early and treat vigorously.

- The **Truelove–Witts criteria** for acute severe colitis are as follows. Stool frequency >6 bloody stools per day, plus one or more of the following.
  - Temperature >37.8 °C.
  - Pulse >90 bpm.
  - Haemoglobin <105 g/l.
  - Erythrocyte sedimentation rate (ESR) >30 mm/h or C-reactive protein >30 mg/l).
- **Flexible sigmoidoscopy or colonoscopy** is used to delineate the disease extent. Long-standing colitis carries a risk for colonic carcinoma. Biopsy may give an indication of chronicity. Reassessment of the extent of disease by colonoscopy is recommended 10 years from diagnosis, with subsequent regular surveillance colonoscopy. In some patients, yearly surveillance may be necessary (those with co-existent primary sclerosing cholangitis and those with a disease history of over 20 years). In acute severe colitis, flexible sigmoidoscopy is useful to confirm the diagnosis and assess severity.
- **Abdominal X-ray**: in acute severe colitis, a plain abdominal X-ray may aid with assessing the extent of disease (inflamed bowel being empty) and allows assessment for 'toxic dilation' of the colon – a life-threatening complication with a high risk of perforation, and which requires consideration of emergency surgery.
- **Stool culture** and ***C. difficile*** **toxin**: to exclude infective diarrhoea which may also complicate inflammatory bowel disease.
- **Faecal calprotectin**: elevated in many causes of bowel inflammation, including UC. Useful as a rule-out test in primary care and may be used to monitor disease activity and response to treatment.

Management

- **Corticosteroids**.
  - Severe acute colitis is a medical emergency which requires hospital admission and *intravenous (IV) steroids* such as hydrocortisone or methylprednisolone, often with rectal corticosteroids. Less severe attacks may be treated with oral corticosteroids such as prednisolone.
  - *Budesonide* as a delayed colonic-release preparation (e.g. budesonide MMX) is effective for less severe flares and has fewer side-effects than prednisolone.
  - Topical corticosteroids such as enemas and suppositories may be effective for flares of proctitis or left-sided disease.
- **Ciclosporin**: may be of benefit for severe acute colitis that fails to respond adequately to initial treatment.
- Tacrolimus may be used topically for resistant proctitis.
- **5-Aminosalicylic acid** compounds such as mesalazine are effective in mild attacks and reduce the risk of subsequent episodes. Thought to reduce malignancy risk.
- **Azathioprine** (or related compound **6-mercaptopurine**) is used to reduce the risk of relapse and to prevent antidrug antibody formation with some biologic agents.
- **Monoclonal antibodies** ('biologics').
  - *Infliximab*: this chimeric anti-tumour necrosis factor (TNF)-α antibody is given intravenously and is useful in acute disease inadequately responding to corticosteroids and also effective in maintaining remission.
  - *Adalimumab*: an alternative anti-TNF-α monoclonal antibody used to maintain remission; given subcutaneously.
  - *Vedolizumab*: monoclonal antibody to α4β7 intergrin which acts to prevent migration of leukocytes into the gut. Used to maintain remission.
  - *Ustekinumab*: monoclonal antibody to interleukins 12 and 23 used to maintain remission.
- **Surgery**: for a colon that is *life-threatening* (i.e. perforation, cancer or severe dysplasia) or one that is *life-limiting* (i.e. incompatible with a reasonable quality of life despite maximal medical therapy). In acute surgery, an ileostomy is typically formed. In planned surgery, or after an interval from acute surgery, consideration is often given to formation of an ileoanal pouch and removal of the ileostomy.

Crohn's disease

A chronic granulomatous inflammatory disease affecting the gut. Pathological features that distinguish it from UC include the following.

- It affects any part of the gut, from the mouth to the anus.
- The inflammation is discontinuous, with 'skip lesions'.
- The inflammation is deep and sometimes transmural, resulting in gut stenosis and penetrating ulcers leading to abscesses and fistulae. Granulomata may be present.
- Uncommon; UK prevalence is up to 100 cases per 100 000 population.

Clinical features

The cardinal symptoms are abdominal pain and systemic upset with weight loss and fever. Bloating and vomiting will be present when stricturing disease is present. Diarrhoea is reported by most patients but has numerous different mechanisms (colonic inflammation, bile salt malabsorption, small bowel bacterial overgrowth). The combination of symptoms will depend upon the following factors.

- **Site of disease**: small bowel disease is more likely to present with malabsorption and features of small bowel obstruction than colonic disease, which causes diarrhoea.
- **Extent and severity of inflammation** are easily underestimated in young adults – many patients present with pronounced fatigue, anorexia and poor general health.

• **Secondary complications**: such as abscess, stricture and fistulae.
• **Extraintestinal manifestations** may be related to disease activity (e.g. aphthous ulceration, erythema nodosum, acute arthropathy, eye complications) or occur independently from disease flares (sacroiliitis, ankylosing spondylitis). These are present in up to 40% of patients.
• **Complications of malabsorption** may be present and include iron deficiency, vitamin B12 deficiency and malnutrition.

The differential diagnosis includes *Yersinia* infection and intestinal tuberculosis.

Investigations

- **Markers of inflammation.**
  - C-reactive protein is useful in monitoring disease activity.
  - Faecal calprotectin is used in some settings to monitor activity.
- **Imaging.**
  - *MRI or CT enterography* may be used to assess small bowel Crohn's disease; these scans have largely superseded barium studies. Such scans allow assessment for fistulation.
  - *Pelvic MRI* may be necessary to assess for fistulation or abscess formation in those with perianal disease.
  - *Small bowel ultrasound* is useful for assessment of distal ileal disease and is risk free with good patient acceptability.
  - *Standard cross-sectional CT* is useful to assess for complications of disease, including obstruction, perforation and abscess formation in those presenting with acute abdominal pain.
- **Endoscopy**: allows for diagnostic biopsy. Colonoscopy with terminal ileoscopy is useful for delineating the extent, severity and disease response of colonic disease.
- **Video capsule endoscopy**: may be of use in identifying subtle mucosal inflammation in the small bowel but the presence of intestinal strictures is a contraindication because of a risk of capsule impaction.

Management and prognosis

Multidisciplinary, involving physicians, surgeons, radiologists and dietitians. Crohn's disease is an incurable illness, follows a remitting/relapsing course, causes considerable morbidity and is estimated to have a standardized mortality ratio of 1.4.

• **Smoking cessation** is important and reduces disease activity as effectively as many drug treatments.
• **Corticosteroids**: remain the most potent medical treatment. Other than in isolated distal colonic disease, these must be administered systemically (e.g. oral prednisolone or IV hydrocortisone), with the attendant long-term risks of adrenal suppression and osteopenia. Budesonide may be used for small bowel and right colon disease and has a reduced side-effect profile owing to its extensive first-pass hepatic metabolism.
• **Monoclonal antibodies**: monoclonal antibodies to TNF-α are used to maintain remission. Vedolizumab and ustekinumab are also used as above.
• **Antimetabolite immunosuppressant agents**: azathioprine, 6-mercaptopurine and methotrexate are antimetabolite medications used as maintenance therapy to reduce relapse and prevent the development of antidrug antibodies.
• **Surgery**: given the patchy and recurrent nature of Crohn's disease, surgery tends to be conservative and reserved for symptoms due to structural disease (such as strictures) not responding to medical therapy and other specific complications (e.g. abscesses, fistulae). In localized small bowel disease, surgical resection may be preferable to drug therapy and provide long-term remission.
• **Nutrition**: nutritional support presents specific challenges, given the combination of the high metabolic demand of acute inflammation with small intestinal dysfunction. Liquid diets are very effective. An 'elemental diet' is a liquid diet in which the nitrogen source is in the form of amino acids and reduces disease activity. A 'polymeric diet' provides short peptides.
• **5-Aminosalicylic compounds**, such as sulfasalazine and mesalazine, were previously used as maintenance treatment for colonic Crohn's disease but are no longer thought to be effective.

129 Gallstone disease

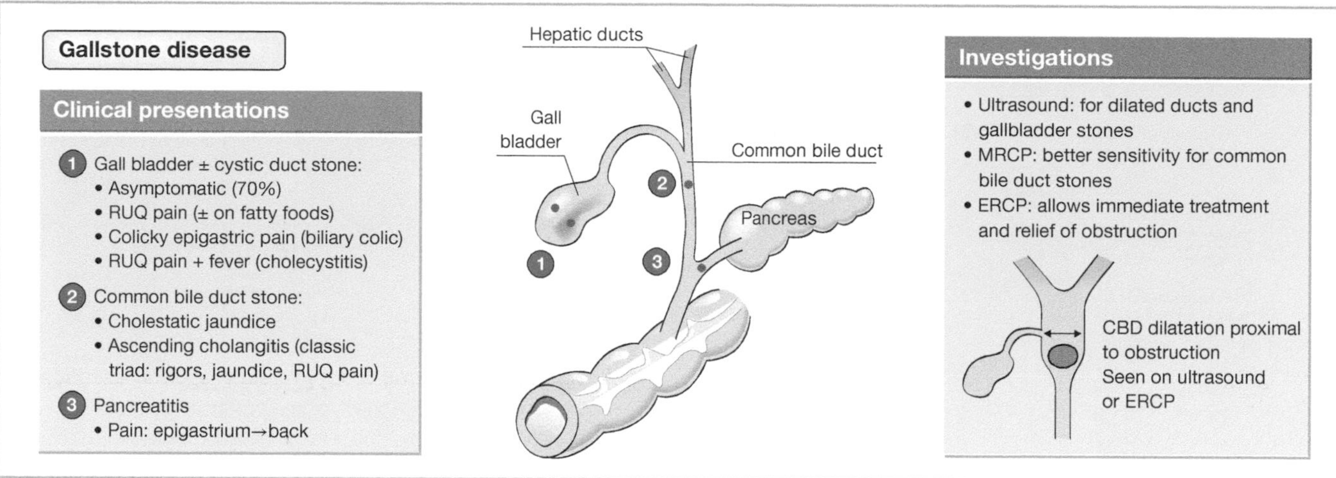

Gallstone disease
Clinical presentations
1 Gall bladder ± cystic duct stone:
• Asymptomatic (70%)
• RUQ pain (± on fatty foods)
• Colicky epigastric pain (biliary colic)
• RUQ pain + fever (cholecystitis)
2 Common bile duct stone:
• Cholestatic jaundice
• Ascending cholangitis (classic triad: rigors, jaundice, RUQ pain)
3 Pancreatitis
• Pain: epigastrium→back
Hepatic ducts
Gall bladder
Common bile duct
Pancreas
Investigations
• Ultrasound: for dilated ducts and gallbladder stones
• MRCP: better sensitivity for common bile duct stones
• ERCP: allows immediate treatment and relief of obstruction
CBD dilatation proximal to obstruction
Seen on ultrasound or ERCP

The prevalence of gallstones is underestimated because around 90% remain asymptomatic. Stones occur in 7% of men and 15% of women aged 18–65 years. There is a 3:1 female predominance in those aged <40 years, which disappears in elderly people.

Pathophysiology

Gallstone formation results from precipitation of cholesterol crystals in supersaturated bile. Stones ultimately contain a combination of calcium salts; they increase in size at a rate of 2.5 mm/year. Less commonly, pigment stones occur from chronic haemolysis (see Chapter 177).

Clinical features

- **Asymptomatic**: gallstones may be an incidental finding.
- **Biliary colic**: recurrent right upper quadrant (RUQ) pain, often precipitated by fatty food. The most common cause of biliary colic is when there is induced contraction against biliary stones, often when these are in the neck of the gall bladder or have moved into the bile ducts.
- **Cholecystitis** typically presents with acute right hypochondral pain and fever. If the neck of the gall bladder becomes obstructed, an empyema of the gall bladder (with a 20–30% mortality rate) may occur.
- **Cholestatic jaundice**: jaundice with pale stools and dark urine indicates biliary obstruction as a result of migration of a stone into the common bile duct (CBD) (choledocholithiasis). With clinical evidence of superadded infection (Charcot triad of jaundice, fever, rigors), this is known as cholangitis.
- **Pancreatitis**: gallstones are a major cause of pancreatitis in the developed world, usually caused by migration of stones down the CBD and through the ampulla of Vater.
- **Carcinoma of the gall bladder**: this is rare and in 90% occurs in association with gallstones. Extensive gall bladder calcification ('porcelain gall bladder') is a particularly powerful risk factor.
- **Rare presentations** and complications include biliary peritonitis, resulting from perforation (30% mortality), and small bowel obstruction (gallstone ileus) caused by a large gallstone being held up at the ileocaecal valve.

Investigations

Fewer than 20% of gallstones are visible on plain X-rays or CT scans.

- **Transabdominal ultrasonography**: most commonly used to identify gallstones. Bile duct dilation (intra- or extrahepatic) raises the possibility of CBD stones although transabdominal ultrasonography can rarely prove or exclude this (30–40% of patients with stones in the CBD have 'normal' ultrasound scans). Endoscopic ultrasonography has greater sensitivity and is now more widely available.
- **Liver chemistry**: should be checked in any patient considered for cholecystectomy. If these are abnormal, magnetic resonance cholangiopancreatography (MRCP) and/or endoscopic retrograde cholangiopancreatography (ERCP) should be considered before surgery, because derangements may reflect stones in the CBD. An alternative is on-table cholangiography.
- **MRCP** is now the first-line investigation for suspected biliary stones; ERCP is an invasive alternative.
- **ERCP**: provides simultaneous imaging of the biliary tree and the opportunity to relieve biliary obstruction by endoscopic sphincterotomy and removal of CBD stones.

Management and prognosis

- **Watchful waiting**: the incidental finding of asymptomatic gallstones requires no treatment.
- **Cholecystectomy**: in patients with symptomatic gallstones or after a significant complication, the definitive treatment is cholecystectomy.
- Ursodeoxycholic acid is occasionally used for stones in patients unsuitable for surgery but takes a long time to have an effect.
- **ERCP**: this is both an investigation and treatment in patients with cholestatic jaundice in the presence of gallstones. For elderly or otherwise unwell patients, ERCP sphincterotomy may be sufficient because the risk of further problems is probably low.

Medicine at a Glance, Fifth Edition. Edited by Patrick Davey and Alex Pitcher.

Companion website: www.wiley.com/go/medicine5e

130 Malabsorption

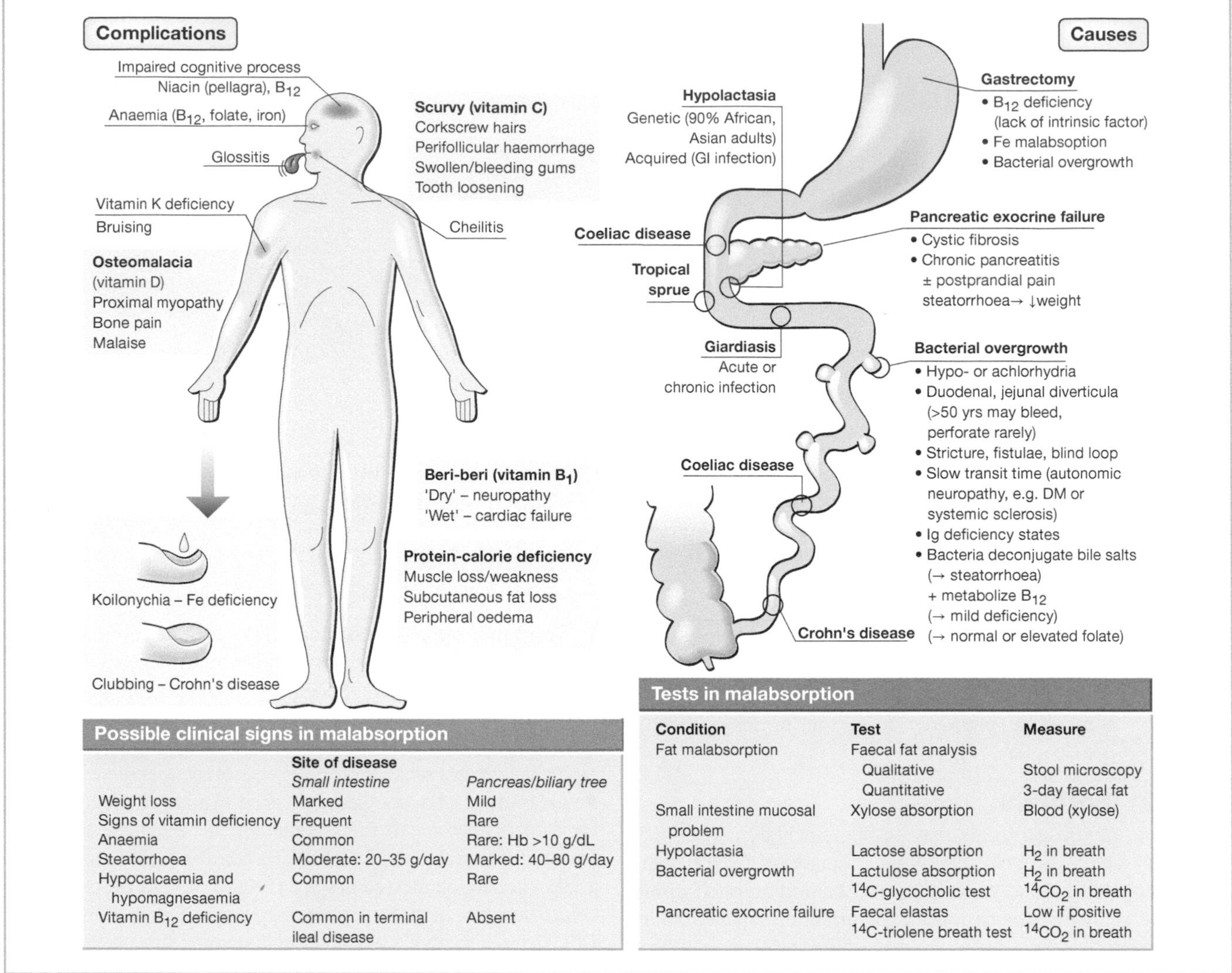

Possible clinical signs in malabsorption

	Site of disease	
	Small intestine	*Pancreas/biliary tree*
Weight loss	Marked	Mild
Signs of vitamin deficiency	Frequent	Rare
Anaemia	Common	Rare: Hb >10 g/dL
Steatorrhoea	Moderate: 20–35 g/day	Marked: 40–80 g/day
Hypocalcaemia and hypomagnesaemia	Common	Rare
Vitamin B_{12} deficiency	Common in terminal ileal disease	Absent

Tests in malabsorption

Condition	Test	Measure
Fat malabsorption	Faecal fat analysis	
	Qualitative	Stool microscopy
	Quantitative	3-day faecal fat
Small intestine mucosal problem	Xylose absorption	Blood (xylose)
Hypolactasia	Lactose absorption	H_2 in breath
Bacterial overgrowth	Lactulose absorption	H_2 in breath
	^{14}C-glycocholic test	$^{14}CO_2$ in breath
Pancreatic exocrine failure	Faecal elastas	Low if positive
	^{14}C-triolene breath test	$^{14}CO_2$ in breath

Malabsorption is suggested by the combination of chronic diarrhoea and weight loss despite preservation of appetite (see Chapter 23). Thyrotoxicosis can also cause these symptoms. The causes of malabsorption include the following.

- **Common**: coeliac disease, pancreatic exocrine insufficiency and Crohn's disease.
- **Uncommon**: hypolactasia, small bowel bacterial overgrowth, giardiasis and HIV.
- **Rare**: tropical sprue, Whipple disease and amyloidosis.

Clinical features and examination

Most patients describe weight loss despite preservation of appetite (and even hunger), general fatigue and diarrhoea – often steatorrhoea (pale offensive stools that float in the toilet pan and require two or more flushes of the toilet because of their fat content). In malabsorption caused by pancreatic exocrine failure, a history of excess alcohol or previous acute pancreatitis may be found. In malabsorption relating to gastrointestinal (GI) infection, a travel history may be relevant. In the physical examination, look specifically for the following.

- Objective evidence of **weight loss**.
- **Markers of malnutrition**: leukonychia, glossitis, cheilitis, anaemia (folate, vitamin B_{12}, protein).
- **Markers of specific nutritional deficiencies**: scurvy (vitamin C), koilonychia (iron), osteomalacia (vitamin D and calcium), bruising (vitamin K).
- Clinical features of **thyrotoxicosis**: tremor, tachycardia, exophthalmos.

Medicine at a Glance, Fifth Edition. Edited by Patrick Davey and Alex Pitcher.

Companion website: www.wiley.com/go/medicine5e

- **Lymphadenopathy**: Troisier's sign of an enlarged Virchow's node – representing intra-abdominal malignancy.
- **Abdominal examination**: a mass may be palpable in ileal Crohn's disease. The stool on rectal examination often appears pale and smells offensively. It may also be 'oily'.

Investigations

Investigations should objectively evaluate the effects of malnutrition and seek to identify the underlying disease.

- **Blood tests.**
  - Determine the severity of malnutrition (full blood count, liver chemistry, albumin, international normalized ratio, calcium, magnesium, zinc, vitamin B_{12}, folate).
  - Exclude certain conditions (thyroxine, thyroid-stimulating hormone, tissue transglutaminase for coeliac disease).
  - Raise the possibility of certain diseases (erythrocyte sedimentation rate/C-reactive protein in Crohn's disease).
- **Endoscopy and duodenal biopsies** are used to exclude coeliac disease and *Giardia*.
- **Small bowel imaging** is used when non-coeliac small bowel mucosal disease is suspected. The range of investigations includes small bowel enema, magnetic resonance or computed tomography (CT) enterography and enteroscopy (either 'push' or 'wireless'/capsule).
- **Testing of stool** for the presence of undigested faecal fat is rarely performed now.
- **Tests of small bowel function**: hydrogen breath tests – H_2 appears in the breath when lactose (hypolactasia) or lactulose (small bowel overgrowth) is given.
- **Pancreatic imaging**: pancreatic ultrasonography, CT and magnetic resonance cholangiopancreatography (MRCP) are indicated when chronic pancreatitis is suspected to underlie pancreatic exocrine failure.
- **Tests of pancreatic function.**
  - *Faecal elastase or chymotrypsin*: low pancreatic elastase activity is found in the stool in moderate–severe pancreatic exocrine failure.
  - *Pancreolauryl test*: fluorescein dilaurate is ingested, and if pancreatic exocrine enzymes are present, fluorescein is split off, absorbed and passed into the urine, where it can be detected.

Management

- Treat the underlying cause: see relevant sections.
- Dietary advice and supplementation, vitamin and nutrient replacement may be indicated (folate, vitamin B_{12}, iron).
- Think about the bones: osteopenia is a significant long-term problem in malabsorption (see Chapter 217).

Diseases causing malabsorption

Coeliac disease

Coeliac disease (gluten-sensitive enteropathy) is the most common cause of small bowel malabsorption in the West. It is common, especially in north-west Europe. The prevalence in western Ireland is over 1:100. The incidence is increasing, although better diagnostic tests may contribute to this. The peak incidence is 20–40 years, although it can present at any age.

Coeliac disease is the result of an immune reaction to gluten. Initially, this causes an increase in the intraepithelial lymphocytes in the small intestinal epithelium. This subsequently progresses to flattening of the intestinal villi (villous atrophy). There are HLA (human leukocyte antigen) associations with HLA-DQ2 and -DQ8; those without these alleles are unlikely to have the disease although only a minority of carriers develop coeliac disease.

Clinical features

- **Iron deficiency**: the diagnosis is often made during investigation of iron deficiency.
- **Malabsorption**: coeliac disease will now rarely present with classic sprue (diarrhoea, weight loss, oedema).
- **Case finding**: although there is no mandate for screening for coeliac disease, the increasing recognition of a strong genetic component has led to a lowered threshold for making the diagnosis in first-degree relatives of affected individuals.
- **Dermatitis herpetiformis**: this rare but characteristic blistering eruption may lead to the diagnosis of coeliac disease.

Investigations

- **Antibodies**: IgA class tissue transglutaminase antibodies are highly sensitive and specific for coeliac disease. However, selective IgA deficiency is present in up to 5% of coeliac patients, rendering the serology relatively 'uninformative' in these individuals. Antiendomysial antibodies are also used. In most cases, antibodies will disappear with successful adherence to a gluten-free diet. In some cases, such as paediatric presentations, positive antibodies alone are sufficient for diagnosis.
- **Endoscopy and distal duodenal biopsy**: traditionally, this is repeated after a period on a gluten-free diet although increasingly the resolution of symptoms and antibodies is considered sufficient evidence of remission.
- **Bone densitometry**: even in the absence of significant weight loss, bone density may be significantly reduced at the time of presentation.

Management and prognosis

- **Gluten-free diet**: completely reverses the histological and nutritional changes.
- **Vitamin and iron replacement** with iron, folate and vitamin B_{12} is needed in malabsorption.
- **Osteopenia**: with effective treatments for osteopenia now available, this important feature should be prospectively monitored and treated.
- **Small intestinal cancers** (enteropathy-associated T-cell lymphoma, adenocarcinoma): these are rare complications for which no surveillance has proven to be effective. They are important to consider in refractory disease or individuals who relapse clinically.

Other causes of malabsorption

- **Small bowel bacterial overgrowth** results from either structural or functional disorders that cause relative stasis (e.g. hypo- or achlorhydria, jejunal diverticulosis, postsurgical blind loops, intestinal strictures, autonomic neuropathy, scleroderma). Diagnosis is confirmed with a lactulose breath test or empirical treatment with antibiotics. Small bowel imaging for structural lesions is usually unnecessary. Treatment is with antibiotics (metronidazole and tetracyline), which may need to be repeated.
- **Giardiasis**: persistent infection with *Giardia lamblia* may cause diarrhoea and malabsorption.
- **Hypolactasia**: loss of lactase from the small intestinal brush border may be primary or secondary following a GI infection. This results in milk intolerance, which causes bloating, nausea, wind and diarrhoea. The diagnosis is confirmed by a lactose breath test. Treatment is with a low-lactose diet.
- **Other diseases**: including pancreatic exocrine failure and Crohn's disease (see Chapter 128).

131 Pancreatitis and pancreatic cancer

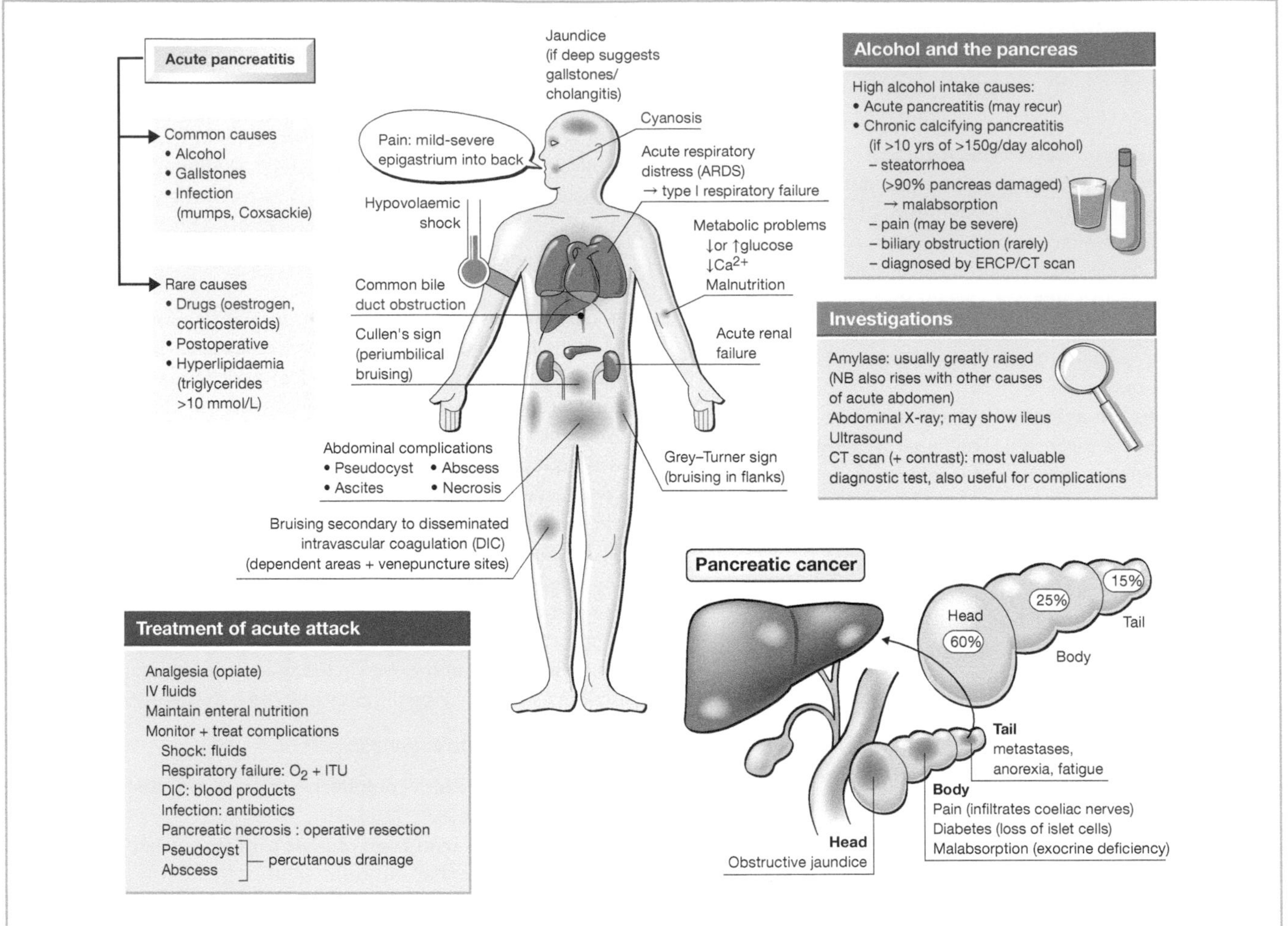

Acute pancreatitis

Acute pancreatitis results from a sudden onset of pancreatic inflammation associated with varying degrees of necrosis and 'autodigestion'. The incidence in the UK is currently 20 per 100 000 population, with a 43% increase in the last decade, probably as a result of increased alcohol consumption nationally. The common causes of acute pancreatitis are as follows.

- **Gallstones**: 30–50%, possibly more if one includes 'microlithiasis' – cholesterol crystals within the bile.
- **Alcohol**: 10–40%.
- **Idiopathic**: 15%.
- Rarer (but important) causes include: trauma (endoscopic retrograde cholangiopancreatography [ERCP], postoperative, blunt trauma), drugs (5%, including loop diuretics and azathioprine), hypertriglyceridaemia, viral (mumps, Coxsackie virus) and genetic causes.

Once the process has started, there is a variable degree of pancreatic necrosis related to proteolytic autodigestion of the gland.

Clinical features

- **Abdominal pain**: characteristically sudden onset, epigastric and radiating through to the back.
- **Hypovolaemia/shock**: the degree of circulating volume depletion may be underestimated and contribute significantly to the associated renal failure.
- **Vomiting**: contributes to hypovolaemia.
- **Jaundice**: suggests the presence of an associated cholangitis.

Various scoring systems are used to grade the severity of pancreatitis (Ranson, Glasgow, APACHE II). In general, prognosis is determined more by markers of shock (acidaemia, hypoxia, etc.) than by the level of serum amylase recorded on admission. Mortality rate varies from 2% in mild attacks to >50% in severe disease.

Management and prognosis

For investigation, see figure and Table 131.1. The key to managing pancreatitis is restoration of euvolaemia and, once stable, determination and treatment of the underlying cause.

Medicine at a Glance, Fifth Edition. Edited by Patrick Davey and Alex Pitcher.

Companion website: www.wiley.com/go/medicine5e

Table 131.1 Glasgow Imrie criteria for severe pancreatitis (most reliable when used at 48 h after the onset of pain; >3 = severe disease).

Assessment of severity of pancreatitis	Criterion
White cell count	$>15 \times 10^9$/l
Urea	>16 mmol/l
Calcium	<2.0 mmol/l
Albumin	<32 g/l
Glucose	>10 mmol/l
PO_2	<8 kPa
Aspartate transaminase	>200 IU/l
Lactate dehydrogenase	>600 IU/l
C-reactive protein	>150 mg/l

- **Resuscitation**: intravenous fluids, central venous pressure monitoring and oxygen. The routine use of broad-spectrum antibiotics is unproven.
- **Electrolyte abnormalities** require replacement, including hypocalcaemia.
- **Nutrition** should be maintained enterally where possible.
- **Treat underlying cause**: clinical features of cholangitis raise the possibility of a gallstone impacted at the ampulla and are an indication to consider early ERCP. If gallstones are confirmed to be the underlying cause of the pancreatitis, early cholecystectomy is recommended.

Complications

Mild cases of pancreatitis usually resolve without complications; the more severe the acute attack, the more likely are complications.

- **Pancreatic pseudocyst/abscess**: suggested by persistent pain and/or fever, diagnosed by computed tomography (CT), and often drained percutaneously.
- **Adult respiratory distress syndrome**.
- **Portal vein/mesenteric thrombosis**.

Chronic pancreatitis

Chronic pancreatitis may result as a consequence of repeated attacks of acute pancreatitis. Some patients present with clinical features of pancreatic insufficiency in the absence of pain. The prevalence is 40–75 per 100 000 and the incidence 8/100 000. Chronic pancreatitis relates to:

- recurrent acute pancreatitis
- alcohol: the most common cause in the UK
- idiopathic: accounts for 20% of cases.

Clinical features

The cardinal features of chronic pancreatitis are as follows.

- **Pain**: in 85%; typical pancreatic pain is epigastric radiating through to the back, often precipitated by eating. The severity is very variable.
- **Exocrine pancreatic insufficiency**: produces steatorrhoea and weight loss.
- **Endocrine pancreatic insufficiency** (i.e. diabetes): in 30%. There are often no abnormal physical signs, despite dramatic symptoms.

Investigations

Pancreatic enzymes raised in attacks of acute pancreatitis are normal in chronic disease.

- **Faecal elastase** (or chymotrypsin) has now largely replaced tests quantifying faecal fat. Tests of exocrine pancreatic function (e.g. pancreolauryl test) are useful in difficult cases, although usually a clinical response to pancreatic enzyme replacement is sufficient.
- **Abdominal CT**: may show pancreatic calcification and small pseudocysts. It might also be used to identify pancreatic masses (i.e. tumour).
- **Magnetic resonance cholaniopancreatography** (MRCP) (or, less commonly, ERCP): demonstrates pancreatic duct irregularity and pseudocystic change.

Management and prognosis

Pancreatic enzyme replacement with preparations such as Creon® and Pancrex® often improves both the pain and the malabsorption of chronic pancreatitis. The diabetes associated with chronic pancreatitis frequently requires insulin therapy. Opioid analgesia is frequently needed where pancreatic pain is dominant; a coeliac axis block may be necessary in selected cases.

Pancreatic cancer

Cancer of the pancreas remains a major source of mortality in the developed world. The incidence is increasing, and is now 11/100 000. The disease is more common in men (1.3:1) and African-Caribbean people (50% higher). Smoking and a high-fat/meat diet are risk factors. Most primary malignant tumours of the pancreas are adenocarcinomas although neuroendocrine tumours are not uncommon.

Clinical features

Pancreatic cancer is notorious for producing few or non-specific signs in the early stages. Painless jaundice caused by biliary obstruction is the most common presentation as the most common location for pancreatic tumours is in the pancreatic head. Tumours in the body or tail of the gland will present with weight loss and abdominal pain.

Investigations

- **Abdominal CT**: this is presently the best first-line investigation in patients where pancreatic cancer is suspected clinically. It is useful in establishing a diagnosis and may identify tumours that are potentially resectable (i.e. no invasion into important local structures such as the superior mesenteric vein or distant metastases).
- **MRCP**: is a valuable adjunct for specific examination of the biliary tree and in assessing for stone disease or strictures.
- **Endoscopic ultrasound**: this affords accurate assessment of pancreatic masses with particular reference to the local vessels (superior mesenteric vein and artery). It also facilitates targeted biopsy.
- **ERCP**: should be reserved until endoscopic therapy is expected/planned.

Management and prognosis

Too often, carcinoma of the pancreas is advanced at the time of presentation and there is no possibility of cure. Overall, 90% of individuals presenting with carcinoma of the pancreas will have succumbed to their disease within a year. Five-year survival is only 2%.

- **Surgery**: in some patients pancreaticoduodenectomy (Whipple procedure) offers the possibility of a surgical cure. Surgery may also be beneficial in patients with advanced disease in providing combined biliary and gastroduodenal bypass.
- **Chemotherapy**: gemcitabine chemotherapy is recommended for use in unresectable pancreatic adenocarcinoma but its role is at present palliative, aiming to slow progression of the disease. Other chemotherapy regimens undergoing clinical trials may yet bring better clinical outcomes.
- **Palliative measures**: stenting of biliary obstruction by either ERCP or percutaneous transhepatic cholangiography may relieve jaundice. Pancreatic pain may require opioid analgesia. Anorexia and weight loss remain major problems.

132 Inflammatory liver disease: viral and immune

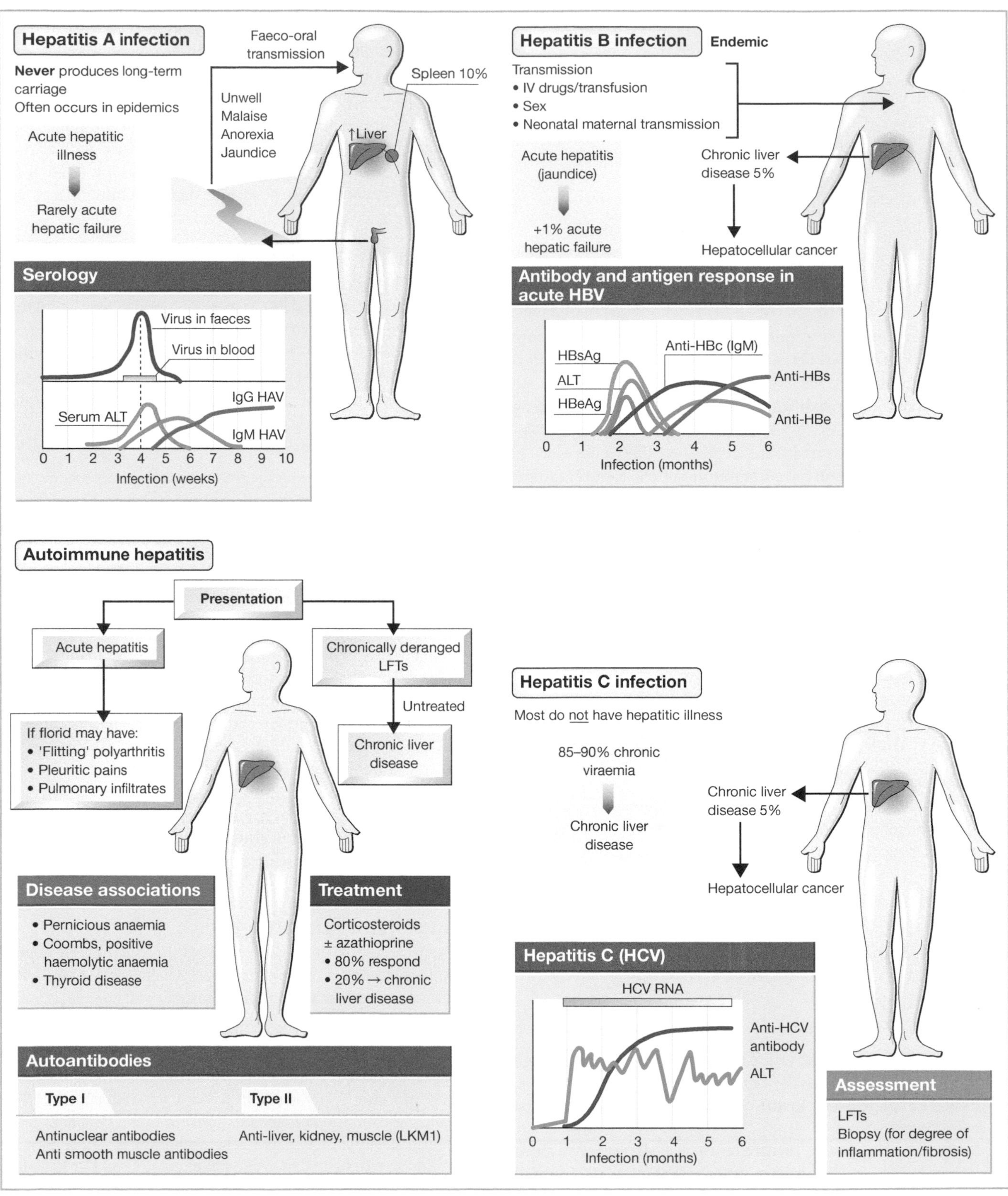

Medicine at a Glance, Fifth Edition. Edited by Patrick Davey and Alex Pitcher.

Companion website: www.wiley.com/go/medicine5e

Viral hepatitis

Hepatitis A virus (HAV)

Common cause of transient hepatitis; faecal–oral transmission.

- **Subclinical**: 50% of adults have IgG antibodies to HAV without previous jaundice.
- **Jaundice/acute hepatitis**: the most common presentation is an acute hepatitis, occasionally with a prolonged cholestatic phase. Fatigue, malaise, anorexia and nausea are prominent.
- **Fulminant liver failure**: very rarely.

Investigations

- **Liver blood tests** usually show an acute hepatocellular abnormality (i.e. predominant rise in aspartate transaminase/alanine aminotransferase, with less marked rises in bilirubin and alkaline phosphatase).
- **HAV IgM serology** in high titre is diagnostic of acute infection.

Management and prognosis

Clinical hepatitis usually settles with symptomatic management and rarely requires hospital admission. Evidence of liver failure (i.e. encephalopathy, coagulopathy) requires referral to a transplant centre. No risk of chronic liver disease/cirrhosis.

- **Similar pathogens**: hepatitis E gives a similar clinical picture, although the risk of acute hepatic failure in pregnancy is particularly high. Cytomegalovirus and Epstein–Barr virus are very rare causes of liver failure.

Hepatitis B virus (HBV)

Worldwide, HBV is the most common cause of chronic liver disease and hepatocellular carcinoma. The incidence of HBV in the UK is increasing, being common among intravenous (IV) drug users, migrant populations and individuals with high-risk sexual practices. It is a parenterally transmitted hepatotropic DNA virus. Genetic factors relating to the host immune response may account for the variability in clinical manifestations.

Clinical features

- **Acute hepatitis**: an acute jaundiced illness occurs in 15% of individuals exposed to HBV; there may be a six-month delay between exposure and illness.
- **Acute liver failure** is rare with HBV but more likely in those co-infected with HCV, human immunodeficiency virus (HIV) or hepatitis D (HDV or δ).
- **Chronic liver disease**: 5% of adults exposed to HBV develop chronic infection, more so in immunocompromised individuals (50% or more) and those acquiring the virus in early childhood (90%).
- **Hepatocellular carcinoma** (HCC) rates are increased 10-fold in HBV carriers.

Investigations

- **Liver biochemistry**: shows a non-specific hepatitic picture and may be normal.
- **HBV serology**: see figure above.
- **Hepatic elastography**: may be useful in detecting and monitoring significant liver fibrosis.
- **Other tests**: liver ultrasonography is needed to screen for focal liver abnormalities (particularly hepatocellular carcinoma). Liver biopsy may guide treatment in patients with chronic HBV.

Management and prognosis

- **Prevention**: individuals at risk (e.g. healthcare workers) should be immunized. Known virus carriers should know the risks to others of exposure to body fluids and should use barrier contraception.
- **General**: acute HBV infection rarely requires hospital admission. Follow-up is necessary to determine whether or not the virus has been cleared.
- **Antiviral therapy**: there is no helpful antiviral therapy during acute infection. Chronic infection may be clinically stable in many patients. Reactivation of disease activity in chronic carriers may require viral suppression with antiviral drugs (e.g. entecavir, tenofovir). Reactivation may also be seen with immunosuppression and close monitoring or prophylactic treatment is necessary. Interferon therapy may induce immune control.
- **Screening** for HCC: typically by six-monthly liver ultrasonography.
- **Liver transplantation**: indicated for decompensated cirrhosis and in selected patients with early hepatocellular carcinoma.

Hepatitis C virus (HCV)

Common; previously accounted for 25% of the liver disease burden in the UK, although this is falling. One of the major causes of chronic liver disease in the world. The RNA HCV virus is transmitted parenterally. It relies on a reverse transcriptase for replication, which has an inherently high error rate, resulting in high rates of viral mutation. This, among other features, means that the virus commonly escapes the immune response, and chronicity of viraemia is the consequence. Recently, however, the power of direct-acting antivirals has led to a fall in rates of transplantation for HCV.

Clinical features

- **Acute hepatitis**: this occurs in only a small number of patients.
- **Asymptomatic carriage**: in the majority of cases, the recipient is oblivious to the fact that they have acquired the virus, yet 85–90% of those exposed will develop chronic viraemia.
- **Chronic liver disease**: 20% of patients with chronic viraemia eventually develop liver fibrosis and clinical chronic liver disease. The rate of progression varies but the clinical course is accelerated by concurrent infection with HBV and excess alcohol consumption.

Investigations

- **Liver blood tests**: show relatively modest elevation in transaminases. The degree of liver blood test derangement bears little relation to the degree of underlying liver fibrosis (scarring).
- **Serological antibody tests** for HCV: the virus is identified in blood by the polymerase chain reaction and levels of viraemia can be quantified. Antibodies to HCV are measurable but persist after viral clearance. Virus genotyping guides selection of antiviral therapy.
- **Elastography**: determines liver stiffness and so fibrosis/cirrhosis.
- **Liver biopsy**: remains the only way to grade the disease in terms of necroinflammatory change in the liver, and also to stage the condition by defining the degree of liver fibrosis. With the advent of newer drugs and techniques to assess fibrosis, liver biopsy is less frequently used.

Management and prognosis

- **Prevention**: public health measures and education are important. There is no vaccine available or likely in the immediate future.
- **Antiviral therapy**.
  - Direct-acting antivirals have been revolutionary and provide all-oral, >95% effective cure. Previously, cure rates were much lower, treatment courses longer and side-effects much greater.
  - All patients with HCV viraemia should be considered for treatment.

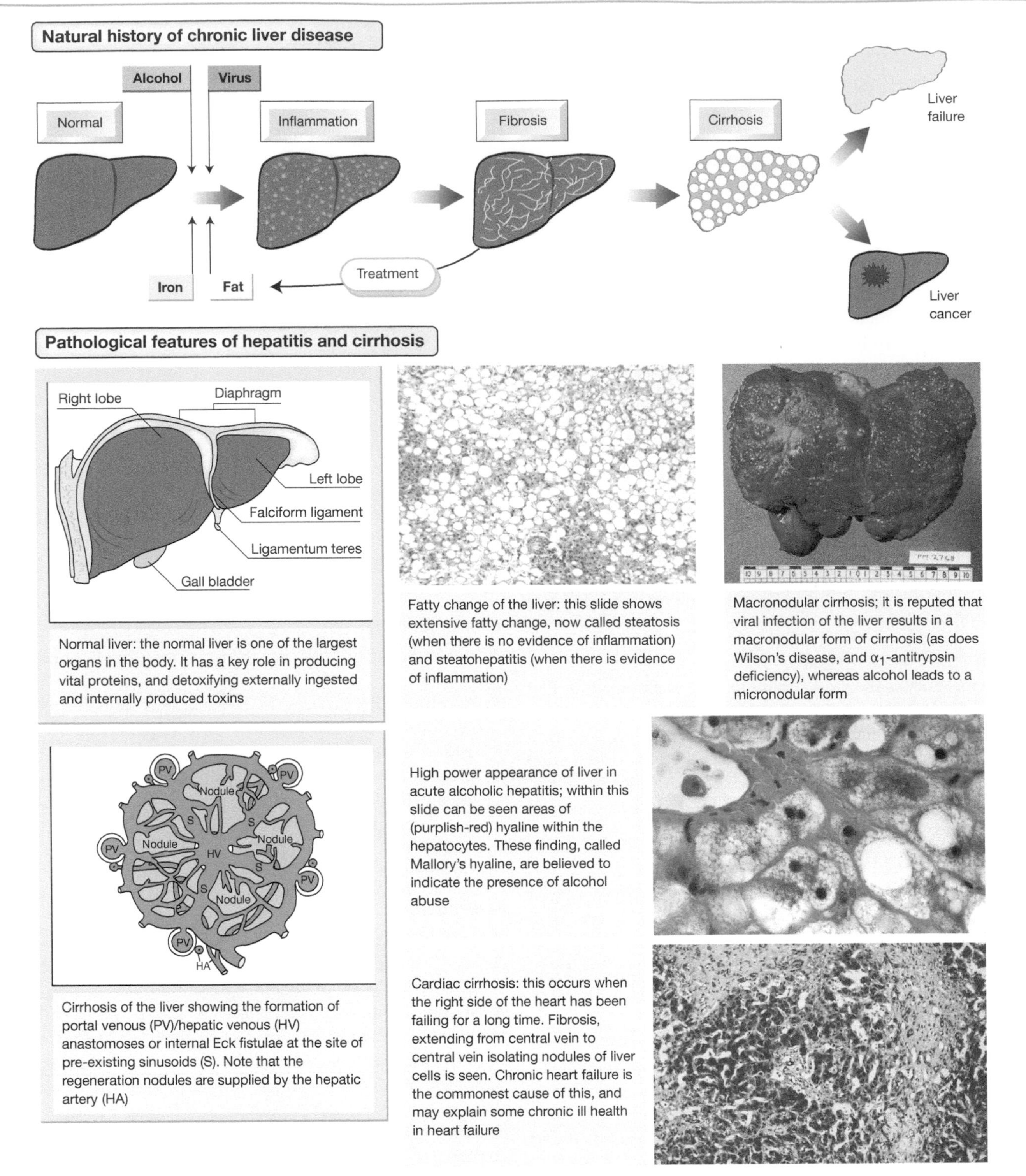

Normal liver: the normal liver is one of the largest organs in the body. It has a key role in producing vital proteins, and detoxifying externally ingested and internally produced toxins

Fatty change of the liver: this slide shows extensive fatty change, now called steatosis (when there is no evidence of inflammation) and steatohepatitis (when there is evidence of inflammation)

Macronodular cirrhosis; it is reputed that viral infection of the liver results in a macronodular form of cirrhosis (as does Wilson's disease, and α_1-antitrypsin deficiency), whereas alcohol leads to a micronodular form

High power appearance of liver in acute alcoholic hepatitis; within this slide can be seen areas of (purplish-red) hyaline within the hepatocytes. These finding, called Mallory's hyaline, are believed to indicate the presence of alcohol abuse

Cirrhosis of the liver showing the formation of portal venous (PV)/hepatic venous (HV) anastomoses or internal Eck fistulae at the site of pre-existing sinusoids (S). Note that the regeneration nodules are supplied by the hepatic artery (HA)

Cardiac cirrhosis: this occurs when the right side of the heart has been failing for a long time. Fibrosis, extending from central vein to central vein isolating nodules of liver cells is seen. Chronic heart failure is the commonest cause of this, and may explain some chronic ill health in heart failure

- Management of cirrhosis etc.; the elevated risk of hepatocellular carcinoma appears to persist after viral clearance.

- **Liver transplantation**: transplantation remains an important mode of therapy for patients with end-stage chronic liver disease. Viral recurrence in the transplanted organ is common.

Autoimmune hepatitis

Rare. Acute autoimmune inflammation is centred predominantly on the hepatic lobule, causing a range of clinical manifestations, ranging from fulminant hepatic failure to chronic liver disease and cirrhosis. Presentation is typically with:

- Jaundice.
- Fatigue.
- Arthralgia.
- Associated autoimmune conditions.

Less commonly autoimmune hepatitis presents with a persistent abnormality of liver blood tests:

- **Liver blood tests** usually show a predominant hepatocellular derangement of transaminases. A high titre of antinuclear antibodies often with smooth muscle (anti-actin) antibodies are found. In a few others, classified as having type II autoimmune hepatitis, autoantibodies may be demonstrable (e.g. liver/kidney microsomal antibody, soluble liver antigen). IgG is usually high.
- **Viral serology** must, given the usual acute presentation, be tested.

- **Liver biopsy** shows an acute lobular inflammation with interface hepatitis and may demonstrate features of chronicity (i.e. fibrosis).

Management and prognosis

- **Immunosuppression**: acute autoimmune hepatitis is very sensitive to high-dose steroids. Longer-term control often requires azathioprine.
- **Liver transplantation**: for fulminant liver failure and decompensated chronic liver disease.

Primary biliary cirrhosis

Rare (prevalence 90–150 per million) disease of mid-life women (male : female ratio 1 : 9). The pathology is of a non-suppurative, granulomatous inflammation centred predominantly on the small interlobular bile ducts, resulting in progressive fibrosis and ultimately cirrhosis. The cause is unknown but genetic loci associated with primary biliary cirrhosis (PBC) have recently been identified by genome-wide association studies.

Clinical features

The typical symptomatic presentation is of chronic progressive (intrahepatic) cholestasis with pruritis, lethargy and fatigue, progressing to steatorrhoea, and possibly with fat-soluble vitamin deficiency (A, D and K) syndromes. Some patients present with established chronic liver disease without prior symptomatic cholestasis. Increasingly, asymptomatic individuals are identified by abnormal liver blood tests with a positive mitochondrial antibody. Associated autoimmune conditions include autoimmune thyroid disease, diabetes and rheumatoid disease.

Investigations

- **Liver blood tests**: demonstrate a cholestatic picture (raised alkaline phosphatase with features of chronic liver disease in the advanced stages [i.e. low albumin]). Elevated (sometimes massively) levels of alkaline phosphatase may be the only abnormality on 'simple' blood tests. The antimitochondrial antibody and the M2 antibody directed at the 2-oxoacid dehydrogenase (E2) complex of the inner mitochondrial membrane are specific autoantibodies, and are found in 95% of patients with PBC. IgM is often raised.
- **Liver imaging** (ultrasonography): should be considered if extrahepatic biliary disease needs to be excluded (gallstones, primary sclerosing cholangitis [PSC]).
- **Liver biopsy**: shows features of PBC and fibrosis, the extent of which has prognostic value.

Management and prognosis

PBC progresses slowly, ultimately resulting in cirrhosis. Treatment of pruritis and fatigue is disappointing, although ursodeoxycholic acid may help. Chronic cholestasis increases the risk of osteopenia (see Chapter 216). Liver transplantation is excellent for persistent jaundice and decompensated chronic liver disease.

Primary sclerosing cholangitis

PSC is an uncommon, complex, probably autoimmune disorder, strongly associated with inflammatory bowel disease. The pattern varies considerably. Inflammation may predominantly involve the intralobular bile ducts – intrahepatic (small duct) PSC – or the extrahepatic biliary strictures – extrahepatic (large duct) PSC. Many patients have both small and large duct disease.

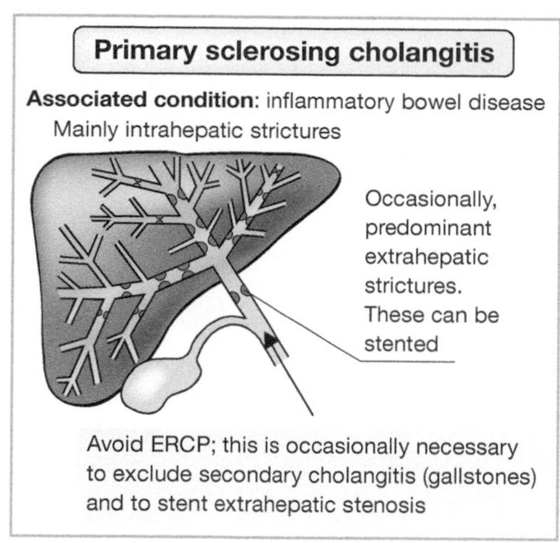

Primary sclerosing cholangitis
Associated condition: inflammatory bowel disease
Mainly intrahepatic strictures
Occasionally, predominant extrahepatic strictures. These can be stented
Avoid ERCP; this is occasionally necessary to exclude secondary cholangitis (gallstones) and to stent extrahepatic stenosis

Clinical features

- **Abnormal LFTs** are the most common presentation (especially increased alkaline phosphatase). Positive antineutrophil cytoplasmic antibody (ANCA) occurs in 80%; antimitochondrial antibodies are not found.
- **Recurrent bacterial cholangitis** with right upper quadrant (RUQ) pain, fever and jaundice may occur in those with dominant extrahepatic disease.
- **Chronic cholestasis and chronic liver disease** are common.
- **Inflammatory bowel disease** may be diagnosed after PSC.

Investigations

- **LFTs**: often demonstrate a mixed pattern of 'hepatitic' and 'cholestatic' abnormalities.
- **Tumour marker CA19-9** may indicate cholangiocarcinoma.
- **ANCA**.
- **Liver ultrasonography** to exclude focal liver lesions (i.e. cholangiocarcinoma).
- **Magnetic resonance cholangiopancreatography** (MRCP) or **endoscopic retrograde cholangiopancreatography** (ERCP) may demonstrate multiple biliary strictures. Dominant strictures should be brushed and bile aspirated for cytology.
- **Liver biopsy** demonstrates features consistent with PSC – the onion-skin lesion around an obliterated bile duct.

Management and prognosis

The clinical course varies considerably and unpredictably. Symptomatic patients are largely dead in 10–15 years, though some 75% of asymptomatic patients are alive after 15 years. Bacterial cholangitis requires antibiotics. Pruritis may improve with ursodeoxycholic acid. There is no specific therapy. Liver transplantation is used for those with a rapidly progressive clinical course and decompensated chronic liver disease. Cholangiocarcinoma risk is increased and has a very poor prognosis.

133 Metabolic liver disease (including alcohol)

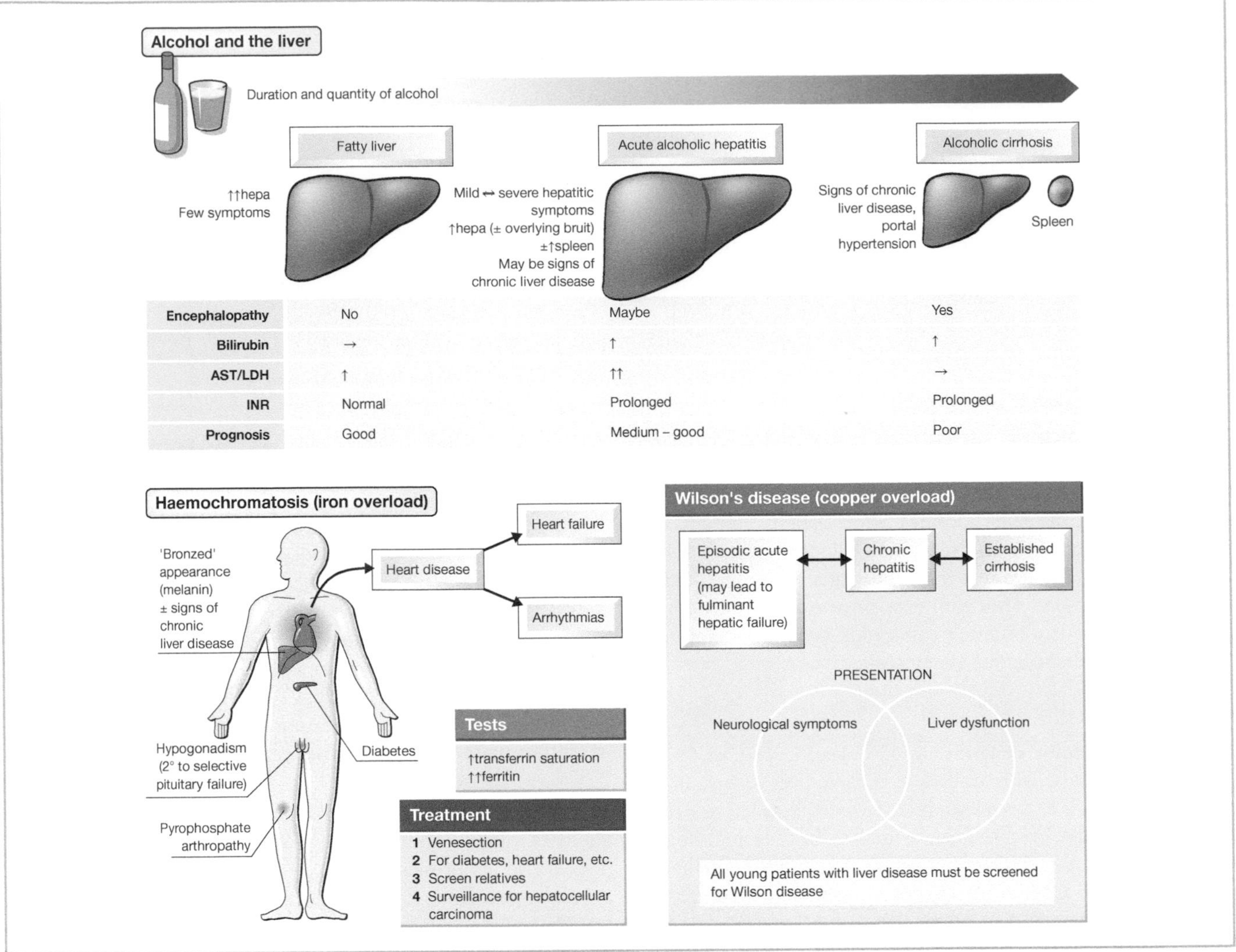

Alcoholic liver disease

The relationship between alcohol and chronic liver disease is complex. Clearly, excess alcohol consumption is a risk factor for chronic liver disease. However, individual susceptibility varies considerably and typical alcohol-related pathology is increasingly seen in individuals who drink modest amounts of alcohol (non-alcoholic steatohepatitis; see Chapter 126).

Incidence

Common. Alcohol remains the most widespread drug of abuse in the world. Despite this, only a fifth of people with alcohol problems develop features of chronic liver disease.

Pathophysiology

Many theories have been proposed to explain alcohol-related liver injury. Many focus on the acetaldehyde derivatives of alcohol. There may be important genetic factors. There are three pathological forms of alcoholic liver disease.

- **Fatty liver**: occurs in 50% of heavy drinkers – reversible on alcohol cessation.
- **Acute alcoholic hepatitis**: occurs in only a proportion of heavy drinkers – most commonly after long periods of heavy drinking. Commonly associated with underlying cirrhosis.
- **Cirrhosis**: a man consuming 210 g ethanol (= 2.5 bottles of wine) a day for 22 years has an approximately 50% chance of developing cirrhosis.

Quantifying of alcohol

Typically, ethanol (ethyl alcohol) is measured in units, often expressed per week.

- In the UK, one unit is 10 ml (8 g) of ethanol; 25 ml of 40% spirit or 250 ml of 4% beer represents one unit. Across the European Union, 10 g of pure ethanol most typically represents one unit but there is a range from 8 to 20 g.

Medicine at a Glance, Fifth Edition. Edited by Patrick Davey and Alex Pitcher.

Companion website: www.wiley.com/go/medicine5e

- Elsewhere, the concept of a standard drink may be used: in the US this has 14 g of ethanol, in Australia 10 g.

Clinical features

Alcohol-related liver injury may present in many different ways.

- Chance finding of abnormal liver blood tests.
- **Decompensated chronic liver disease** (gastrointestinal [GI] bleeding, ascites).
- **Acute alcoholic hepatitis**: this presentation is particularly challenging. Often, there is a long history of alcohol use and then, the apparently sudden onset of jaundice often with anorexia, nausea, malaise, fever and neutrophil leukocytosis.

Investigations

Although clinicians have previously relied on γ-glutamyl transferase and mean cell volume as indicators of alcohol abuse, these are unreliable. A good clinical history (often with corroborative testimonies of relatives) is still the best method for determining alcohol dependence, possibly supported with random ethanol levels. Additional methods such as ethyl glucuronide testing have limited availability but are used in some centres.

Management and prognosis

Management of patients with alcohol-related liver injury involves the following aspects.

- Addressing the difficult challenge of total abstinence from alcohol.
- In alcoholic cirrhosis, five-year survival is 70% in abstinent patients and only 35% in drinkers.
- Objectively assessing the degree of chronic liver disease (biopsy for fibrosis).
- Hepatocellular carcinoma occurs in 15% of people with alcoholic cirrhosis; surveillance for this may be indicated.

Haemochromatosis

Haemochromatosis is the term used to describe primary iron overload (total body iron of >5 g vs normal stores of <3 g). In most cases, iron overload is the result of increased GI absorption of iron. The excess iron is deposited in many organs, resulting in damage.

Incidence

The mutation in the *HFE* gene on chromosome 6, responsible for a large majority of cases of haemochromatosis (*C282Y*), is common in white people, with a prevalence of up to 1:150 in populations with a strong Celtic ancestry (e.g. the Irish). This makes haemochromatosis the most common single gene disorder to affect north-west European populations. Despite this, symptomatic presentation remains rare and even biochemical penetrance, the development of increased ferritin, is variable. The reason for these disparities is not clear.

Pathophysiology

The *C282Y* mutation in the *HFE* gene prevents cell surface expression of the protein. How this leads to the demonstrable increase in GI iron absorption is still not clear. Once absorbed, excess iron is deposited in the liver and other organs (pancreas, heart, joints). This leads to liver fibrosis and ultimately a risk of hepatocellular carcinoma. Penetrance is, however, variable even in *C282Y* homozygotes.

Clinical features

The original 'classic' description of haemochromatosis was of bronzed diabetes with a pigmented cirrhosis and heavy iron deposition in the liver, pancreas (provoking diabetes) and heart (leading to heart failure). Joint involvement, often producing a pyrophosphate arthropathy, was in many cases the most disabling symptom. The bronzed discoloration of the skin was due to excess secretion of melanocyte-stimulating hormone from the pituitary. This 'full-blown' clinical presentation is rarely seen today and increasingly the diagnosis is made in patients without distinctive clinical symptoms or physical signs.

Secondary haemochromatosis may also be seen in patients who have received multiple transfusions over years, e.g. those with haemoglobinopathies or myelodysplasia.

Investigations

- **Liver blood tests**: non-specific hepatitis usually with a raised alanine transaminase.
- **Iron indices**: ferritin and transferrin saturation increased. Ferritin levels are often very high, not infrequently >1000 mg/L (normal <300 mg/L).
- **Assessment of fibrosis**: liver biopsy shows a characteristic distribution of iron and provides important information on staging (i.e. the degree of liver fibrosis). Elastography is useful.
- Assessment of iron overload, e.g. with T2* MRI.
- **Genetic mutation analysis**: 90% of haemochromatosis patients of European descent are homozygous for the *C282Y* mutation in *HFE*. The other key mutation of note is *H63D*.

There are rarer forms of haemochromatosis to be considered in patients with otherwise unexplained iron overload.

Management and prognosis

- **Venesection**: 500 g of whole blood removed regularly until excess iron stores are removed (which takes up to 12–18 months in heavily iron-loaded individuals). Thereafter, venesection is adjusted to control ferritin.
- **Surveillance for hepatocellular carcinoma**: in patients who have developed cirrhosis before the diagnosis has been made, there remains a risk of developing hepatocellular carcinoma and in these cases it may be appropriate to regularly test α-fetoprotein and undertake liver ultrasonography.
- **Screening first-degree relatives**: this process has been greatly facilitated by *HFE* mutation analysis.

Wilson disease

Rare (worldwide incidence 1–30 per million), autosomal recessive disorder of copper metabolism resulting in copper overload. Arises when mutations in the gene coding for a copper transport protein (*ATP7B*, chromosome 13q14.3) lead to failure of biliary excretion of copper and thus progressive copper accumulation. This often results in hepatic and neurological damage. It usually presents in children and young adults; there is an equal sex incidence. Kayser–Fleischer rings may be identified in the eyes by slit-lamp examination. There are various presentations.

- **Hepatic**: acute hepatitis. Fulminant liver failure or chronic liver disease/cirrhosis.
- **Neuropsychiatric**: extrapyramidal disturbance/psychosis.
- **Haematological**: acute intravascular haemolysis.

Investigations

- **Copper studies**: serum copper (low); caeruloplasmin (low in 80%); 24-hour urinary copper (increased).
- **Liver biopsy**: defines degree of fibrosis as well as quantifying copper load.
- **Cerebral computed tomography/magnetic resonance imaging**.
- **Genetics**: although there is a wide variety of mutations, these are increasingly well defined.

Management and prognosis

- **Liver disease**: penicillamine is used to chelate copper, which is then excreted in the urine. Other chelating agents include zinc and trientine. Severe liver disease has been successfully treated with liver transplantation.
- **Neuropsychiatric disease** is often permanent.
- **Screening** of first-degree relatives.

134 Acute and chronic liver disease

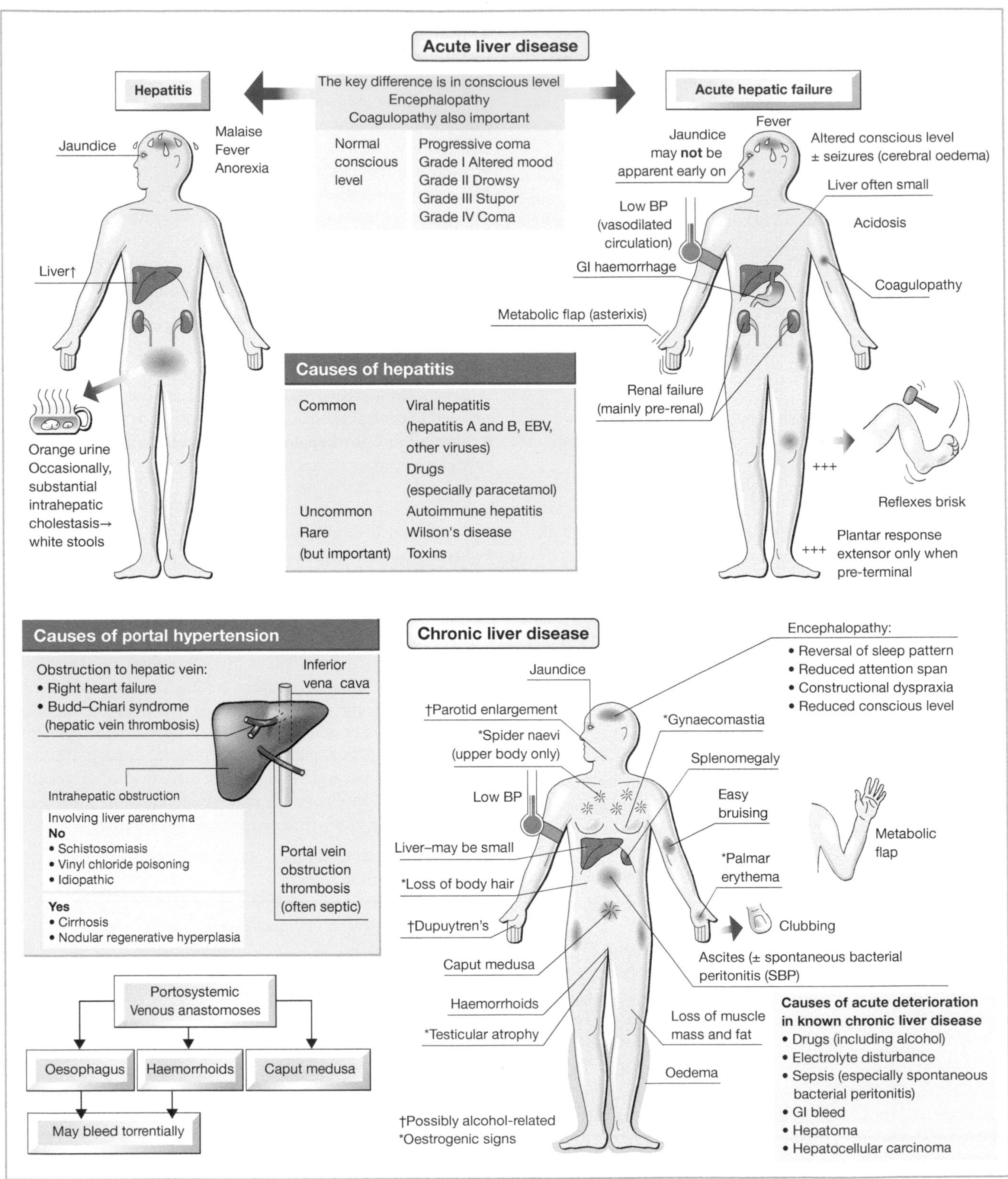

Medicine at a Glance, Fifth Edition. Edited by Patrick Davey and Alex Pitcher.

Companion website: www.wiley.com/go/medicine5e

Acute hepatitis

This non-specific term refers to a short-term (self-limiting) liver inflammation. There are many causes (see figure above). Jaundice, nausea and anorexia, right upper quadrant discomfort, fever and fatigue occur.

Investigations

- **Liver biochemistry**: hepatitic enzymes, alanine transaminase; cholestatic enzymes – alkaline phosphatase; synthetic function tests – prothrombin time, albumin.
- **Tests to determine cause**: viral serology, immunoglobulins and autoantibody profile, iron indices, α_1-antitrypsin, copper.
- **Liver ultrasonography**: to exclude structural lesions (e.g. neoplasia, biliary disease, etc.).

Management and prognosis

Stop all potentially harmful drugs. Prognosis is usually good but a minority require liver transplantation to survive.

Acute liver failure

The term 'acute liver failure' traditionally describes the progression from jaundice to hepatic encephalopathy within 12 weeks. In the King's/O'Grady definition, this is subdivided into hyperacute at <1 week (e.g. from paracetamol), acute 2–4 weeks (e.g. from a viral infection), or subacute 4–12 weeks.

Other classifications use the terms 'fulminant' or 'severe' which may be defined as acute liver failure occurring between two and eight weeks from jaundice.

Clinical features

- **Encephalopathy** is the clinical hallmark of liver failure, characterized by a progressive deterioration in cognitive function from a shortened attention span through a reversal of sleep pattern to deep coma. The characteristic clinical sign is the metabolic flap (or asterixis), a coarse and irregular flapping tremor of the hands.
- **Jaundice**: depending on the rate of deterioration, jaundice may not initially be clinically evident.
- **Haemorrhage** may be confined to the gastrointestinal (GI) tract or occur widely as a result of haemostatic failure.
- **Acidosis (typically with high lactic acid), hypoglycaemia and renal failure**.

Investigations

- **Prothrombin time** is the single best prognostic marker. Coagulopathy should not be corrected (with blood products) unless bleeding is otherwise life-threatening.
- **Blood glucose** should be measured frequently. Hypoglycaemia is an ominous sign.
- **Electrolytes**: renal impairment most commonly relates to a degree of acute tubular necrosis on admission, rather than reflecting a true hepatorenal syndrome.
- **Arterial blood gases**: lactic metabolic acidosis is a poor sign.
- **Paracetamol level** should be measured in all cases and is a common cause of acute liver failure in the UK; it may be amenable to medical treatment (*N*-acetylcysteine).

Management and prognosis

- **Airway management**: patients can deteriorate quickly. Those with progressive coma should undergo early intubation and ventilation, especially if between-hospital transfer occurs.
- **Optimize circulatory state**: patients have a hyperdynamic circulation with lowered systemic vascular resistance. The degree of volume depletion on admission is often underestimated.

Table 134.1 Indications for referral to a liver transplant unit in acute liver failure.

Paracetamol-induced acute liver failure	Non-paracetamol-induced acute liver failure
Arterial pH <7.3 or HCO_2 <18	Arterial pH <7.3 or HCO_2 <18
INR >3.0 on day two or >4.0 thereafter	INR >1.8
Oliguria and/or AKI	Oliguria and/or AKI or Na <130 mmol/l
Altered level of consciousness Hypoglycaemia	Encephalopathy, hypoglycaemia or metabolic acidosis
Elevated arterial lactate >4.0 mmol/l unresponsive to fluid resuscitation	Bilirubin >300 micromol/l

AKI, acute kidney injury; INR, international normalized ratio.

- ***N*-acetylcysteine** is the antidote to paracetamol poisoning, although increasing evidence suggests that it might benefit patients with acute liver failure from all causes.
- **Broad-spectrum antibiotics** and systemic antifungals.

Indications for liver transplant unit referral and possible transplantation are as follows (see also Table 134.1).

- Encephalopathy or raised intracranial pressure (ICP). Signs of CNS oedema include BP >160/90 mmHg (sustained) or brief rises (systolic >200 mmHg), bradycardia, decerebrate posture, extensor spasms and poor pupil responses. ICP monitoring can help.
- INR >2.0 at or before 48 hours or >3.5 at or before 72 hours (so measure INR every 12 hours). Peak elevation occurs around 72–96 hours. Liver chemistry is not a good marker of hepatocyte death.
- Renal impairment (creatinine >200 μmol/l). Monitor urine flow and daily U&E and serum creatinine (use haemodialysis if >400 μmol/l).
- Blood pH <7.3 (lactic acidosis results in tissue hypoxia).
- Systolic BP <80 mmHg despite adequate fluid resuscitation.
- Hypoglycaemia.
- Metabolic acidosis (pH <7.3 or bicarbonate <18 mmol/l).

Chronic liver disease

Much liver pathology follows an indolent course and presents with clinical features of chronic liver disease. Compensated chronic liver disease implies a (relatively) well patient, whereas those with 'decompensated' chronic liver disease have substantial symptoms and/or signs.

Pathophysiology and clinical features

Long-term, low-grade liver damage results in progressive liver fibrosis, which presents with a combination of reduced liver cell mass and function, and portal hypertension. These cause the clinical features – the relative dominance of one over the other varies between patients.

- Weakness, anorexia and muscle loss.
- GI bleeding from portosystemic venous anastomoses (i.e. varices).
- Ascites: possibly complicated by spontaneous bacterial peritonitis.
- Jaundice.
- Encephalopathy.

Problems caused by reduced liver cell mass

- **Encephalopathy**: the hallmark of liver cell failure and a common, albeit subtle, feature of most patients with chronic liver disease, causing a reduced attention span and reversed sleep pattern (insomnia and daytime somnolence). A metabolic flap may be found (asterixis). With more advanced encephalopathy, patients demonstrate a constructional dyspraxia and ultimately progress to hepatic coma. Encephalopathy can be worsened by portosystemic shunting (which is sometimes used as a treatment, e.g. in transjugular intrahepatic portosystemic shunt placement).
- **Loss of lean body mass** is usually most evident at the shoulders. The accumulation of body water (oedema and ascites) means that the extent of muscle loss is underestimated.
- **Coagulopathy**.
- **Hypoalbuminaemia** and **immune dysfunction.**

Problems caused by portal hypertension

- **Varices**: form at sites of portosystemic communication, most commonly in the lower oesophagus but also including the stomach, small bowel and rectum. GI bleeding, sometimes torrential, may be the first presentation of chronic liver disease and can provoke decompensation of the chronic liver disease.
- **Ascites**: the result of sodium retention, possibly contributed to by high portal pressure and low albumin. It is important to exclude spontaneous bacterial peritonitis, as this commonly complicates low protein ascites resulting from cirrhosis.
- **Shunting:** from the portal to systemic circulations, may provoke encephalopathy.

Investigations

These are directed to identify the cause of the underlying liver disease and identify the triggers for decompensation (infection, bleeding, drugs, electrolyte disturbance, hepatocellular carcinoma).

- **Haematology**: haemoglobin may be low, as a result of bleeding and hypersplenism. The prothrombin time is prolonged, as a result of synthetic failure ± disseminated intravascular coagulation (DIC).
- **Autoimmune profile**/immunoglobulins.
- **Iron** studies (haemochromatosis) and **copper** studies (Wilson disease).
- **Viral serology** (hepatitis B surface antigen and C virus antibody ± PCR).
- α_1**-Antitrypsin levels**, to exclude α_1-antitrypsin deficiency.
- **Liver biopsy** in selected cases.

Management

Identify and treat the cause of the clinical decompensation (see figure above).

Treatment of acute complications

- **Variceal bleeding**: blood product support, urgent endoscopy, with band ligation of the varices. Vasoconstrictors (terlipressin) are a short-term but complementary measure. In overwhelming haemorrhage, balloon tamponade (Minnesota or Sengstaken–Blakemore tube) may be tried. Acute percutaneous portosystemic shunting (transjugular intrahepatic portosystemic shunt [TIPS]) can also control bleeding. In the long term, injection/banding of varices and/or non-cardioselective β-blockers such as propranolol reduce the risk of haemorrhage.
- **Ascites**: spironolactone and salt restriction are useful.
- **Encephalopathy:** provoking factors are removed/treated (opioids, benzodiazepines, constipating agents). Minimize absorption of dietary nitrogenous substances using lactulose. Enemas may be useful to speed bowel transit acutely.

Long-term management and prognosis

Prognosis is unpredictable but relates to the Child–Turcotte–Pugh class (see Table 134.2).

- If a clear aetiology is identified, treatment can restore good health even if cirrhosis is present (e.g. haemochromatosis, hepatitis C virus or autoimmune hepatitis).
- **Hepatocellular carcinoma**: may complicate long-standing cirrhosis from some aetiologies (viral hepatitis, haemochromatosis, alcohol). Regular liver ultrasonography is recommended for early tumour detection.
- Treatment-refractory symptoms may be relieved by **liver transplantation** in selected cases.
- Varices should be sought with endoscopy and considered for pharmacological or banding prophylaxis.
- Bone density assessment should be considered.
- Immunizations should be completed, including to hepatitis A and B.
- Encephalopathy management may require lactulose, enemas and/or rifaximin.

EASL Clinical Practice Guidelines for the management of patients with decompensated cirrhosis, 2018.

EASL Clinical Practical Guidelines on the management of acute liver failure, 2018.

Bernal W, Wendon J. (2013) Acute liver failure. N Engl J Med 26: 2525–2534. http://doi.org/10.1056/NEJMra1208937

Table 134.2 Child–Turcotte–Pugh scoring system.

Criterion	1 point	2 points	3 points
Bilirubin	<34 µmol/l <2 mg/dl	34–51 µmol/l 2–3 mg/dl	>51 µmol/l >3 mg/dl
Albumin (g/L)	>35 g/l	28–35 g/l	<28 g/l
Ascites	None	Controlled	Poorly controlled
Encephalopathy	None	Minimal	Advanced
Prothrombin time prolongation	<4 s (INR <1.7)	4–6 s (INR 1.7–2.3)	>6 s (INR >2.3)

Child–Turcotte–Pugh score: A = 5–6 points; B = 7–9 points; C = ≥10 points

CTP A ~ 95% 1-year survival (98% for A5; 90% for A6)
CTP B ~ 80% 1-year survival
CTP C ~ 45% 1-year survival

135 Functional gastrointestinal disorders

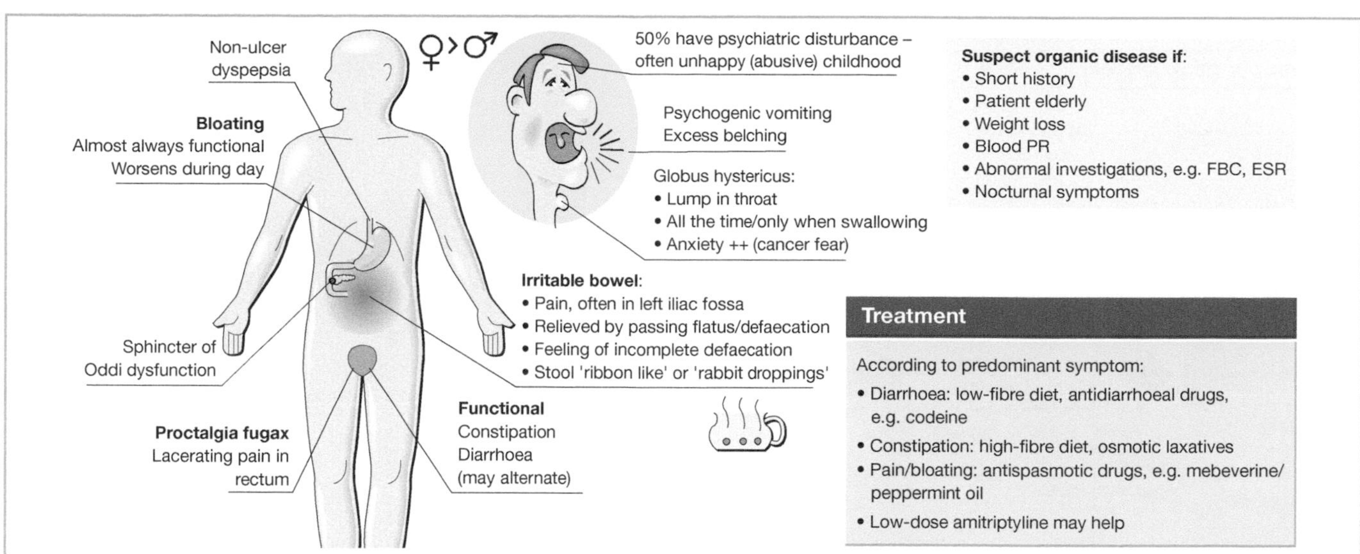

Irritable bowel syndrome is a widely used term with relatively limited clinical value. It represents one of many functional syndromes of gut sensitivity and/or motility that affect any part of the gastrointestinal (GI) tract. Examples include globus hystericus, non-ulcer dyspepsia, irritable bowel syndrome, functional diarrhoea, functional constipation, proctalgia fugax and sphincter of Oddi dysfunction.

The common link between these conditions is that they have characteristic symptom complexes without clinical or laboratory features to suggest progressive intestinal pathology.

Incidence and pathophysiology

The prevalence depends on definition. Ten percent of the population consults doctors with functional GI complaints; 20% who consider themselves normal admit to symptoms consistent with irritable bowel. Other overlapping symptom complexes include chronic fatigue syndrome, fibromyalgia, headache and functional gynaecological symptoms. In some individuals, episodes of gut insult (e.g. severe gastroenteritis) may have triggered the problem (postinfective irritable bowel). Sufferers may have heightened visceral sensory awareness.

Clinical features

Although the symptoms vary enormously, there are some patterns that dominate.

- **Bloating**.
- **Marked gastrocolic reflex** (the need to defaecate shortly after eating).
- **Identifiable dietary precipitants**: specific foods may cause symptoms, e.g. dairy products, fatty or spicy foods and alcohol.
- **Pain** relieved by defaecation.
- **Chaotic bowel habit**: patients often describe an increased frequency of defaecation with clustering in the morning – the 'cork out of the champagne bottle' effect.
- **Stress** may be an overt feature even if this is not recognized by the patient.

Some symptoms should not be put down to a functional cause without further investigation.

- Dysphagia.
- Anorexia and/or weight loss.
- Nocturnal diarrhea.
- Rectal bleeding.

Management and prognosis

The extent of clinical investigation to exclude a progressive intestinal pathology must be individually tailored. A detailed history (including dietary) from the patient is central to correct diagnosis and management. A full and thorough examination should be undertaken. Thereafter, investigations depend largely on the patient's particular symptom complex. As a minimum, a basic blood screen including haematology, biochemistry and inflammatory markers should be performed.

The process of undergoing an in-depth history and physical examination can be therapeutic and often the qualified reassurance of being told that there is no objective evidence of physical disease is sufficient to improve symptoms (or at least the resulting concern). It is important to avoid unnecessary over-investigation in the absence of concerning clinical features.

- **Antispasmodic drugs**: mebeverine or alverine are useful for colicky abdominal pain.
- **Anticholinergics**: low doses of amitriptyline help those with depressive features (low mood, anhedonia, rumination, poor sleep, etc.). Relaxation therapy may also help.
- **Antidiarrhoeal** drugs: e.g. loperamide.
- **Dietary measures**: patients resistant to the above measures or those with clearly identifiable dietary intolerances may benefit from dietary intervention (reduction in insoluble fibre, low-lactose diet, exclusion diet). Paradoxically, many patients with an irritable bowel find that their symptoms worsen with a high-fibre diet.

Medicine at a Glance, Fifth Edition. Edited by Patrick Davey and Alex Pitcher.

Companion website: www.wiley.com/go/medicine5e

136 Upper gastrointestinal cancer

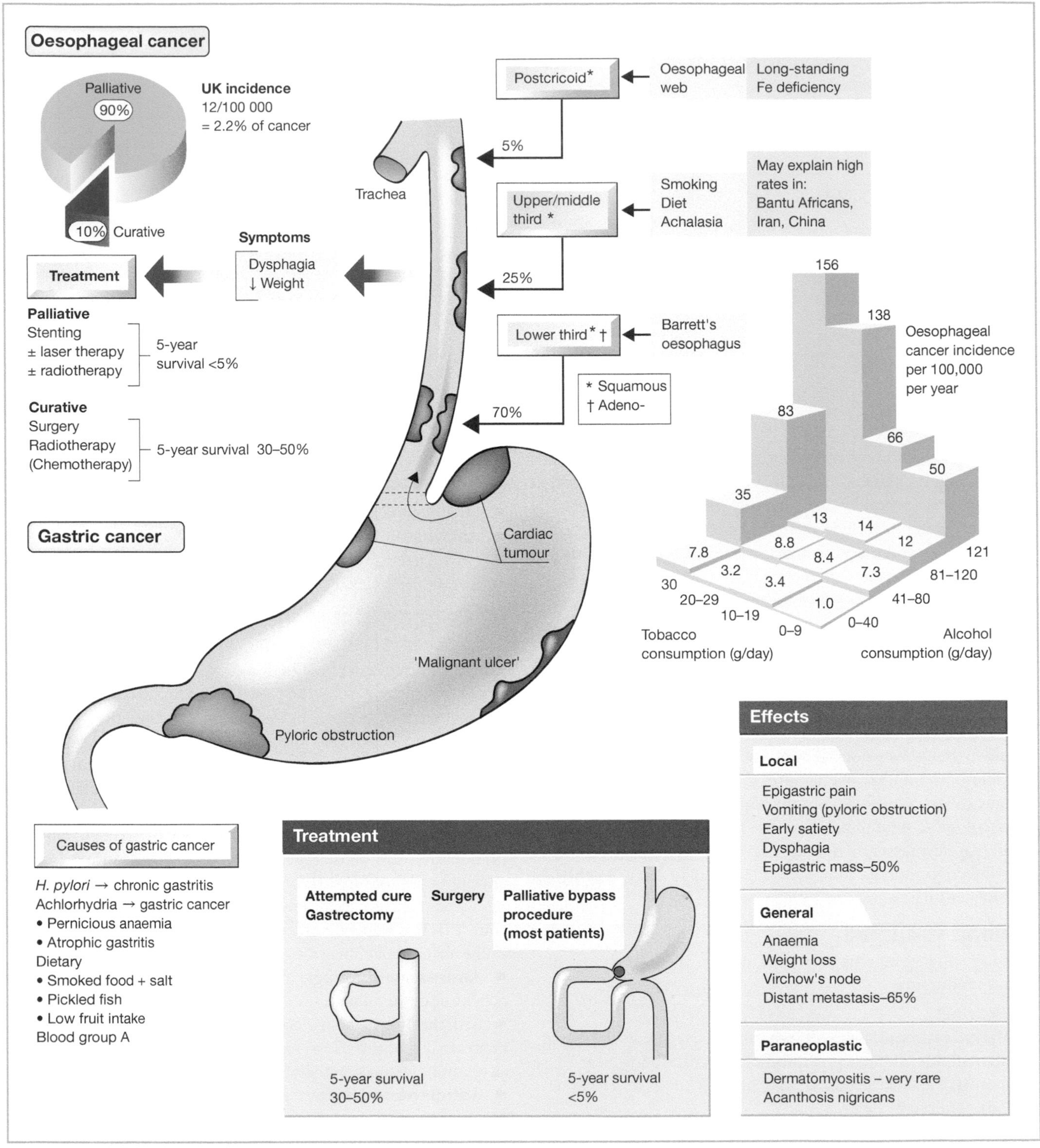

Causes of gastric cancer

H. pylori → chronic gastritis
Achlorhydria → gastric cancer
- Pernicious anaemia
- Atrophic gastritis

Dietary
- Smoked food + salt
- Pickled fish
- Low fruit intake

Blood group A

Treatment

Attempted cure Gastrectomy	Surgery	Palliative bypass procedure (most patients)
5-year survival 30–50%		5-year survival <5%

Effects

Local

Epigastric pain
Vomiting (pyloric obstruction)
Early satiety
Dysphagia
Epigastric mass–50%

General

Anaemia
Weight loss
Virchow's node
Distant metastasis–65%

Paraneoplastic

Dermatomyositis – very rare
Acanthosis nigricans

Medicine at a Glance, Fifth Edition. Edited by Patrick Davey and Alex Pitcher.

Companion website: www.wiley.com/go/medicine5e

Oesophageal carcinoma

Incidence

Although squamous carcinoma is declining in the western world, in keeping with the reduction in cigarette smoking, adenocarcinoma of the distal oesophagus/gastric cardia is increasing throughout the world. The UK incidence is 12 per 100 000, with a 50% increase in incidence over the last 20 years.

Pathophysiology

The two different tumour types behave very differently.

- **Squamous carcinoma** most commonly affects the middle third of the oesophagus. There is a strong association with cigarette smoking.
- **Adenocarcinoma** most commonly affects the lower third of the oesophagus and merges pathologically with carcinoma of the gastric cardia. Most theories on the cause of distal oesophageal adenocarcinoma involve chronic gastro-oesophageal reflux of both acid and possibly bile.

Clinical features

The major clinical feature relating to oesophageal malignancy is **dysphagia**. Rapidly progressive dysphagia (i.e. dysphagia to solids progressing to dysphagia to soft food and liquids) and weight loss at the time of presentation are particularly worrying features.

Investigations

Progressive dysphagia always requires urgent investigation (see Chapter 29).

- **Endoscopy** will achieve a histological diagnosis and allows symptom relief (oesophageal dilation).
- **Computed tomography** (CT): in patients suitable for consideration of surgery (bearing in mind the high prevalence of significant co-morbidity), a CT of the chest and upper abdomen will exclude gross pulmonary and/or hepatic metastases and may identify local invasion into other important structures such as the pericardium or aorta.
- **Positron emission tomography** scanning is being used increasingly in the preoperative assessment of oesophageal patients being considered for surgery.
- **Endoscopic ultrasonography** is more sensitive than CT for detecting local tumour invasion.
- **Staging laparoscopy**: occasionally undertaken before attempted curative surgery, because malignant spread to lymph nodes may be missed on CT scan.

Management and prognosis

The prognosis is poor, with a five-year survival of 9%.

- **Endoscopic resection** may be possible for very localized disease and is associated with fewer adverse events.
- **Surgery**: this offers the best chance of cure, which justifies the efforts put into preoperative staging, although even with 'curative' resection the five-year survival rate is <20%.
- **Radiotherapy and chemotherapy**: squamous carcinoma of the oesophagus is sensitive to radiotherapy and newer combination regimens are proving beneficial in adenocarcinoma as well.
- **Palliative procedures**: even without the possibility of cure, it is possible to alleviate the distressing symptom of dysphagia.
- **Stenting**: in tumours causing mediastinal encasement, stenting with self-expanding metal stents provides reasonable palliation.

Gastric carcinoma

Incidence

The incidence of gastric carcinoma (other than that of the gastric cardia) is decreasing (17 per 100 000). There is a higher incidence in males than in females.

Pathophysiology

Predisposing factors include atrophic gastritis and previous surgery for peptic ulcer disease. The role of *Helicobacter pylori* in the aetiopathogenesis of upper gastrointestinal (GI) malignancy is controversial. There is an association between *H. pylori* infection and the development of gastric lymphoma (MALToma, where MALT is mucosa-associated lymphoid tissue), but the relationship with adenocarcinoma is less clear.

Clinical features

Gastric cancer often presents late because there are no early clinical symptoms. Although dyspepsia remains a common prompt for diagnostic endoscopy, ironically patients with gastric cancer often have reduced gastric acid output (e.g. gastric atrophy). Many gastric cancers will prove to be at an advanced stage at the time they are identified.

- **Anaemia**: occult GI bleeding and the resulting iron deficiency are probably the most common ways in which gastric carcinoma presents (see Chapter 125).
- **Weight loss** is common and suggests advanced or metastatic disease.
- **Vomiting**: indicates impending gastric outflow obstruction.

Investigations

- **Endoscopy**: including biopsies for histological confirmation of the diagnosis.
- **Abdominal CT** for staging, i.e. to detect hepatic and other metastasis.
- Occasionally **laparoscopy ± PET.**

Management and prognosis

The prognosis is poor, with a five-year survival of 12%.

- **Surgery** should be considered in most cases because, even in tumours that are advanced at the time of presentation, a surgical bypass (i.e. gastrojejunostomy) can provide good palliation. Increasingly, laparoscopy is being used to stage the tumour before any attempted resection.
- **Chemotherapy and radiotherapy**: these modalities tend to be less useful in gastric carcinoma.
- **Immunotherapy** is being explored as part of trials.

137 Colorectal cancer

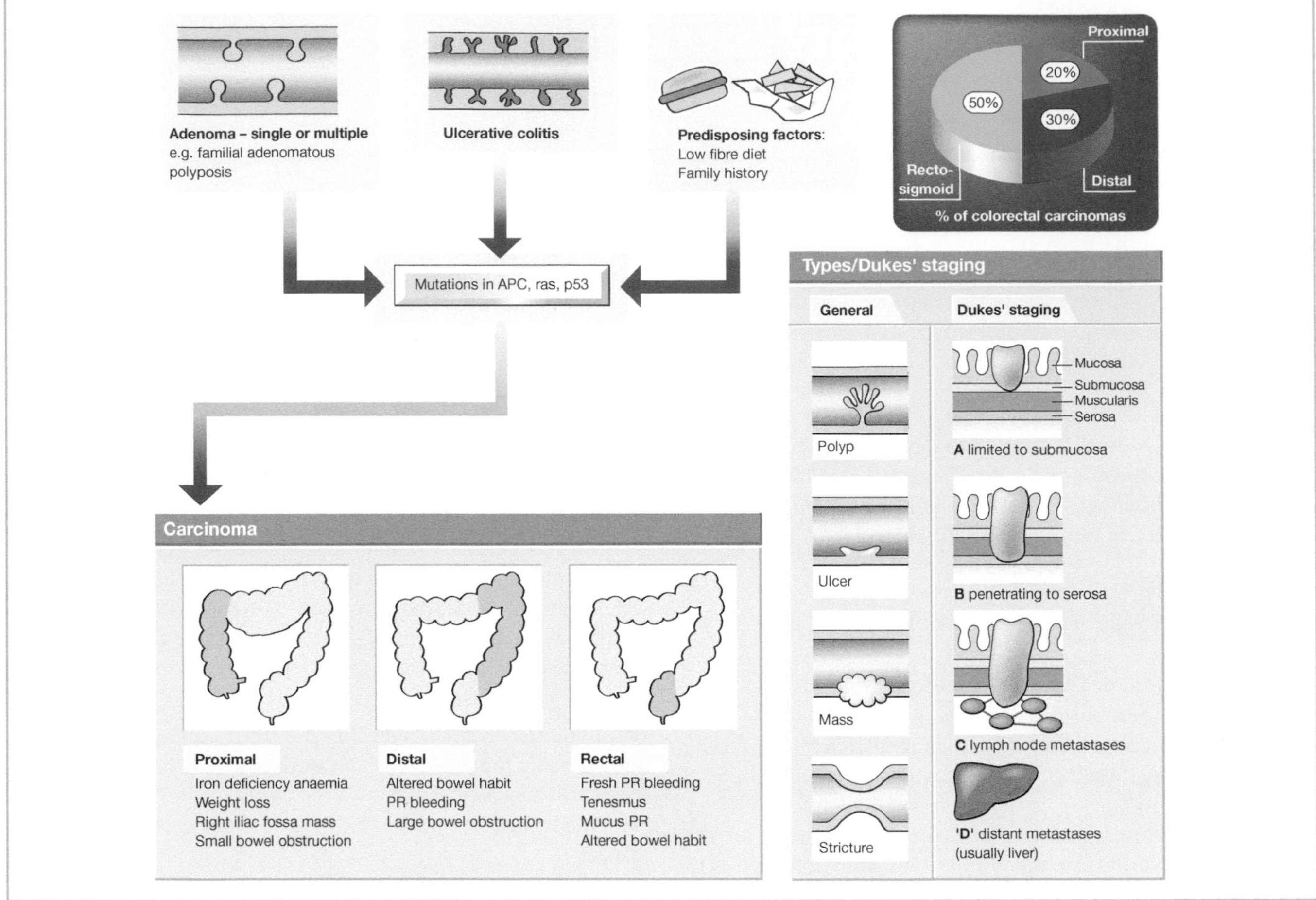

Colorectal cancer is a major public health problem in the developed world and increasingly efforts are being directed to identifying the condition early in individuals considered to be at risk.

Incidence

The incidence of colorectal cancer increases with age and is higher in men than women (1 in 15 males and 1 in 18 females will be diagnosed with bowel cancer in their lifetime). Colorectal cancer is the fourth most common cancer in the UK; it accounts for 10–15% of all cancer deaths, being responsible for over 16 000 deaths/year in the UK. Five-year survival is almost 60% and has increased over the last 40 years. Probably the single greatest determinant of prognosis is early detection, which has led to the principle of screening the population for colorectal cancer.

Pathophysiology

There are several conditions that are recognized to predispose to colorectal cancer.

Adenomatous polyps of the colon

Colorectal cancer usually develops in pre-existing adenomatous polyps in the colon. The risk of finding cancer depends upon the size of the polyp (<1 cm = 1–10% cancer risk, >2 cm = 35–55% cancer risk).

Ulcerative colitis

Long-standing total ulcerative colitis predisposes to colorectal cancer and patients with a 10-year history of total colitis should be offered colonoscopic surveillance and colonic biopsies taken to detect severe dysplasia.

Family history

A greater understanding of the genetic predisposition to colorectal cancer is resulting in an increasing number of individuals being referred for colonoscopic screening/surveillance. Risks vary, from no family history = 1 in 40 lifetime risk, to two first-degree affected relatives = 1 in 8 lifetime risk. Surveillance colonoscopy is beneficial at risk ratios of ≥1:12.

Familial cancer syndromes

There are some rare but important hereditary cancer syndromes. The most important of these are familial adenomatous polyposis and Lynch syndrome (hereditary non-polyposis colon cancer, HNPCC). In the former, affected individuals have hundreds of adenomatous polyps throughout the colon evident from an early age. The risk of neoplasia is such that prophylactic colectomy is performed before the age of 20. Lynch syndrome is inherited in an autosomal dominant fashion and is the result of mutations in DNA mismatch repair genes;

Medicine at a Glance, Fifth Edition. Edited by Patrick Davey and Alex Pitcher.

Companion website: www.wiley.com/go/medicine5e

the life-time risk of developing colorectal cancer is 50–80%. Individuals at risk are offered genetic screening, discussion about risk-reducing measures for other malignancies in addition to colonoscopic surveillance. Aspirin can be considered to reduce cancer risk.

Clinical features

The clinical presentation of sporadic colorectal cancer depends to a degree on the site of the tumour. Proximal colonic cancers may present with features of subacute bowel obstruction or may be identified during the investigation of iron deficiency anaemia. Distal colon cancers will often cause a change in bowel habit (either constipation or diarrhoea) or present with overt rectal bleeding. Other symptoms include abdominal pain and weight loss without a specific cause or symptoms due to metastatic disease.

Investigations

Investigations should aim to achieve a diagnosis, establish stage of cancer (degree of spread) and assess patient fitness.

- **Full clinical examination and baseline blood tests**: including full blood count (may identify iron deficiency anaemia), biochemistry and liver function tests (may be abnormal in the presence of liver metastatic disease).
- **Colonoscopy**: the most sensitive and specific investigation for patients suspected of having colorectal cancer.
- **Computed tomography (CT) colonography**: could be used if full colonoscopy is not possible.
- **MRI (contrast enhanced)**: to evaluate local spread of disease and involvement of local structures; particularly used in planning treatment for rectal cancer and may also be used to more fully assess liver lesions.
- **Search for metastatic disease**: CT of chest, abdomen and pelvis is most often used to look for metastatic disease. FDG-PET can be helpful in some cases. Although surgery is required in most cases, it is useful to identify whether or not the patient has metastatic disease before laparotomy.
- **Carcinoembryonic antigen**: this tumour marker is not useful for diagnosis, but is useful in monitoring the patient's response to treatment and for the identification of disease relapse.

Management and prognosis

- **Surgery** is required in most cases of colorectal cancer. The extent of bowel resection depends on the site of the tumour. Attempts are made to resect at least 5 cm of normal bowel either side of the tumour, and regional lymph nodes should also be resected. Prognosis after surgery depends on a number of factors, including the stage of the tumour (Table 137.1), degree of lymph node sampling, histological grade of the tumour, presence of lymphovascular invasion, involvement of resection margins and serum CEA. All colorectal adenocarcinomas should be assessed for presence of microsatellite instability/mismatch repair protein status. Mismatch repair deficiency/microsatellite instability is a prognostic factor and can help determine the benefit of adjuvant treatment. Results may also suggest that further tests are required to assess for Lynch syndrome (see familial cancer syndromes above). Genetic counselling and screening can then be offered.
- **Chemotherapy**: adjuvant fluoropyrimidine-based chemotherapy (e.g. 5-fluorouracil, given with folinic acid, or the oral chemotherapy agent capecitabine) for 3–6 months has been shown to improve survival in stage III disease (and high-risk stage II). The decision to proceed with adjuvant chemotherapy is determined by predicted benefit balanced against risk of complications. Dihydropyrimide dehydrogenase (DPD) is the main enzyme involved in the metabolism of fluoropyrimidines. DPD gene testing is performed prior to treatment with fluoropyrimidines as genetic polymorphism leading to DPD deficiency can lead to life-threatening toxicity.
- **Radiotherapy**: preoperative chemo-irradiation to 'down-stage' rectal tumours is gaining popularity.
- **Follow-up/secondary prevention**: patients with a prior history of colorectal cancer should undergo clinical and CEA assessment every 3–6 months, colonoscopy every 3–5 years and CT scan every 6–12 months for five years.
- **Palliative approaches**: although surgery has been considered the appropriate treatment for patients with impending colonic obstruction, stenting of tumours with self-expanding metal stents offers an alternative approach for the palliative relief of obstruction.
- **Management of metastatic disease**: colorectal cancers commonly metastasize to the peritoneum, liver and lung. Treatment is determined by patient factors (including performance status), tumour factors (e.g sequencing for specific tumour mutations) and pattern of spread. Systemic anticancer treatment includes chemotherapy (often fluoropyrimidine-based). Other systemic treatment options that have been investigated include antiangiogenic agents (bevacizumab, aflibercept), anti-EGFR antibodies (e.g. cetuximab, in tumours which do not harbour a RAS mutation) and immune checkpoint inhibition (e.g. pembrolizumab) in tumours with mismatch repair deficiency (miscrosatellite instability).
- **Liver resection** may be considered in the case of resectable liver metastatic disease. In some cases with lung metastatic disease surgical resection, ablation or stereotatic radiotherapy can be considered.

Table 137.1 Five-year survival after resection of colorectal cancer.

Stage		Five-year survival rate (%), approximately
I	Limited to bowel wall	90
II	Cancer has grown into or penetrated bowel wall, no metastases	80
III	Cancer has spread to lymph node	60–70
IV	Distant metastases	5–10

Screening

Following a successful feasibility study, a national programme for bowel cancer screening was launched in England. This now takes the form of screening the UK population over the age of 60 (over 50 in Scotland) by faecal immunochemical testing (FIT) (previously faecal occult blood [FOB] testing) every two years until age 74. Patients identified as positive are invited to attend for colonoscopy. This process identifies patients with early-stage (Dukes' A) cancer, resulting in improved survival, though up to 30% of colonic cancers are FOB negative. Furthermore, the process will identify colonic polyps, which if removed endoscopically will not develop into cancer (i.e. the process might actually *prevent* rather than just detect cancer). In time, flexible sigmoidoscopy or even total colonoscopy might increasingly be seen as the best primary screening tool although there are issues of safety, quality assurance, staffing and patient acceptability that will need to be addressed.

138 Nutrition

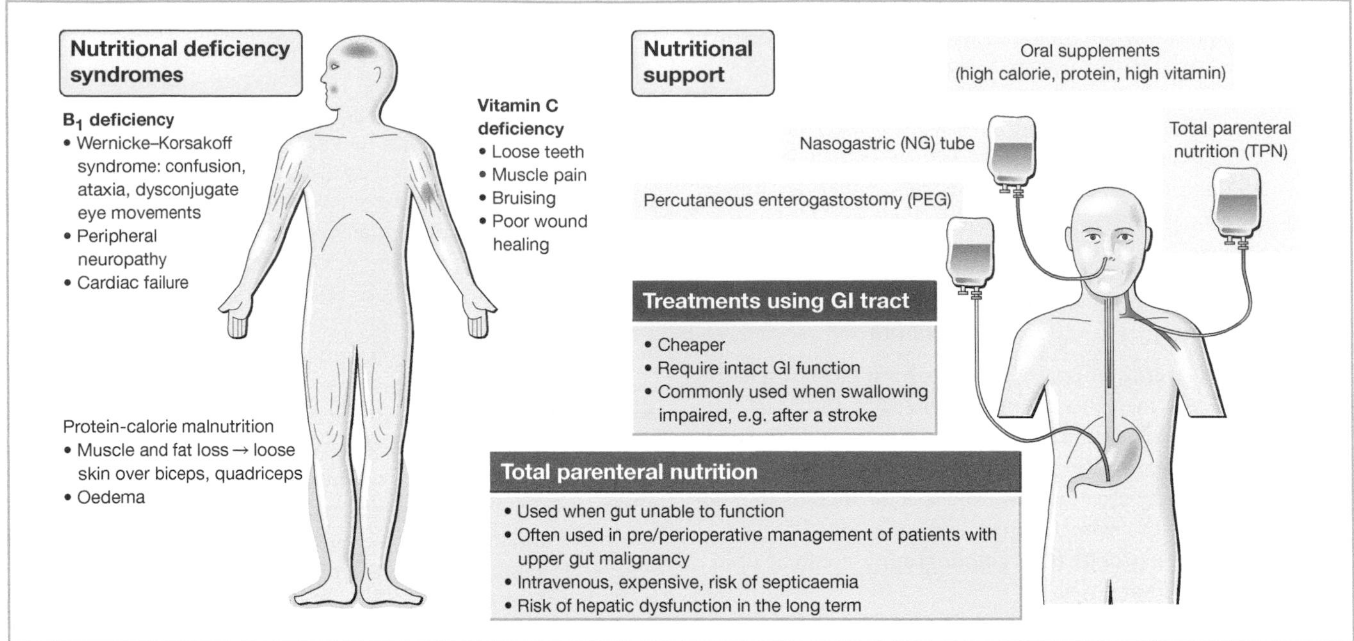

Nutritional deficiency syndromes
B1 deficiency
• Wernicke–Korsakoff syndrome: confusion, ataxia, dysconjugate eye movements
• Peripheral neuropathy
• Cardiac failure
Vitamin C deficiency
• Loose teeth
• Muscle pain
• Bruising
• Poor wound healing
Protein-calorie malnutrition
• Muscle and fat loss → loose skin over biceps, quadriceps
• Oedema
Nutritional support
Oral supplements (high calorie, protein, high vitamin)
Nasogastric (NG) tube
Total parenteral nutrition (TPN)
Percutaneous enterogastostomy (PEG)
Treatments using GI tract
• Cheaper
• Require intact GI function
• Commonly used when swallowing impaired, e.g. after a stroke
Total parenteral nutrition
• Used when gut unable to function
• Often used in pre/perioperative management of patients with upper gut malignancy
• Intravenous, expensive, risk of septicaemia
• Risk of hepatic dysfunction in the long term

The extent of malnutrition in hospital inpatients is often underestimated. Many diseases lead to anorexia and a reduction in calorific intake, and this is especially relevant when placed in the context of the increased nutritional requirements resulting from the catabolic state of malignant or inflammatory disease.

Identification of malnutrition in hospital patients

General (protein-calorie malnutrition)

Protein-calorie malnutrition is easy to miss in the hospitalized patient because the primary disease often dominates the clinical picture. Starvation is, however, very common, and can be recognized by weight loss of >10% in <3 months (when the body mass index or BMI is <19 kg/m^2), muscle wasting, peripheral oedema (with an albumin <35 g/l) and lymphocytes <1.5 × 10^9/l.

Specific (vitamin and mineral deficiencies)

Acute vitamin deficiency is much more frequent with the water-soluble vitamins (particularly vitamin B_1 [thiamine] and vitamin C) (Table 138.1), rather than those that are fat-soluble, for which there are substantial body stores.

- **Thiamine deficiency** can develop quickly (within three weeks), and leads to Wernicke encephalopathy. People with alcohol problems are particularly predisposed, but so are patients with prolonged (>3 weeks) vomiting.
- **Folate** stores are relatively small and deficiency can occur quickly, causing a macrocytic anaemia.
- B_{12} deficiency presents with megaloblastic anaemia with or without neuropathy and neurocognitive impairment.
- **Vitamin C deficiency** (scurvy) is much more common than realized, and impairs wound healing. If prolonged, classic scurvy may occur, with the development of unusual 'corkscrew'-shaped hair, haemorrhages around the hair follicle, swollen spongy gums, leading to loose teeth, spontaneous bruising and bleeding. Anaemia, which is usually hypochromic but can be normochromic, occurs. Vitamin C levels can be measured in the plasma, and also in the leukocyte–platelet layer of centrifuged blood – the 'buffy' layer. Treatment is with ascorbic acid.
- **Iron** (microcytic anaemia, glossitis, cheilosis, koilonychia), **calcium** (proximal myopathy, perioral paraesthesia, tetany) and **magnesium** (myopathy not responding to calcium) deficiency can all occur in hospitalized patients.

Nutritional support

Indications

In patients considered to be malnourished, attention should always be given to nutritional support.

Forms of nutritional support

See figure above.

Therapeutic diets

Many diets are useful for the treatment of specific gastrointestinal (GI) conditions and for non-specific symptoms. Some common diets and their indications are: Gluten-free for coeliac disease, with total gluten withdrawal; low lactose in hypolactasia, low in dairy products; high fibre in constipation/diverticular change, high insoluble fibre (e.g. bran); low residue for subacute small bowel obstruction e.g. Crohn's disease, low in fibre to reduce obstructive symptoms; exclusion diet for intractable irritable bowel, bland diet; low salt for cirrhosis or heart failure, a useful adjunct to diuretics in control of oedema and/or ascites; elemental/peptide for Crohn's disease, a liquid diet with nitrogen as either short peptides or amino acids. Low-protein diets tend not to be advised nowadays for either renal failure or hepatic encephalopathy.

Refeeding syndrome

The refeeding syndrome is a potentially lethal condition characterized by metabolic abnormalities and rapid fluid and electrolyte shifts in malnourished patients receiving increased calorific intake. Typically, patients are underweight and have had minimal nutrition for a prolonged period. Patients with psychiatric and eating disorders, malignancies, alcohol and drug addiction, and those recovering from surgery or chemotherapy may be at particular risk.

- Salt and water retention leading to oedema and potentially cardiac failure.
- Rapid decreases in key electrolyte concentrations including hypokalaemia, hypocalcaemia, hypomagnesaemia and hypophosphataemia.
- Rapid depletion of the glycolysis co-factor thiamine. This is associated with neuropathy and the Wernicke–Korsakoff syndrome.
- Hypo- or hyperglycaemia.
- Severe cases can be complicated by sepsis that is not necessarily accompanied by fever and raises in inflammatory markers, and can be particularly associated with hypothermia.

Management

- Pre-emptive identification of patients at risk with a measure such as the Malnutrition Universal Screening Tool (MUST).
- Replacement of thiamine.
- Replacement of electrolytes.
- Cardiac monitoring where appropriate.
- Slow and graduated introduction of nutrition, supervised when necessary.

Table 138.1 Features of water-soluble vitamin deficiency (for features of vitamin C deficiency, see text; folate deficiency and B_{12} deficiency, see Chapter 176).

	Vitamin B_1	Vitamin B_2	Vitamin B_3	Vitamin B_6
Solubility	Water			
Common name	Thiamine	Riboflavin	Niacin	Pyridoxine
Occurrence	• Cereals • Beans • Nuts • Pork, duck	• Dairy products • Offal • Leafy vegetables	• Plants • Meat • Fish	Found widely in plant- and animal-derived foods
Function	Essential co-factor in many enzyme systems, especially involving carbohydrate metabolism		Hydrogen acceptor in many oxidative reactions	Co-factor in metabolism of many amino acids
Cause of deficiency	• Dietary deficiency, e.g. milled rice • Alcoholism (usually due to dietary deficiency) • Prolonged vomiting, e.g. hyperemesis gravidarum, cancer especially with chemotherapy	Low dietary intake	Lost during the milling process of cereals – unless replaced, deficiency occurs in those with cereal-only diet • Isoniazid therapy • Malabsorption syndromes (rare) • Carcinoid syndrome	• Dietary deficiency is very rare • Drugs can produce deficiency (e.g. isoniazid, hydralazine, penicillamine)
Consequence of deficiency	• 'Dry' beriberi; polyneuropathy, ± cerebral involvement with Wernicke-Korsokoff syndrome (causing dementia, ataxia, external ophthalmoplegia, nystagmus) • 'Wet' beriberi: oedema of legs, ascites, pleural effusions (largely due to cardiac failure) • Vasodilation (due to lactic acid), bounding pulse	Clinical deficiency very rare: • Angular stomatitis • Red inflamed tongue • Seborrhoeic dermatitis • Conjunctivitis	Pellagra (→ the 3 Ds): • **Dermatitis**: in sun-exposed areas of the skin → thickening, dry, hyperpigmentation • **Diarrhoea**: other GI symptoms include a red raw tongue, glossitis, angular stomatitis • **Dementia**: in severe cases; in milder cases, depression, apathy and thought disorders	• Polyneuropathy • Rarely, some sideroblastic anaemias respond to B_6 • Some premenstrual tension symptoms may respond to B_6 supplementation
Diagnosis	• Clinical response to thiamine • Red cell (transketolase) before and after added thiamine		Clinical features	Clinical features
General treatment	Most vitamin deficiencies are not isolated, and accordingly multiple different vitamin supplements should be given, along with protein and calories			
Treatment	Supplemental thiamine – if due to alcohol abuse, thiamine must be given prior to carbohydrates	Riboflavin supplementation	Niacin supplementation	Vitamin B_6
Excess	Ataxia	No data		

139 Renal physiology and function tests

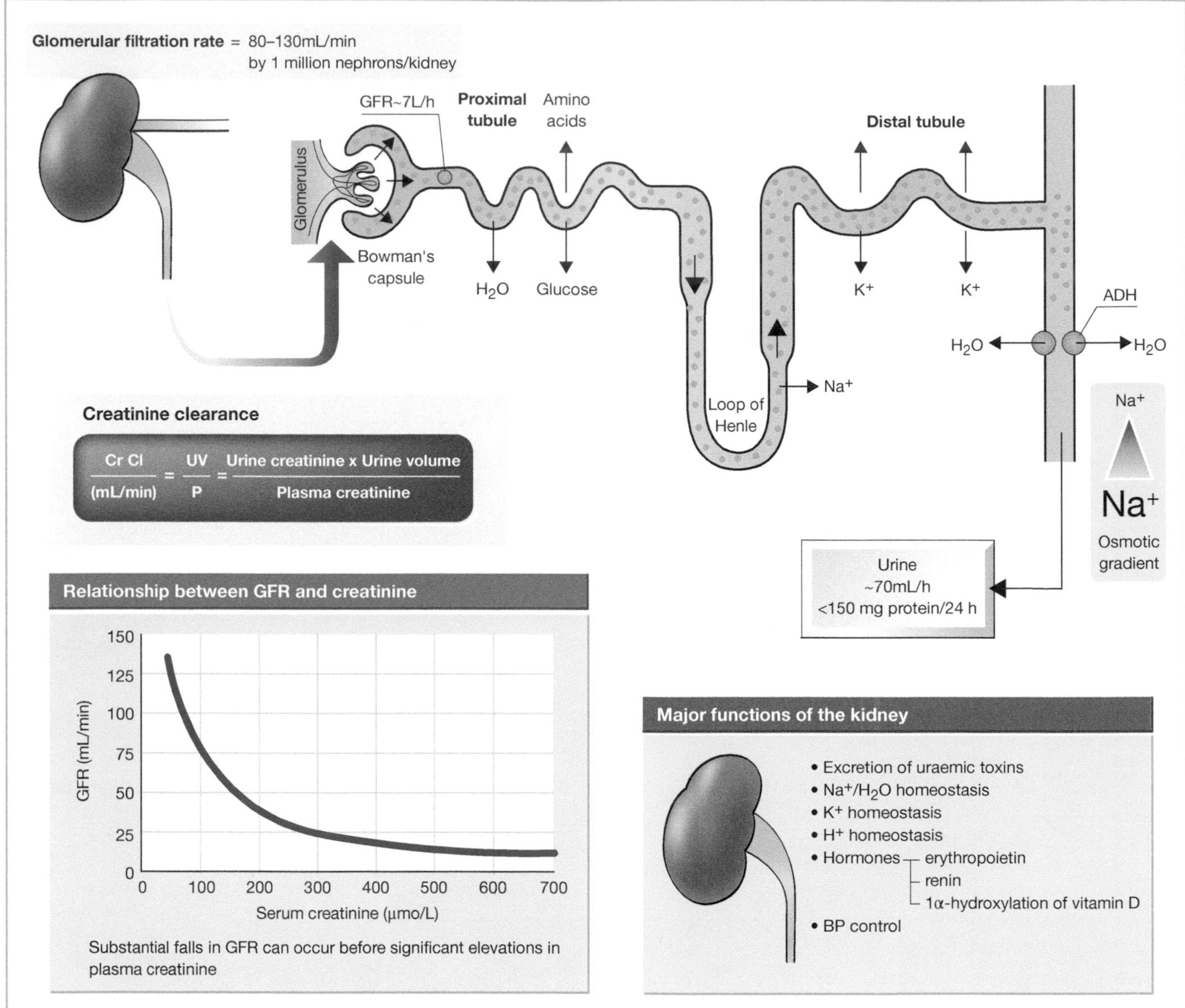

Each kidney consists of approximately 1 million nephrons. Each nephron has a glomerulus, which is located mainly in the renal cortex and filters into a renal tubule. The tubule consists of proximal and distal tubules, and the loop of Henle in which reabsorption of water, electrolytes and other important solutes occurs; this produces urine, which drains into the collecting ducts, undergoes further water absorption and then drains into the renal pyramids. The thick ascending limb of the loop of Henle possesses a specialized plaque of cells that attaches to the extraglomerular mesangium and afferent arteriole to form the juxtaglomerular apparatus; this secretes renin and is involved in the regulation of glomerular blood flow and filtration rate. The kidneys receive 20% of the cardiac output and filter 7 l of fluid per hour to produce 50–100 ml of urine per hour, showing the efficiency with which water and other solutes are reabsorbed by the renal tubules.

The key functions of the kidney are therefore to excrete/secrete the waste products of metabolism, and other substances harmful to the body, while conserving useful constituents of blood. In addition, the kidney has major endocrine functions including the secretion of erythropoietin, the α_1-hydroxylation of vitamin D and the production of renin. Although often renal disease leads to failure in all three of these key functions, diseases can affect the first two functions independently. It is convenient to consider how the different functions of the kidney can be assessed according to anatomical location.

Medicine at a Glance, Fifth Edition. Edited by Patrick Davey and Alex Pitcher.

Companion website: www.wiley.com/go/medicine5e

Glomerular function

Toxin/metabolic waste product elimination

The key variable reflecting the efficiency of the kidney in waste product disposal is the glomerular filtration rate (GFR). The most commonly used measure of GFR is serum creatinine, an end-product of skeletal muscle metabolism (higher in those with large muscle bulk). The relationship between GFR and serum creatinine is not linear (see figure above), and it is important to emphasize that highly significant falls in GFR can occur before serum creatinine rises. If impairment of GFR is suspected, it is insufficient to rely on plasma creatinine; a more accurate measure of GFR should be used instead, such as the creatinine clearance. The principle underlying this measure is that creatinine is an inert molecule, passively filtered by the kidney. A knowledge of urine creatinine quantity ($Urine_{Cr}$) and plasma creatinine concentration (P_{Cr}) (over 24 h) allows calculation of the GFR, from:

$$GFR = \left(Urine_{Cr} \times \text{urine volume}\right) / P_{Cr}$$

Increasingly, laboratories are quoting estimated GFR (eGFR) using calculations that require serum creatinine. Creatinine clearance measurements are usually sufficiently accurate for day-to-day clinical practice, although the GFR measured this way may overestimate the true GFR by up to 100% in severe renal disease, as a result of renal tubular secretion of creatinine (thus overestimating the amount of urine creatinine derived from glomerular filtration). More precise measurement of GFR can be undertaken with radioisotope scans (diethylene triamine penta-acetic acid [DTPA]), and cystatin clearance is increasingly used.

Conservation of normal blood constituents

Glomerular function can be disturbed such that plasma protein is no longer conserved. This leak of protein can range from mild, significant as a marker of renal disease, to substantial (greater than 3.5 g in 24 hours), associated with profound hypoalbuminaemia and substantial oedema (the nephrotic syndrome). In addition to defective glomerular function, mild proteinuria also results from defects in tubular function (see Table 139.1) and as an overflow phenomenon (e.g. multiple myeloma, immunoglobulin κ or λ light chains: acute leukaemia, lysozymuria). These three different kinds of mild proteinuria are distinguished on the basis of electrophoretic properties. Urine dipsticks primarily detect albumin, which is found in glomerular disease and not in tubular disease or multiple myeloma. If these conditions are suspected, urine electrophoresis should be performed.

Renal concentrating ability

The loop of Henle, via the countercurrent mechanism, establishes an osmotic gradient that increases from the cortex to the inner medulla. Water excretion is adjusted in the collecting ducts, which pass through the medulla and where permeability of water is controlled by the antidiuretic hormone (ADH). The ability of the kidney to concentrate urine is disturbed in many intrinsic renal diseases, particularly tubulointerstitial ones, as well as in actual or functional deficiency of ADH (diabetes insipidus).

The renal concentrating power can be measured by: (i) osmolality of early morning urine, which is the easiest and safest test; and (ii) concentrating ability when faced with 24-hour fluid deprivation, which is uncomfortable (so compliance is an issue), rarely undertaken and which may induce hypovolaemic renal failure. It is usual to admit patients to hospital for this.

Amino acid conserving function

Amino acids are filtered at the glomerulus, and reabsorbed in the proximal tubules. Diffuse proximal tubular damage results in generalized aminoaciduria, whereas specific lesions cause specific patterns of amino acid loss. The pattern of aminoaciduria is detected by two-dimensional chromatography.

Renal acid–base control

A major function of the proximal and distal tubules is acid–base balance. Advanced renal failure gives rise to retention of metabolic acids (exacerbating renal bone disease), which may provoke myocardial depression and death. Specific tubular lesions may, in the absence of filtration failure, produce retention of metabolic acid – so-called renal tubular acidosis.

Electrolyte control

The kidney is central in the control of potassium, as a result of secretion of potassium into the tubular fluid in exchange for sodium or hydrogen ions, and in the regulation of urinary pH. Aldosterone (which is stimulated by angiotensin II and potassium levels) promotes reabsorption of sodium and water and excretion of potassium. In advanced renal failure, the distal tubule cannot exchange plasma K^+/H^+ for tubule Na^+, leading to hyperkalaemia, which when profound may lead to cardiac arrest.

Hormonal function

The kidney has hormonal functions, notably in the production of renin and erythropoietin, and the α_1-hydroxylation of vitamin D from an inactive to an active form. When renal function is globally disturbed, renal hormone production is usually diminished, provoking anaemia (erythropoietin deficiency) and exacerbating renal bone disease. Other hormones, especially the renin–angiotensin system, are involved in blood pressure control. Renal diseases such as renal ischaemia (e.g. unilateral renal artery stenosis) or glomerulonephritis are commonly associated with hypertension.

Table 139.1 Proteinuria in renal disease.

	Glomerulonephritis	Tubular disease	Overflow proteinuria
Amount of proteinuria	+ to ++++	+ to ++	+ to ++++
Dipstick positive for protein	Yes	No	No

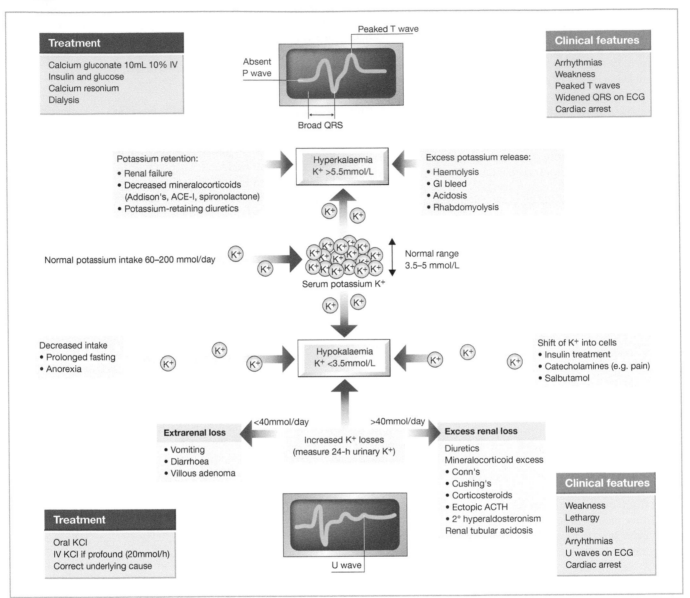

140 Hypokalaemia and hyperkalaemia

Treatment

Calcium gluconate 10mL 10% IV
Insulin and glucose
Calcium resonium
Dialysis

Absent P wave
Peaked T wave
Broad QRS

Clinical features

Arrhythmias
Weakness
Peaked T waves
Widened QRS on ECG
Cardiac arrest

Potassium retention:
- Renal failure
- Decreased mineralocorticoids (Addison's, ACE-I, spironolactone)
- Potassium-retaining diuretics

Hyperkalaemia
K^+ >5.5mmol/L

Excess potassium release:
- Haemolysis
- GI bleed
- Acidosis
- Rhabdomyolysis

Normal potassium intake 60–200 mmol/day

Serum potassium K^+

Normal range
3.5–5 mmol/L

Decreased intake
- Prolonged fasting
- Anorexia

Hypokalaemia
K^+ <3.5mmol/L

Shift of K^+ into cells
- Insulin treatment
- Catecholamines (e.g. pain)
- Salbutamol

Increased K^+ losses
(measure 24-h urinary K^+)

<40mmol/day

Extrarenal loss
- Vomiting
- Diarrhoea
- Villous adenoma

>40mmol/day

Excess renal loss

Diuretics
Mineralocorticoid excess
- Conn's
- Cushing's
- Corticosteroids
- Ectopic ACTH
- 2° hyperaldosteronism

Renal tubular acidosis

Treatment

Oral KCl
IV KCl if profound (20mmol/h)
Correct underlying cause

U wave

Clinical features

Weakness
Lethargy
Ileus
Arryhthmias
U waves on ECG
Cardiac arrest

Hypokalaemia

Hypokalaemia is a serum potassium of less than 3.5 mmol/l. It is the most common electrolyte disorder in hospitalized patients, mostly attributable to diuretic therapy. It can occur as a result of increased losses from the urinary or gastrointestinal (GI) tract, poor intake (such as in eating disorders) or a shift to the intracellular compartment (insulin treatment or very rarely familial periodic paralysis; see Chapter 209). GI losses may occur as a result of diarrhoea, vomiting, laxative abuse or villous adenomas of the colon. Renal losses may occur as the result of diuretic therapy, mineralocorticoid excess (Conn syndrome or primary hyperaldosteronism, Cushing syndrome, ectopic adrenocorticotrophic hormone [ACTH]), secondary hyperaldosteronism (renal artery stenosis, hypertension, heart failure) or renal tubular acidosis. β-Receptor stimulation moves potassium into cells, which explains why hypokalaemia is common in the sick and in those treated with salbutamol.

Common causes

- Diuretic therapy.
- Acute illness.
- Gastrointestinal losses.

Medicine at a Glance, Fifth Edition. Edited by Patrick Davey and Alex Pitcher.

Companion website: www.wiley.com/go/medicine5e

Clinical features

Often asymptomatic when mild, hypokalaemia can produce weakness, intestinal ileus, decreased renal-concentrating ability and electrocardiogram (ECG) changes of T-wave flattening, the appearance of U waves and an increased incidence of tachyarrhythmias. Long-standing hypokalaemia can lead to (poorly reversible) damage to the distal tubule, leading to a failure of renal-concentrating properties, and polyuria, with compensatory polydipsia.

When severe (K^+ <2 mmol/l), skeletal muscle weakness, which may be profound, dominates the clinical picture and flaccid paralysis may be seen. Very rarely, respiratory failure can occur in this situation.

Management

Treat the underlying cause. If potassium is <2.5 (or <3.0 mmol/l in a patient at risk of arrhythmias, e.g. post myocardial infarction), give intravenous (IV) potassium chloride (KCl) as an infusion not exceeding 20 mmol/h at a concentration not exceeding 40 mmol/l because concentrated potassium will damage peripheral veins. If potassium is between 2.5 and 3.5 mmol/l, give oral replacement therapy (unless the patient is nil by mouth or vomiting) at 80–120 mmol/day in divided doses. Once hypokalaemia is present, total body depletion of potassium may be substantial and require significant replacement. Check for hypomagnesaemia and replace if low.

Hyperkalaemia

The main cause of hyperkalaemia is renal failure (because potassium excretion is impaired). Other causes include reduced mineralocorticoids, such as in Addison disease, spironolactone (aldosterone antagonist), angiotensin-converting enzyme (ACE) inhibitors, angiotensin receptor blockers (ARBs) or potassium-retaining diuretics such as amiloride. Cell destruction in haemolysis, cytotoxic therapy and rhabdomyolysis can liberate large amounts of potassium and cause hyperkalaemia. The hyperkalaemic effects of ACE inhibitors or potassium-retaining diuretics such as amiloride can be very marked in patients with renal impairment. Hyperkalaemia can be artefactual as a result of the haemolysis of blood during venepuncture, so treat an unsuspected/anomalous finding of hyperkalaemia with suspicion, and repeat the measurement.

Common causes

- Renal failure.
- Drugs in those with borderline or frankly abnormal renal function, e.g. ACE inhibitors and/or spironolactone in elderly people or those with heart failure.

Clinical features

Even very severe hyperkalaemia is usually asymptomatic although it can very rarely be accompanied by muscular weakness. It may be associated with ECG abnormalities of T-wave peaking, QRS widening, prolonged PR interval, loss of P waves and a sine wave appearance, leading to cardiac arrest.

Management

In mild hyperkalaemia (potassium <6.0 mmol/l), oral or IV potassium should be restricted. Severe hyperkalaemia (potassium >6.5 mmol/l or hyperkalaemic ECG changes) is a medical emergency, particularly if the rate of rise of potassium has been rapid. The patient should receive IV calcium chloride or calcium gluconate (10 ml of 10% over 2 min), which stabilizes the myocardium. Measures to lower potassium should be instituted: the administration of IV glucose with insulin (50 ml of 50% glucose and 10 units of short-acting insulin), the potassium-binding resin calcium resonium, and dialysis may be required. Newer potassium binders such as patiromer are being introduced.

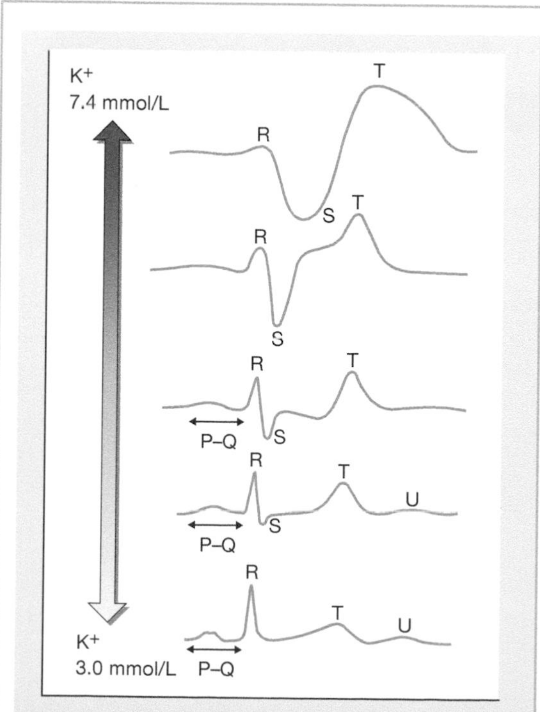

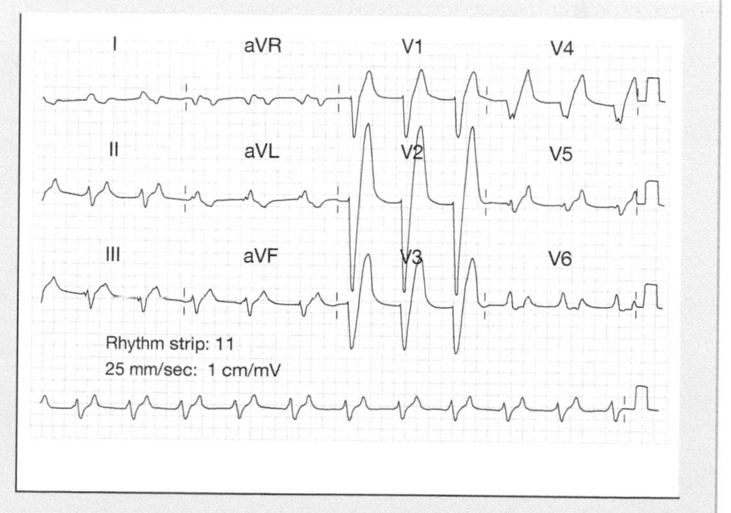

An ECG of a middle-aged woman with acute renal failure, and a K+ of 8.0 mmol/L. This ECG shows absent P waves, very broad QRS complex and tall 'peaked' T waves, especially in leads V1 to V4

Hyponatraemia and hypernatraemia

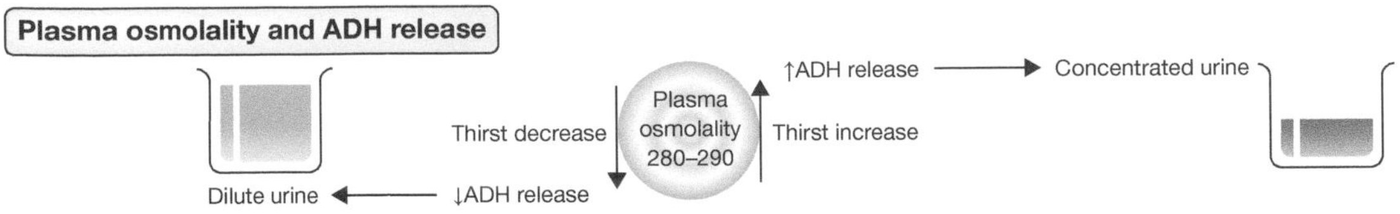

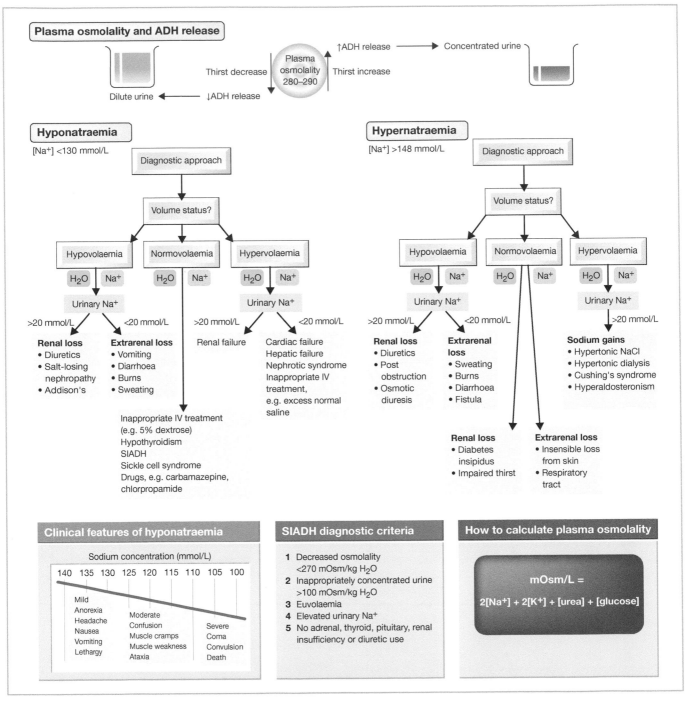

Plasma osmolality and ADH release

Plasma osmolality 280–290

- Thirst increase → ↑ADH release → Concentrated urine
- Thirst decrease → ↓ADH release → Dilute urine

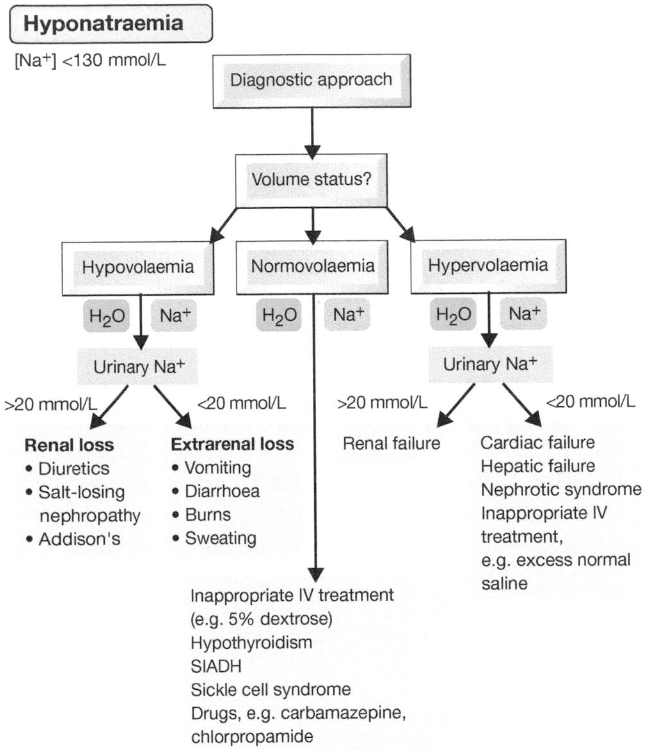

Hyponatraemia

$[Na^+]$ <130 mmol/L

Diagnostic approach → Volume status?

Hypovolaemia (H_2O, Na^+) → Urinary Na^+

- >20 mmol/L: **Renal loss**
  - Diuretics
  - Salt-losing nephropathy
  - Addison's
- <20 mmol/L: **Extrarenal loss**
  - Vomiting
  - Diarrhoea
  - Burns
  - Sweating

Normovolaemia (H_2O, Na^+) →

Inappropriate IV treatment (e.g. 5% dextrose)
Hypothyroidism
SIADH
Sickle cell syndrome
Drugs, e.g. carbamazepine, chlorpropamide

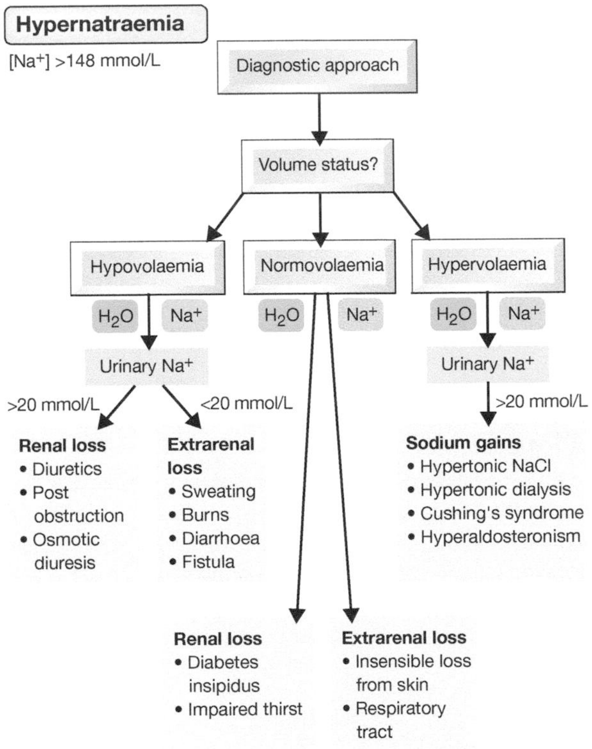

Hypervolaemia (H_2O, Na^+) → Urinary Na^+

- >20 mmol/L: Renal failure
- <20 mmol/L: Cardiac failure
  Hepatic failure
  Nephrotic syndrome
  Inappropriate IV treatment, e.g. excess normal saline

Hypernatraemia

$[Na^+]$ >148 mmol/L

Diagnostic approach → Volume status?

Hypovolaemia (H_2O, Na^+) → Urinary Na^+

- >20 mmol/L: **Renal loss**
  - Diuretics
  - Post obstruction
  - Osmotic diuresis
- <20 mmol/L: **Extrarenal loss**
  - Sweating
  - Burns
  - Diarrhoea
  - Fistula

Normovolaemia (H_2O, Na^+) →

- **Renal loss**
  - Diabetes insipidus
  - Impaired thirst
- **Extrarenal loss**
  - Insensible loss from skin
  - Respiratory tract

Hypervolaemia (H_2O, Na^+) → Urinary Na^+

- >20 mmol/L: **Sodium gains**
  - Hypertonic NaCl
  - Hypertonic dialysis
  - Cushing's syndrome
  - Hyperaldosteronism

Clinical features of hyponatraemia

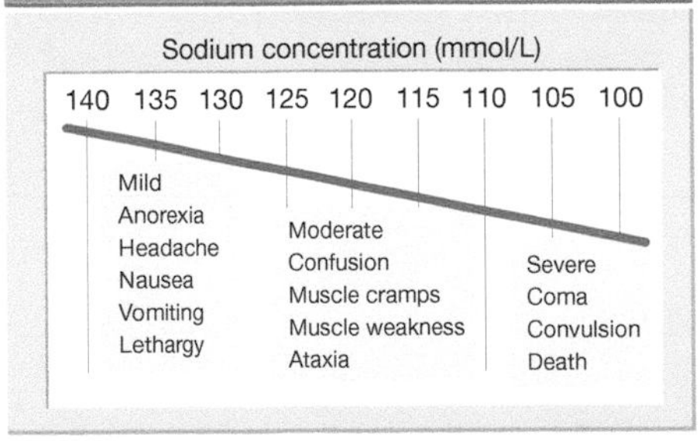

Sodium concentration (mmol/L)

140 135 130 125 120 115 110 105 100

Mild	Moderate	Severe
Anorexia Headache Nausea Vomiting Lethargy	Confusion Muscle cramps Muscle weakness Ataxia	Coma Convulsion Death

SIADH diagnostic criteria

1. Decreased osmolality <270 mOsm/kg H_2O
2. Inappropriately concentrated urine >100 mOsm/kg H_2O
3. Euvolaemia
4. Elevated urinary Na^+
5. No adrenal, thyroid, pituitary, renal insufficiency or diuretic use

How to calculate plasma osmolality

$$\text{mOsm/L} = 2[Na^+] + 2[K^+] + [\text{urea}] + [\text{glucose}]$$

Medicine at a Glance, Fifth Edition. Edited by Patrick Davey and Alex Pitcher.

Companion website: www.wiley.com/go/medicine5e

Abnormalities of serum sodium are closely linked to water balance. The most common causes of altered serum sodium are the result of excessive losses or administration of water.

Hyponatraemia

Hyponatraemia is defined as a serum sodium <130 mmol/l and is found in 5% of hospital inpatients. Hyponatraemia may be asymptomatic, but can produce confusion, coma and convulsions.

In hyponatraemia, there is an excess of extracellular water relative to the sodium content of the extracellular compartment. This can occur in three different circumstances.

1 **Hypovolaemia** (body Na^+ and water deficit).
2 **Normovolaemia** (no change in body Na^+ but a modest increase in water).
3 **Hypervolaemia** (increase in body Na^+ and water).

Common causes

- Syndrome of inappropriate antidiuretic hormone secretion (SIADH).
- Heart failure (severity of hyponatraemia relates to severity of heart failure and prognosis).
- Inappropriate overvigorous intravenous dextrose in postoperative patients.
- Iatrogenic Addison disease (over-rapid corticosteroid withdrawal in elderly patients on large doses of steroids or with failure to increase corticosteroids when ill).
- Diuretics.

Management

The underlying aetiology should be sought and corrected where possible. The volume status of the patient should be determined. If signs of hypovolaemia are present (thirst, tachycardia, hypotension, postural fall in blood pressure, reduced skin turgor, etc.) then sodium chloride (NaCl) should be administered intravenously. In mild hyponatraemia, (serum sodium 130–134 mmol/l), patients do not usually have symptoms due to hyponatremia, and do not require intravenous treatment. However, such patients should undergo monitoring to detect a further decrease in serum sodium. If there is no evidence of hypovolaemia, the patient's fluid intake should be restricted. If there is evidence of hypervolaemia (oedema, elevated jugular venous pressure, hypertension), diuretics and water restriction may be necessary. Cautious correction of Na^+ is essential to avoid central pontine myelinolysis, a syndrome of encephalopathy, cranial nerve palsies and quadriplegia, which occurs after rapid correction of Na^+. In chronic hyponatraemia, the Na^+ should be corrected at less than 0.5 mmol/l/h, although in acute hyponatraemia, if neurological symptoms are present, more rapid correction may be appropriate.

Syndrome of inappropriate ADH secretion

This is a relatively common cause of hyponatraemia in hospital patients. However, the diagnosis requires the exclusion of adrenal, thyroid, pituitary or renal insufficiency, no diuretic usage and euvolaemia. For the plasma tonicity, there is inappropriate elevation of ADH (vasopressin) levels which leads to an inappropriate urinary concentration. There are a large number of possible causes (see Table 141.1) which can be broadly grouped into carcinomas (particularly of the lung), pulmonary disorders including pneumonia, central nervous system disorders such as meningitis and head trauma, and drugs.

Treatment of SIADH involves removing the precipitating cause wherever possible. Fluid restriction, of increasing degree with increasingly lower sodium, is usually effective and tolerable. Demeclocycline (which inhibits the action of ADH on the distal tubule) may be used if these simple manoeuvres are ineffective. ADH antagonists such as tolvaptan are now available though their therapeutic role is unclear.

Table 141.1 The common causes of the syndrome of inappropriate antidiuretic hormone release.

Idiopathic	
Postoperative	Pain Lung infection + COPD Drugs (see below)
CNS causes	Infection Stroke Neoplasia
Lung causes	Infection Tumour
Oncological causes	Lung cancer – most common Prostate, GI tract, haematological malignancies
Drugs	↑ H_2O permeability of nephron, e.g. vasopressin ↑ ADH release, e.g. carbamazepine ↑ ADH action, e.g. cyclophosphamide ↓ Prostaglandin synthesis, e.g. aspirin

ADH, antidiuretic hormone; CNS, central nervous system; COPD, chronic obstructive pulmonary disease; GI, gastrointestinal.

Hypernatraemia

Hypernatraemia is defined as a serum sodium >145 mmol/l caused by a relative water deficit, and the major defence against it is thirst. It therefore occurs more commonly in patients who are unable to increase their water intake. The causes can be grouped into three categories depending on volume status.

1 **Hypovolaemia** (low body sodium with loss of water exceeding that of Na^+).
2 **Normovolaemia** (normal body Na^+ but water loss).
3 **Hypervolaemia** (increased total body Na^+).

As with hyponatraemia, assessment of volume status and determination of urinary sodium are central to the diagnostic approach.

Common causes

- Fluid (water) deprivation, particularly in elderly people.
- Hyperosmolar diabetic coma.

Management

The underlying cause requires identification and correction. In patients with hypovolaemia, the volume deficit should be corrected with physiological saline until haemodynamics are normalized; water may then be required. In hypervolaemic hypernatraemia, the excess sodium requires removal, often with diuretics. In euvolaemic hypernatraemia, water is given intravenously as 5% dextrose. In all cases, careful monitoring of volume status and serum sodium concentration is necessary and correction of Na^+ should be made at a rate of less than 0.5 mmol/l/h.

Diabetes insipidus is characterized by polyuria and polydipsia and is the result of defects in ADH action. It can produce hypernatraemia and is discussed in greater detail in Chapter 162.

142 Disorders of acid–base balance

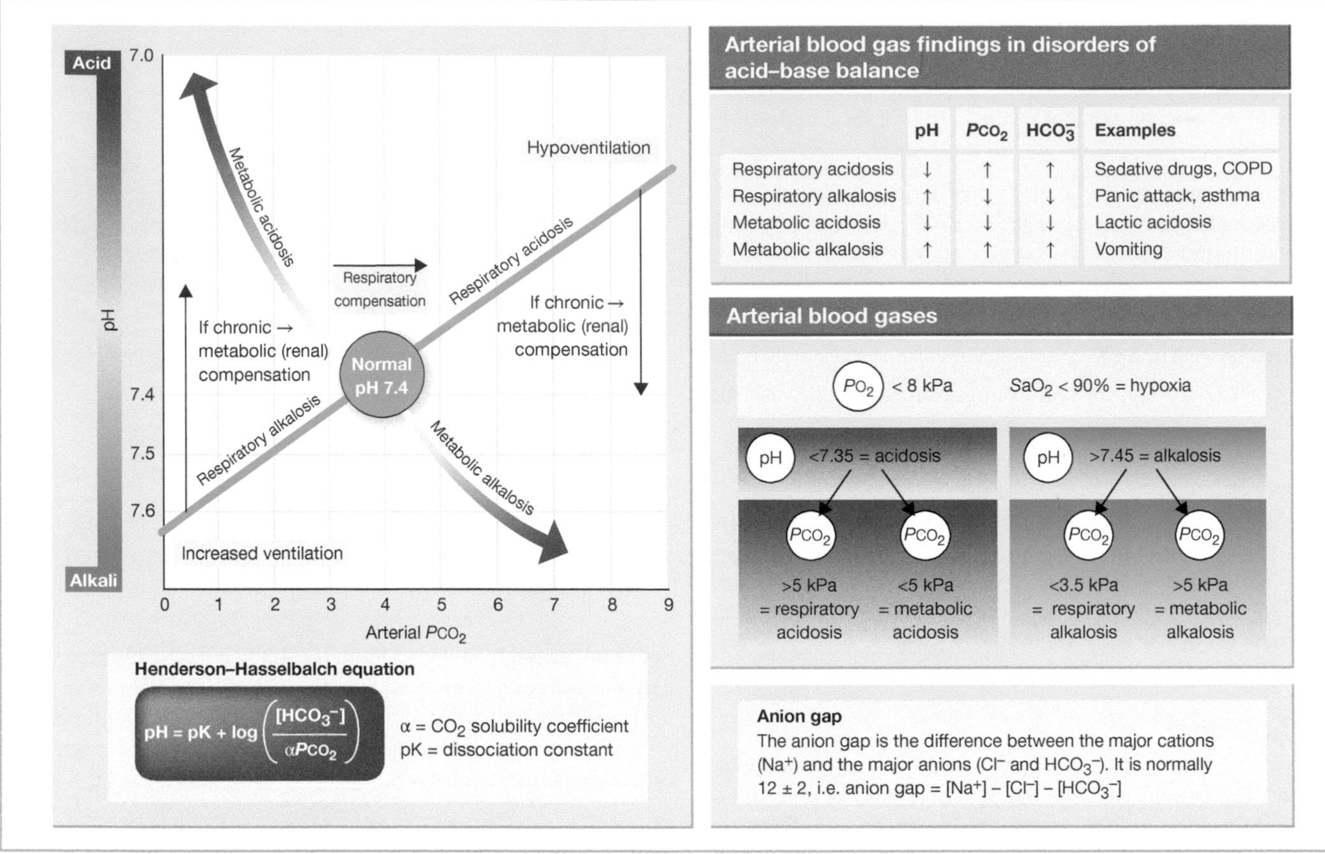

In many ill patients, important acid–base disturbances occur. They may lack specific symptoms, and in any seriously ill patient arterial blood gases should be determined. The type of acid–base disturbance can be determined from the pH and P_{CO_2}. When interpreting arterial blood gases, ask the following questions.

1 Is there hypoxia?
2 Is there acidosis, alkalosis or normal pH?
3 Is there low normal or elevated pCO_2?

Metabolic acidosis

Metabolic acidosis is seen most commonly in diabetic ketoacidosis (DKA), lactic acidosis and renal failure. The presence of a significant metabolic acidosis is important and requires urgent diagnosis and treatment. It can be grouped into four major categories by aetiology.

1 Ingestion of acid, such as salicylate, methanol or ethylene glycol poisoning.
2 Accumulation of endogenous acids, such as lactic acid in tissue hypoperfusion or ketones in DKA.
3 Loss of alkali in severe diarrhoea, with biliary or enteric fistulae or renal loss in proximal renal tubular acidosis.
4 Failure of elimination of acid in renal failure and distal tubular acidosis.

Severe acidosis results in cardiac depression and death.

The anion gap can be useful in the diagnosis of metabolic acidoses. The anion gap is the difference between the major cation (sodium) and the major measured anions (chloride and bicarbonate). It is normally 12 ± 4 (some laboratories include potassium levels in the calculation, giving a normal range of 16 ±4). An elevated anion gap suggests the presence of additional anions such as lactate (in lactic acidosis) or ketones (in DKA), whereas a normal or reduced anion gap (or hyperchloraemic acidosis) suggests bicarbonate loss or renal tubular acidosis (see Tables 142.1 and 142.2).

The body will usually respond to the acidaemia with respiratory compensation, an increase in respiratory rate causing a fall in carbon dioxide, which in turn increases the blood pH. Metabolic acidosis may be associated with the signs or symptoms of the precipitating cause – the increased rate and depth of respiration, sometimes described as Kussmaul respiration – or if severe, it may itself be associated with the signs of shock.

Medicine at a Glance, Fifth Edition. Edited by Patrick Davey and Alex Pitcher.

Companion website: www.wiley.com/go/medicine5e

Table 142.1 Anion gap and metabolic acidosis.

Anion gap	Disease
Normal (= hyperchloraemic acidosis)	Renal tubular acidosis
	Extrarenal HCO_3^- loss Hyperparathyroidism Hypoaldosteronism ± Diabetic ketoacidosis
Increased (>20 mmol/l)	Renal parenchymal disease Ingestion of acid Acid metabolized from endogenous substances Lactic acidosis ± Diabetic ketoacidosis

Diabetic ketoacidosis may give rise to either normal or high anion gap acidosis.

Table 142.2 Causes of lactic acidosis.

Mechanism	Disease
Increased rate of lactate production	Any cause of decreased tissue perfusion, either cardiovascular in origin or ischaemia of a large tissue mass, e.g. the gut, or a limb Hypoxia Increased skeletal muscle activity (e.g. status epilepticus or marathon runners) Destruction of large tumour masses (e.g. lymphoma or leukaemia) Poisoning (e.g. CO or cyanide)
Decreased lactate transport	Decreased cardiac output due to any cause
Decreased lactate metabolism	Liver failure (any cause) Intoxication (metformin or alcohol) Diabetes mellitus Liver hypoxia
Miscellaneous	Haemofiltration with lactate buffer

Traditionally lactic acidosis is divided into type A (clinical evidence of poor tissue perfusion/oxygenation) and type B (no clinical evidence of poor tissue perfusion/oxygenation). B1 is associated with underlying diseases; B2 is due to drugs and toxins; B3 is due to inborn errors of metabolism.

The treatment should be directed towards reversing the underlying cause. In exceptional circumstances, sodium bicarbonate may be administered and haemodialysis or haemofiltration used.

Metabolic alkalosis

Metabolic alkalosis rarely gives rise to symptoms from the alkalosis alone. The aetiologies of metabolic alkalosis include:

- loss of acid such as in vomiting, particularly with pyloric stenosis
- increased renal reabsorption of bicarbonate which can occur with hyperaldosteronism or severe hypokalaemia
- excess intake of alkali (e.g. the milk–alkali syndrome, where large quantities of alkaline antacids are ingested, often with milk).

There may be respiratory compensation with a reduction in respiratory rate, a rise in carbon dioxide and a fall in pH.

Treatment involves the identification and treatment of the underlying cause.

Respiratory acidosis

The primary control of ventilation is achieved by monitoring of blood pH by the respiratory centre, and appropriate changes in ventilatory rate to alter the blood partial pressure of carbon dioxide, which in turn leads to changes in blood pH. The development of respiratory acidosis is a concern and may indicate the need for ventilatory support (see Chapter 100).

A reduction in ventilation leads to an accumulation of carbon dioxide and the development of acidosis. This may be the result of a wide variety of causes of ventilatory impairment and commonly includes:

- sedation, particularly with opiates
- respiratory muscle weakness, e.g. Guillain–Barré syndrome, poliomyelitis or myasthenia gravis
- severe chronic obstructive pulmonary disease (COPD).

The accumulation of carbon dioxide can sometimes be associated with clinical signs, which include a bounding pulse, papilloedema or a metabolic flap. If the carbon dioxide retention has been chronic, there may be metabolic renal compensation with an elevated blood bicarbonate concentration.

Treatment usually involves attempts to improve the underlying ventilatory defect. Rarely, respiratory stimulants may be used, whereas in particular patients with acute ventilatory failure artificial ventilation may be appropriate.

Respiratory alkalosis

This arises as a consequence of increased ventilation causing the partial pressure of carbon dioxide in the blood to fall, with a resultant rise in blood pH. The causes include:

- a response to hypoxaemia or tissue hypoxia
- increased ventilation, e.g. in panic attacks
- excessive artificial ventilation
- stimulation of respiration by drugs, central nervous system stimulation or pulmonary disease in which there is stimulation of chest receptors.

The fall in carbon dioxide and rise in pH can be associated with a fall in ionized calcium which can produce symptoms of peripheral and circumoral paraesthesia, light-headedness and carpopedal spasm. Chvostek's sign may be present (tapping of the facial nerve elicits a brief facial muscle contraction, reflecting latent hypocalcaemic tetany).

Treatment is directed towards ensuring that there is correction of any concomitant hypoxaemia and reversal of the underlying cause.

Mixed acid–base disorders

The ability of the body to compensate for pH disturbances with respiratory or metabolic compensations and the presence of more than one cause of acid–base disturbance in a particular patient can produce complex disturbances. In such cases, a detailed history, complete examination, consideration of the blood gases and determination of the anion gap are critical in establishing the correct diagnosis.

143 Urinary calculi

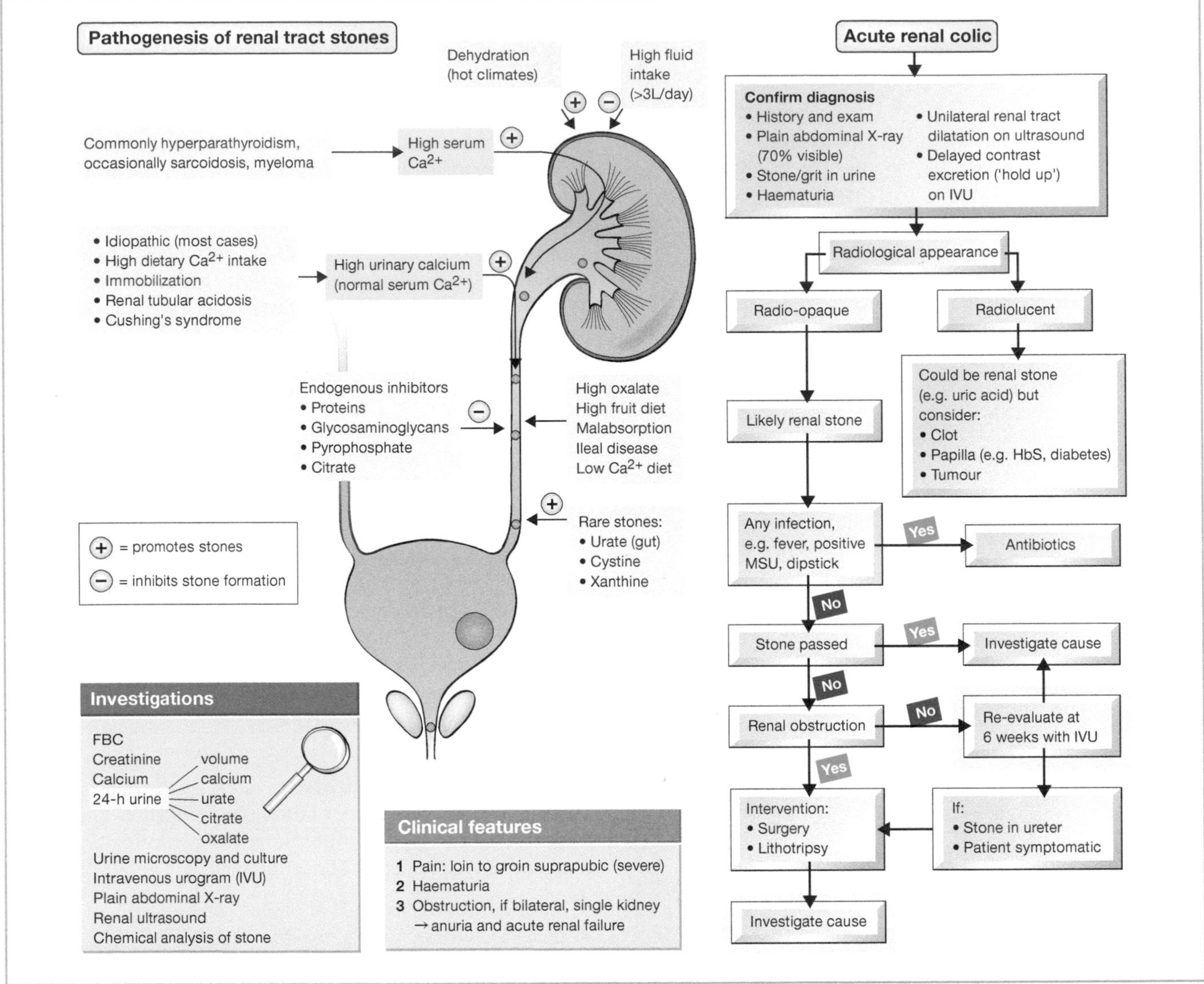

Urinary calculi are very common, with a prevalence of 5%. There is a peak prevalence at age 30–40 years and a 3:1 male predisposition. Most calculi contain calcium oxalate; the remainder consists of mixed calcium and ammonium phosphate (usually caused by infection), urate and cystine stones.

Aetiology

Most calculi are idiopathic; the remainder may be associated with hypercalciuria, hypercalcaemia, recurrent urinary tract infection (UTI), hyperuricosuria or cystinuria. Urinary calculi form when urinary solutes exceed their maximum urinary solubility. Conditions producing excretion of a high solute load or reduced urine volume will promote calculus formation (see Table 143.1). Urine is usually supersaturated for some solutes and crystallization inhibitors such as citrate tend to prevent calculus formation.

Presentation

Urinary calculi can cause haematuria (both macroscopic and microscopic), loin pain, renal colic, suprapubic pain, dysuria, UTIs, urinary tract obstruction, and acute or chronic renal failure as a result of obstruction ± infection. The pain of renal colic may be excruciating and commonly localizes to the flank, although radiation to the anterior abdomen, groin or scrotum can occur. Beware of important differential diagnoses including aortic aneurysm.

Medicine at a Glance, Fifth Edition. Edited by Patrick Davey and Alex Pitcher.

Companion website: www.wiley.com/go/medicine5e

Table 143.1 Conditions predisposing to renal stones.

- Metabolic syndromes
- Hypercalciuria: present in 50% of patients with renal stones
- Hyperoxaluria: idiopathic, genetic (type I or II) or secondary to gastrointestinal disease
- Hypocitraturia: distal renal tubular acidosis, K^+ depletion, renal failure
- Chronic hypercalcaemia: usually hyperparathyroidism
- Rare genetic metabolic diseases (e.g. cystinuria, etc.)
- Repeated infection
- Concentrated urine
- Chronically low fluid intake (<2 l/day)/high insensible losses (e.g. in hot countries)
- High dietary intake of animal protein
- Structural abnormality
- Renal tract obstruction (e.g. sloughed papilla, prostate, neurogenic bladder)
- Nephrocalcinosis: renal tubular acidosis (distal – type 1)

Investigations

- Full blood count to exclude the very rare association with haematological malignancies (urate stones).
- Creatinine, urea, electrolytes, plasma calcium and urate.
- 24-hour urine collection for urine volume, urine pH, calcium, urate, citrate and oxalate.
- Urine microscopy and culture because recurrent UTIs may be the cause or consequence of urinary calculi.
- Computed tomography (CT) urogram, renal tract ultrasonography and plain abdominal X-ray (AXR) to exclude obstruction and demonstrate the position of calculi.
- Chemical analysis of calculi.

Imaging of calculi

- **Ultrasonography**: 20% sensitivity, 97% specificity. Accessible, good for diagnosing hydronephrosis and renal stones, and requires no ionizing radiation. Poor at visualizing ureteral stones.
- **Plain radiography**: 50% sensitive, 75% specific. Accessible and inexpensive. Problems: stones in the middle section of the ureter, phleboliths, radiolucent calculi, extraurinary calcifications and non-genitourinary conditions.
- **Intravenous pyelography**: 65% sensitive, 90% specific. Accessible; provides information on anatomy and functioning of both kidneys. Problems: variable quality imaging, requires bowel preparation and use of contrast media, poor visualization of non-genitourinary conditions, delayed images required in high-grade obstruction.
- **Non-contrast CT**: 95% sensitive, 95% specific. Most sensitive and specific and preferred radiological test (i.e. facilitates fast, definitive diagnosis). Provides information on non-genitourinary conditions. Problems: indirect signs of degree of obstruction, less accessible and relatively expensive, no direct measure of renal function.

Management

Renal colic can be particularly painful, so adequate analgesia is important, often requiring non-steroidal anti-inflammatory drugs and/or opiate analgesia. Fluid intake should be increased to >3 l/day. Surgical treatment (required in 20%) of calculi or extracorporeal shock wave lithotripsy – where ultrasonic energy sufficient to fragment the calculus is transmitted from a probe placed on the skin over the renal tract – may prove necessary if the calculus is causing renal obstruction, particularly if infection is present. Renal failure (anuria) can occur if ureteric obstruction to a sole remaining kidney occurs. This is a medical emergency and requires immediate diagnosis and treatment. Several treatments facilitate the passage of stones (particularly <10 mm in diameter), notably α-blockers (e.g. tamsulosin) and calcium channel blockers (e.g. nifedipine).

Prevention

The most important measure is increasing fluid intake to promote a dilute urine. Other measures can include increasing endogenous inhibitors of stone formation, by giving oral potassium citrate and lemon juice and reducing sodium and animal protein in the diet. Specific preventive treatments include the following.

- **Infection** associated with stones: prophylactic antibiotics.
- **Hypercalciuria**: the amount of calcium in the urine can be lessened with thiazide diuretics, and by reducing the amount of sodium in the diet.
- **Urate calculi**: can be prevented with allopurinol.
- **Oxalate stones**: in oxalate stones, the amount of oxalate in the diet (e.g. rhubarb or spinach) should be reduced, while maintaing normal dietary calcium intake to bind oxalate in the gut. Increasing dietary vitamin B_6 intake decreases urinary oxalate.
- **Cystinuria**: treated with urinary alkalinization or dissolution with penicillamine (although side-effects limit its use) or captopril.

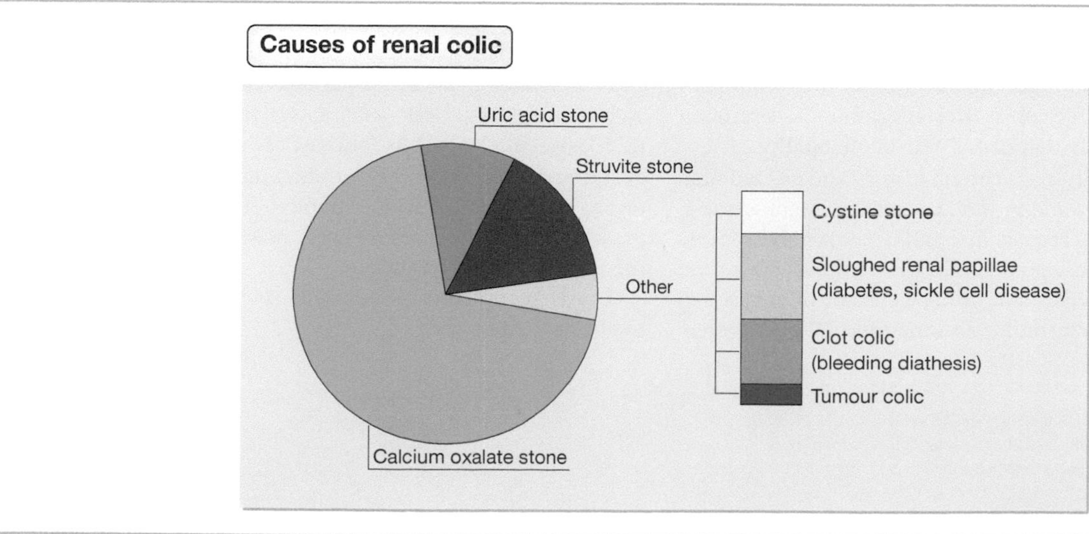

144 Nephrotic and nephritic syndromes

Normal urinary protein

<150 mg/day

Microalbuminuria

30–300 mg/day
Early sign of diabetic nephropathy

Proteinuria

300 mg–4.5g/day

If >2g/day, + microscopic haematuria or + renal impairment consider renal biopsy

Nephrotic syndrome

>4.5g/ day
Oedema
Hypoalbuminaemia
Renal biopsy usually indicated

Common causes
- Glomerulonephritis
- Diabetes
- Amyloid

Histology in glomerulonephritis associated with the nephrotic syndrome

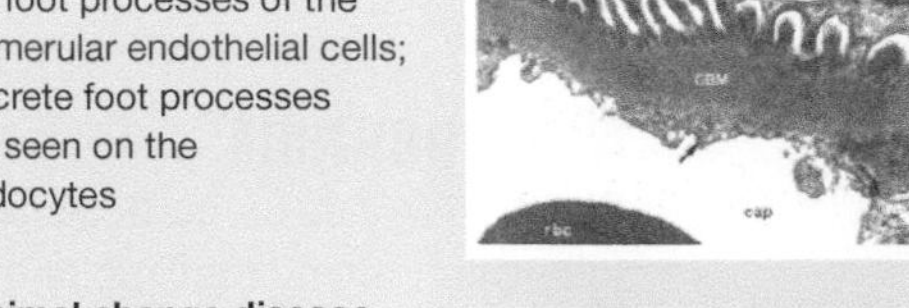

Normal kidney
Normal electron micrograph of the foot processes of the glomerular endothelial cells; discrete foot processes are seen on the podocytes

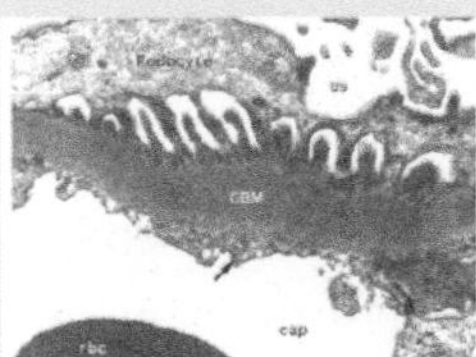

Minimal change disease
Whereas in minimal change GN, the light microscope shows no change, the EM image shows fusion of the foot processes

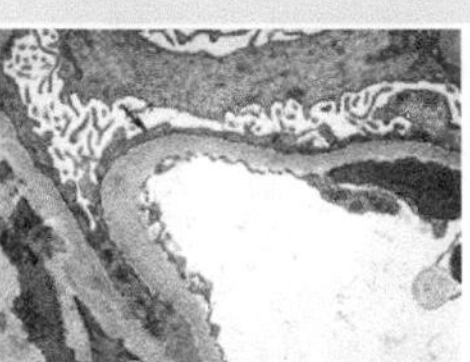

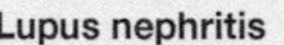

Lupus nephritis
A large number of different histological appearances occur in lupus nephritis – this image shows staining for the C1q component of complement

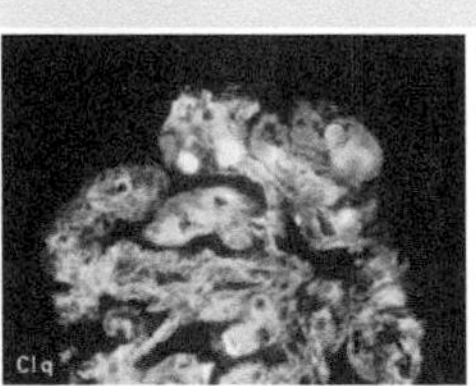

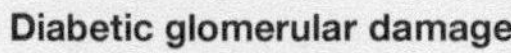

Diabetic glomerular damage
This image shows the characteristic sclerotic lesions found in diabetic glomerular damage. Early on, diabetes leads to glomerular hyperfiltration; later proteinuria and decreases in GFR occur, often culminating in renal failure with the nephrotic syndrome

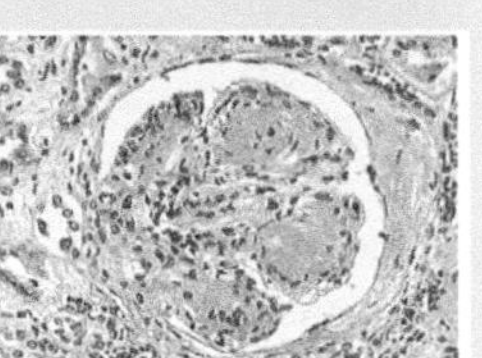

Cause of proteinuria as related to quantity

Daily protein excretion	Cause
0.15 to 2.0 g	Mild glomerulopathies Tubular proteinuria Overflow proteinuria
2.0 to 4.0 g	Usually glomerular
>4.0 g	Always glomerular

Features of the nephrotic syndrome

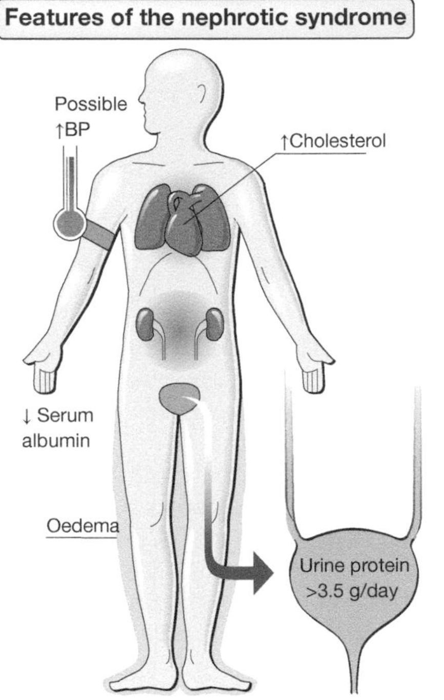

Proteinuria and the nephrotic syndrome

The normal amount of protein in urine is <150 mg/day. Most of this is the result of a physiological, rather viscous glycoprotein that is secreted by tubular cells, termed 'Tamm–Horsfall protein'. The presence of higher amounts of protein may indicate significant renal disease, often **glomerulonephritis** (GN). Dipsticks detect mainly albumin and will not detect pathological proteins, such as immunoglobulin light chains (Bence-Jones protein) in myeloma. Microalbuminuria (urinary albumin excretion 30–300 mg/day) is an early sign of **diabetic nephropathy**.

In patients with proteinuria, a careful history and examination should be performed, looking for causes of renal disease. Hypertension, evidence of renal failure and oedema may be found on examination. Renal function should be assessed with serum creatinine and electrolytes, and a 24-hour urine collection performed to determine creatinine clearance and 24-hour protein excretion. A 'spot' urine protein:creatinine (or albumin:creatinine ratio [ACR]) ratio correlates well with 24-hour protein excretion, and can be used as a simple estimate of renal protein loss.

If these results confirm significant proteinuria (see Table 144.1) or renal dysfunction, further investigations should include ultrasonography of the renal tract, blood glucose (to exclude diabetes, a common cause of the nephrotic syndrome) and immunological investigations to exclude myeloma and autoimmune conditions such as systemic lupus erythematosus (SLE), systemic vasculitis (antinuclear factor and antineutrophil cytoplasmic antibody), or membranous nephropathy (consider testing for the anti-PLA2R antibody). If significant proteinuria is present (>2 g/day), a renal biopsy may be appropriate to define the cause of the proteinuria.

Levels of proteinuria >3.5 g in 24 hours may produce the **nephrotic syndrome**.

Medicine at a Glance, Fifth Edition. Edited by Patrick Davey and Alex Pitcher.

Companion website: www.wiley.com/go/medicine5e

Table 144.1 Classification of proteinuria.

Type	Pathophysiological features	Cause
Glomerular	Increased glomerular capillary permeability to protein	Primary or secondary glomerulopathy
Tubular	Decreased tubular reabsorption of proteins in glomerular filtrate	Tubular or interstitial disease
Overflow	Increased production of low molecular weight proteins	Monoclonal gammopathy

The nephrotic syndrome

The nephrotic syndrome is characterized by the following.

- Proteinuria (usually 3–4+ on dipstick testing; 24 h urine excretion of protein is often >4 g/24 h).
- Hypoalbuminaemia (usually albumin <30 g/dl).
- Peripheral oedema.
- Unlike the nephritic syndrome, haematuria is rare and blood pressure (BP) is normal or only mildly elevated.

Causes

The nephrotic syndrome is usually a consequence of one of the following.

- Glomerular disease, commonly GN. The types of GN most commonly found to be responsible for the nephrotic syndrome on renal biopsy are minimal change disease (overwhelmingly the most likely cause for nephrotic syndrome in childhood), membranous nephropathy and focal segmental glomerulosclerosis.
- Diabetes.
- Renal amyloid, which may relate to primary or secondary amyloidosis, or multiple myeloma.
- Drugs (particularly those used in rheumatology, such as non-steroidal anti-inflammatory agents, penicillamine and gold) are occasionally the cause.
- Other causes include SLE.

Complications

Complications of the nephrotic syndrome relate in part to the low albumin, and partly to more complex pathophysiological changes induced by the nephrotic condition.

- **Oedema**: found in dependent sites (i.e. the lower limbs in ambulant patients and the sacral area in bed-bound patients), but can also be found in the face (e.g. periorbitally) and hands.
- **Hypercoagulability**: may lead to renal vein thrombosis and a dramatic worsening of renal function, or may produce deep venous thrombosis. Prophylactic anticoagulation should be considered in patients with severe nephrotic syndrome.
- **Hypercholesterolaemia**: may play a large role in the accelerated atheroma that can be found in long-standing nephrotic syndrome. The reason why hypercholesterolaemia occurs is not clear; it may relate to hypersynthesis of apolipoproteins, resulting from the general increase in protein synthesis found in many nephrotic patients.
- **Infection**: the nephrotic syndrome is associated with hypogammaglobulinaemia and impairment of the immune system. Infection, which may be overwhelming, can occur, particularly with pneumococci. Immunization against the pneumococcus should be given.

Treatment

Any underlying cause should be fully diagnosed and treated with specific therapy. General management includes the use of diuretics to reduce oedema (although their use must be balanced against the possibility of diuretic-induced hypovolaemia, which itself will worsen renal function) and angiotensin-converting enzyme (ACE) inhibitors may be used to reduce proteinuria and treat hypertension aggressively to slow the progression of renal impairment, particularly in diabetes. Anticoagulation may be instituted for thrombotic episodes and hyperlipidaemia commonly requires treatment. Specific treatment exists for certain types of GN, e.g. minimal change disease commonly responds well to corticosteroids. Unfortunately, some diseases are very resistant to treatment, such as the nephrotic syndrome related to renal amyloid.

The nephritic syndrome

This is an acute renal illness with the following features.

- Haematuria (occasionally macroscopic) and mild proteinuria, i.e. usually only 1–2+ on dipstick testing, which is insufficient to cause a depression in serum albumin, unlike the nephrotic syndrome.
- Inability of the kidney to excrete fluids, leading to fluid retention (oedema), hypertension and occasionally oliguria.
- Decreased glomerular filtration rate (GFR), producing varying degrees of uraemia.

This term was previously more widely used when streptococcal infection was common, because the nephritic syndrome not infrequently followed 2–3 weeks after a throat infection with group A β-haemolytic streptococci. The prognosis of post-streptococcal GN is excellent, the need for dialysis in the acute stage is low, and the likelihood of spontaneous and full recovery of renal function is very high. The differential diagnosis of the nephritic syndrome is wide and includes most of the diseases capable of producing GN (see Chapter 145). Immunological tests and a renal biopsy are usually indicated.

Treatment

It is important to treat any underlying cause with specific therapies. Oedema, hypertension and renal impairment should be treated as for the nephrotic syndrome, although as hypertension is more common and more severe, it should be looked for assiduously and treated aggressively with antihypertensive drugs (often ACE inhibitors). Dialysis is more likely to be needed for uraemia than in the nephrotic syndrome.

145 Glomerulonephritis

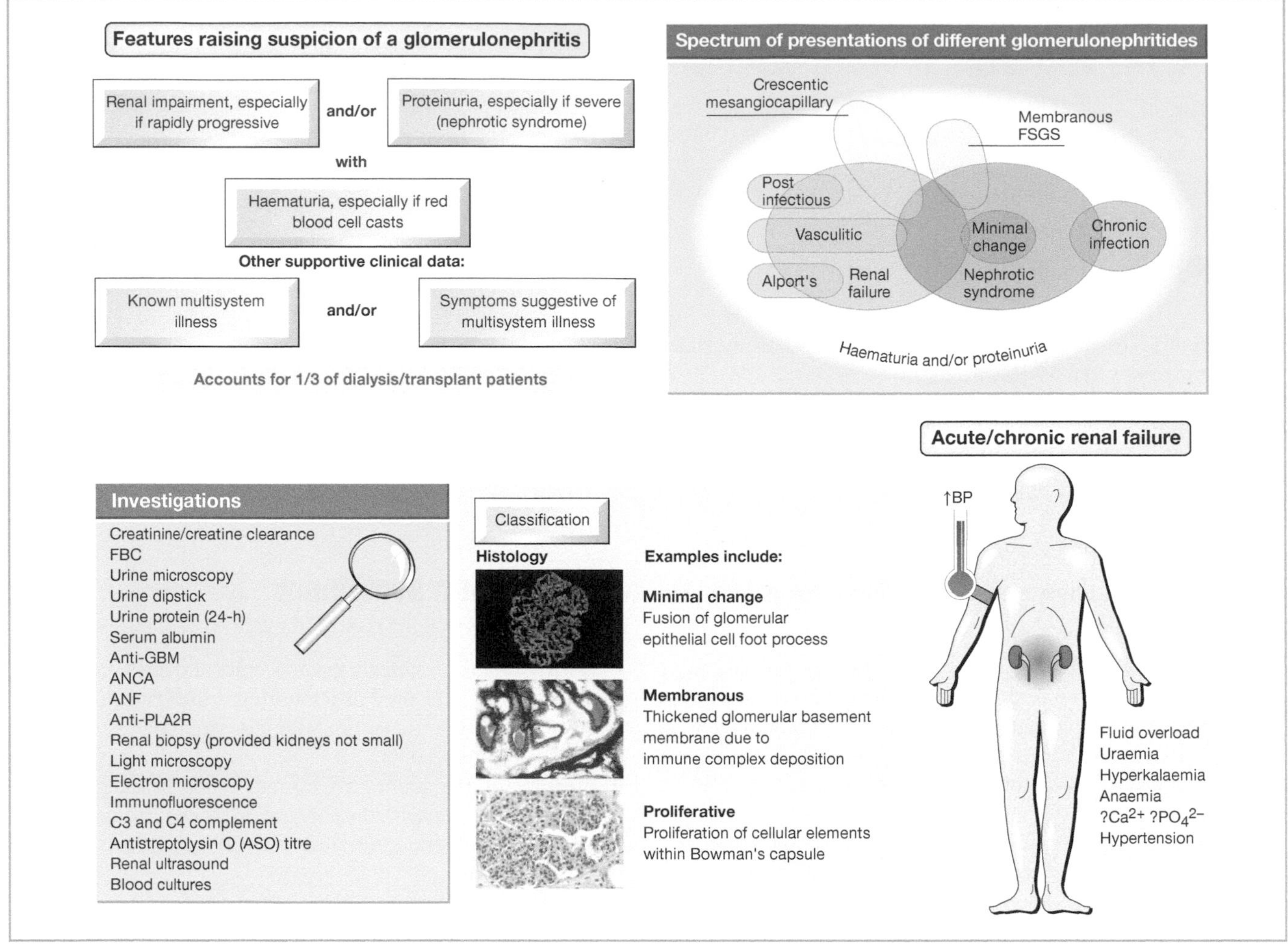

Features raising suspicion of a glomerulonephritis
Renal impairment, especially if rapidly progressive
and/or
Proteinuria, especially if severe (nephrotic syndrome)
with
Haematuria, especially if red blood cell casts
Other supportive clinical data:
Known multisystem illness
and/or
Symptoms suggestive of multisystem illness
Accounts for 1/3 of dialysis/transplant patients
Spectrum of presentations of different glomerulonephritides
Crescentic mesangiocapillary
Membranous FSGS
Post infectious
Vasculitic
Minimal change
Chronic infection
Alport's
Renal failure
Nephrotic syndrome
Haematuria and/or proteinuria
Acute/chronic renal failure
↑BP
Fluid overload
Uraemia
Hyperkalaemia
Anaemia
?Ca2+ ?PO42−
Hypertension
Investigations
Creatinine/creatine clearance
FBC
Urine microscopy
Urine dipstick
Urine protein (24-h)
Serum albumin
Anti-GBM
ANCA
ANF
Anti-PLA2R
Renal biopsy (provided kidneys not small)
Light microscopy
Electron microscopy
Immunofluorescence
C3 and C4 complement
Antistreptolysin O (ASO) titre
Renal ultrasound
Blood cultures
Classification
Histology
Examples include:
Minimal change
Fusion of glomerular epithelial cell foot process
Membranous
Thickened glomerular basement membrane due to immune complex deposition
Proliferative
Proliferation of cellular elements within Bowman's capsule

Glomerulonephritis (GN) can present in a variety of ways: (i) acute or chronic renal failure; (ii) the nephrotic syndrome (oedema, proteinuria, hypoalbuminaemia); (iii) haematuria; and (iv) proteinuria and hypertension.

It is the cause of renal failure in up to one-third of patients requiring dialysis or transplantation. The cardinal features of glomerular abnormalities are:

- proteinuria
- haematuria
- urinary casts.

Glomerulonephritis affects both kidneys symmetrically. The disease may affect primarily the kidneys (primary GN) or be associated with systemic illnesses such as granulomatosis with polyangiitis (GPA), systemic lupus erythematosus (SLE) and other vasculitides (secondary GN). The type of GN is usually established by renal biopsy (light microscopy, immunofluorescence, electron microscopy [EM]). The different histological types of GN each have a different spectrum of presentation, and vary in their prognosis and response to treatment.

Acute glomerulonephritis

A confusing aspect of glomerular disease is that many different histological subtypes can produce the same clinical syndrome and, conversely, each histological form can produce different clinical patterns. It is therefore usual to classify glomerulonephritis in terms of both the clinical syndrome and the pathological diagnosis. The different pathological forms underlying the different clinical syndromes are as follows.

- **Acute renal failure**: GN can underlie acute renal failure, when it is termed 'rapidly progressive GN'. This is usually characterized by the presence of crescents (a crescentic-shaped proliferation of cells in Bowman's capsule) and is most commonly seen with the

Medicine at a Glance, Fifth Edition. Edited by Patrick Davey and Alex Pitcher.

Companion website: www.wiley.com/go/medicine5e

GN associated with the vasculitic conditions such as granulomatosis with polyangiitis (GPA), Goodpasture syndrome (acute renal failure and pulmonary haemorrhage caused by a circulating antiglomerular basement membrane [anti-GBM] antibody) and postinfectious GN after a streptococcal infection. Time is of the essence, because many patients progress from normal renal function to dialysis-dependent renal failure within days, and rapidly progressive GN is therefore a medical emergency. Early aggressive treatment often stabilizes or improves renal function, whereas late (i.e. occurring by the time renal support is needed, or when the patient is oliguric) treatment is usually much less effective.

- **Nephrotic syndrome**: the most common causes of the nephrotic syndrome in adults are shown in the chart below.

Renal histology

- **Membranous GN**: the light microscopic appearances are of a thickened basement membrane, which on EM is the result of numerous subepithelial immune complex deposits of IgG and complement C3. Although usually idiopathic, it can be secondary to underlying malignancy in 10% of cases, and can relate to SLE, drugs or infections. A circulating antibody, antiphospholipid A2 receptor (anti-PLA2R), is been found in over two-thirds of patients with idiopathic membranous GN.

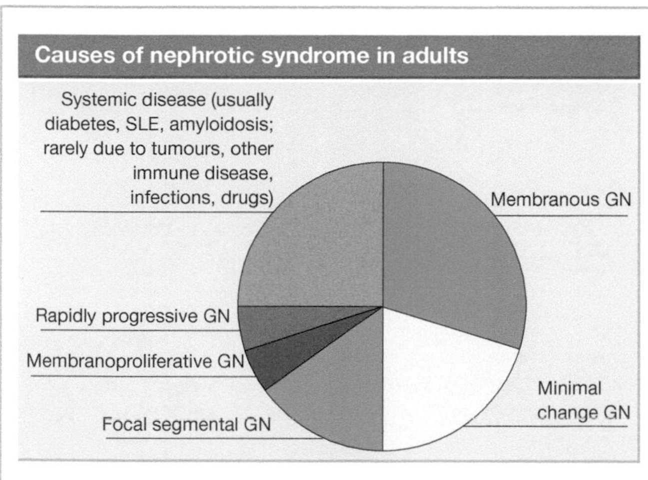

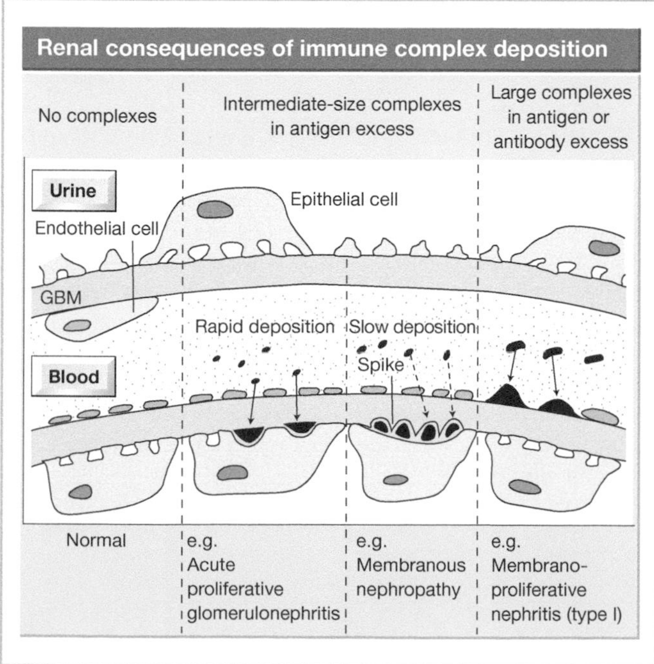

- **Minimal change GN**: light microscope and immunological studies are normal, but podocyte foot processes are fused on EM. Focal segmental glomerulosclerosis (FSGS) is similar, except some glomeruli have segmental sclerotic lesions.
- The renal histology in **incidental haematuria** and/or **proteinuria** varies. The most common finding at renal biopsy is of IgA nephropathy (Berger disease). Clinically, patients often have visible haematuria after upper respiratory tract infections. Histologically, the condition is characterized by mesangial deposition of IgA with variable segmental mesangial proliferation. Although most patients have a benign prognosis, 20–40% of patients progress to renal failure. IgA nephropathy also occurs in people with longstanding alcohol problems who have liver disease.

Chronic glomerulonephritis

Patients presenting with chronic renal failure may have small, shrunken kidneys on ultrasonography and chronic fibrotic changes with glomerulosclerosis on biopsy. The disease underlying the renal failure is then presumed to be a GN, particularly if there is a history of previous proteinuria or haematuria. The process is usually burnt out and does not respond to any treatment. Renal biopsy does not usually alter treatment and is contraindicated when small kidneys are found in view of the risks posed by renal biopsy.

Management

Important investigations in a patient with suspected GN include assessment of renal function with serum creatinine and creatinine clearance, urine dipstick and microscopy (examining particularly for red cells and casts), 24-hour urinary protein excretion and renal ultrasonography for renal size. Significant proteinuria (>1 g/day) is strongly suggestive of a GN. Immunological tests are essential in establishing whether the GN is secondary and should include antineutrophil cytoplasmic antibody (ANCA) (granulomatosis with polyangiitis [GPA], microscopic polyangiitis), antinuclear factor (ANF), anti-PLA2R (membranous GN), complement C3 and C4 (SLE), anti-GBM antibodies (Goodpasture syndrome) and antistreptolysin O (ASO) titre (poststreptococcal GN) (see Chapter 146) and hepatitis B and C serologies. Renal biopsy is necessary to establish an accurate diagnosis; however, this will not usually be undertaken if the kidneys are small.

In GN, aggressive blood pressure treatment, usually including ACEi or ARB, can reduce the speed of disease progression, control of lipids is important and nephrotoxic drugs should be avoided.

The **treatment** of GN depends on the precise type.

- **Minimal change GN**: corticosteroid treatment can often produce remission. Half of adult patients relapse once after initial remission; a second course of steroids is then indicated. It is the most common cause of the nephrotic syndrome in children and young adults. Further relapses or failure to induce remission are indications for more aggressive immunosuppression.
- **Membranous GN**: the prognosis is variable. At 10 years, 25% have remitted spontaneously, 25% have persistent non-nephrotic proteinuria, 25% have nephrotic proteinuria and 25% have renal failure. In those with deteriorating renal function, regimens including steroids and cyclophosphamide, ciclosporin or rituximab may be beneficial. Drug-induced membranous GN may remit after drug cessation.
- **Rapidly progressive GN**: more aggressive immunosuppressive regimens are commonly advocated and include corticosteroids, cyclophosphamide, rituximab and plasmapheresis.

146 Renal involvement in systemic disease

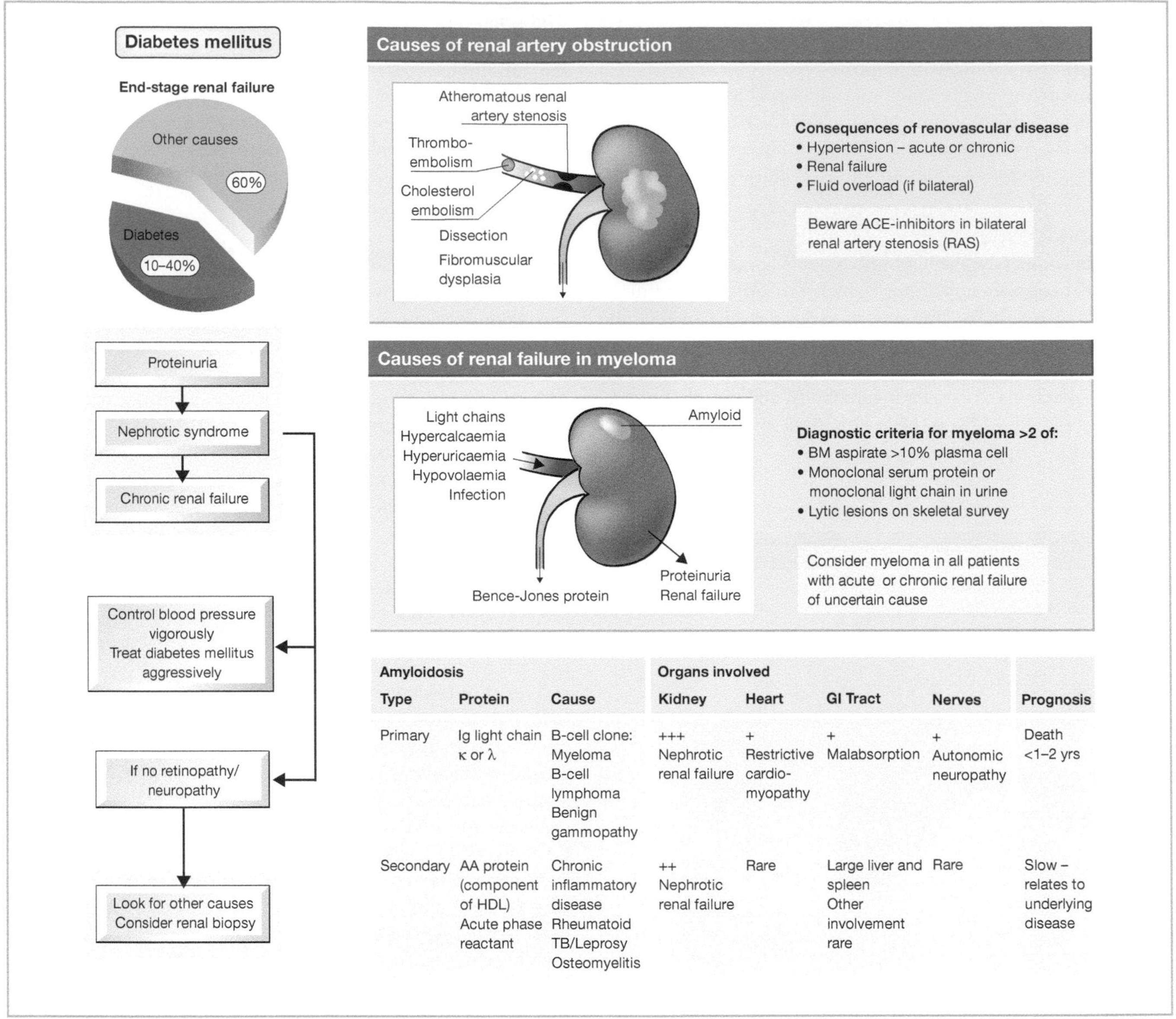

Amyloidosis			Organs involved				
Type	Protein	Cause	Kidney	Heart	GI Tract	Nerves	Prognosis
Primary	Ig light chain κ or λ	B-cell clone: Myeloma B-cell lymphoma Benign gammopathy	+++ Nephrotic renal failure	+ Restrictive cardio-myopathy	+ Malabsorption	+ Autonomic neuropathy	Death <1–2 yrs
Secondary	AA protein (component of HDL) Acute phase reactant	Chronic inflammatory disease Rheumatoid TB/Leprosy Osteomyelitis	++ Nephrotic renal failure	Rare	Large liver and spleen Other involvement rare	Rare	Slow – relates to underlying disease

Diabetes mellitus

Diabetes mellitus causes renal disease; the incidence increases with longer duration of disease, with 30% having nephropathy 20 years after diagnosis. It accounts for 40% of patients on renal replacement therapy. The initial diabetic renal lesion is manifest as microalbuminuria, which progresses to increasing levels of proteinuria or even the nephrotic syndrome. There may be a gradual loss of excretory function manifest as rising creatinine and urea. Patients with diabetic nephropathy commonly suffer from diabetic retinopathy or neuropathy. If absent, this should prompt a search for alternative causes of renal impairment or nephrotic syndrome. If doubt remains about whether the renal dysfunction is attributable to diabetes, a renal biopsy should be performed.

In diabetes, very aggressive blood pressure lowering, often with angiotensin-converting enzyme (ACE) inhibitors or angiotensin II receptor blockers, can slow progression of the renal disease. Similarly, excellent glycaemic control may reduce the development and progression of renal disease. Smoking cessation, control of lipids and antiplatelet agents are important. Increasing evidence is accumulating for beneficial roles of sodium-glucose co-transporter 2 (SGLT2) inhibitors such as empaglifozin in slowing the progression of renal disease and reducing mortality.

Medicine at a Glance, Fifth Edition. Edited by Patrick Davey and Alex Pitcher.

Companion website: www.wiley.com/go/medicine5e

Myeloma

Myeloma commonly produces renal impairment. In patients with acute or chronic renal impairment of unknown cause, myeloma should be considered in the differential diagnosis and protein electrophoresis (for paraproteinaemia), urine electrophoresis (for Bence-Jones proteins) and immunoglobulin estimations undertaken. Renal impairment in myeloma has several causes, including the direct toxicity of immunoglobulin light chains to the tubular cells, hypercalcaemia, dehydration, hyperuricaemia, renal amyloid, hyperviscosity and infection. Treatment involves that of the underlying myeloma and rapid correction of hypovolaemia and hypercalcaemia. Plasma exchange has a role in rapidly removing myeloma protein in some patients with renal failure, and treatment of the underlying myeloma with newer agents, such as bortezomib and lenalidomide, may improve the chances of renal recovery. Monoclonal gammopathies may also contribute to renal impairment.

Amyloidosis

Amyloidosis is characterized by the deposition of protein fibrils in many organs, including the kidney. It may be primary in association with myeloma (amyloid AL) or secondary to chronic infections or inflammation or have a hereditary cause (amyloid AA). The most common renal presentation is with proteinuria, often sufficient to produce the nephrotic syndrome. Renal biopsy demonstrates an eosinophilic tissue infiltration that stains positive with Congo red and exhibits green birefringence under polarized light. The prognosis for renal function is usually poor.

Haemolytic uraemic syndrome

Haemolytic uraemic syndrome (HUS) is characterized by haemolysis, platelet consumption and acute renal failure. It may be associated with diarrhoea, particularly in children, when *Escherichia coli* serotype O157 produces verocytotoxin which causes endothelial damage. Atypical HUS may occur in patients with inherited or acquired deficiencies of complement regulatory proteins such as factor H. Investigations reveal haemolysis, thrombocytopenia and renal failure. Renal biopsy shows fibrin thrombi occluding glomerular tufts. In diarrhoea-associated disease, spontaneous remission is common, but in severe forms plasmapheresis is often advocated. There may be benefit from the anti-C5a antibody, eculizumab.

Renovascular disease

There are two main pathologies causing renovascular disease.

1 **Atherosclerotic renal artery stenosis**: this presents with hypertension, renal impairment or, if bilateral, fluid overload manifesting as pulmonary oedema. A renal bruit may rarely be audible and renal ultrasonography may show small or asymmetrical kidneys. Renal angiography or magnetic resonance angiography can demonstrate the stenosis. Cardiovascular risk factors should be treated. Angioplasty and/or stenting has no definite benefit on subsequent renal function and hypertension; they are usually reserved for patients with resistant hypertension or deteriorating renal function. Obstruction of renal blood flow can also occur with embolism of the renal arteries or renal artery dissection, and classically presents with loin pain and impairment of renal function. Atherosclerosis of intrarenal vessels may occur with or without renal artery stenosis and contributes to renal impairment and hypertension.

2 **Fibromuscular dysplasia**: produces a beaded appearance of the renal artery on angiography, occurs more commonly in younger females and is an important cause of hypertension.

Renal vasculitis

The UK prevalence of systemic vasculitis affecting the kidney is 30/100 000 (see Table 146.1). Vasculitis is a difficult disease to diagnose because of its ability to affect many parts of the body. It should be considered in patients with unexplained renal failure, rash, fever, weight loss and upper and lower repiratory symptoms.

Table 146.1 Renal vasculitis.

			Organ involvement							
	Incidence	F : M	Kidney	Lung	Heart	Skin	URT/sinus	GI tract	Diagnostic test	Treatment
Goodpasture syndrome	±	1 : 1	+++	+++	0	0	0	0	GBM antibody	St, CyP, PE
Microscopic polyarteritis	+	1 : 1	+++	+	0	+	0	+	pANCA (MPO)	St, CyP, PE
Churg–Strauss syndrome	±	1 : 1	++	+++	++	++	++	0	Eosinophils/CXR	St
Henoch–Schönlein purpura	+++	1 : 2	+	0	0	+++	0	++	None	None
Granulomatosis with polyangiitis (GPA)	+(+)	1 : 2	+++	++	0	0	+++	0	cANCA (PR3)	St, CyP, PE
SLE	++	9 : 1	++	+	+	++	+	+	Anti-dsDNA	St, AM, CyP
Scleroderma	++	4 : 1	+	++	+	+++	0	+++	ANA, Scl-70	ACE inhibitors, none
Cryoglobulinaemia	+	1 : 1	++	0	0	+++	0	0	See text	St, PE

ACE, angiotensin-converting enzyme; AM, antimalarials (chloroquine); ANA, antinuclear antibodies; ANCA, antineutrophil cytoplasmic antibodies; CyP, cyclophosphamide; CXR, chest X-ray; GI, gastrointestinal; GBM, glomerular basement membrane; MPO, myeloperoxidase; PE, plasma exchange; PR3, proteinase 3; SLE, systemic lupus erythematosus; St, corticosteroids; URT, upper respiratory tract.

Granulomatosis with polyangiitis (GPA)

This rare condition (600 new cases/year in the UK) is characterized by granulomatous disease of the upper airway (including nose, sinuses, trachea) and lung, and renal impairment resulting from a focal necrotizing glomerulonephritis (GN). It is part of the differential diagnosis in patients with upper airway disease, lung masses or rapidly progressive GN. If suspected, an antineutrophil cytoplasmic antibody (ANCA) test should be performed, where the pattern of staining of the cytoplasmic components of neutrophils after applying serum IgG antibodies is studied. Two patterns of staining are found: one where staining is principally cytoplasmic (cANCA – the antigen is principally proteinase-3 [PR3]) and the other where staining is principally perinuclear (pANCA – the antigen is predominantly myeloperoxidase [MPO]) and can be confirmed with specific enzyme-linked immunosorbent assay (ELISA). pANCA is found in microscopic polyangiitis and cANCA is positive in over 90% of cases of GPA, in which its titre can reflect disease activity. A renal biopsy shows a focal necrotizing GN, sometimes with crescent formation and granuloma. Treatment should be prompt because patients can deteriorate rapidly, and involves aggressive immunosuppression with corticosteroids, cyclophosphamide (or rituximab) and plasmapheresis.

Microscopic polyangiitis

This rare vasculitis (400 new cases/year in the UK) produces inflammation of the small blood vessels and can present with multisystem or single-organ involvement. The kidneys, skin, brain and nerves are the most common organs affected. Rapidly progressive renal impairment can result. Testing for ANCA usually reveals a positive staining with a perinuclear pattern (pANCA). Treatment is as for granulomatosis with polyangiitis (GPA).

Goodpasture syndrome

Very rare (50 new cases/year in the UK). This syndrome is characterized by pulmonary haemorrhage (which is more common in people who smoke), haematuria and rapidly progressive renal failure. It is caused by an autoantibody directed against a collagen found only in basement membrane – the antiglomerular basement membrane (anti-GBM) antibody. The antibody can be detected in blood. Renal biopsies demonstrate a crescentic GN with linear antibody staining along the GBM on immunofluorescence. Lung function tests may reveal an elevated carbon monoxide transfer factor (*K*co), consistent with pulmonary haemorrhage because haemoglobin binds CO very avidly. Treatment is with plasmapheresis to remove the antibody, and immunosuppression with corticosteroids ± cyclophosphamide to reduce its production.

Polyarteritis nodosa

This vasculitis (150 cases/year in the UK) affects larger blood vessels and presents with non-specific symptoms such as weight loss, fever, malaise and abdominal pain. Arteriography demonstrates microaneurysms and arterial narrowing, and biopsies of affected tissue may be diagnostic. ANCA tests are usually negative. There can be an association with hepatitis B infection. Renal involvement causes haematuria and proteinuria or renal impairment. Treatment is immunosuppression.

Systemic lupus erythematosus

Renal disease occurs in half of patients with systemic lupus erythematosus (SLE), with an annual incidence of 3000 patients in the UK. Involvement ranges from mild, with proteinuria and haematuria, to severe, with nephrotic syndrome or rapidly progressive renal failure. In determining the nature of renal involvement, urine microscopy is important. The presence of significant haematuria, proteinuria or red cell casts implies a significant glomerular lesion. Renal biopsy is then undertaken to define the glomerular pathology. Several patterns of renal involvement are seen, including a focal and segmental proliferative GN, a membranous GN or a diffuse proliferative GN with crescents. The immunology varies: 90% of patients have a positive ANA test (i.e. IgG staining of the nucleus, often of discrete nuclear or nucleolar elements). Although antibodies to double-stranded DNA (anti-dsDNA antibodies) are highly specific for SLE, in renal

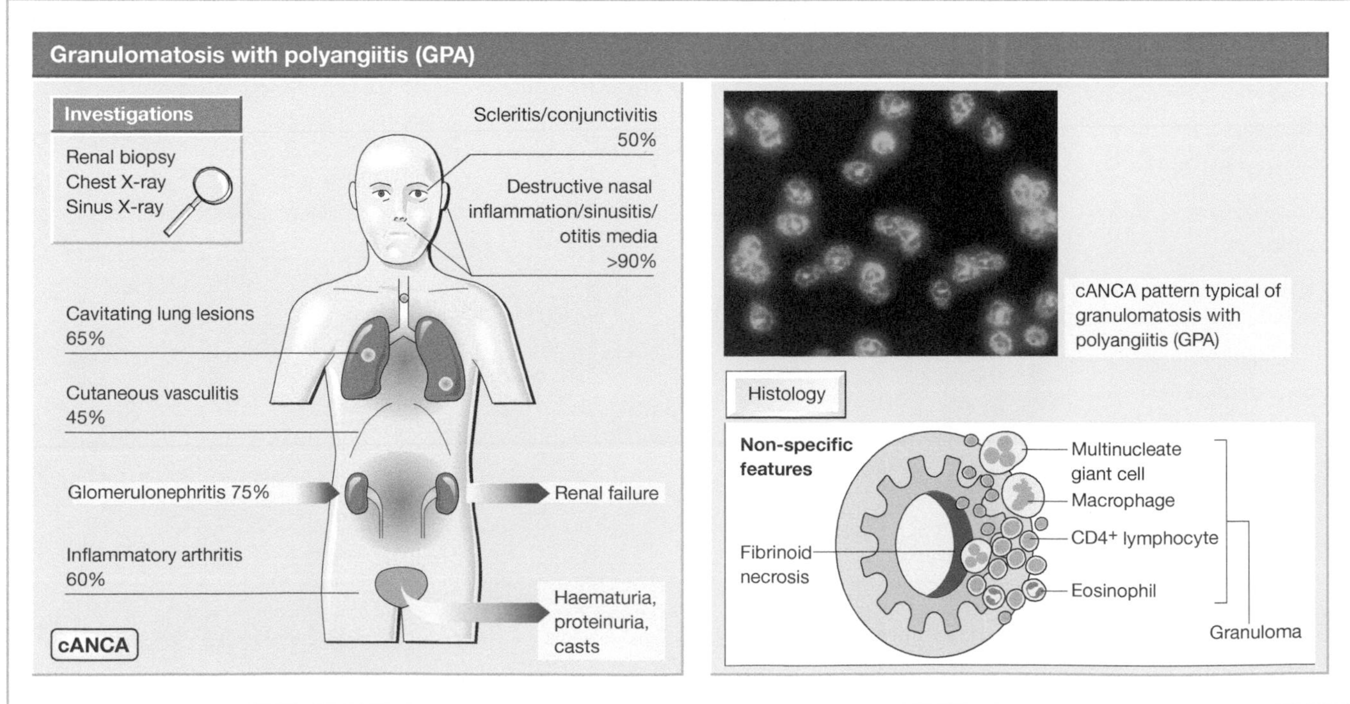

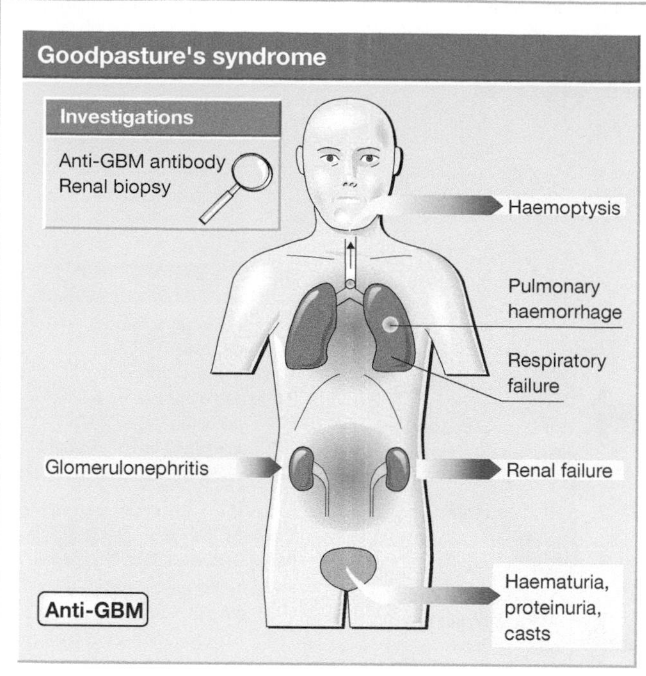

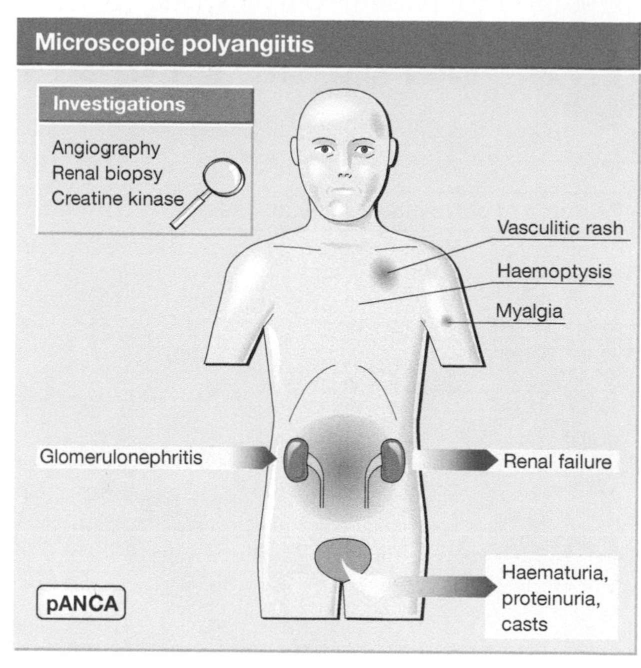

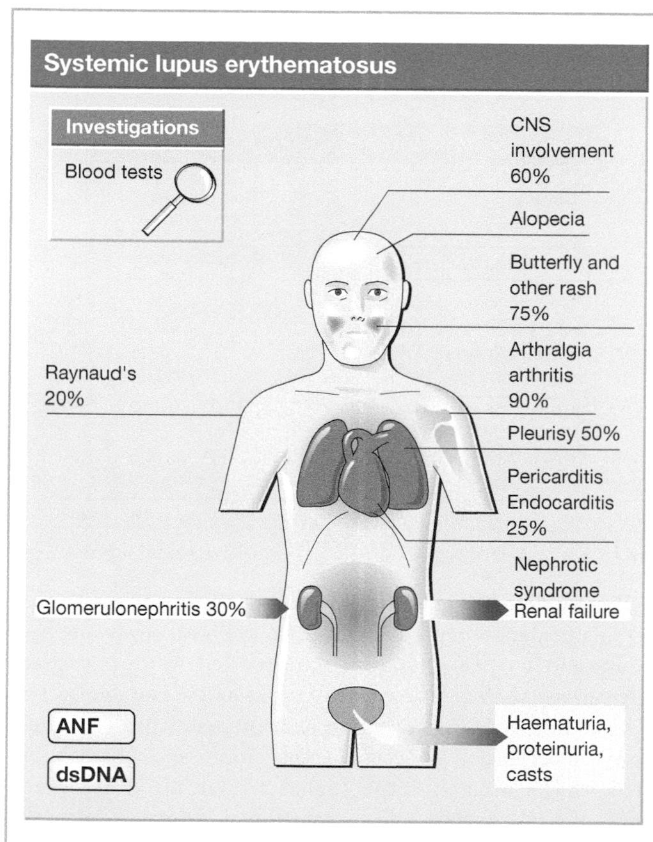

disease their titre may paradoxically be depressed. Some 40% have antibodies to extractable nuclear antigens (such as Smith Sm or Ro-SS-A). Antibodies to platelets, red cells and phospholipid are also common. There is often complement consumption with lowered levels of C3 and C4. The erythrocyte sedimentation rate (but not the C-reactive protein) is elevated. Treatment depends on histology but often involves corticosteroids and immunosuppressive agents such as cyclophosphamide, mycophenolate and azathioprine.

Henoch–Schönlein purpura

Although common in children, Henoch–Schönlein purpura is rare in adults (<300 new cases/year in the UK). The aetiology is not known, but it may reflect an autoimmune response to an infective agent, which in part explains the seasonal variation and that one-third have a preceding upper respiratory tract infection. Malaise, arthralgia, abdominal pain and, most typically, a purpuric rash on the extensor surfaces (elbows, buttocks, knees) characterize the illness. Renal involvement consists of a usually self-limiting focal GN. Occasionally progressive renal failure occurs.

Scleroderma

Renal involvement complicates 25% of scleroderma, occurs early or late on in the course of the disease, and accounts for 40% of deaths. Incidence is about 200 new cases/year. It may present as an active sediment (i.e. haematuria, sometimes severe enough to produce 'red cell casts') or ominously as a 'scleroderma renal crisis', with treatment-resistant hypertension, rapidly progressive uraemia and a characteristic 'onion skin' appearance of blood vessels on renal histology. Immunological tests show antibodies to Scl-70 (the enzyme topoisomerase I) and often to RNA polymerases 1–3. Anticentromere antibodies are associated with mild cutaneous disease. ACE inhibitor therapy may help.

Cryoglobulinaemia

Cryoglobulins are abnormal immunoglobulins that precipitate when cooled. Blood must be transported to the laboratory at 37 °C for testing for the presence of a cryoglobulin. If cooling occurs in superficial blood vessels, then obstruction of the vessel and tissue necrosis may occur. Type I cryoglobulins are monoclonal proteins, and found in association with myeloma, Waldenstrom macroglobulinaemia and lymphoma. Type II cryoglobulins comprise a monoclonal component that has rheumatoid factor activity and binds to normal immunoglobulins. These are found in chronic infections such as hepatitis C and bacterial endocarditis, as well as connective tissue disease and myeloma or lymphoma. Type III cryoglobulins are polyclonal with rheumatoid factor activity and are usually associated with SLE and rheumatoid arthritis.

147 Hereditary renal disorders

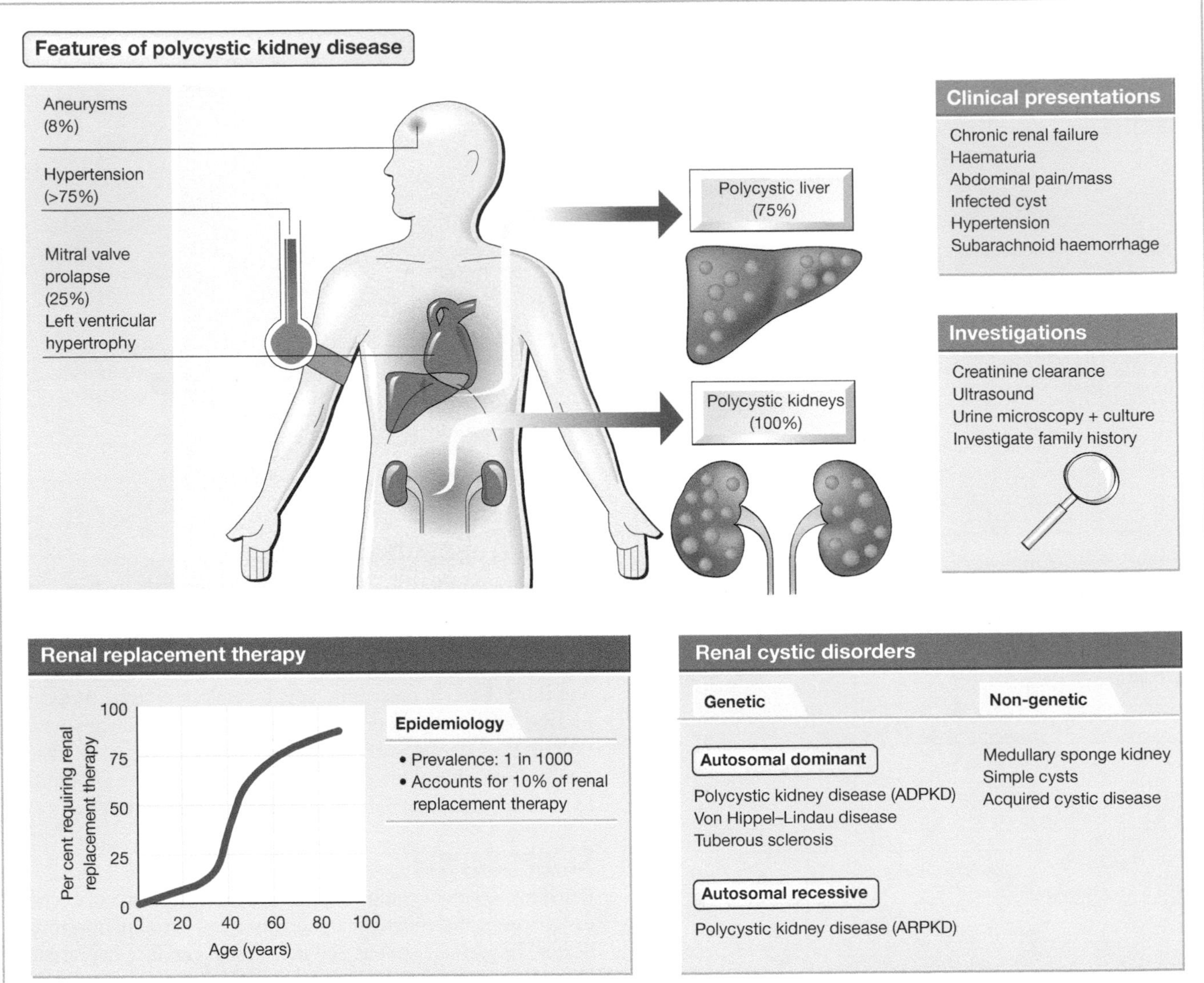

Features of polycystic kidney disease
Aneurysms (8%)
Hypertension (>75%)
Mitral valve prolapse (25%)
Left ventricular hypertrophy
Polycystic liver (75%)
Polycystic kidneys (100%)
Clinical presentations
Chronic renal failure
Haematuria
Abdominal pain/mass
Infected cyst
Hypertension
Subarachnoid haemorrhage
Investigations
Creatinine clearance
Ultrasound
Urine microscopy + culture
Investigate family history
Renal replacement therapy
Per cent requiring renal replacement therapy
100
75
50
25
0
0 20 40 60 80 100
Age (years)
Epidemiology
• Prevalence: 1 in 1000
• Accounts for 10% of renal replacement therapy
Renal cystic disorders
Genetic
Autosomal dominant
Polycystic kidney disease (ADPKD)
Von Hippel–Lindau disease
Tuberous sclerosis
Autosomal recessive
Polycystic kidney disease (ARPKD)
Non-genetic
Medullary sponge kidney
Simple cysts
Acquired cystic disease

Autosomal dominant polycystic kidney disease

A variety of inherited conditions affect the kidney, but adult polycystic kidney disease (APKD) is by far the most common, affecting one in 1000 individuals and accounting for 8–10% of patients with end-stage renal disease. It usually presents in adult life (the rarer autosomal recessive form presents in infancy). Inheritance is autosomal dominant so children of an affected parent have a 50% chance of inheriting the condition. About 25% of cases are the result of spontaneous mutation. The genetic defect is on chromosome 16 (*PKD1*, which accounts for 95% of cases) or more rarely on chromosome 4 (*PKD2*).

The condition is characterized by a progressive appearance and enlargement of renal cysts. These may bleed, producing haematuria and loin pain, or may become infected. As the cysts gradually enlarge, there is a slowly progressive and inexorable decline in renal function. Patients may also present with abdominal masses, hypertension and chronic renal failure, and subarachnoid haemorrhages occur in some 10% as a result of the associated berry aneurysms that affect intracranial arteries. Polycystic kidneys may be found incidentally on ultrasonography during investigations for other indications. Cysts also occur in the liver, pancreas, spleen and ovaries, although these rarely cause clinical problems.

Medicine at a Glance, Fifth Edition. Edited by Patrick Davey and Alex Pitcher.

Companion website: www.wiley.com/go/medicine5e

Investigations

The condition is usually suspected from the clinical features and family history and confirmed with ultrasonography or computed tomography (CT). Renal function should be determined with serum creatinine and creatinine clearance, and urinary infection excluded.

There are no specific treatments to slow the disease progression but there is some evidence for benefit of the ADH antagonist tolvaptan, though its role is not completely established. It is important to control any hypertension. Infections require appropriate antibiotic treatment and pain caused by haemorrhage may require analgesia. As renal failure progresses, renal replacement therapy with dialysis or transplantation is required, at a mean age in *PKD1* of 55–60 years. Sometimes nephrectomy is required to permit space so that peritoneal dialysis or transplantation can be undertaken. Genetic counselling is important and screening of children of affected individuals should be delayed until cysts are identifiable on ultrasonography – usually >18 years unless there is renal impairment or hypertension.

Simple cysts

These become increasingly common with age and can be detected in >12% of individuals aged over 50 years. They are usually asymptomatic and are detected incidentally. It is important to distinguish them from the multiple cysts of APKD, other cystic diseases and renal cell carcinoma. On ultrasonography, simple cysts have smooth walls and no intracystic debris. If doubt exists then CT scanning is necessary.

Other inherited disorders affecting the kidney

Alport syndrome

This syndrome is characterized by haematuria, sensorineural deafness (overt in 40%) and progressive renal impairment with proteinuria in most and ocular abnormalities in 15%. It is caused by mutations in the basement membrane type IV collagen gene (most commonly *COL4A5*); 20% are the result of new mutations. It is X-linked in 80% of patients, producing a more severe phenotype in males. The diagnosis is confirmed on renal biopsy, where thickening and splitting of the glomerular basement membrane on electron microscopy is found. End-stage renal failure (i.e. disease requiring dialysis) develops usually between 16 and 35 years of age in virtually all affected males with X-linked Alport syndrome, and males and females with the autosomally inherited form. Transplantation, although not contraindicated, can very rarely result in a Goodpasture disease-like syndrome caused by the immunological reaction to the previously 'unseen' type IV collagen in the transplanted kidney.

Medullary sponge kidney

This condition, which is often inherited, is characterized by dilated medullary collecting ducts and can affect both, one or part of one kidney. It is often asymptomatic, but small calculi can form which may produce haematuria and predispose to urinary tract infection, or larger calculi may produce obstruction. Renal failure is unusual.

Tuberous sclerosis

In this rare (1–2/100 000), autosomal dominant condition, tumour-like malformations called hamartomas develop in the central nervous system (often causing learning disorders and epilepsy) and produce skin lesions including facial angiofibromas and hypomelanotic macules. The kidneys can develop angiomyolipomas, cysts and renal malignancies. The mTOR inhibitor everolimus can be used in treatment.

Von Hippel–Lindau syndrome

This is a very rare, autosomal dominantly inherited condition characterized by tumours affecting the kidney (renal cell carcinoma), brain (haemangioblastomas) and adrenals (phaeochromocytoma). Occasionally, bilateral nephrectomy for tumours leads to the patient requiring dialysis. Mutations in the von Hippel–Lindau gene are also commonly found in cells from patients with sporadic renal cell carcinomas.

Anderson–Fabry disease

This X-linked recessive disorder is the result of mutations in the gene encoding α-galactosidase A. Anderson–Fabry disease results in the intracellular accumulation of glycosphingolipids, which leads to progressive renal failure, autonomic dysfunction and skin lesions called angiokeratomas (dark red macules or papules). Diagnosis is confirmed by the demonstration of reduced urinary α-galactosidase A. It occurs in two forms: typical Anderson–Fabry disease, where there is no α-galactosidase A activity, and atypical Anderson–Fabry disease, where there is some, albeit greatly reduced, α-galactosidase A activity. Patients with typical Anderson–Fabry disease develop symptoms when very young, in many organs, whereas patients with atypical Anderson–Fabry disease develop symptoms later, typically only affecting the heart.

Typical Anderson–Fabry disease

This affects about 1200 patients in the UK. The first symptoms usually occur around the age of 10 years; unfortunately, they are often ignored or misdiagnosed, and in the typical patient the actual diagnosis of Anderson–Fabry disease is not made until 18 years later. Patients can, however, present at any age: symptoms include pain (especially of the hands and feet) and painful crises (often starting in the hands and feet, spreading to other parts of the body, lasting minutes to days), angiokeratomas, peripheral vasospasm and ophthalmological abnormalities. Later (age 10–30 years) the following can occur: renal dysfunction, fever, reduced sweating, heat sensitivity, exercise intolerance, diarrhoea and abdominal pain, and an increase in angiokeratomas. In later adulthood (age >30 years), heart disease, impaired renal function, stroke and epilepsy can occur.

Atypical Anderson–Fabry disease

This affects many thousands in the UK (maybe 6000–10 000). Atypical Anderson–Fabry disease usually presents in adulthood (20–70 years). It is increasingly recognized, and the most common manifestation is left ventricular (LV) hypertrophy. Typically, the heart is the only organ affected. Atypical Anderson–Fabry disease should be considered in all with unexplained LV hypertrophy, especially if LV outflow tract gradient is present. Indeed, atypical Anderson–Fabry disease may account for some 3% of all cases of LV hypertrophy (and a higher percentage in those suspected of having hypertrophic cardiomyopathy). Electrocardiogram evidence of LV hypertrophy (sometimes with pre-excitation) is usually present and is confirmed by cardiac ultrasound. Some (1–30%) α-galactosidase A activity is found.

Treatment

To treat, consider α-galactosidase A enzyme replacement therapy.

148 Tubulointerstitial disease

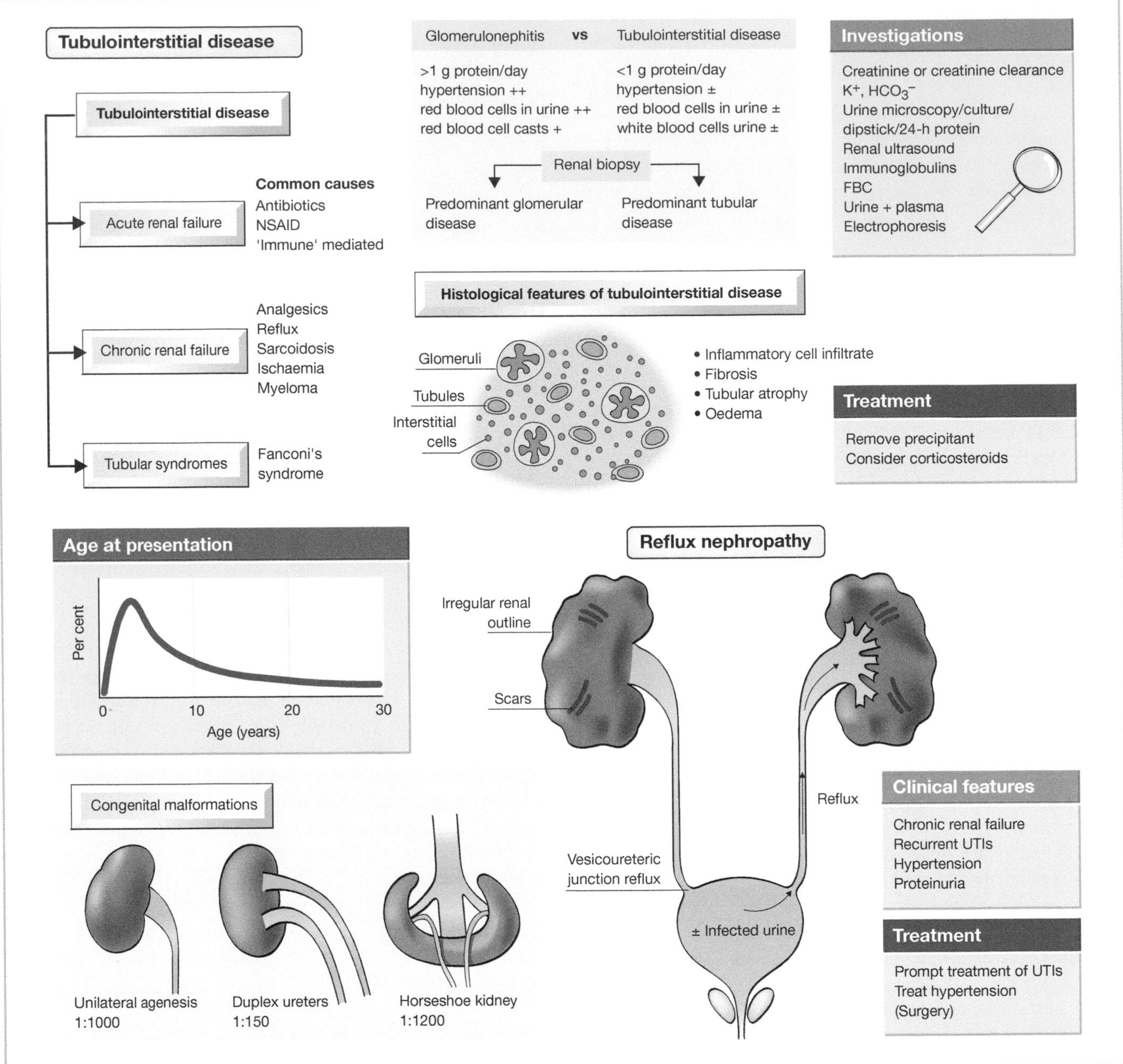

Diseases affecting the renal interstitium and tubules can present with renal impairment, proteinuria, haematuria or tubular syndromes and, in some, prominent abnormalities in electrolyte balance. The most common of these conditions is interstitial nephritis which, in its chronic form, accounts for up to 15% of end-stage renal failure and in its acute form is a common cause of acute renal failure.

Acute interstitial nephritis

Acute inflammation of the renal interstitium is a common consequence of drug hypersensitivity, particularly to antibiotics and non-steroidal anti-inflammatory drugs (NSAIDs). Some 30% of those with drug-induced acute interstitial nephritis have fever, rash and eosinophilia. Acute interstitial nephritis may also relate to infection (leptospirosis, cytomegalovirus, hantavirus). It can

Medicine at a Glance, Fifth Edition. Edited by Patrick Davey and Alex Pitcher.

Companion website: www.wiley.com/go/medicine5e

also occur in conjunction with other illnesses such as Sjögren disease or with uveitis (tubulointerstitial nephritis and uveitis or 'TINU syndrome').

Cholesterol emboli

Cholesterol emboli can produce renal failure, and result when an atheromatous plaque in the aorta ruptures, either spontaneously (in elderly people) or after angiography, with systemic emboli resulting in fever, myalgia, skin rash, livedo reticularis, retinal emboli (amaurosis fugax), high white blood cell count and C-reactive protein, and a variable decline in renal function.

Chronic interstitial nephritis and chronic pyelonephritis

Chronic interstitial nephritis may present more insidiously with a progressive decline in renal function, small kidneys on ultrasonography, severe electrolyte disturbance and, in a minority, a salt-losing nephropathy leading to sodium depletion and hypotension. Causes include the following.

- **Analgesics**: analgesic nephropathy used to be a very common cause of chronic renal failure though its incidence has declined with the withdrawal of phenacetin-containing analgesics. It is four times more common in women than in men. Features include polyuria, mild proteinuria, insidious progressive renal failure and hypertension (in 60% of cases), often complicated by renal papillary necrosis and renal colic.
- **Reflux nephropathy** and **obstructive uropathy**, either of which may be complicated by infection. When chronic interstitial nephritis results primarily from chronic infection, it is termed 'chronic pyelonephritis'.
- **Primary glomerular disease**.
- **Other causes** (in 15%) include sarcoidosis, ischaemia, hyperuricaemia, myeloma and chronic hypokalaemia. Long-standing hypercalcaemia produces chronic interstitial inflammation, possibly related to calcium salt deposition. Medullary sponge kidney and hyperoxaluria (genetic, high ascorbic acid consumption, long-standing gastrointestinal disease) also occur.
- **Chronic poisoning with heavy metals** (lead, cadmium, mercury): common in industrial workers, especially in certain developing countries, and in Chinese herbs (aristolochic acid), which are often found in over-the-counter herbal preparations.

Features that can help distinguish glomerulonephritis from tubulointerstitial disease are that, in glomerulonephritis, there is usually >1 g of proteinuria/day, hypertension is more common, red blood cells and casts are found in the urine and, in the renal biopsy (which is the diagnostic test), the glomeruli are primarily affected.

Isolated/specific tubular defects

Other rare disorders exist in which there are specific tubular defects, including distal tubular syndromes such as nephrogenic diabetes insipidus and proximal tubular syndromes (Fanconi defects) which are often congenital, such as renal tubular acidoses. There may be other tubular defects associated with Fanconi syndrome resulting in aminoaciduria, glycosuria, phosphaturia and bicarbonaturia.

Investigations and treatment

In investigating the patient in whom interstitial nephritis is suspected, important investigations include examining for peripheral blood eosinophilia (which when present may suggest a drug allergy), immunoglobulins, urine and plasma electrophoresis to exclude myeloma, urine microscopy and culture, renal ultrasonography and renal biopsy.

Treatment consists of removing the precipitating cause. There is no effective treatment for many forms of interstitial nephritis but in others, corticosteroids can produce important responses. Spontaneous improvement of interstitial nephritis does occur.

Reflux nephropathy

The vesicoureteric junction normally prevents reflux of urine up the ureter; congenital incompetence at this junction can lead to renal damage. 'Reflux nephropathy' is the term given to the scarred and shrunken kidney with chronic tubulointerstitial nephritis that results. This can present during childhood with urinary tract infection (UTI), hypertension, proteinuria or renal failure. For unknown reasons, it is more common in females. UTI is important in the genesis of damage by the refluxing urine.

Investigations

Renal function should be assessed, proteinuria quantified and urine culture performed to exclude active infection. CT or intravenous urograms (IVUs) characteristically show an irregular renal outline with clubbed calyces, and kidney size is often reduced. A micturating cystogram can demonstrate vesicoureteric reflux whereas DMSA ([99mTc] mercaptosuccinic acid) scanning can reveal scars. A renal biopsy is not usually appropriate but would show chronic tubulointerstitial nephritis.

Treatment

Any acute UTI should be treated promptly, although in some individuals there may be a role for prophylactic antibiotics. Any associated hypertension should be treated aggressively, asymptomatic infection should be looked for and renal function carefully monitored. The role of surgical ureteric reimplantation to prevent reflux is controversial. There is a strong familial predisposition to reflux and it may be sought in family members.

If there has been substantial scarring, progressive renal failure may develop. However, if renal function is normal during adolescence, the development of renal failure in adulthood is unusual.

Other congenital malformations of the urinary tract

Congenital malformations may affect the kidney, ureter or bladder.

- **Kidney**: unilateral renal agenesis occurs in 1:1000 of the population and is not normally associated with renal impairment. Horseshoe kidneys are fused at their lower pole and are found in 1:1200 individuals and sometimes present with reflux or obstruction.
- **Ureters**: duplex ureters are the most common congenital malformation of the renal tract, occurring in 1:150 individuals, but they rarely cause clinical problems. Pelviureteric junction obstruction is a common cause of urinary tract obstruction in children and young adults. There may be hyperplasia of the smooth muscle of the renal pelvis. It may present with loin pain after high fluid intake or even with hydronephrosis. An IVU may suggest the diagnosis and surgical treatment may be necessary.
- **Bladder**: congenital disorders of the bladder include a neuropathic bladder, prune belly syndrome (abdominal muscle agenesis, undescended testes and urinary tract malformations, including renal dysplasia and bladder dilation) and posterior urethral valves in males.

149 Acute renal failure

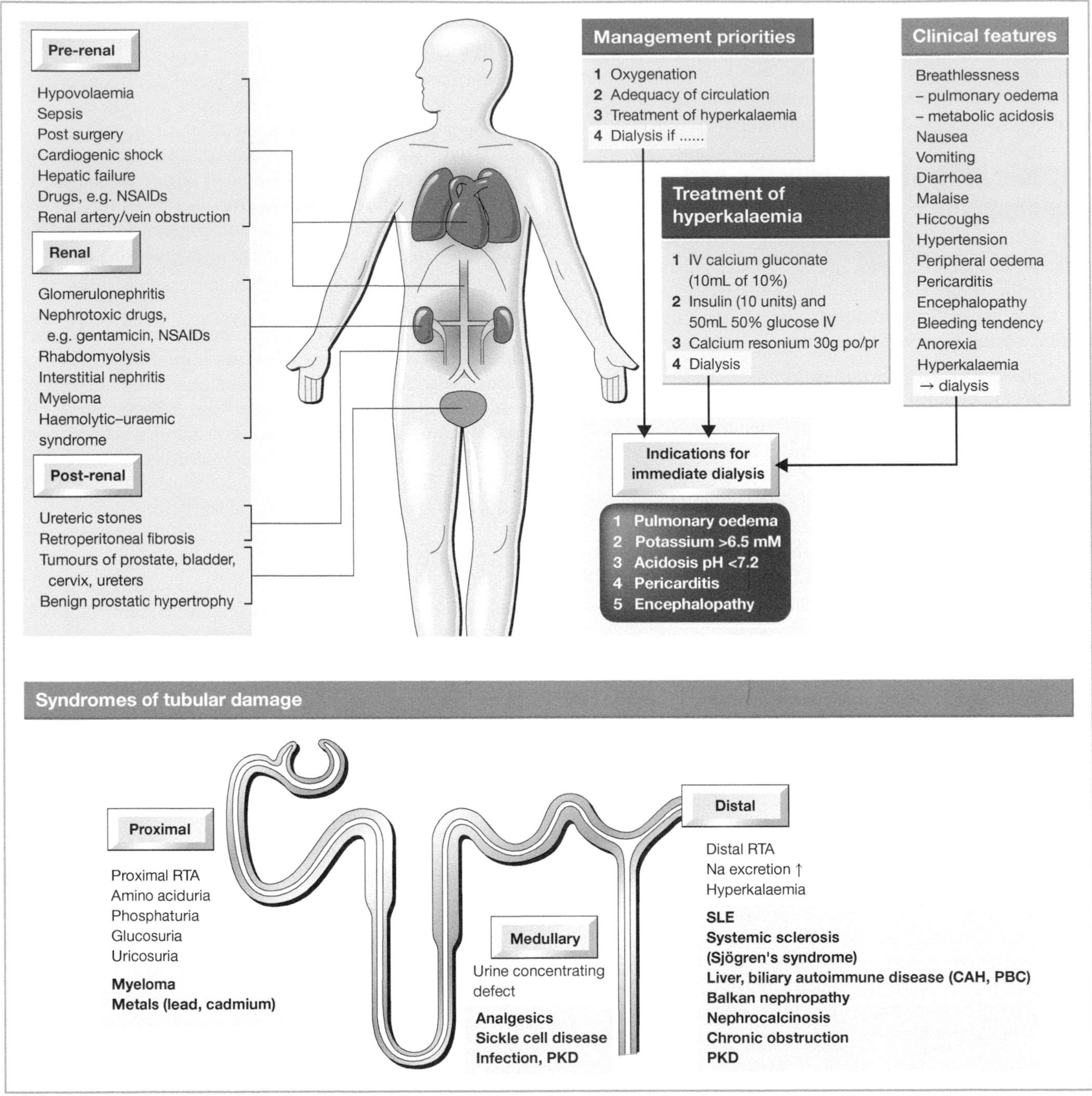

Pre-renal
Hypovolaemia
Sepsis
Post surgery
Cardiogenic shock
Hepatic failure
Drugs, e.g. NSAIDs
Renal artery/vein obstruction
Renal
Glomerulonephritis
Nephrotoxic drugs, e.g. gentamicin, NSAIDs
Rhabdomyolysis
Interstitial nephritis
Myeloma
Haemolytic–uraemic syndrome
Post-renal
Ureteric stones
Retroperitoneal fibrosis
Tumours of prostate, bladder, cervix, ureters
Benign prostatic hypertrophy
Management priorities
1 Oxygenation
2 Adequacy of circulation
3 Treatment of hyperkalaemia
4 Dialysis if ......
Treatment of hyperkalaemia
1 IV calcium gluconate (10mL of 10%)
2 Insulin (10 units) and 50mL 50% glucose IV
3 Calcium resonium 30g po/pr
4 Dialysis
Clinical features
Breathlessness
– pulmonary oedema
– metabolic acidosis
Nausea
Vomiting
Diarrhoea
Malaise
Hiccoughs
Hypertension
Peripheral oedema
Pericarditis
Encephalopathy
Bleeding tendency
Anorexia
Hyperkalaemia
→ dialysis
Indications for immediate dialysis
1 Pulmonary oedema
2 Potassium >6.5 mM
3 Acidosis pH <7.2
4 Pericarditis
5 Encephalopathy
Syndromes of tubular damage
Proximal
Proximal RTA
Amino aciduria
Phosphaturia
Glucosuria
Uricosuria
Myeloma
Metals (lead, cadmium)
Medullary
Urine concentrating defect
Analgesics
Sickle cell disease
Infection, PKD
Distal
Distal RTA
Na excretion ↑
Hyperkalaemia
SLE
Systemic sclerosis
(Sjögren's syndrome)
Liver, biliary autoimmune disease (CAH, PBC)
Balkan nephropathy
Nephrocalcinosis
Chronic obstruction
PKD

Acute renal failure is a syndrome characterized by a rapid decline in glomerular filtration rate over days to weeks with the accumulation of nitrogenous waste and failure to correctly regulate extracellular volume and electrolytes. It is often recognized by a rapidly rising serum urea and creatinine. It may be accompanied by reduced urine output. It is a common and important complication in unwell hospitalized patients. The symptoms of acute renal failure include those of the precipitating aetiology (e.g. shock or sepsis) and those resulting from renal failure itself, including fluid overload, nausea, malaise and encephalopathy. The annual incidence of acute renal failure in developed countries is 180 cases/million. The causes of renal failure are conventionally divided into pre-renal, renal and postrenal.

Medicine at a Glance, Fifth Edition. Edited by Patrick Davey and Alex Pitcher.

Companion website: www.wiley.com/go/medicine5e

Pre-renal causes

The kidneys need an adequate perfusion pressure for normal function. This depends on the systemic blood pressure (BP) being high enough, and the postglomerular arteriole being able to constrict. If either the systemic BP falls too low (the most common cause) or the postglomerular arteriole dilates inappropriately, glomerular perfusion falls and the kidneys fail. Pre-renal renal failure usually occurs in the context of a seriously ill patient. There are often several systemic insults which produce renal hypoperfusion sufficient to lead to renal failure, including:

- hypovolaemia from haemorrhage, severe diarrhoea or vomiting
- cardiogenic shock
- sepsis
- drugs such as angiotensin-converting enzyme inhibitors and non-steroidal anti-inflammatory drugs (NSAIDs)
- severe liver disease leading to renal failure, termed the 'hepatorenal syndrome'.

The common histological pattern seen in the kidney in response to severe injury of this nature is acute tubular necrosis (ATN), now known as acute kidney injury (AKI), which usually recovers over several weeks. In very severe and prolonged hypotensive insults, acute cortical necrosis can also occur, from which recovery is less certain. In established renal failure caused by ATN, the concentrating ability of the kidney is lost and urinary sodium is >40 mmol/l. This contrasts with early pre-renal failure which may be reversible, with attention to haemodynamics and fluid balance when the urine is concentrated (urinary sodium usually <40 mmol/l).

Renal causes

There are many causes of renal failure as a result of disease affecting the kidney itself. These include glomerulonephritis, vasculitis, nephrotoxic drugs (e.g. gentamicin), rhabdomyolysis, interstitial nephritis, haemolytic uraemic syndrome and myeloma.

Postrenal causes

Urinary tract obstruction can occur at any site in the urinary tract and produce renal failure. Common causes include prostatic hypertrophy, carcinoma of the prostate, ureteric stones, tumours of the renal pelvis, ureters or bladder, external compression of the ureters by tumour or retroperitoneal fibrosis. Advanced renal failure will only occur with the obstruction of both kidneys.

Diagnostic approach

The rapid diagnosis of the cause of acute renal failure is important because a reversible cause may be present that will respond to specific treatment. A careful history and examination often point towards the likely cause of acute renal failure. Examination should include palpation and percussion of the bladder, the prostate gland in men and the pelvis for a mass in women. In pre-renal failure, the insults are often apparent, such as significant surgical operation, shock, sepsis or perhaps all three! In any patient with pre-renal failure, examination for hypovolaemia is vital, and the diagnosis is suggested by:

- **decreased skin turgor** (an unreliable sign)
- **tachycardia**, often >100 bpm
- **hypotension**, with systolic BP <100 mmHg, and a postural systolic BP fall between lying and sitting/standing of >20 mmHg
- **low venous pressure**: if the jugular venous pressure is not reliably seen, the central pressure can be measured invasively.

In patients in whom the history and clinical examination suggest the possibility of hypovolaemia, the response (urine output and haemodynamic observations) to an intravenous (IV) bolus of fluid (e.g. 500 ml physiological saline) should be undertaken. Any other pre-renal precipitants should be rapidly corrected. Renal ultrasonography is important to examine for urinary tract obstruction which will manifest as urinary tract dilation, particularly hydronephrosis. It will also provide information about renal size and symmetry (small kidneys indicating chronic renal disease).

If the renal size is normal, the kidneys are not obstructed and the history and examination do not suggest a pre-renal cause, further blood tests including immunology should be undertaken and the urine examined for the presence of red cells, protein and casts, which may suggest a renal cause such as glomerulonephritis. A renal biopsy may be necessary for accurate definition of the cause of the acute renal failure.

Management

As in any seriously ill patient, the priorities in acute renal failure are ensuring adequate oxygenation and circulation. In acute renal failure, the most dangerous threat to oxygenation is fluid overload resulting in pulmonary oedema. The accurate assessment of the fluid status of the patient is thus crucial. In patients with fluid overload who are in established renal failure, oxygen should be administered and fluid removed. Diuretics will not work, vasodilators such as IV nitrates may provide temporary benefit, but definitive treatment with haemodialysis, haemofiltration or peritoneal dialysis should be performed. As above, evidence of hypovolaemia should result in treatment with IV fluids.

The other major life-threatening complication of acute renal failure is the presence of hyperkalaemia, which can result in cardiac dysrhythmias (especially ventricular fibrillation and cardiac asystole). The potassium should be measured urgently, electrocardiogram (ECG) changes of hyperkalaemia sought (peaked T waves, widened QRS, absent P waves, sine wave appearance) and, if the potassium is >6 mmol/l or if ECG abnormalities are present, treatment with IV calcium (with ECG monitoring), insulin and glucose, and oral or rectal calcium resonium, and urgent dialysis treatment arranged.

Other serious complications of acute renal failure that may require urgent treatment with dialysis include metabolic acidosis, encephalopathy and pericarditis.

Once these priorities have been addressed, specific treatments for the cause of the renal failure may be necessary. These might include the relief of obstruction, the treatment of sepsis or the administration of immunosuppression for a rapidly progressive glomerulonephritis.

150 Chronic renal failure and the dialysis patient

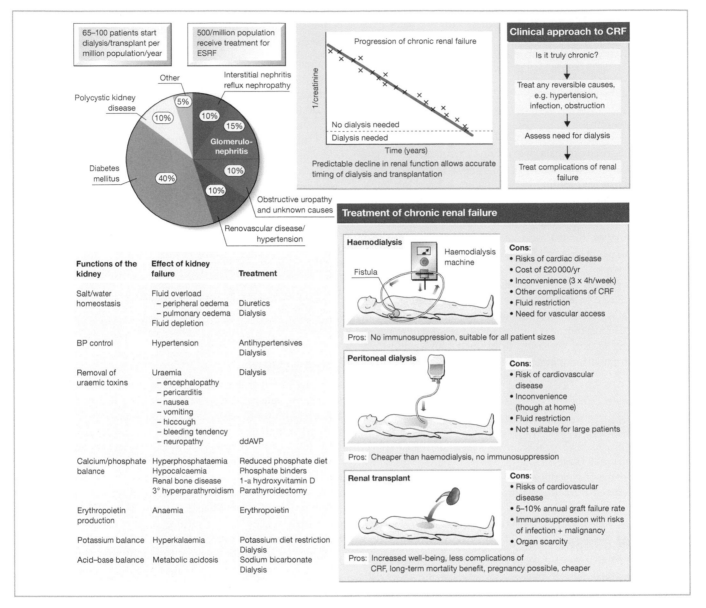

65–100 patients start dialysis/transplant per million population/year

500/million population receive treatment for ESRF

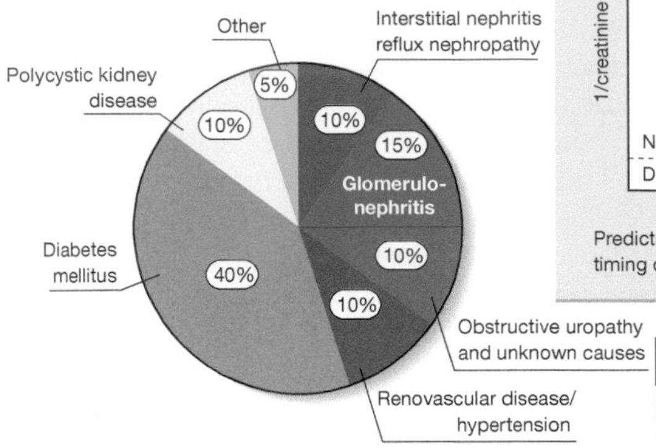

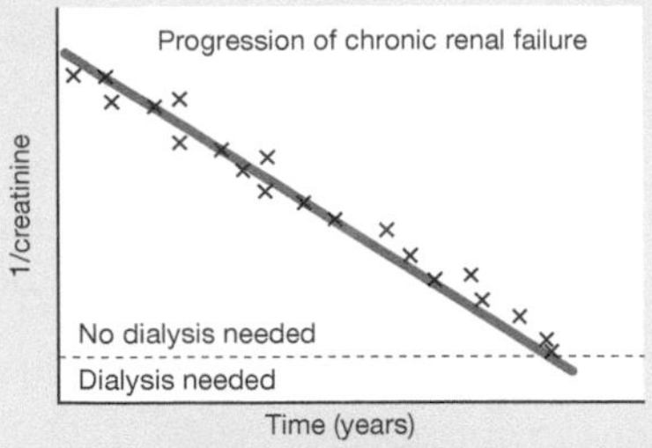

Other 5%

Interstitial nephritis reflux nephropathy 10%

Polycystic kidney disease 10%

Glomerulo-nephritis 15%

Diabetes mellitus 40%

Obstructive uropathy and unknown causes 10%

Renovascular disease/hypertension 10%

Progression of chronic renal failure

1/creatinine

No dialysis needed

Dialysis needed

Time (years)

Predictable decline in renal function allows accurate timing of dialysis and transplantation

Clinical approach to CRF

Is it truly chronic?

↓

Treat any reversible causes, e.g. hypertension, infection, obstruction

↓

Assess need for dialysis

↓

Treat complications of renal failure

Functions of the kidney	Effect of kidney failure	Treatment
Salt/water homeostasis	Fluid overload – peripheral oedema – pulmonary oedema Fluid depletion	Diuretics Dialysis
BP control	Hypertension	Antihypertensives Dialysis
Removal of uraemic toxins	Uraemia – encephalopathy – pericarditis – nausea – vomiting – hiccough – bleeding tendency – neuropathy	Dialysis ddAVP
Calcium/phosphate balance	Hyperphosphataemia Hypocalcaemia Renal bone disease 3° hyperparathyroidism	Reduced phosphate diet Phosphate binders 1-a hydroxyvitamin D Parathyroidectomy
Erythropoietin production	Anaemia	Erythropoietin
Potassium balance	Hyperkalaemia	Potassium diet restriction Dialysis
Acid–base balance	Metabolic acidosis	Sodium bicarbonate Dialysis

Treatment of chronic renal failure

Haemodialysis

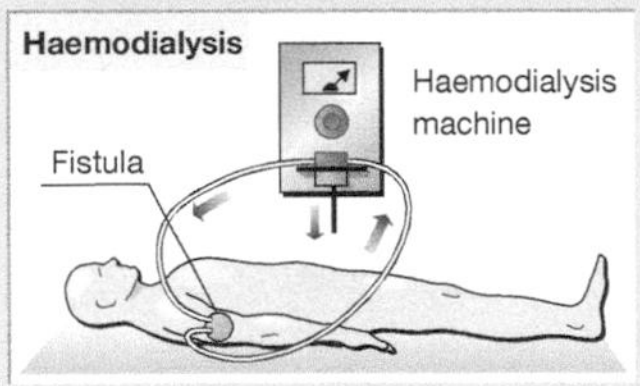

Haemodialysis machine

Fistula

Cons:
- Risks of cardiac disease
- Cost of £20 000/yr
- Inconvenience (3 x 4h/week)
- Other complications of CRF
- Fluid restriction
- Need for vascular access

Pros: No immunosuppression, suitable for all patient sizes

Peritoneal dialysis

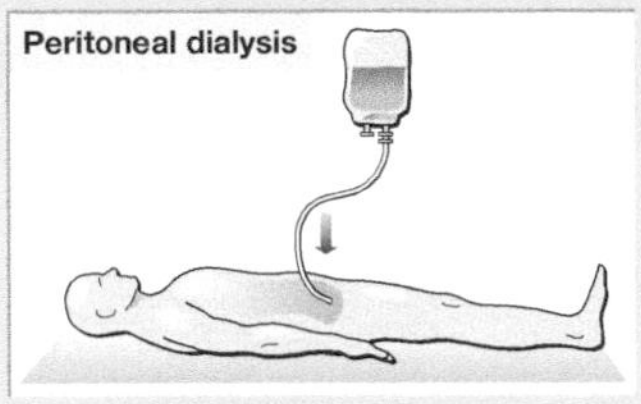

Cons:
- Risk of cardiovascular disease
- Inconvenience (though at home)
- Fluid restriction
- Not suitable for large patients

Pros: Cheaper than haemodialysis, no immunosuppression

Renal transplant

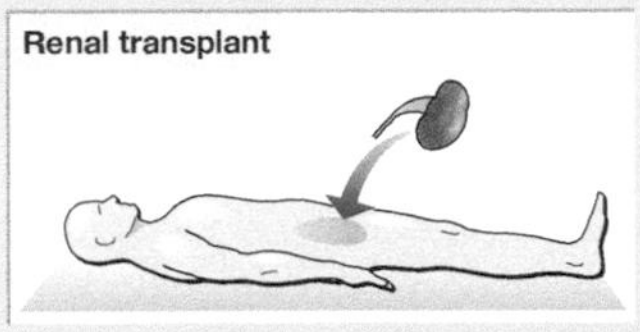

Cons:
- Risks of cardiovascular disease
- 5–10% annual graft failure rate
- Immunosuppression with risks of infection + malignancy
- Organ scarcity

Pros: Increased well-being, less complications of CRF, long-term mortality benefit, pregnancy possible, cheaper

Chronic renal failure (CRF) or chronic kidney disease (CKD) is defined as an abnormally low glomerular filtration rate (GFR) for >3 months. Numerous disorders produce CRF including diabetes mellitus (40%), polycystic kidney disease (10%), interstitial nephritis and reflux nephropathy (10%), obstructive uropathy and unknown causes (10%), glomerulonephritis (15%), renovascular disease and hypertension (10%). The incidence of chronic renal failure suitable for renal replacement therapy is 100/million population/year, with 500/million patients receiving end-stage renal failure (ESRF) treatment.

In CRF, the normal functions of the kidney are perturbed, resulting in the following conditions.

- Failure of regulation of salt and water excretion which can produce oedema (peripheral and pulmonary) or more rarely fluid depletion. Failure of concentrating power leads to nocturia.
- Hypertension is common and occasionally severe enough to cause encephalopathy. Premature cardiovascular disease (particularly coronary artery disease) accounts for much of the excess mortality of CRF; this may relate to dyslipidaemia (commonly found in CRF), hypertension, chronic anaemia, abnormalities of calcium metabolism and renin–angiotensin system activation.
- Accumulation of nitrogenous waste products in the blood (and of metabolic products with molecular weight of 500–2000: the 'middle molecules') produces symptoms that include

Medicine at a Glance, Fifth Edition. Edited by Patrick Davey and Alex Pitcher.

Companion website: www.wiley.com/go/medicine5e

encephalopathy, hiccough, pericarditis, nausea, vomiting, pruritus, malaise, impotence, menstrual irregularities and (mixed motor/sensory) neuropathy. Uraemia causes anorexia and complex disturbances in protein metabolism, resulting in malnutrition, so maintenance of lean body mass is difficult. Muscle wasting causes weakness, inactivity and further muscle loss.

- Metabolic acidosis and hyperkalaemia.
- Anaemia, mainly from erythropoietin deficiency, with contributions from a reduced red cell lifespan, occasionally iron deficiency from gastrointestinal bleeding, etc. Anaemia is milder than expected in polycystic kidney disease and can be more severe than expected in diabetics.
- Renal bone disease: this can be profound and disabling. This relates to osteomalacia (failure of renal hydroxylation [1α] of vitamin D), secondary hyperparathyroidism driven by chronic hypocalcaemia (caused by high phosphate and low vitamin D), adynamic bone disease and nutritional osteoporosis.
- There is an increased bleeding tendency, largely as a result of platelet dysfunction and depressed activity of von Willebrand factor.
- Infection is common, because immunity is impaired.

The symptoms of CRF may have an insidious onset, or may present as a uraemic emergency with life-threatening complications.

Management (see Table 150.1)

A full history and examination may provide important clues to the aetiology of the renal failure. A history of frequent urinary tract infections in childhood may suggest a diagnosis of reflux nephropathy, whereas a family history may suggest polycystic kidney disease. Haematuria found at previous medical examinations might point towards chronic glomerulonephritis. It is important to establish that the renal failure is truly chronic to ensure that there is no acute and reversible cause of renal failure. Previous estimations of renal function are of the greatest help in determining this; furthermore, the absence of anaemia usually suggests that the renal failure is acute rather than chronic, whilst small kidneys are usually found in chronic (irreversible) disease.

The investigation of patients with CRF includes renal tract ultrasonography to exclude obstruction and document renal size. If the cause is unclear and the kidneys are of normal size, a renal biopsy is undertaken. Tests to exclude myeloma and autoimmune disease (systemic lupus erythematosus, vasculitis) and urinalysis for proteinuria, haematuria and urinary infection are indicated. The severity of the renal failure is determined from creatinine, urea and creatinine clearance.

Once significant renal dysfunction develops, there is usually an inexorable deterioration in renal function over several years (possibly caused by hyperfiltration in the remaining glomeruli). Apart from treatments directed against the specific cause of the renal failure, the main therapy reducing the speed of deterioration is aggressive blood pressure control. ESRF is a term used when patients would not survive without renal replacement therapy (haemodialysis, peritoneal dialysis, renal transplantation).

Patients are prepared for renal replacement therapy by creating dialysis access before the renal failure progresses to cause uraemic symptoms. In patients with severe CKD, calcium and phosphate balance are corrected, using 1α-hydroxycholecalciferol and phosphate binders, anaemia is improved by erythropoietin, acidosis is ameliorated with sodium bicarbonate, hypertension is treated and sodium and water retention are controlled with diuretics.

Indications for dialysis are:

- uraemic symptoms: the usual indication, often when creatinine is >500 μmol/l
- life-threatening complications (hyperkalaemia, acidosis, fluid overload, uraemic pericarditis or encephalopathy).

In **haemodialysis** vascular access is achieved by forming an arteriovenous fistula (which needs eight weeks to 'mature' before use) or by using double-lumen jugular, subclavian or femoral lines. The diffusion of solutes and water occurs across a semipermeable membrane, which separates blood and dialysate flow in opposite directions. The major difficulties with haemodialysis are cardiovascular instability (from concurrent cardiovascular disease and drugs used for its treatment, as well as the major fluid shifts that occur during dialysis), difficulties in adhering to the dietary and fluid intake restrictions and difficulties with vascular access. Dialysis membranes can activate the clotting cascade, so heparin is used to prevent this. Most membranes do not allow the removal of β_2-microglobulin, which can accumulate chronically causing carpal tunnel syndrome and arthropathy. Over-rapid removal of toxic metabolites can cause a profound illness – dialysis 'disequilibrium' – particularly during the first dialysis treatments, and can be prevented by frequent 'small' dialysis schedules.

In **continuous ambulatory peritoneal dialysis** patients instill several litres of isotonic or hypertonic glucose solution four times a day into the peritoneal cavity via a permanent catheter or connect to a machine which does this at night (automated peritoneal dialysis). The peritoneal lining acts as the dialysis membrane. After several hours, the fluid containing solutes and waste products is drained out. Excess body fluid is removed by using hypertonic solutions. Infection of the peritoneal fluid (peritoneal dialysis peritonitis) is the most common complication requiring treatment with intraperitoneal or intravenous antibiotics.

Table 150.1 Management of chronic renal failure.

Glomerular filtration rate (GFR)	Management
<15 ml/min	Severe renal failure: if new → urgent specialist referral
>15 and <30 ml/min	Significant impairment of renal function → prompt assessment and referral
>30 and <60 ml/min	May reflect age, biological variation or renal disease (suggested by proteinuria, haematuria ± ↑ BP). Evaluate, repeat after 1 week in unwell patients and 1 month in the well. Refer all those with renal damage and any with a GFR <3rd centile for age

The GFR can be estimated from the serum creatinine using the following formulas:

MDRD	GFR (ml/min/1.73 m²) = 186 × (creatinine (μmol/l)/88.4)$^{-1.154}$ × (age)$^{-0.203}$ × (0.742 if female) × (1.210 if African American)
Cockcroft–Gault	$\frac{(140-\text{age})\times\text{weight}\times1.23\times(0.85\text{ if female})}{\text{Creatinine}(\mu\text{mol/l})}$

Normal GFR in male/female (ml/min):

Centile	40 years	50 years	60 years	70 years
50th	95/85	85/75	70/65	65/55
10th	75/65	65/60	55/50	45/40
3rd	65/55	60/50	45/40	35/35

151 The renal transplant recipient

Management of a rise in creatinine in the renal transplant patient

History and examination

Investigations
- Ultrasound
- Ciclosporin level
- Renal biopsy
- Renal arteriogram

Major causes of graft dysfunction
- Rejection
- Obstruction
- Ciclosporin toxicity
- Renal artery stenosis
- Recurrent disease
- Urinary tract infection

Medical problems

Increased incidence of cardiovascular disease
- Twenty-fold increase in risk of death from MI compared with age-matched control
- Hypertension

Increased incidence of malignancies
- Skin (increased 20-fold)
- Lymphoma (increased 20–50-fold)
- Other, e.g. colon/lung (increased 1.5-fold)

Drug side effects

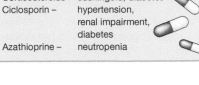

Corticosteroids – cushingoid, diabetes
Ciclosporin – hypertension, renal impairment, diabetes
Azathioprine – neutropenia

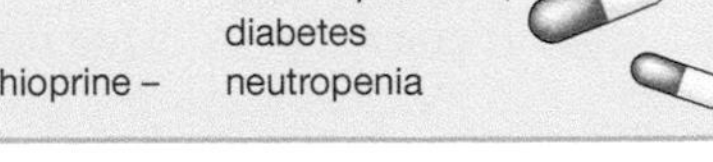

Brainstem death criteria

Patient apnoeic and in deep coma due to irreversible, structural damage to brain

No depressant drugs, neuromuscular blockers, hypothermia, gross metabolic or endocrine disturbance

Lack of brainstem function
No reaction of pupils to light
No corneal reflex
No facial response to pain
No caloric reflex (vestibulocular)
No cough/gag reflex
No respiratory movement after disconnection from ventilator and $PaCO_2$ >6.7kPa whilst oxygenated
Repeat x 2 >1/2 h apart

Post-transplant infections

0–1 month: 'conventional'

Postoperative chest infections/pneumonia
UTIs, wound infections

1–4 months: 'opportunistic'

Viral, e.g. CMV, VZV
Fungal, e.g. *Aspergillus*
Bacterial, e.g. TB, *Listeria*
Parasitic, e.g. *Pneumocystis, Toxoplasma*

3–4 months: 'late-opportunistic'

Cryptococus, zoster, CMV retinitis
Viral-associated malignancy, e.g. lymphoma (EBV), Kaposi's (HHV-8)

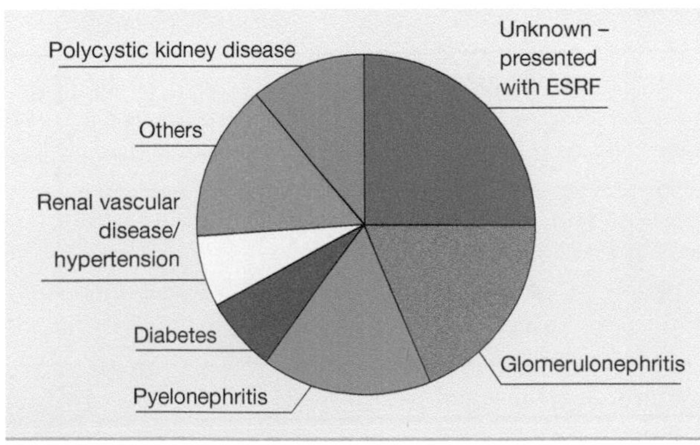

Indications for renal transplantation

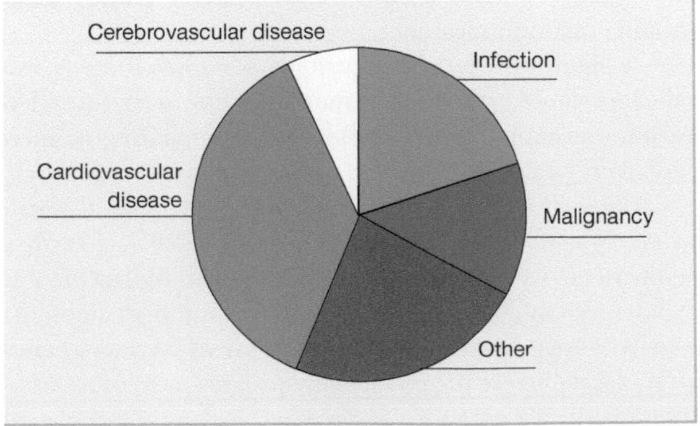

Causes of mortality following renal transplantation

Medicine at a Glance, Fifth Edition. Edited by Patrick Davey and Alex Pitcher.

Companion website: www.wiley.com/go/medicine5e

Stages of renal dysfunction

Stage	Description	Creatinine clearance (~GFR) (mL/min/1.73 m^2)	Metabolic consequences
1	Normal or increased GFR – people at increased risk or with early renal damage	>90	
2	Early renal insufficiency	60–89*	Concentration of parathyroid hormone starts to rise (GFR ~ 60–80)
3	Moderate renal failure (chronic renal failure)	30–59*	Decrease in calcium absorption (GFR <50) Lipoprotein activity falls Malnutrition Onset of left ventricular hypertrophy Onset of anaemia (erythropoietin deficiency)
4	Severe renal failure (pre-end-stage renal disease)	15–29	Triglyceride concentrations start to rise Hyperphosphataemia Metabolic acidosis Tendency to hyperkalaemia
5	End-stage renal disease (uraemia)	<15	Azotaemia develops

* May be normal for age (see Chapter 151)

Adapted from National Kidney Foundation—K/DOQI

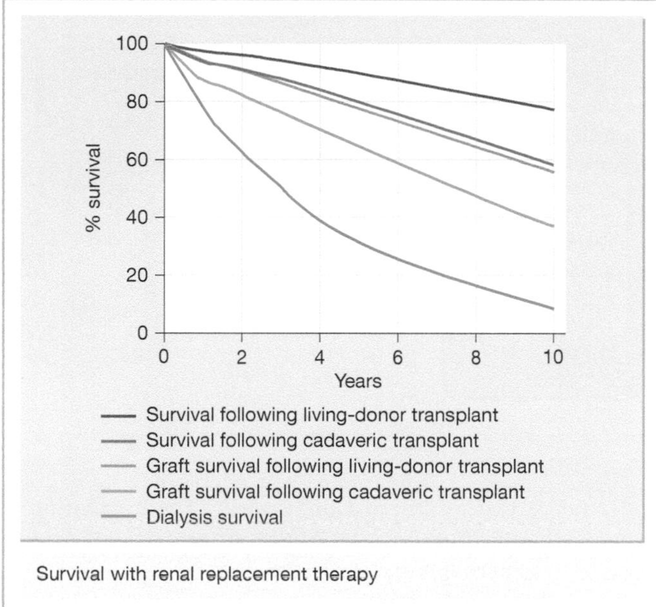

Survival with renal replacement therapy

Table 151.1 Relative contraindications to transplantation.

- Age >70 years
- Bacterial infection
- Recent/current malignancy
- Severe cardiac disease
- Renal disease with high risk of recurrence

In the UK, 3500 patients receive renal transplants every year, compared with the 8000 who are taken on for renal replacement treatment. Not all patients with end-stage renal failure (ESRF) are suitable for renal transplantation (see Table 151.1). Transplantation is limited by the availability of donor organs. Organs are most commonly obtained from donors in whom brainstem death has been diagnosed. Increasingly, kidneys are being transplanted from living related (or spouse) donors. In type 1 diabetic patients, dual kidney–pancreas transplants may be undertaken.

The kidney is usually transplanted into the iliac fossa and anastomosed to the iliac vessels. In the immediate postoperative period, the patient faces the risks of the operation and of infection resulting from heavy immunosuppression. Common infections include cytomegalovirus (CMV) disease, herpes zoster and BK nephropathy. In the longer term, the renal transplant recipient faces a variety of medical problems, including those related to immunosuppression, the increased incidence of cardiovascular and cerebrovascular disease, hypertension, increased incidence of a variety of malignancies, notably of the skin and lymphoma, the consequences of previous chronic renal failure, the underlying renal disorder and the problems of graft failure.

Recipients of renal transplants are commonly immunosuppressed with a combination of drugs, including prednisolone, azathioprine, mycophenolate, ciclosporin, tacrolimus, everolimus and specific therapeutic antibodies (e.g. anti-IL2 receptor). These agents share the general side-effects of an increased incidence of infections resulting from immunosuppression, but each has important unique side-effects. Examples of these include the cushingoid features that occur with corticosteroid administration; the hypertension, tremor, increased incidence of diabetes mellitus and renal impairment that can occur with ciclosporin and tacrolimus; and the neutropenia that can occur with azathioprine and mycophenolate.

The survival of renal transplants at one, five and 10 years is 90%, 70% and 55%, respectively. Graft survival is enhanced by careful human leukocyte antigen matching of donor and recipient.

The success of renal transplantation is largely the result of the ability to follow renal function precisely and frequently with measurements of serum creatinine. Any significant rise in creatinine should prompt investigation for rejection, ciclosporine/tacrolimus toxicity, problems with the renal vasculature or the obstruction of urine flow. Rejection is usually diagnosed with renal biopsy and is treated with high-dose methylprednisolone or anti-T-cell antibodies. Obstruction can usually be diagnosed with ultrasonography; ciclosporin/tacrolimus levels determined to exclude toxicity and angiography may be required to demonstrate normal renal blood supply.

Drugs and renal failure

The following categories contain examples only and are not exhaustive

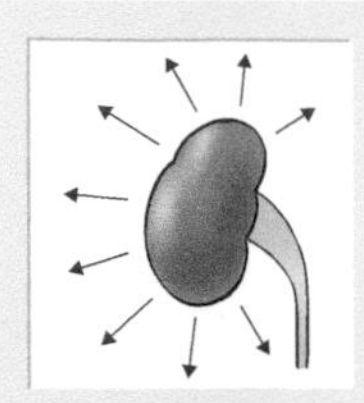

Drugs usually excreted by the kidney which can accumulate in renal failure

- Digoxin
- Lithium
- Morphine (+ metabolites), pethidine (+ metabolites)
- Penicillins, gentamicin, vancomycin, erythromycin, aciclovir

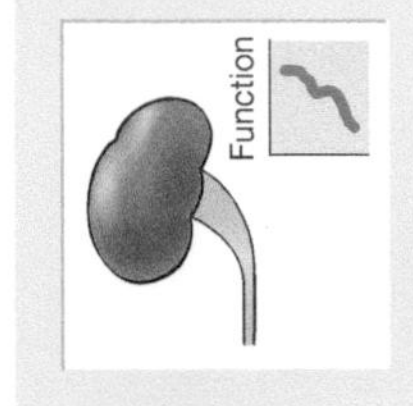

Drugs which can reduce renal function and should be used with caution in renal failure

- NSAIDs
- Angiotensin-converting enzyme inhibitors
- Ciclosporin, aciclovir
- Contrast media

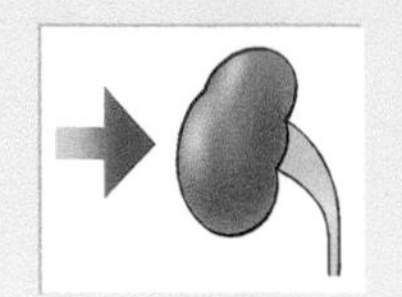

Drugs which require higher dosage in renal failure

- Furosemide (frusemide)

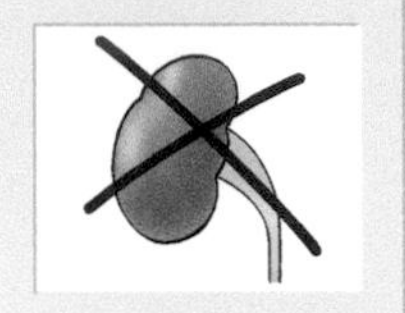

Drugs which can produce renal failure in overdose

- Gentamicin
- Paracetamol
- Ethylene glycol

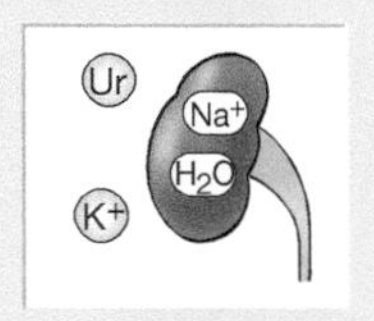

Drugs which can exacerbate metabolic effects in pre-existing renal failure

- K^+ sparing diuretics → hyperkalaemia
- Corticosteroids → ↑uraemia
- NaCl, $NaHCO_3$ → Na^+/ H_2O retention

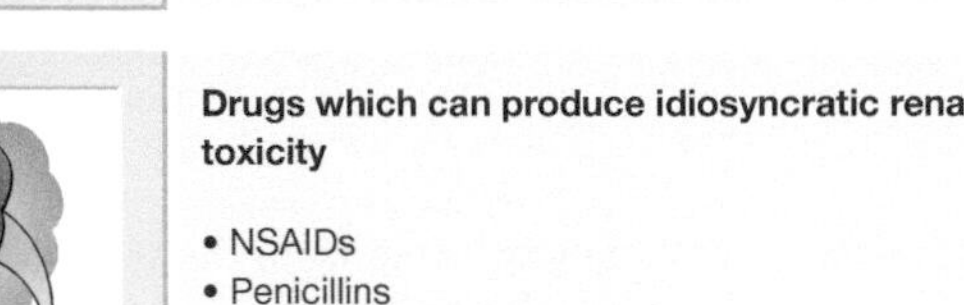

Drugs which can produce idiosyncratic renal toxicity

- NSAIDs
- Penicillins
- Gold, penicillamine

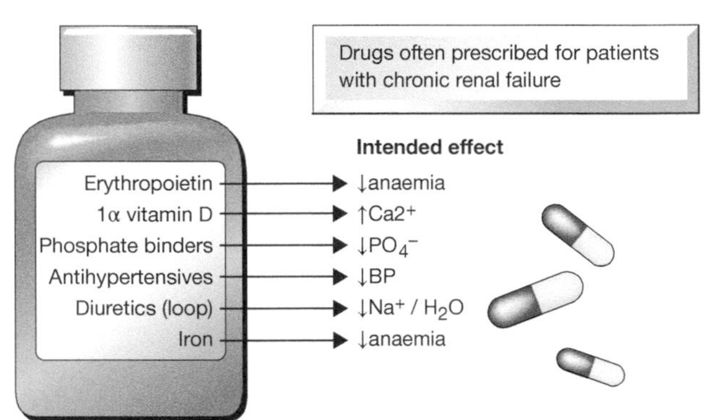

When prescribing a drug for a patient with renal failure, several issues need to be addressed.

- What is the effect of the renal impairment on renal excretion of the drug?
- What is the effect of the renal impairment on drug action?
- What is the effect of the drug on the kidneys?
- How should the prescription be altered in view of the renal impairment?

The golden rules when prescribing in all patients with renal failure are to 'use drugs sparingly' and 'always check the dose in a pharmacopoeia such as the *BNF*.'

Effect of renal impairment on excretion

Nearly all drugs are excreted to some extent by the kidneys. Furthermore, in patients with renal impairment, there may be differing bioavailability, and alterations in volume of distribution and in plasma protein binding. If there is significant renal impairment, appropriate dosing should be prescribed based on recommended guidelines. For some drugs, such as morphine and pethidine, active drug metabolites may be excreted by the kidney and produce toxicity in renal impairment. The monitoring of blood levels (for drugs such as digoxin or gentamicin) may be essential to achieve appropriate dosing.

Effect of renal impairment on drug action

Uraemia may produce increased or decreased end-organ sensitivity; for example, loop diuretics such as furosemide (frusemide) must be prescribed in much larger doses in renal impairment to achieve the same therapeutic effect.

Effect of drug on the kidneys

Drugs may produce an idiosyncratic renal toxicity such as the interstitial nephritis produced by antibiotics and non-steroidal anti-inflammatory drugs (NSAIDs), or have a predictable adverse effect such as the exacerbation of renal hypoperfusion by angiotensin-converting enzyme inhibitors and NSAIDs.

In patients undergoing dialysis treatment, it is also necessary to know whether the drug is removed by dialysis. In transplant recipients, there are many important and potentially dangerous interactions with the immunosuppressive agents.

Medicine at a Glance, Fifth Edition. Edited by Patrick Davey and Alex Pitcher.

Companion website: www.wiley.com/go/medicine5e

Benign prostatic hypertrophy

Prostatic hypertrophy

- 50% in >60-year-olds

Symptoms:

From bladder outflow obstruction:
- Poor urinary stream
- Hesitancy
- Terminal dribbling
- Frequency
- Nocturia
- Overflow incontinence

From metabolic complications:
- Acute renal failure
- Chronic renal failure

Treatment

α-adrenergic blockers
5α-reductase inhibitors
Transurethral resection of prostate (TURP)

? Enlarged bladder

Enlarged smooth prostate

Nodule craggy mass

Prostatic cancer

- Rare in <60-year-olds
- Common in elderly

Symptoms:
- Often asymptomatic
- Bladder outflow obstruction
- Systemic symptoms (malaise, weight loss)
- Pain from metastatic deposits
- From renal failure

± local pain
metastases especially bone (sclerotic)

Treatment

Antiandrogen therapy
Radiotherapy
Occasionally prostatectomy (open or TURP)

Investigations

Transrectal/abdominal ultrasound
Renal function
Prostate-specific antigen:
- ↑ in cancer – confirm by biopsy
- ↑↑ if metastasis (confirm by bone scan)

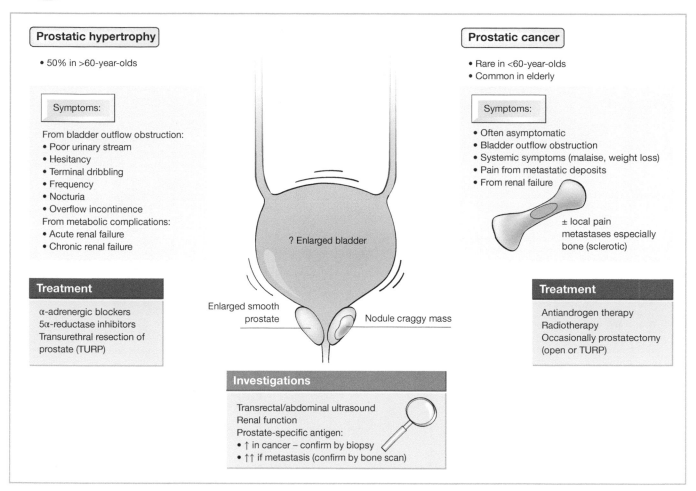

Benign prostatic hypertrophy is characterized by enlargement of the prostate gland and is very common, being present in over 50% of men aged over 60 years, and 80% over the age of 80. It most commonly presents with features of bladder outflow obstruction/poor urinary stream, hesitancy, terminal dribbling and frequency. Other symptoms can include dysuria and overflow incontinence. Alternatively, patients may present with symptoms of chronic renal failure or acute urinary retention. Cancer of the prostate is common, affecting one in six men, though only 3% of men die from prostate cancer.

Examination

On examination, a bladder may be palpable or detected by percussion. An enlarged smooth prostate is found on digital rectal examination.

Investigations

These may include measurement of serum creatinine, ultrasonography of the renal tract, urodynamics and determination of prostate-specific antigen (PSA) levels because these are raised in prostate malignancy (see Chapter 194). PSA can also be elevated with prostatitis, rises with age and only has a limited specificity (*c.* 70%) and sensitivity (*c.* 70%) for the diagnosis of prostate cancer.

Management

Medical management includes the use of α-adrenergic blockers such as terazosin, α_1-adrenoceptor antagonists such as tamsulosin (which relax the smooth muscle of the prostate and bladder neck) or finasteride (a 5α-reductase inhibitor that inhibits the conversion of testosterone to its active metabolite dihydrotestosterone, thus reducing prostatic hypertrophy). Surgery is often necessary to improve urine flow and transurethral resection of the prostate (TURP) is undertaken endoscopically. Laser-based endoscopic therapy (called HoLEP – holmium laser enucleation of the prostate), steam therapy (REZUM), and pinning segments of the hypertrophied prostate back (urolift) are all contemporary surgical treatments.

Medicine at a Glance, Fifth Edition. Edited by Patrick Davey and Alex Pitcher.

Companion website: www.wiley.com/go/medicine5e

154 Urinary tract infection

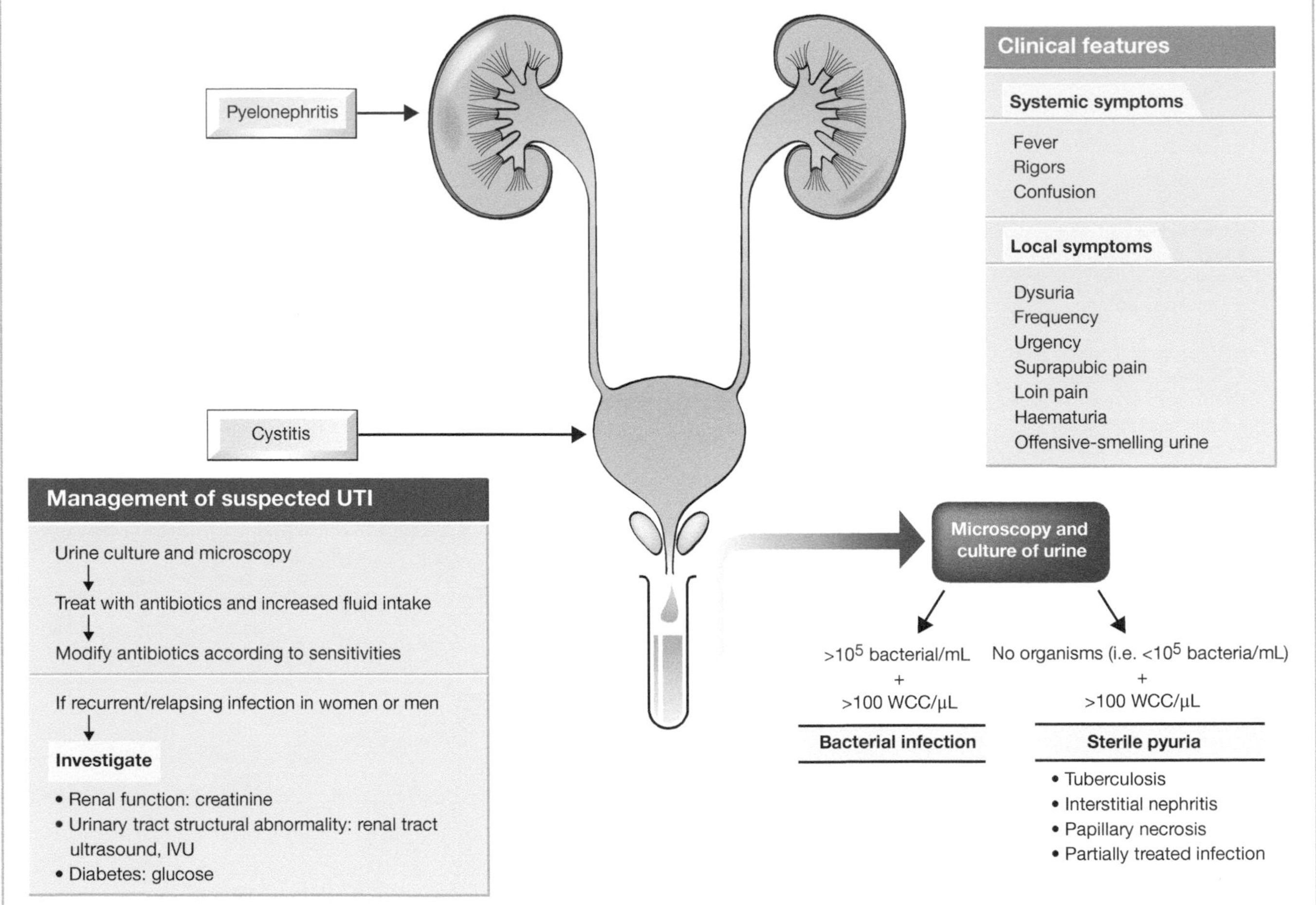

Pyelonephritis
Cystitis
Clinical features
Systemic symptoms
Fever
Rigors
Confusion
Local symptoms
Dysuria
Frequency
Urgency
Suprapubic pain
Loin pain
Haematuria
Offensive-smelling urine
Management of suspected UTI
Urine culture and microscopy
Treat with antibiotics and increased fluid intake
Modify antibiotics according to sensitivities
If recurrent/relapsing infection in women or men
Investigate
• Renal function: creatinine
• Urinary tract structural abnormality: renal tract ultrasound, IVU
• Diabetes: glucose
Microscopy and culture of urine
>10^5 bacterial/mL + >100 WCC/μL
Bacterial infection
No organisms (i.e. <10^5 bacteria/mL) + >100 WCC/μL
Sterile pyuria
• Tuberculosis
• Interstitial nephritis
• Papillary necrosis
• Partially treated infection

Urinary tract infections (UTIs) are very common, accounting for 1–2% of general practice consultations. They occur much more commonly in females and in young, sexually active women, in whom the annual incidence may be as high as 0.5/woman/year. Most infections arise from the introduction of bowel flora via the urethra into the bladder. The increased frequency of UTIs in women is attributed to short urethral length, and a UTI can commonly follow sexual intercourse. Other host factors associated with an increased risk of UTI include (i) pregnancy; (ii) incomplete bladder emptying (e.g. neurogenic bladder in multiple sclerosis, spinal cord injury); (iii) urinary calculi; (iv) diabetes mellitus (all suspected UTIs should have urine dipstick tested for glucose); (v) structural abnormality of the urinary tract (e.g. reflux); and (vi) instrumentation of the urinary tract (e.g. urethral catheterization).

The causative organisms are usually coliforms (70%) but other bacterial pathogens include *Proteus mirabilis*, *Staphylococcus epidermidis* and *Streptococcus faecalis*. Certain cell surface antigens may enhance pathogenicity by aiding the adhesion of bacteria to uroepithelial surfaces.

The typical symptoms of a UTI are dysuria, urinary frequency and urgency, suprapubic discomfort, loin pain, fever, haematuria and offensive smelling urine. Sometimes, particularly in the elderly, local symptoms may be absent but the patient may present with confusion or general deterioration. If the infection primarily causes symptoms in the bladder, it can be termed 'cystitis', whereas infection affecting the kidney is termed 'pyelonephritis'.

Investigations

A number of investigations are helpful.

- **Urine dipsticks**: most Gram-negative bacteria, the most common organisms implicated in UTIs, convert nitrate, a normal constituent of urine, to nitrite, which is detected by dipstick. The presence of nitrite is therefore a useful guide to the presence of pathogenic Gram-negative organisms. Finding leukocytes in the urine suggests an inflammatory process in the renal/urinary tract. The most common cause of this is infection

Medicine at a Glance, Fifth Edition. Edited by Patrick Davey and Alex Pitcher.

Companion website: www.wiley.com/go/medicine5e

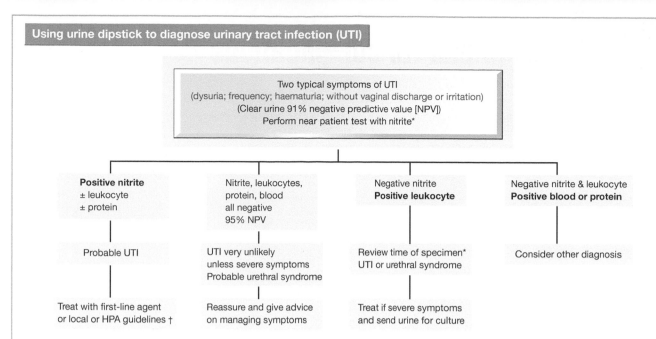

Using urine dipstick to diagnose urinary tract infection (UTI)

Two typical symptoms of UTI
(dysuria; frequency; haematuria; without vaginal discharge or irritation)
(Clear urine 91% negative predictive value [NPV])
Perform near patient test with nitrite*

Positive nitrite ± leukocyte ± protein	Nitrite, leukocytes, protein, blood all negative 95% NPV	Negative nitrite **Positive leukocyte**	Negative nitrite & leukocyte **Positive blood or protein**
Probable UTI	UTI very unlikely unless severe symptoms Probable urethral syndrome	Review time of specimen* UTI or urethral syndrome	Consider other diagnosis
Treat with first-line agent or local or HPA guidelines †	Reassure and give advice on managing symptoms	Treat if severe symptoms and send urine for culture	

*Nitrite is produced by the action of bacterial nitrate reductase in urine. As contact time between bacteria and urine is needed, morning specimens are most reliable. Leukocyte esterase detects intact and lysed leukocytes produced in inflammation. Haematuria and proteinuria occur in UTI but are also present in other conditions. When reading test **WAIT** for the time recommended by manufacturer.

HPA, Health Protection Agency guidelines † = www.hpa.org.uk/infections/topics_az/antimicrobial_resistance/guidance.htm

Urethral syndrome: a syndrome characterized by symptoms identical to urinary tract infection (e.g. frequency, suprapubic pain, dysuria) but in which no microbes are found to colonize the urinary tract. Other conditions affecting the uro-gynaecological tract need to be ruled out; in many the cause remains unclear

From Health Protection Agency www.hpa.org.uk

Microorganisms causing hospital-acquired UTIs

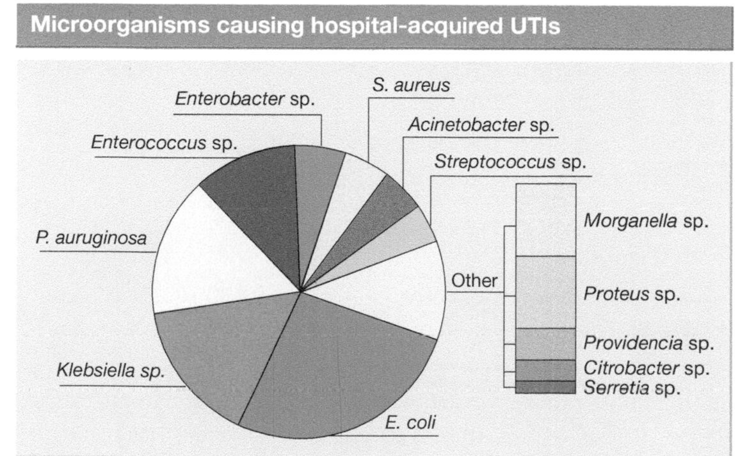

Causes of community-acquired UTIs

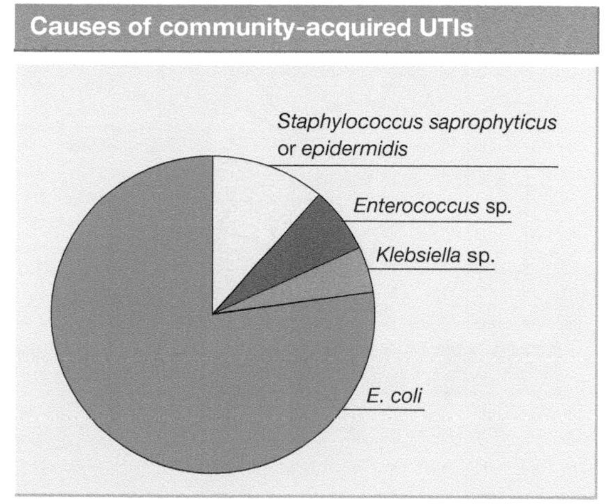

by conventional bacteria; if these cannot be found (so-called sterile pyuria), other causes should be considered, such as tuberculosis of the renal tract, cancer and renal or bladder stones.

- **Microscopy and culture of a midstream specimen of urine**: if a UTI is suspected, a sample of urine (preferably obtained as a 'clean catch' from midstream urine) should be microscoped and cultured. A finding of more than 10^5 organisms/ml urine is significant. Culture enables the causative organism to be identified and its antibiotic susceptibilities defined. Organisms may be cultured from urine without being of pathogenic significance, e.g. because of perineal contamination; but the presence of >100 leukocytes/mm^3 of urine usually characterizes significant bacterial infections.
- **Renal tract imaging**: investigations for a predisposing cause should be undertaken if there are multiple infections in a woman, or a first UTI in a child or man, and these may include tests of renal function (any structural abnormality of the kidneys or renal tract can predispose to infection), glucose, CT urogram or ultrasonography (to detect renal calculi, abnormalities of the urinary tract and incomplete bladder emptying) and micturating cystogram (particularly in children to exclude reflux).

Management

Urine should be sent for microscopy and culture before starting antibiotic treatment. In uncomplicated UTIs, short-duration (five-day or even single-dose) antibiotic therapy is usually adequate. Trimethoprim, nitrofurantoin or amoxicillin are commonly prescribed, but the prescription may need to be altered in the light of the antibiotic sensitivities of the causative organism. Acute pyelonephritis or prominent systemic symptoms of infection may require intravenous antibiotics. A high fluid intake (>3 l/day) is recommended to prevent urinary stasis in the bladder and to decrease bacterial replication.

Diabetes and its complications

Type 1 diabetes – pancreatic islet β-cell deficiency

≈10%

Autoimmune Beta-cell & insulin deficiency

Can present at any age
- But more common when <30 years
- Peak incidence at 14 years

Presents with:
- Polyuria, polydipsia, weight loss
- DKA

Usually free from complications for 5–10 years

Personal or family history of other autoimmune disease, coeliac, thyroid, Addison, etc.

Treatment
- Subcutaneous insulin delivered by multiple daily injections or continuous subject insulin infusion
- Carbohydrate counting
- Self-monitoring for capillary glucose and ketones
- Treat cardiovascular risk factors

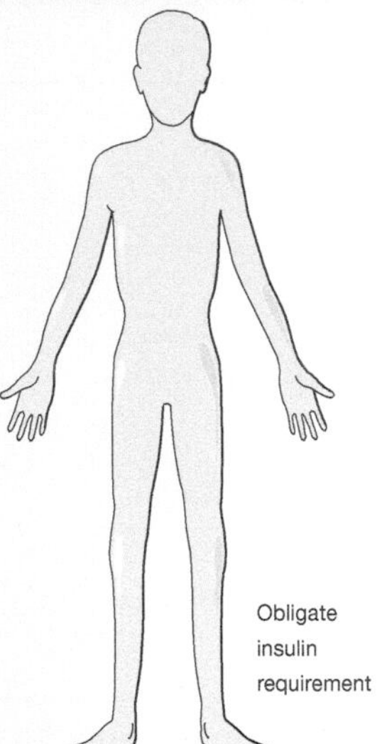

Type 2 diabetes – defective insulin action or secretion

≈85%

Insulin resistance + gradual Beta-cell & insulin deficiency

Usually presents >40 years age

Presents with:
- Insidious onset osmotic symptoms
- Asymptomatic on screening
- Hyperosmolar hyperglycaemic state (HHS)

Often have established complications at diagnosis:
- Macrovascular atherosclerotic disease
- Microvascular: retinopathy, nephropathy, neuropathy

Family history of T2DM or personal history of GDM is typical

Treatment
- Diet
- Treat cardiovascular risk factors
- Hypoglycaemic agents
- Insulin

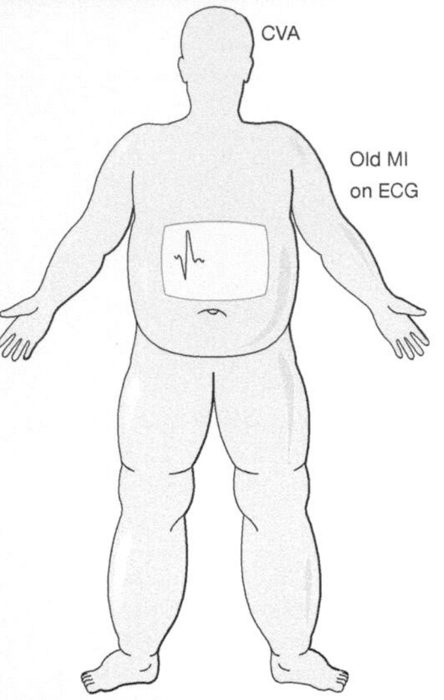

Insulin treatment

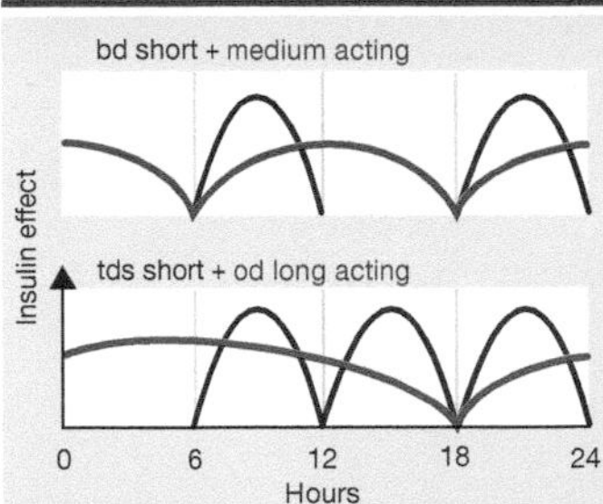

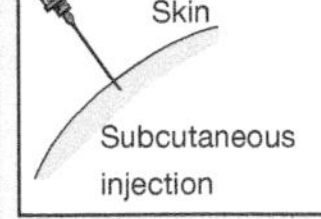

Usual injection sites

Side effects
- Pain
- ↑Weight
- Hypoglycaemia
- Infection/abscess – very rare
- Lipohypertrophy – prevented by rotating site

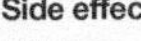

	Mode of Action	Hba1c Reduction (mmol/mol)	Advantages	Disadvantages	Specia Considerations
Biguanides - Metformin	Reduces hepatic glucose output and increases peripheral glucose uptake.	15 – 20	Potent Inexpensive CV Risk Reduction Modest weight loss	GI upset	Dose reduction in renal impairment
Sulphonylureas - Gliclazide - Glibenclamide - Glimepiride	Binds to the Sulfonylurea receptor on the beta-cell, stimulating insulin release.	c. 15	Potent Inexpensive	Hypoglycaemia Modest weight gain	Accumulation in renal impairment with increased risk of hypoglycaemia
GLP1 Analogues - Semaglutide - Dulaglutide - Liraglutide - Exenetide	Resists degradation by DPP4. Activation of the GLP1 receptor, potentiates insulin, inhibits glucagon and promotes satiety.	15 – 20	Potent CV Risk Reduction Weight loss	Expensive GI upset	Administered by subcutaneous injection given daily or weekly
DPP4 inhibitors - Sitagliptin - Saxagliptin - Linagliptin	Delays the degradation of native GLP1, potentiating its effects.	c. 5	Well tolerated	Minimal Hba1c lowering	Contraindicated in combination with GLP1 Analogues
SGLT2 inhibitors - Empagliflozin - Dapagliflozin - Canagliflozin	Inhibits SGLT2 mediated glucose reabsorption from the proximal tubular, promoting glycosuria	5 – 10	CV Risk Reduction Renoprotective Modest weight loss	Genitourinary thrush Euglycaemic DKA	Modest BP lowering effect
Thiazolidinediones - Pioglitazone	Alters transcription of genes involved in carbohydrate and lipid metabolism.	c. 15	Potent	Weight gain Fluid retention	Possible Renal Cell Carcinoma risk Possible Osteoporosis risk
Insulin - Detemir - Glargine - Aspart - Lispro	Activation of the insulin receptor reduces hepatic glucose output and increases peripheral skeletal muscle glucose uptake.	≥25	Uncapped potency	Hypoglycaemia Weight gain	Variety of agents and individualised regimens available

Annual assessment of the patient with DM

Eyes
- Screen for retinopathy
- Dilated ophthalmoscopy
- Visual acuity for maculopathy

Blood pressure
- Target BP <140/90 in all, tighter in some
- Orthostatic hypotension may indicate autonomic neuropathy

Consider occult IHD silent angina

Kidneys
- Screening for nephropathy
- Persistent UACR >30 mg/g
- Serum creatinine climbing/GFR falling

Feet
- Screen for neuropathy and PVD
- Protective sensory threshold
- Vibration sensation/proprioception
- Absent ankle jerks
- Symptoms of PVD and pedal pulses
- ABIs with toe pressures if PVD suspected

Also check
- Glucose control HbA1c
- Ask about frequency and symptoms of hypoglycaemia
- Consider if statin indicated (if calculated 10 yr cardiovascular risk >10%)
- Monitor weight and consider assessment for associated conditions (e.g. OSA) and suitability for weight lowering/weight neutral therapies

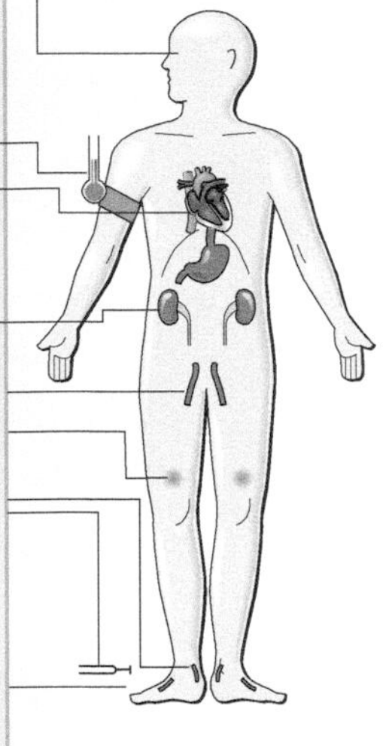

Medicine at a Glance, Fifth Edition. Edited by Patrick Davey and Alex Pitcher.

Companion website: www.wiley.com/go/medicine5e

Definition

Diabetes mellitus (DM) is a chronic disease characterized by persistently elevated blood glucose (hyperglycaemia), resulting from either absolute insulin deficiency or relative insulin insufficiency in the context of insulin resistance. Diabetes mellitus affects ≈10% of the adult population and may result in chronic micro-/macrovascular complications or acute metabolic emergencies (see Chapter 156).

Diagnosis

Random plasma glucose, fasting plasma glucose (FPG), plasma glucose two hours post 75 g oral glucose tolerance test (2-h OGTT) or glycated hemoglobin (HbA1c) can be used to diagnose DM. HbA1c correlates with mean plasma glucose over the previous three months. Asymptomatic patients should be confirmed by repeat testing. A random plasma glucose ≥11.1 mmol/l is sufficient to diagnose if symptomatic.

	Normal	Intermediate	Diabetes mellitus[a]
FPG (mmol/l)	≤5.5	5.6–6.9 (IFG)	≥7.0
2-h OGTT (mmol/l)	≤7.8	7.9–11.0 (IGT)	≥11.1
HbA1c (mmol/mol) (%)	≤42 (6.0%)	43–47	≥48 (6.5%)

[a] The diagnosis is made if any one parameter is above the threshold in the right column.

These diagnostic thresholds represent the degree of hyperglycaemia associated with microvascular complications, specifically retinopathy. Patients with intermediate hyperglycaemia (often referred to as 'pre-diabetes') are still at risk of macrovascular complications, and of developing overt DM in the future. Risk can be reduced through lifestyle modification and weight loss. Gestational diabetes is diagnosed as the degree of hyperglycaemia associated with worse maternal and fetal outcomes; the exact protocol for testing and thresholds for diagnosis are not universally agreed.

Classification and pathophysiology

Type 1 diabetes mellitus (rapid β-cell failure, absolute insulin deficiency)

Five percent to 10% of adult cases, 90% of paediatric cases. Presents at any age, but most common when aged <30 years. Absolute insulin deficiency results from antibody-mediated, autoimmune β-cell destruction in the genetically predisposed. Up to 30% also have evidence of insulin resistance. Antibodies (e.g. anti-GAD) can be measured in the serum and aid classification; without insulin therapy, T1DM is fatal. Commonly associated with other autoimmune conditions (coeliac, hypothyroidism, vitiligo, Addison disease, etc.).

Presentation: acute-onset polyuria, polydipsia and weight loss. Many present in ketoacidosis. Patients present at disease onset, without established complications.

Type 2 diabetes mellitus (insulin resistance, relative insulin insufficiency)

Eighty-five percent of adult cases. Obesity drives insulin resistance; disordered fatty acid metabolism is implicated. Most patients also demonstrate progressive loss of β-cell function over decades. Historically considered a disease of adults but, due to childhood obesity, now accounts for 10% of paediatric cases. Substantial polygenic contribution; identical twin concordance is 90%.

Presentation: insidious polyuria and polydipsia, or picked up on routine testing of the asymptomatic patient; 20% have established complications at diagnosis.

LADA (latent autoimmune diabetes of adults, slow autoimmune β-cell destruction)

Diabetes-associated autoantibodies are detected in 10% of patients classified as T2DM based on presentation and phenotype. Such patients are said to have LADA. The antibodies signify underlying autoimmune β-cell destruction, though at a much slower rate than in T1DM, and predict an eventual need for insulin therapy.

Gestational diabetes (new-onset diabetes in the second or third trimester)

Similar pathophysiology to T2DM, which 30–50% develop within 10 years. Maternal glucose crosses the placenta and the fetal pancreas increases insulin secretion, resulting in macrosomia, which complicates delivery. The babies are at increased risk of obesity and T2DM later in life. Dietary modification is first line, followed by metformin and insulin.

MODY (maturity-onset diabetes in the young, i.e. monogenetic diabetes)

One percent to 2% of cases of DM are caused by autosomal dominant gene mutations. Over a dozen different subtypes of MODY have now been described. Consider MODY in any patient with a strong family history of diabetes mellitus, and in all diagnosed aged <6 months. Treatment may be impacted; MODY1 (HNF4α) and MODY3 (HNF1α) are extremely sensitive to sulfonylureas, whereas MODY2 (GCK) results in only mild hyperglycaemia, without the potential for complications, and thus usually requires no treatment.

Other specific causes of diabetes (secondary diabetes mellitus, miscellaneous)

- *Exocrine pancreas failure:* post pancreatitis, post pancreatectomy, carcinoma, etc.
- *CFRD:* cystic fibrosis-related diabetes; exocrine pancreas failure is common in CF.
- *Endocrine disease:* Cushing, acromegaly, glucagonoma, haemochromatosis, etc.
- *Chemical-induced diabetes:* e.g. glucocorticoids, or HAART for the treatment of HIV.
- *NODAT:* new-onset diabetes after transplant; glucocorticoids, ciclosporin, tacrolimus, etc.
- *Flatbush diabetes:* a type of ketosis-prone T2DM, affecting patients of African descent.
- *Lipodystrophy syndromes:* abnormal adipose deposition with severe insulin resistance.
- *Progeroid syndromes:* such as Werner syndrome and Bloom syndrome.
- *Rabson–Mendenhall syndrome:* severe insulin resistance, autosomal recessive.

Management

The goals of management, in order of priority, are to (1) prevent metabolic emergencies, (2) eliminate symptoms, and (3) reduce the risk of long-term complications. These need to be achieved while avoiding an undue burden from treatment. Prevention of complications is discussed later in this chapter while options for glucose-lowering therapy are discussed below.

Patient education: specialist diabetes nurses and dieticians teach patients to self-manage their diabetes. Structured education courses (e.g. carbohydrate counting) are beneficial.

Dietary advice: aim for moderate, sustainable weight loss to lessen insulin resistance. Control portion sizes. Minimize confectionery and alcohol.

Specific treatments (including oral agents, GLP-1 analogues and insulin)

Metformin is first line in almost all patients with T2DM. The choice of second-line agent can be individualized. All patients with T1DM require insulin, as do other patients with absolute β-cell failure (e.g. post pancreatectomy, late-stage T2DM, etc.).

Metformin: the remaining available biguanide. Reduces insulin resistance and hepatic gluconeogenesis. Mild anorexic effect results in modest weight loss. 10% report transient GI upset. Reduce dose in renal impairment to avoid lactic acidosis. Contraindicated in renal failure and hepatic insufficiency. Associated with contrast-induced nephropathy.

Sulfonylureas: gliclazide, glibenclamide, glimepride, tolbutamide. Act via the sulfonylurea receptor on the β cell to close K^+ channels, cause cell depolarization and thus insulin release. Usually cause modest weight gain. Hypoglycaemia can be problematic, particularly in the elderly. Dose reduction is required in renal impairment.

GLP-1 analogues: exenatide, liraglutide, semaglutide, dulaglutide. GLP-1 (a gut hormone released on nutrient ingestion) stimulates insulin, inhibits glucagon and acts on the hypothalamus to induce satiety. GLP-1 is rapidly inactivated ($t_{1/2} \approx 2$ minutes) by the enzyme DPP-4. GLP-1 analogues, injected subcutaneously, resist DPP-4 and have a prolonged duration of action. Some patients achieve significant weight loss. Newer agents demonstrate cardiovascular risk reduction. GI upset is common.

DPP-4 inhibitors: sitagliptin, saxagliptin, linagliptin, vildagliptin. Extend the half-life of endogenous GLP-1. Well tolerated and weight neutral.

SGLT-2 inhibitors: canagliflozin, dapagliflozin, empagliflozin. The sodium-glucose transporter reabsorbs glucose from the glomerular filtrate; inhibition causes glucose disposal in the urine. Some achieve moderate weight loss. Cardiovascular outcome data have been very encouraging. Polyuria is inevitable. Urinary tract infections and genital thrush are common. Euglycaemic DKA is reported and limits the utility of this class in certain at-risk groups: pancreatitis, alcohol excess, long duration of diabetes, etc.

Pioglitazone: the remaining available thiazolidinedione; rosiglitazone and troglitazone were withdrawn. A potent insulin sensitizer; activates the PPAR-γ receptor which stimulates transcription of glucose transporter molecules. Associated with increased fractures and bladder carcinoma. Avoid in heart failure as fluid retention is common.

Meglitinides: repaglinide, nateglinide. Similar to sulfonylureas, but act directly on the K^+ channel. Short duration of action makes hypoglycaemia less common.

Acarbose: inhibits α-glucosidase, limiting carbohydrate digestion and thus reducing intestinal glucose absorption. Bloating and diarrhea result in poor tolerability.

Insulin: given by subcutaneous injection. Insulin analogues are chemically modified to alter absorption from the subcutaneous tissue; rapidly absorbed analogues (lispro, aspart, glulisine) are taken with food (bolus), whereas slowly absorbed, long-acting analogues (detemir, glargine, degludec) are taken once or twice daily to provide a steady background insulin level (basal). Premixed preparations are available. Hypoglycaemia and weight gain are common. Lipohypertrophy can occur at injection sites.

CSII: rapid-acting analogues may be delivered via continuous subcutaneous insulin infusion pump. This allows for variable basal rates and frequent boluses. Pumps may be linked to a continuous glucose sensor, which predicts impending hypoglycaemia and suspends the infusion. Fully automated 'closed-loop' systems are being developed.

Transplantation: islet cell transplantation may be used in T1DM. Combined pancreas and kidney transplant may be performed in patients with T1DM and renal failure.

Bariatric surgery: procedures designed to reduce stomach capacity and/or nutrient absorption, but altered appetite due to gut hormone changes seems to be important; ≥40% of excess weight can be lost, often resulting in long-term remission of T2DM.

Monitoring glycaemic control in diabetes

Patients on insulin are encouraged to monitor capillary blood glucose by finger prick testing. Based on the results, insulin doses can be adjusted. Continuous glucose monitors and flash glucose sensors measure subcutaneous interstitial fluid glucose as a surrogate for plasma glucose. These devices facilitate frequent testing and provide additional information on glucose trends. Glucose monitoring is less important in patients not on insulin, where HbA1c is the primary measure of glucose control, but should be encouraged in all patients on agents which cause hypoglycaemia, especially if driving. Patients at risk of ketosis can measure capillary blood ketones.

Complications of diabetes

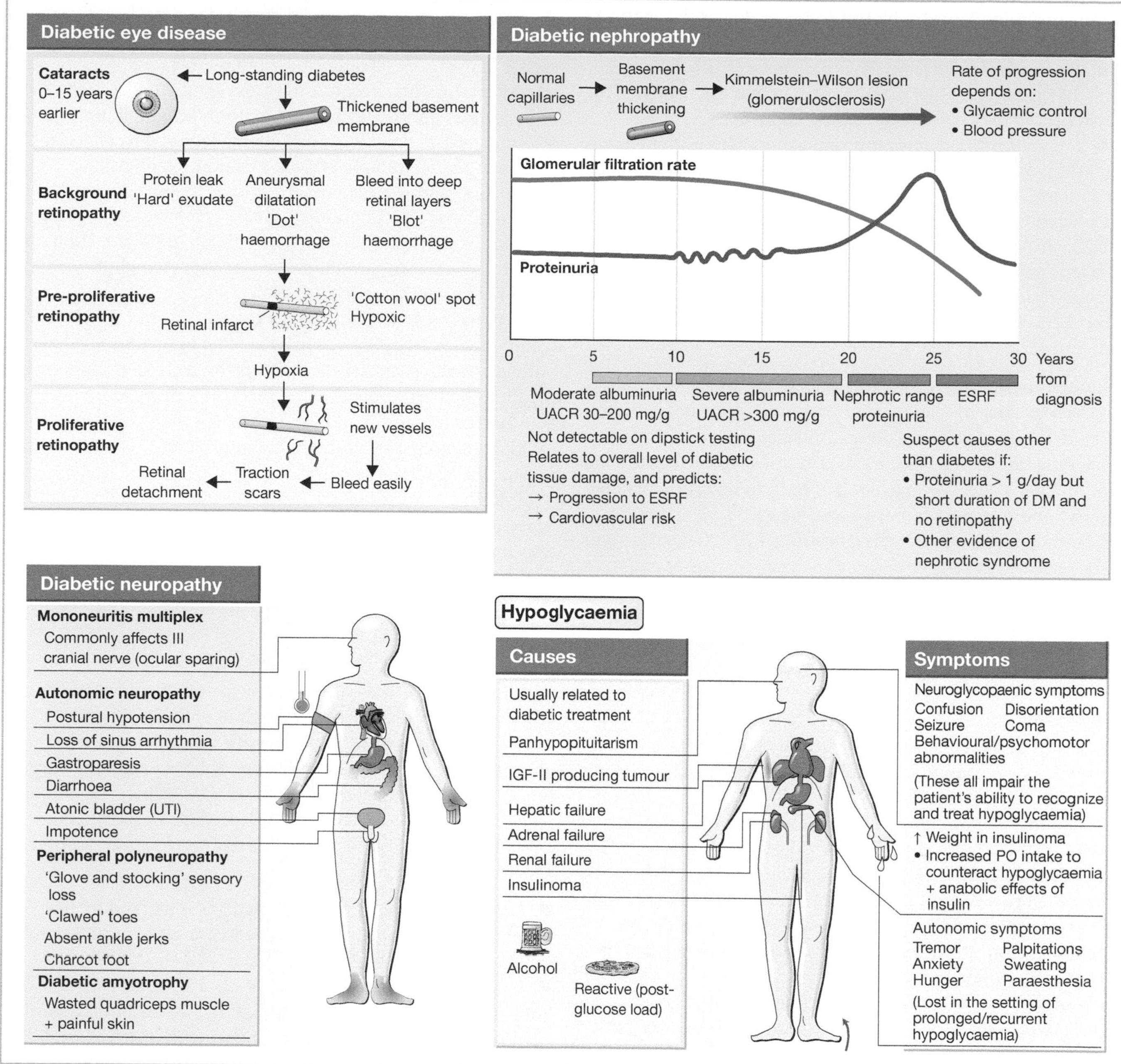

Burden and classification

The ultimate goal of treating DM is the prevention of complications. Yet, despite widely available therapies with proven benefit, DM still remains a major cause of morbidity and mortality worldwide. The WHO estimated that 1.5 million deaths in 2012 were directly attributable to DM and resulting complications.

The potential complications of DM are broadly divided into two categories.

- **Macrovascular complications** refer to the development of atherosclerotic disease within the larger blood vessels: cardiovascular disease, cerebrovascular disease, peripheral vascular disease, renovascular disease, mesenteric ischaemia, etc.
- **Microvascular complications** refer to retinopathy, nephropathy and neuropathy. These complications are grouped together as damage to the small blood vessels (arterioles and capillaries) is implicated in their pathogenesis. The risk of developing microvascular complications is directly linked to both the duration of DM and the magnitude of hyperglycaemia, and is higher in the setting of concomitant hypertension.

Microvascular complications

Retinopathy

Several pathways have been proposed to explain how hyperglycaemia causes the initial retinal injury, but it is the subsequent development of new blood vessels within the retina that most commonly leads to sight-threatening retinopathy. Thus retinopathy is often classified into two main phases.

- **Non-proliferative retinopathy** (sight is not impaired unless the macula is involved).
  - *Background retinopathy*: microaneurysms (dots), intraretinal haemorrhages (blots) and hard exudates not involving the macula (lipid-rich, waxy-appearing deposits).
  - *Preproliferative retinopathy*: retinal nerve fibre layer infarcts (cotton wool spots). Venous beading and tortuous, dilated capillaries.
- **Proliferative retinopathy** (can follow NPDR, or arise without NPDR). Growth factors, such as VEGF, promote new vessels that are fragile and prone to bleeding. Pre-retinal and vitreous haemorrhages result in acute loss of sight that may recover as blood is reabsorbed. Subsequent fibrosis causes traction retinal detachment and permanent loss of vision.

Maculopathy: the macula is responsible for the central, sharp, color vision. Any of the above-mentioned features can impair vision if the macula is involved. Macular oedema is a sight-threatening change that occurs as a result of protein and fluid accumulating under the macula. It is hard to detect on ophthalmoscopy and requires specialist assessment.

Cataract: a non-vascular complication of DM. Cataracts occur 10–15 years earlier in DM.

Management: aim for tight glucose control and treat hypertension. Annual screening allows early detection and treatment. Anti-VEGF therapy and laser photocoagulation reduce the risk of hemorrhage from new blood vessels and are potentially sight saving.

Nephropathy

Diabetes mellitus remains a major cause of end-stage renal disease (ESRD), contributing to up to 80% of cases. The other major contributor is hypertension.

Screening: albuminuria is the earliest clinical evidence of nephropathy. The urinary albumin to creatinine ratio (UACR), measured on a spot (random) urine sample, should be assessed annually. Normal UACR is generally defined as <30 mg/g. False positives can occur, but a persistent UACR ≥30 mg/g indicates DN. A serum creatinine should also be measured and the glomerular filtration rate should be calculated.

Progression: the natural history of nephropathy is quite predictable in patients with T1DM (see figure). Patients with T2DM are older, more likely to have concomitant hypertension, and often have hyperglycaemia for years before diagnosis; the rate of progression of DN in these patients is less predictable, and may advance rapidly.

Management: aim for tight glucose control and treat hypertension with a regimen that includes either an ACE inhibitor or an angiotension II receptor blocker, but not both. SGLT2 inhibitors and GLP1 analogues delay progression of diabetic nephropathy. ACE-Is and ARBs reduce albuminuria and delay progression to ESRD, but combination treatment increases the risk of acute kidney injury and hyperkalaemia. The complications of chronic kidney disease need to be addressed as the GFR falls. Once ESRD is established, renal replacement therapy with dialysis or kidney transplantation is required.

Neuropathy

Diabetes mellitus results in nerve damage through multiple mechanisms. Inflammatory damage to the small blood vessels that supply the nerves, mediated by advanced glycosylation end-products (AGEs), seems to play an important role. There are several manifestations.

- *Peripheral polyneuropathy*: symmetrical, mixed sensorimotor neuropathy affecting the longest nerves in the body. Results in the classic 'glove and stocking' distribution sensory loss. Loss of vibration sensation occurs early; loss of pain sensation, thermosensation, proprioception and motor reflexes follows.
- *Autonomic neuropathy*: a debilitating neuropathy affecting the nerves of the autonomic system. Postural hypotension, erectile dysfunction and gastroparesis (resulting in chronic nausea and vomiting) may be prominent. Gustatory sweating, nocturnal diarrhoea and bladder dysfunction with retention, infections and incontinence can occur. Absent cardiac vagal tone leads to a loss of sinus arrhythmia – a helpful clinical sign.
- *Mononeuropathies*: cranial nerves III, IV and VI are most commonly affected. CN VII palsy is often idiopathic (Bell palsy) but can result from diabetic neuropathy. Peripheral mononeuropathies such as peroneal nerve palsy (foot drop) also occur.
- *Mononeuropathy multiplex*: describes the occurrence of multiple mononeuropathies in the same patient. The differential is usually DM versus vasculitis.
- *Treatment-induced neuropathy*: formally 'insulin neuritis'. A systemic polyneuropathy associated with autonomic dysfunction and cachexia. Very rare, but can occur with rapid correction of chronic, severe hyperglycaemia. Tends to resolve in time.
- *Amyotrophy*: painful wasting of the thigh muscles. Rare.

Macrovascular complications

Risk factors: DM is a major risk factor for the development of atherosclerosis. Risk is relatively high in both T1DM and T2DM, but the great majority of atherosclerotic risk is conferred by other factors: age, male sex, family history, tobacco smoking, hypertension and dyslipidaemia. However, DM synergizes strongly with these other macrovascular risk factors. Thus patients with DM who have additional risk factors require aggressive risk factor modification.

- *Hypertension*: target blood pressure is <140/90 mmHg in all patients with DM and in selected patients a target of <130/80 mmHg (or even <120/80 mmHg) is appropriate.
- *Dyslipidaemia*: statins should be offered to all patients with known atherosclerotic disease or high risk of cardiovascular disease. In practice, this means all patients with diabetes aged ≥50 years and younger patients with additional risk factors (including albuminuria).
- *Glucose control*: macrovascular risk, while less amenable than microvascular risk, is reduced by tight glucose control. However, it appears that a significant proportion of the macrovascular risk is conferred directly by insulin resistance. As such, even patients with 'pre-diabetes' should probably be offered aggressive risk factor modification.
- *Smoking*: every patient encounter should be an opportunity to discuss smoking cessation.
- *Albuminuria*: a strong independent risk factor for cardiovascular disease. Other risk factors should be managed aggressively once albuminuria develops.

Screening: screening for asymptomatic cardiovascular disease in DM is controversial. At a minimum, patients should be assessed annually for symptoms of cardiovascular disease, but due to myocardial neuropathy, angina in DM may be silent. Peripheral vascular disease should be assessed for annually (see below).

Diabetic foot disease

Diabetic foot disease is usually multifactorial, resulting from neuropathy and peripheral vascular disease. Unfortunately, foot disease often begets more foot disease.

Pathogenesis: neuropathy diminishes the sensory pain threshold and thus predisposes to injury. A patient may not recognize, for example, that shoes are tight and causing trauma. This leads to ulceration. In the absence of pain, the causative trauma may not be removed. Ongoing trauma, poor blood supply and persistent hyperglycaemia prevent ulcer healing and eventually infection develops. Infection can spread to adjacent bone, resulting in osteomyelitis, which is very difficult to treat, requiring an extended course of antibiotics and often amputation. Amputation results in foot deformity and abnormal weight bearing in the affected foot, the contralateral foot, or both. Deformity thus leads to further trauma, ulceration, infection and amputation. Input from a multidisciplinary foot team can break this vicious cycle.

Screening: patients with DM should be assessed annually for the following.

- *Neuropathy*: assessment of the protective sensation threshold is with a 10 g monofilament, or a finger as per the Ipswich touch test. Assessment of vibration sensation with a 128 Hz tuning fork is highly sensitive for detecting early neuropathy.
- *Peripheral vascular disease*: examine the pedal pulses and ask about symptoms of intermittent claudication. Formal assessment of the ankle brachial pressure index with toe pressures is indicated if peripheral vascular disease is suspected.

Prevention: patient education and vigilance are vital. Sources of potential injury should be avoided – walking barefoot, hot water bottles, etc. Patients should examine their feet daily. Detected ulcers should be cleaned, dressed and monitored. Ulcers that are slow to heal require prompt assessment for occult infection. Good footwear is essential.

Management: infections require antibiotics. Vascular surgery can restore blood supply. Debridement and offloading of ulcers encourage healing. The multidisciplinary foot team must include an experienced podiatrist. Amputation may ultimately be required.

Charcot foot: the acute Charcot foot is typically swollen, warm and erythematous, with a bounding pedal pulse. Loss of proprioception results in increased range of joint movement, instability and trauma. Fractures (or microfractures) may occur, but loss of pain sensation allows for continued weight bearing and further trauma. An initial osteolytic phase is followed by a hypertrophic repair phase. The architecture of the foot becomes deformed and often the classic 'rocker-bottom' foot of chronic Charcot develops. As above, deformity leads to amputation, thus the acute Charcot foot should be managed aggressively. Offloading to prevent repetitive trauma is vital.

Prevention of complications

A target HbA1c of ≤53 mmol/mol (≤7.0%) is appropriate in most patients with DM and balances favourable long-term microvascular protection against the short-term risk of hypoglycaemia. It is important to understand that microvascular complications take years to develop, and thus it takes years to realize benefit from tight control. The strongest predictor of microvascular risk is the duration of diabetes. A looser target may thus be appropriate in an older patient, with long duration of disease and already established complications. Such patients are the least likely to achieve benefit from tight control and the most likely to suffer harm from hypoglycaemia. Conversely, younger patients could target tighter control, especially if it can be achieved without undue side-effects and cost. Treatment must be individualized.

Hypoglycaemia

Hypoglycaemia is a common iatrogenic complication of diabetes. Many glucose-lowering medications, especially insulin and sulfonylureas, increase the risk of hypoglycaemia.

Definition and classification: in the setting of glucose-lowering medication, hypoglycaemia is arbitrarily defined as blood glucose <4.0 mmol/l. Hypoglycaemia can be classified as mild if the patient is able to self-correct, or severe if they require assistance from a third party. Glucometers can be inaccurate at this lower range.

Symptoms of hypoglycaemia:

- *Autonomic symptoms*: can occur at any blood glucose level below that which the patient is accustomed to. Tremor, palpitations, anxiety, sweating, hunger and paraesthesia, though distressing, alert the patient to the presence of hypoglycaemia and thus encourage treatment. Arrhythmias can occur at lower levels of blood glucose.
- *Neuroglycopenic symptoms*: once blood glucose is <2.8 mmol/l, confusion, disorientation and behavioural changes may impair the patient's ability to treat hypoglycaemia. Psychomotor abnormalities, seizure and coma may follow.

Treatment: hypoglycaemia should be promptly treated with oral glucose. In the unconscious patient, IM glucagon should be administered. Buccal glucose gel is also available. In the hospitalized patient, IV glucose can be given.

Risk of hypoglycaemia: prolonged or recurrent hypoglycaemia can result in attenuation of the autonomic symptoms (loss of hypoglycaemic awareness). This means that the neuroglycopenic symptoms may be the only symptoms that the patient experiences. This is a dangerous situation. Without early warning, hypoglycaemia can result in road traffic accidents, falls, seizures or even fatal cardiac arrhythmia.

Hypoglycaemia in the absence of glucose-lowering medication

True hypoglycaemia is uncommon in patients who are not on glucose-lowering medications. In such cases, Whipple's triad must be demonstrated.

1. Symptoms consistent with hypoglycemia.
2. Low plasma glucose measured at the time of the symptoms.
3. Relief of symptoms when the glucose is raised to normal.

In this cohort, the more common causes of hypoglycaemia include alcohol, hepatic failure, renal failure and sepsis. The cause of hypoglycaemia is usually obvious. Adrenal insufficiency is a potentially life-threatening cause of hypoglycaemia and should always be considered. An extensive work-up is only required when the cause is not immediately apparent. Blood insulin and c-peptide levels paired with a low plasma glucose assist the diagnosis. Rare causes include the following.

- *Postprandial hypoglycaemia*: rebound hypoglycaemia after an oral glucose load.
- *Insulinoma*: neuroendocrine tumour producing inappropriate insulin.
- *Paraneoplastic*: tumors secreting insulin-like growth factor II (IGF-II).
- *Other*: surreptitious use of insulin or sulfonylureas is occasionally encountered.

156 Diabetic emergencies

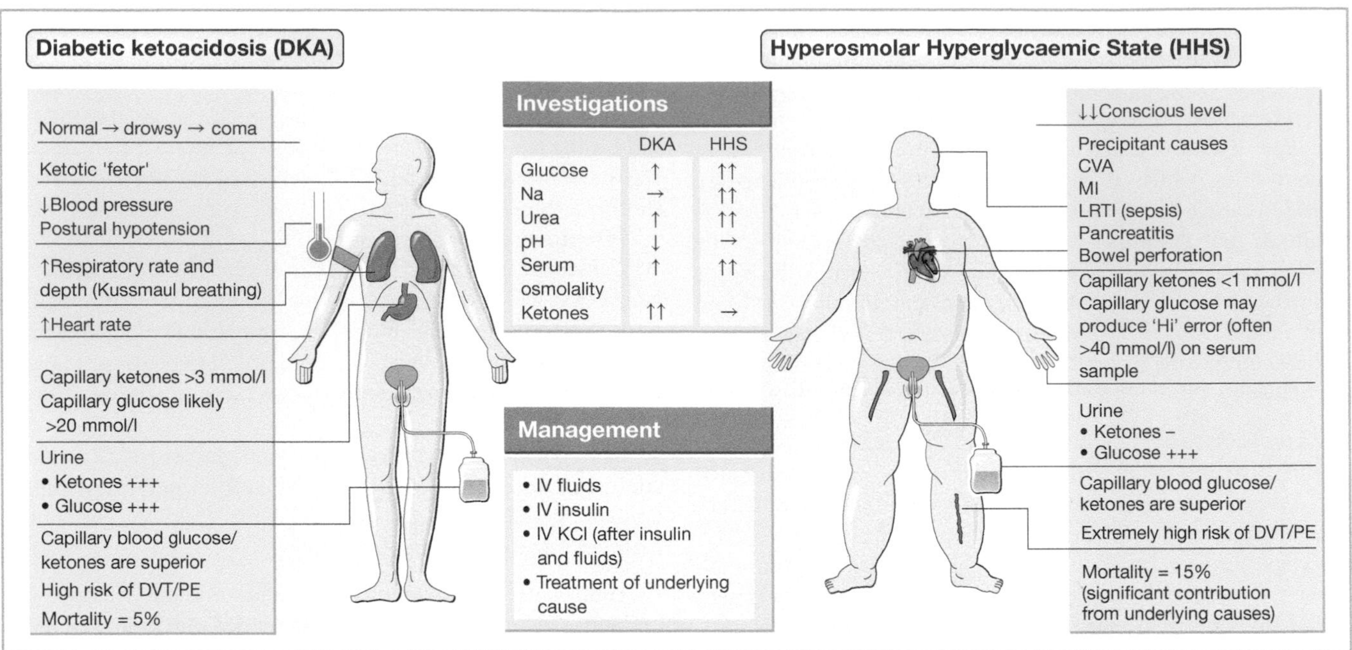

Diabetes mellitus may result in acute, life-threatening, metabolic emergencies. Diabetic ketoacidosis (DKA) is commonly encountered, with an estimated incidence of 80/10 000 patient years. The precise incidence of hyperosmolar hyperglycaemic state (HHS) is not known, but it is encountered much less often than DKA in clinical practice. Mortality rates in DKA and HHS are high, at 5% and 15% respectively.

Diabetic ketoacidosis

- **Pathogenesis**: ketone bodies are an alternative energy source for the central nervous system when glucose is not readily available. Serum ketone levels are elevated during periods of prolonged fasting or carbohydrate restriction. Insulin inhibits ketogenesis following carbohydrate ingestion. In states of absolute insulin deficiency, ketone body production becomes unregulated, and life-threatening ketoacidosis develops. Hyperglycemia and high ketone levels cause a profound osmotic diuresis.
- **Precipitants**: all patients with T1DM are at risk of DKA. Insulin omission (missed doses) is a frequent precipitant. Even patients fully adherent to subcutaneous insulin regimens can develop DKA in the setting of intercurrent illness, where high levels of counter-regulatory hormones (glucagon, catecholamines, cortisol) inhibit the effective action of insulin. Thus, an underlying precipitating cause (infection, sepsis, myocardial infarction, stroke, etc.) should always be sought. Frequently, new cases of T1DM present in DKA.
- **Clinical features:** polydipsia, polyuria, weight loss and dehydration are typical. Hypotension is often exacerbated by nausea and vomiting, and can result in organ dysfunction (shock). Abdominal pain usually indicates an underlying cause (e.g. appendicitis) but occasionally there is no cause other than the DKA itself. Kussmaul breathing and tachypnoea result from acidosis. CNS depression is seen in severe cases.

Diagnosis

Diabetic ketoacidosis is diagnosed when the following criteria are present.

- *Diabetes:* usually glucose will be >11 mmol/l (and often >20 mmol/l) but patients with T1DM may administer rapid-acting insulin prior to presentation, so a normal glucose level does not exclude DKA.
- *Ketosis*: β-hydroxybutyrate can be measured in capillary blood on a point-of-care ketone meter, and has superseded measurement of urinary ketones. Levels >3 mmol/l are consistent with DKA.
- *Metabolic acidosis*: pH <7.3 and/or serum bicarbonate <15 mmol/l. In the setting of acidosis, hyperkalaemia often features but falls rapidly with treatment.

Management

- *Fluid resuscitation*: rapid correction of hypovolaemia/shock is the priority.
- *Intravenous insulin*: promotes clearance of ketones and normalization of acid–base balance. Blood glucose is brought into the asymptomatic range, but the priority is clearing ketones; IV glucose may be administered to allow ongoing IV insulin infusion while avoiding hypoglycaemia.

Medicine at a Glance, Fifth Edition. Edited by Patrick Davey and Alex Pitcher.

Companion website: www.wiley.com/go/medicine5e

- *Potassium supplementation*: correction of acidosis, fluid resuscitation and IV insulin combine to cause a precipitous decline in serum potassium. Fatal arrhythmia can result if potassium is not proactively replaced.
- *Precipitant*: identify and treat the underlying cause. Sepsis is common and the threshold for commencing empirical antibiotics should be low.
- *Thromboembolic prophylaxis*: the risk of thromboembolism is high. Prophylactic low molecular weight heparin should be commenced unless there is a contraindication.
- *Monitoring*: close monitoring of vital signs, fluid balance and biochemistry is required. Ideally, DKA should be managed in a high-dependency setting.
- *Subcutaneous insulin*: once ketones are cleared, pH is normalized and the patient is tolerating oral diet, SC insulin can be initiated and IV insulin can be discontinued. Patients with known T1DM should continue on their prescribed basal insulin regimen while on IV insulin. This allows easier transition back to SC insulin and reduces the risk of recurrence of DKA should IV insulin delivery be interrupted; IV cannulas are easy to dislodge.

Prevention

At-risk patients should be educated on precipitating factors and 'sick-day rules' for monitoring and correction of hyperglycaemia and ketosis. Patients can self-monitor capillary blood ketones with a ketone meter.

Iatrogenic DKA

Diabetic ketoacidosis as a result of omission of insulin therapy during inpatient admission is an alarmingly frequent occurrence in T1DM patients. It is never appropriate to stop/hold basal insulin in a patient with T1DM, especially when they are unwell/sick; perhaps the one exception would be in the setting of a large-volume insulin overdose.

DKA in other subtypes of DM

Diabetic ketoacidosis can occur in other conditions of absolute or near absolute insulin deficiency.

- *T2DM*: patients with long-standing T2DM eventually experience β cell failure and can be prone to DKA, especially during intercurrent illness.
- *Exocrine pancreas failure:* post pancreatitis, post pancreatectomy, carcinoma, etc.
- *Flatbush diabetes:* ketosis-prone T2DM, mainly affects patients of African descent. The phenotype is similar to T2DM, but DKA can develop quickly during intercurrent illness.
- *SGLT2 inhibitors*: euglycaemic DKA is a recognized side-effect. The pathogenesis is not entirely clear. Risk factors include excessive alcohol intake, history of pancreatitis and long duration of T2DM.

Hyperosmolar hyperglycaemic state

Pathogenesis

Hyperosmolar hyperglycaemic state can develop in conditions of relative insulin insufficiency, where insulin levels are inadequate to maintain normoglycemia but sufficient to prevent ketogenesis. HHS most commonly occurs in patients with T2DM during intercurrent illness, when counter-regulatory hormones result in severe hyperglycaemia and a profound osmotic diuresis.

Biochemical features

- *Hyperglycaemia*: >35 mmol/l (usually >40 mmol/l).
- *Hyperosmolality*: plasma osmolality (concentration) can be measured on a laboratory osmometer, or can be calculated. Normal serum osmolality is ≈ 275–290 mOsm/kg. Osmolality >320 mOsm/l is consistent with HHS.

$$\text{Osmolality} = \left(2 \times \left[\text{Na}\right]\right) + \left[\text{Glu}\right] + \left[\text{Urea}\right].$$

- *Acid–base balance*: usually the plasma pH and $HCO3^-$ will be normal, unless there is a co-existent cause of acidosis (e.g. lactic acidosis due to shock). Ketones may be modestly elevated (due to starvation, etc.) but not in the range associated with DKA.
- *Hypernatraemia*: water losses outpace sodium losses and, even with the osmotic shift of intracellular fluid to the extracellular space, plasma sodium may be moderately elevated.

Clinical features

Polydipsia, polyuria, weight loss, dehydration and shock. Neurological symptoms such as drowsiness, delirium, seizures, hemiparesis or even coma may feature.

Management

Aggressive fluid resuscitation and IV insulin to gradually lower serum glucose to the asymptomatic range. Identify and treat the precipitating cause. Close monitoring of fluid balance and electrolytes; avoid hypoglycaemia and hypokalaemia. Cardiovascular, pulmonary, renal and CNS function may need to be supported. Thromboembolic risk is extremely high and prophylactic low molecular weight heparin should be commenced unless there is a contraindication.

Lactic acidosis

Lactic acidosis (LA) results from organ hypoperfusion and is frequently encountered during sepsis and shock. Patients with DM have an increased risk of LA compared to non-diabetic patients. Additionally, LA is a very rare side-effect of metformin though often there is a precipitating cause (such as sepsis). Metformin should generally be held if serum lactate is elevated but can usually be safely restarted if another precipitating cause is identified and treated, and lactate levels have normalized.

157 Hyperprolactinaemia and acromegaly

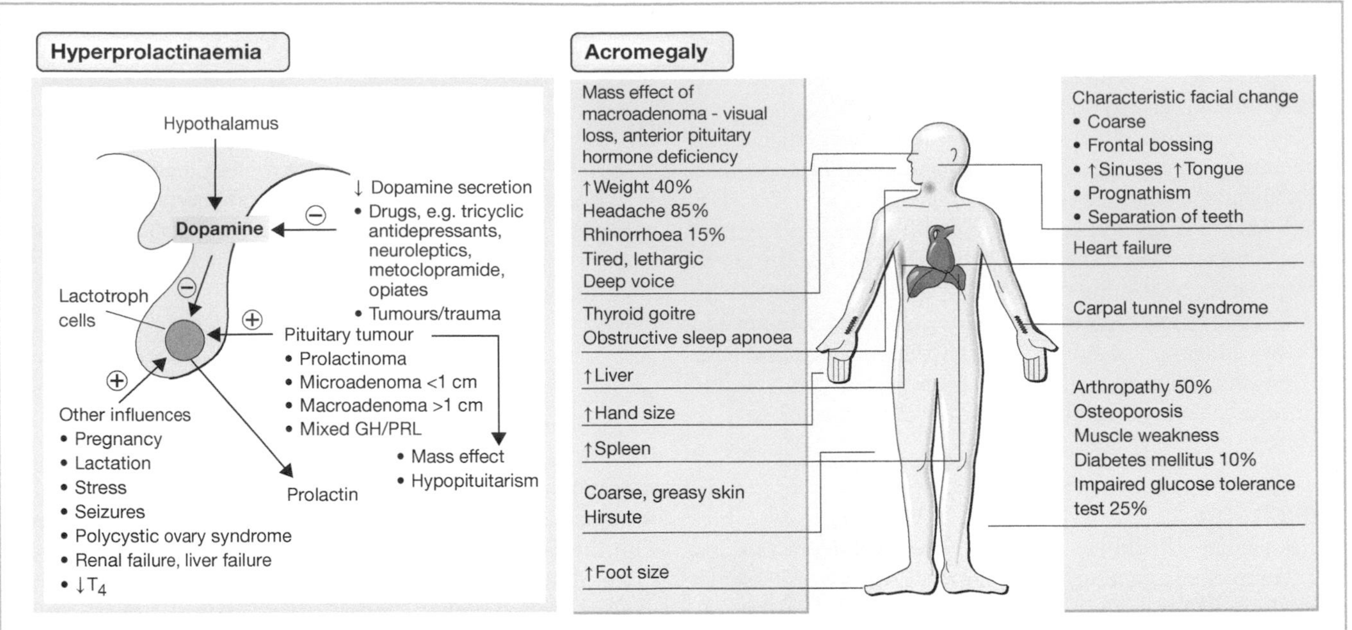

Hyperprolactinaemia

This is more obvious in women, because of presentation with menstrual disturbance or infertility.

- **Females**: milk production (galactorrhoea) in 30–80%, menstrual irregularity (oligo-/amenorrhoea), infertility.
- **Males**: galactorrhoea (<30%), erectile impotence, infertility.
- **Males and females**: ± features of a macroadenoma (mass effect, see Chapter 163).

Investigations

- Exclude drugs, stress (even of venipuncture) renal failure, liver failure, PCOS and primary hypothyroidism.
- Visual fields and MRI pituitary (microprolactinoma – moderate elevation of prolactin and normal visual fields [f>>>m], macroprolactinoma – marked elevation in prolactin and often abnormal visual fields).
- Anterior pituitary function investigations (usually normal with microprolactinoma, deficiency common with macroprolactinoma).

Management of prolactinomas

- **Drug treatment**: dopamine agonists (bromocriptine or cabergoline) inhibit prolactin (PRL) secretion and cause tumour shrinkage. Side-effects include nausea, vomiting and postural hypotension. More rarely, cabergoline is associated with cardiac valvulopathy and echo monitoring is required. In addition, patients should be warned about disinhibition syndrome, e.g. excessive spending, extreme behaviours, abnormal diet. Sex hormone replacement and bone protection if required. Pituitary hormone replacement if impaired.
- **Surgery**: trans-sphenoidal removal if there is drug intolerance or if the tumour fails to shrink on dopamine agonist therapy.
- **Radiotherapy**: to prevent tumour regrowth after drug treatment or surgery for macroadenoma.

Acromegaly

This is the clinical condition resulting from prolonged excessive growth hormone (GH) secretion in adults (prepubertal excessive GH results in gigantism). Rare: 5/10^6 population; males = females; usually diagnosed at age 40–60 years. The underlying pathology is (i) benign pituitary tumour (macroadenomas more common than microadenomas); (ii) pituitary carcinoma (very rare); and (iii) GH-releasing hormone-secreting carcinoid tumours (very rare). Occasionally familial; consider in young patients/fh. The clinical syndrome results from insulin-like growth factor (IGF)-I which mediates the effects of GH: increased sweating, headache (independent of tumour size), tiredness and lethargy; joint pains; effects of a mass in the pituitary fossa (visual field defects, hypopituitarism).

- **Examination**: characteristic facial appearance, deep voice, carpal tunnel syndrome, hand and foot enlargement and organomegaly (goitre, hepatosplenomegaly).
- **Complications**: acromegaly increases cardiovascular morbidity and mortality, from hypertension, impaired glucose tolerance and diabetes mellitus. Cardiac failure (heart muscle disease),

Medicine at a Glance, Fifth Edition. Edited by Patrick Davey and Alex Pitcher.

Companion website: www.wiley.com/go/medicine5e

ischaemic heart and cerebrovascular disease are all increased. Obstructive sleep apnoea occurs. There may be an increased risk of colonic polyps and carcinoma.

Investigations and management

- **Laboratory tests**: lack of GH suppression on oral glucose tolerance test (often undiagnosed diabetes too) and IGF-I is high.
- **Other investigations**: MRI scan of the pituitary and visual field assessment.

The aim of treatment is to normalize GH and reduce the associated high mortality.

- **Surgery**: trans-sphenoidal adenomectomy is often curative.
- **Pituitary radiotherapy (including targeted radiosurgery)**: useful if the tumour is not fully removed and reduces GH progressively over years.
- **Drugs**: long-acting somatostatin analogues (octreotide, lanreotide) suppress GH in 60%. Dopamine agonists (bromocriptine, cabergoline) lower but rarely normalize GH. GH receptor antagonist (pegvisomant) normalizes IGF-I in >90% of patients.

158 Hypothyroidism

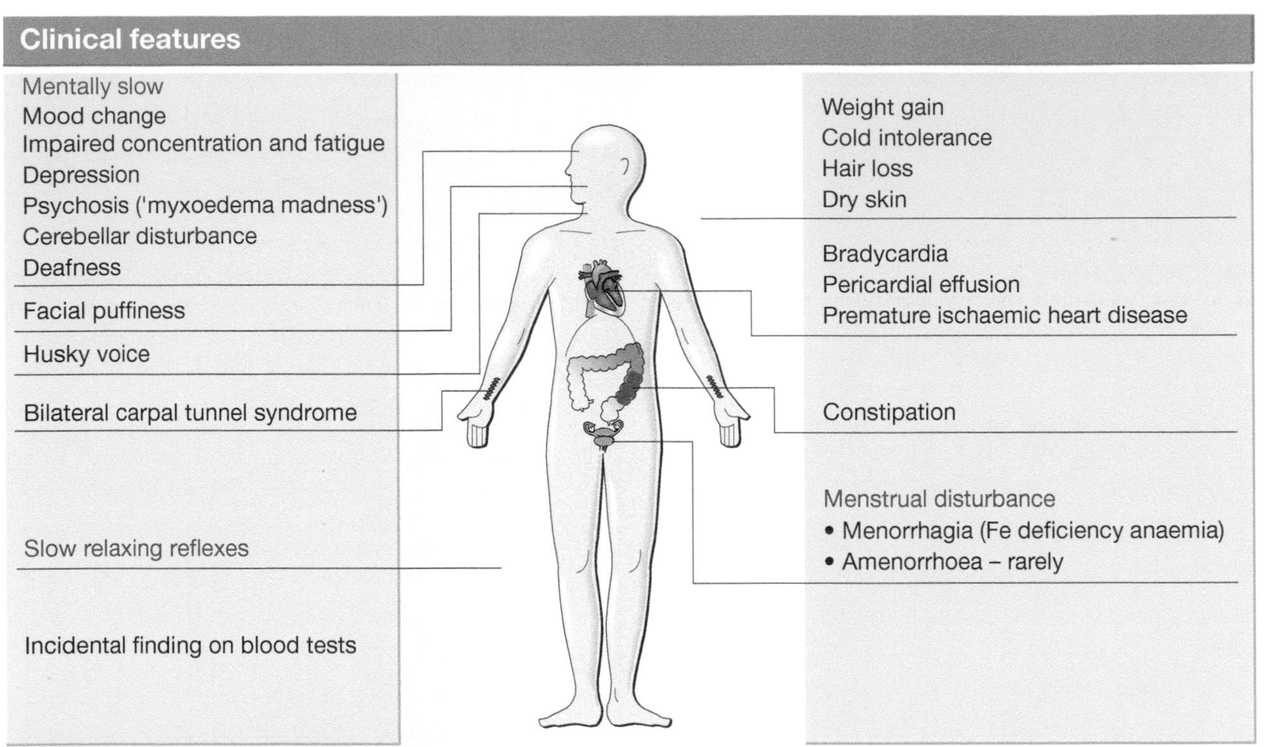

Causes of hypothyroidism

Hypothalamo–pituitary disease (rare)

Thyroid synthetic failure

- Iodine excess, e.g. amiodarone
- Congenital – 1/3-4000
- Iodine deficiency → epidemic goitrous hypothyroidism

Iatrogenic

- Drugs: amiodarone, interferon alpha, immunotherapy (pembrolizumab, nivolumab)
- Post surgery
- Post radio-iodine (50% hypothyroid at 10 years)
- Sick euthyroid syndrome (severe illness leads to abnormal and low thyroid hormones – usually no treatment indicated)

Thyroid destruction (chronic inflammation)

- Hashimoto's (autoimmune) thyroiditis: very common, familial, with other autoimmune illnesses.
- Silent and postpartum thyroiditis (transient/permanent in 30%)
- Atrophic (autoimmune) hypothyroidism: elderly people, inhibitory autoantibody to TSH receptor. No goitre. Common
- Riedel's thyroiditis: woody sclerosis of thyroid, related to other sclerosing retroperitoneal fibrosis. Very rare

Medicine at a Glance, Fifth Edition. Edited by Patrick Davey and Alex Pitcher.

Companion website: www.wiley.com/go/medicine5e

Hypothyroidism is the clinical state arising from decreased production of thyroid hormones. Primary hypothyroidism (commonly) is due to insufficient thyroid production from the thyroid gland. Secondary hypothyroidism (rare) is due to inadequate TSH (from pituitary) or TRH (from hypothalamus) production.

Epidemiology

The female:male ratio is 6:1 in primary hypothyroidism. The prevalence is 1–5% in the adult population, and the incidence 2/1000. It is most common from middle age onwards and is often associated with a family history of autoimmune disease.

Causes

Thyroid failure can be caused by disease of the thyroid (primary hypothyroidism), pituitary gland (secondary) or hypothalamus (tertiary). Primary hypothyroidism is common and in Europe/ North America is usually the result of autoimmune disease or previous radioiodine treatment for hyperthyroidism (50% hypothyroid at 10 years). Worldwide, the most common cause is iodine deficiency.

Although hypothyroidism can be congenital, the important causes in adult life are as follows.

- **Autoimmune**: there are two forms of autoimmune thyroiditis, distinguished by the presence (Hashimoto thyroiditis/lymphocytic) or absence (atrophic) of a goitre. Circulating autoantibodies are common, and there is frequently a family history of hypothyroidism, or less commonly Addison's disease, pernicious anaemia or diabetes. Occasionally Hashimoto's thyroiditis gives rise to pain during the acute phase and, rarely, to transient hyperthyroidism.
- **Post-thyrotoxicosis treatment**: radioiodine (50% at 10 years), surgery, antithyroid drugs.
- **Iodine deficiency**: endemic goitre (e.g. Derbyshire neck) is the most common worldwide cause of hypothyroidism.
- **Iodine excess**: chronic excess (e.g. amiodarone) may cause hypothyroidism.
- **Drugs**: lithium, immunotherapy (causes thyroiditis with transient hyperthyroidism followed by hypothyroidism), tyrosine kinase inhibitors and interferon.
- **Thyroiditis**: usually silent but sometimes acute and painful, common post pregnancy – subsequent hypothyroidism may be temporary.

Clinical features

See figure above.

Investigations

- **Haematology**: a full blood count may show a mild macrocytic anaemia (mean cell volume (MCV) 95–110 fl). If haemoglobin is <10 g/dl, suspect an additional cause; if MCV is >115 fl, this may be pernicious anaemia (associated autoimmune condition, see Chapter 174), and if MCV is <85 fl it may be iron deficiency anaemia (menorrhagia).
- **Thyroid function tests**: low free Thyroxine (fT_4) and elevated thyroid-stimulating hormone (TSH) – primary hypothyroidism; low or inappropriately normal TSH – secondary/tertiary hypothyroidism.
- **Cortisol**: to exclude co-existent hypoadrenalism (Addison's disease or reduced adrenocorticotrophic hormone reserve in secondary hypothyroidism).
- **Thyroid antibodies**: positive thyroid peroxidase antibodies in autoimmune primary hypothyroidism.
- **Other biochemistry**: cholesterol levels may be raised, as may be muscle enzyme levels (e.g. aspartate transaminase and creatine kinase).
- **Electrocardiogram**: bradycardia, low voltage complexes.

Management

Levothyroxine replacement therapy, often starting at 50 μg/day and increasing to 125–150 μg/day, with the dose titrated against clinical and biochemical (normal TSH) response. Lower starting doses may be used in elderly patients and patients with ischaemic heart disease because higher doses may provoke angina or myocardial infarction. *NB: Levothyroxine replacement should be delayed until cortisol is known if there is concern about co-existent Addison's/ cortisol deficiency, as this could precipitate an adrenal crisis.*

Myxoedema coma

This is a rare complication with a mortality rate >50%. It should be suspected in any patient with hypothermia and coma. It is difficult to distinguish from other causes of hypothermia, because the same risk factors (sedatives, age, etc.) are present. Cortisol deficiency due to pituitary failure or Addison's disease should be excluded, with serum cortisol and hydrocortisone (100 mg 6 hourly) commenced. It is vital to start treatment immediately (before diagnostic biochemistry is available) with intravenous or nasogastric thyroxine. Management should be in the ITU. Supportive therapy, including space blankets, antibiotics, fluids and correction of acidosis, may also be needed.

Congenital hypothyroidism

Though essentially beyond this textbook, it is nonetheless important to mention congenital hypothyroidism. The incidence varies from one per 1300 (Middle East) to one per 4000 births. Worldwide, this results most commonly from low environmental iodine levels. In the developed world, where iodine supplementation of the drinking water is common, endemic congenital hypothyroidism does not occur; sporadic congenital hypothyroidism does, however, and is commonly due to thyroid gland agenesis (50%), ectopia (25%), errors of metabolism (10%), and rarely (15%) from disorders in the hypothalamic–pituitary axis.

While *in utero*, the fetus receives thyroid hormone through the placenta from the mother, and so develops normally. However, after birth, this exogenous supply disappears – the infant is then deprived of thyroid hormone. This results in failure of the brain to develop, leading to profound developmental retardation and a syndrome previously called 'cretinism'. Treatment must be given early or permanent damage occurs. Many (though not all) of the deleterious effects of thyroid hormone deficiency can be prevented by early diagnosis and treatment (i.e. diagnosis by day 13 with normalization of thyroid hormone status by week 3). Since the clinical features can be far from obvious in infants, the best means of diagnosis is by biochemical assay. All children in the UK and developed countries are screened at birth for congenital hypothyroidism by assaying TSH levels.

159 Hyperthyroidism

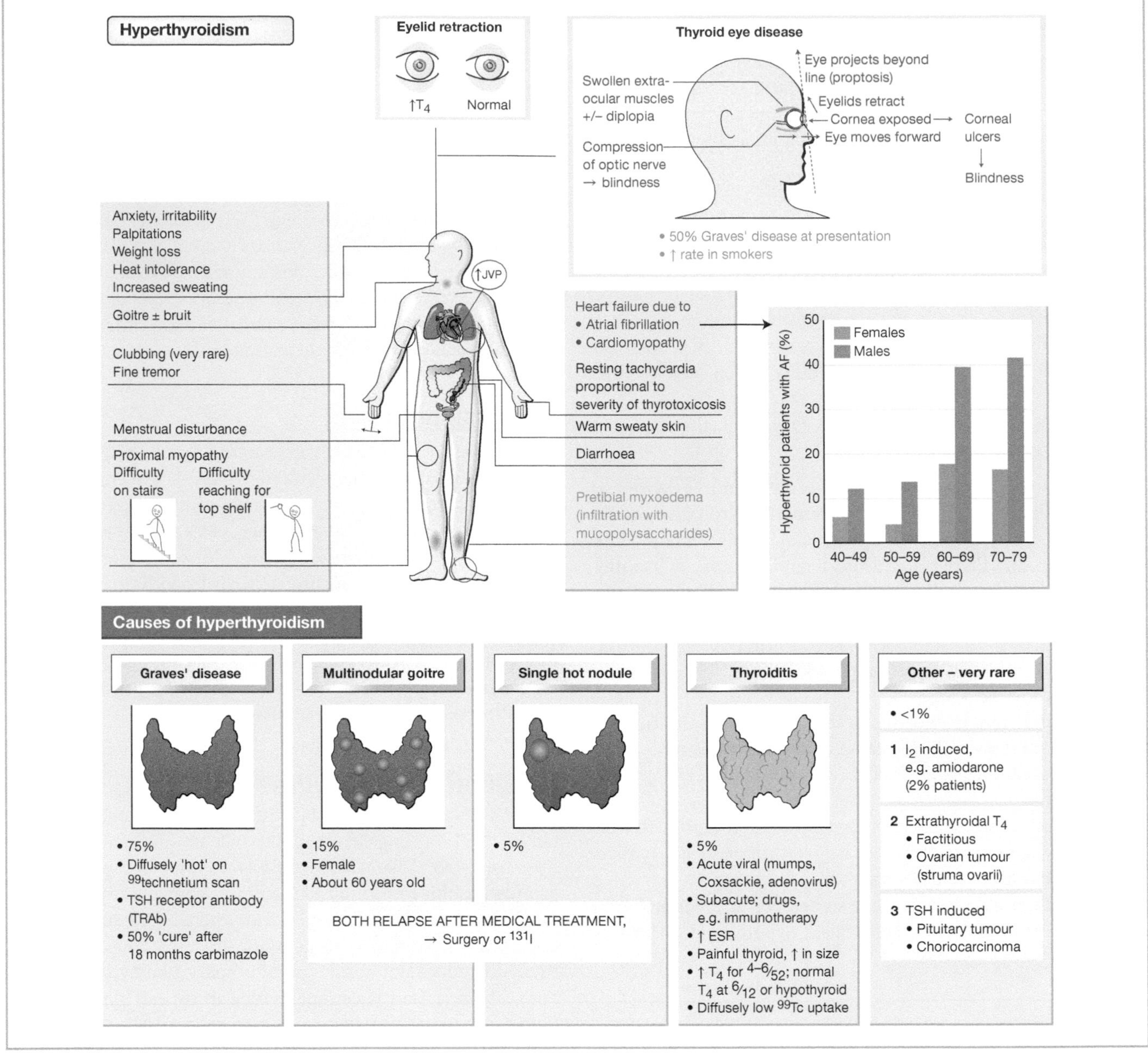

Definition and epidemiology

The clinical condition is caused by increased synthesis and secretion of thyroid hormone leading to increased circulating free levels of thyroid hormones. The prevalence is 2%. The male:female ratio is 1:5. It is most common in middle age.

Causes

The most common causes of hyperthyroidism are autoimmune thyroid disease (usually Graves' disease), a toxic nodular goitre and a toxic adenoma.

- **Graves' disease**: 75% of cases. An autoimmune disorder in a genetically susceptible person (associated with CTLA4), resulting from the interaction of antibodies to immunoglobulin IgG thyroid-stimulating hormone (TSH) receptors with the thyroid gland TSH receptor, leading to thyroid gland stimulation, increased thyroxine (T_4) secretion and thyroid growth. Associated with Graves' disease is eye disease (ophthalmopathy) and organ-specific autoimmune disease.
- **Toxic multinodular goitre**: 15% of cases. Hyperthyroidism may develop in a long-standing goitre. Relapses after antithyroid drug therapy, so definitive surgery/radiotherapy is required.

Medicine at a Glance, Fifth Edition. Edited by Patrick Davey and Alex Pitcher.

Companion website: www.wiley.com/go/medicine5e

- **Toxic adenoma** (single nodular goitre): 5% of cases. An autonomous hyperfunctioning nodule that produces excess thyroid hormones and suppresses TSH secretion.
- **Hashimoto thyroiditis**: autoimmune (thyroid peroxidase antibody related), smooth thyroid enlargement; may produce hyper- and then hypothyroidism.
- **Postpartum thyroiditis**: usually self-limiting.
- **Rare causes**: viral (de Quervain) thyroiditis, drugs such as amiodarone, immunotherapy (nivolumab and pembrolizumab, excessive T_4 replacement, iodine excess (Jod–Basedow effect), hypothalamic–pituitary disease (TSH-secreting tumour or pituitary resistance to thyroid hormones) or hyperemesis gravidarum (human chorionic gonadotrophin-mediated stimulation of the thyroid). Ingestion of contaminated food (hamburger) or surreptitious administration of thyroid hormone.

Clinical features

- Heat intolerance, increased sweating.
- Palpitations ± dyspnoea. Atrial fibrillation.
- Weight loss.
- Hyperactivity, insomnia.
- Increased stool frequency.
- Oligo-/amenorrhoea, reduced libido.

In Graves' disease, the following also occur.

- *Ophthalmopathy.*
- Gritty eyes and lid lag (50%).
- Retro-orbital pain.
- Periorbital oedema, chemosis.
- Diplopia due to extraocular muscle dysfunction (severe 5%).
- Poor vision due to optic neuropathy.
- *Pretibial myxoedema* (rare, <0.5%) and raised indurated lesions on shins, occasionally elsewhere.
- *Thyroid acropachy* (very rare), appearance of finger clubbing.

Investigations

- **Thyroid function tests**: increased free T_4 and tri-iodothyronine (T_3), suppressed TSH (primary hyperthyroidism). Increased T4, with unsuppressed/elevated TSH (secondary).
- **Thyroid autoantibodies**: thyroid stimulating hormone receptor antibodies raised in Graves' disease, thyroid peroxidase and antithyroglobulin antibodies suggest an autoimmune aetiology.
- **Imaging**: thyroid uptake scan differentiates Graves' disease (diffusely increased uptake) from toxic adenoma (single hot spot), multinodular goitre (multiple hot spots) and thyroiditis (minimal tracer uptake).

Management

- **Drug treatment**: first-line therapy in all patients regardless of diagnosis. Carbimazole decreases thyroid hormone synthesis; initial dose 20–60 mg/day, later reduced to a maintenance dose. The dose is titrated according to thyroid function and continued for 18 months, after which up to 50% patients with Graves' disease remain cured on discontinuation of treatment. An alternative approach is to give a large dose of carbimazole with additional replacement T_4 to avoid hypothyroidism ('block and replace' technique). Carbimazole causes agranulocytosis in 0.1%; it should be immediately stopped if sore throat or fever occurs. Propylthiouracil is an alternative antithyroid drug that is often preferred in the first trimester of pregnancy. It is associated with ANCA vasculitis and acute liver failure (1 in 10 000). It is essential to give written warning to all patients on antithyroid drugs regarding the risk of agranulocytosis, very rare risk of severe pancreatitis, advice to avoid pregnancy.
- **Surgery**: thyroidectomy for multinodular goitre, toxic adenoma or relapses of Graves' disease after antithyroid drug therapy. The risks are small but include vocal cord palsy (recurrent laryngeal nerve damage), hypothyroidism and hypoparathyroidism (temporary or permanent).
- **Radioiodine** is concentrated in the thyroid gland, so destroying thyroid tissue. Antithyroid drugs are stopped 7–10 days before administration to allow uptake of radioiodine. Occasionally repeated doses are required. Side-effects: worsening of thyroid eye disease (may be the result of the aggravating effect of hypothyroidism), transient/permanent hypothyroidism (50% at 10 years), thyrotoxic crisis (if hyperthyroidism is poorly controlled before administration), pain. Radiation protection issues: no pregnancy for six months, avoid close contact with people in first few days.

Treatment of thyroid-associated ophthalmopathy

- **Supportive**: elevation of head of bed, artificial tears and prismatic glasses for diplopia, selenium supplementation and discontinuation of smoking.
- **Definitive**: medical with high-dose steroids ± other immunosuppressants, e.g. rituximab (to decompress orbit), surgical orbital decompression or orbital radiotherapy.

Thyroid storm

This is a rare life-threatening emergency (mortality rate of 10% or more). Fever, anxiety, agitation, confusion and tachycardia, and occasionally heart failure, can also occur.

- Affects <2% of patients with hyperthyroidism.
- Treatment *must* be started before biochemical diagnosis (which takes too long).
- Mortality 10–20%.
- 50% of patients have lost >15 kg.
- Storm often provoked by minor physical stress.
- Severe symptoms of hyperthyroidism in most, though not always in the elderly (apathetic hyperthyroidism).
- Examination shows tachycardia, often very marked, sweating and sometimes confusion.
- Intensive care unit admission may be required, and should be anticipated.
- β-blockers, often in high dose, are the mainstay of therapy.
- Give carbimazole or propylthiouracil immediately, by nasogastric tube if necessary.
- One hour later give iodide.
- Intravenous glucocorticoids may be given in large doses to inhibit the synthesis of new circulating thyroid hormone.
- Fluid and electrolyte replacement as appropriate.

160 Calcium metabolism

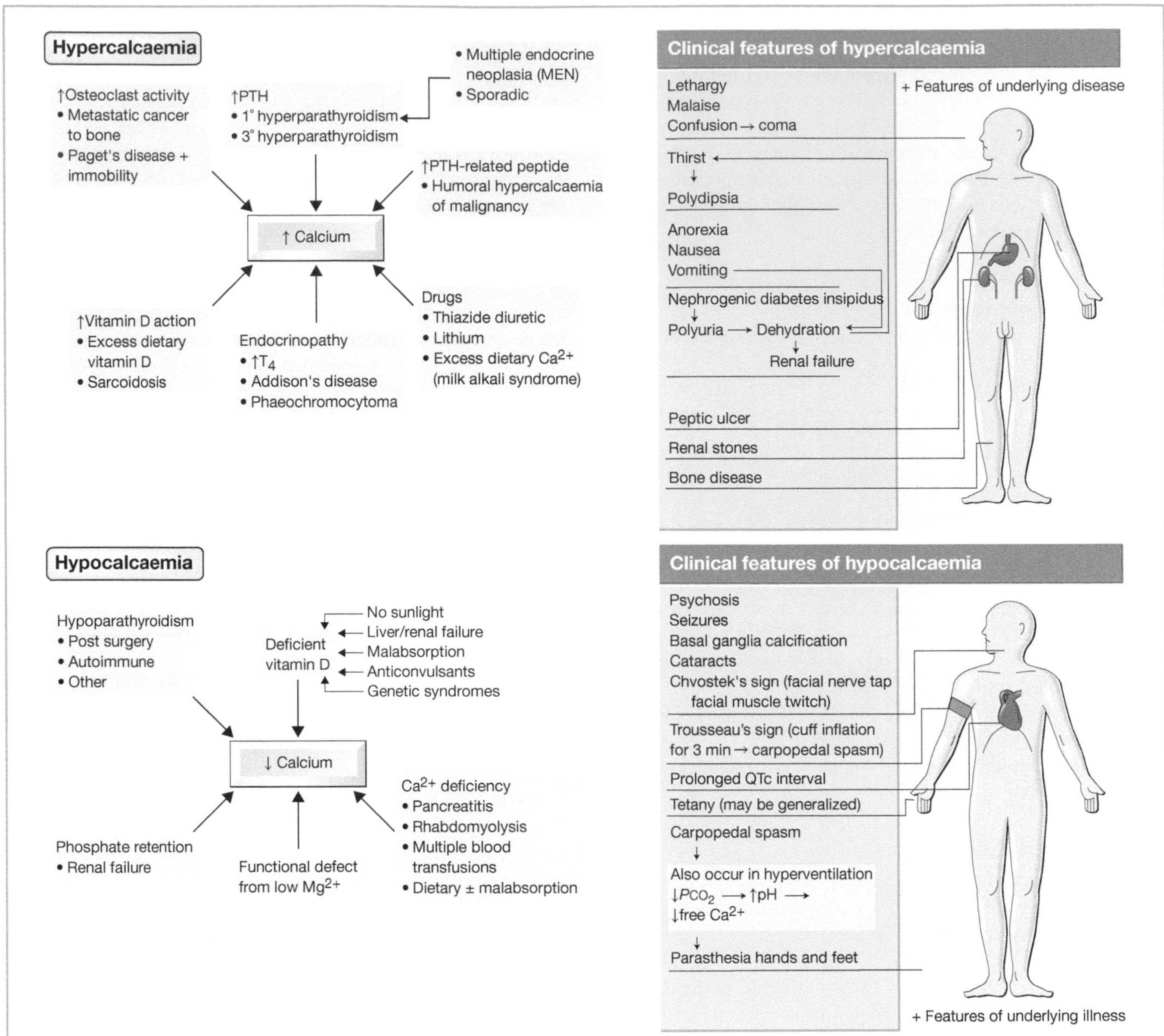

Acute hypercalcaemia

The more rapid the rise and the higher the calcium level, the more likely are patients to present with an acute brain syndrome, comprising confusion, drowsiness and coma (rarely muscle weakness or psychosis). In less marked hypercalcaemia, there can be thirst and polyuria, from calcium-induced nephrogenic diabetes insipidus and abdominal symptoms such as anorexia, nausea and vomiting, abdominal pain and constipation. Chronic hypercalcaemia also produces renal stones and bone disease.

Aetiology

Hypercalcaemia occurs in 5–50 per 10 000.

- Is malignancy present or likely clinically or on routine investigations?
- Is the parathyroid hormone (PTH) level high or suppressed?

Investigations

- Dietary and drug history (vitamin D excess, thiazides, lithium)
- U and E (?renal failure)

Medicine at a Glance, Fifth Edition. Edited by Patrick Davey and Alex Pitcher.

Companion website: www.wiley.com/go/medicine5e

- PTH (elevated in primary hyperparathyroidism, suppressed in malignancy, drug associated, or sarcoidosis)
- TFTs (?primary hyperthyroidism)
- Angiotensin converting enzyme levels (?sarcoid)
- Alkaline phosphatase (malignancy or Paget disease)
- Immunoglobulin electrophoresis (myeloma)
- Chest X-ray (malignancy/bilateral hilar lymphadenopathy [sarcoid])
- PTHrP (parathyroid-related peptide in malignancy)

Causes

Primary hyperparathyroidism

This is the most common cause of hypercalcaemia; the female:male ratio is 2:1 and 90% of patients are >50 years (female incidence is 3/1000). Symptoms of hypercalcaemia may occur, although 50% are asymptomatic patients undergoing biochemical assessment for other reasons. In 80%, the pathology is a single parathyroid adenoma; occasionally diffuse hyperplasia of all four glands occurs. Very rarely, multiple endocrine neoplasia (MEN) 1, 2 or 4 is present (see Chapter 162). In asymptomatic patients with mild hypercalcaemia, an expectant course may be followed. In others, definitive treatment is surgical resection, following imaging studies (sestamibi nuclear and ultrasound scan) to localize the adenoma. Postoperative hypocalcaemia is usually transient and treated with calcium supplements and 1α-hydroxy vitamin D. Cinacalcet (increases sensitivity of calcium-sensing receptor to reduce PTH secretion) is reserved for patients who are unsuitable for surgery/unsuccessful surgery.

Hypercalcaemia of malignancy

- **Tumour deposits in bone**: most (>95%) hypercalcaemia in malignancy relates to widespread metastatic disease. The most common neoplasms are lung, breast and myeloma. Patients are usually highly symptomatic both from the cancer and, as calcium levels are high and have risen quickly, from hypercalcaemia.
- **Humoral hypercalcaemia of malignancy** relates to PTH-related peptide, a 144 amino acid peptide which is structurally related to PTH and mimics its action. The responsible neoplasm is most likely to be squamous carcinoma of the lung, although it can be a genitourinary or gynaecological malignancy. Although humoral hypercalcaemia of malignancy is rare, its clinical importance is that *not all patients with malignancy and hypercalcaemia necessarily have metastatic disease*. This point is vital in deciding whether or not the primary should be resected.

Sarcoidosis and other granulomatous diseases

These are associated with hypercalcaemia, which responds readily to steroids.

Other causes of hypercalcaemia

Thyrotoxicosis and thiazide diuretics can induce hypercalcaemia. Familial hypocalciuric hypercalcaemia is an autosomal dominant inherited condition in which hypercalcaemia is associated with low renal excretion of calcium. Paget disease can also induce hypercalcaemia.

Management

Acute/symptomatic hypercalcaemia is a medical emergency and requires urgent treatment, principally aggressive rehydration with 0.9% **saline**, which alone readily lowers calcium. **Intravenous bisphosphonates** are effective regardless of the underlying pathology. **Steroids** may be added in hypercalcaemia of malignancy and vitamin D-related hypercalcaemia. **Calcitonin** helps in Paget disease. Definitive therapy varies according to the underlying disease.

Hypocalcaemia

Acute hypocalcaemia results in neuromuscular excitability, circumoral tingling, tetany, especially in the muscles supplied by long nerves, and seizures. Chvostek's sign (a tap to the facial nerve just anterior to the ear causes a brief facial muscle contraction) and Trousseau's sign (inflation of a blood pressure cuff resulting in carpopedal spasm) occur. Chronic hypocalcaemia in addition results in neuropsychiatric symptoms, basal ganglia calcification and cataracts.

Aetiology

Hypocalcaemia is rare, and usually relates to one of four diseases.

- **Secondary hyperparathyroidism**: the most common cause of hypocalcaemia, occurring in acute or chronic renal failure. Failure of renal vitamin D hydroxylation, together with phosphate retention (through the calcium phosphate double product), depresses serum Ca^{2+}, stimulating PTH release in an attempt to normalize serum Ca^{2+}. This leads to osteoclast activation, cyst formation and bone marrow fibrosis (osteitis fibrosa cystica), which together with aluminium toxicity contribute to renal bone disease. Characteristic X-ray findings are found in the hand, skull ('pepper pot') and spine ('rugger jersey'). The diagnosis is usually obvious from creatinine and phosphate levels and the characteristic radiology. Treatment is with vitamin D and phosphate binders. If secondary hyperparathyroidism is left untreated, parathyroid gland hyperplasia leads to autonomous production of PTH, resulting in tertiary hyperparathyroidism with frank hypercalcaemia.
- **Post-thyroid/parathyroid surgery**: transient or less commonly permanent hypocalcaemia may occur.
- **Idiopathic autoimmune parathyroid failure**: very rare. Rare genetic and also idiopathic. Parathyroid autoantibodies may be found. Genetic screening is available. Other autoimmune conditions (vitiligo, etc.) may occur.
- **Osteomalacia**: resulting from inadequate active vitamin D. It is associated with low calcium levels, although these are usually not so low as to cause symptoms. Osteomalacia may be compounded by dietary calcium deficiency or relate to malabsorption.

Treatment

- **Acute symptoms** (Ca^{2+} <1.9 mmol/l): intravenous (IV) bolus of 10% calcium gluconate 10–20 ml with electrocardiogram monitoring followed by IV infusion if necessary. Oral calcium and vitamin D as soon as possible. IV magnesium sulphate may be required.
- **Chronic disease**: vitamin D metabolites (calcitriol or α-calcidol) and oral calcium.

161 Adrenal disease

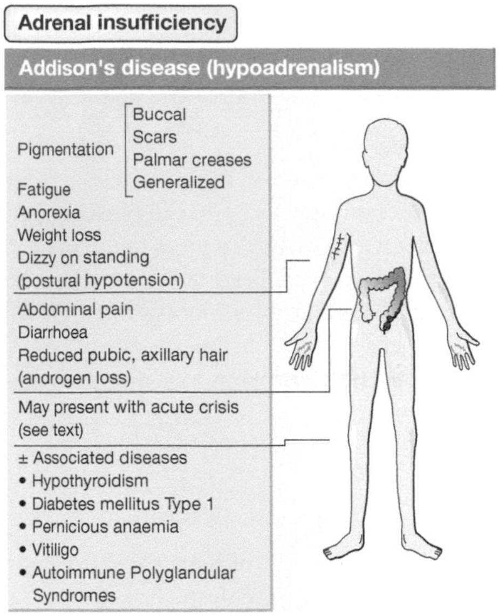

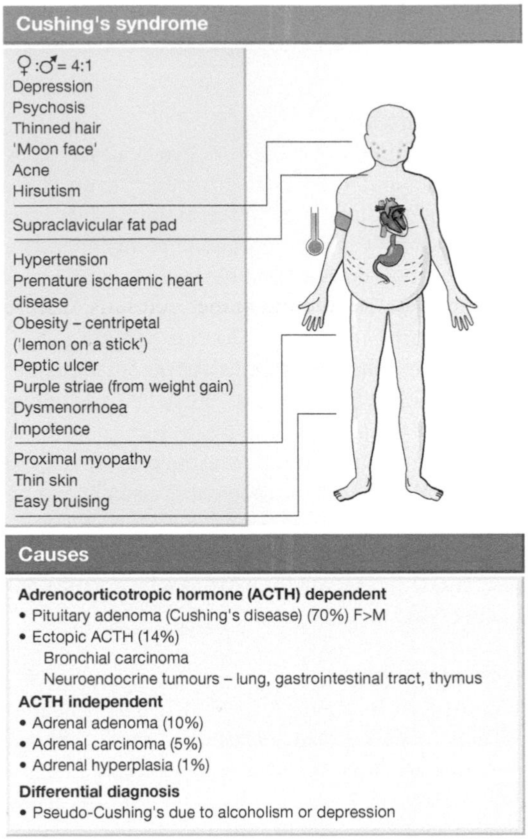

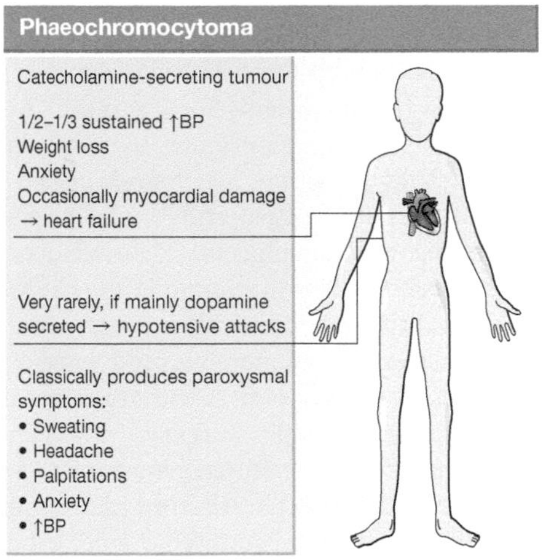

Adrenal failure

- **Primary adrenal failure** (= destruction of adrenal glands, leading to reduced glucocorticoids, mineralocorticoids, androgens, increased ACTH): rare, occurring in 50/1 000 000 population. Autoimmune (Addison's disease) adrenal destruction, associated with vitiligo, premature ovarian failure and hypothyroidism. Females > males; gradual onset of symptoms; worldwide; tuberculosis destruction of the adrenal glands is more common. Other causes are very rare.
  - Malignancy – usually metastases (lymphoma, breast, lung).
  - Infection (TB, HIV, fungi).
  - Haemorrhage: anticoagulants, Waterhouse–Friderichsen syndrome from meningococcal septicaemia-induced disseminated intravascular coagulation – adrenal failure occurs days/weeks after the initial haemorrhage-induced cortisol release.
  - Infiltration (amyloid, sarcoid, haemochromatosis).
  - Congenital adrenal hyperplasia.
  - Adrenalectomy or drugs, e.g. ketoconazole, immunotherapy (nivolumab, pembrolizumab).
- **Secondary adrenal failure** (= loss of ACTH leading to adrenal atrophy, loss of glucocorticoids). Common; chronic steroid therapy (oral, topical, inhaled, nasal) suppresses ACTH levels, producing adrenal cortex atrophy. Physical stress or over-quick steroid withdrawal can then provoke acute adrenal failure.

Clinical features of Addison disease

- Chronic adrenal failure often presents with vague symptoms, including fatigue, pigmentation, weight loss, anorexia, abdominal pain, diarrhoea and postural hypotension (due to mineralocorticoid deficiency). Androgen deficiency leads to loss of pubic hair and libido.

Medicine at a Glance, Fifth Edition. Edited by Patrick Davey and Alex Pitcher.

Companion website: www.wiley.com/go/medicine5e

- Acute adrenal failure presents with hypovolaemic shock precipitated by intercurrent stress. Untreated, this leads to refractory shock, profound hypoglycaemia and death.

Investigations

U and E (↑potassium, ↓sodium). Glucose↓. FBC: ↓ HB, ↑eosinophils. Random cortisol (do not wait for result before treating empirically if acutely unwell). ACTH ↑ (primary) ↔/↓(secondary). Acute adrenal failure should always be suspected when the patient is in shock with hyponatraemia (± hyperkalaemia and hypoglycaemia). Hyponatraemia occurs late in the disease, but only in primary adrenal failure (mineralocorticoid deficiency) as usually in secondary adrenal failure the renin–angiotensin system remains intact. Cortisol is low or inappropriately normal; ACTH is high in primary failure and low in secondary failure.

- **Short synacthen test**: adrenal stimulation using synthetic ACTH fails to produce cortisol. (NB: may be misleading and normal if recent onset of secondary adrenal failure.)
- **Adrenal autoantibodies** (autoimmune Addison's disease – may disappear in time).
- **CT adrenal** (?metastases, infiltration, haemorrhage).

Management

- **Chronic adrenal failure**: glucocorticoid replacement with hydrocortisone 20 mg/day in divided doses, doubled with treatment of infection or intercurrent illness, or surgery. Mineralocorticoid replacement (fludrocortisone) only in primary adrenal failure.
- **Acute adrenal failure**: a medical emergency. Large volumes of intravenous fluid (physiological saline) and hydrocortisone are given at high doses. The precipitant (infection, etc.) may also need treating. Monitor electrolytes and glucose.
- Education is essential so patients recognize adrenal crises, mentioning compliance, steroid card and MedicAlert, and advice if vomiting or undergoing a procedure or major surgery; see endocrinology.org/media/3873/steroid-card.pdf.

Hyperaldosteronism

This causes treatment-resistant hypertension (up to 10% of hypertension) with hypokalaemia. Occasionally K^+ is normal if salt intake is low. The causes are:

- benign adenoma (Conn syndrome) (66%)
- bilateral adrenal hyperplasia (30%)
- rarely, glucocorticoid remedial aldosteronism or adrenal carcinoma.

Investigations

U and E (hyperkalaemia), urinary potassium secretion (increased), renin and aldosterone (suppressed renin, elevated aldosterone, elevated renin/aldosterone ratio); note, affected by drugs, e.g. ACEI and β-blockers. CT adrenals (for adenoma/bilateral hyperplasia). Saline suppression test (lack of suppression of aldosterone). Adrenal vein sampling.

Treatment

Laparoscopic adrenalectomy (adenoma). Aldosterone antagonists (spironolactone or eplerenone) for hyperplasia.

Phaeochromocytoma

This is a catecholamine-producing tumour of the adrenal medulla. It accounts for <0.5% of hypertension and has an equal sex incidence. It is most common at age 30–50 years. A genetic cause is increasingly recognized (>30% of cases, e.g. RET mutations in MEN2 with coincident medullary carcinoma, von Hippel–Lindau, with coincident angiomas, or SDHB mutations and their potential for recurrent and malignant tumours, as well as many newer genetic syndromes which can be screened for). Characteristically, it produces paroxysmal symptoms: labile hypertension (crises precipitated by exercise, abdominal examination, surgery, general anaesthesia, β-blockade), palpitations, sweating, headache, pallor or flushing, anxiety and glucose intolerance.

Investigations, management and prognosis

Plasma or urinary metanephrines are elevated. Adrenal imaging with magnetic resonance imaging (MRI) shows a bright hyperintense lesion. MIBG or PET scan can be helpful.

- **Initial management**: at diagnosis α-adrenoreceptor blockade (phenoxybenzamine) before β-blockade (propranolol).
- **Definitive management**: laparoscopic adrenalectomy for tumour removal. Preoperative α- and β-blockade are vital because tumour handling may precipitate a crisis. Surgery is curative in >90% in benign disease; recurrence occurs in <10%. The five-year survival rate is ≥95% for treated benign tumours but <50% for malignant tumours.

Cushing's syndrome

This is the clinical condition resulting from prolonged exposure to excessive glucocorticoids from:

- exogenous glucocorticoid administration
- endogenous hypersecretion of glucocorticoids: very rare ($1–4/10^6$).

Investigations

- **Confirm Cushing's syndrome**: diagnosed when there is lack of cortisol suppression on overnight dexamethasone testing, and elevated 24h urine free cortisol secretion.
- **Determine the cause**: ACTH levels are normal/increased in ACTH-dependent cases or low in ACTH-independent cases. Serum K^+ <3.2 mmol/l suggests ectopic ACTH secretion. In pituitary-dependent cases (termed Cushing's disease), CRH testing is helpful and high dose dexamethasone suppression test is occasionally useful.
- **Venous sampling**: inferior petrosal sinus sampling to confirm pituitary-dependent disease. Body sampling to locate ectopic source of ACTH.
- **Imaging**: Cushing's disease is usually the result of a microadenoma, which may not be visible on MRI. CT of chest or elsewhere used to locate ectopic sources of ACTH.

Management and prognosis

- **Drug treatment**: metyrapone (blocks cortisol synthesis) or ketoconazole (inhibits cytochrome P450 enzyme; NB: careful monitoring of liver biochemistry is essential) lower cortisol levels short term before surgery or long term when surgery is inappropriate.
- **Pituitary adenoma**: trans-sphenoidal adenomectomy produces remission in >70% cases; radiotherapy is used for uncured relapse. Bilateral adrenalectomy may be required if the patient remains uncured but may rarely lead to aggressive pituitary tumour enlargement and hyperpigmentation as a result of excessive ACTH secretion (Nelson syndrome) unless pituitary radiotherapy is also given.
- **Adrenal adenoma**: adrenalectomy is curative.
- **Adrenal carcinoma**: surgery is usually not curative. Drug treatment with mitotane, an adrenolytic agent, can be helpful.
- **Ectopic secretion**: surgical removal of tumour if possible, otherwise medical treatment or adrenalectomy.

Untreated, Cushing syndrome has a survival of <5 years as a result of cardiovascular disease or infection. Long-term management includes monitoring for increased cardiovascular risk and psychological complications as well as osteoporosis and increased risk of fracture.

Miscellaneous endocrine disorders

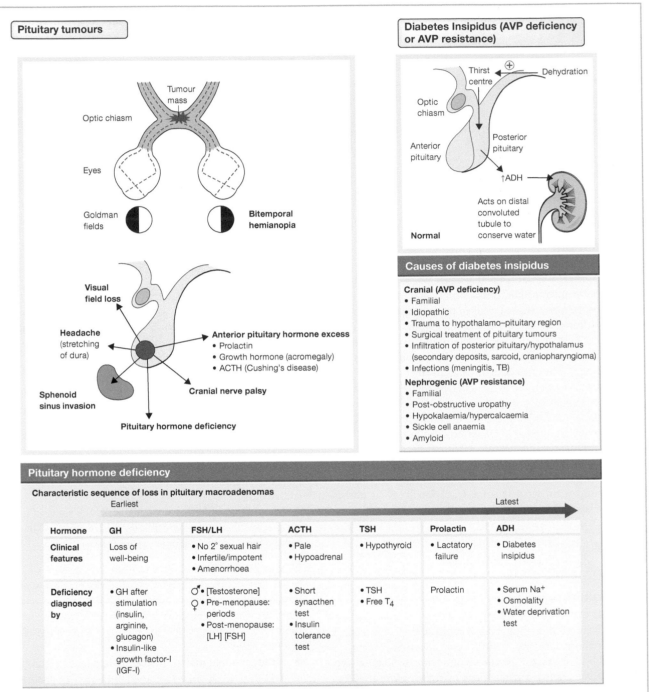

Pituitary tumours

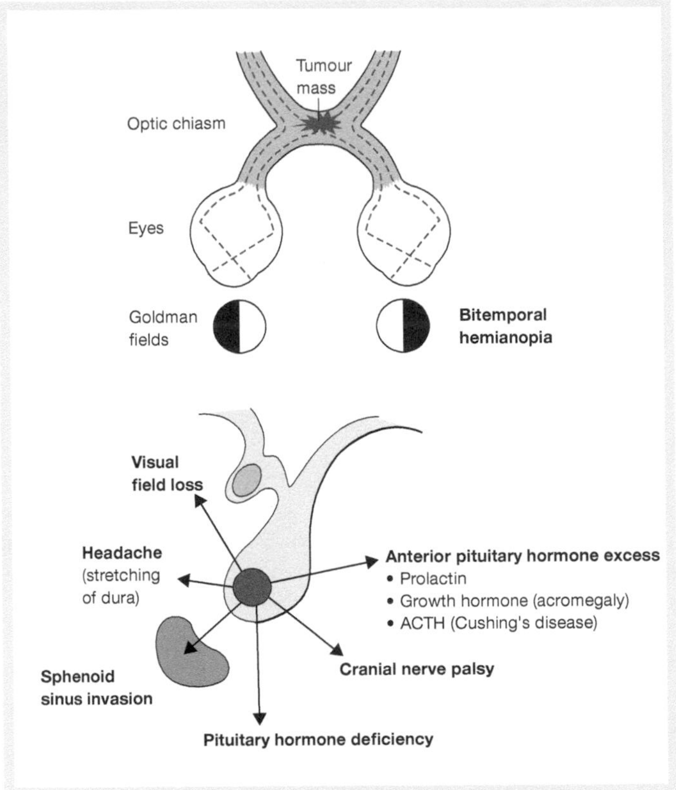

Tumour mass
Optic chiasm
Eyes
Goldman fields
Bitemporal hemianopia

Visual field loss
Headache (stretching of dura)
Anterior pituitary hormone excess
• Prolactin
• Growth hormone (acromegaly)
• ACTH (Cushing's disease)
Sphenoid sinus invasion
Cranial nerve palsy
Pituitary hormone deficiency

Diabetes Insipidus (AVP deficiency or AVP resistance)

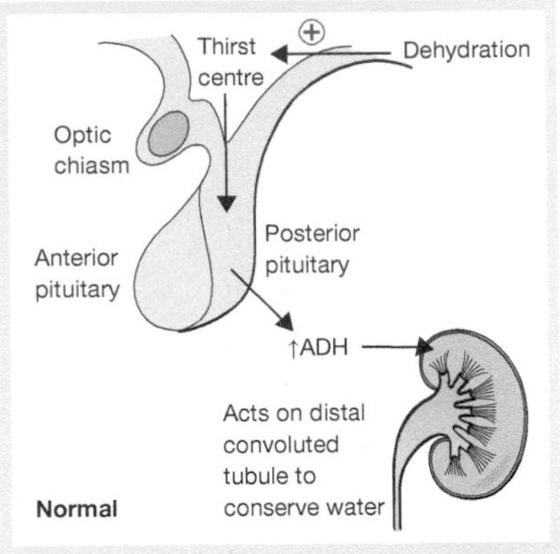

Thirst centre
Dehydration
Optic chiasm
Anterior pituitary
Posterior pituitary
↑ADH
Acts on distal convoluted tubule to conserve water
Normal

Causes of diabetes insipidus

Cranial (AVP deficiency)
- Familial
- Idiopathic
- Trauma to hypothalamo–pituitary region
- Surgical treatment of pituitary tumours
- Infiltration of posterior pituitary/hypothalamus (secondary deposits, sarcoid, craniopharyngioma)
- Infections (meningitis, TB)

Nephrogenic (AVP resistance)
- Familial
- Post-obstructive uropathy
- Hypokalaemia/hypercalcaemia
- Sickle cell anaemia
- Amyloid

Pituitary hormone deficiency

Characteristic sequence of loss in pituitary macroadenomas

Earliest → Latest

Hormone	GH	FSH/LH	ACTH	TSH	Prolactin	ADH
Clinical features	Loss of well-being	• No 2° sexual hair • Infertile/impotent • Amenorrhoea	• Pale • Hypoadrenal	• Hypothyroid	• Lactatory failure	• Diabetes insipidus
Deficiency diagnosed by	• GH after stimulation (insulin, arginine, glucagon) • Insulin-like growth factor-I (IGF-I)	♂ • [Testosterone] ♀ • Pre-menopause: periods • Post-menopause: [LH] [FSH]	• Short synacthen test • Insulin tolerance test	• TSH • Free T_4	Prolactin	• Serum Na^+ • Osmolality • Water deprivation test

Diseases of the pituitary gland

Pituitary gland diseases are rare, and may be characterized by selective or total (panhypopituitary) pituitary failure, visual failure, selective excess in pituitary-dependent hormones (tumours) and hyperprolactinaemia (from mass lesions). Causes of pituitary gland disease include the following.

- Benign pituitary adenoma: may result in pituitary failure, mass effects if macroadenoma (headaches, visual failure, hyperprolactinaemia due to stalk compression), and a selective increase in a pituitary-dependent hormone.
- Craniopharyngioma (associated with mass effect).
- Inflammation (tuberculosis, sarcoidosis or autoimmune hypophysitis) and invasion by extrinsic tumours result in pituitary failure and, occasionally, in hyperprolactinaemia, by disruption of the tonic dopamine-mediated inhibition to prolactin release.
- Drug induced, e.g. checkpoint inhibitor drugs (ipilimumab, nivolumab, pembrolizumab).
- Pituitary apoplexy: haemorrhage/infarction.
- Head injury.

Table 162.1 Pathophysiology of insipidus (AVP deficiency or AVP resistance depending on aetiology).

	[Na⁺]	Osmolality of plasma	Urine	Urine osmolality on water deprivation	Response to synthetic ADH	Treatment
AVP deficiency						
Cranial DI	↑	↑	↓	Fails to concentrate	Normal	Desmopressin
AVP resistance						
Nephrogenic DI	↑	↑	↓	Fails to concentrate	Fails to concentrate	Of underlying cause/high-dose desmopressin/thiazides
Primary polydipsia	↓	↓	↓	Concentrates	Normal	Reduce fluid intake

ADH, antidiuretic hormone.

- Pituitary atrophy: infarction related to hypotension, often postpartum (Sheehan syndrome). Pituitary failure occurs early or up to two years after the hypotensive event.

Pituitary tumours

Pituitary tumours are the most common pituitary disorder and account for 10% of intracranial neoplasms. Tumours are classified according to size.

- **Microadenoma**: <1 cm in diameter; do not cause mass effects or hypopituitarism.
- **Macroadenoma**: >1 cm; can produce mass effects and hypopituitarism. Non-functioning pituitary adenomas are the most common but macroadenomas secreting prolactin (PRL), growth hormone (GH) and rarely adrenocorticotrophic hormone (ACTH) are not uncommon. Usually non-functioning, but can cause excessive hormonal secretion, e.g. macroprolactinoma.

The clinical features of pituitary tumours are predictable, based on which hormones have been lost or gained.

Investigations aim to determine the following.

- Pituitary function and/or excess secretion from adenomas: pituitary hormones (and their target endocrine gland hormone) are measured: GH during OGTT, insulin-like growth factor I (IGF-I); follicle-stimulating hormone (FSH) and luteinizing hormone (LH) (testosterone/oestradiol); ACTH (cortisol ± dynamic stimulation [synacthen, insulin tolerance] or suppression [dexamethasone] tests); thyroid-stimulating hormone (TSH) (thyroxine [T_4]) and PRL. Antidiuretic hormone (ADH) is assessed from osmolality, copeptin, serum Na^+ and fluid deprivation tests.
- Underlying disease process: assessed by magnetic resonance imaging ± biopsy (rarely).
- Visual field loss (bitemporal hemianopia from compression of the optic chiasma), headache (dural stretching), cranial nerve palsies (lateral extension) or cerebrospinal fluid rhinorrhoea/secondary meningitis (downward erosion into sphenoid sinus).

Management

- **Replacement of anterior pituitary hormones**: hydrocortisone and T_4 to replace ACTH and TSH deficiency; sex hormone and GH therapy.
- **Treatment of underlying cause**: non-functioning tumours are treated surgically (trans-sphenoidally) and may need postoperative radiotherapy. Functioning tumours are treated by a combination of drugs, surgery and radiotherapy, either cranial or targeted.
- **Functioning tumours**: prolactin (hyperprolactinaemia, see Chapter 157), GH (acromegaly, see Chapter 157) and ACTH (Cushing disease, see Chapter 161).

Arginine Vasopressin Deficiency (AVP-D) or Arginine Vasopressin Resistance (AVP-R)

This is the passage of large volumes of inappropriately dilute urine in the presence of concentrated plasma. It is uncommon, and has to be differentiated from other causes of polyuria (urine volume >2.5 l/day) and polydipsia, which include the following.

- Diabetes mellitus.
- Renal failure.
- Primary polydipsia, usually psychogenic in origin.
- Diabetes insipidus: cranial (AVP-D) (relative/absolute vasopressin ADH deficiency) or AVP-R (renal resistance to vasopressin, e.g. as a result of lithium toxicity) diabetes insipidus. Pathophysiology and causes are shown in the figure above and investigations and management are shown in Table 162.1.

Treatment

In AVP-D unrestricted access to fluid is essential, and desmopressin (a long-acting ADH analogue) is given.

Syndrome of inappropriate ADH secretion

The syndrome of inappropriate ADH secretion (SIADH) is a common cause of hyponatraemia. For a full discussion see Chapter 141.

Multiple endocrine neoplasia

Multiple endocrine neoplasia (MEN) syndromes are very rare conditions in which a single gene defect causes multiple endocrine tumours within a patient. MEN syndromes most commonly present with disorders of calcium metabolism (see Chapter 160). Probands and their families need to be regularly screened for new malignancies.

- **MEN 1 (autosomal dominant germline mutation in MEN 1 gene 11q13 encoding the tumour suppressor gene menin)**: parathyroid hyperplasia 90%, pituitary adenoma 30–40%, pancreatic islet tumour 30–70%, neuroendocrine tumours 15%, adrenal adenomas. Clinical condition arises from germline inherited mutation and subsequent inactivating somatic mutation.
- **MEN 2 (mutation in RET oncogene 10q11.2 encoding a signalling membrane receptor)**: medullary thyroid cancer 95%, parathyroid tumours/hyperplasia (30%), phaeochromocytoma 70% bilateral.
- **MEN 2b (or 3)**: also has marfanoid habitus and mucosal neuromas. Dominant oncogene on chromosome 10 (ret proto-oncogene).
- **MEN 4 CDK inhibitor gene mutation encoding p27**: very rare. Primary hyperparathyroidism, pituitary adenomas, testicular tumours, neuroendocrine tumours.

163 Hypogonadism

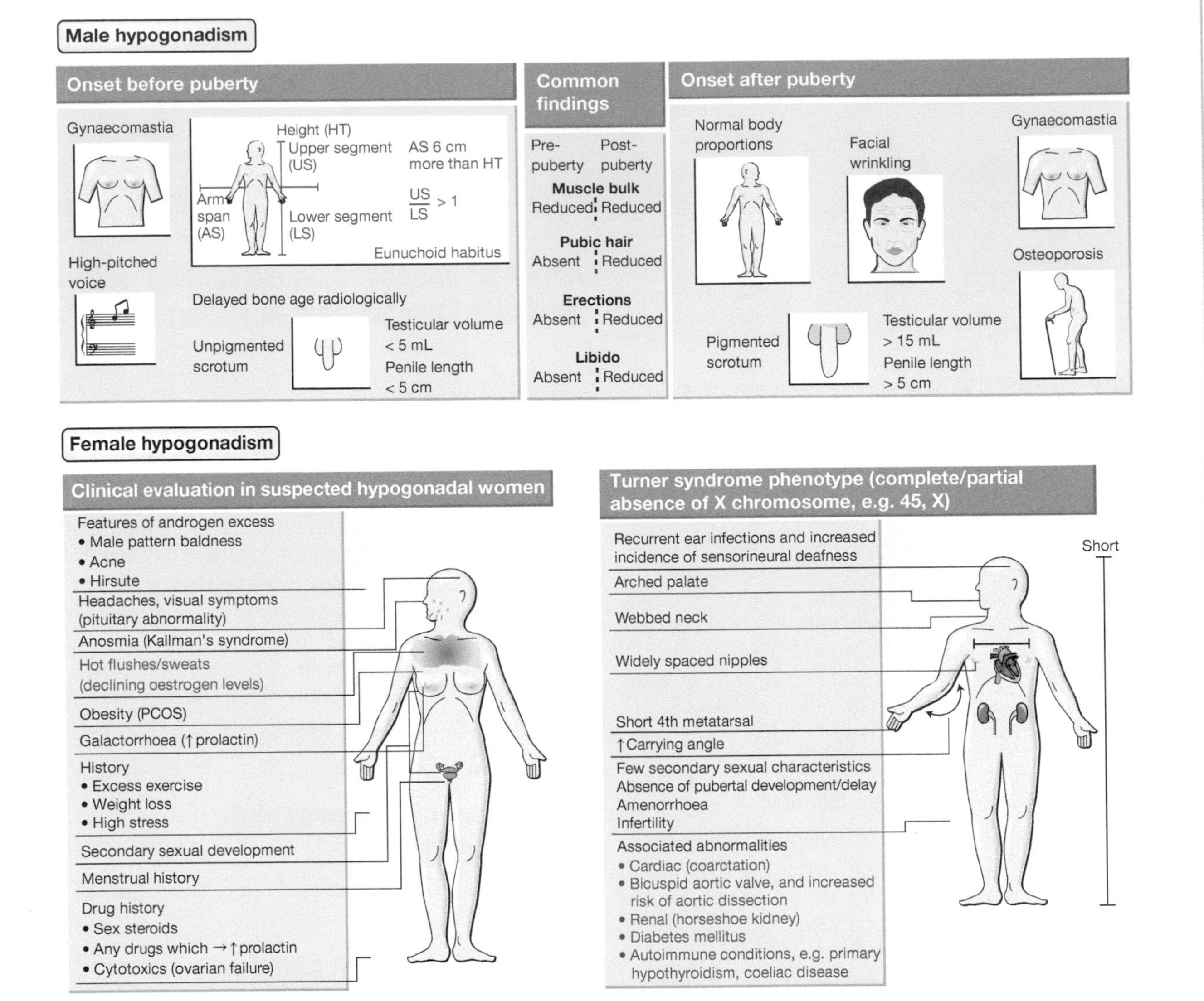

Hypogonadism is the failure of the ovaries or testes to produce sex steroids (oestrogen or testosterone) due to either gonadal failure (primary hypogonadism) or hypothalamic–pituitary failure (secondary hypogonadism). The key difference between primary and secondary hypogonadism is whether luteinizing hormone (LH)/follicle-stimulating hormone (FSH) levels are high (intact hypothalamic–pituitary axis) or low (damaged hypothalamic–pituitary axis) (see Table 163.1).

Male hypogonadism

The clinical features of pre- and postpubescent male hypogonadism are shown in the figure above. Acquired hypogonadism affects 20% of all men. Causes are shown in Table 163.2.

Management

Androgen replacement therapy will relieve symptoms and prevent osteoporosis, but will not improve fertility, which is irreversible in primary hypogonadism. Gonadotrophins or gonadotrophin-releasing hormone (GnRH) are used to induce fertility in secondary hypogonadism. Assisted reproductive techniques such as intracytoplasmic sperm injection (ICSI), testicular sperm extraction (TESE) and microdissection TESE (mTESE) are increasingly of value.

Female hypogonadism

The symptoms of female hypogonadism are amenorrhoea (primary or secondary), failure of pubertal development and

Medicine at a Glance, Fifth Edition. Edited by Patrick Davey and Alex Pitcher.

Companion website: www.wiley.com/go/medicine5e

Table 163.1 Differences between primary and secondary hypogonadism.

	LH/FSH	Testosterone or oestrogen	Other tests
Primary hypogonadism	↑	↓	Karyotype
Secondary hypogonadism	↓ or normal	↓	Prolactin MRI of pituitary fossa/hypothalamus Genetic screen for KAL1, FGFR1

FSH, follicle-stimulating hormone; LH, luteinizing hormone; MRI, magnetic resonance imaging.

Table 163.2 Primary and secondary male hypogonadism.

Primary	Secondary
Congenital	**Congenital**
Kleinfelter syndrome 47XXY Other chromosomal abnormalities	Idiopathic hypogonadotrophic hypogonadism (Kallmann syndrome if associated anosmia [absent olfactory bulbs]), sporadic/XL/AD/AR
Cryptorchidism/anorchia	
Acquired	**Acquired**
Orchitis (viral, e.g. mumps)	Hypothalamic/pituitary disease (tumour, hyperprolactinaemia, haemochromatosis, head injury, irradiation)
Testicular torsion/trauma	Acute critical illness
Radiation	Chronic illness (type 2 diabetes, obesity)
Drugs (ketoconazole, chemotherapy, alcohol)	Drugs (anabolic steroids, opiates)
Systemic disease (renal failure, cirrhosis)	Exercise and weight loss
	Syndromic (Prader–Willi, Laurence–Moon–Biedl)

infertility (Table 163.3). In primary hypogonadism, oestrogen withdrawal symptoms also occur: hot flushes and sweats, mood changes, vaginal dryness and pain on intercourse. The signs of established female hypogonadism include fine facial wrinkling, breast involution and a general reduction in body hair.

Management

In ovarian insufficiency, treatment is with oestrogens, which alleviate deficiency symptoms and prevent long-term complications, such as osteoporosis. Progestogens are added for women with an intact uterus to avoid endometrial hyperplasia and subsequent endometrial carcinoma. Oocyte donation is needed for fertility. In secondary hypogonadism, it is vital to have a full assessment of the hypothalamic–pituitary axis functionally and structurally, to diagnose and treat any underlying disease. Gonadotrophins (FSH/human menopausal gonadotrophin + human chorionic gonadotrophin [hCG], or pulsatile GnRH therapy) are used to induce fertility in hypogonadotrophic hypogonadism.

Table 163.3 Primary and secondary female hypogonadism.

Primary female hypogonadism (affects 1% aged <40 years)	Secondary female hypogonadism
Genetic (Turner syndrome 45, X 1/2000)	Weight loss, excess exercise, stress
Autoimmune (isolated or associated with autoimmune polyglandular syndrome (primary hypothyroidism, Addison disease, type 1 diabetes)	Structural (hypothalamic or pituitary disorder, e.g. pituitary adenoma or infiltration)
Iatrogenic (treatment of childhood malignancy, pelvic surgery)	Endocrine (hyperprolactinaemia)
Idiopathic	

Menstrual failure (amenorrhoea)

Menstrual failure is associated with infertility and oestrogen deficiency (increased osteoporosis and cardiovascular disease risk). Menstrual failure can be primary amenorrhoea (failure of menarche by 16 years), secondary amenorrhoea (failure of menstruation for >6 months in women who have previously menstruated, affecting 3–9% of women of reproductive age) or oligomenorrhoea (fewer than nine menstrual periods/year). Important causes of amenorrhoea are as follows.

- **Pregnancy**: should always be excluded by measuring hCG in the urine.
- **PCOS**: symptoms may be mild or severe (Stein–Leventhal syndrome). In PCOS, excess androgen production occurs, mainly from the ovary (where multiple small cysts are found), but also from the adrenal glands, resulting in disruption of the menstrual cycle (mild to profound) and mild androgenization, mainly hirsutism (see Chapter 40) or acne. More profound virilization suggests pathology other than PCOS (particularly virilizing ovarian or adrenal tumours). Insulin resistance and dyslipidaemia are also common features. Examination often shows marked obesity, with hirsutism and acne. Cushing disease and late-onset congenital adrenal hyperplasia may need to be excluded.

  Investigations show mildly elevated androgen levels, normal oestrogen and normal/elevated LH. Ovarian ultrasonography may demonstrate multiple small (3–5 mm) cysts. Androgen levels are mildly elevated, oestrogen levels are usually normal and LH levels may or may not be raised. There is no completely satisfactory treatment. Weight reduction, metformin (insulin sensitizer), antiandrogens (spironolactone, cyproterone) with contraception, ovarian suppression with the combined oral contraceptive pill, and ovarian diathermy all have a role.
- **Illness, malnutrition and overexercise**: all are usually readily apparent.
- **Endocrine disease** such as hyperthyroidism or excess of androgens (see Chapter 40).
- **Primary or secondary hypogonadism**, investigated as outlined above.
- **Hyperprolactinaemia**: most commonly due to a microadenoma, and less commonly, due to drugs, hypothyroidism, PCOS or substantial physical or psychological stress.
- Rarely, **structural disease** such as an imperforate hymen or absent uterus underlies primary amenorrhoea.

164 Bacteraemia and septic shock

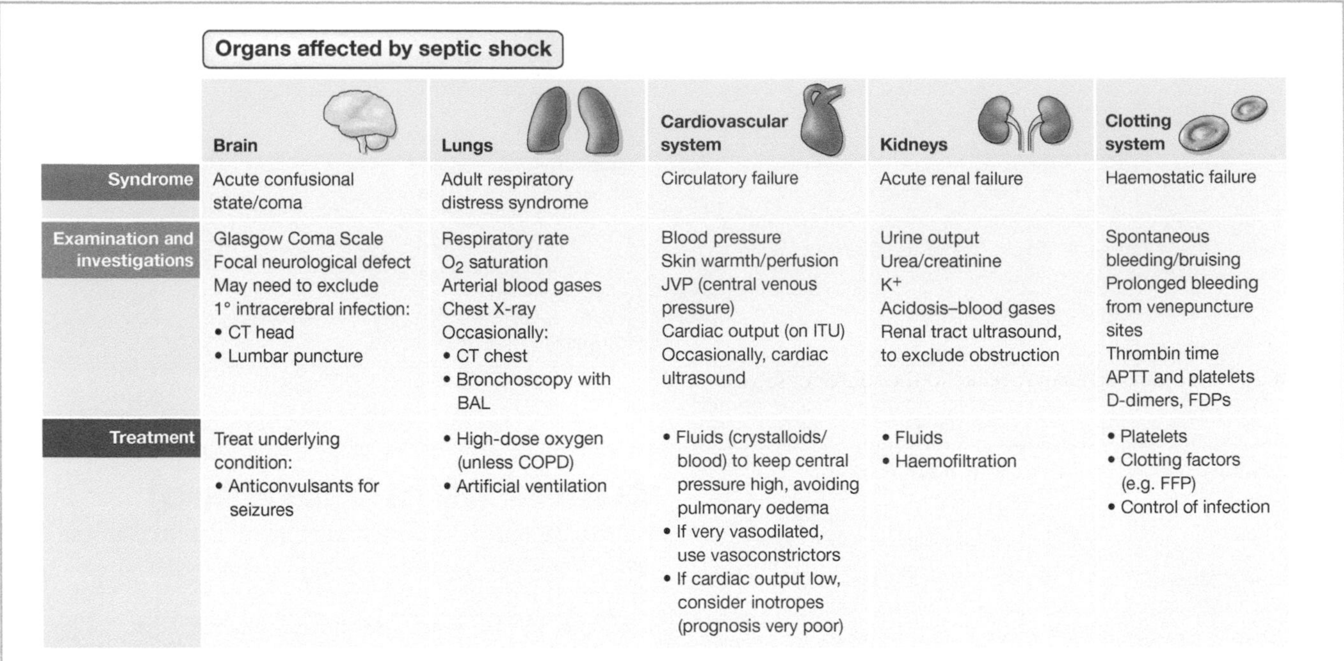

Organs affected by septic shock

	Brain	Lungs	Cardiovascular system	Kidneys	Clotting system
Syndrome	Acute confusional state/coma	Adult respiratory distress syndrome	Circulatory failure	Acute renal failure	Haemostatic failure
Examination and investigations	Glasgow Coma Scale Focal neurological defect May need to exclude 1° intracerebral infection: • CT head • Lumbar puncture	Respiratory rate O_2 saturation Arterial blood gases Chest X-ray Occasionally: • CT chest • Bronchoscopy with BAL	Blood pressure Skin warmth/perfusion JVP (central venous pressure) Cardiac output (on ITU) Occasionally, cardiac ultrasound	Urine output Urea/creatinine K^+ Acidosis–blood gases Renal tract ultrasound, to exclude obstruction	Spontaneous bleeding/bruising Prolonged bleeding from venepuncture sites Thrombin time APTT and platelets D-dimers, FDPs
Treatment	Treat underlying condition: • Anticonvulsants for seizures	• High-dose oxygen (unless COPD) • Artificial ventilation	• Fluids (crystalloids/blood) to keep central pressure high, avoiding pulmonary oedema • If very vasodilated, use vasoconstrictors • If cardiac output low, consider inotropes (prognosis very poor)	• Fluids • Haemofiltration	• Platelets • Clotting factors (e.g. FFP) • Control of infection

Some infections result in locally contained pathology but others trigger a systemic inflammatory response known as sepsis. This is a clinical syndrome thought to be caused by dysregulation of pro-inflammatory mediators, which cause tissue damage. The result is a chain of clinical deterioration:

Infection → sepsis → septic shock

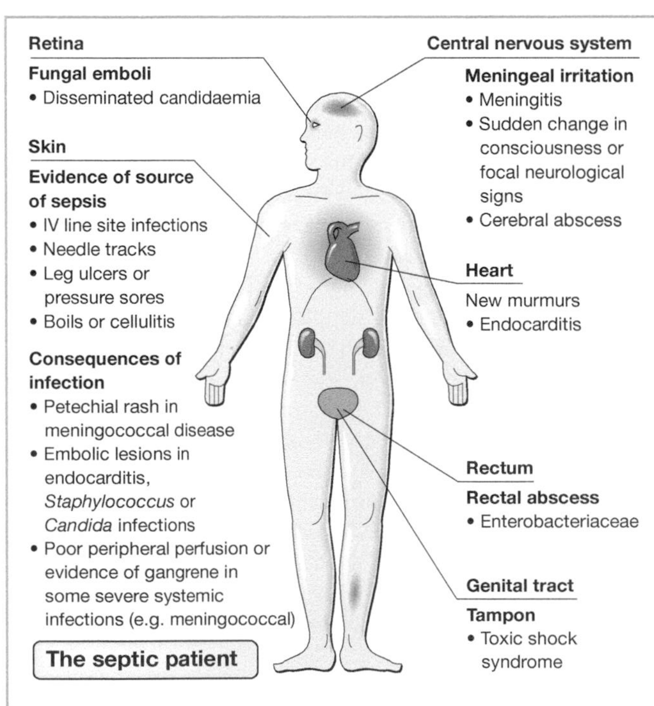

Definitions

- **Bacteraemia**: presence of viable bacteria in the blood, diagnosed by blood culture. Sustained bacteraemia may result in a systemic response (bacteraemia can also occur transiently with little or no clinical effect, e.g. after an operation, dental extraction or even simply teeth brushing).
- Other infections e.g. fungaemias and localized infections, which result in significant immune activation, can also trigger sepsis responses.
- Sepsis is defined as life-threatening organ dysfunction caused by a dysregulated host response to an infection.
- **Septic shock**: a subset of sepsis, in which there is co-existence of: persistent hypotension requiring vasopressors to maintain mean arterial pressure ≥65 mmHg; and serum lactate >2 mmol/L (>18 mg/dL). This occurs when endotoxins from pathogens or a cytokine-mediated immune response cause vasodilation and increased vascular permeability ('leaky' capillaries). The result is failure to maintain circulating volume and accumulation of fluid in the extravascular spaces, including peripheral and pulmonary oedema.

Sepsis is the most common cause of death in intensive care units. Mortality rates in critical care are 30–40%, and may be much higher if there is septic shock or multiorgan failure. Rates are increasing as there are:

- more unwell patients with diminished resistance to infections. Septic shock most often occurs in patients with underlying conditions, making them susceptible to infection
- increased numbers of surgical procedures
- more invasive procedures, intravascular lines, etc.

An inflammatory response syndrome identical to sepsis can be triggered by a wide variety of causes, including non-infectious conditions e.g. pancreatitis, burns or cardiopulmonary bypass.

Epidemiology

Only 50% of patients with septic shock have bacteria found in their bloodstream. The most common organisms are as follows: 1) **Gram positive**: 55–65% (*Staphylococcus* sp., enterococci, pneumococci). 2) **Gram negative**: 35–45% (*Escherichia coli, Pseudomonas sp., Klebsiella* sp.). 3) **Fungi**: 5–10% (*Candida* sp. in particular).

Clinical manifestations of sepsis

Fever and chills are common, non-specific signs. Patients with severe sepsis can be apyrexial, particularly if elderly – a poor prognostic sign. Symptoms/signs may relate to the source of sepsis.

Clinical assessment

1 Look for signs of sepsis in all patients who are unwell.
2 Aim to identify a source to guide antibiotics.
3 Assess severity using response to fluids and vital organ function, including the following aspects.

- *Heart and cardiovascular system*: skin and core temperature, arterial and venous pressures.
- *Peripheral perfusion*: patients may be warm and vasodilated in initial stages, cold and poorly perfused in severe refractory septic shock.
- *Mental state*: confusion is common, especially in elderly people.
- *Kidneys*: urinary catheterization should be performed to measure hourly urine output as the best minute-to-minute indication of renal function.
- *Lung function*, as measured by respiratory rate, oxygenation and alveolar–arterial (A–a) O_2 gradient (from arterial blood gases). These should be measured frequently, and if deterioration occurs, the patient should receive mechanical ventilation.
- *Vital organ perfusion*, as reflected by tissue hypoxia and arterial blood gas acidaemia and lactate levels.
- *Haemostatic function*: spontaneous bleeding, e.g. from venepuncture sites, suggests haemostatic failure, which requires blood product support.

Meningococcal septicaemia

Meningococcaemia is now a relatively rare cause of community-acquired sepsis, in children or young adults, and results in a characteristic illness, with fever, malaise and myalgia and a non-blanching rash, proceeding to hypotension and disseminated intravascular coagulation (DIC). Symptoms and signs of meningitis may or may not be present.

Toxic shock syndrome

Toxic shock syndrome is a specific syndrome produced by exotoxins of *Staphylococcus* or *Streptococcus* spp. The syndrome is characterized by fever, vomiting and diarrhoea, desquamation of skin, hypotension and multisystem involvement, leading to a high mortality. Treatment is antibiotics and supportive care (IV fluids).

Management

Key components of early management are as follows.

- Oxygenation: ventilatory support, for respiratory failure.
- Blood cultures and other antimicrobial sampling.
- Broad-spectrum antibiotics should be started immediately after taking blood for culture and any other relevant samples. Each hour of delay is associated with additional mortality.
- Intravenous fluid resuscitation, guided by monitoring of urine output and central venous pressure (in critically unwell patients).
- Measurement of lactate, as a marker of severity, can guide decisions on escalation of care.
- High-quality nursing care is crucial.

'Sepsis bundles' such as the UK's 'Sepsis 6' remind clinical staff of these initial steps and can improve clinical outcomes in patients.

Other vital measures include the following:

- Localization of site/origin of sepsis, using clinical pointers, chest X-ray and computed tomography (CT) of the abdomen in selected cases. Infected intravascular lines are a common source of hospital-acquired sepsis and should be removed/exchanged.
- Abscesses and dilated urinary systems should be drained urgently.
- Renal support for acute renal failure.
- Blood product support for anaemia, thrombocytopenia and coagulopathy.

Antimicrobial therapy

Antibiotics should be started immediately. Empirical therapy, i.e. treatment for suspected rather than proven infection, should be commenced, according to local antibiotic stewardship guidelines. Later, antibiotics should be rationalized according to the results of cultures (blood, urine and other appropriate fluid/tissue culture) or on the basis of the most likely organism if an obvious source exists. Antibiotic therapy should be reviewed regularly, taking clinical response into account. Suitable choices in the absence of an obvious focus include the following. 1) **Community-acquired sepsis**: penicillin combined with β-lactamase inhibitor (co-amoxiclav) 2) **Hospital-acquired sepsis**: broad spectrum penicillin combined with β-lactamase inhibitor (piperacillin-tazobactam) or carbapenem (meropenem).

Aminoglycosides should be added for critically ill patients or if resistant organisms are suspected. Vancomycin or teicoplanin should be used for suspected staphylococcal sepsis in a patient at risk of methicillin-resistant *Staphylococcus aureus* (MRSA) (e.g. recent hospitalization).

Prognosis

Gram-negative sepsis has a mortality of 25–40%; Gram-positive sepsis has a lower death rate of 10–20%. Mortality rates are highly dependent on age and pre-existing medical conditions.

165 Herpes virus infections in adults

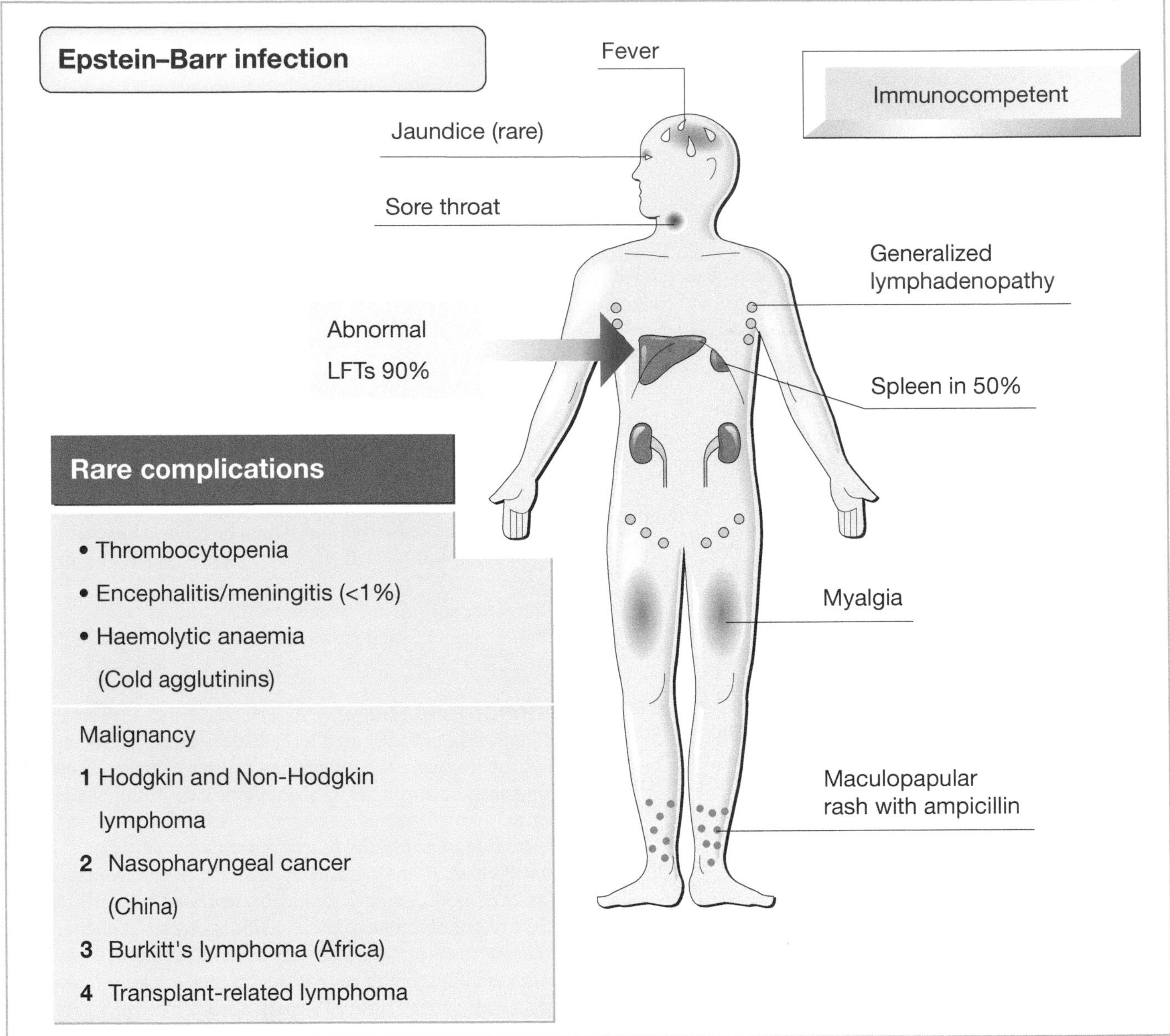

Once acquired, all herpes virus infections are lifelong and hence disease is caused by primary infection but also secondary reactivation, the latter typically occurring when immunity wanes (as a result of immunosuppression or simply ageing).

Epstein–Barr virus

Epstein–Barr virus (EBV) is common – 90% of people are infected by adulthood. Half of infections occur asymptomatically in childhood. Infection in adolescent life is more commonly associated with clinical disease. EBV occurs in oropharyngeal secretions and many cases result from intimate contact (hence the name 'kissing disease').

Symptoms are fever, sore throat, headache, myalgia, anorexia and chills, and signs are lymphadenopathy, prominent pharyngitis and splenomegaly in 50% – the **glandular fever syndrome.** A maculopapular rash often occurs if the patient is given amoxicillin. Symptoms usually resolve spontaneously over 2–3 weeks, but prolonged fatigue is not unusual. Complications are: (i) abnormal liver function tests (LFTs) (common) and occasional jaundice; (ii) haemolytic anaemia; (iii) rare neurological: encephalitis or aseptic meningitis; and (iv) lymphoproliferative disorder. EBV-related

Medicine at a Glance, Fifth Edition. Edited by Patrick Davey and Alex Pitcher.

Companion website: www.wiley.com/go/medicine5e

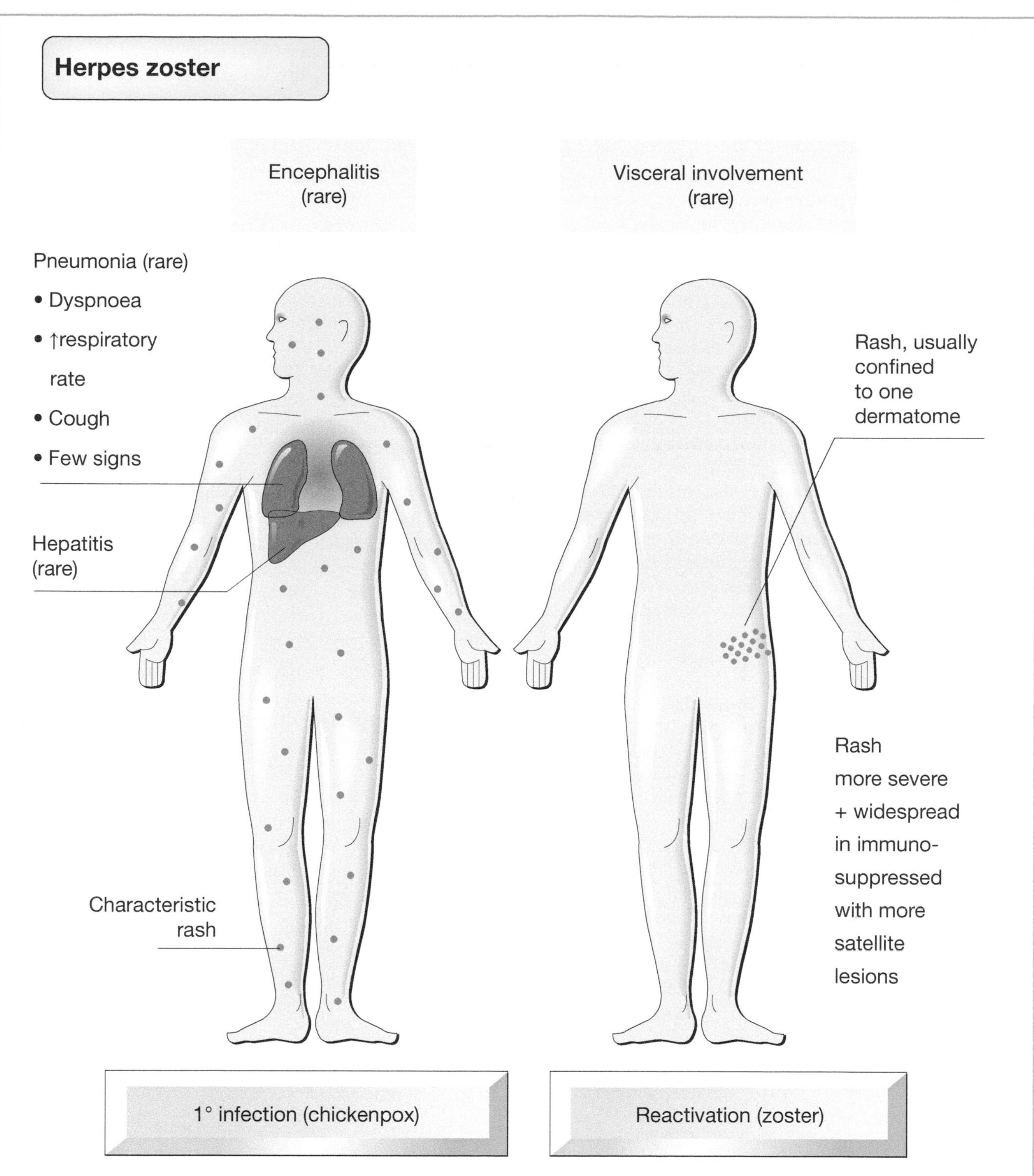

lymphoproliferative syndromes (including malignancy) are associated with prolonged immunodeficiency, e.g. can occur with prolonged immunodeficiency transplant patients and late-stage human immunodeficiency virus (HIV) and carry a poor prognosis.

Diagnosis and treatment

- Full blood count: mononucleosis, >10% atypical lymphocytes. Thrombocytopenia is common. Serology: IgM antibodies to EBV or detection of heterophile antibodies (serum antibodies against red blood cells of other species) – monospot or Paul–Bunnell test.
- Differential diagnosis is from other agents causing a 'glandular fever' type syndrome, principally HIV, cytomegalovirus (CMV) or toxoplasmosis. Streptococcal pharyngitis may give similar symptoms.
- No specific antiviral treatment is available. Steroids may be considered in severe pharyngitis, thrombocytopenia and haemolytic anaemia.

Herpes simplex virus

Herpes simplex virus (HSV) infection is common. It has a predilection for mucocutaneous sites, affecting both normal and immunocompromised hosts, and is transmitted by direct oral or genital contact. Two types – HSV-1 and HSV-2 – have differing epidemiology and clinical patterns, although there is considerable overlap. Most people encounter HSV1 infection in childhood, whereas acquisition of HSV-2 depends on sexual contact. Recurrent infections are common as a result of latency of the virus in sensory nerve ganglia. Identified triggers of recurrence include stress, sunlight and bacterial infection (especially pneumococcal pneumonia).

- **Oral mucocutaneous HSV**: most primary infections are asymptomatic; fever and pharyngitis or gingivostomatitis may occur. The usual manifestation is of recurrent herpes labialis (cold sores). There is a prodrome of tingling or burning, followed by painful vesicles at the edge of lip. Oral lesions may occur. Vesicles heal with crusting within 10 days.
- **Genital HSV**: in the UK this is now more commonly caused by HSV-1, although HSV-2 is more likely to cause recurrent anogenital symptoms. Many infections are asymptomatic. Painful vesicles occur on the glans, penis shaft or vulva, perineum and vagina, 2–7 days after contact. There is dysuria. It is more common in women. Fever, malaise and tender inguinal lymphadenopathy may occur. Vesicles often ulcerate and may persist for several weeks; recurrence is common. Asymptomatic viral shedding can occur and cause transmission to sexual partners.
- **HSV proctitis**: this is a significant cause of proctitis in men who have sex with men (MSM).
- **HSV eye infection (keratoconjunctivitis)**: this is a common problem in immunosuppressed patients or older patients e.g. when recovering from pneumonia. The key clinical marker of keratitis (corneal infection) is the presence of a 'red eye' associated with **reduced visual acuity** (distinguishing it from bacterial or viral conjunctivitis). If HSV keratitis is suspected, urgent referral to ophthalmology for slit-lamp examination is needed.
- **HSV-1 encephalitis**: this is a devastating disease caused by HSV-1, and typically occurs in patients with at least moderate immunosuppression. Early recognition, diagnosis (PCR of CSF) and treatment (with high-dose intravenous aciclovir) are critical (see Chapter 207).
- **HSV-2 meningitis**: a pure meningitis, without clinical evidence of encephalitis, is more associated with HSV-2 and can be recurrent.
- **Other clinical syndromes**: (i) herpetic whitlow (infection of the finger); (ii) eczema herpeticum: skin infection in atopic dermatitis, which can cause severe illness.

Herpes simplex

- Mouth (cold sores)
- Eye (keratitis)
- Genitalia (genital sores)
- Encephalitis (HSV-1)
- Meningitis (HSV-2)

Treatment

Intravenous (IV) aciclovir is useful for severe systemic illness, e.g. encephalitis. Oral aciclovir used early in oral or genital disease leads to fewer lesions and quicker healing. Topical antivirals are also vital when there is eye disease. Suppressive aciclovir can be helpful for patients who are distressed by frequently recurrent herpes lesions but it does not eliminate viral shedding so sexual partners still need protection.

Immunocompromised hosts

Severe mucocutaneous lesions are common in people with advanced HIV disease or transplant recipients. HSV may affect other parts of the gut and, rarely, disseminates to involve organs such as the liver.

Varicella-zoster virus

Varicella-zoster virus (VZV) causes both varicella (chickenpox) and herpes zoster (shingles); varicella reflects the primary infection and zoster the recurrent infection. Spread of the virus occurs through respiratory droplets, and 90% of primary cases occur in childhood. VZV becomes latent in the dorsal root ganglia after primary infection.

Varicella is usually a disease of children; chickenpox in adults is much more severe, with a 15-fold higher mortality. Fever and malaise precede the development of maculopapular lesions on the face and trunk, which become vesicular and crust over. In adults, particularly pregnant women, complications include:

- varicella pneumonitis: occurs in one in 400 adults. Tachypnoea, cough and dyspnoea. Chest signs may not be prominent
- varicella encephalitis: depressed consciousness and progressive headaches; fatal in up to 15%
- varicella hepatitis.

Herpes zoster is associated with immunosuppression, typically occurring in older people, those with advanced HIV disease or organ transplants or on immunosuppressive drugs. A prodrome of pain is followed by a unilateral rash in a dermatomal distribution. Vesicles develop over 2–3 days, crust over and then heal.

- The lumbar or thoracic dermatomes are most commonly involved.
- Trigeminal nerve involvement may lead to ocular involvement (herpes zoster ophthalmicus). Urgent ophthalmology review is necessary.
- Ramsay Hunt syndrome: the seventh cranial nerve is involved; vesicles may be hidden in the auditory canal. Hearing loss and facial paralysis may occur.

Rare neurological complications include meningoencephalitis, delayed contralateral hemiparesis after herpes zoster ophthalmicus and transverse myelitis. Postherpetic neuralgia is distressing and occurs in up to half of elderly patients.

Immunocompromised hosts

Chickenpox causes significant morbidity and mortality; 30% of bone marrow transplant recipients without prophylaxis have infections in the first year. Dissemination occurs in 50%: lung, central nervous system and liver.

Zoster rash is more severe and lesions may occur outside the dermatome or be disseminated over the skin. Visceral involvement is rare.

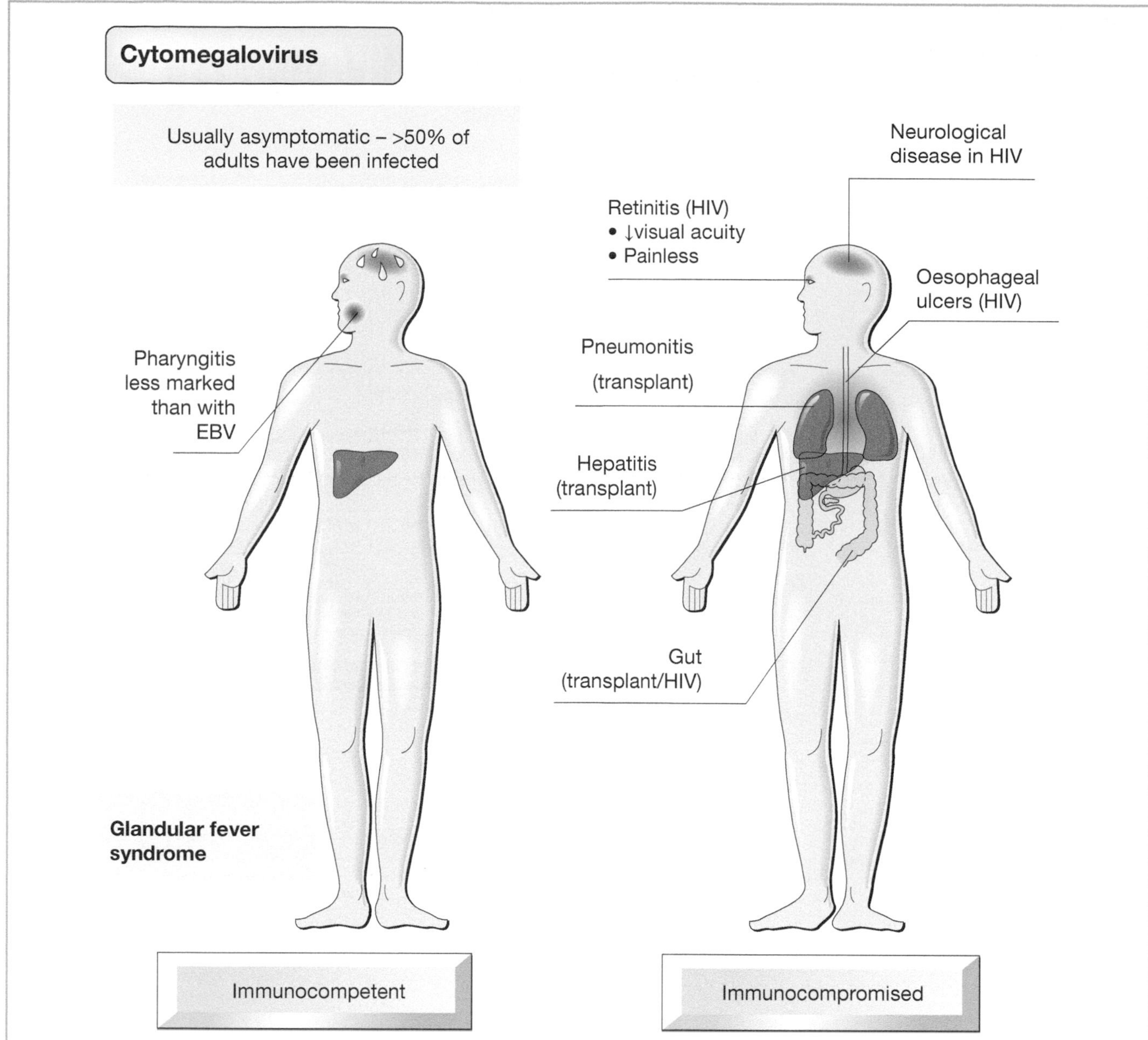

Diagnosis and management

The diagnosis is usually clinical. Vesicle fluid can be analysed using polymerase chain reaction to confirm or rule out VZV. IV aciclovir or the highly bioavailable valaciclovir are used to treat immunocompromised individuals (including those on high-dose steroids) with varicella or zoster. Treatment of chickenpox in adults may reduce complications. Early treatment reduces the number of lesions and subsequent pain in zoster.

Infection during pregnancy

Varicella infection in the first two trimesters of pregnancy is associated with a small but significant increase in the rate of birth defects. Non-immune expectant mothers should avoid contact with chickenpox and shingles patients.

Post-exposure prophylaxis with antivirals or immunoglobulin is recommended for individuals with significant exposure to chickenpox (varicella) or shingles (zoster) who are at increased risk of severe chickenpox (i.e. immunosuppressed individuals, neonates and pregnant women) and have no antibodies to varicella-zoster virus (VZV).

Cytomegalovirus

Infection with CMV is common but rarely causes clinical disease: 50–95% of adults have been infected. It is, however, a major pathogen in immunocompromised individuals. Disease occurs because of: (i) reactivation or (ii) transplantation of a CMV-positive organ into a CMV-negative recipient. The clinical features of infection are as follows.

- A glandular fever-like syndrome, with increased monocytes and abnormal liver function tests may occur.
- Transplant recipients: CMV pneumonitis, hepatitis and gastrointestinal disease, such as diarrhoea.
- HIV infected: CMV retinitis, neurological infection and gut disease.

Prophylaxis is often indicated in advanced HIV with evidence of replicating virus and some groups of transplant recipients. Diagnosis is challenging; high titres of CMV in the blood are suggestive of active infection but definitive diagnosis that CMV is causing pathology in an organ requires biopsy and demonstration of typical inclusion bodies. Treatment is with CMV antivirals such as valganciclovir.

166 HIV infection and advanced HIV disease

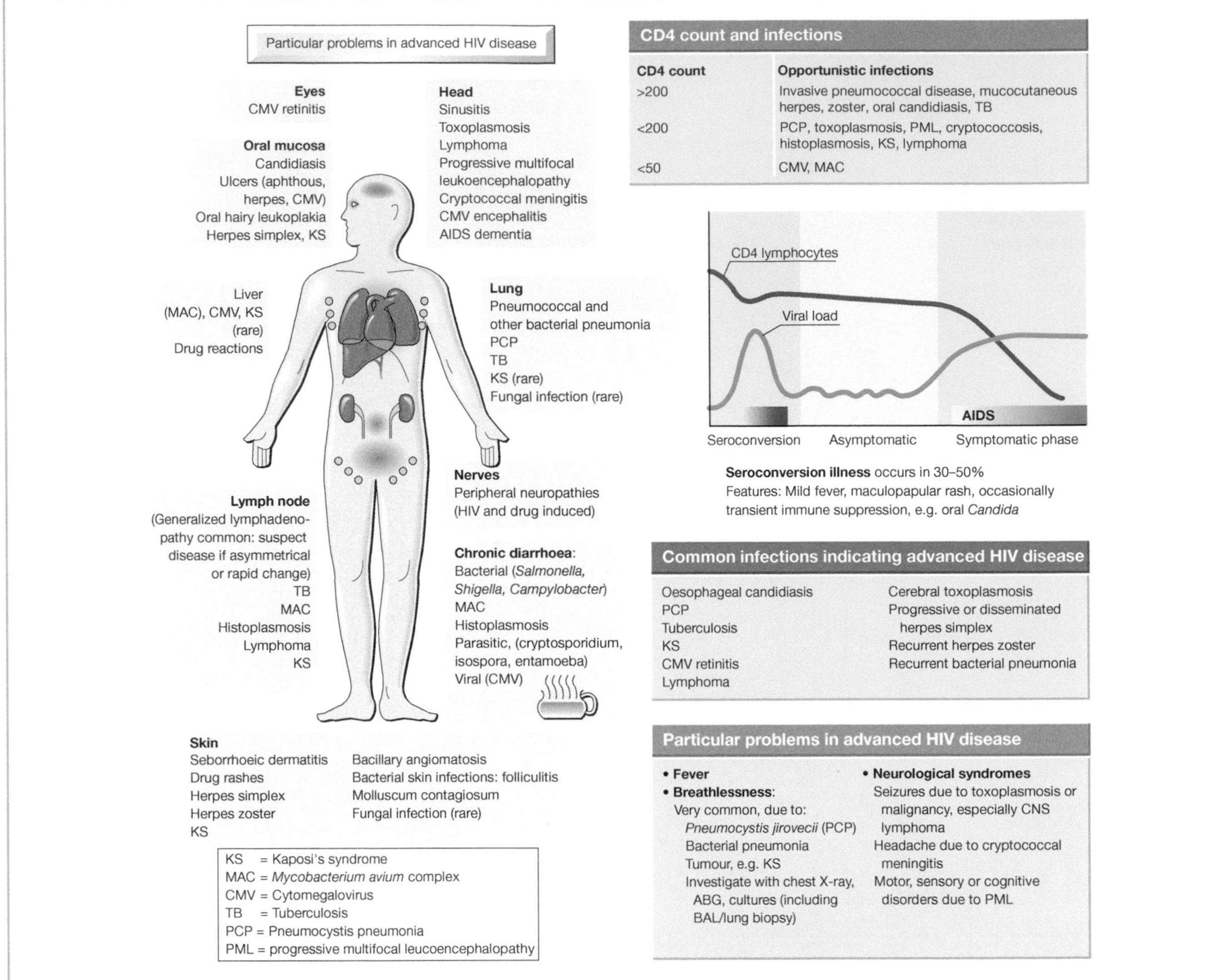

Human immunodeficiency virus (HIV) infection causes a clinical syndrome characterized by the development of progressive immunodeficiency following a long asymptomatic period. Cellular immunodeficiency eventually leads to severe opportunistic infection and, more rarely, malignancy.

Epidemiology

An estimated 37.7 million people across the globe were living with HIV infection in 2020. Approximately 3000 new diagnoses of HIV are made in the UK per year. Transmission of the blood-borne RNA retrovirus occurs predominantly by four mechanisms.

- Sexual contact.
- Intravenous drug abuse.
- Maternal–child (vertical) transmission.
- Transfusion of blood products (although much less common with improved transfusion screening).

Pathogenesis

After transmission, HIV enters lymphoid tissue where it infects CD4-bearing T lymphocytes and monocyte/macrophages. The virus enters the cell by binding to the CD4 molecule and chemokine receptors, and then replicates and integrates itself into host DNA. Latent infection or virus production follows. A total of 10^{10}–10^{11} virions are produced each day with considerable turnover of HIV-infected cells. Ultimately, progressive loss of CD4 cells leads to impairment of the immune function.

Clinical patterns

- **Primary HIV infection**: 30–80% patients experience an acute clinical syndrome when viral replication occurs after HIV infection. Symptoms typically occur 2–4 weeks after infection and include fever, malaise, lymphadenopathy and a maculopapular rash. A small proportion have transient immunosuppression with clinical features such as oral *Candida* infection.
- **Asymptomatic HIV**: after seroconversion, most patients have a prolonged asymptomatic period (median 10 years without treatment) before any further clinical manifestations.
- **Advanced HIV disease**: this term is now more commonly used than 'acquired immune deficiency syndrome' (AIDS). As HIV infection progresses, patients become symptomatic with certain opportunistic diseases defining advanced HIV disease along with systemic features such as significant weight loss, persistent fever or persistent diarrhoea.

- **Stage of disease** is most easily considered in terms of the CD4 count, expressed as cells/μl, which reflects the degree of immunosuppression and the likelihood of particular opportunistic infections.

Diagnosis of HIV infection

HIV tests have now reached their 'fourth generation' involving detection of both HIV antibodies and p24 antigen. Using such tests, 99% of HIV-infected individuals have a positive test within 44 days of exposure. Point-of-care tests are increasingly used but always require confirmation with a formal laboratory test.

HIV should be considered in anyone presenting with recurrent infections, especially shingles, unexplained fever or lymphadenopathy. In the 2000s routine antenatal testing became standard practice in the UK. Given the range of syndromes which result from HIV and associated opportunistic infections, there are strong arguments for routine HIV testing in patients attending emergency departments and specialist medicine clinics (e.g. respiratory, gastroenterology, hepatology, neurology) as well as for new patients in GP practices.

Treatment of HIV infection

Use of antiretroviral drugs in combination has led to a significant decrease in mortality and reversal of HIV disease progression, so that a person living with HIV has a similar life expectancy to an HIV-negative person, providing they are diagnosed early, and have good access and adherence to treatment. Even in advanced disease, antiretroviral drugs can restore good immune function and improve health in the great majority of patients.

Most combination regimens are made up of drugs from the following classes. 1) Nucleoside reverse transcriptase inhibitors (NRTIs); 2) Protease inhibitors (PIs); 3) Non-nucleoside reverse transcriptase inhibitors (NNRTIs); 4) Integrase strand transfer inhibitors (INSTIs).

There are additional classes of drug (e.g. CCR5 antagonists) that may be appropriate in certain situations.

A combination of three or four drugs is used to reduce the viral load (ideally below the detection limit of the assay). The viral load and CD4 response reflect the efficacy of treatment.

Common antiretroviral treatment (ART) problems:

- Resistance to antiretroviral drugs: common in patients who have experienced several different drugs already. Resistance to one drug often limits use of the whole class. New drugs continue to be developed to treat such patients.
- Side effects (e.g. neuropathy, lipodystrophy) and drug intolerance.
- Adherence issues from complex multidrug regimens.
- Antiretrovirals can interact with other drugs.
- Limited drug access for patients in developing countries with a high HIV burden due to drug costs and health system limitations.

Common opportunistic infections

Patients with HIV are susceptible to both standard pathogens and unusual opportunistic infections; although ART and routine primary prophylaxis have reduced the incidence of many opportunistic infections, they still present considerable problems. In addition, a third of new patients in the West present late with advanced immunosuppression. The major clinical syndromes are shown in the figure.

- *Pneumocystis jirovecii* pneumonia (PCP) is a common mode of presentation of advanced HIV. Risk increases once the CD4 count drops below 200. Primary prophylaxis with co-trimoxazole (e.g. Septrin®) is effective. PCP usually presents with a non-productive cough, fever and dyspnoea; it is usually subacute, with a mean duration of symptoms of 3–4 weeks. Physical examination is often unremarkable. Blood gases often show a moderate hypoxaemia. The chest X-ray (CXR) is abnormal in 90%, classically showing fine interstitial perihilar shadowing, although the spectrum of abnormalities is wide. Confirmation by immunofluorescence microscopy or polymerase chain reaction (PCR) of induced sputum (although this introduces an infection control risk) or bronchoalveolar lavage (BAL) fluid establishes the diagnosis. Treatment is with high-dose co-trimoxazole; the addition of steroids improves the prognosis in severe disease.
- Cytomegalovirus (CMV) occurs in late-stage infection (CD4 <50). The major problem is progressive retinitis (85%), but gut, nervous system and lung infections also occur. It is asymptomatic early on, so proactive ophthalmological screening is useful in advanced HIV. Retinitis is diagnosed clinically; white fluffy retinal lesions with perivascular haemorrhages and exudates. Treatment is with CMV antiviral agents and treatment of HIV; long-term maintenance therapy is necessary, as relapse is common until the CD4 count has improved.
- Toxoplasmosis is a protozoal infection, which most commonly causes encephalitis (80%) in late HIV (CD4 <100). Patients present with fever, headache, confusion, fits and focal neurological signs. Magnetic resonance imaging (MRI) is more sensitive than computed tomography (CT) in demonstrating ring-enhancing lesions, which are often multiple and classically in the basal ganglia or corticomedullary junction. Toxoplasmosis is rare in patients with no serological evidence of previous exposure. Treatment is with pyrimethamine and sulfadiazine, with clinical and radiological response typically confirming the diagnosis.
- Tuberculosis (see also Chapter 170): this can of course present at any CD4 count, although in advanced HIV, TB presentation is different from that in immunocompetent patients. For example, patients with advanced HIV with active pulmonary TB tend to have more subtle radiological signs and sputum that is smear negative but culture positive. A high index of suspicion for TB therefore needs to be maintained for patients living with HIV who have spent time in regions of high TB endemicity. Mycobacterial culture of blood and urine can contribute to diagnosis.
- Disseminated non-tuberculous mycobacterial (NTM) disease, of which *Mycobacterium avium* complex (MAC) causes the majority of cases. This presents as fever, lymphadenopathy and hepatosplenomegaly in patients with CD4 counts <50. Definitive diagnosis is via culture from biopsy specimens (as well as blood and bone marrow).
- Kaposi sarcoma (KS) is caused by human herpes virus 8 and is associated with very low CD4 counts. Skin lesions are initially macular and progress to reddish-purplish indurated plaques; there can also be oral, lymph node, gastrointestinal tract or lung involvement. Diagnosis is clinical or by skin biopsy. Skin disease may completely regress following a good immune response to ART. Localized radiotherapy and chemotherapy are occasionally needed for problematic lesions or disseminated disease.
- Non-Hodgkin lymphoma occurs in late-stage disease – 20% are in the central nervous system (CNS). It presents with fever, sweats and organ-related symptoms; extranodal involvement is common. Treatment is with chemotherapy. Prognosis has improved in recent years.
- Progressive multifocal leukoencephalopathy (PML) is a demyelinating disease presenting with insidious onset of focal neurological defects; it is caused by the polyoma virus (JC virus). While it usually occurs at low CD4 counts, cases are described with relatively preserved counts (>200). Diagnosis is by imaging (white matter lesion) and PCR of the cerebrospinal fluid for JC virus. The only effective treatment is improving immune function with ART.
- Disseminated fungal diseases: cryptococcal meningitis is a reasonably common presentation of advanced HIV disease (see Chapter 167) while histoplasmosis and talaromycosis (in patients from south-east Asia) are increasingly recognized causes of severe illness.

Immune reconstitution inflammatory syndrome (IRIS) is the paradoxical worsening of symptoms of an opportunistic infection following commencement of HIV treatment, or the unmasking of an undiagnosed opportunistic infection. IRIS can be life-threatening and particularly complicates treatment of TB/HIV co-infection, where steroids are beneficial.

167 Common fungal infections

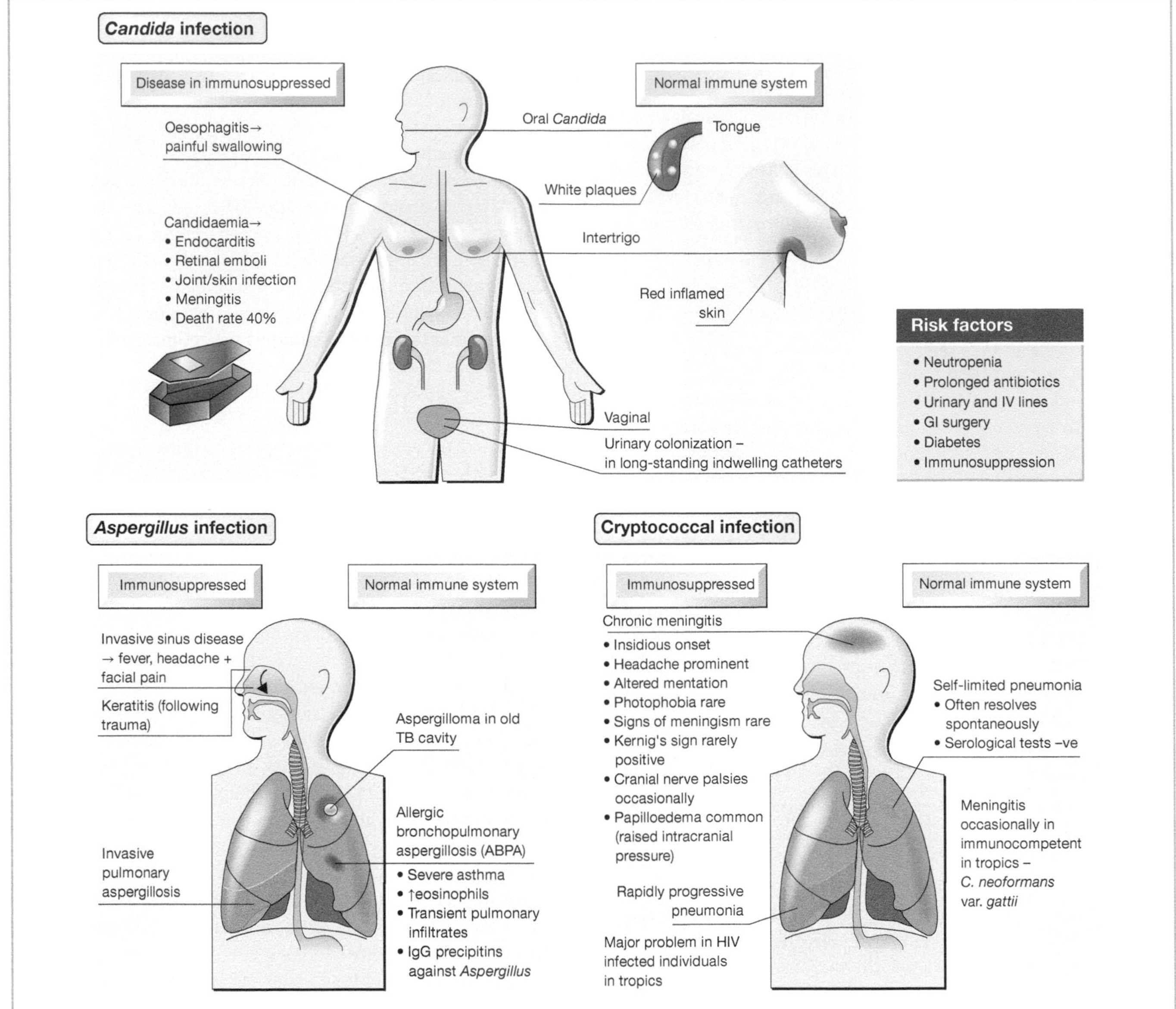

In the immunologically competent host, fungi generally cause only mild disease, whereas in the immunocompromised individual, severe or life-threatening disease can result. Thus, fungal infections have assumed increasing importance as the number of immunocompromised patients increases. Many different species cause significant disease; only the main fungal infections encountered in the UK are discussed here.

Candida species

These yeasts are the most common invasive fungal species in the UK. The organisms are found readily in the environment and are commensals on mucous membranes in the gastrointestinal (GI), respiratory and genitourinary tracts. *Candida albicans* is the most important species, although non-*albicans* species are becoming more common. *Candida* spp. can cause both mucocutaneous and invasive disease.

Mucocutaneous candidiasis

This may occur in immunocompetent and immunocompromised individuals; it is particularly common in those with diabetes or with altered cellular immunity such as HIV.

- **Oral *Candida* infection**: the most common clinical manifestation is creamy-white 'curd-like' patches on the mucosa and tongue. The underlying surface is raw if the exudate is scraped off.

Medicine at a Glance, Fifth Edition. Edited by Patrick Davey and Alex Pitcher.

Companion website: www.wiley.com/go/medicine5e

The diagnosis is usually made clinically, although hyphae can be demonstrated in lesions.

- **Candidal oesophagitis**: usually in advanced HIV or haematological malignancy. May occur without oral lesions, and produces symptoms of dysphagia, odynophagia and retrosternal pain. Diagnosed by appearance on endoscopy and biopsies.
- **Vaginal candidiasis**: see Chapter 49.
- **Intertrigo**: infection in the warm damp environment between skinfolds – red macerated skin with satellite lesions.
- **Chronic mucocutaneous candidiasis**: the syndrome is associated with specific T-cell deficiency. There is infection of the skin, mucous membrane and scalp, which may be disfiguring.

Invasive candidiasis

Invasive infections usually arise from endogenous colonization. Entry occurs through damaged skin or mucosa or direct access to the circulation. Both neutrophils and cell-mediated immunity are important in defence against *Candida* spp. The following are risk factors for invasive disease.

- Neutropenia increases the risk of candidaemia.
- Prolonged use of antibiotics.
- Indwelling urinary or intravenous (IV) catheters.
- GI surgery.
- IV drug abuse.

Candidaemia

Candida spp. are commonly isolated from blood cultures. Although this sometimes reflects colonization of indwelling lines rather than disseminated candidal disease, candidaemia also occurs in disseminated candidiasis, especially in immunosuppressed patients. All patients should be carefully evaluated for metastatic infection, including examination of the fundi, the heart for endocarditis, the joints and skin. Candidaemia has a 40% mortality rate.

Disseminated candidiasis

Blood-borne spread can lead to infection in most organs, including the central nervous system, respiratory tract, joints, kidneys and peritoneum. Only 50% of patients with disseminated candidiasis have demonstrated candidaemia. The presence of skin or eye lesions (present in 10%) confirms the diagnosis. *Candida* spp. in the urine occurs in both invasive and disseminated candidiasis.

Treatment

- Oral or vaginal candidiasis: topical therapy or short-term systemic therapy.
- Serious mucocutaneous disease: systemic therapy.
- Candidaemia: usually treated with azoles or echinocandins (e.g. caspofungin). Amphotericin can also be used. IV catheters should be removed.
- Disseminated candidiasis: aggressive antifungal therapy.
- Surgery is usually required for endocarditis.

Antifungal prophylaxis

This is used in HIV patients with recurrent disease, and in high-risk bone marrow and most solid organ transplantations.

Aspergillus species

These mould species are found readily in the environment. Systemic infection is acquired by inhalation of spores. Disease may be caused in three ways.

- Allergic reactions: allergic bronchopulmonary aspergillosis (see Chapter 117).
- Colonization of cavities (aspergillomas) (see Chapter 117).
- Invasive aspergillosis.

Invasive aspergillosis is a disease of immunocompromised patients. Important risk factors include prolonged neutropenia, high-dose steroids and prolonged antibiotic therapy.

Clinical patterns of invasive disease

- Sinus disease: in neutropenic patients, colonizing organisms may become invasive in the nose and sinuses. Patients present with fever, headache and sinus symptoms. Soft tissue and bony invasion may lead to vascular invasion and brain involvement. Diagnosis is suspected when computed tomography shows loss of the normal bony sinus margins, and confirmed by tissue biopsy.
- Invasive pulmonary aspergillosis: a pneumonic process in immunosuppressed patients.
  - Fever, cough (±blood), chest pain, dyspnoea.
  - Rapidly progressing pneumonia, sometimes with cavitation.

A working diagnosis is often made from a combination of radiology and culture of respiratory samples; definitive diagnosis requires lung biopsy (rarely undertaken). Serum galactomannan testing adds further support to the diagnosis. *Aspergillus* is rarely found in blood cultures in pneumonia.

Treatment

Amphotericin has been replaced by voriconazole as the drug of choice for invasive aspergillosis. Caspofungin may be used in refractory disease. Response rates in invasive aspergillosis remain poor and the mortality rate is about 40%.

Cryptococcal disease

Cryptococcus neoformans is a yeast-like fungus that affects both normal and immunocompromised hosts. The organism is acquired through inhalation; there are three main clinical syndromes.

- **Pulmonary disease**: occurs in both normal and immunocompromised hosts.
- **Meningitis**: occurs in immunosuppressed individuals, particularly with HIV but also poorly controlled diabetes. There is a long, non-specific history; the most common symptoms are headache and a change in mentation. There may be surprisingly few signs and neck stiffness may not be present. Papilloedema and cranial nerve palsies may occur, and visual impairment and deafness are common sequelae. Management of the raised CSF pressure, as well as the infection itself, is critical.

  Diagnosis is achieved via sampling of CSF. General findings are predominant lymphocytes, low glucose, high protein and high pressure. An Indian ink stain demonstrates yeast and capsule in the CSF, with diagnosis confirmed by culture of *C. neoformans*. Cryptococcal antigen titres are raised in the serum and CSF.
- **Cryptococcaemia** (positive culture from blood): may present with fever alone in the immunocompromised or can be associated with meningitis. Skin lesions occur in 10%.

Treatment

- **Normal immune system**: pulmonary disease may not need treatment and can be observed. Treat meningitis as below.
- **Immunocompromised**: liposomal amphotericin combined with flucytosine as 'induction' therapy, followed by fluconazole. Prolonged therapy is required and long-term secondary prophylaxis required. The mortality rate in meningitis in HIV is around 25%.

168 Specific bacterial infections

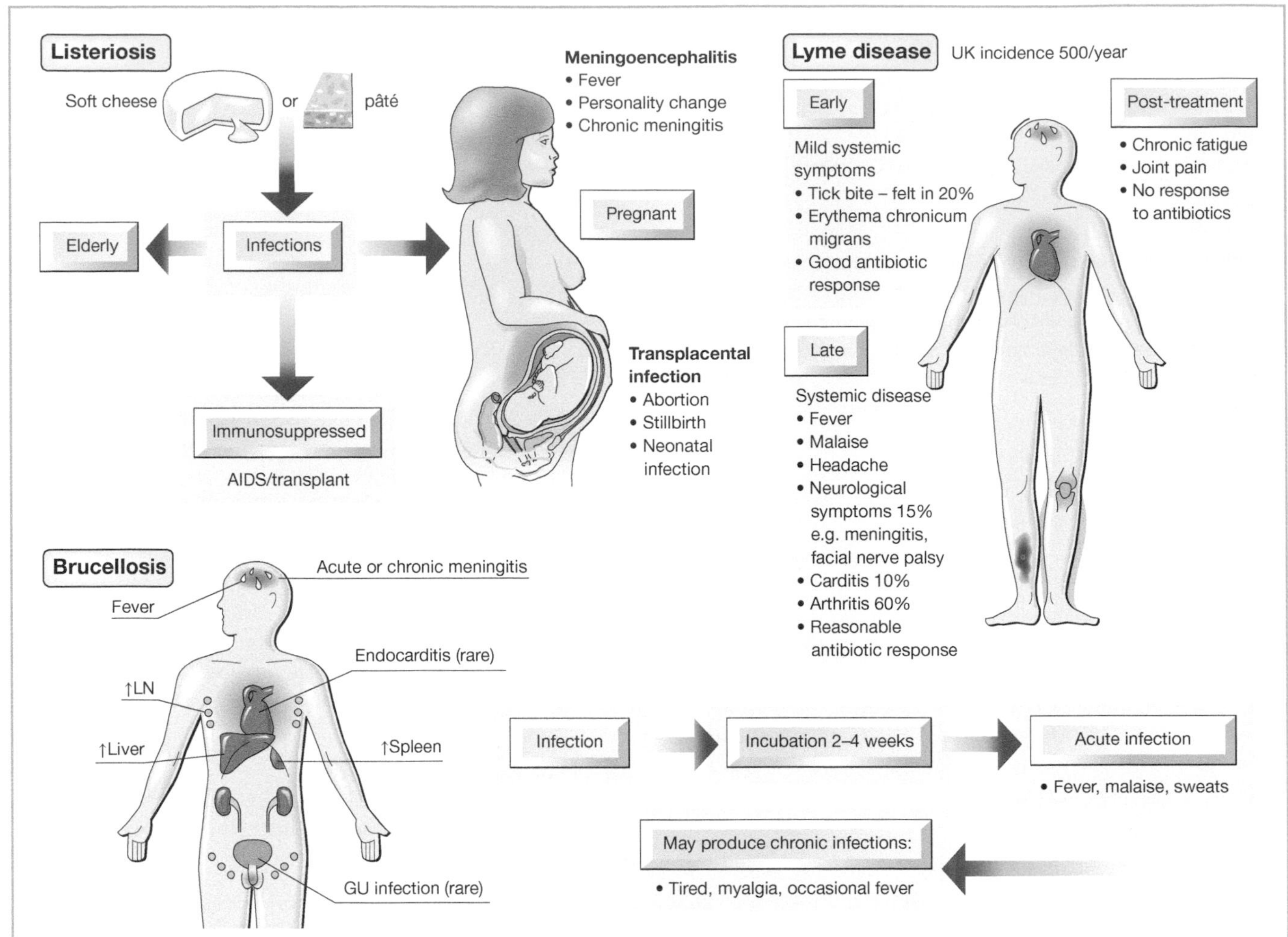

Listeriosis

Listeria monocytogenes is a Gram-positive bacillus causing disease in pregnant women, immunocompromised individuals and neonates. Infection is usually acquired through food, particularly soft cheeses and pâté. Clinical manifestations include the following.

- **Pregnancy associated**: bacteraemia producing a flu-like illness, and sometimes transplacental infection or ascending infection leading to abortion, stillbirth or neonatal sepsis. Very rarely maternal meningitis.
- **Neonatal infection**: acute meningitis with high mortality.
- **Immunocompromised / older adults**: Neurological illness with a wide clinical spectrum including meningitis/meningoencephalitis, brain stem infection with cranial nerve involvement and cerebritis with abscess formation.

Diagnosis and treatment

In meningitic syndromes, few organisms are present in the cerebrospinal fluid (CSF), so Gram staining may be difficult. PCR and CSF cultures are positive. Blood cultures may be positive. The mainstay of treatment is ampicillin.

Brucellosis

This is caused by four species of a Gram-negative coccobacillus: *Brucella abortus*, *B. melitensis*, *B. suis* and *B. canis*. It is acquired from contact with infected animals or milk products or by inhalation of infected aerosols. The vast majority of UK infections are imported. Systemic spread leads to granuloma formation in different organs. The incubation period is 2–4 weeks. Fever, malaise, sweats and other non-specific symptoms occur; nausea, vomiting and gastrointestinal complaints are frequent; hepatosplenomegaly is common; and lymphadenopathy occurs in 20%. It may cause:

- bone and joint infection: particularly sacroiliitis and spondylitis
- respiratory infection: bronchitis and abscesses
- acute or chronic meningitis
- rarely endocarditis and genitourinary (GU) infection.

Diagnosis and management

Diagnosis requires a very high clinical suspicion because brucellosis can mimic many other diseases. The mainstay of diagnosis is culture from blood or bone marrow (which is more sensitive) but prolonged culture is necessary and laboratory staff need to be warned of the potential diagnosis as *Brucella* is highly contagious. Serology may contribute also to diagnosis.

Doxycycline is the drug of choice in combination with rifampicin or an aminoglycoside or both to prevent relapse. Treatment is for six weeks or longer in serious infection.

Tetanus

Tetanus is caused by infection with the anaerobic Gram-positive bacillus *Clostridium tetani*. Spores from soil infect a wound and germinate under anaerobic conditions, producing the toxin tetanospasmin, which is transported via neurons to the central nervous system (CNS), where it inhibits presynaptic transmitter release from inhibitory neurons, leading to muscular rigidity.

Clinical features

The incubation period is usually 1–21 days.

- **Neonatal tetanus**: common in the developing world; results from infection of the umbilical stump. Initially poor feeding, trismus and spasms; high mortality.
- **Generalized tetanus**: initially spasm of the masseter muscles causing trismus and 'risus sardonicus', gradually spreading to spasms involving the whole of the trunk and body, which can lead to arching of the back – opisthotonos. Spasms may be precipitated by noise or tactile stimuli and may be severe enough to tear muscle or break bones. Autonomic instability – arrhythmias or blood pressure changes may occur.

Diagnosis and management

Tetanus is diagnosed clinically. Human tetanus immunoglobulin is administered intramuscularly to neutralize circulating toxin. Wounds should be debrided thoroughly and metronidazole or penicillin given to eradicate the organism. Supportive care consists of benzodiazepines to reduce rigidity and spasms; ventilation may be required. Autonomic disturbances are difficult to treat and may require inotropic support or α- and β-blockade. Mortality (20%) occurs from respiratory problems or autonomic instability. Tetanus can be prevented by primary immunization and boosting with tetanus toxoid. Dirty wounds should be debrided and a booster dose given if five or more doses of toxoid have not been given previously.

Lyme disease

This is an infection with the spirochaete *Borrelia burgdorferi*, transmitted by the tick *Ixodes* sp., found on infected deer or mice. Foci of disease occur in the USA and Europe and cases are also reported in areas of Russia, China, Japan and Australia. The number of new cases has increased over the last 30 years as diagnostic methods and awareness have improved. The clinical features are the presence of a tick and/or tick bite, followed by the following stages.

- **Localized early disease** (3–30 days after tick bite): an annular lesion (erythema chronicum migrans) with central clearing usually develops at the site of the bite; present in 60–85% of all cases. Mild systemic symptoms.
- **Disseminated disease** (days to months after bite): some patients develop disseminated disease. Blood spread may lead to a fluctuating flu-like illness. Secondary skin lesions may occur. Subsequent development of arthritis occurs in 60% (monoarticular, affecting large joints), neurological symptoms in 15% (meningitis, cranial neuropathy, myelitis, painful radiculopathy) and carditis in 10% (atrioventricular block, myopericarditis). Symptoms and signs are often self-limiting.
- **Post-treatment Lyme syndrome:** patients can have symptoms of pain, fatigue, or difficulty thinking lasting for more than 6 months after completion of treatment.

Diagnosis and treatment

A clinical diagnosis of erythema chronicum migrans should prompt immediate treatment with doxycycline. Serology (IgG testing) can take several weeks to become positive but is sensitive and specific in late disease.

Early disease may be treated with oral doxycycline, amoxicillin or ceftriaxone. Cephalosporins are indicated for arthritis or neurological involvement. There is good evidence that 14–21 days of treatment is adequate and that longer courses of intravenous antibiotics do not give benefit. Treatment of disseminated disease has been shown to stop the development of new symptoms but residual tissue damage may persist.

Syphilis

Syphilis is a sexually transmitted disease caused by the spirochaete *Treponema pallidum*. Having once been rare in the UK, recent decades have seen a substantial increase in incidence across all population groups, with the disease disproportionately affecting gay, bisexual and other men who have sex with men (MSM). Organisms enter the body of a sexual partner through breaches in the skin or epithelium. *T. pallidum* is disseminated via the blood. The clinical features of syphilis, the 'great mimicker', are diverse.

- **Primary syphilis**: median incubation period of three weeks. An ulcerated, painless papule – the primary chancre – develops at the site of inoculation on the penis or cervix and labia. Painless inguinal lymphadenopathy occurs. The lesion heals spontaneously after several weeks.
- **Secondary syphilis**: 2–12 weeks later, with a generalized maculopapular rash (involving the palms and soles), generalized lymphadenopathy (50%) and condylomata lata (moist, broad, highly infectious plaques in warm intertriginous areas). Systemic symptoms include fever, headache and sore throat. Neurological involvement may occur with cranial nerve palsies (facial nerve) and meningitis. The eyes are affected in around 10% of cases, common syndromes including uveitis, keratitis and optic neuritis.
- **Latent syphilis**: symptoms and signs disappear. The only manifestation of infection is positive serology. Asymptomatic CNS infection is common.
- **Tertiary syphilis**: gummata (hard granulomatous lesions) occur after 3–10 years in many sites, including the skin, in which ulceration with damage to the underlying cartilage or connective tissue occurs. Aortitis is a rare complication which develops after 10–30 years and causes ascending aortic aneurysms. Neurosyphilis produces a wide spectrum of disease including:
    - meningovascular: 4–7 years
    - general paresis of the insane: 10–20 years
    - tabes dorsalis: 15–25 years.

Diagnosis and management

Diagnosis is made through the identification of *T. pallidum* on dark-ground microscopy of primary or secondary syphilis lesions. Serology: combination of non-treponemal tests (e.g. rapid plasma regain test) and specific treponemal antibody tests (e.g. *T. pallidum* haemagglutination test). CSF should be examined in suspected neurosyphilis; elevation of mononuclear cells and protein may occur and the rapid plasma reagin test is usually positive on CSF. Penicillin is the drug of choice; the regimen and dose depend on the stage. Alternative drugs include doxycycline and ceftriaxone. Steroids are needed to prevent the Jarisch–Herxheimer reaction (anaphylaxis to dead/dying spirochaetes) after treatment in late syphilis. Contacts should be traced and treated.

169 Malaria

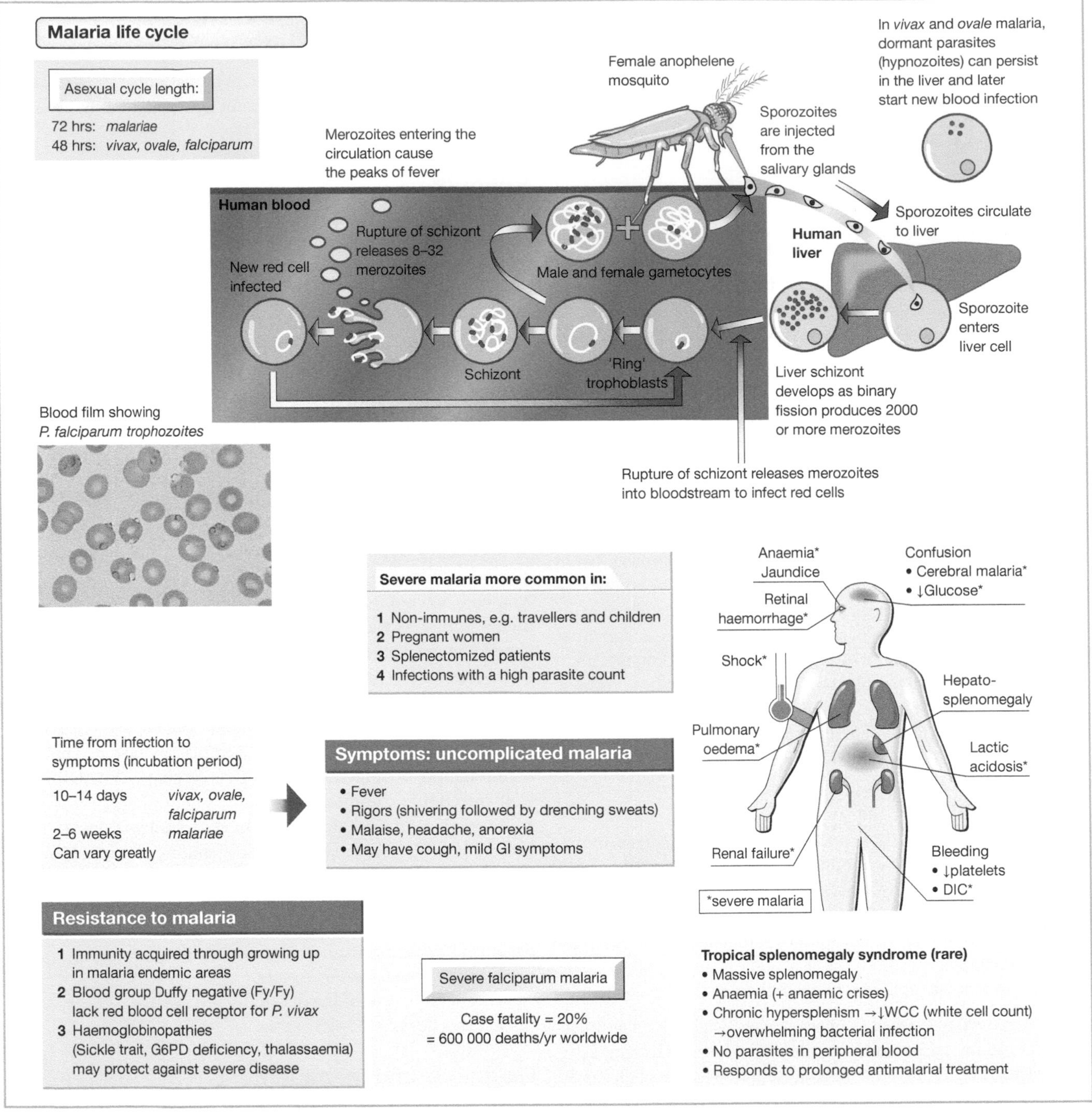

Malaria life cycle
Asexual cycle length:
72 hrs: malariae
48 hrs: vivax, ovale, falciparum
Female anophelene mosquito
In vivax and ovale malaria, dormant parasites (hypnozoites) can persist in the liver and later start new blood infection
Merozoites entering the circulation cause the peaks of fever
Sporozoites are injected from the salivary glands
Human blood
Rupture of schizont releases 8–32 merozoites
Sporozoites circulate to liver
Human liver
New red cell infected
Male and female gametocytes
Sporozoite enters liver cell
Schizont
'Ring' trophoblasts
Liver schizont develops as binary fission produces 2000 or more merozoites
Blood film showing P. falciparum trophozoites
Rupture of schizont releases merozoites into bloodstream to infect red cells
Severe malaria more common in:
1 Non-immunes, e.g. travellers and children
2 Pregnant women
3 Splenectomized patients
4 Infections with a high parasite count
Anaemia*
Jaundice
Confusion
• Cerebral malaria*
• ↓Glucose*
Retinal haemorrhage*
Shock*
Hepato-splenomegaly
Pulmonary oedema*
Lactic acidosis*
Time from infection to symptoms (incubation period)
10–14 days vivax, ovale, falciparum
2–6 weeks malariae
Can vary greatly
Symptoms: uncomplicated malaria
• Fever
• Rigors (shivering followed by drenching sweats)
• Malaise, headache, anorexia
• May have cough, mild GI symptoms
Renal failure*
Bleeding
• ↓platelets
• DIC*
*severe malaria
Resistance to malaria
1 Immunity acquired through growing up in malaria endemic areas
2 Blood group Duffy negative (Fy/Fy) lack red blood cell receptor for P. vivax
3 Haemoglobinopathies (Sickle trait, G6PD deficiency, thalassaemia) may protect against severe disease
Severe falciparum malaria
Case fatality = 20%
= 600 000 deaths/yr worldwide
Tropical splenomegaly syndrome (rare)
• Massive splenomegaly
• Anaemia (+ anaemic crises)
• Chronic hypersplenism →↓WCC (white cell count) →overwhelming bacterial infection
• No parasites in peripheral blood
• Responds to prolonged antimalarial treatment

Epidemiology

Malaria is primarily a disease of the tropics and subtropics, but it is also the most common imported infection in the UK. It is still estimated to cause more than half a million deaths per year worldwide, particularly in children in sub-Saharan Africa. In highly endemic areas, malaria mainly causes morbidity and mortality in children, but where transmission is less intense it is a disease of both adults and children. The severity of clinical illness is highly modified by the degree of immunity of an individual. Malaria in an expatriate traveller is far more likely to be life-threatening than in someone who has grown up in an endemic malarial area.

Medicine at a Glance, Fifth Edition. Edited by Patrick Davey and Alex Pitcher.

Companion website: www.wiley.com/go/medicine5e

Pathogenesis

Malaria is a protozoal infection transmitted by the bite of the mosquito *Anopheles* spp. Injected sporozoites initially multiply in the liver and then invade red blood cells. Classically, four species of *Plasmodium* infect humans: *P. falciparum*, *P. vivax*, *P. ovale* and *P. malariae*; a primate parasite, *P. knowlesi*, has also been shown to cause zoonotic cases in parts of Asia. *P. ovale* and *P. vivax* have forms that remain dormant in the liver for a number of years ('hypnozoites') and cause subsequent relapsing infection. *P. falciparum* is the main cause of severe disease as a result of its ability to infect red blood cells of all ages, and most critically to 'sequester', i.e. adhere to vascular endothelium in vital organs such as the brain, liver, kidneys and muscles, leading to multiorgan failure.

Clinical features

The incubation period for *P. falciparum* is typically 10–42 days, but is highly variable for other species. Prophylaxis may delay onset of symptoms with *P. falciparum*. The predominant symptoms are:

- malaise, headache, fever and rigors
- occasionally gastrointestinal (GI) or respiratory symptoms dominate, making the clinical diagnosis difficult.

Irregular fever occurs in the acute stages of malaria; classic periodic fever tends only to occur in untreated non-*falciparum* malaria. Examination is often unremarkable apart from mild hepatosplenomegaly. Malaria does not cause rashes, although patients with rashes from other causes, e.g. drugs, may have malaria.

Severe malaria

P. falciparum causes the vast majority of severe malaria cases; case fatality rates may be 20% or higher.

- **Cerebral malaria**: coma, often with seizures. Risk of long-term damage in adults, with a greater risk in children (hemiplegia, cortical blindness, mental handicap).
- **Severe anaemia**: due to haemolysis and a depressed marrow response.
- **Respiratory distress**: particularly prominent in children, associated with acidosis and sometimes with severe anaemia.
- **Hypoglycaemia**: as a result of increased glucose consumption, impaired gluconeogenesis and quinine-induced hyperinsulinaemia.
- **Acute renal failure**: multifactorial in origin. Rare in children. Rarely, 'blackwater' fever occurs: intravascular haemolysis, producing haemoglobinuria and deep jaundice. Dialysis is needed in 10% of cases of severe malaria.
- **Jaundice**: caused by haemolysis and hepatic dysfunction, particularly in adults.
- **Disseminated intravascular coagulation** (DIC; see Chapter 186).
- **Non-cardiogenic pulmonary oedema/ARDS** (adult respiratory distress syndrome), which can be life-threatening.
- **Shock** ('algid malaria'): concomitant Gram-negative bacteraemia is common.

Diagnosis

Malaria films

The gold standard of diagnosis is the demonstration of malaria trophozoites on a blood film using stains such as Giemsa or Field.

- Thick blood films are used to screen for the presence of parasites.
- Thin films demonstrate detail of parasites, allowing determination of the species.

Patients may have a low parasite burden, especially if malaria prophylaxis has been used. Repeated thick blood films may be needed to make the diagnosis.

Lateral flow tests

Commercial rapid diagnostic lateral flow tests require less expertise to perform and provide a result in a few minutes. Most kits have a band for detection of the PfHRP2 antigen (specific to *P. falciparum*) and a separate band for detection of LDH from all human malaria species, thereby allowing differentiation of *P. falciparum* from non-*falciparum* malaria. Following treatment of *falciparum* malaria with artemisinin-based combination therapies (ACT), the test often remains positive for several weeks (despite negative blood films) due to circulation of once-infected red cells containing residual PfHRP2.

Other tests

Even in uncomplicated malaria, the platelet count is almost invariably low (although rarely associated with bleeding).

Differential diagnosis

Uncomplicated malaria needs to be distinguished from the long list of tropical and non-tropical diseases that can cause a fever (see Chapter 43). The differential diagnosis of cerebral malaria includes bacterial, viral and fungal meningitis, arbovirus and other viral causes of encephalitis, and non-infectious causes of coma.

Treatment and management

Treatment of malaria depends on the malaria species.

- **Uncomplicated *P. falciparum***: first-line treatment is artemisinin-containing combination therapy (ACT) for children and adults including pregnant women at all trimesters, which is generally given over three days. Alternatives include oral quinine and doxycycline for seven days, mefloquine and atovaquone-proguanil.
- **Severe *P. falciparum* infection**: parenteral therapy should be given to those with severe malaria or in high-risk subgroups (parasitaemia >2% and pregnancy). Parenteral artesunate is now the first-line drug of choice in both adults and children, being superior to quinine. A full course of ACT should always follow initial doses of artesunate. Supportive care is crucial, including careful fluid balance that avoids pulmonary oedema. Hypoglycaemia is common, and should be anticipated. Exchange transfusion in severe malaria can be considered when there are high parasite counts, although there is no proven benefit.
- ***P. ovale*, *P. vivax*, *P. malaria* and *P. knowlesi***: these infections can be treated with chloroquine or ACT, to eliminate red blood cell infection. Primaquine is required for *P. vivax* and *P. ovale* malaria to eliminate hepatic forms. Glucose-6-phosphate dehydrogenase (G6PD) status should be checked before prescribing primaquine to avoid primaquine-induced haemolysis.

Course and prognosis

Most patients become afebrile and aparasitaemic within 2–3 days. There is a significant case fatality rate from severe malaria, especially in non-immune patients. Antimalarials must be continued for their full course; if inadequate treatment courses are given or if parasites are partially resistant to the drug, then recrudescence of infection can occur.

Preventing infection

Avoid mosquito bites by physical measures: long-sleeved shirts and trousers, mosquito nets, insect repellents, etc. Chemoprophylaxis against *P. falciparum* infection is highly effective (although never 100%); atovaquone-proguanil, doxycycline and mefloquine are generally effective globally (chloroquine is ineffective in most areas due to resistance). In South-east Asia and increasing areas of Africa, *P. falciparum* shows extensive resistance to antimalarial drugs and specialist advice is necessary.

170 Tuberculosis

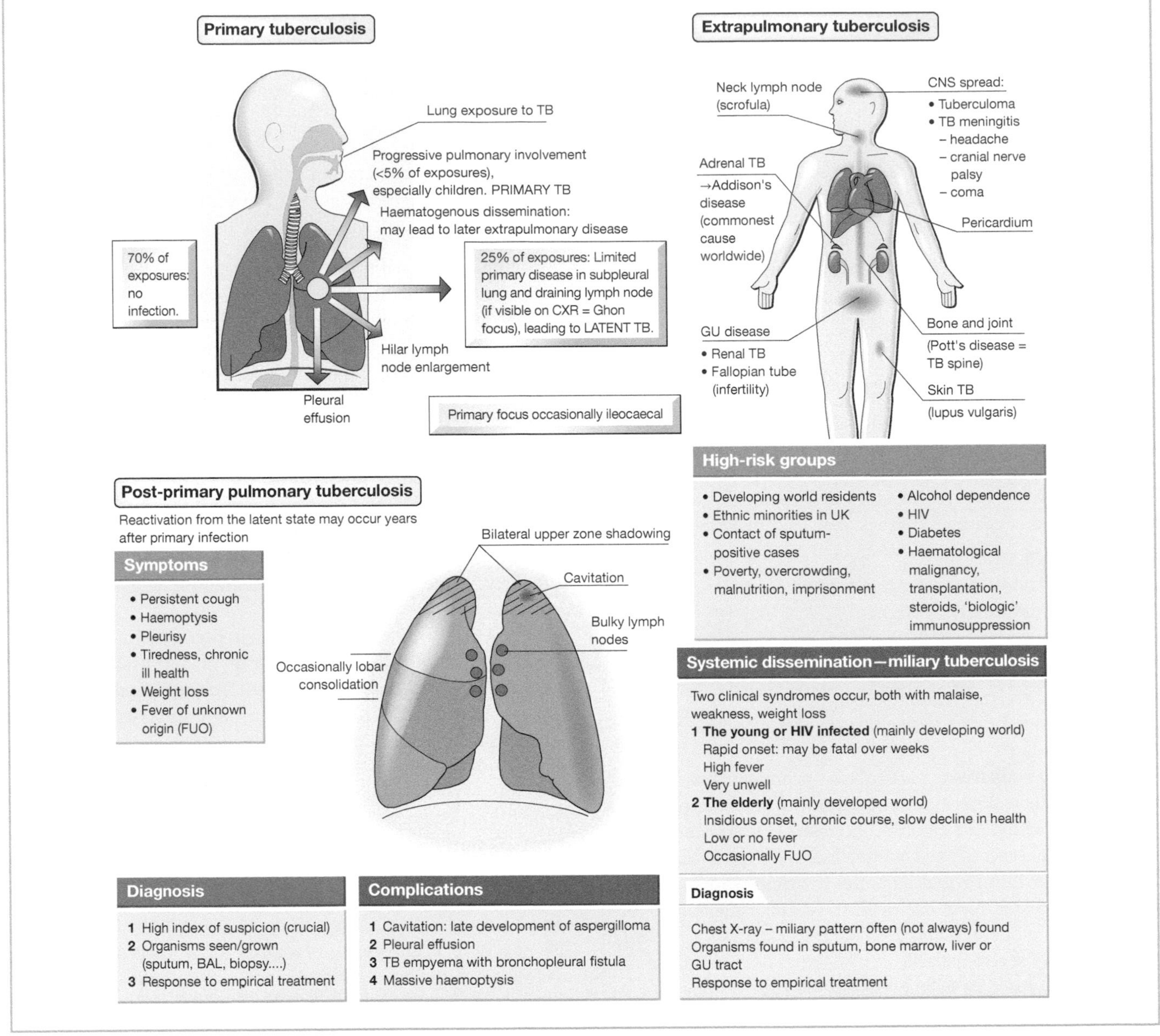

Primary tuberculosis
Lung exposure to TB
Progressive pulmonary involvement (<5% of exposures), especially children. PRIMARY TB
Haematogenous dissemination: may lead to later extrapulmonary disease
70% of exposures: no infection.
25% of exposures: Limited primary disease in subpleural lung and draining lymph node (if visible on CXR = Ghon focus), leading to LATENT TB.
Hilar lymph node enlargement
Pleural effusion
Primary focus occasionally ileocaecal
Extrapulmonary tuberculosis
Neck lymph node (scrofula)
CNS spread:
• Tuberculoma
• TB meningitis
– headache
– cranial nerve palsy
– coma
Adrenal TB →Addison's disease (commonest cause worldwide)
Pericardium
GU disease
• Renal TB
• Fallopian tube (infertility)
Bone and joint (Pott's disease = TB spine)
Skin TB (lupus vulgaris)
High-risk groups
• Developing world residents
• Ethnic minorities in UK
• Contact of sputum-positive cases
• Poverty, overcrowding, malnutrition, imprisonment
• Alcohol dependence
• HIV
• Diabetes
• Haematological malignancy, transplantation, steroids, 'biologic' immunosuppression
Post-primary pulmonary tuberculosis
Reactivation from the latent state may occur years after primary infection
Symptoms
• Persistent cough
• Haemoptysis
• Pleurisy
• Tiredness, chronic ill health
• Weight loss
• Fever of unknown origin (FUO)
Bilateral upper zone shadowing
Cavitation
Bulky lymph nodes
Occasionally lobar consolidation
Systemic dissemination – miliary tuberculosis
Two clinical syndromes occur, both with malaise, weakness, weight loss
1 The young or HIV infected (mainly developing world)
Rapid onset: may be fatal over weeks
High fever
Very unwell
2 The elderly (mainly developed world)
Insidious onset, chronic course, slow decline in health
Low or no fever
Occasionally FUO
Diagnosis
Chest X-ray – miliary pattern often (not always) found
Organisms found in sputum, bone marrow, liver or GU tract
Response to empirical treatment
Diagnosis
1 High index of suspicion (crucial)
2 Organisms seen/grown (sputum, BAL, biopsy....)
3 Response to empirical treatment
Complications
1 Cavitation: late development of aspergilloma
2 Pleural effusion
3 TB empyema with bronchopleural fistula
4 Massive haemoptysis

Tuberculosis (TB) remains the cause of over 1.5 million deaths per year, a figure somewhat lower than that seen at the millennium. Most infection occurs in tropical regions but there are also a significant number of infections in Europe and the USA, often in poorer, homeless populations and in HIV-infected patients. The HIV pandemic caused a huge global increase in cases, particularly in sub-Saharan Africa. The emergence of multidrug-resistant (MDR) and extensively drug-resistant (XDR) TB is a major challenge to global control.

Epidemiology

Mycobacterium tuberculosis is spread by respiratory droplets; transmission occurs from close proximity to an infected individual. Household contacts of patients with *M. tuberculosis* in their sputum have a one in four chance of becoming infected. Clinical disease develops in 5–15% of those infected; this risk is higher in HIV.

Pathogenesis

Following inhalation of organisms, multiplication occurs in subpleural and midzone terminal airspaces. Bacteria ingested by alveolar macrophages survive and spread to local lymph nodes. Bloodstream spread occurs to the lung apices and other organs, where latent infection may persist for many years. The slow development of a cellular immune response leads to tuberculous granulomata in tissues and cutaneous hypersensitivity to mycobacterial antigens.

Primary infection

Exposure occurs in childhood in endemic areas, but in later life in most western regions. The immune response limits damage to a localized area of the lung with hilar node involvement, termed the primary or Ghon focus; calcification may subsequently be visible on a chest X-ray (CXR). Clinical disease is rare at the time of primary infection in adolescents and adults, although primary pulmonary TB does occur.

Pulmonary TB

Eighty percent of TB used to be pulmonary, but the proportion of extrapulmonary disease is increasing and is over 50% in HIV patients. Most cases are the result of reactivation; reinfection also occurs. The major symptoms are cough, weight loss, malaise, fever and night sweats. Haemoptysis occurs in a third. Examination is often unremarkable. The CXR is usually abnormal – classically, apical disease with infiltration and cavitation that heals with fibrotic changes. Complications include severe haemoptysis, bronchopleural fistula and aspergilloma within cavities.

Extrapulmonary disease

- **Pleural TB**: commonly occurs after primary infection. There are systemic symptoms, cough and pleuritic pain. Unilateral effusions are common. Often self-limiting, sometimes with resolution of symptoms. Most develop active disease within three years.
- **Lymph node TB**: occurs after primary infection, reactivation and contiguous spread. Cervical in 70%. Systemic symptoms occur in 30–60%. Painless discrete nodes enlarge in size and become matted. Nodes eventually break down with discharging sinuses and chronic skin lesions.
- **Bone/joint TB**: affects any bone or joint. Most common form is spinal (Pott disease). Vertebral destruction leads to collapse and, sometimes, severe angulation of the spine (gibbus). Paravertebral abscesses may occur. Watch for cord compression; most can be treated medically.
- **TB meningitis**: typically presents with the insidious development of fever, vomiting and headache (often without neck stiffness), symptoms which continue for several weeks before complications start to develop. During this period, patients often seek medical help but are reassured as they 'look well' and general blood tests are normal (although sodium is often low due to SIADH). Hence a high index of suspicion is needed and the diagnosis needs to be considered when any patient with a high epidemiological risk of TB experiences the above symptoms for more than a few days, as lumbar puncture can quickly demonstrate (or rule out) classic CSF findings (lymphocytic meningitis, high protein, very low glucose).
- **Complications of TB meningitis** include cranial nerve palsies (independent of or secondary to hydrocephalus), papilloedema and brainstem stroke, all due to the basal distribution of TB meningitis. Seizures are common in children and can also be seen in the distinct tuberculomatous form of cerebral infection. Mortality is high if the diagnosis has been delayed.
- **Pericardial TB**: usually caused by spread from the lungs or mediastinal lymph nodes. There are three clinical syndromes: acute pericarditis ± effusion, chronic pericardial effusion and chronic constrictive pericarditis. Systemic symptoms, shortness of breath and signs of effusion or constriction occur; tamponade due to effusion may occur. Pericardial calcification (late) on CXR may be seen in constrictive pericarditis. Echocardiography is helpful.
- **Miliary TB**: disseminated disease from haematogenous spread in those with underlying chronic disease or immunosuppression. Insidious symptoms: weight loss, fever, malaise. Pulmonary, central nervous system (CNS) and liver involvement are most frequent. Choroidal tubercles (15%) are pathognomonic. Classic CXR; multiple 1–2 mm nodules in lung fields.

Diagnosis

Definitive diagnosis depends upon demonstrating or culturing the organism.

- **Pulmonary TB** is normally diagnosed by 1) Ziehl–Neelsen staining of acid-fast bacilli (AFB) in the sputum and 2) culture of samples on selective media (takes up to eight weeks).
- **Open TB** describes the presence of AFB in sputum.
- **Extrapulmonary TB**: sputum culture is occasionally positive, but the diagnosis is usually made from the culture of appropriate samples (needle aspiration of lymph node or marrow and liver biopsy in miliary TB) or by histology (pleural or pericardial biopsy) showing granulomata or AFB. Classic X-ray changes (in Pott disease) may be diagnostic. The CSF in TB meningitis (lymphocytes, high protein, low sugar) likewise may be highly suggestive. Polymerase chain reaction (PCR) techniques are increasingly used to make a more rapid diagnosis and assessment of rifampicin resistance. Whole-genome sequencing on cultured isolates reduces the time taken to confirm sensitivity to the standard range of antituberculous drugs.
- **Tuberculin skin test (Mantoux)**: measures the delayed hypersensitivity reaction to intradermal purified protein derivative. Positive tests indicate previous exposure; they do not confirm active disease. Anergy occurs in systemic illness such as miliary TB, and immunosuppression can also obtund the response. In the UK, patients may react because of previous BCG (bacille Calmette–Guérin) immunization.
- **Interferon γ release assays** also indicate exposure rather than active disease; they are used in clinical practice to test for latent TB in individual patients prior to planned immunosuppression, or for screening of recent migrants (e.g. employment, refugee health programmes). Unlike tuberculin skin tests, they are unaffected by previous BCG.

Treatment

Short-course chemotherapy (6 months) is given for most TB using 1) **isoniazid** (side-effects of liver toxicity, neuropathy prevented by vitamin B6); 2) **rifampicin** (liver reactions, drug interactions); longer courses are needed for TB meningitis and miliary TB. A combination of four drugs is used to ensure a high cure rate, with 2 drugs added for the first 2 months, **pyrazinamide** (liver reactions), and **ethambutol** (retrobulbar neuritis, so check colour vision before and during treatment). The clinical response to therapy is important in confirming the diagnosis; reductions in fever, and weight gain are helpful markers. Steroids are of benefit in pericardial disease and TB meningitis.

Resistance to individual TB drugs is a major problem, and isolates that are resistant to multiple drugs are associated with higher mortality (multidrug resistant [MDR] = resistance to rifampicin and isoniazid; extensively resistant [XDR] = additional resistance to a fluoroquinolone and at least one of three injectable second-line drugs). The risk of MDR-TB is increased in patients who have had previous treatment, contact with resistant disease or who are from the prison population, and those from China, India, Pakistan, a number of former Soviet states and several African countries. Prolonged treatment for at least 18 months is necessary, involving a more complex array of second and third-line agents.

Surgery is sometimes needed for Pott disease (spinal TB) if there is severe cord compression or spinal instability. Surgery can also be indicated in chronic constrictive pericarditis and for extensive pulmonary cavitatory disease.

Infection control issues need to be considered; those with smear-positive TB should be isolated for the first two weeks of treatment and if factors suggest the possibility of MDR-TB (previous TB treatment or birth in a foreign country), special precautions must be taken.

Tropical infectious diseases

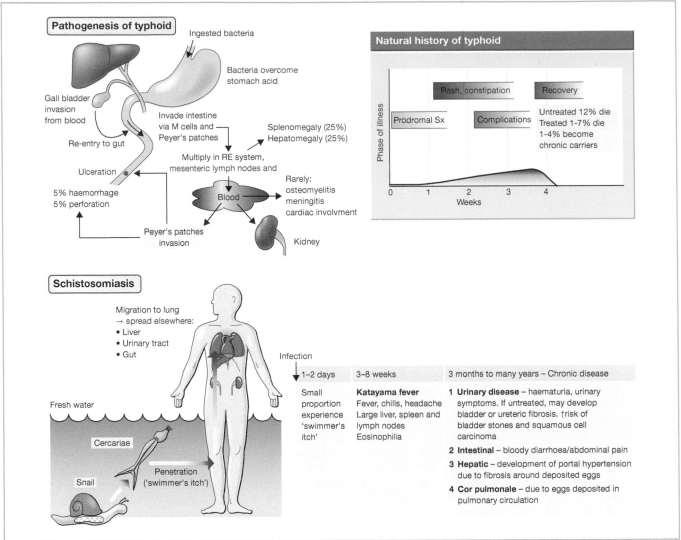

Pathogenesis of typhoid

Ingested bacteria
Bacteria overcome stomach acid
Gall bladder invasion from blood
Re-entry to gut
Invade intestine via M cells and Peyer's patches
Splenomegaly (25%)
Hepatomegaly (25%)
Multiply in RE system, mesenteric lymph nodes and
Ulceration
5% haemorrhage
5% perforation
Blood
Rarely: osteomyelitis meningitis cardiac involvment
Peyer's patches invasion
Kidney

Natural history of typhoid

Phase of illness
Prodromal Sx
Rash, constipation
Complications
Recovery
Untreated 12% die
Treated 1-7% die
1-4% become chronic carriers
0 1 2 3 4
Weeks

Schistosomiasis

Migration to lung → spread elsewhere:
• Liver
• Urinary tract
• Gut
Fresh water
Cercariae
Snail
Penetration ('swimmer's itch')
Infection

1–2 days	3–8 weeks	3 months to many years – Chronic disease
Small proportion experience 'swimmer's itch'	**Katayama fever** Fever, chills, headache Large liver, spleen and lymph nodes Eosinophilia	1 **Urinary disease** – haematuria, urinary symptoms. If untreated, may develop bladder or ureteric fibrosis. ↑risk of bladder stones and squamous cell carcinoma 2 **Intestinal** – bloody diarrhoea/abdominal pain 3 **Hepatic** – development of portal hypertension due to fibrosis around deposited eggs 4 **Cor pulmonale** – due to eggs deposited in pulmonary circulation

Enteric fever

Enteric fever occurs from infection with the Gram-negative bacteria *Salmonella typhi* or *S. paratyphi* through ingestion of contaminated food or water. The bacteria enter through the gut, multiply within the mesenteric lymph nodes and macrophages and enter the bloodstream to be disseminated to many sites where further replication occurs.

Clinical features

The incubation period is 10–14 days. There is a gradually rising fever, reaching 39–40 °C at the end of the first week of symptoms, which also include abdominal pain and altered bowel habit (constipation or diarrhoea) and headache, malaise and a dry cough. Examination may reveal tender hepatosplenomegaly, abdominal distension and a diffuse abdominal tenderness. Classically, the heart rate is relatively low compared to the high fever. Rose spots (erythematous maculopapular lesions on the trunk) are sometimes reported. Later complications of untreated disease include encephalopathy, intestinal perforation or bleeding, colitis and finally shock. Rare complications include osteomyelitis (more common in sickle cell disease), cholecystitis and myocarditis.

Diagnosis

Leukopenia is common and elevated transaminases may occur. Enteric fever is most commonly confirmed by positive blood culture (bone marrow is more sensitive but rarely performed); positive culture from stool may indicate carriage rather than disease. Serology (Widal's test) is rarely helpful, even in non-immunized cases.

Treatment

Resistance to previous mainstays of treatment (chloramphenicol, co-trimoxazole, ciprofloxacin or ampicillin) is now very common, with rates of resistance to fluoroquinolones particularly high in South Asia. Oral azithromycin is first-line empirical treatment for non-severe disease, with ceftriaxone used for severe disease (oral switch can be guided by sensitivities). Complete resolution of fever takes at least five days so the presence of fever for up to a week is not necessarily an indication to change treatments. Steroids can be considered when there are severe complications. Relapse occurs in 10%. Long-term asymptomatic carriage may occur from persistence of the organism in the gall bladder (1–4%). Isolation of cases is necessary.

Dengue

Dengue is caused by an arbovirus transmitted by the mosquito *Aedes* sp.; it is increasingly common as its geographical distribution expands. Two main clinical syndromes occur. 1) Dengue fever, seen mostly in travellers. 2) Dengue haemorrhagic fever/dengue shock syndrome (DHF/ DSS), usually seen in children in endemic areas as a result of an immunological response to a second infection.

Clinical features (3–8-day incubation)

These are sudden fever, severe headache, backache, muscle pains and rigors. Fever may be biphasic, i.e. it disappears then reappears. Maculopapular rash occurs late on in the illness. In DHF/ DSS (rare in the UK) increased vascular permeability results in shock, petechiae and bleeding.

Diagnosis and treatment

Leukopenia and thrombocytopenia are common. In DHF/DSS, severe thrombocytopenia, raised haematocrit and abnormal liver enzymes are found. Diagnosis is clinical because virus isolation is not routinely available. Serology is useful for retrospective diagnosis.

No specific treatment is available. DHF/DSS requires supportive therapy and fluids and has a high case fatality.

Schistosomiasis

More than two hundred million people are infected worldwide and it is common in returned travellers, although patients are rarely systemically unwell. Schistosomal cerceriae penetrate the skin after freshwater exposure and migrate via the lungs to the vessels of the bladder or gut (depending on the species), where eggs are produced. Eggs migrate back into the gut lumen or urinary tract, where they cause local inflammation. Worm burdens are low in expatriates, in whom severe disease is rare. The clinical features of disease are as follows.

- **Swimmer's itch**: transient rash 1–2 days after exposure, often unrecognized.
- **Katayama fever**: 3–8 weeks after exposure in a small proportion of patients. Acute fever, sweats, malaise – sometimes lymphadenopathy, hepatosplenomegaly or bronchospasm; it is self-limiting.
- **Urinary schistosomiasis** (*Schistosoma haematobium*): often asymptomatic and diagnosed because of eosinophilia. May have haematuria, urinary symptoms or altered ejaculate. Long-term complications are unusual in travellers.
- **Intestinal/hepatic schistosomiasis**: vague abdominal symptoms/bloody diarrhoea or asymptomatic. The long-term complication of non-cirrhotic portal hypertension is rare in travellers, but is very common worldwide.

Diagnosis and treatment

Diagnosis is supported by eosinophilia and demonstration of eggs in urine, ejaculate, stool or rectal/bladder biopsies. Schistosomal serology is useful, but may not be positive until several months after exposure. **Praziquantel** is effective for all species.

Rickettsial/other tick-borne infections

A wide range of Rickettsiae and other arthropod-borne zoonoses can affect travellers, particularly those spending time in rural areas. Consideration of these infections is particularly important given their intrinsic resistance to penicillins. Most typically cause fever, myalgia, headache and maculopapular rash.

African tick typhus is the most common rickettsial disease seen in the UK, and presents with an eschar (black scab due to necrosis at the tick bite) which confirms the diagnosis; there is usually lymphadenopathy localized to the region of the eschar but severe systemic illness is rare. **Scrub typhus** is a more severe rickettsial disease found in many Asian countries and parts of Australia; it is transmitted by mites living in vegetation, so is typically acquired after adventurous hiking trips involving sections of dense undergrowth. The key clinical features are eschar (sometimes in non-exposed parts of the body), rash and fever. **Mediterranean spotted fever** is a tick-borne infection with many of the same features and is acquired in southern Europe (France and Iberian peninsula). **Rocky Mountain spotted fever**, from the United States, is also tick-borne and can cause severe illness (but no eschar). **Tularaemia** is a distantly related bacterial infection acquired by several routes in rural areas of northern Europe and North America.

Diagnosis and treatment

Doxycycline is extremely effective as treatment; indeed, a clinical response to empirical doxycycline, particularly when standard antibiotics (e.g. pencillins) have failed, provides strong evidence for a rickettsial (or related bacterial) disease. Retrospective serological confirmation of infection is possible but usually takes weeks to achieve in practice.

Leptospirosis

This occurs after contact with water infected by animal urine containing leptospires. It may be contracted in the UK (sewer workers, river/ lake swimming) and is common in many parts of the tropics. Leptospires penetrate the skin and mucosa, multiply in the blood and then localize in the liver, central nervous system, muscle and renal cortex.

Clinical features

There is a wide spectrum of illness from fever, headache and muscle pains to severe sepsis with conjunctivitis, pneumonitis, jaundice, renal failure and extensive haemorrhages.

Diagnosis and treatment

Leukocytosis and thrombocytopenia are common. Creatine kinase is elevated in moderate or severe cases. There is abnormal liver function and renal function. Clinical suspicion may be confirmed by identification of leptospires on dark-ground microscopy of the blood. Serology gives retrospective diagnosis. Some cases of leptospirosis are clearly self-limiting. For mild disease doxycycline and azithromycin are effective. Severe disease necessitates intravenous antibiotics (usually penicillin or ceftriaxone).

Viral haemorrhagic fevers

Viral haemorrhagic fevers (VHF) are caused by a number of different RNA viruses, are predominantly zoonoses and occur on every continent apart from Australia. Diseases include Ebola, Marburg, Lassa fever, yellow fever, Hanta and Crimean-Congo haemorrhagic fever.

Although uncommon, high mortality and potential for transmission to others mean that such fevers should be considered in sick patients returning from the tropics. In the UK, the Advisory Committee on Dangerous Pathogens (ACDP) algorithm provides a practical framework for considering whether a patient might have such a disease (by considering ongoing outbreaks and risk factors for acquisition such as contact with healthcare facilities and exposure to rural environments, ticks or certain animals). Clinically, VHFs present with fever, severe myalgia and increasing prostration. Pharyngitis is prominent in Lassa fever. Petechiae and bleeding gums may progress to shock and frank haemorrhage.

Diagnosis and treatment

All samples need to be treated with appropriate precautions. Severe malaria is the major differential diagnosis and must be excluded urgently. Diagnosis of VHF is by viral PCR or serology. Patients with suspected VHF are isolated until the diagnosis has been excluded. Ribavirin is often used in Lassa fever while monoclonal antibody treatment reduces mortality in Ebola. Supportive care is crucial.

172 Diseases predisposing to infection

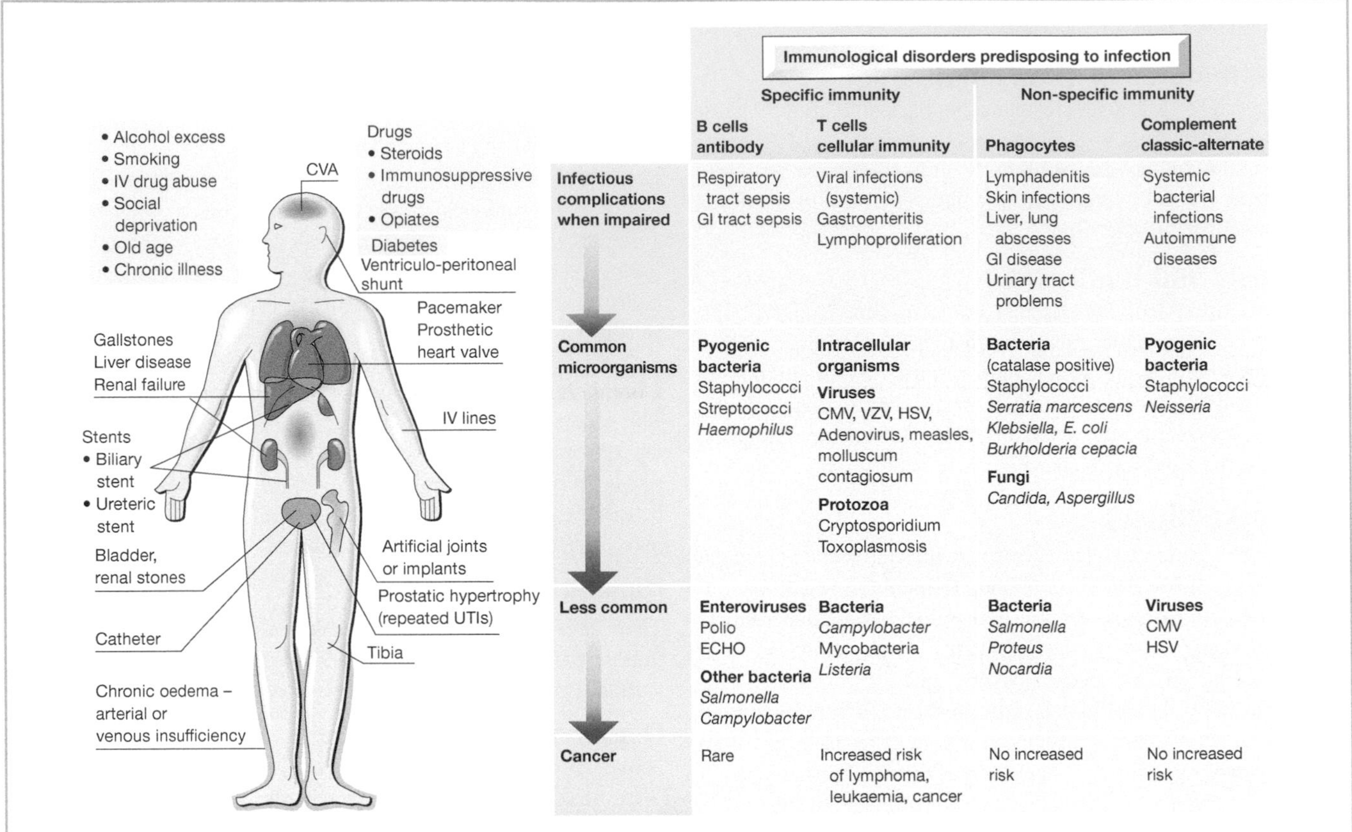

	Specific immunity		Non-specific immunity	
	B cells antibody	**T cells cellular immunity**	**Phagocytes**	**Complement classic-alternate**
Infectious complications when impaired	Respiratory tract sepsis GI tract sepsis	Viral infections (systemic) Gastroenteritis Lymphoproliferation	Lymphadenitis Skin infections Liver, lung abscesses GI disease Urinary tract problems	Systemic bacterial infections Autoimmune diseases
Common microorganisms	**Pyogenic bacteria** Staphylococci Streptococci *Haemophilus*	**Intracellular organisms** **Viruses** CMV, VZV, HSV, Adenovirus, measles, molluscum contagiosum **Protozoa** Cryptosporidium Toxoplasmosis	**Bacteria** (catalase positive) Staphylococci *Serratia marcescens* *Klebsiella, E. coli* *Burkholderia cepacia* **Fungi** *Candida, Aspergillus*	**Pyogenic bacteria** Staphylococci *Neisseria*
Less common	**Enteroviruses** Polio ECHO **Other bacteria** *Salmonella* *Campylobacter*	**Bacteria** *Campylobacter* Mycobacteria *Listeria*	**Bacteria** *Salmonella* *Proteus* *Nocardia*	**Viruses** CMV HSV
Cancer	Rare	Increased risk of lymphoma, leukaemia, cancer	No increased risk	No increased risk

Abnormalities of host immunity predispose to:

- unusually severe infection
- infection in unusual sites
- recurrent infection
- infection with unusual pathogens, or organisms not usually regarded as pathogenic.

In a patient with any of the above, a search for diseases that alter immunity is crucial. The type of pathogen, site and extent of infection sometimes help to identify the underlying disease.

Diseases predisposing to infections with common bacterial pathogens

- Diabetes mellitus predisposes to infection, which may be recurrent or more severe in most tissues, especially the lung, urinary tract and soft tissues (particularly the feet).
- Renal failure is a potent factor predisposing to infection. Not only does uraemia impair immunity, but those with renal failure also have recurrent instrumentation (particularly dialysis lines) which introduces infection. Infective endocarditis, often caused by *Staphyloccoccus aureus*, occurs annually in 0.1% of the dialysis population. The nephrotic syndrome predisposes even more powerfully to infection, possibly as the renal protein loss includes IgG and some complement proteins, although not IgM.
- Chronic liver disease impairs immunity (e.g. bacterial uptake by the reticuloendothelial system), and contributes to infection in those with chronic alcohol dependence, as well as other forms of chronic hepatitis.
- Steroid therapy, especially in high dose, impairs immunity and, although it may lead to unusual infections, more frequently infection is with common pathogens (e.g. pneumococci, herpes zoster, etc.). The same is true for many other drugs that impair immunity, such as azathioprine, cyclophosphamide, ciclosporin A, etc. Anticonvulsants impair antibody synthesis and cause secondary hypogammaglobulinaemia.
- Chronic inflammatory illness itself also impairs immunity. For example, patients with active rheumatoid arthritis, Crohn's disease or disseminated malignancy have impaired nutritional status, producing hypoalbuminaemia and hypogammaglobulinaemia.

Structural factors predisposing to infection

- Structural abnormalities should be considered in repeated infections of the same structure, e.g. bladder and renal stones or prostatic hypertrophy may cause recurrent urinary tract infections

Medicine at a Glance, Fifth Edition. Edited by Patrick Davey and Alex Pitcher.

Companion website: www.wiley.com/go/medicine5e

(UTIs). An obstructing bronchial carcinoma may underlie recurrent/severe pneumonia. Lymphoedema predisposes to cellulitis.

- Prosthetic implant infection is a growing problem in resource-rich settings given the increasing prevalence of joint replacement, permanent pacemaker, vascular grafts, etc. (see Chapters 43 & 44). Niduses of infection form on prosthetic material and cause persistent/recurrent local complications or spread to produce bacteraemia/septicaemia. Typical bacterial pathogens such as staphylococci and streptococci may be involved, although infection can also be with relatively indolent bacteria, e.g. *Staphylococcus epidermidis*, *Enterococcus faecalis*, etc. Once colonized by certain bacteria (staphylococci) or yeast (*Candida*), prosthetic material can rarely be sterilized because of 'biofilm' formation, and usually needs to be **removed or exchanged**. Prosthetic valve endocarditis carries a mortality of approximately 25%.
- The impact of prosthetic infections is particularly high in immunosuppressed or otherwise vulnerable patients, e.g. prosthetic joint infection in patients with rheumatoid arthritis on long-term immunosuppression, VP shunt infection in patients with neurological illness.
- Stroke is unfortunately frequently complicated by pneumonia, particularly in its acute phase, although this can be reduced by protocols that screen for swallowing difficulty and modify oral intake accordingly. Urinary tract infection is also a significant problem.
- Many long-term neurological illnesses are associated with respiratory infection, including multiple sclerosis, myasthenia gravis and motor neuron disease. Patients with paraplegia do not experience the pain of conditions like appendicitis or soft tissue infection so tend only to present when systemic features of their infection become prominent.
- Gastroenterological pathology such as dysphagia (especially if the result of neurological disease) or gastro-oesophageal reflux can underlie recurrent pneumonia.
- Lack of a spleen (congenital, traumatic, elective removal) or poor splenic function (e.g. in coeliac disease) predisposes to overwhelming sepsis with encapsulated organisms (*Pneumococcus*, *Haemophilus*).

Miscellaneous conditions

- Opiate dependence lowers immunity and is a risk factor for systemic bacterial infections, including pneumonia. In addition, people who inject drugs are at risk from blood-borne viruses (particularly hepatitis C) and a range of injection-related bacterial infections including skin abscess, septic thrombophlebitis, endocarditis (right- or left-sided), septic pulmonary embolism leading to lung abscess, and osteomyelitis.
- Alcohol excess, even in the absence of chronic liver disease, predisposes to many infections, particularly those involving the respiratory tract, e.g. pneumococcal pneumonia and tuberculosis (TB).
- Smoking has a clear role in repeated respiratory tract infections.
- People experiencing homelessness are at risk of a range of infections associated with the physical and social challenges they face, including pneumonia, TB and sexually transmitted infections.
- Cachexia impairs the ability of the body to fight infection and underlies infections in terminal illness. Milder degrees of malnutrition, such as those relating to undiagnosed inflammatory or neoplastic illness, social deprivation or psychiatric illness, are relatively easy to miss and can underlie some repeated infections. Iron is essential to host defence and iron deficiency increases infection risk.
- Immobility predisposes to UTIs because a low fluid intake (deliberate, to avoid unnecessary visits to the toilet) fails to 'flush' the urinary tract free of pathogens.
- Failure of the immune system predisposes to infection with opportunistic pathogens (see following section), as well as with common pathogens – illness in this situation is likely to be more severe and progress more rapidly. Many viral infections depress immunity transiently, predisposing to subsequent bacterial infection, e.g. influenza in elderly people predisposing to bacterial pneumonia, and measles in malnourished individuals leading on to infective diarrhoea. Previous haematological cancer or autologous bone marrow transplantation predisposes, even many years later, to infection with many common pathogens.

Diseases predisposing to infection with unusual pathogens

Defects in immune function should be considered when infection involves unusual organisms (e.g. normally non-pathogenic organisms), or if common pathogens infect patients at unexpected ages (e.g. *Neisseria meningitidis* in adults), in unusual sites (e.g. fungal pneumonia) or are particularly severe or recurrent (e.g. extensive pyogenic abscesses). Underlying conditions include diabetes, immunosuppressive drugs and the conditions listed here.

Complement defects

Complement defects predispose to infection with bacteria and, particularly, *Neisseria meningitidis*.

- Acquired complement defects, e.g. as a result of systemic lupus erythematosus or treatment with Eculizumab, a monoclonal antibody which inhibits activation of C5 (used to treat aytpical haemolytic-uraemic syndrome and paroxysmal nocturnal haemoglobinuria). The latter is associated with neisserial meningitis, and recipients should be immunized against this organism.
- Inherited deficiency is very rare. C5, C6, C7 or C8 deficiency predisposes to *N. meningitidis*. C3 deficiency behaves like antibody deficiency, with susceptibility to common pathogenic bacteria.

Neutrophil defects

Neutrophil defects predispose to overwhelming sepsis with *Staphylococcus aureus*, *Serratia marcescens* and fungi, typically *Aspergillus*.

- **Neutropenia**: inadequate neutrophil numbers (see Chapter 53). The most common causes are drugs and haematological cancer and its treatment. Rare causes include genetic neutropenias, including cyclic neutropenia.
- **Defects in neutrophil function**: myelodysplasia and haematological cancer depress neutrophil counts and the function of any remaining cells. Other functional defects include the rare inherited ones (see Chapter 173).

Antibody deficiencies

Antibody deficiency predisposes to bacterial infection, especially with staphylococci, streptococci and *Haemophilus influenzae*. Infections, particularly those caused by pneumococci, may be overwhelming.

- Multiple myeloma is a relatively common cause of acquired hypogammaglobulinaemia. There will be a large amount of monoclonal immunoglobulin, but non-clonal immunoglobulins will be reduced.
- Chronic lymphocytic leukaemia and other haematological malignancies and their treatment, particularly rituximab (anti-CD20), depress B-cell counts, both during and after treatment, and cause hypogammaglobulinameia.
- Primary antibody deficiencies are all extraordinarily rare (see Chapter 175).
- Some drugs may cause hypogammaglobulinaemia, such as anti-epileptics, and drugs used to treat rheumatoid arthritis.

Defects in cell-mediated immunity

Defects in cell-mediated immunity include:

- HIV infection (see Chapter 166)
- haematological cancer (including chronic lymphocytic leukaemia) and its treatment
- primary defects (see Chapter 173).

173 Immunological deficiency syndromes

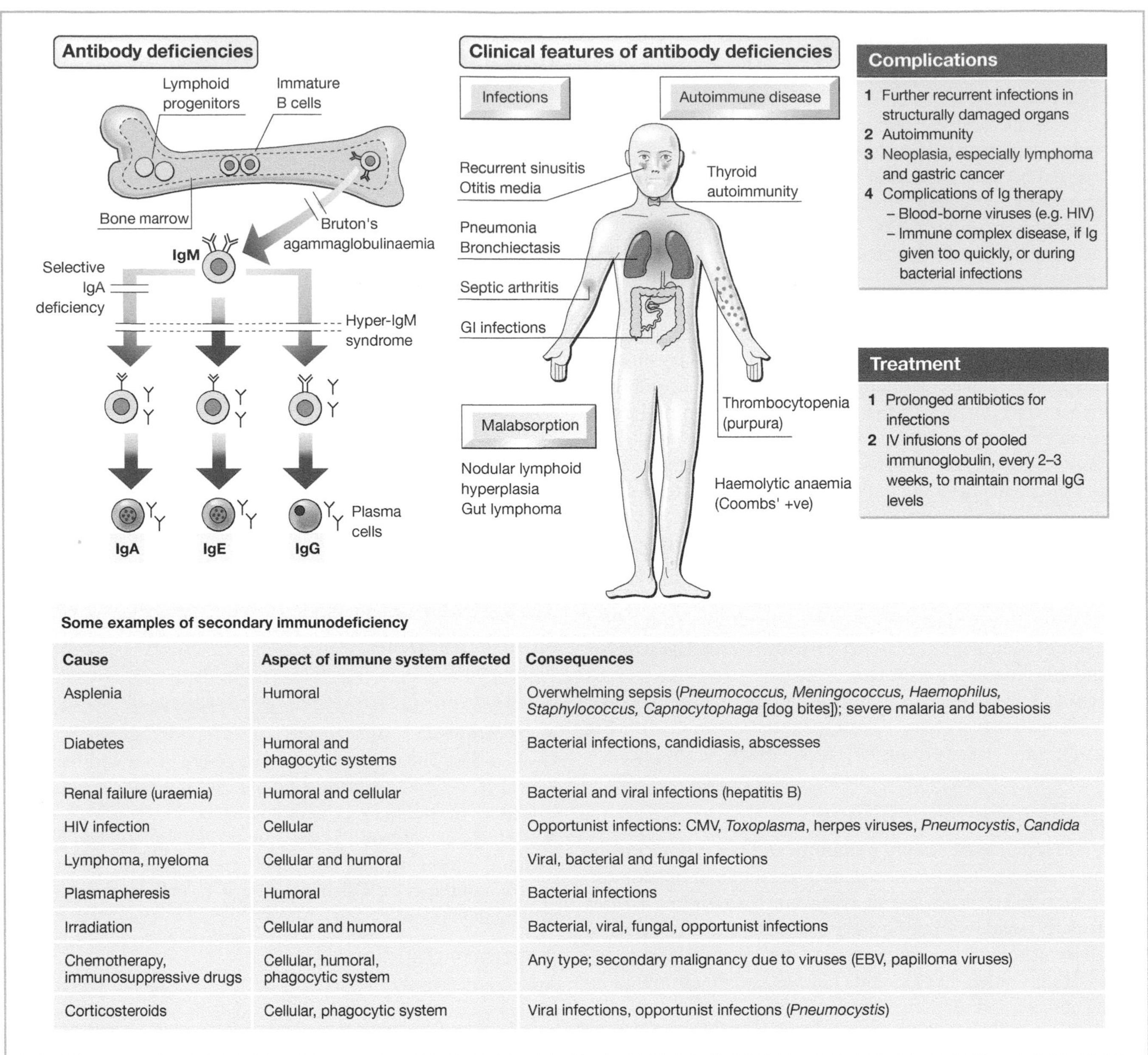

Some examples of secondary immunodeficiency

Cause	Aspect of immune system affected	Consequences
Asplenia	Humoral	Overwhelming sepsis (*Pneumococcus, Meningococcus, Haemophilus, Staphylococcus, Capnocytophaga* [dog bites]); severe malaria and babesiosis
Diabetes	Humoral and phagocytic systems	Bacterial infections, candidiasis, abscesses
Renal failure (uraemia)	Humoral and cellular	Bacterial and viral infections (hepatitis B)
HIV infection	Cellular	Opportunist infections: CMV, *Toxoplasma*, herpes viruses, *Pneumocystis*, *Candida*
Lymphoma, myeloma	Cellular and humoral	Viral, bacterial and fungal infections
Plasmapheresis	Humoral	Bacterial infections
Irradiation	Cellular and humoral	Bacterial, viral, fungal, opportunist infections
Chemotherapy, immunosuppressive drugs	Cellular, humoral, phagocytic system	Any type; secondary malignancy due to viruses (EBV, papilloma viruses)
Corticosteroids	Cellular, phagocytic system	Viral infections, opportunist infections (*Pneumocystis*)

Immunodeficiency should be suspected whenever there is evidence of increased susceptibility to infection. The most common causes of immunodeficiency are secondary to other medical or surgical problems or their therapy. Symptomatic primary immunodeficiency is rare. There are no hard and fast rules indicating that immunodeficiency is likely to be present, but two or more serious (requiring intravenous antibiotics) infections in a year are highly suspicious. Infections in unusual sites, for example liver or brain abscesses, osteomyelitis, septic arthritis, where there is no obvious structural reason, and infection with unusual or normally non-pathogenic organisms are highly suspicious of immunodeficiency. Primary immunodeficiency may also be accompanied by evidence of immune dysfunction such as autoimmune disease.

The immune system is very adaptable and often the severity of the clinical problem is less extreme than one might predict because of compensatory mechanisms. The nature of the infection gives a clue to the underlying defect (see Table 173.1). Cases of suspected primary or secondary immunodeficiency should be referred to an immunologist for formal investigation; suspected

Medicine at a Glance, Fifth Edition. Edited by Patrick Davey and Alex Pitcher.

Companion website: www.wiley.com/go/medicine5e

Table 173.1 Classification of immunological deficiency syndromes.

Type of defect	Typical infections	Type of defect	Typical infections
B-cell defect (reduced antibody)	Bacterial infections: • *Streptococcus pneumoniae* • *Haemophilus influenzae* • *Moraxella* species • *Neisseria meningitidis* • *Staphylococcus aureus* • *Campylobacter* species • *Salmonella* species and other enteric pathogens • *Mycoplasma* species • *Ureaplasma* species Viral infections: • Enteroviruses (polio, echoviruses, Coxsackie viruses) Protozoal infections: • *Giardia lamblia*		Fungal infections: • *Candida* • *Aspergillus* • *Pneumocystis carinii (jirovecii)* Protozoal infections: • *Toxoplasma gondii* • Cryptosporidium • Microsporidium
		Combined T- and B-cell defect	As for B- and T-cell defects Pattern may be variable
		Neutrophil defects	Bacterial infections: • Catalase-positive organisms (*Staphylococcus aureus*) • *Pseudomonas* species Fungal infections: • Any fungus (typically *Aspergillus*)
T-cell defect	Bacterial infections: • May be some increase in bacterial infections due to poor T-cell help for B-cell responses Viral infections: • All types, often persistent • Enteric viruses (rotavirus) • Respiratory viruses (respiratory syncytial virus, parainfluenza viruses, adenoviruses) • Herpes viruses (EBV, CMV, HHV6) • Papillomaviruses (warts) • JC and BK viruses (progressive multifocal leukoencephalopathy)	Complement deficiency	Bacterial infections: • *Neisseria* species As for antibody deficiency (C3 deficiency only)
		Cytokine and cytokine receptor defects; TLR defects	• Bacterial infections • Recurrent mycobacterial infection • Viruses (herpes viruses; corona viruses)

CMV, cytomegalovirus; EBV, Epstein–Barr virus; HHV, human herpes virus; JC, John Cunningham; TLR, toll-like receptors.

human immunodeficiency virus (HIV) infection should be referred to a consultant in infectious diseases or genitourinary medicine experienced in the management of the condition.

Antibody deficiency syndromes

In antibody deficiencies recurrent bacterial infections occur, usually with common organisms (e.g. *Haemophilus influenzae*, *Streptococcus pneumoniae*), although less usual organisms (e.g. *Mycoplasma*) are also important. Infections most frequently involve the upper and lower respiratory tract, but may involve the gastrointestinal (GI) tract (e.g. *Giardia*) and other sites. Malabsorption may be due to infection, a coeliac-like condition, nodular lymphoid hyperplasia or malignancy. If the underlying disorder is untreated, the frequency and severity of the infections result in structural end-organ damage including bronchiectasis and growth retardation in children. Deficiencies are classified into primary and secondary antibody deficiencies.

Primary antibody deficiency

Primary antibody deficiency is a reduction or absence of one or more immunoglobulin isotypes when no other contributory disorder is present. There are four major forms. All are rare – a prevalence of 12 per million. In primary antibody deficiencies both infections and antibody-mediated autoimmune disease occur.

- **X-linked agammaglobulinaemia** (Bruton agammaglobulinaemia): mutation in the X chromosome (*Btk* gene) prevents normal B-cell maturation. Presents in patients aged 3–12 months; milder forms present later.
- **Hyper-IgM syndrome**: presents in childhood with recurrent bacterial infections and autoimmune disease (neutropenia, thrombocytopenia). The X-linked form (70% of cases) is a deficiency of the CD40 ligand on T cells (a lymphocyte communication molecule). The IgM antibody response is intact. B cells cannot produce mature IgG or IgA antibody. There is very high IgM, low/undetectable IgG and IgA, and an increased risk of IgM lymphomas.
- **Common variable immunodeficiency** (CVID): the aetiology is unknown but is partly genetic (50% have a family history of IgA deficiency). There are heterogeneous laboratory findings. Serum IgG levels may be only marginally reduced, but specific antibody production is invariably poor or absent. IgM levels may be normal. Patients present at any age, particularly in adolescence and early adulthood. Autoimmune disease is common. There is a 40-fold increased risk of lymphoma, and also an increased risk of gastric cancer.
- **Selective IgA deficiency**: this affects one in 400–800. Most are asymptomatic, but there is an increased incidence of allergic disease and connective tissue disease. Recurrent infections are rarely a problem unless additional immune defects are present. The diagnosis is made based upon *absent* serum IgA (not just low levels).
- **Specific antibody deficiency (with normal immunoglobulins)**: this is linked to CVID and selective IgA deficiency and represents a failure of immune responsiveness to a single class of antigens such as bacterial polysaccharides. Serum immunoglobulins and IgG subclasses are normal.

Secondary antibody deficiency

Secondary antibody deficiency syndromes are the most common cause of antibody deficiency and relate to conditions such as the nephrotic syndrome (protein leak), protein-losing enteropathies/ malabsorption (protein leak), immunosuppressive drug therapy, multiple myeloma (negative feedback), lymphoproliferative disease (especially chronic lymphocytic leukaemia) and (probably) malignancy.

Investigations

The initial investigations in suspected primary antibody deficiency are serum immunoglobulins and protein electrophoresis. These measure the ability to produce antibodies, although not their 'usefulness'. The absence of immunoglobulins is always significant, but specific antibody deficiency can occur with normal serum immunoglobulins and functional tests of antibody production may be required. The diagnosis in CVID is complicated, as while serum IgG may be absent or very low, this is not invariable. In such cases, it is important to measure specific antibodies to antigens to which the patient has been exposed, e.g. tetanus/ diphtheria vaccinations. If specific antibodies are undetectable or very low, the patient may be test immunized with a (killed) vaccine and serology repeated 4–6 weeks later. Failure to mount a response may indicate an antibody deficiency. Secondary antibody deficiencies should be excluded. Lymphocyte subpopulations (T, B, NK cells) should be measured: B cells (CD19+) are severely reduced or absent in XLA. Genetic screening for known immunodeficiency-causing mutations is required for confirmation on monogenic disorders.

Management and prognosis

The mainstay of treatment is long-term replacement therapy with pooled immunoglobulin, which provides passive protection from bacterial infections. Once diagnosed and treated, patients usually lead normal active lives, although recurrent infections can occur despite adequate replacement therapy if there is pre-existing structural damage. If an infection becomes established, early and prolonged treatment with antibiotics is essential, usually for 10 days. Autoimmune diseases usually require corticosteroids. There is an increased incidence of malignancies, particularly lymphoma.

T-cell deficiencies

These are usually secondary to another disease process (haematological malignancy, its treatment or HIV infection) but can be primary. Most are evident in childhood but may present in early adult life.

- **22q11 deletion syndrome** (DiGeorge syndrome): complex genetic disorder (chromosome 22) with major cardiac, facial and parathyroid gland defects. Intellectual impairment is common. There is a high risk of blood-borne infection from transfusions during cardiac surgery. The degree of immunodeficiency is very variable: severe cases have a small, atrophic thymus and no T cells and can mimic severe combined immunodeficiency (SCID). Autoimmune diseases often develop later in life. Survival into adult life is common. Bone marrow and thymic transplants have been used.
- **Chronic mucocutaneous candidiasis**: a common, mainly T-cell defect, leading to chronic candidiasis, typically of the mouth and nails. Fifty percent have an autoimmune endocrinopathy (associated with defects in the autoimmune regulator gene, *AIRE*). Bacterial, viral and mycobacterial infections may also occur.
- **Other syndromes**: other predominantly T-cell syndromes include Wiskott–Aldrich syndrome (eczema, thrombocytopenia with small platelets, immune deficiency), due to mutations in the *WASP* gene on the X chromosome, and ataxia telangiectasia (progressive cerebellar degeneration, immune deficiency), due to mutations in the *ATM* gene. The IPEX syndrome is due to a genetic deficiency of the FOXP3 protein required for regulatory T-cell function; severe autoimmune disease, with bowel involvement, is common.

Severe combined immunodeficiency

This only rarely presents in adult life. Features are those of bacterial, viral, fungal and opportunist infections. Genetic defects include mutations affecting the cytokine common γ chain, JAK-3, adenosine deaminase genes. The bare lymphocyte syndrome often presents slightly later and may be due to defects in genes controlling major histocompatibility complex (MHC) antigen expression.

Investigations

Measurement of T-cell subpopulations (CD4, CD8) and MHC antigens (MHC class I and class II) and functional assays of T cells are required. This can only be undertaken in specialist laboratories and early referral to an immunologist is required.

Management of severe combined and T-cell disorders

Prevention of infection is critical in all T-cell deficiencies.

- Live vaccines (e.g. BCG) should not be given.
- Concomitant antibody deficiency can be treated with immunoglobulin replacement therapy.
- Blood transfused should be cytomegalovirus negative and irradiated to avoid graft vs host disease (mediated by donor lymphocytes).
- Prophylaxis against *Pneumocystis jirovecii* infection should be given.
- Human stem cell transplantation (HSCT) is indicated in severe primary disease, including all patients with SCID and the Wiskott–Aldrich syndrome. This is also being undertaken in adults with severe primary immunodeficiencies.
- Gene therapy is available for some conditions.

Neutrophil disorders

The most common neutrophil disorders in adults are secondary, but primary neutrophil disorders may also present in adults for the first time. They typically present with recurrent abscesses (liver), unusual granulomatous disease (mimicking sarcoidosis) and atypical Crohn's disease.

- **Chronic granulomatous disease**: occurs due to defects in neutrophil oxidative metabolism, caused by mutations in genes for the components of the multiprotein NADPH (reduced nicotinamide adenine dinucleotide phosphate) oxidase enzyme. X-linked and autosomal recessive forms may occur. Involvement of the bowel with consequent malabsorption and hepatosplenomegaly is common.
- **Other inherited neutrophil defects**: other genetic diseases interfere with chemotaxis (hyper-IgE syndrome, Chediak–Higashi syndrome), phagocytosis (leukocyte adhesion deficiency) or neutrophil numbers (cyclic neutropenia).
- **Acquired defects**: neutrophil abnormalities include deficient numbers (neutropenia, see Chapter 53 – often drug or leukaemia related) or quality (e.g. in myelodysplasia, see Chapter 183).

Investigations

Diagnosis of chronic granulomatous disease is made using the nitroblue tetrazolium test or a flow cytometric assay of neutrophil oxidative metabolism.

Management

Prevention of infection is critical.

- Prophylactic co-trimoxazole (active in neutrophil phagocytic granules).
- Prophylactic itraconazole to prevent fungal infections.
- γ-interferon may be helpful for treating infection in combination with antibiotics.
- Investigate for bowel involvement.
- HSCT (any age), as long-term outlook without is poor.

Complement deficiency

Complement deficiency is strongly associated with recurrent neisserial infection and atypical connective tissue disease (systemic lupus erythematosus) and glomerulonephritis. Any component may be deficient. Investigate every patient with more than one episode of bacterial meningitis.

Investigations

Complement deficiency can be proved by demonstration of the absence of haemolytic complement activity in fresh serum (CH100 and alternate pathway CH100). Individual components can then be tested.

Management

- Prophylactic penicillin V 500 mg bd for adults.
- Immunize against *Meningococcus* (quadrivalent conjugate vaccine) and *Pneumococcus*.

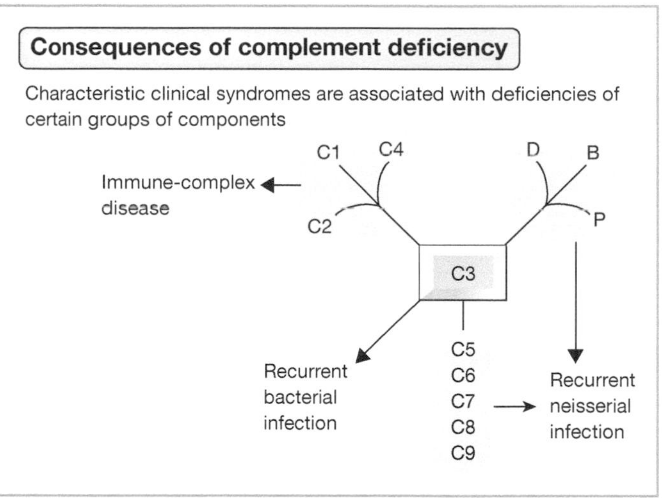

174 Haematinic deficiency anaemias

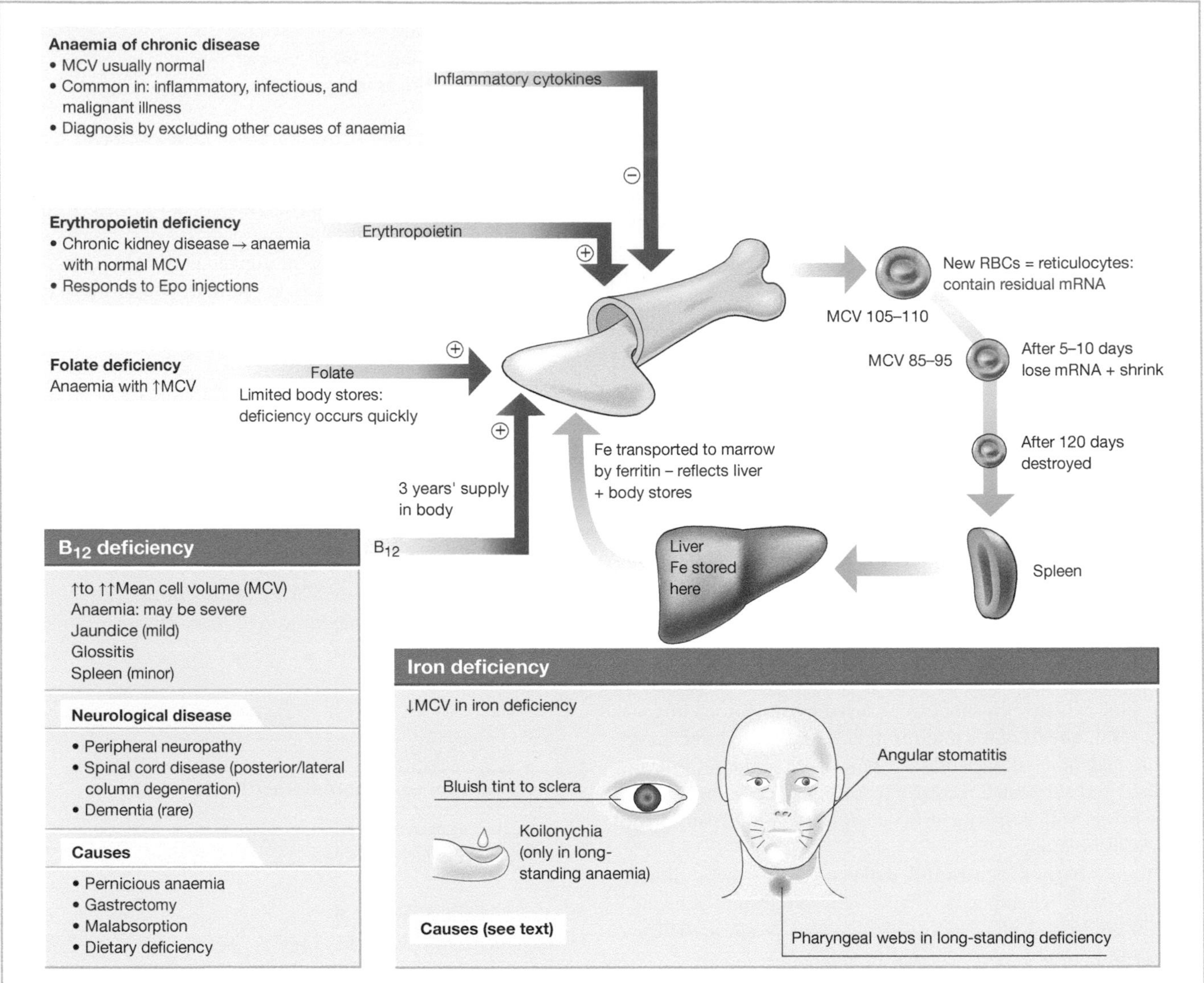

Iron deficiency

Iron deficiency is the most common cause of anaemia, with 500 million affected individuals worldwide. Women of childbearing age are more commonly affected than men because of menstrual blood loss. Iron is absorbed from the upper small intestine, with a normal Western diet providing around 15 mg/day. Adult men have a daily iron requirement of 1 mg, menstruating females 1.5 mg and an extra 5–6 mg/day are needed in pregnancy. Iron is transported in the blood by transferrin, and stored bound to ferritin.

Causes

Iron deficiency solely caused by an inadequate diet is uncommon in the West, though circumstances of increased iron demand (e.g. pregnancy) may promote deficiency. Instead, blood loss from the gastrointestinal or genitourinary tracts is the most common cause of iron deficiency (causes include ulcers, inflammation and cancers). Malabsorption (e.g. due to coeliac disease) is also an important cause.

Clinical features

The important clinical features relate to anaemia (fatigue, breathlessness, swollen feet and ankles, pale mucous membranes) and, more rarely, as the result of tissue iron deficiency (angular stomatitis, glossitis and, very rarely, koilonychia – spoon-shaped nails).

Medicine at a Glance, Fifth Edition. Edited by Patrick Davey and Alex Pitcher.

Companion website: www.wiley.com/go/medicine5e

Diagnosis

Iron deficiency anaemia is characterized by microcytic and hypochromic red cells. Typically serum iron and ferritin are low and the total iron-binding capacity (transferrin) is high, but iron studies are not always easy to interpret. Serum iron is also expected to be low in inflammation and infection, and ferritin is an acute phase protein which can be raised in patients with inflammation, infection or malignancy – even in the presence of iron deficiency.

Management

- It is vital to diagnose the underlying illness and manage it appropriately. Blood loss is identified from the history, examination and investigation. Occult gastrointestinal malignancy may be found.
- Oral iron supplementation is given to replace and replenish body iron stores; it should be given until the haemoglobin and mean cell volume (MCV) are normal, then continued for a further three months to build up adequate body iron stores. Side-effects include nausea, diarrhoea or constipation. Intravenous iron is rarely needed.
- Blood transfusion is seldom appropriate unless the patient is severely symptomatic with angina or breathlessness.

Vitamin B_{12} deficiency

The most common cause of vitamin B_{12} deficiency in the UK is pernicious anaemia. Other causes include malabsorption of vitamin B_{12} in the terminal ileum (e.g. Crohn's disease), after a total gastrectomy, pancreatic disease, bacterial overgrowth as a result of blind loop syndrome, gut infection with the fish tapeworm and, very occasionally, dietary deficiency, usually in strict vegans.

Pernicious anaemia

This is the failure to absorb B_{12} because of immune attack on intrinsic factor or the gastric parietal cells that produce it. It is more common in older individuals, and may be associated with other autoimmune diseases.

Pathophysiology

Vitamin B_{12} is obtained from food of animal origin. Vitamin B_{12} absorption requires intrinsic factor (made by gastric parietal cells), and occurs in the terminal ileum. In pernicious anaemia there is an autoimmune gastritis and antibodies occur against:

- gastric parietal cells, diminishing intrinsic factor secretion
- intrinsic factor, preventing vitamin B_{12} binding.

In addition to vitamin B_{12}, methyltetrahydrofolate is needed as a coenzyme in the methylation of homocysteine to methionine – the first step in intracellular folate production. Thus, vitamin B_{12} deficiency results in intracellular folate deficiency. Given this biochemical background, it is not surprising that the haematological features are the same in both vitamin B_{12} and folate deficiency.

Clinical features

Common clinical features are symptoms of anaemia, mild jaundice, glossitis and weight loss. Features of other autoimmune diseases such as vitiligo may be present. Neurological disturbances (peripheral neuropathy or subacute combined degeneration of the cord) are rare now, as a result of earlier diagnosis. Dementia may very occasionally be caused by vitamin B_{12} deficiency in the absence of a macrocytic anaemia.

Diagnosis

Most patients have a macrocytic anaemia with a megaloblastic bone marrow (delay in nuclear maturation of red cell precursors). Mild/moderate thrombocytopenia and leukopenia are common. A small increase in the plasma bilirubin is found. The diagnosis is confirmed by finding:

- low serum vitamin B_{12}
- antibodies against gastric parietal cells and intrinsic factor: found in 50% of patients with pernicious anaemia. Also check thyroid antibodies and thyroid function in view of the close association between pernicious anaemia and thyroid disease.

Treatment and prognosis

Intramuscular vitamin B_{12} (with ongoing treatment for life) should be given. Hypokalaemia can occur within the first few days of starting treatment so close monitoring and consideration of potassium supplements are advisable. Iron deficiency can develop because the patient responds to the vitamin B_{12} with a huge increase in red cell production. The prognosis for treated patients is excellent, although there is a slightly higher incidence of gastric cancer.

Folate deficiency

Folate deficiency is a common cause of a macrocytic anaemia. Folate is found in green vegetables and is mainly absorbed in the upper part of the small intestine. Folate deficiency may be the result of:

- dietary deficiency
- malabsorption, such as in coeliac disease
- excessive requirement, e.g. haemolytic anaemia
- increased requirement, i.e. pregnancy
- folate antagonist drugs, such as methotrexate.

Diagnosis

A macrocytic anaemia associated with a low serum folate establishes the diagnosis. The marrow will be megaloblastic.

Treatment

Treatment is with folic acid supplementation. The underlying cause should be investigated and treated.

175 Haemolytic anaemia

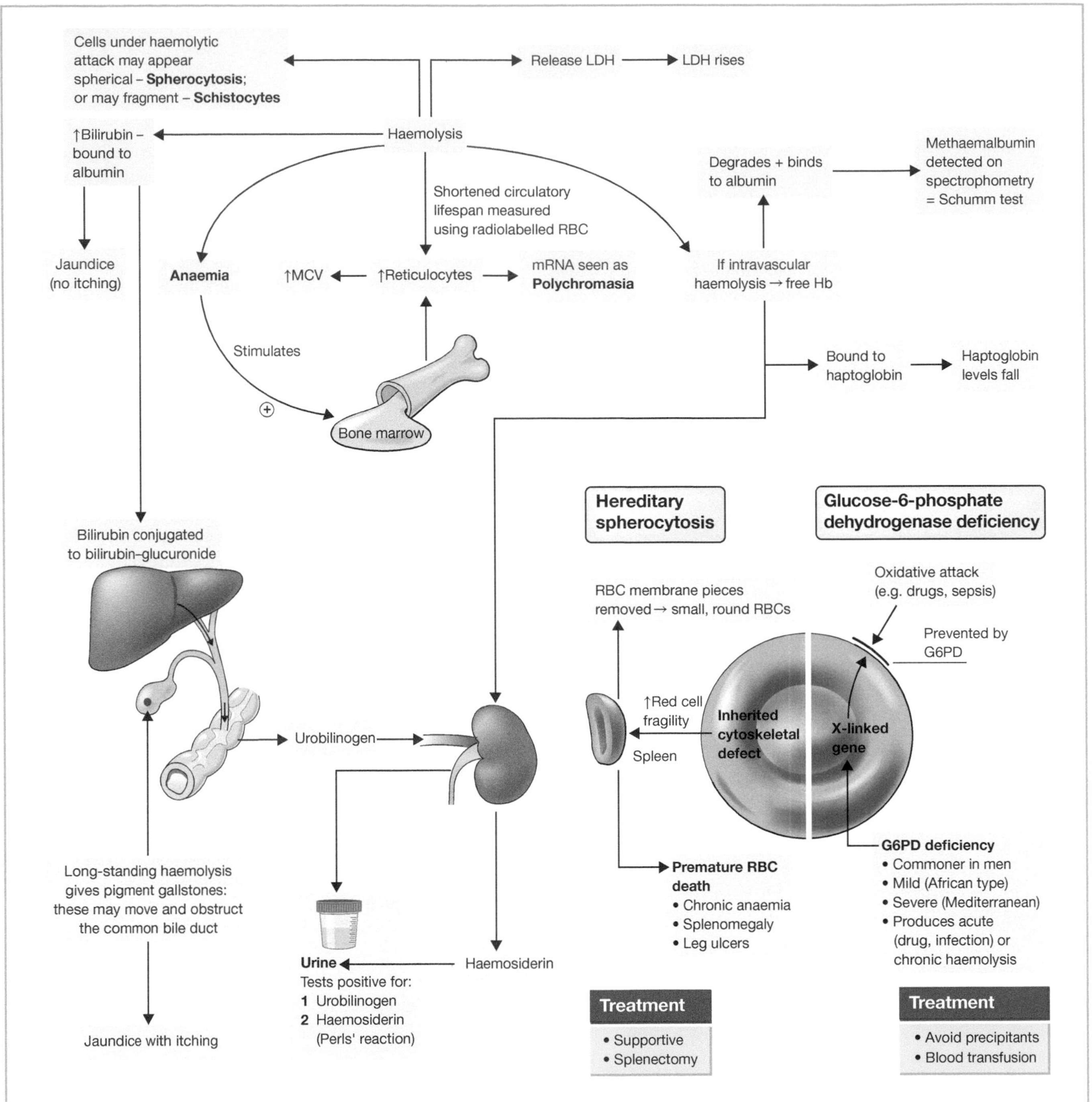

Medicine at a Glance, Fifth Edition. Edited by Patrick Davey and Alex Pitcher.

Companion website: www.wiley.com/go/medicine5e

Table 175.1 Common causes of haemolytic anaemia.

Congenital

- Hereditary spherocytosis
- Glucose-6-phosphate dehydrogenase deficiency
- Pyruvate kinase deficiency
- Sickle cell disease
- Thalassaemia (NB: ineffective erythropoiesis in addition to haemolysis)

Acquired

- Infection
- Autoimmune
- Drug induced
- Cardiac (typically across a defective prosthetic heart valve)
- Haemolytic transfusion reaction
- Microangiopathic (e.g. haemolytic uraemic syndrome, thrombotic thrombocytopenic purpura)
- Paroxysmal nocturnal haemoglobinuria

Haemolysis is the accelerated destruction of red blood cells such that their lifespan is reduced below the expected 120 days. The bone marrow can increase red cell production to several times the normal level, but when marrow synthesis cannot fully compensate for the increased red cell destruction, haemolytic anaemia results. Such an increase in red cell production increases folate requirements, which if unmet can provoke folate deficiency. Haemolysis may be congenital or acquired (see Table 175.1). General clinical features include pallor, jaundice (increased unconjugated bilirubin due to haem breakdown) and variably splenomegaly. Pigment gallstones can occur in those who are chronically hyperbilirubinaemic, and may lead to obstructive jaundice.

General laboratory abnormalities in haemolysis

Laboratory tests show evidence of increased red cell breakdown.

- Increased unconjugated plasma bilirubin (from haem metabolism).
- Raised plasma lactate dehydrogenase (LDH), released from damaged red cells.
- Low or absent plasma haptoglobin (binds avidly to free plasma haemoglobin).

The bone marrow response will cause an increased reticulocyte count, manifest on the blood film as polychromasia (an increase in slightly larger more basophilic red cells, with more residual RNA). Intravascular haemolysis (e.g. due to shear damage to the red cells over a prosthetic heart valve) gives free plasma haemoglobin which is filtered by the glomerulus. Iron is taken up by the urothelial cells, which are then sloughed off into the urine and can be detected as haemosiderinuria, a characteristic finding in intravascular haemolysis.

Further laboratory tests will define the underlying cause of haemolysis and are discussed below.

Hereditary haemolytic anaemias

Hereditary spherocytosis

This typically autosomal dominant inherited illness results in an abnormal red cell membrane and usually presents in childhood with pallor and jaundice. There is usually, but not always, a family history. Splenomegaly is very common. The diagnosis is made from the history, physical findings (splenomegaly) and the general laboratory features of haemolysis and finding spherocytes (small, spherical, darkly staining red cells with no central area of pallor) on the blood film. Many patients do not need treatment but if anaemia is severe and symptomatic, it can be successfully treated by splenectomy. As those without a spleen are at increased risk of infection by encapsulated bacteria, vaccines against *Pneumococcus* and *Haemophilus influenzae* type B and the meningococcal vaccines should be given beforehand. After surgery, lifelong prophylactic penicillin should be given and annual influenza vaccination given.

Red cell enzyme deficiency

The deficiency of almost any enzyme involved in red cell glucose metabolism can result in a haemolytic anaemia. The most important (and common) are glucose-6-phosphate dehydrogenase (G6PD) deficiency and pyruvate kinase deficiency.

G6PD deficiency

NADPH (reduced nicotinamide adenine dinucleotide phosphate) protects against oxidative damage to the red cell, and is therefore essential to the maintenance of functional haemoglobin. It is generated by the catalysis of glucose-6-phosphate by G6PD as part of the pentose phosphate shunt. A deficiency of G6PD leads to oxidative damage to the red cell and therefore to a haemolytic anaemia. G6PD deficiency results from a variety of mutations, and is common in people of African and Mediterranean ethnicity. The gene for G6PD is on the X chromosome, so G6PD deficiency is much more common in males. Most people with G6PD deficiency are asymptomatic until an acute haemolytic episode occurs, triggered by a number of oxidative challenges including infection, some drugs (e.g. sulfonamides, primaquine) or the ingestion of fava beans. An acute haemolytic attack is usually self-limiting and supportive care only is required. A chronic haemolytic anaemia is rare.

Diagnosis and treatment: The general features of haemolysis are found. Heinz bodies (caused by denaturation of unstable haemoglobin) are detected in the red blood cells. Red cell G6PD activity is low (<20% of normal). Treatment is by transfusion if needed and by avoidance of triggers.

Pyruvate kinase deficiency

Pyruvate kinase deficiency is an autosomal recessive disease with a prevalence of 1:10 000. The clinical features vary but most present in childhood with anaemia and jaundice. Typically, haemoglobin is 60–100 g/l. Splenomegaly is usually only mild. The diagnosis is made by finding a haemolytic anaemia, bizarre 'prickle cells' in the blood and a significantly reduced red cell pyruvate kinase activity. Treatment is usually supportive. Folic acid is recommended. Patients may need blood transfusion on occasion, and splenectomy may be useful for patients with significant anaemia.

Haemoglobin defects

Sickle cell anaemia – see Chapter 176.

Acquired haemolytic anaemias

Autoimmune haemolytic anaemia

Autoimmune haemolytic anaemia (AIHA) is the accelerated destruction of red cells caused by autoantibodies binding to red cell surface antigens. It may be warm (IgG) or cold (IgM) antibody mediated. The key diagnostic test is the direct antiglobulin test, or Coombs test, which detects antibody or fixed complement on the red cell surface.

Warm antibody-mediated haemolysis

This is usually caused by IgG binding to red cells, resulting in either complete or partial phagocytosis of the cell by splenic macrophages (partial phagocytosis producing spherocytes, visible on the blood film). Some complement-mediated cell death also occurs. In many cases, no underlying causative pathology is found, but causes of warm AIHA include:

- lymphoproliferative diseases
- autoimmune disease (e.g. systemic lupus erythematosus)
- drugs (e.g. methyldopa, mefenamic acid, penicillin).

The direct antiglobulin test (Coombs test), which detects the presence of antibody and complement on the red cell surface, is usually positive. Most patients respond to prednisolone. Blood transfusions are avoided where possible but may be required for severe, symptomatic anaemia. The anti-CD20 antibody rituximab is also used, as are other immunosuppressive agents.

Cold antibody-mediated haemolysis

The antibody (usually IgM) may be polyclonal and arises as a consequence of infection, or monoclonal secondary to a lymphoproliferative disorder.

- **Cold antibody-mediated haemolysis and infection**: polyclonal IgM antibodies causing haemolysis sometimes occur 1–2 weeks after infection, usually with either *Mycoplasma pneumoniae* or infectious mononucleosis. The disorder is usually self-limiting. Avoidance of the cold and, where needed, blood transfusion (given through a blood warmer) are appropriate measures.
- **Cold haemagglutin disease**: here, an often occult clone of lymphocytes produces an IgM antibody, which binds to red blood cells in the cooler peripheries, activates complement and destroys red cells. Typically pallor, mild jaundice and occasionally mild splenomegaly occur. Acrocyanosis of the extremities (purplish discoloration from red cell agglutination in small distal vessels) is common. Diagnosis is by finding a mild-to-moderate anaemia, red cell agglutination in the blood film and a positive Coombs test for complement, but not for antibody (IgM antibodies elute from the red cell into the serum *in vitro*). The concentration of IgM antibodies may be too low for detection by serum electrophoresis – they are instead found because of their ability to agglutinate red cells in the cold (cold agglutinins). Avoidance of the cold, folic acid supplements and treatment of the underlying lymphoproliferative disorder are usually effective.

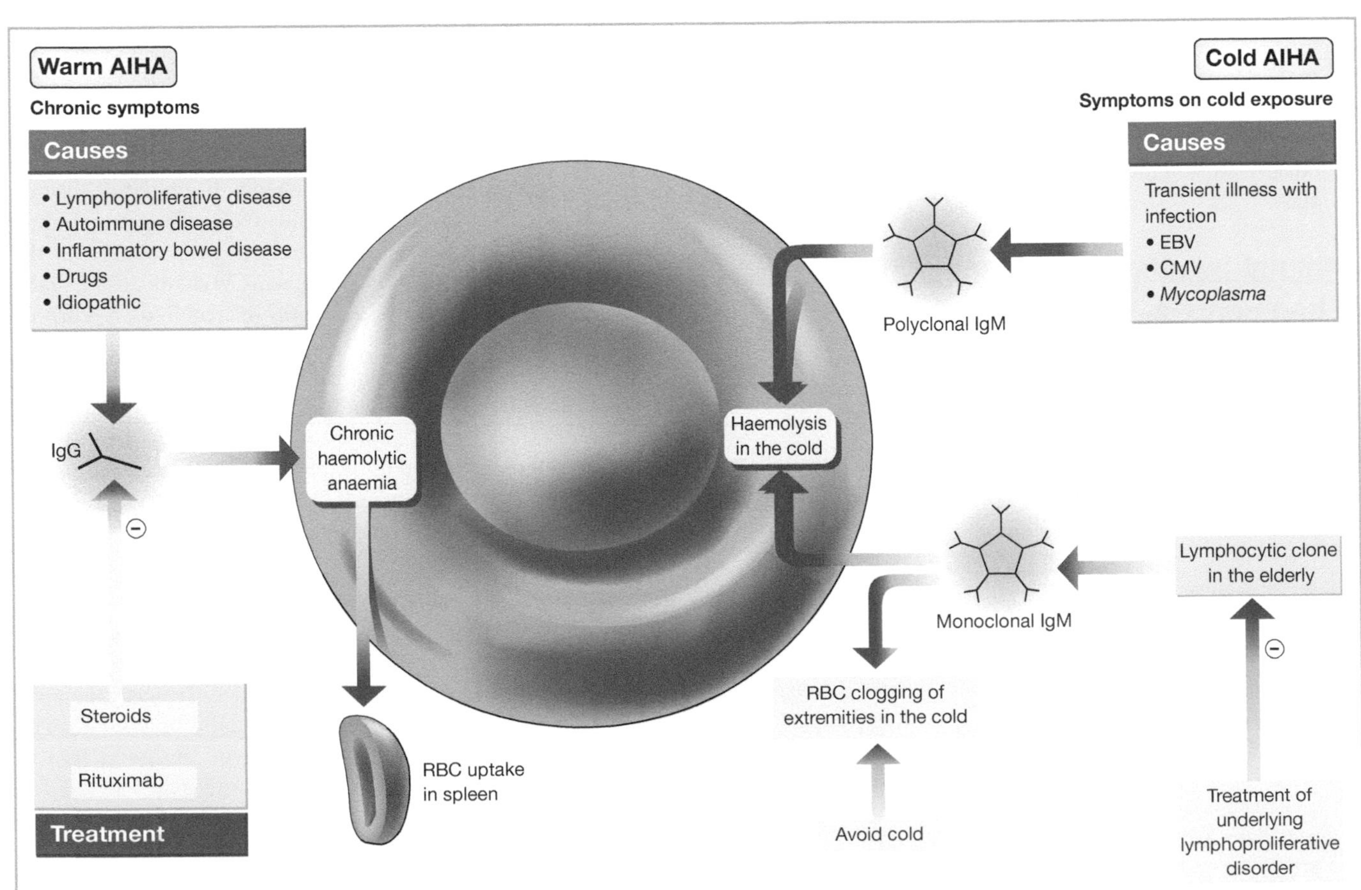

Microangiopathic haemolytic anaemia

In this group of conditions, there is direct damage to the red cell in the vasculature, with red cell rupture, release of free haemoglobin, and the formation of red cell fragments which can be seen on the blood film.

Cardiac haemolysis

This usually occurs only after prosthetic heart valve replacement and is caused by a small leak around the valve. The shear forces caused by the abnormal flow result in red cell damage. Affected patients are anaemic and found to have red cell fragments in the blood film. The haemolysis is usually mild but reoperation is sometimes needed. Other causes of haemolysis need to be excluded.

Thrombotic thrombocytopenic purpura (TTP)

This uncommon acquired disorder is characterized by a pentad of microangiopathic haemolytic anaemia, thrombocytopenia, neurological abnormalities, renal impairment and fever. The onset is often abrupt and the disease is usually fatal without treatment. An antibody occurs against a metalloprotease which is normally responsible for cleaving the high molecular weight polymers of von Willebrand factor (vWF). The persisting high molecular weight multimers bind platelets and also induce red cell damage. Plasmapheresis, which removes antibody, and infusion of fresh frozen plasma (FFP), which contains the metalloprotease, are the mainstays of successful treatment. Occasional patients have a relapsing/remitting course, caused by an inherited deficiency of the metalloprotease enzyme or by recurrence of the antibody.

Haemolytic uraemic syndrome

This condition is often seen as part of a clinical spectrum with TTP. It is also characterized by a microangiopathic haemolytic anaemia, thrombocytopenia and renal impairment, but does not manifest the metalloprotease deficiency seen in TTP. The aetiology is often obscure but infection with *Escherichia coli* O157 is sometimes responsible and may cause small clusters of cases. Haemolytic uraemic syndrome (HUS) is associated with a deficiency of complement factor H. Although most clinical and laboratory features of TTP and HUS are similar, neurological injury is unique to TTP. The treatment involves supportive care. Dialysis may be required. Most patients recover, although some patients are left with persistent renal impairment.

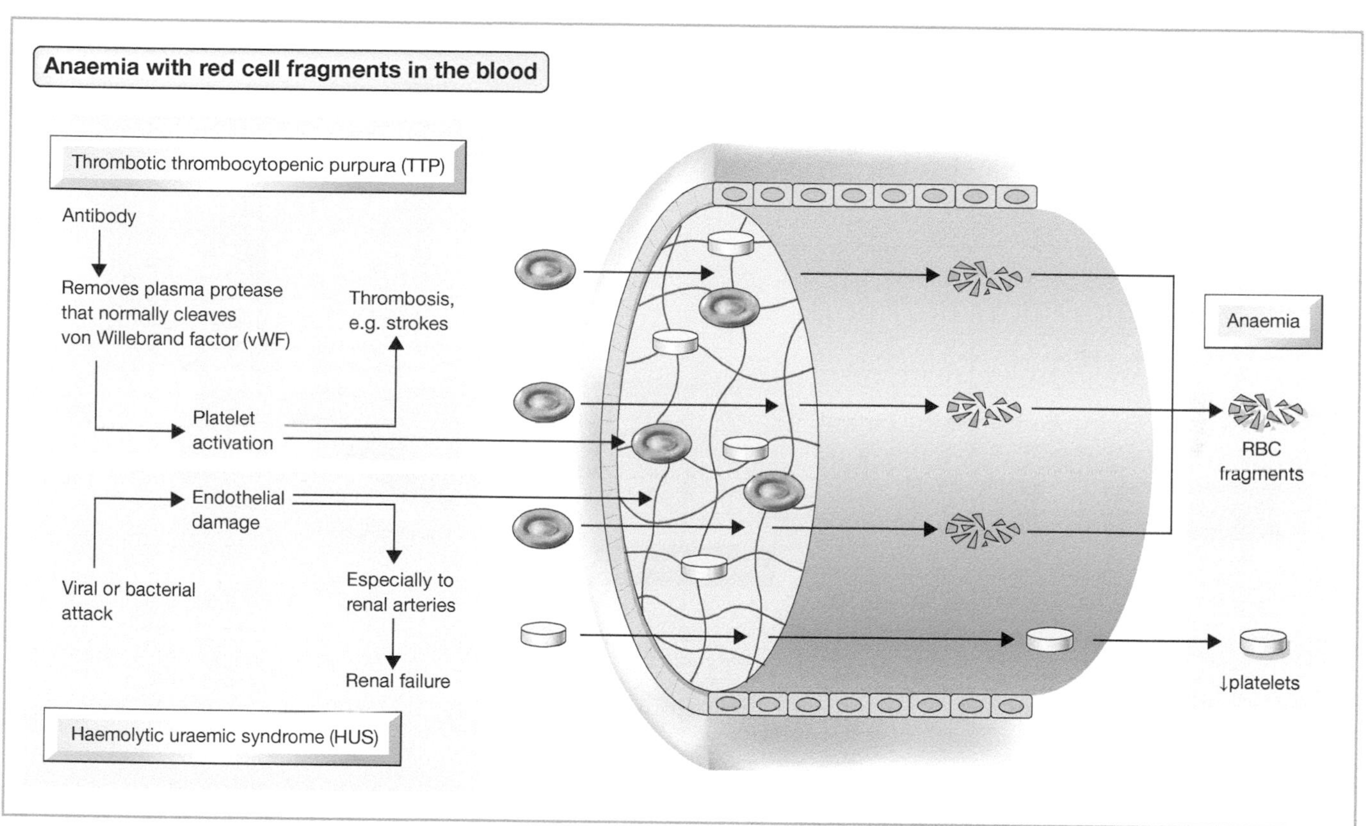

176 Thalassaemia and sickle cell disease

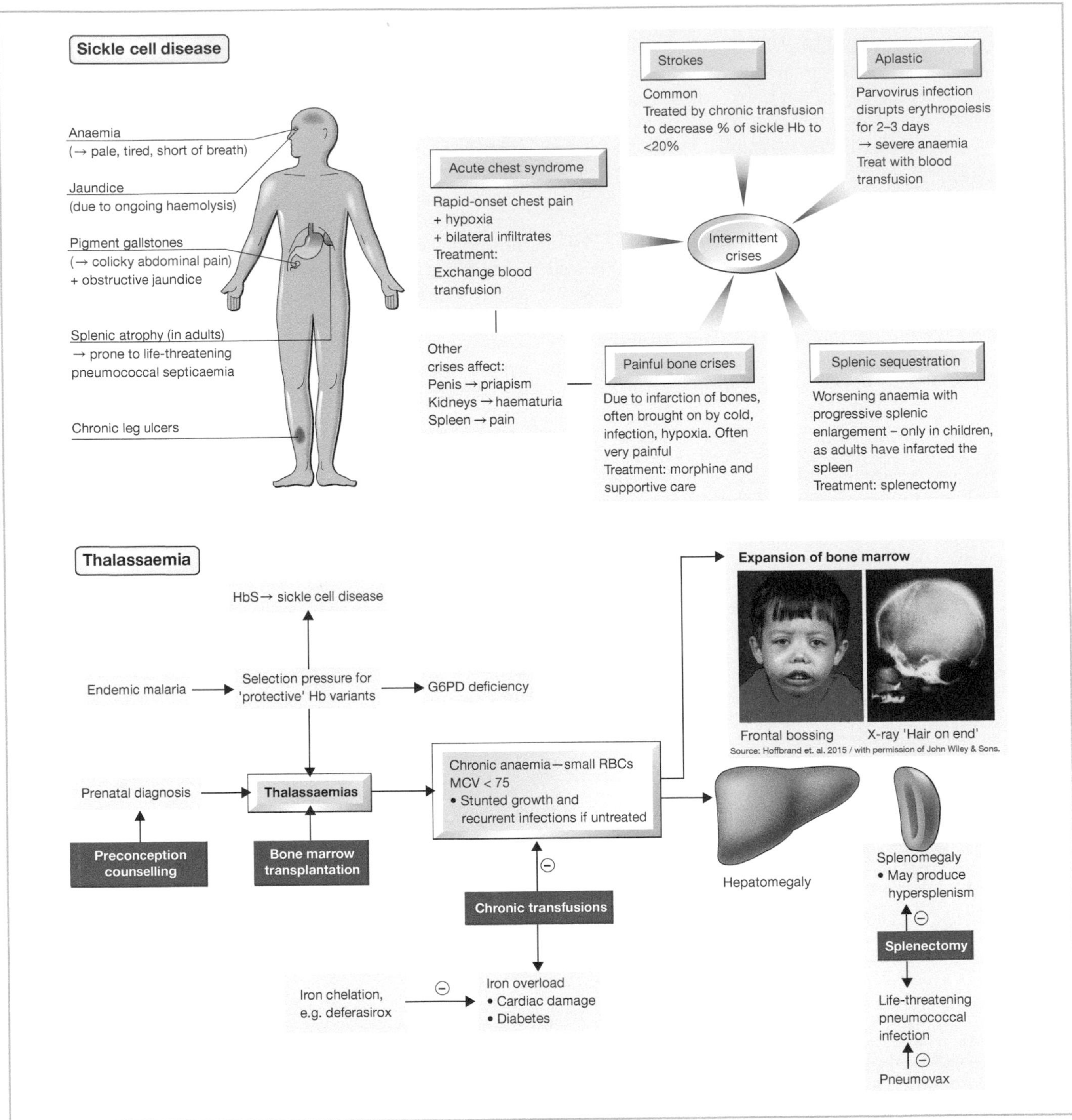

The genetic disorders of haemoglobin synthesis are classified by whether there is an imbalance between α and β globin chain production (the thalassaemias) or a functional defect in the resulting haemoglobin (e.g. sickle cell disease). Thalassaemia can be further divided genetically into α-thalassaemia (where α-globin genes are affected) and β-thalassaemia (where the β-globin genes are affected). Heterozygous thalassaemia and sickle cell disease offer some protection against malaria explaining the high gene frequency in the Mediterranean, sub-Saharan Africa and the Far East.

Thalassaemia

Thalassaemia trait

- In **β-thalassaemia trait,** the β globin gene on one copy of chromosome 11 is mutated, and there is a mild imbalance between α and β globin production. Most haemoglobin produced in patients with β-thalassaemia trait, as for unaffected individuals, is HbA ($\alpha_2\beta_2$), but there is also a mild increase in HbA2 ($\alpha_2\delta_2$). This can be detected by haemoglobin high-performance liquid chromatography (HPLC) or haemoglobin electrophoresis.

- Since there are two copies of the α globin gene on each copy of chromosome 16, **α-thalassaemia trait** may be either α_0 trait, where both copies are deleted, or α_+ thalassaemia trait in which only one of the two genes on a single copy of chromosome 16 is lost. HPLC is normal.

In both cases, thalassaemia trait is characterized by either a normal haemoglobin or a mild anaemia (Hb 100–120 g/l); the red cells have microcytic, hypochromic indices, and the red cell count is typically raised. Diagnosis is important to avoid unnecessary iron supplementation (as the main differential is iron deficiency) and to permit genetic counselling.

Thalassaemia major/transfusion-dependent thalassaemia

Thalassaemia major, also known as transfusion-dependent thalassaemia, is an imbalance between α and β globin chain production so significant that endogenous erythropoiesis is too ineffective to support life without regular transfusion support.

- **β-Thalassaemia major**, caused by point mutations in both copies of the β-globin genes, results in symptomatic anaemia at 6–12 months, as fetal haemoglobin ($\alpha_2\gamma_2$) levels fall. Untransfused infants and young children fail to thrive. The continued drive to erythropoiesis, met with an ineffective response due to the α:β imbalance, leads to marrow expansion and bony deformity, and splenomegaly with the typical 'hair on end' skull X-ray appearance. Laboratory tests show a severe microcytic anaemia, target and nucleated red cells in the peripheral blood, and no HbA ($\alpha_2\beta_2$). Without transfusion, affected children would die. Blood transfusion, to maintain a normal haemoglobin level and suppress abnormal red cell production, results in normal physical development, though iron overload from frequent transfusions causes cardiac, hepatic and endocrine dysfunction and death by 25 years, unless prevented by chelation. Bone marrow transplantation can be considered if a suitable sibling donor is found.
- **α-Thalassaemia major** is better known as Hb Barts hydrops fetalis, and results from deletion of all four α globin genes. As α globin is required for the production of fetal haemoglobin (HbF, $\alpha_2\gamma_2$) as well as adult haemoglobins, Barts hydrops fetalis typically causes death *in utero*. Rarely, the diagnosis is made prenatally, when intrauterine blood transfusions may be life saving. In these cases, life-long transfusion is necessary.

Thalassaemia intermedia

The severity of thalassaemia intermedia lies between thalassaemia trait and thalassaemia major. Several different genetic disorders underlie this condition. The most common is homozygous β-thalassaemia where one or both genes still produce small amounts of HbA. Deletion of three of the four α globin genes (HbH disease) causes a similar picture, with a moderately severe anaemia of 70–90 g/l and splenomegaly. By definition, these patients are not transfusion dependent.

Sickle cell disease

Sickle cell haemoglobin results from a point mutation in the β globin gene (βS). It is common in Africa, the Arabian peninsula and southern Europe. Heterozygous carriers have one normal β and one βS globin gene – sickle cell trait (AS).

Sickle cell trait is usually asymptomatic. The blood count is normal. The diagnosis is made on finding a positive sickle solubility test (in which a reducing agent is added to lysed red cells in the laboratory, prompting precipitation of the sickle component of haemoglobin), along with one peak for HbA (normal adult haemoglobin) and one of HbS (sickle haemoglobin) on HPLC or haemoglobin electrophoresis.

Sickle cell disease occurs in those homozygous for HbS (SS). Sickle haemoglobin precipitates in conditions of low oxygen tension, and forms long polymers or 'tactoids'. These distort the red cell into the characteristic 'sickle' shape. This distortion means the cells tend to lodge in the microvasculature with downstream ischaemia and infarction. The blood count shows evidence of a moderate haemolytic anaemia (Hb 50–90 g/l), with sickling on the blood film and a HbS peak on HPLC but no peak for HbA. The sickle solubility test is positive. The natural history of this condition is variable, but is characterized by recurrent crises.

- Painful crisis is the most common and may be precipitated by cold, infection or hypoxia. Treatment is with simple analgesia, hydration, oxygen antibiotics for infection. Most episodes settle in a few days.
- Acute chest syndrome, in which there is a vicious cycle of sickling in the pulmonary vasculature, hypoxia, and further sickling, may be fatal. It is characterized by the rapid onset and progression of chest pain associated with hypoxia, cough and bilateral lung infiltrates. Exchange blood transfusion is the treatment of choice.
- Splenic sequestration is commoner in children than in adults, as splenic atrophy from autoinfarction occurs by the age of 5–6 years. Typical features are a rapidly worsening anaemia and progressive splenomegaly. Blood transfusion is used as necessary. It is usually short-lived.
- Aplastic crises are caused by infection by erythrovirus (parvovirus) B19, which temporarily prevents erythroid maturation. This is clinically unnoticed in normal individuals, but in patients with haemolytic anaemia where the red cell lifespan is very short, temporary cessation of red cell production causes an abrupt, potentially life-threatening fall in haemoglobin, with a near absence of reticulocytes. Red cell transfusion is usually required.
- Sickle cell disease is the most common cause of strokes in children; adults are also affected, and can suffer either haemorrhagic or occlusive strokes. An exchange blood transfusion programme is usually initiated, to maintain the HbS concentration <30%. Monitoring of the cerebral blood flow has been shown to be a useful method for identifying children at high risk of stroke so that prophylactic transfusions can be given.

Chronic complications of sickle cell disease demonstrate that there is ongoing subclinical sickling even in the absence of acute crisis. Sickle nephropathy is common with some patients requiring renal replacement therapy. Avascular necrosis of the femoral head is common, due to its single, vulnerable blood supply. Chronic sickling in the lungs can induce pulmonary hypertension which is challenging to treat.

Treatment

Most patients with sickle cell disease are treated supportively with specific treatment for crises. Hyposplenism from splenic infarction is common, so immunization and prophylaxis against encapsulated bacteria with penicillin are essential. Folic acid is prescribed. Disease severity is very variable: those with the highest concentration of HbF have the mildest clinical course. Hydroxycarbamide is used in severe disease to increase HbF concentration and decrease the frequency of crises. Bone marrow transplantation may be used in young people with severe disease.

Other haemoglobin variants

Other haemoglobin variants include haemoglobins C, D and E. Heterozygous patients are asymptomatic. In combination with haemoglobin S or β-thalassaemia trait, more serious disorders can occur, e.g. the combination of haemoglobins S and C – haemoglobin SC disease. The clinical course is milder than SS, although proliferative retinopathy is much more common.

Bone marrow failure

Pancytopenia

Septic illness
- Usually severe and obvious
- Poor prognosis

Myelodysplasia

Malignant infiltrate
- Haematologic
- Other (esp. breast, bronchus)

B_{12} deficiency

Alcohol

Pancytopenia: ↓Hb ↓WCC ↓platelets

Cytotoxic drugs

Bone marrow failure

High dose radiation

Aplastic anaemia

Pale (anaemic)

Sepsis (neutropenia)
- Minimal febrile response
- Usual pathogens are:
  - Gram –ve rods
  - fungi

Bleeding (thrombocytopenia)

Aplastic anaemia

Hypo- or acellular marrow

Causes

1 Idiopathic (most)
2 Hepatitis
3 Drugs
4 Chemical, e.g. benzene
5 PNH

Treatment

- Supportive
- Bone marrow transplant
- Immunomodulation (anti-lymphocyte globulin, ciclosporin)

Paroxysmal nocturnal haemoglobulinuria (PNH)

GPI – anchors proteins DAF and MIRL which inhibit complement

Normal

PNH

no GPI

Complement attack

Intravascular haemolysis
- Dark urine
- Anaemia
- Recurrent venous thrombosis (e.g. Budd–Chiari)

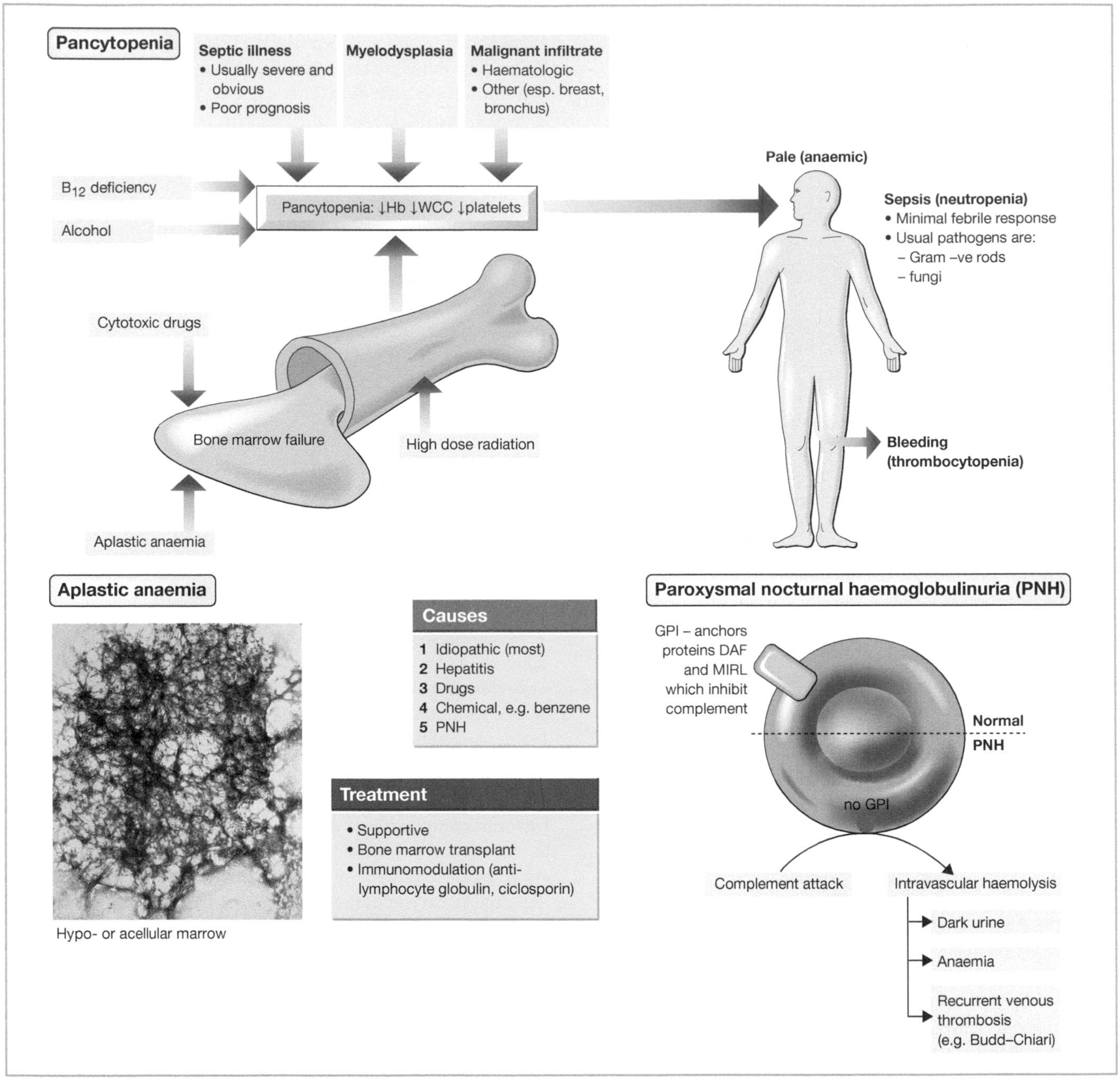

Bone marrow failure may develop from both congenital and acquired causes, or may arise as the consequence of cytotoxic chemotherapy or radiotherapy. The clinical features of bone marrow failure relate to the absence of:

- haemoglobin (symptoms of anaemia)
- neutrophils (bacterial or fungal sepsis)
- platelets (petechiae, purpura and bleeding).

Although one cell line may be more severely affected than another, the peripheral blood film shows variable depression of all three cell lines, i.e. pancytopenia. It is important to realize that a peripheral blood pancytopenia does not necessarily mean that there is an underlying marrow failure caused by an aplastic anaemia. Thus, the differential diagnosis of a peripheral blood pancytopenia includes the following.

Medicine at a Glance, Fifth Edition. Edited by Patrick Davey and Alex Pitcher.

Companion website: www.wiley.com/go/medicine5e

- Sepsis: usually clinically obvious and severe.
- Hypersplenism
- Vitamin B_{12} or folate deficiency (see Chapter 174).
- A clonal haematopoietic disorder, such as acute leukaemia, myelodysplasia or marrow infiltration by lymphoproliferative disease.
- Bone marrow failure as a result of drug toxicity.
- Immune attack on haematopoietic stem cells (aplastic anaemia).
- Marrow fibrosis.
- Infiltration of the marrow by metastatic malignancy.
- Severe malnutrition such as that associated with severe anorexia nervosa.

The key investigation in peripheral blood pancytopenia is the bone marrow examination, which will diagnose aplastic anaemia or an underlying haematological disease process. Bone marrow is usually obtained by aspirating cells from the posterior iliac crest or the sternum, and from a biopsy – termed a 'trephine' – where the architecture of the bone marrow is preserved. In pancytopenia caused by aplastic anaemia, a hypocellular marrow is seen. Aplastic anaemia may be idiopathic (primary) or secondary to another disease process or drugs.

Acquired aplastic anaemia

Epidemiology

This is a rare disorder occurring in three per million people per year, defined as a peripheral blood pancytopenia in conjunction with a hypocellular bone marrow in which there are no malignant cells.

Aetiology

In most patients (70–80%), no cause is found and the condition is thought to be an autoimmune disorder targeting the haematopoietic stem cell. In the rest, causes include:

- viral infections (e.g. hepatitis C)
- an idiosyncratic reaction to some drugs (e.g. gold, chloramphenicol)
- chemicals such as benzene
- paroxysmal nocturnal haemoglobinuria: see next section.

Clinical features

Most patients present with bleeding as a result of thrombocytopenia, bacterial and fungal infection because of neutropenia, and symptoms of anaemia. Splenomegaly is not a feature.

Diagnosis

The blood count will show a decrease in haemoglobin, platelet and neutrophil counts, i.e. a pancytopenia of variable severity. A bone marrow aspirate and trephine biopsy show a hypocellular marrow.

Treatment and prognosis

Patients should be given supportive care with blood products (red cells, platelets) and antibiotics in the first instance, and then withdrawal of any relevant drug, or specific treatment for hepatitis C. In primary aplastic anaemia, immunosuppressive treatment with antilymphocyte globulin, ciclosporin and the TPO mimietic eltrombopag is effective in improving blood counts in most patients. Bone marrow transplantation is used for younger patients with severe disease who have an appropriate donor.

Paroxysmal nocturnal haemoglobinuria

This is a rare, acquired, clonal disease of bone marrow, which may arise during the course of aplastic anaemia. The abnormal blood cells lack a series of proteins (glycosyl-phosphatidylinositol [GPI] anchored proteins), which normally anchor complement regulatory proteins on to the cell. The absence of such proteins encourages complement attack on red cells, with the net result being complement-mediated haemolysis.

The clinical features are the result of an intravascular haemolytic anaemia – with characteristic haemoglobinuria. Haemolysis is worse with infection/inflammation, even when minor (e.g. colds and surgical trauma). Patients develop insidious symptoms of anaemia and many (although not all) have intermittently dark urine. Large vessel thrombosis is a feature and abdominal pain as a result of bowel ischaemia or infarction may occur. Occasionally Budd–Chiari syndrome occurs.

The physical signs are pallor (from anaemia), mild jaundice (from intravascular haemolysis), minor splenomegaly and brown/black urine. Urine testing reveals haemosiderinuria. The blood film shows a pancytopenia, with the red cells having a normal or high mean cell volume (MCV) – a low MCV suggests complicating iron deficiency from urinary iron loss. The diagnosis is made by immunophenotyping of the red and white cells showing a deficiency on GPI-linked proteins.

Treatment is mainly supportive with blood products. Treatment with a monoclonal antibody (eculizumab) against the complement protein C5 has resulted in significant improvement in patients' anaemia and general health.

Congenital aplastic anaemia

These disorders are rare and include conditions such as Fanconi anaemia and dyskeratosis congenita. Fanconi anaemia is an autosomal recessive disease in which – in addition to aplastic anaemia, which usually develops in the first few years of life – there may be other abnormalities such as small stature, skeletal defects and hyperpigmentation. In dyskeratosis congenita, learning disability, skin, nail and hair abnormalities, and growth failure may complicate the aplastic anaemia.

178 Acute leukaemia

Figure 178.1

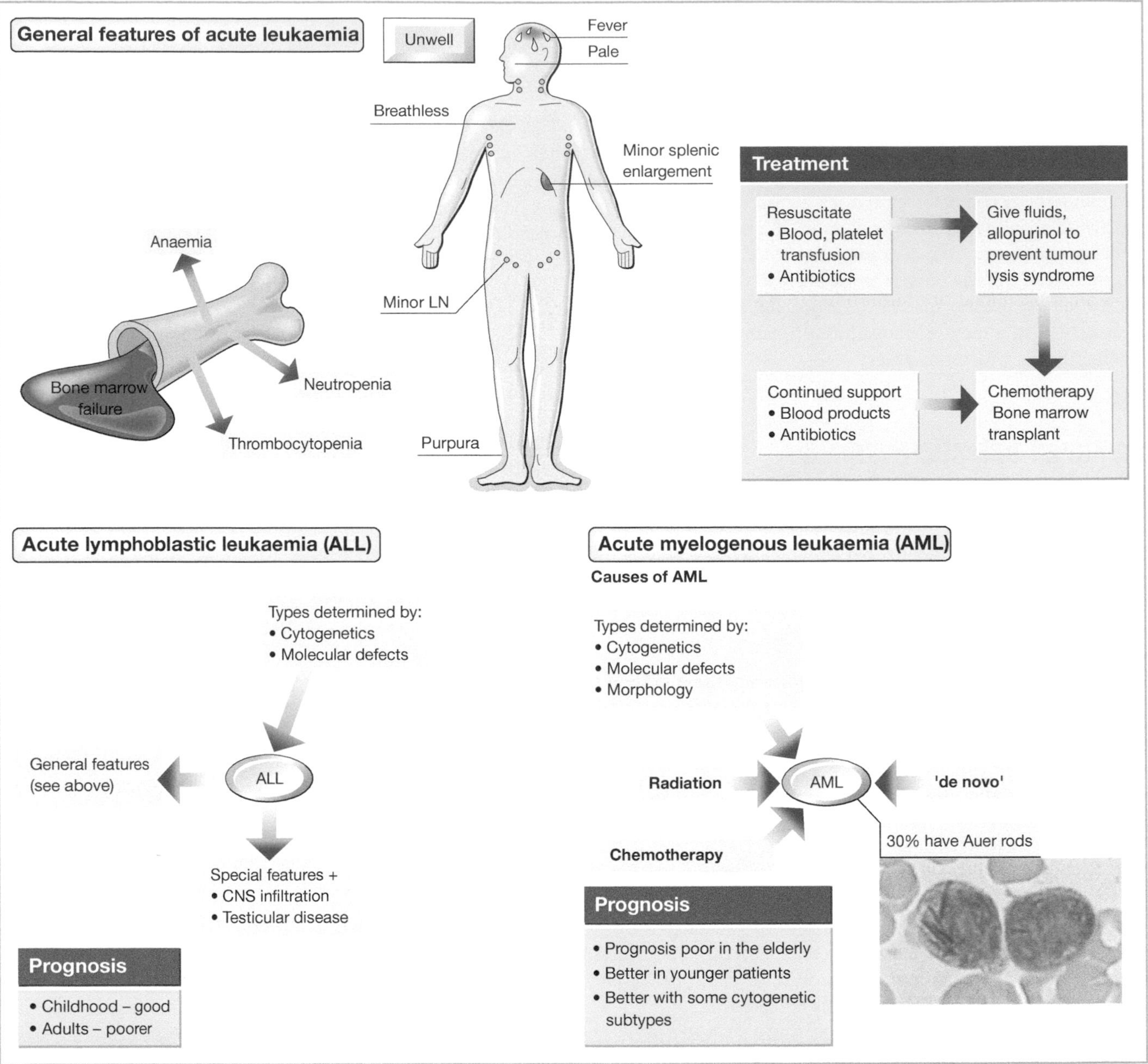

Acute leukaemia is a clonal haematopoietic stem cell/progenitor disorder characterized by the rapid accumulation of immature progenitor cells (blasts) with a failure of maturation, leading to severe bone marrow failure. In the absence of treatment, this results in the death of the patient within a few weeks or months. Acute leukaemia may affect the lymphoid cell line (acute lymphoblastic leukaemia, ALL) or the myeloid cell line (acute myeloid leukaemia, AML).

Epidemiology

ALL is more common in children, with a peak age of onset of four years. In contrast, AML occurs more commonly with increasing age, with a peak age of onset of 70 years (Figure 178.2). For most patients the cause of acute leukaemia cannot be determined, although exposure to cytotoxic drugs, radiation and some chemicals such as benzene increases the likelihood of acute leukaemia developing. The clonal haematological disorder myelodysplasia

Medicine at a Glance, Fifth Edition. Edited by Patrick Davey and Alex Pitcher.

Companion website: www.wiley.com/go/medicine5e

Figure 178.2

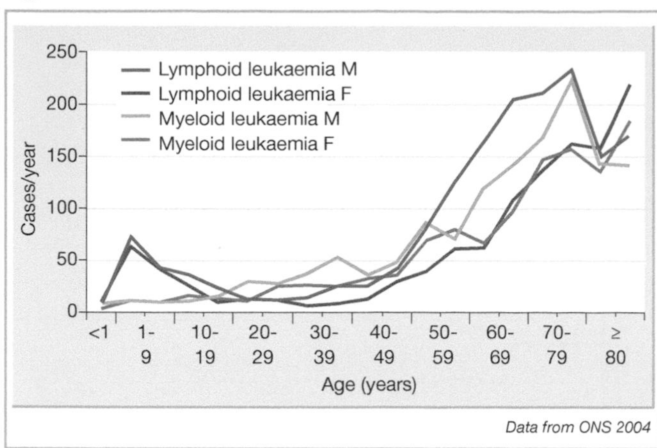

Data from ONS 2004

has a high likelihood of transforming to AML; there is a lesser risk posed by the chronic myeloproliferative neoplasms, especially myelofibrosis.

Symptoms and signs

Symptoms of acute leukaemia usually develop over weeks and can be divided into three types.

1 **Bone marrow failure symptoms**: these are the most common presentation complaints. Leukaemia suppresses normal bone marrow function, causing any combination of anaemia, neutropenia and thrombocytopenia. Typical symptoms are fatigue and breathlessness (from anaemia), bacterial infection (from neutropenia) and bleeding (from thrombocytopenia and sometimes from disseminated intravascular coagulation [DIC]). Examination often reveals pallor, some bruising and bleeding. Fever suggests infection, although in some it may be caused by the leukaemia itself. It is, however, dangerous to assume this (see Management). Lymphadenopathy, when present, is usually small volume and more typical of ALL than AML.

2 **Systemic symptoms** of malaise, weight loss, sweats and anorexia are common.

3 **Local symptoms**: occasional patients present with symptoms or signs of leukaemic infiltration of skin, gums or the central nervous system.

Investigations

- Full blood count: usually shows anaemia and thrombocytopenia. The neutrophil count is decreased but the total white blood count may be low, normal or raised: when normal or raised, most of the cells are primitive white cells (blasts).
- Biochemistry: may show renal dysfunction and high bilirubin levels.
- Coagulation profile: may show prolonged clotting times and reduced fibrinogen suggestive of DIC.
- Blood cultures because of the risk of infection.
- Chest X-ray (CXR): patients with ALL of T-cell lineage often have a mediastinal mass.
- Blood group and antibody screen because transfusion of blood and platelets will be needed.
- Specific diagnostic investigations include a bone marrow aspirate and trephine biopsy, with cell marker studies (immunophenotyping) and cytogenetic studies for accurate distinction of ALL from AML. Auer rods in the cytoplasm of blast cells are pathognomonic for AML, but are found in only a minority of cases. Immunophenotyping can help distinguish B- from T-lineage ALL as well as helping to differentiate the various subtypes of AML (see Figure 178.1). Chromosome analysis gives key prognostic information, and molecular diagnostic tests are important in allowing the monitoring of minimal residual disease as well as directing therapy in some cases.

Management

Resuscitation

A newly diagnosed patient with acute leukaemia is often very ill and vulnerable to severe infection and/or bleeding. The priority is resuscitation using broad-spectrum intravenous antibiotics for infection, platelets and fresh frozen plasma for bleeding, and blood transfusion to correct anaemia.

Chemotherapy

The definitive treatment of acute leukaemia is with cytotoxic chemotherapy using multiple drugs given in combination. The precise protocols differ for ALL and AML, but side-effects in both cases result in hair loss, nausea and vomiting, mucositis, and bone marrow failure as a result of bone marrow toxicity. One of the major consequences of chemotherapy-induced neutropenia is severe infection. Patients are treated for months (AML) or for 2–3 years (ALL). A subtype of AML (promyelocytic leukaemia) associated with t(15:17) responds very well to a combination of a vitamin A analogue (all trans retinoic acid) and low-dose chemotherapy.

Stem cell transplantation

This is a treatment option for patients with high-risk disease and those who relapse following standard cytotoxicity chemotherapy. The haematopoietic cells are typically obtained from an HLA (human leukocyte antigen) matched donor (allogeneic transplantation). High-dose 'conditioning' treatment ablates the patient's bone marrow, and the infused stem cells restore bone marrow function. However, it is the immunological antitumour effect of the donor marrow (the graft vs leukaemia effect) mediated by transplanted T lymphocytes that is thought to mediate much of the therapeutic benefit of allogeneic transplantation.

Prognosis

The prognosis worsens with increasing age; complex karyotypic abnormalities are also associated with a poorer response. For adults less than 50 years old with ALL or AML, around 30–40% will be cured. For children with ALL, survival rates are very significantly higher, with nearer 90% being cured.

179 Lymphoma

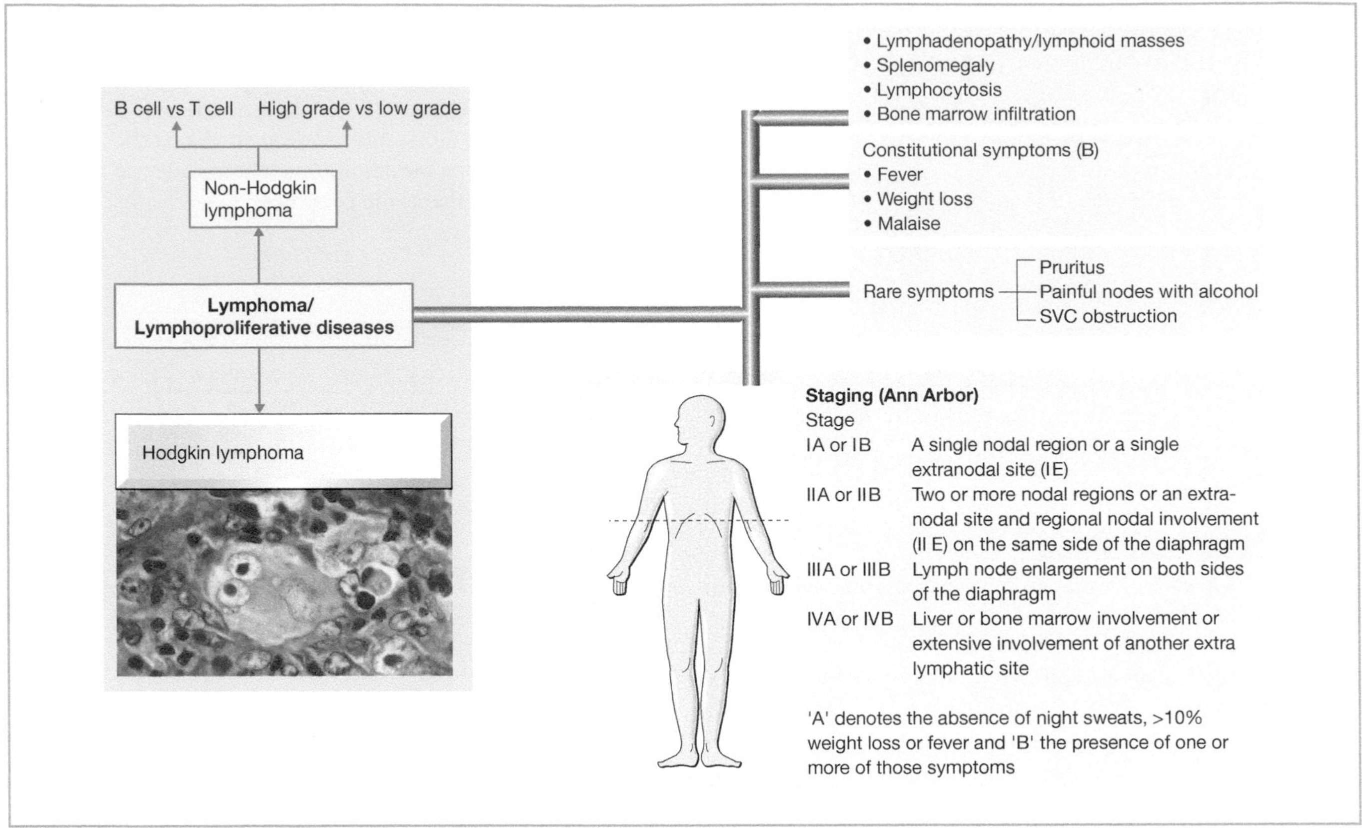

General principles

The WHO classification identifies different types of lymphoma based on clinical, histological, genetic and molecular features. Lymphomas are malignancies derived from lymphoid cells which include precursor lymphoblasts (lymphoblastic leukaemia/lymphoma) and more differentiated B and T cells.

There are two main groups of lymphoma: Hodgkin lymphoma (HL) and non-Hodgkin lymphoma (NHL). Whilst Hodgkin is confined to two main entities (classical HL and nodular lymphocyte predominant HL), there are many different subtypes of non-Hodgkin lymphoma.

Suspecting and investigating malignant lymphoid diseases

Hodgkin lymphoma typically presents with enlargement of lymph nodes. Non-Hodgkin lymphoma may also present with enlargement of lymph nodes, but in many cases infiltration of other organs – extranodal sites – may be present. Common sites of extranodal involvement are the gastrointestinal tract and the skin though almost any other organ of the body can be affected, including the brain. Both types of lymphoma can manifest with B-symptoms (fever, sweats and weight loss). Pruritus is also a common clinical feature.

Investigation of a possible lymphoma starts with a biopsy, either an excision biopsy or a core biopsy of an enlarged lymph node or mass. The histology is complex and uses immunostains to identify and characterize the malignant lymphoid cells and their cellular context. Once a diagnosis of lymphoma is made, radiological staging using a PET-CT scan is performed. Both the type of lymphoma and the staging determine treatment.

There are a number of types of NHL which may involve the blood, including chronic lymphocytic leukaemia. This condition arises from B-lymphocytes; it is rare in young people and is often diagnosed by a chance finding of an increased number of lymphocytes in the blood. The diagnosis is made using immunophenotyping of lymphocytes in the blood by flow cytometry, which identifies a characteristic pattern of cell marker expression on the circulating abnormal B cells. Other NHL subtypes can also present with involvement of the blood, including Waldenstrom macroglobulinaemia, hairy cell leukaemia and various forms of

Medicine at a Glance, Fifth Edition. Edited by Patrick Davey and Alex Pitcher.

Companion website: www.wiley.com/go/medicine5e

splenic lymphoma. Flow cytometry may separate these different types of lymphocytosis by identifying characteristic patterns of cell markers on circulating cells, though biopsy may still be required for a definitive diganosis.

Classical Hodgkin lymphoma

Histologically, HL is characterized by the presence of malignant Reed–Sternberg cells lying within a variable reactive mix of lymphocytes, neutrophils, eosinophils and fibroblasts. The reactive cells fall into four common patterns: lymphocyte rich, nodular sclerosing, mixed cellularity and lymphocyte depleted. These histological patterns confer some prognostic information but are generally not used to determine therapy.

Hodgkin lymphoma occurs in all ages with a peak in adolescence and a second peak later in life. It may be accompanied by systemic symptoms such as fever, sweats, weight loss or pruritus. The enlarged lymph nodes are usually painless. A common presentation of nodular sclerosing HL in young patients is with a mediastinal mass, causing cough and breathlessness. A chest X-ray is therefore an important investigation in patients presenting with systemic symptoms but without lymphadenopathy. The cause is unknown.

Treatment and prognosis

Treatment depends on stage. Early stage disease (stage I and II) is treated with a short course of combination chemotherapy sometimes followed by radiotherapy. Over 90% of patients may be cured. Advanced disease (stage III–IV) is treated with longer courses of chemotherapy, with radiotherapy sometimes given to sites of bulk at presentation. Treatment results show that many patients with advanced-stage disease can be cured. As HL affects young patients, considerable weight is given to trying to reduce the risk of secondary malignancies and preserving fertility when deciding on a treatment regimen.

Nodular lymphocyte-predominant HL

This is a rare type of HL which often presents with lymphadenopathy in young people. It can be managed in a similar way to low-grade NHL (see Chapter 180). It is distinguished from classical HL on biopsy.

180 Non-Hodgkin lymphoma

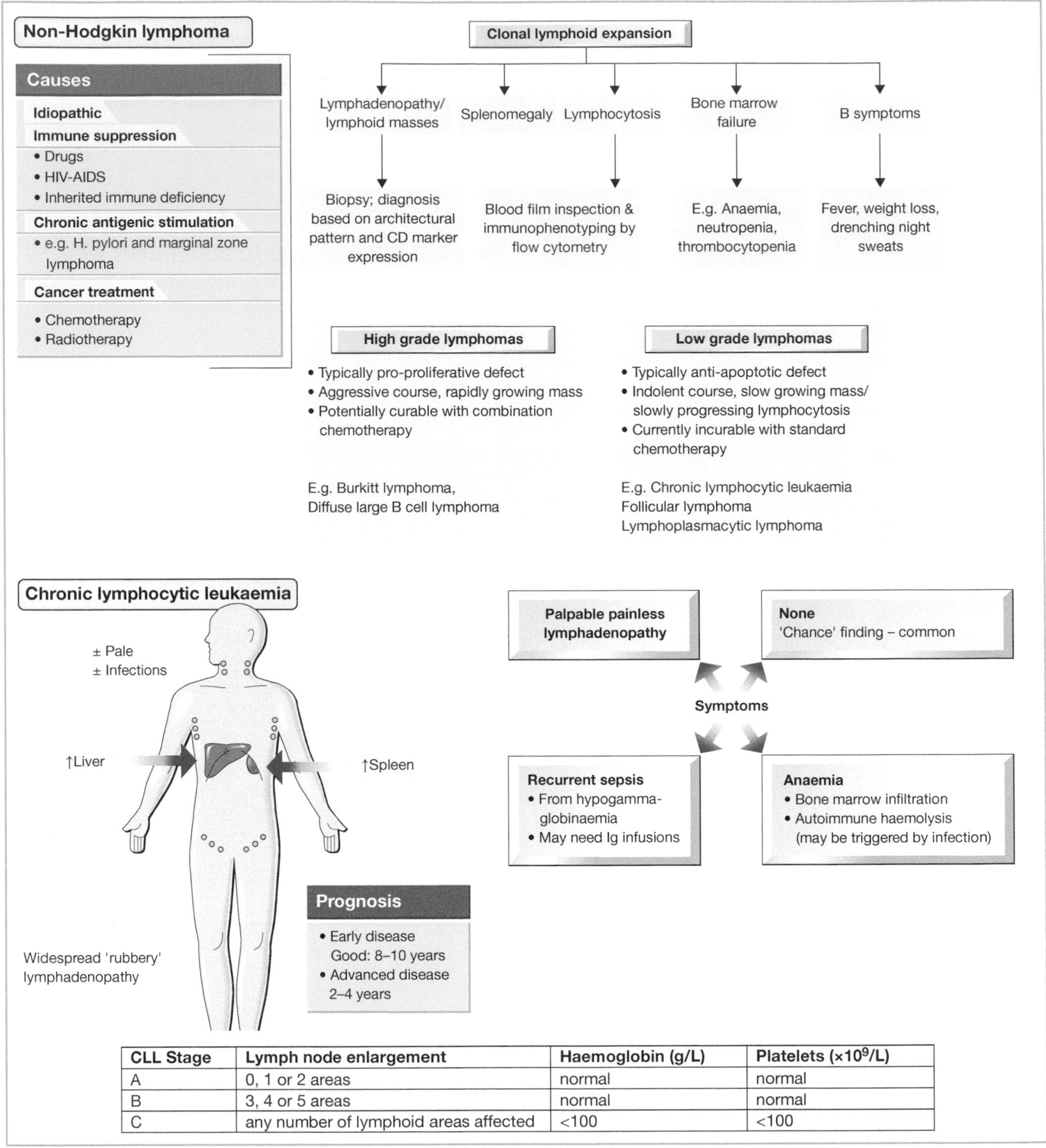

CLL Stage	Lymph node enlargement	Haemoglobin (g/L)	Platelets ($\times 10^9$/L)
A	0, 1 or 2 areas	normal	normal
B	3, 4 or 5 areas	normal	normal
C	any number of lymphoid areas affected	<100	<100

Non-Hodgkin lymphoma (NHL) is divided in the World Health Organization classification into B-cell and T-cell malignancies. B-cell lymphomas are much more common than T-cell lymphomas in the Western world, and T-cell lymphomas generally have a worse prognosis. Lymphomas derived from precursor lymphoblasts are discussed in Chapter 178 on acute leukaemias, since

Medicine at a Glance, Fifth Edition. Edited by Patrick Davey and Alex Pitcher.

Companion website: www.wiley.com/go/medicine5e

their basis and management are similar to those of acute lymphoblastic leukaemia.

Aetiology

The causes of most NHLs are still poorly understood, though there are some well-recognized causative factors, and some forms of NHL for which the pathophysiology is better defined. Chronic antigen simulation is implicated particularly in a group of indolent NHLs derived from lymphocytes found in the marginal zone of lymphoid tissue. Marginal zone lymphomas are much more common in patients with autoimmune disorders such as systemic lupus erythematosus, Sjögren syndrome and Hashimoto thyroiditis. Chronic infection with *Helicobacter pylori* can lead to the development of gastric extranodal marginal cell lymphoma, also known as gastric MALT (mucosa-associated lymphoid tissue) lymphoma. Treatment with *H. pylori* eradication therapy will lead to regression in the majority of cases of gastric MALT lymphoma.

Immunosuppression is also associated with NHL. In situations where there is profound immunosuppression such as after organ transplantation, aggressive Epstein–Barr virus-generated lymphomas can arise. Post-transplant lymphomas (PTLDs) can resolve spontaneously on withdrawal of immunosuppression but may require combination chemotherapy. In a similar way, patients with HIV-AIDS are at a higher risk of developing lymphoma, with the risk related to the degree of immunosuppression.

Genetic and genomic analysis has identified a wide range of oncogenic mutations in many types of lymphoma. Mutations or translocations affecting genes implicated in apoptosis, such as BCL-2, can lead to a failure of cell death, causing the accumulation of lymphocytes normally programmed to die. This mechanism is thought to be important in lymphomas such as chronic lymphocytic leukaemia and follicular lymphoma. In addition, mutations in B-cell signalling pathways may lead to uncontrolled proliferation of lymphoid cells.

Clinical classification

Clinically, NHLs can be divided into those which run an indolent course, termed low-grade NHL, and those that are aggressive, termed high-grade NHL. The low-grade NHLs include chronic lymphocytic leukaemia, follicular lymphoma, marginal zone lymphoma and lymphoplasmacytic lymphoma. Low-grade lymphomas are generally controllable with chemotherapy but are not curable with conventional therapies. High-grade lymphomas, including entities such as diffuse large B-cell lymphoma and Burkitt lymphoma, require aggressive combination chemotherapy and will lead to early death if progressive despite therapy; they are, however, curable in a proportion of cases. All indolent lymphomas are uncommon in young people whereas high-grade lymphomas occur at any age.

Low-grade NHL

Chronic lymphocytic leukaemia

Chronic lymphocytic leukaemia (CLL) is a indolent low-grade NHL affecting the blood (see above). CLL is a disorder of older persons and presents with lymphocytosis which progresses to lymphadenopathy, splenomegaly and finally in advanced stages to bone marrow failure. A subgroup of patients present with lymphadenopathy without involvement of the blood, often referred to as **small lymphocytic lymphoma**, though this is otherwise pathologically indistinguishable from CLL. Many patients can be managed on a 'watch and wait' basis with simple monitoring of the blood count. Some patients will have acquired hypogammaglobulinaemia resulting in recurrent infections, usually respiratory. Replacement immunoglobulin infusions and judicious antibiotic use reduce the risk of bronchiectasis and frequency of infections.

Patients with progressive CLL require therapy, the nature of which is the subject of ongoing clinical research. Treatment may involve the use of agents targeting a specific component of the B-cell signalling pathway, Bruton's tyrosine kinase, such as ibrutinib or acalabrutinib, or a BCL-2 inhibitor, venetoclax. The choice of treatment will take into account the patient's clinical picture as well as the genetic characteristics of their disease (e.g. *TP53* mutation).

Lymphoplasmacytic lymphoma

Lymphoplasmacytic lymphoma (LPL) is a low-grade NHL which commonly presents with bone marrow infiltration causing anaemia and other low blood counts. It may also present with lymphadenopathy and, in common with many indolent lymphomas, splenomegaly. The malignant cells share some features of plasma cells and often secrete monoclonal IgM. When monoclonal IgM paraprotein is detected, the condition is known as **Waldenstrom macroglobulinaemia**. The large molecular weight of IgM means that as IgM levels rise, some patients will develop hyperviscosity, leading to headaches, confusion and stroke if left untreated. Patients presenting with signs of hyperviscosity require urgent plasma exchange and subsequent chemotherapy. A mutation in the *MYD88* gene is found in many patients with this disease.

Follicular lymphoma

Follicular lymphoma characteristically presents with lymphadenopathy. Patients are often well and even with advanced stage disease may require no immediate treatment. Early (stage I) stage disease can be treated with low-dose radiotherapy which results in prolonged remissions in some patients. In patients with progressive disease or who develop systemic symptoms, combination chemotherapy plus rituximab will result in 80% achieving a response. Maintenance rituximab, given every 2–3 months after completion of R-chemotherapy, will lengthen the time to progression. Patients who fail first-line therapy can be treated with second-line chemotherapy usually followed by autologous or allogeneic transplantation in young fit patients. Modern management has resulted in an average 18-year survival.

High-grade NHL

Diffuse large B-cell lymphoma (DLBCL)

This is the most common high-grade lymphoma. The biopsy shows sheets of large B cells with effacement of normal lymph node architecture. The disease commonly presents with lymphadenopathy but involvement of extranodal sites is present in almost half of patients. Night sweats, weight loss and fever are common. Treatment of this aggressive lymphoma involves administration of a combination of rituximab and multiagent chemotherapy. Response rates are high (80%) and many patients with DLBCL can be cured.

Burkitt lymphoma (BL)

Burkitt lymphoma is a highly proliferative and therefore a rapidly progressive lymphoma. Involvement of extranodal sites such as the GI tract, ovaries, breast and central nervous system is common. In Africa, it is a disorder of childhood and has been strongly linked to EBV and malaria infection. This endemic type often presents with involvement of the jaw and facial bones, and is very sensitive to chemotherapy. Sporadic Burkitt lymphoma occurs in the West, affects all ages, and is less associated with EBV infection. Sporadic BL is treated with sequential high-dose chemotherapy. Many patients will be cured, depending on disease stage at presentation. Central nervous system involvement is common and patients require imaging of the brain and cerebrospinal examination at presentation. Patients with HIV have a higher risk of Burkitt lymphoma.

181 Myeloproliferative neoplasms

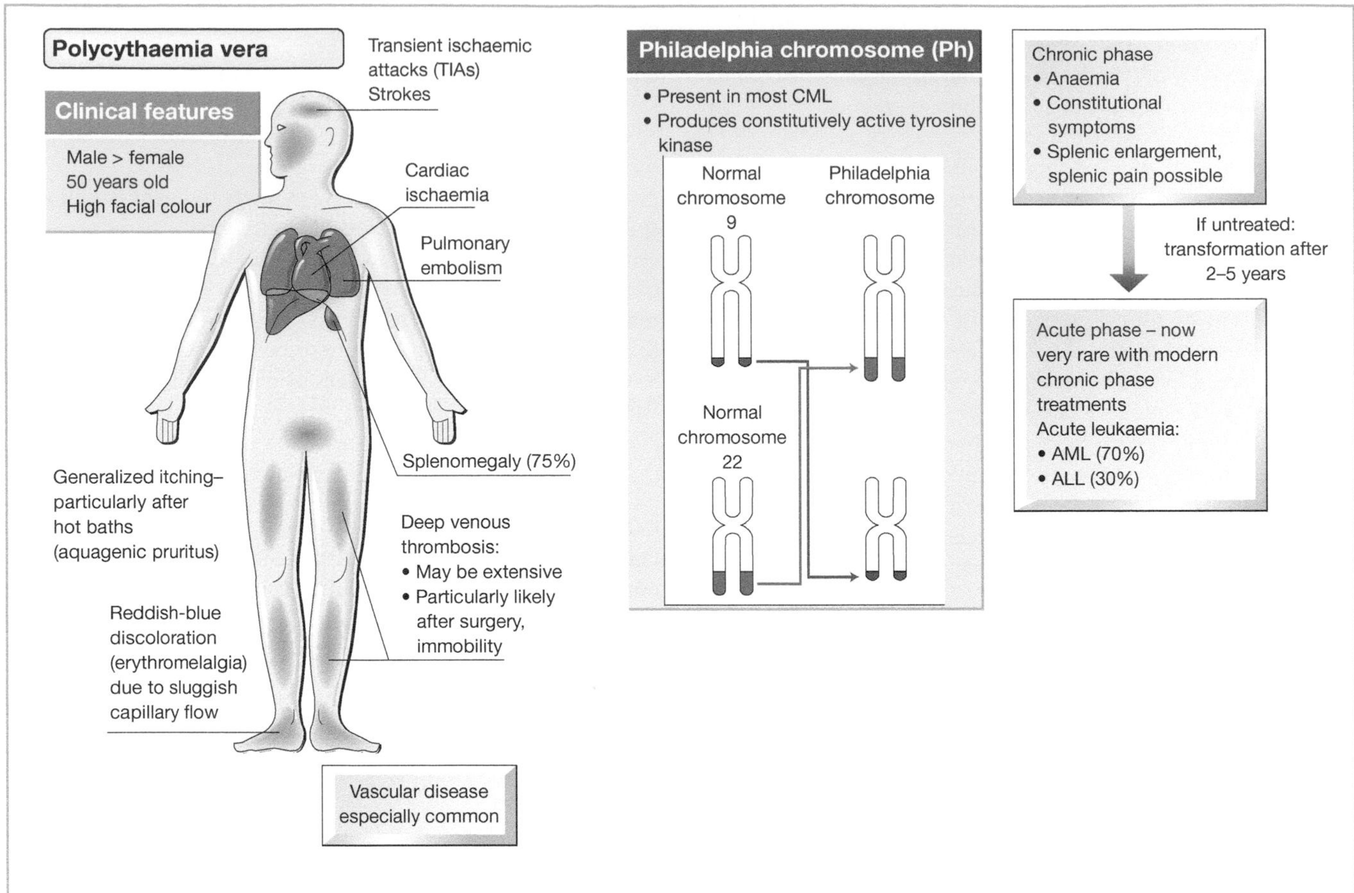

The myeloproliferative neoplasms are a group of four diseases caused by clonal proliferation of haematopoietic stem cells.

- Chronic myeloid leukaemia (CML)
- Myelofibrosis
- Polycythaemia vera (PV)
- Essential thrombocythaemia

Chronic myeloid leukaemia

CML has an incidence of 1/100 000 per year and is most common in middle age. Children are rarely affected. It is a clonal disorder arising in a pluripotential stem cell. The cells contain the Philadelphia chromosome, a translocation between chromosomes 9 and 22, which produces the oncogene *BCR-ABL*. This encodes a constitutively active tyrosine kinase which underlies the pathophysiology of this condition, with excess and uncontrolled granulocytic proliferation and maturation.

Clinical features

Systemic symptoms of weight loss, sweating and anorexia are common at presentation. Abdominal pain as a result of splenomegaly is frequent and symptoms from anaemia may occur. However, in some cases the disease is detected incidentally on a full blood count, which will demonstrate a marked excess of mature and maturing granulocytes (neutrophils, eosinophils, basophils). The platelet count may be normal or high, and the Hb is typically slightly low. A bone marrow biopsy will be hypercellular with a significant excess of myeloid cells. Diagnosis requires demonstration of the Ph chromosome by karyotype or fluorescence *in situ* hybridization (FISH), or detection of the *BCR-ABL* fusion gene by polymerase chain reaction (PCR).

Treatment and prognosis

Imatinib blocks the adenosine triphosphate (ATP) binding site on the constitutively active tyrosine kinase encoded by the *BCR-ABL* fusion gene. The great majority of patients will achieve a complete haematological remission within three months. Around 80% will achieve a complete cytogenetic remission (i.e. no Ph chromosome detected in the bone marrow by FISH), and deeper remission can be assessed molecularly using reverse transcriptase PCR for the fusion transcript. Resistance to imatinib occurs in a small percentage of patients over the first few years of treatment and newer tyrosine kinase inhibitors (nilotinib and dasatinib amongst others) can be used in this situation.

Bone marrow transplantation is used infrequently because of the effectiveness of imatinib but it may still be considered for young patients or those who do not respond well to serial tyrosine kinase inhibitors.

Myelofibrosis

Myelofibrosis is caused by a clonal abnormality of megakaryocyte precursor cells which causes these cells to release growth factors, including platelet-derived growth factor and other cytokines. This results in a polyclonal marrow fibrotic reaction, which gives the disease its name. The clinical consequences include anaemia and leukoerythroblastic change on the blood film (a mix of mature and immature granulocytes, with nucleated red blood cells, suggesting marrow stress). Teardrop-shaped red cells are also classically seen. The bone marrow is often inaspirable as a result of the fibrosis, but the trephine biopsy is hypercellular with increased marrow fibrosis. Splenomegaly is typically found, and can be massive.

Diagnosis is often helped by detection of the *JAK2* V617F mutation which is found in approximately 50% of cases. Other clonal molecular markers can be found in many of the remaining cases, including mutations in *MPL* and *CALR*.

The prognosis varies significantly with the genetic basis of the disorder, and a combination of clinical, laboratory and genetic indices determine the treatment used. High-risk patients may undergo stem cell transplantation or can be treated with the *JAK2* inhibitor ruxolitinib. Patients with lower-risk disease may be treated supportively or with hydroxycarbamide.

Polycythaemia vera (PV)

This is a clonal stem cell disorder characterized in >95% of cases by mutation of the *JAK2* gene and constitutive activation of JAK-STAT signalling pathways. The effect is dysregulation of erythropoiesis with an increase in red cell production.

Clinical features

The common complications of PV relate to the increased haematocrit. These include transient ischaemic attacks (TIAs), strokes, myocardial infarction, deep venous thrombosis and pulmonary emboli. Such events are more common in those with other risk factors for vascular disease. Other common features are facial plethora; itching, particularly after a hot bath or shower (aquagenic pruritus); and a burning discomfort, usually occurring in the fingers or toes associated with a reddish/blue discoloration (erythromelalgia). The latter is caused by sluggish blood flow and platelet aggregation in the small arterioles, which may lead to gangrenous digits. There is a small increased risk of haemorrhage as a result of abnormal platelet function. Bruising is common but more serious gastrointestinal or central nervous system bleeding may occur. Splenomegaly occurs in 75% of patients.

Investigations

The haemoglobin (Hb) and RBC count are high, and there may be a mild neutrophilia and thrombocytosis. PV must be distinguished from other causes of polycythaemia: secondary polycythaemia caused by hypoxaemia (e.g. lung disease, cyanotic heart disease, high altitude); tumours releasing erythropoietin (e.g. renal, cerebellar haemangioblastoma, etc.) – all of which are characterized by a high serum erythropoietin level, unlike the EPO suppression seen in PV. A further differential is apparent polycythaemia in which the red cell mass is not increased but rather the plasma volume contracted.

Treatment and prognosis

Venesection to reduce the haematocrit to <45% is a simple and usually safe treatment. Treatment with hydroxycarbamide may be effective where adequate control of the red cell count cannot be achieved by venesection or in those with high platelet counts. Excellent control of the red cell mass and the platelet count will reduce the risk of vascular events. Antiplatelet drugs such as aspirin are also indicated prophylactically.

The prognosis for well-treated patients with PV is good. The median survival is 10 years. Some patients' PV transforms into secondary myelofibrosis and a small percentage of patients develop acute leukaemia.

Essential thrombocythaemia (ET)

Epidemiology, aetiology and pathogenesis

Again, this clonal myeloid disorder is a manifestation of *JAK2* mutation in some 50% of cases (and the exact mechanisms by which an identical mutation can produce these distinct clinical phenotypes remain unclear). *CALR* and *MPL* mutations are seen in *JAK2*-negative patients, as in myelofibrosis. In ET, the predominant feature is a raised platelet count, and the main differential is a reactive thrombocytosis. The peripheral blood platelet count will be >400 × 10^9/l and often >1000 × 10^9/l. The differential diagnosis includes:

- other myeloproliferative neoplasms
- illnesses associated with a reactive thrombocytosis, where the platelet count is usually 400–1000 × 10^9/l, but may be higher, and where cytoreductive treatment is not needed.

Clinical features

Most patients are diagnosed as an incidental finding. In the remainder, the most common presenting symptoms are thrombotic events from the raised platelet count, such as cardiac ischaemia/infarction, strokes and venous thrombosis. The risk of a thrombotic event is increased by coincidental risk factors such as hypertension, diabetes and cigarette smoking. There is also an increased risk of bleeding in these patients because of impaired platelet function.

Investigations

There is no single diagnostic test for essential thrombocythaemia, although about 50% will be found to have a *JAK2* mutation. *MPL* and *CALR* mutations should also be sought. Exclusion of other myeloproliferative neoplasms, such as polycythaemia and CML, and of a reactive cause is important.

Treatment and prognosis

High-risk patients are treated with hydroxycarbamide as a cytoreductive agent (with anagrelide as an alternative). Antiplatelet agents may be used. If the platelet count is maintained within the normal range, the risk of vascular events drops to close to normal. Most patients have a normal life expectancy, though a small percentage go on to develop acute myeloid leukaemia.

182 Myeloma

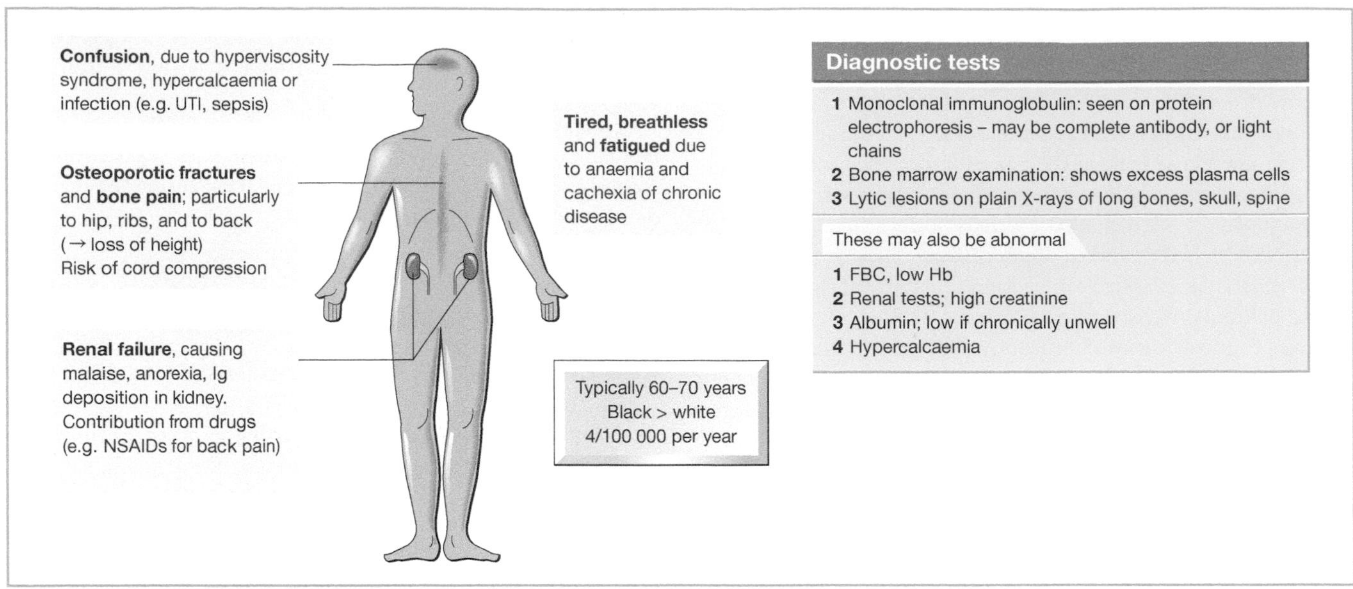

Myeloma is a malignancy of plasma cells in the bone marrow, with an incidence of 4/100 000. It is more common in elderly people and in people of Afro-Caribbean/African American ethnicity.

Pathophysiology

In myeloma, a clone of malignant plasma cells forms, filling the bone marrow, and producing just a single (monoclonal) immunoglobulin type, known as an M band or a paraprotein. Normal immunoglobulin production is suppressed, i.e. immunoparesis occurs, responsible for the increased risk of infection. Anaemia is common from tumour infiltration, a cytokine-mediated anaemia of chronic disease, and from the often co-existent renal impairment. Kidney failure affects 50% of patients at some time during their illness and is most frequently the result of the renal deposition of Bence-Jones protein (i.e. the light chains of an immunoglobulin molecule), although it can be the result of dehydration, sepsis, drugs (especially non-steroidal anti-inflammatories) and hypercalcaemia.

The latter is found in 25% of patients at diagnosis, and is caused by the release of cytokines by malignant plasma cells, which stimulate osteoclastic bone resorption and release of calcium from the bony cortex into the circulation.

Clinical features and investigations

The mean age of presentation is 65–70 years. Common complications are bacterial infection (from hypogammaglobulinaemia), bone pain and fractures resulting from lysis and resorption of cortical bone (also visible as lytic lesions on skeletal survey or whole-body MRI); nausea, thirst, polyuria, constipation and confusion from hypercalcaemia, anaemia and renal impairment. Diagnosis depends on demonstrating a monoclonal immunoglobulin band on serum electrophoresis, with depression of the other immunoglobulins and/or finding a monoclonal light chain excess (Bence-Jones protein) in the urine. Monoclonal free light chains can also be detected in the blood using the Freelite® assay. The bone marrow aspirate shows >10% plasma cells.

Treatment and prognosis

The standard treatment is with chemotherapy, usually a combination of proteosome inhibitor (e.g. bortezomib, carfilzomib), lenalidomide and dexamethasone. High-dose therapy and stem cell rescue (autologous bone marrow transplantation) can achieve more substantial remissions in patients who are able to tolerate this.

Overall survival has been shown to depend on a number of prognostic factors including chromosomal translocations, but is between 5 and 7 years for patients with intermediate risk disease.

Monoclonal gammopathy of undetermined significance

This condition, increasingly common with rising age, is sometimes referred to as benign paraproteinaemia, but is better termed monoclonal gammopathy of undetermined significance (MGUS). Patients have a monoclonal paraprotein but no other features of myeloma, e.g. bone lesions, anaemia or renal impairment. In these patients, the risk of developing myeloma or similar disorder is about 1% per year.

Medicine at a Glance, Fifth Edition. Edited by Patrick Davey and Alex Pitcher.

Companion website: www.wiley.com/go/medicine5e

183 Myelodysplasia

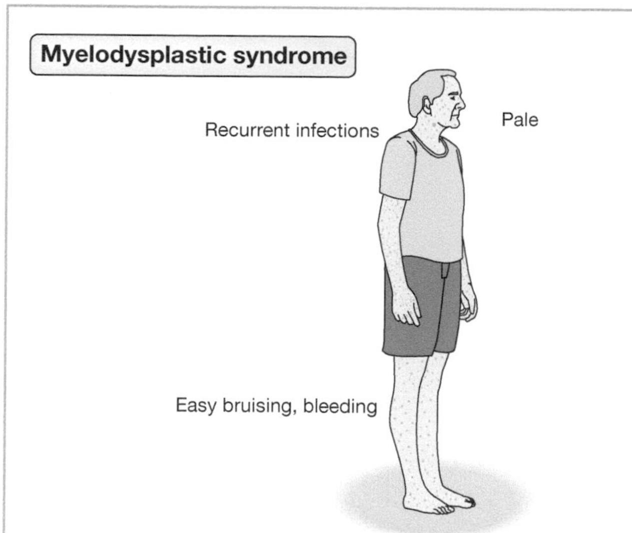

Clinical features

- Common
- Usually older patients
- FBC shows ↓Hb (↑MCV) ↓neutrophil and ↓platelets
- Bone marrow exam with karyotype and genetics is diagnostic

Treatment

- Mainly supportive (blood, platelets, antibiotics)
- Newer treatment agents can slow progression and improve outcomes

Prognosis

- After a variable period, may transform to AML (difficult to treat)

Myelodysplasia is a clonal disorder of the bone marrow in which morphologically and functionally abnormal blood cells are produced. It occurs with increasing frequency with rising age. Most patients have a macrocytic anaemia; neutropenia and thrombocytopenia are also very common. In most, no cause can be identified, though in some cases myelodysplasia develops after exposure to cytotoxic drugs or radiotherapy. Importantly, myelodysplasia is seen as a preleukaemic condition, with the transformation to acute myeloid leukaemia being part of its natural history.

Clinical features

The clinical features can be predicted from the pathological findings. Symptoms of anaemia are common. There is an increased risk of bacterial infection resulting from the neutropenia and because the neutrophils are functionally abnormal. Haemorrhagic complications are common as a result of thrombocytopenia and because platelet function is usually abnormal. The World Health Organization defines several subtypes, defined by cytogenetic abnormalities, number of cytopenias, and the percentage of blasts in the bone marrow; each type has a different prognosis, and prognostic scoring systems provide further information about the expected course of the disease.

Diagnosis

Most patients have a macrocytic anaemia without vitamin B_{12} or folate deficiency. Abnormal-looking (dysplastic) cells in the blood film are commonly found. The bone marrow is hypercellular and dysplastic.

Treatment and prognosis

The treatment for myelodysplasia remains unsatisfactory although there are some agents which have been found to have a positive effect on the disease's course.

- **Drug treatment**: azacytidine is a hypomethylating agent which has benefits in both high- and low-risk myelodysplasia with a survival benefit. Lenalidomide is an immunomodulatory drug which seems particularly effective in a subtype of myelodysplastic syndrome (MDS) associated with loss of the long arm of chromosome 5 (so-called 5q-syndrome).
- **Erythropoeitin treatment**: erythropoietin can be beneficial in anaemic patients with myelodysplasia, especially where the endogenous epo level is relatively low.
- **Supportive care:** this may involve transfusions for anaemia; infections should be promptly treated with antibiotics. Platelet transfusions help in haemorrhage caused by thrombocytopenia, but are not recommended for uncomplicated low platelet counts because platelet antibodies may develop and lessen the effectiveness of future platelet transfusions. Transfused platelets have a lifespan of 24–48 hours.
- **Allogeneic bone marrow transplantation**: this can be curative in young patients when a donor can be found. Patients with an increased blast count may benefit from AML-type chemotherapy regimens, although the remission rate and survival are worse than in *de novo* AML.

The prognosis for patients with myelodysplasia varies enormously depending on the risk stratification of the disease (i.e. blast percentage, cytogenetic features, degree and number of cytopenias). In poor risk disease, survival may be <1 year, with transformation to AML expected; in better risk disease, much longer survival can be expected.

Medicine at a Glance, Fifth Edition. Edited by Patrick Davey and Alex Pitcher.

Companion website: www.wiley.com/go/medicine5e

The blood in systemic disease

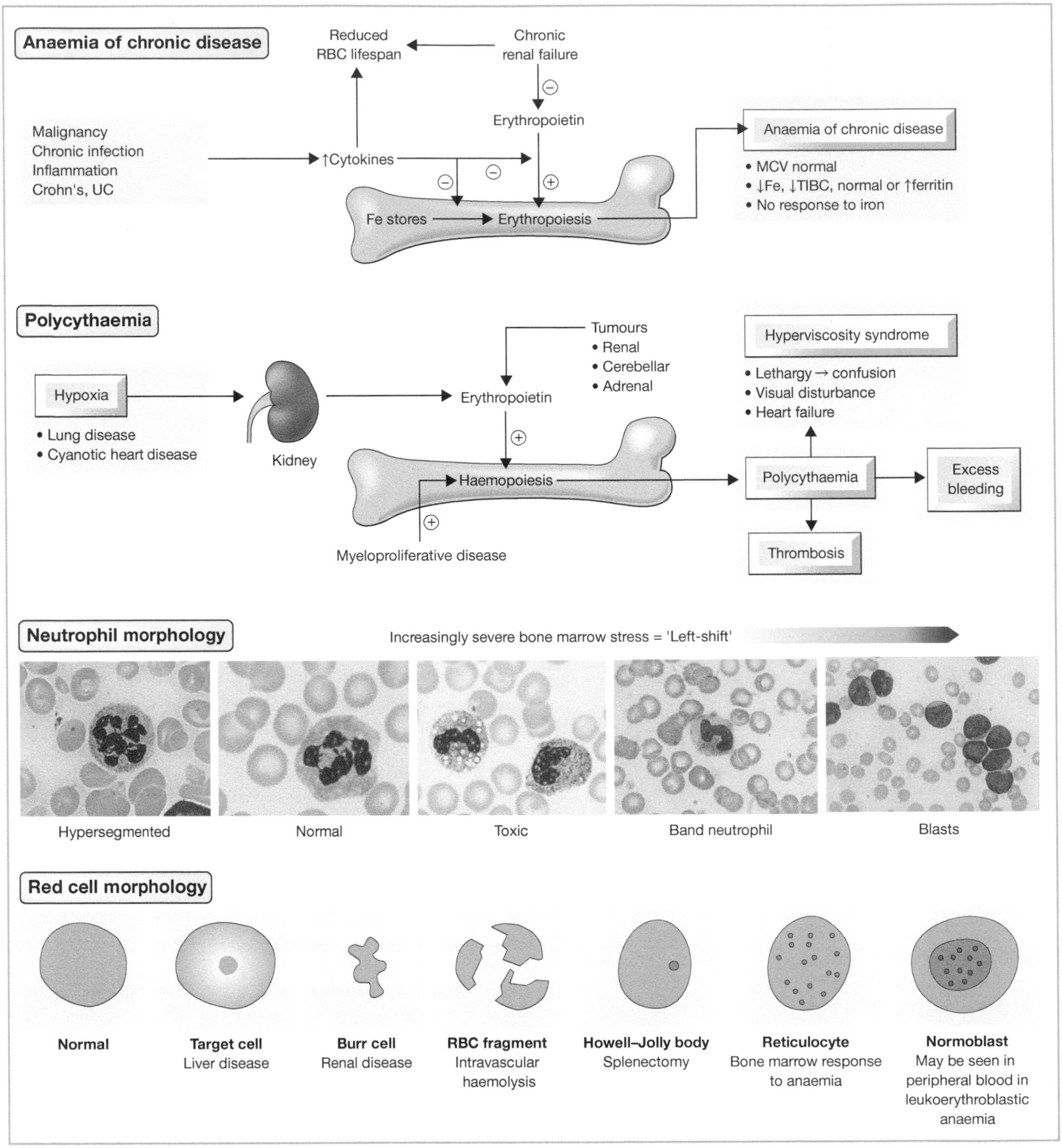

Anaemia of chronic disease

Reduced RBC lifespan

Chronic renal failure

Erythropoietin

Malignancy
Chronic infection
Inflammation
Crohn's, UC

↑Cytokines

Fe stores → Erythropoiesis

Anaemia of chronic disease

- MCV normal
- ↓Fe, ↓TIBC, normal or ↑ferritin
- No response to iron

Polycythaemia

Hypoxia

- Lung disease
- Cyanotic heart disease

Kidney

Erythropoietin

Tumours
- Renal
- Cerebellar
- Adrenal

Haemopoiesis

Myeloproliferative disease

Hyperviscosity syndrome

- Lethargy → confusion
- Visual disturbance
- Heart failure

Polycythaemia

Excess bleeding

Thrombosis

Neutrophil morphology

Increasingly severe bone marrow stress = 'Left-shift'

Hypersegmented

Normal

Toxic

Band neutrophil

Blasts

Red cell morphology

Normal

Target cell
Liver disease

Burr cell
Renal disease

RBC fragment
Intravascular haemolysis

Howell–Jolly body
Splenectomy

Reticulocyte
Bone marrow response to anaemia

Normoblast
May be seen in peripheral blood in leukoerythroblastic anaemia

Medicine at a Glance, Fifth Edition. Edited by Patrick Davey and Alex Pitcher.

Companion website: www.wiley.com/go/medicine5e

The blood is commonly affected by systemic disease.

Anaemia of chronic disease

Many chronic disease processes produce inflammatory cytokines, which depress haematopoiesis by reducing iron transfer to developing red cells and diminishing the effects of erythropoietin on the bone marrow. Red cell survival is also shortened. Underlying disease processes include the following.

- Chronic infection, e.g. infective endocarditis, abscesses (particularly in the lung) and osteomyelitis.
- Chronic inflammation, e.g. rheumatoid arthritis, temporal arteritis and other vasculitides (e.g. systemic lupus erythematosus [SLE], polyarteritis nodosa).
- Inflammatory bowel disease, which causes both chronic disease and iron deficiency anaemia.
- Malignancy.
- Chronic renal failure, which causes anaemia principally by impairing the production of erythropoietin, although other mechanisms are also implicated.

The anaemia is usually mild (Hb usually ≥8 g/dl), and the mean cell volume (MCV) is normal (80–90 fl). Serum iron is low, as are iron transfer proteins (as measured by the total iron-binding capacity [TIBC]). Bone marrow examination, indicated when iron deficiency cannot be excluded non-invasively, shows plentiful supplies of iron. The anaemia does not respond to iron supplementation, but does to treatment of the underlying disease. Erythropoietin helps in renal failure and in some other diseases, e.g. anaemia of malignancy. Blood transfusions may help symptomatic patients.

Anaemia of acute disease

Anaemia can occur within a few days in severe acute illnesses.

- Acute severe infection pneumonia, septicaemia, etc.
- Acute renal failure from any cause although especially from vasculitis.

It is vital to actively exclude acute gastrointestinal haemorrhage, a common cause of anaemia in sick patients. In addition to treating the underlying disease, blood transfusion has a role.

Leukoerythroblastic anaemia

Leukoerythroblastic anaemia is anaemia with immature white and red blood cells found in the blood film. Leukoerythroblastic anaemia is a common reaction to severe bone marrow stress in:

- severe gastrointestinal haemorrhage
- severe haemolytic anaemia
- overwhelming sepsis
- bone marrow malignancy, commonly metastatic, although also intrinsic haematological malignancy, such as myelofibrosis and myeloma.

If the underlying diagnosis is unclear, bone marrow examination is usually diagnostic. The treatment is of the underlying condition and blood transfusion.

Polycythaemia

Polycythaemia is an increase in haemoglobin level by ≥2 standard deviations from the mean. Increased haemoglobin occurs in myeloproliferative disease (see Chapter 181), though these are rare. Much more common is polycythaemia secondary to the following.

- Chronic hypoxaemia from lung disease, usually chronic obstructive pulmonary disease (COPD).
- Heavy cigarette smoking associated with systemic hypertension (Gaisböck syndrome); this occurs mainly in men. Premature death from coronary or lung disease is common.
- Cyanotic heart disease.
- Rare causes include excess erythropoietin-secreting tumours in the kidney or, rarer still, cerebellar haemangioblastomas, uterine fibroids and other tumours.
- Spurious causes: dehydration is a common cause of a transient polycythaemia.

Polycythaemia may be asymptomatic or produce a hyperviscosity syndrome (tiredness, effort intolerance, headaches, visual disturbance). Thrombosis, usually venous and occasionally arterial, may occur. As most polycythaemia is secondary or relative, investigation should include blood gases and lung function tests. Other tests include estimation of red cell mass using radioactive chromium and occasionally bone marrow biopsy. Renal, abdominal and cerebellar imaging may demonstrate a tumour. Treatment is of the underlying disease.

Leukocytosis

A neutrophil leukocytosis most commonly occurs in patients with bacterial infection and a lymphocytosis in those with a viral infection. A neutrophil leukocytosis also occurs in: (i) tissue necrosis, e.g. myocardial or pulmonary infarction, associated with a mild fever; (ii) malignancy; (iii) non-infectious inflammatory causes, including connective tissue disease; (iv) corticosteroid usage; and (v) diabetic ketoacidosis.

Investigations to exclude infection, vasculitis and malignancy may be needed if the cause is not obvious. Rarely neutrophil or lymphocytic leukocytosis is leukaemic in origin.

An increase in the eosinophil count is defined as $>0.5 \times 10^9$ eosinophils/l. It is uncommon and occurs in the following.

- Drug allergy: a common cause.
- Skin diseases: atopic eczema, urticaria.
- Asthma: complicating allergic bronchopulmonary aspergillosis should be considered.
- Parasitic infection, often intestinal, although infection elsewhere may be responsible, such as in the skin (cutaneous larva migrans).
- Vasculitis, especially polyarteritis nodosa.
- Malignancy such as Hodgkin disease.
- More rarely found in the hypereosinophilic syndrome.

Patients usually do not have symptoms from the excess eosinophils, and treatment is of the underlying condition. Occasionally very high eosinophil counts occur, usually with tropical infections (tropical eosinophilia), causing myocardial and endocardial damage (restrictive cardiomyopathy).

Thrombocytosis

Although increases in platelet counts occur in myeloproliferative diseases (see Chapter 181), most increases are secondary to:

- bleeding, especially chronic blood loss anaemia
- infection
- post surgery, especially after splenectomy
- malignancy
- inflammatory disease, including vasculitis.

Mild increases ($400–700 \times 10^9$/l) are usually asymptomatic, but the higher the platelet count, the more likely is thrombosis, both arterial and venous. Treatment is of the underlying cause; if this is not possible, aspirin is used for thrombosis prophylaxis.

Table 184.1 Causes of a macrocytosis (MCV >100 fl).

Cause	Clues from full blood count and film	Other blood results	Causes/comment
Drug-induced	Usually unremarkable	No specific abnormality	Many drugs, e.g. azathioprine, zidovudine
B_{12}/folate deficiency	Oval macrocytic red cells, hypersegmented neutrophils, pancytopenia	Low serum B_{12}/red cell folate Positive intrinsic factor antibodies in pernicious anaemia	B_{12} deficiency: pernicious anaemia/malabsorption Folate deficiency: inadequate dietary intake/malabsorption
Haemolysis	See Table 184.2. Haemolytic anaemia is usually normocytic but can be macrocytic if there is marked reticulocytosis		
Primary bone marrow disorder	MCV usually >110 fl Other cytopenias Leukocytosis Monocytosis Thrombocytosis Blast cells	No specific abnormality	Myelodysplasia, leukaemia
Alcohol	Alcohol may also cause lymphopenia and thrombocytopenia	Abnormal liver function tests, with raised AST (>ALT) and γ-GT	Macrocytosis due to alcohol usually indicates a chronic intake of 80 units/day or more
Hypothyroidism	Usually unremarkable	Raised TSH, low free T_4/free T_3	Hypothyroidism may also cause normocytic anaemia
Chronic liver disease	Associated thrombocytopenia may be seen in cirrhosis with portal hypertension and splenomegaly	Abnormal liver function tests/ prothrombin time	Anaemia may also be due to acute or chronic gut bleeding (e.g. from oesophageal varices)

Table 184.2 Causes of a normocytic anaemia (MCV 78–100 fl).

Cause	Clues from full blood count and film	Other blood results	Causes/comment
Bleeding	Polychromasia Anisocytosis	Falling haemoglobin without evidence of haemolysis	Occult bleeding may occur from gut or into retroperitoneal space
Haemolysis	Polychromasia (reflecting increased reticulocyte count) Spherocytes Keratocytes ('bite' cells, due to acute haemolysis induced by oxidant damage, as may occur in G6PD deficiency) Fragmented red cells seen in microangiopathic haemolytic anaemia	Increased unconjugated bilirubin, increased LDH and reduced serum haptoglobin seen in haemolysis of all causes	Haemolysis is due either to intrinsic red cell abnormalities (e.g. G6PD deficiency, sickle cell anaemia) or to extrinsic factors (immune and non-immune causes)
Anaemia of chronic disease	Film usually unremarkable	Low iron Low/normal transferrin Normal/increased ferritin Abnormalities related to underlying cause	Seen in acute and chronic infection, cancer, renal failure, inflammatory disorders (e.g. rheumatoid arthritis, SLE), endocrine disorders and chronic rejection after solid-organ transplantation
Bone marrow disorder	Other cytopenias Leukocytosis Monocytosis Thrombocytosis Blast cells	Paraproteinaemia in myeloma	Myelodysplasia, myeloma, leukaemia

Table 184.3 Causes of a microcytic anaemia (MCV <78 fl).

Cause	Clues from full blood count and film	Other blood results	Causes/comment
Iron deficiency	Increased red cell distribution width Anisocytosis Increased platelet count	Low iron Increased transferrin Low ferritin	Most common cause of microcytic anaemia; caused by inadequate dietary intake, malabsorption (e.g. coeliac disease) or blood loss
Anaemia of chronic disease (ACD)	Film usually unremarkable	Low iron Low/normal transferrin Normal/increased ferritin Abnormalities related to underlying cause	c. 20% of ACDs are microcytic: causes include Hodgkin disease and renal cell carcinoma (see Table 184.2)
Thalassaemia	Polychromasia Target cells	Normal ferritin Haemoglobin electrophoresis normal in α-thalassaemia trait and abnormal in β-thalassaemia trait and other thalassaemia syndromes	Haematocrit usually >30% and MCV <75 fl in β-thalassaemia trait
Sideroblastic anaemia	Siderocytes may be seen: hypochromic red cells with basophilic stippling that stains positive for iron (Pappenheimer's bodies)	Increased ferritin	Rare Hereditary and acquired forms

Table 184.4 White blood cell abnormalities.

Finding	Possible causes	Finding	Possible causes
Neutrophilia	Sepsis Metastatic cancer Acidosis Corticosteroid therapy Trauma, surgery, burn Myeloproliferative disorders	Lymphopenia	Infections (e.g. viral, HIV, severe bacterial) Immunosuppressive therapy Systemic lupus erythematosus Alcohol excess Chronic renal failure
Neutropenia	Drugs (e.g. carbimazole) Infections (e.g. viral, severe bacterial, HIV) B_{12} and folate deficiency Systemic lupus erythematosus Felty syndrome Haematological disorders (e.g. leukaemia)	Monocytosis	Infections Myeloproliferative disorders (e.g. chronic myelomonocytic leukaemia) Metastatic cancer
Lymphocytosis	Infections (e.g. infectious mononucleosis) Chronic lymphocytic leukaemia	Eosinophilia	Drug allergy Parasitic infestation Haematological disorders (e.g. lymphoma, leukaemia) Churg–Strauss vasculitis Disorders with eosinophilic involvement of specific organs Adrenal insufficiency Atheroembolism

Table 184.5 Common causes of thrombocytosis (platelet count >350 × 10^9/l).

Setting	Common causes
Acute admission	Acute blood loss/iron deficiency Acute infection Cancer
Inpatient	After surgery or trauma Acute infection Acute pancreatitis Cancer Chronic inflammatory disorders
Outpatient	Chronic infection Post splenectomy Cancer Chronic inflammatory disorders Chronic myeloproliferative or myelodysplastic disorder

Table 184.6 Causes of pancytopenia (red cell, white cell and platelet counts all low).

- Aplastic anaemia
- Idiopathic
- Cytotoxic drugs and radiation
- Idiosyncratic drug reaction
- Viral infections
- Acute leukaemia
- Marrow replacement
- Cancer
- Myelofibrosis
- Miliary tuberculosis
- B_{12}/folate deficiency
- Paroxysmal nocturnal haemoglobinuria
- Myelodysplasia
- Human immunodeficiency virus infection

185 Platelet disorders

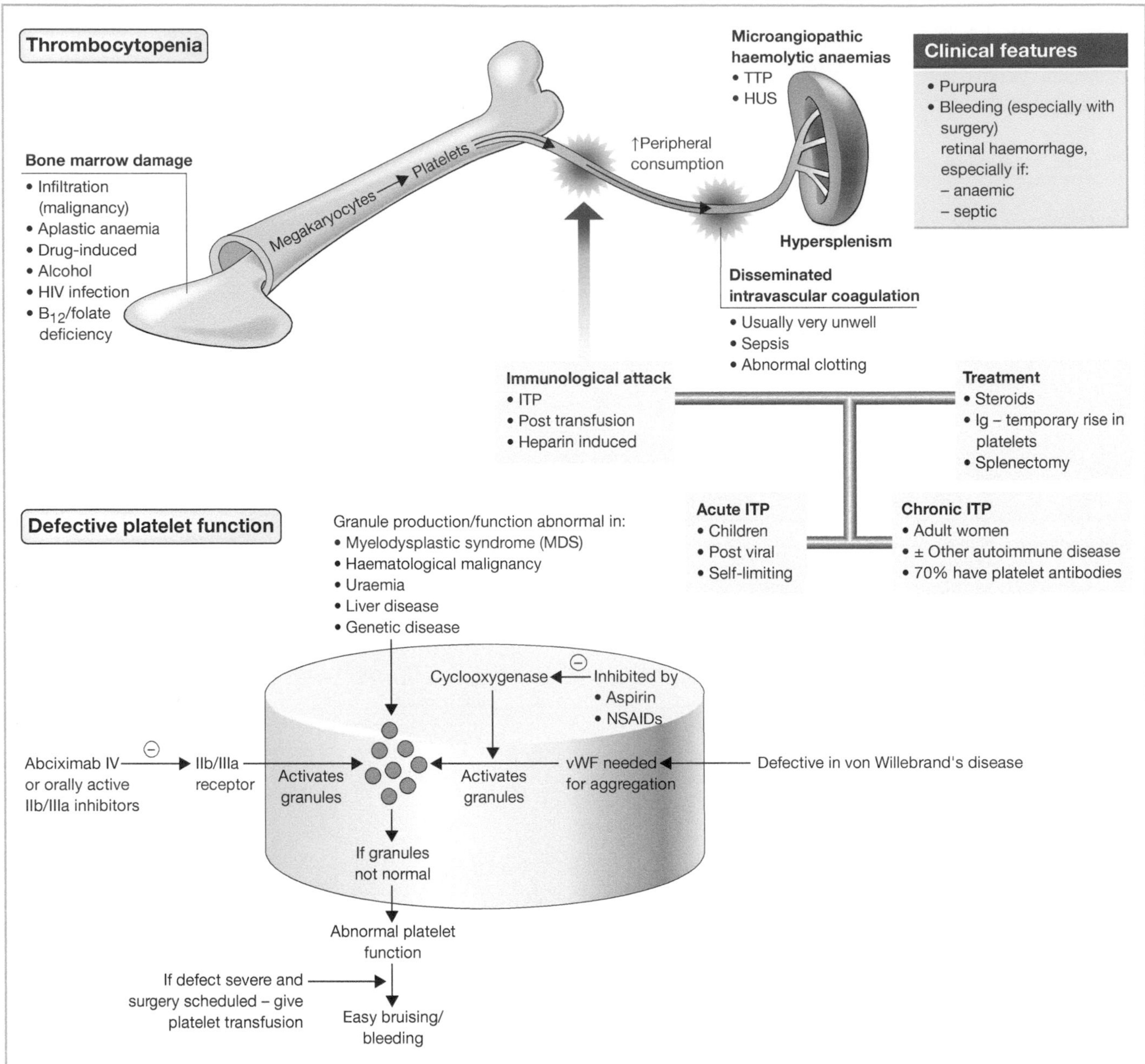

Physiology of haemostasis

When there is injury to a blood vessel, a series of five events are initiated to control haemostasis. The first three processes are: (1) local vasoconstriction, (2) adhesion and aggregation of platelets, and (3) activation of the clotting cascade to create a fibrin clot. Coagulation inhibitors are then activated (4) to restrict coagulation to the site of injury and (5) fibrinolysis occurs later to restore vessel patency. Step 2 (platelet adhesion/aggregation) requires that platelets adhere to the exposed collagen in damaged blood vessels via von Willebrand factor (vWF), a large polymeric molecule, individual subunits of which possess collagen- and platelet-binding sites (for platelet glycoprotein Ib). The platelets aggregate to each other by cross-linking with fibrinogen, which binds to specific fibrinogen-binding sites on the platelet surface (glycoprotein IIb/IIIa). Upon activation, platelets release agents (including adenosine diphosphate [ADP]) from their dense granules to recruit other platelets to the site plus thromboxane, a potent platelet agonist, which provides positive feedback.

Medicine at a Glance, Fifth Edition. Edited by Patrick Davey and Alex Pitcher.

Companion website: www.wiley.com/go/medicine5e

Platelet disorders

Platelet disorders are quantitative or qualitative. They present clinically with purpura, petechiae, mucosal bleeding, epistaxis and menorrhagia.

Thrombocytopenia

The causes of thrombocytopenia are summarized in Table 185.1.

Immune thrombocytopenic purpura

Immune thrombocytopenic purpura (ITP) is an autoimmune disorder in which antibodies are directed against antigens on the platelet surface, causing platelet removal from the circulation by reticuloendothelial cells, largely in the spleen. An acute self-limiting form occurs in children, typically after a viral infection and often not needing treatment. In adults, ITP is a chronic disorder that is most common in middle-aged women. The diagnosis is largely one of exclusion, the bone marrow being normal or having an increased number of normal megakaryocytes. Treatment with steroids is only given to maintain the platelet count at safe levels and there is usually no need for therapy if the platelet count is above 30×10^9/l. Alternative therapies if steroids fail or if too high a dose is needed include rituximab or the thrombopoietin receptor agonist romiplostim. Intravenous IgG gives a good, rapid, albeit temporary, response and is useful for emergencies.

Thrombotic thrombocytopenic purpura

Thrombotic thrombocytopenic purpura (TTP) has a classic pentad of thrombocytopenia, microangiopathic haemolytic anaemia, neurological disturbance, fever and renal failure. The defect is the absence of a vWF-cleaving protease (ADAMTS-13) normally present in plasma. This results in abnormally large vWF polymers in the circulation, which induce platelet microthrombi, resulting in end-organ ischaemia. The common sporadic form is the result of cleaving protease-directed autoantibodies. The rare autosomal recessive familial form of TTP is caused by an inherited deficiency. Treatment is with plasma exchange which replaces the enzyme and removes antibody and ultra-large vWF multimers. The patient is simultaneously started on steroids and rituximab if there is neurological or cardiac involvement.

Disseminated intravascular coagulation

See Chapter 186.

Table 185.1 Causes of thrombocytopenia.

Decreased production

- Marrow aplasia or infiltration
- Megaloblastic anaemia
- Acute alcohol toxicity

Increased consumption

- Immune:
  - Immune thrombocytopenic purpura
  - Thrombotic thrombocytopenic purpura
  - Post-transfusion purpura
  - Heparin-induced thrombocytopenia
  - Drug induced thrombocytopenia
  - Antiphospholipid antibody syndrome
- Non-immune:
  - Disseminated intravascular coagulation
  - Haemolytic uraemic syndrome
  - Hypersplenism

Bone marrow infiltration

Bone marrow infiltration (by tumour) or aplasia (particularly chemotherapy induced) may cause thrombocytopenia.

Post-transfusion purpura

Post-transfusion purpura is suspected if thrombocytopenia occurs about 10 days after a blood transfusion. The patient's own platelets lack the HPA-1a antigen, which is present on the platelets in 98% of the population. When transfused with HPA-1a-positive platelets, the recipient makes antibodies against HPA-1a and these, bizarrely, cross-react with the recipient's own HPA-1a-negative platelets, resulting in thrombocytopenia. Treatment is with intravenous immunoglobulin and the avoidance of HPA-1a-positive platelets.

Heparin-induced thrombocytopenia

Heparin-induced thrombocytopenia is a rare but serious adverse reaction to heparin. The patient makes IgG antibodies to heparin–platelet factor 4 complexes. This antibody then interacts with the platelet Fcγ receptor, resulting in platelet activation, thrombocytopenia and arterial and venous thrombosis. Heparin must be stopped and an alternative such as argatroban, danaparoid or fondaparinux substituted.

Haemolytic uraemic syndrome

Haemolytic uraemic syndrome (HUS) presents with thrombocytopenia, renal failure and microangiopathic haemolytic anaemia. Although clinically similar to TTP, the pathology is different and is the result of endothelial damage with subsequent platelet activation. It is often seen in children after infection with verotoxin-producing strains of *Escherichia coli*. Treatment is supportive.

Qualitative platelet defects

Disorders of platelet function (see Table 185.2) are rare other than those caused by drugs.

- **Aspirin** irreversibly and **non-steroidal anti-inflammatory drugs** (NSAIDs) reversibly inhibit the cyclo-oxygenase 1 enzyme in platelets, preventing thromboxane synthesis and so ameliorating platelet aggregation.
- **Myelodysplastic platelets** have major functional defects, as do those from uraemic patients.
- **Bernard–Soulier disease** and **Glanzmann thrombasthenia** are rare, inherited, autosomal recessive disorders caused by the absence of platelet glycoproteins (Gp Ib and Gp IIb/IIIa, respectively). Bleeding can be severe and treatment is with platelet transfusions as required.
- **Storage pool disease** is generally a mild disorder resulting from an inherited defect in the platelets' storage granules. The inability to release ADP and other agents from the granules reduces platelet activation and recruitment.

Table 185.2 Disorders of platelet function.

Inherited

- Storage pool disease
- Glycoprotein (Gp) Ib deficiency: Bernard–Soulier disease
- Gp IIb/IIIa deficiency: Glanzmann thrombasthenia

Acquired

- Drugs: aspirin and NSAIDs
- Hypergammaglobulinaemia
- Myeloproliferative disorders
- Uraemia

186 Disorders of coagulation

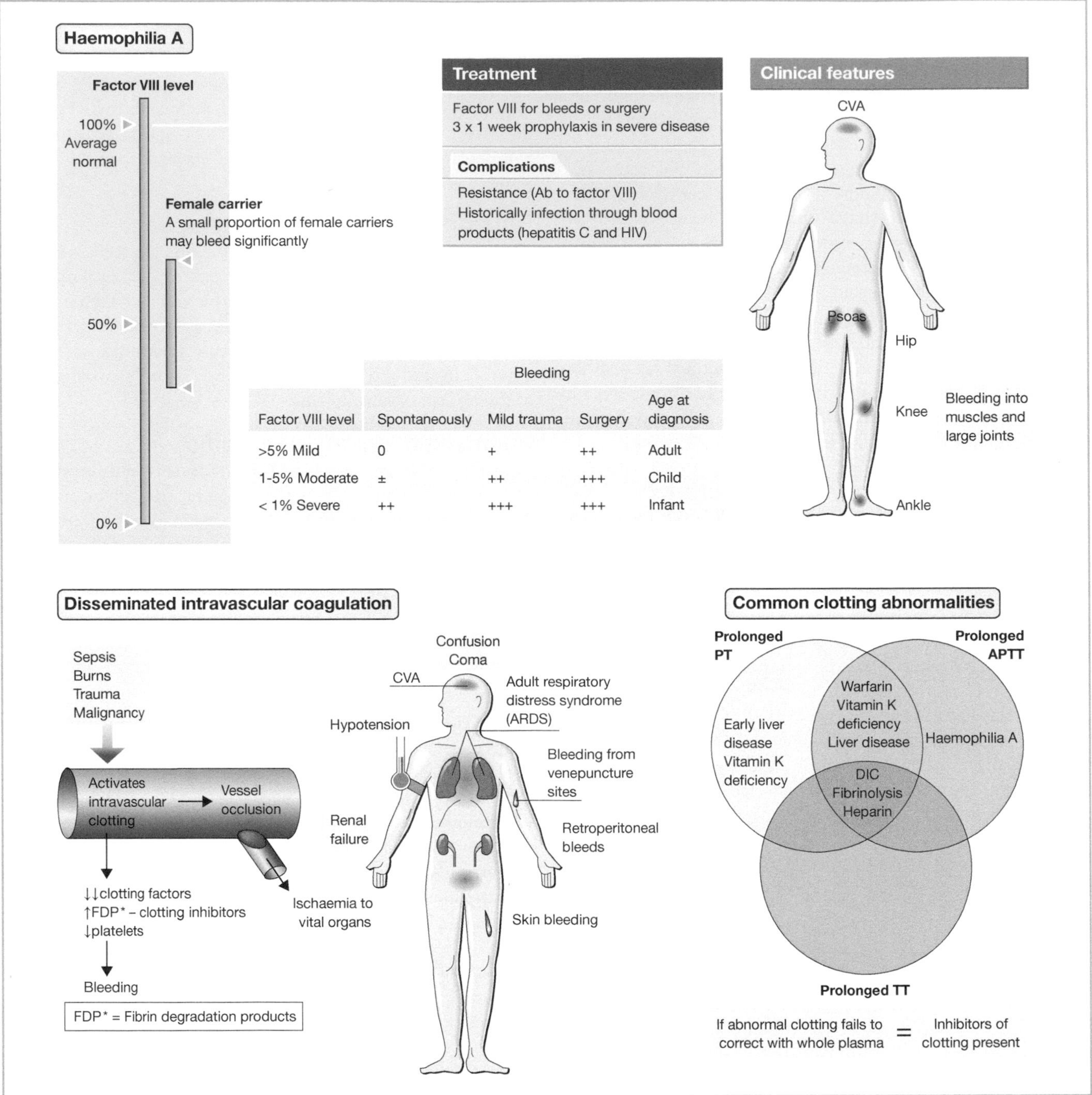

	Bleeding			
Factor VIII level	Spontaneously	Mild trauma	Surgery	Age at diagnosis
>5% Mild	0	+	++	Adult
1-5% Moderate	±	++	+++	Child
< 1% Severe	++	+++	+++	Infant

In vitro tests of clotting

The coagulation cascade has classically been divided into the intrinsic pathway, which was thought to be initiated by contact between denuded endothelium and coagulation factors (contact activation), and the extrinsic pathway initiated by the tissue factor/factor VIIa complex. Both pathways activate factor X, which then cleaves prothrombin (II) to release thrombin (IIa). This simplified version is still the most useful for interpreting routine coagulation tests, which comprise the activated partial thromboplastin time (APTT), the prothrombin time (PT) and occasionally the thrombin time (TT). Characteristic abnormalities in PT, APTT and TT occur in different diseases.

Medicine at a Glance, Fifth Edition. Edited by Patrick Davey and Alex Pitcher.

Companion website: www.wiley.com/go/medicine5e

- PT prolonged, APTT normal: factor VII deficiency (early liver disease or vitamin K deficiency).
- PT normal, APTT prolonged: factor VIII, IX, XI or contact factor deficiency. Lupus anticoagulant; heparin and direct thrombin inhibitors (PT may also be prolonged).
- PT prolonged, APTT prolonged: interpretation depends on whether or not the TT is abnormal.
  - Normal TT: factor II, V or X deficiency; frank vitamin K deficiency or warfarin therapy; liver disease, anti-Xa inhibitors (though effect is variable).
  - Prolonged TT: deficiency of fibrinogen and disseminated intravascular coagulation (DIC), especially as a result of fibrin degradation products (FDPs) interfering with fibrin polymerization; fibrinolysis; heparin and direct thrombin inhibitors (PT may not be significantly prolonged).

In vivo coagulation

In vivo, it is the tissue factor/factor VIIa pathway that initiates coagulation, largely by activation of factor IX. Factor IXa in conjunction with its co-factor, factor VIII, then activates factor X. The centrality of factors VIII and IX to clotting explains why haemophilia A (deficient factor VIII) and haemophilia B (deficient factor IX) are such severe coagulation disorders. This clotting cascade also explains why patients deficient in contact factors do not bleed abnormally. Factor XI is activated by thrombin, which then activates more factor IX in a positive feedback loop. Patients with factor XI deficiency exhibit a variable bleeding disorder.

Inherited disorders of coagulation

Deficiency of coagulation factors presents with haemarthroses and muscle haematomas (in contrast with platelet disorders which present principally with skin bleeds), although gastrointestinal, genitourinary and intracranial bleeds can occur. The most common inherited deficiencies are of factors VIII and IX and von Willebrand factor (VWF); other inherited coagulation disorders are rare.

Haemophilia A

Haemophilia A is caused by a deficiency of factor VIII. It is an X-linked recessive disorder affecting 1 in 5000 males. In severe disease (<1% factor VIII), spontaneous bleeding into large joints and muscles (e.g. psoas) occurs, unless regular prophylactic treatment with factor VIII concentrate is given. Moderate (1–5% factor VIII) and mild (5–40% factor VIII) disease is associated with bleeding on mild or moderate trauma. Factor VIII is given here only in response to trauma or in anticipation of surgery. Historically, plasma-derived FVIII concentrates resulted in infection with hepatitis C and HIV. Although virally screened and inactivated plasma derived FVIII products may still be used, they have largely been replaced by recombinant FVIII products. Novel therapies are also in late-phase clinical trials (such as gene therapy) or already available (emicizumab, a monoclonal antibody which mimics the action of factor VIII).

Haemophilia B

Haemophilia B is caused by a deficiency of factor IX. Factor IX acts with factor VIII to activate factor X, and like factor VIII is encoded on the X chromosome. Haemophilia A and haemophilia B (which is only one-fifth as common) are clinically indistinguishable.

Von Willebrand disease

Von Willebrand disease (VWD) is the most common inherited bleeding disorder – mild autosomal dominant forms may affect up to 1% of the population. The VWF is either deficient (partial: type 1 VWD; complete: type 3 VWD) or defective (type 2 VWD). The VWF circulates as large polymers and serves two functions. Its principal function is to form the bridge that allows platelets to adhere to damaged endothelial surfaces. Thus, in VWD clinical presentation is with the same pattern of bleeding as in patients with platelet disorders, e.g. skin bruising, epistaxis and menorrhagia. A secondary function of VWF is to stabilize circulating factor VIII. Plasma factor VIII levels therefore parallel those of VWF – although severe factor VIII deficiency occurs only in the rare type 3 disease. Treatment is with desmopressin (which raises VWF and factor VIII) in mild disease, and factor VIII/VWF concentrate in more severe disease.

Acquired disorders of coagulation

The most common acquired coagulation disorders are DIC, liver disease and vitamin K deficiency. Rarely, men or women can develop autoantibodies to factor VIII and so develop an acquired haemophilia.

Disseminated intravascular coagulation

This describes pathological activation of coagulation resulting in widespread microvascular thrombosis. Although consumption of coagulation factors often results in bleeding, it is the end-organ damage from thrombosis, rather than the bleeding itself, that leads to the very high mortality. Many insults can trigger DIC, e.g. septicaemia, malignancy and obstetric emergencies. The key to management is to treat the underlying disease. Blood products, fresh frozen plasma and platelets are given to support the patient if bleeding.

Liver disease

Coagulation factors are synthesized in the liver and deficiency occurs as liver disease progresses. The situation is often compounded by thrombocytopenia, caused by splenic uptake in the large spleen occurring in portal hypertension. As a result of the short half-life of factor VII, the PT is a sensitive marker of liver damage.

Vitamin K deficiency

Vitamin K is required as a coenzyme for the γ-carboxylation of the coagulation factors II, VII, IX and X. This post-translational modification is necessary for efficient secretion from the liver and in order for these factors to bind Ca^{2+}, which then enables them to bind to phospholipid surfaces. Vitamin K deficiency may present with easy bruising and occurs in malnutrition, and especially in the malabsorption resulting from obstructive jaundice. Patients with obstructive jaundice should receive vitamin K before any surgical procedure, including endoscopic retrograde cholangiopancreatography.

187 Anticoagulation and antiplatelet drugs

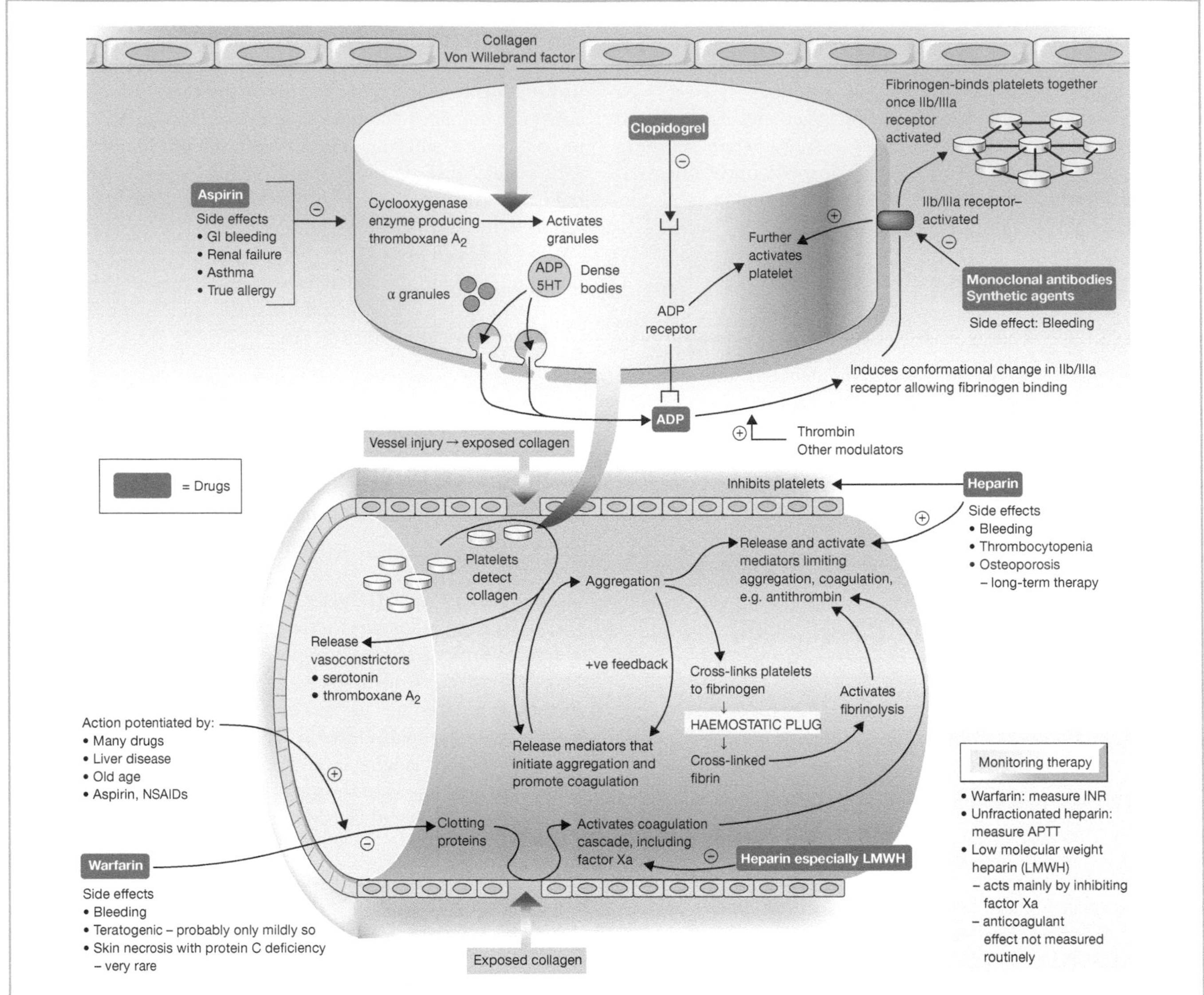

Anticoagulant and antiplatelet drugs are frequently used to prevent/treat abnormal clotting. Which is chosen depends on whether the mechanism underlying the clotting process is platelet or clotting protein dependent.

Antiplatelet agents

Diseases primarily involving platelet activation include most *in situ* arterial thrombosis, i.e. acute coronary syndromes (unstable angina, acute myocardial infarction [MI]), transient ischaemic attacks (TIAs) and strokes secondary to atherosclerosis. Drugs with antiplatelet action include the following.

Aspirin

Aspirin is powerful and cheap, and inhibits platelet function by irreversibly acetylating platelet cyclo-oxygenase. The duration of action is several days, until new platelets are produced. It is effective in stable angina (reduces MI rates), unstable angina (reduces MI and death rates), MI (reduces death rate by 15%) and TIAs (reduces stroke rate). If immediate action is required (e.g. MI or stroke), 300 mg should be chewed (absorbed from the mouth). Otherwise, it is given orally in a daily dose of 75 mg. Side-effects include upper gastrointestinal (GI) ulceration and bleeding and renal dysfunction (especially if there is pre-existing renal impairment). True allergy (rash or frank anaphylaxis) is very rare and is found more frequently in those with recurrent nasal polyps.

Medicine at a Glance, Fifth Edition. Edited by Patrick Davey and Alex Pitcher.

Companion website: www.wiley.com/go/medicine5e

Dipyridamole

Dipyridamole inhibits the uptake of adenosine into platelets and inhibits phosphodiesterase in various tissues. Aspirin plus sustained-release dipyridamole is more effective than aspirin alone in secondary stroke prevention.

Clopidogrel and other ADP receptor antagonists

Clopidogrel irreversibly inhibits the platelet adenosine diphosphate (ADP) receptor. It has a role in acute coronary syndromes, and after implantation of intracoronary stents. It is used as monotherapy in aspirin allergy/intolerance and has an expanding role in primary prevention of acute MI in high-risk patients. Prasugrel and ticagrelor are alternative ADP receptor antagonists (the latter binds reversibly).

Platelet IIb/IIIa receptor inhibitors

The platelet glycoprotein Gp IIb/IIIa binds to fibrinogen. Fibrinogen binding plays a critical role in thrombosis through both cross-linking of platelets in a growing thrombus and also further inducing platelet activation. There are two classes of IIb/IIIa receptor inhibitors.

- Abciximab is a monoclonal antibody to the IIb/IIIa receptor, given intravenously, and useful in percutaneous coronary intervention (percutaneous coronary angioplasty, intracoronary stenting), reducing MI rate and increasing procedural success rates. It is very expensive. Side-effects are bleeding around the groin (entry site for the catheter to the arterial circulation) and retroperitoneally. Abciximab binds very strongly to the IIb/IIIa receptor and prevents fibrinogen binding; in severe haemorrhage, fresh platelet transfusion is given to stem the bleeding.
- Intravenous, synthetic, small molecule IIb/IIIa receptor inhibitors (eptifibatide, tirofiban) improve the outcome in high-risk unstable angina (i.e. ongoing angina despite drug therapy, pulmonary oedema during angina, persisting major abnormalities on the resting electrocardiogram, or elevation in troponin ≥10 the detect limit). Side-effect: excess bleeding (e.g. intracranial or retroperitoneal haemorrhage).

Anticoagulants

Most venous clotting involves clotting cascade activation, e.g. deep vein thrombosis, pulmonary embolus, paradoxical right-to-left embolus, left atrial thrombosis (predisposition through atrial fibrillation) and any resulting emboli. Clotting on artificial heart valves also involves the clotting cascade. For sagittal venous sinus thrombosis, see Chapter 202. Warfarin and heparin have been used to treat and prevent venous thrombosis for decades, and the direct oral anticoagulants (DOACs) more recently.

Warfarin

Warfarin is a vitamin K antagonist and so inhibits the γ-carboxylation of clotting factors II, VII, IX and X. Its effect is measured by the international normalized ratio (INR), which is the patient's prothrombin time (PT; see Chapter 186), divided by the mean normal PT, raised to the power of the international sensitivity index of the reagent used.

- INR = 2.0–3.0 is usually therapeutic; some heart valves (e.g. Starr–Edwards) require an INR of 3.0–4.0.
- INR ≤2.0 provides inadequate therapeutic action and excess thrombosis.
- INR >3.0 is associated with an increased risk of bleeding.

Although warfarin rapidly inhibits vitamin K epoxide reductase, the clotting proteins whose production is inhibited have various half-lives. This 'buffer' delays the onset of therapeutic action (and the prolongation of the INR) by several days. Thus, if an anticoagulant is required to have immediate effect, heparin rather than (or as well as) warfarin should be used. Side-effects of warfarin therapy include the following.

- **Bleeding**, often from overanticoagulation, i.e. an INR ≥3.0. Bleeding can occur anywhere (intracranially, into the GI tract, etc.). Bleeding into the urinary tract, unless the INR is very prolonged (i.e. ≥6.0), often indicates intrinsic urinary tract pathology, e.g. urinary epithelial tumour.
- **Drug interactions** are very important and can increase or decrease warfarin metabolism, leading to over- or underanticoagulation. Antibiotics can decrease gut vitamin K production, so increasing the action of warfarin. Concomitant antiplatelet drugs may lead to bleeding. As there are so many drugs that interact with warfarin, it is recommended that before prescribing additional drugs, possible interactions are identified from the *British National Formulary*.
- **Skin necrosis** is an exceptionally rare side-effect, and often a manifestation of protein C deficiency.

Heparin

Heparin is a powerful, naturally occurring anticoagulant, which potentiates the action of antithrombin. It has an immediate onset of action, unlike warfarin.

- **Unfractionated heparins** (UFHs) are a mixture of different molecular weights (5000–35 000, average 13 000), which inhibit activated serine protease coagulation factors by promoting their irreversible union with antithrombin. They are usually given by continual intravenous infusion, with the dose titrated against the activated partial thromboplastin time (APTT; see Chapter 186). It is difficult to obtain ideal anticoagulation. Side-effects: bleeding, thrombocytopenia and osteoporosis in long-term therapy.
- **Low molecular weight heparins** (LMWHs) are unfractionated heparins chemically or physically reduced in size to a molecular weight of 2000–8000. Their principal action is also via antithrombin, although they have a higher anti-Xa:IIa ratio. LMWHs have a much more predictable anticoagulant effect in an individual and are given subcutaneously as a body weight-adjusted dose once/twice a day. The APTT does not satisfactorily measure factor Xa inhibition, but fortunately anticoagulant action does not need to be monitored routinely. Side-effects: bleeding and thrombocytopenia, both rarer than with UFHs.

Direct oral anticoagulants (DOACs)

The DOACs have many advantages compared to warfarin: oral, fixed dose, no monitoring routinely required, few drug and food interactions, and a short onset/offset of action (similar to LMWHs). They are not suitable for all patients (for example, they are not suitable for patients who need anticoagulation for metallic heart valves) but they can be considered as an alternative to warfarin in patients with atrial fibrillation or venous thromboembolism. Apixaban, edoxaban and rivaroxaban act by directly inhibiting factor Xa. Dabigatran etexilate is orally available and is metabolized rapidly by non-specific esterases in the blood to dabigatran, which is a direct thrombin inhibitor.

Parenteral thrombin inhibitors

Bivalirudin and argatroban are parenteral direct thrombin inhibitors and are used occasionally in hospital in patients with heparin-induced thrombocytopenia when heparin is contraindicated.

188 Thrombophilia

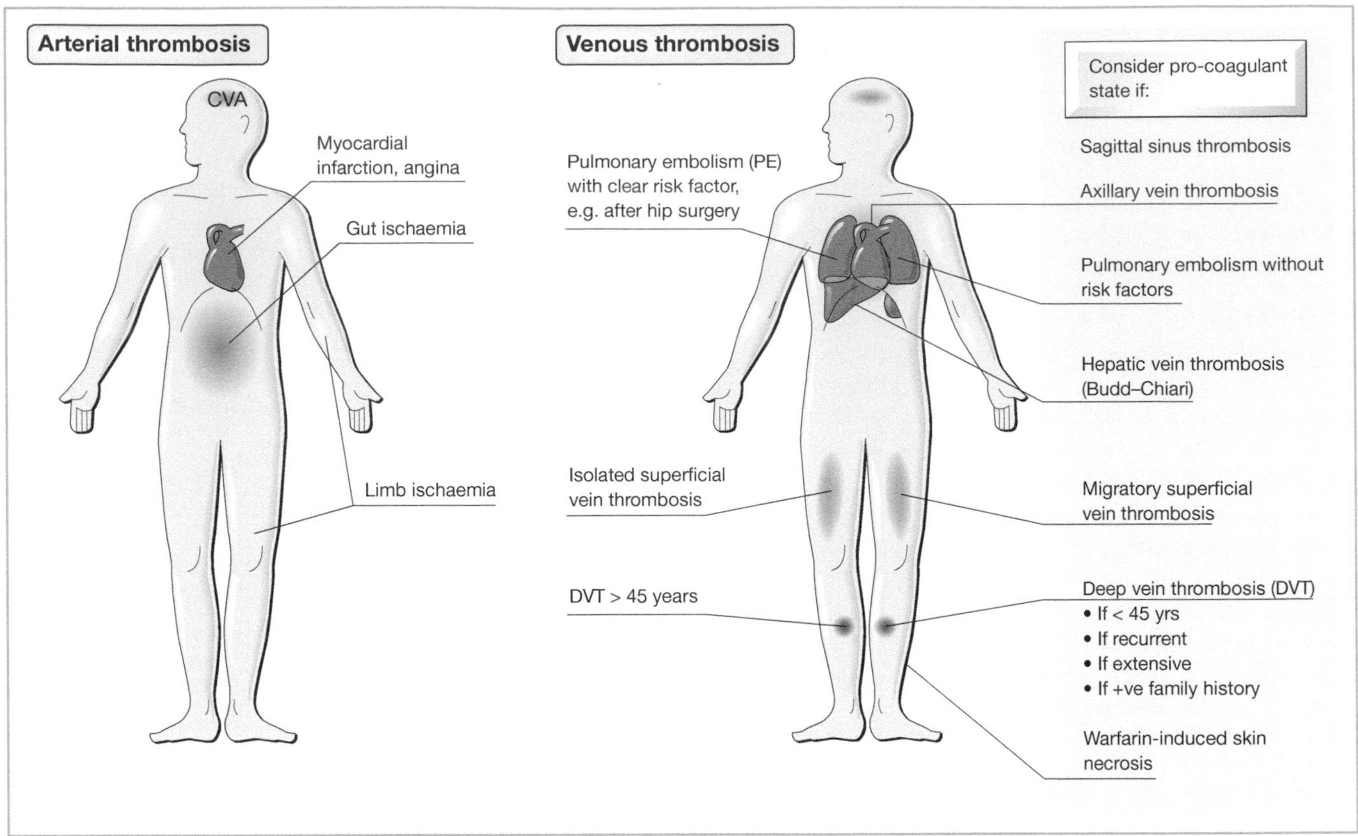

Two natural anticoagulant pathways prevent excess thrombus forming *in vivo*.

- **Antithrombin** is a serine protease inhibitor or serpin. Many coagulation proteins are serine proteases and antithrombin, through the formation of a 1:1 stoichiometric complex, has substantial inhibitory activity against such proteases. Antithrombin's main effect is to neutralize thrombin, although it does also have inhibitory activity against factor Xa.
- **Protein C pathway**: the zymogen protein C is activated by thrombin in the presence of an endothelial cell co-factor, thrombomodulin. Activated protein C (APC) is a serine protease that acts as a natural anticoagulant by cleaving the two co-factors in the coagulation pathway, factors V and VIII, for which it needs its own co-factor, protein S. Both protein C and protein S are vitamin K-dependent proteins.

Inherited thrombophilia

Inherited mutations increasing the risk of thrombosis are common, affecting 5–7% of the population (see Table 188.1). The inherited forms of thrombophilia are associated only with venous thrombosis, not (in adults) with arterial disease.

Table 188.1 Prevalence of inherited thrombophilia.

Deficiency/abnormality	Population prevalence
Factor V Leiden	1 in 20
Prothrombin G20210A	1 in 50–100
Protein C	1 in 300
Protein S	1 in 300
Antithrombin	1 in 3000

Deficiencies of antithrombin, protein C or protein S predispose to thrombosis. Heterozygotes for these deficiencies with approximately 50% of normal levels are at risk, so the thrombotic tendency is inherited in an autosomal dominant fashion. Homozygous antithrombin deficiency is not seen and is presumably fatal *in utero*, whereas homozygosity for protein C or protein S deficiency leads to the very rare condition of neonatal purpura fulminans. Until 1993, these three deficiencies were the only well-characterized forms of inherited thrombophilia.

Medicine at a Glance, Fifth Edition. Edited by Patrick Davey and Alex Pitcher.

Companion website: www.wiley.com/go/medicine5e

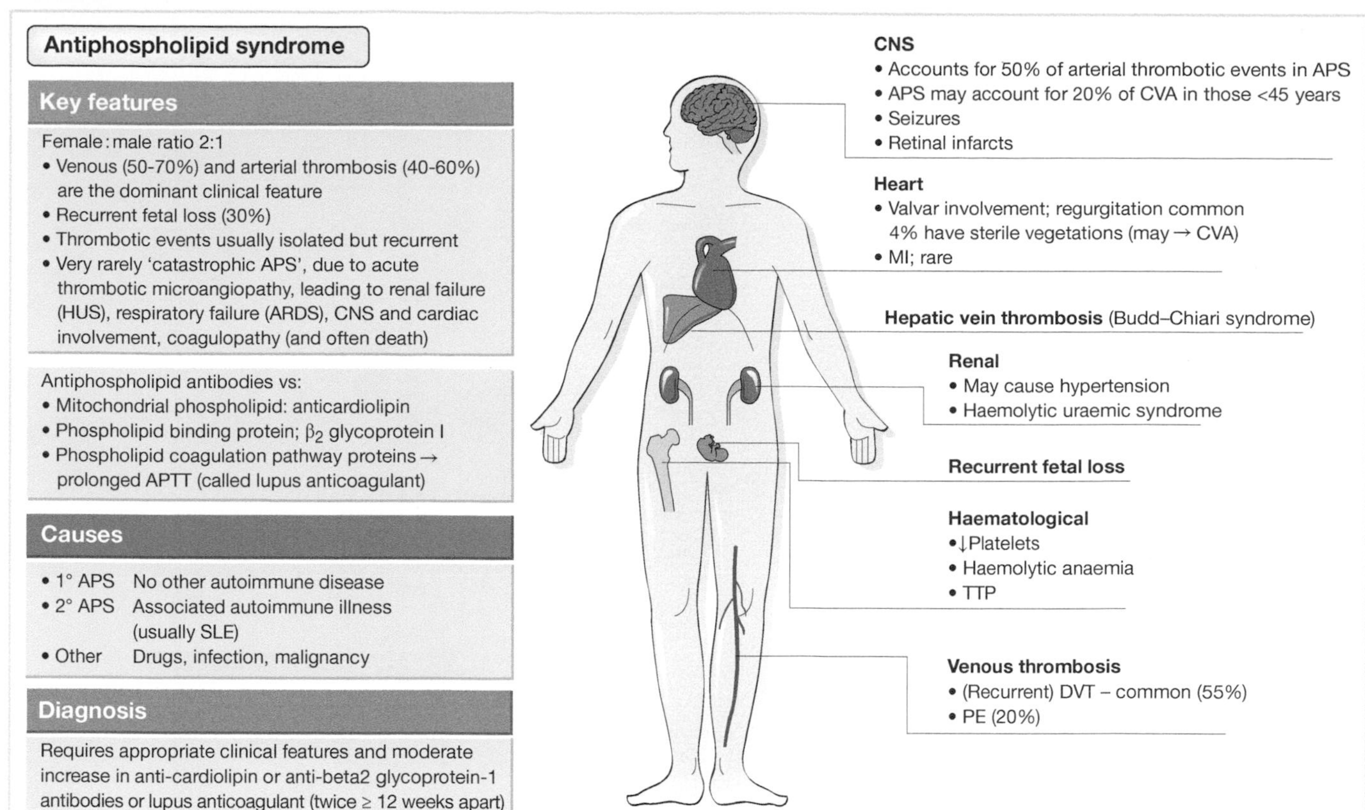

Antiphospholipid syndrome
Key features
Female : male ratio 2:1
• Venous (50-70%) and arterial thrombosis (40-60%) are the dominant clinical feature
• Recurrent fetal loss (30%)
• Thrombotic events usually isolated but recurrent
• Very rarely 'catastrophic APS', due to acute thrombotic microangiopathy, leading to renal failure (HUS), respiratory failure (ARDS), CNS and cardiac involvement, coagulopathy (and often death)
Antiphospholipid antibodies vs:
• Mitochondrial phospholipid: anticardiolipin
• Phospholipid binding protein; β2 glycoprotein I
• Phospholipid coagulation pathway proteins → prolonged APTT (called lupus anticoagulant)
Causes
• 1° APS No other autoimmune disease
• 2° APS Associated autoimmune illness (usually SLE)
• Other Drugs, infection, malignancy
Diagnosis
Requires appropriate clinical features and moderate increase in anti-cardiolipin or anti-beta2 glycoprotein-1 antibodies or lupus anticoagulant (twice ≥ 12 weeks apart)
CNS
• Accounts for 50% of arterial thrombotic events in APS
• APS may account for 20% of CVA in those <45 years
• Seizures
• Retinal infarcts
Heart
• Valvar involvement; regurgitation common 4% have sterile vegetations (may → CVA)
• MI; rare
Hepatic vein thrombosis (Budd–Chiari syndrome)
Renal
• May cause hypertension
• Haemolytic uraemic syndrome
Recurrent fetal loss
Haematological
• ↓Platelets
• Haemolytic anaemia
• TTP
Venous thrombosis
• (Recurrent) DVT – common (55%)
• PE (20%)

Factor V Leiden

In 1993, the phenomenon of resistance to APC was described and one year later the defect was identified as a point mutation in factor V (G to A substitution at nucleotide position 1691), resulting in the arginine at position 506 being replaced by a glutamine. The abnormal factor is referred to as factor V Leiden after the Dutch town where it was identified. This substitution occurs at the site where protein C inactivates factor V. Normally factor V is inactivated by an initial cleavage of the peptide bond on the carboxyl side of arginine 506. Thus, the mutation here renders factor V resistant to APC. Factor V Leiden is present in 5% of the population; in heterozygotes it increases the risk of venous thrombosis seven-fold, whereas in homozygotes (one in 1600 of the population) there is a 50–100-fold increase in risk.

The prothrombin G20210A mutation

A polymorphism in the 3′-untranslated region of the prothrombin gene was identified in 1996; it is present in 1–2% of the population and is associated with a four-fold increased risk of venous thromboembolism. The mechanism seems to be higher prothrombin levels in individuals with the mutation.

Investigation of inherited thrombophilia

Testing for inherited thrombophilia in a patient who has had a venous thrombosis rarely changes clinical advice, and for the majority of people it is therefore not helpful. The indications for inherited thrombophilia screening are therefore limited and studies should be confined to those in whom testing will affect management or usefully inform relatives (in conjunction with careful counselling around VTE risk). Consider testing:

- patients with unprovoked venous thromboembolism who have a positive family history or are young with children/siblings (especially daughters/sisters)
- relatives (especially females of child-bearing age) of a patient with proven venous thromboembolism and an identified heritable thrombophilia.

In addition to testing for the five causes of inherited thrombophilia in Table 188.1, patients could also be tested for antiphospholipid antibodies, which are acquired risk factors for both venous and arterial disease.

Acquired thrombophilia

See figure at the beginning of this chapter.

189 Aetiology of cancer

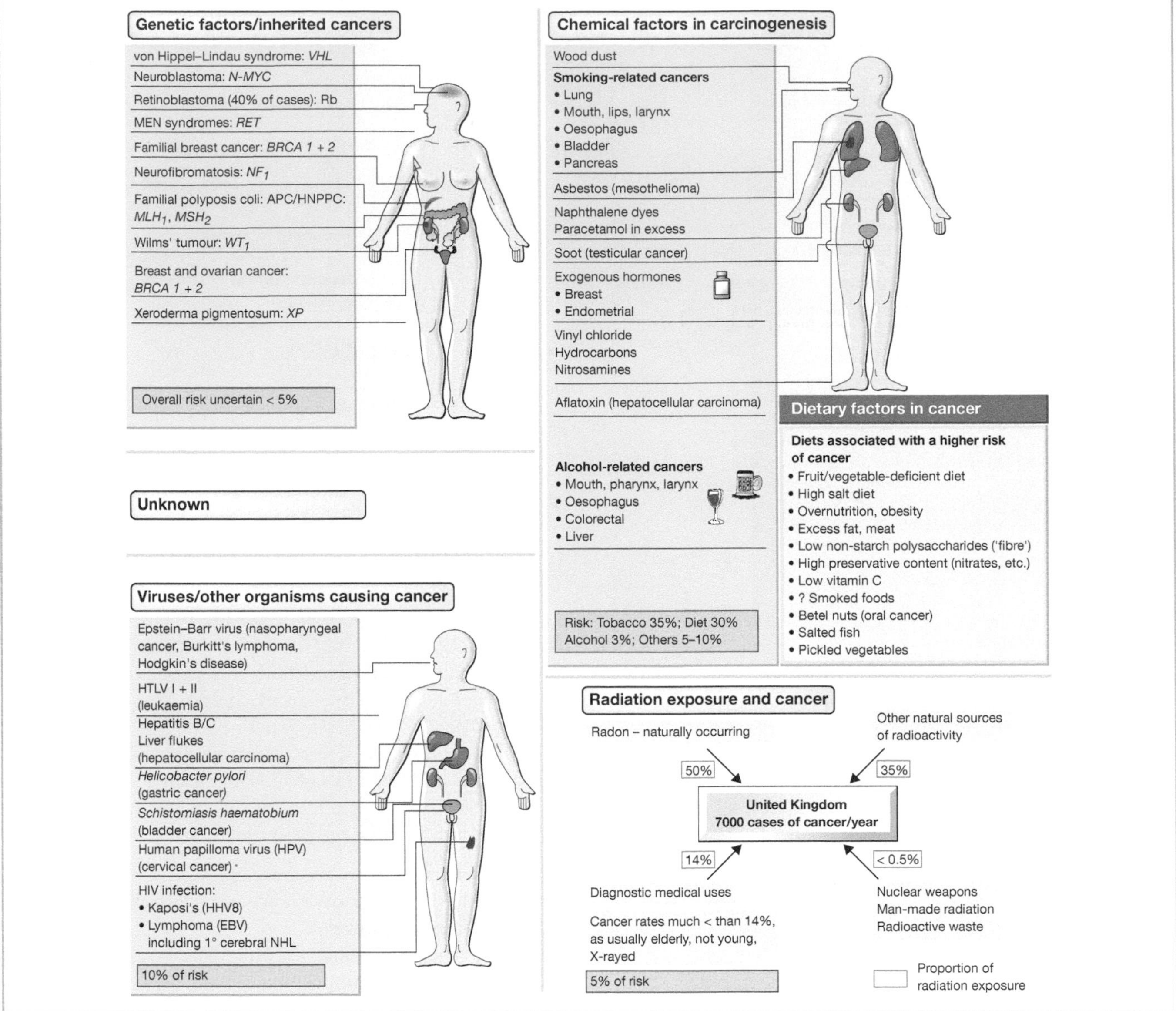

Genetic factors/inherited cancers
von Hippel–Lindau syndrome: *VHL*
Neuroblastoma: *N-MYC*
Retinoblastoma (40% of cases): Rb
MEN syndromes: *RET*
Familial breast cancer: *BRCA 1 + 2*
Neurofibromatosis: NF_1
Familial polyposis coli: APC/HNPPC: MLH_1, MSH_2
Wilms' tumour: WT_1
Breast and ovarian cancer: *BRCA 1 + 2*
Xeroderma pigmentosum: *XP*
Overall risk uncertain < 5%
Unknown
Viruses/other organisms causing cancer
Epstein–Barr virus (nasopharyngeal cancer, Burkitt's lymphoma, Hodgkin's disease)
HTLV I + II (leukaemia)
Hepatitis B/C
Liver flukes (hepatocellular carcinoma)
Helicobacter pylori (gastric cancer)
Schistomiasis haematobium (bladder cancer)
Human papilloma virus (HPV) (cervical cancer)
HIV infection:
• Kaposi's (HHV8)
• Lymphoma (EBV) including 1° cerebral NHL
10% of risk
Chemical factors in carcinogenesis
Wood dust
Smoking-related cancers
• Lung
• Mouth, lips, larynx
• Oesophagus
• Bladder
• Pancreas
Asbestos (mesothelioma)
Naphthalene dyes
Paracetamol in excess
Soot (testicular cancer)
Exogenous hormones
• Breast
• Endometrial
Vinyl chloride
Hydrocarbons
Nitrosamines
Aflatoxin (hepatocellular carcinoma)
Alcohol-related cancers
• Mouth, pharynx, larynx
• Oesophagus
• Colorectal
• Liver
Risk: Tobacco 35%; Diet 30%
Alcohol 3%; Others 5–10%
Dietary factors in cancer
Diets associated with a higher risk of cancer
• Fruit/vegetable-deficient diet
• High salt diet
• Overnutrition, obesity
• Excess fat, meat
• Low non-starch polysaccharides ('fibre')
• High preservative content (nitrates, etc.)
• Low vitamin C
• ? Smoked foods
• Betel nuts (oral cancer)
• Salted fish
• Pickled vegetables
Radiation exposure and cancer
Radon – naturally occurring
Other natural sources of radioactivity
50%
35%
United Kingdom
7000 cases of cancer/year
14%
< 0.5%
Diagnostic medical uses
Nuclear weapons
Man-made radiation
Radioactive waste
Cancer rates much < than 14%, as usually elderly, not young, X-rayed
5% of risk
Proportion of radiation exposure

Cancer causes 20–25% of deaths. The development of cancer is a multistep process of genetic alterations. Many cancers are age-related, reflecting this accumulation of genetic damage. Cancer cells can grow in defiance of the normal restraints on cell growth and they can invade and colonize areas normally reserved for other cells. Carcinogenesis is the term for the genetic events producing malignant transformation and metastasis.

Environmental causes of carcinogenesis

- **Chemical carcinogenesis**: there are two stages to chemical carcinogenesis – tumour initiation and tumour promotion. Initiation means permanent, potentially inheritable (passed in the germline, i.e. gonadal) DNA damage from carcinogens (direct) or metabolites (indirect). Promotion can produce malignancy only in previously initiated cells and reflects increased cellular proliferation rather than direct effects on DNA (mitogenic as opposed to mutagenic). Common carcinogens include aromatic hydrocarbons and amines and nitrosamines. Aflatoxin B_1 induces a point mutation in *p53* (G to T transversion in codon 249) and causes hepatocellular carcinoma. Although the mechanisms are less clear, carcinogens in tobacco smoke are overwhelmingly the most important, probably causing 30% of cancers.
- **Radiation carcinogenesis**: ultraviolet irradiation, mainly UVB, produces pyrimidine dimers in DNA, normally repaired by the nucleotide excision–repair system. Excess UVB exposure

Medicine at a Glance, Fifth Edition. Edited by Patrick Davey and Alex Pitcher.

Companion website: www.wiley.com/go/medicine5e

overwhelms this pathway, resulting in DNA damage. Mutations in this repair pathway in xeroderma pigmentosa result in high rates of skin malignancy. UVB also causes mutations in oncogenes or tumour suppressor genes, e.g. *p53*. Ionizing radiation damages DNA by direct ionization or through the production of highly reactive free radicals from the ionization of adjacent water.

- **Viral carcinogenesis**: >15% of cancer incidence worldwide is attributed to infectious agents. Viruses are the most significant infectious causes and cause cancer by integrating genetic material into the host cell genome, which then activates oncogenes or inactivates tumour suppressor genes. RNA viruses may cause malignancy by the insertion of proviral DNA near a proto-oncogene, inducing a structural change and so conversion to a cellular oncogene (*c-onc*). This is termed 'insertional mutagenesis'. Epidemiologically, the most important viruses are human papillomavirus (HPV) (cervical cancer) and hepatitis B (liver cancer).

Inherited factors contributing to the development of cancer

An inherited predisposition occurs in 5–10% of cancers. Inheritance of a single mutant gene in germ cells (e.g. disrupting a tumour suppressor gene) increases the risk of tumour development (e.g. retinoblastoma). Subsequent mutation of the remaining tumour suppressor gene in somatic cells causes transformation. There are several well-characterized familial cancer syndromes linked to a specific inherited mutant gene, e.g. familial breast and ovarian cancer (*BRCA* genes) and familial adenomatous polyposis (*APC* gene). Although these are autosomal dominantly inherited, there are autosomal recessive syndromes (e.g. xeroderma pigmentosa). Subtle inherited variations in enzyme activity (genetic polymorphisms) and differences in gene expression profiles (epigenetics) affect the development and growth of cancers.

Genetic mechanisms underlying carcinogenesis

The genetic mechanisms underlying carcinogenesis are crucial to tumour development and growth. Most human tumours so far studied show activation of several oncogenes and the loss of two or more tumour suppressor genes. The important gene groups are as follows.

- **Oncogenes** (cancer-causing genes) are derived from proto-oncogenes, normal cellular genes that promote and control normal growth and differentiation. Cellular oncogenes are normal cellular genes that have become oncogenic through structural changes inducing altered *in situ* behaviour. Typically changes in the gene sequence produce an abnormal gene product with an aberrant function. Alternatively, changes in gene expression (protein production) by gene amplification (multiple copies) or overexpression cause high levels of normal growth-promoting proteins (often receptors). Oncoproteins (proteins encoded by oncogenes) include growth factors and their receptors, signal transduction proteins, nuclear transcription factors (regulating gene expression), cyclins and cyclin-dependent kinases (regulating cell cycle progression from synthesis of new DNA to mitosis).
- **Tumour suppressor gene products** regulate cell growth by inhibition of cellular proliferation. Their loss is the key event in most, if not all, human cancers. Mutated tumour suppressor genes are mostly recessive – that is, carcinogenesis requires inactivation of both normal alleles, e.g. the protein product of the retinoblastoma gene (*pRb*), which controls cell cycle progression, and *p53*, which monitors for genetic damage, halting cell cycle progression and triggering apoptosis if damage is not repaired.
- **Caretaker genes** are a class of tumour suppressor genes but their inactivation is not directly responsible for cancer development. For example, genes regulating DNA repair are not themselves oncogenic when defective, but allow mutations in other genes to develop during replication, thereby increasing the likelihood of tumour development, e.g. the defective mismatch repair genes in Lynch syndrome, the breast and ovarian cancer predisposition genes *BRCA-1* and *-2*, and the defective DNA repair mechanism in xeroderma pigmentosum.
- **Genes regulating apoptosis**: apoptosis or programmed cell death is the orchestrated involution of redundant cells. Many genes regulate apoptosis. If these genes are damaged, there is a steady inappropriate accumulation of cells, e.g. overexpression of *bcl-2* in lymphoma or mutations in *bax* associated with failure of apoptosis in several solid tumours.
- **Ageing telomerase**: it is increasingly clear that cancer is a correlate of ageing, and the regulation of cellular longevity through telomere length has an important anticancer role.

Factors underlying the growth and spread of tumours

The key processes in cancer are growth and metastasis.

- **Growth**: clonal expansion of a transformed cell. Cancer cells are no longer dependent on normal mitogenic growth signals, they exhibit insensitivity to antigrowth signals and have developed mutations to evade apoptosis. Speed of growth is determined by the balance between cycle time and cell apoptosis, and by the proportion of tumour cells progressing through the cell cycle (growth fraction).
- **Invasion**: malignant cells invade locally (using collagenases and metalloproteases) or metastasize, by invading lymphatic channels and blood vessels, from where they embolize to distant sites. Adhesion molecules, vascular supply, vessel calibre, tumour cell size and target tissue characteristics determine the distribution of metastases. Initial metastatic growth relates to tumour angiogenesis, which in turn depends on the production of various cytokines, including vascular endothelium growth factor (VEGF).
- **Cellular immortality**: cancer cells evade the normal mechanisms of cell death and are able to continuously replicate. Malignant cells have (express) the enzyme telomerase, which allows the ends of the chromosomes (telomeres – the cellular clock) to be elongated and so avoid the senescence (crisis death) of typical cellular ageing.
- **Angiogenesis**: tumours need to develop a blood supply to grow beyond 1–2 mm. Angiogenesis is an important part of embryology and healing, is disordered in malignancy and is driven by VEGF, inhibition of which is a potential cancer treatment.
- **Metabolism**: cancer cells use alternative metabolic pathways to generate their energy (for example, upregulation of glycolysis and lactic acid fermentation, the Warburg effect).
- **Host factors**: the interaction between the cells of the immune system and tumour is complex, with evidence to suggest that tumour cells evade immune surveillance. Increasingly, there is evidence to suggest that the host environment (particularly inflammation) in which the tumour grows contributes to the growth and spread of cancers.
- **Genomic instability**: cancers continually evolve and develop, gaining genomic alterations. This results in an individual's cancer often being a heterogeneous disease; different metastasis or different areas of a single tumour may have different genomic expression and may display different sensitivity to anticancer therapies.

Knowledge of the underlying biology of cancer is vital; it is guiding potential treatment options in the rapidly developing field of cancer medicine.

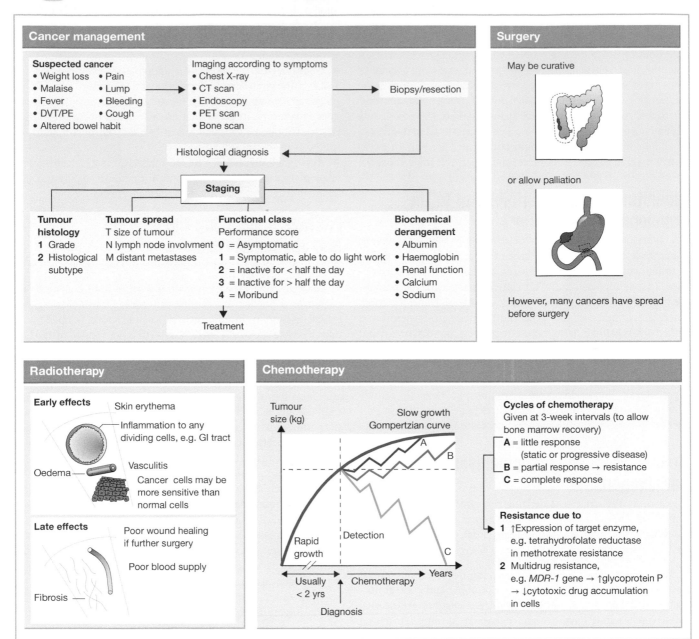

Diagnostic strategies and basic principles of cancer management

Cancer management

Suspected cancer
- Weight loss
- Pain
- Malaise
- Lump
- Fever
- Bleeding
- DVT/PE
- Cough
- Altered bowel habit

→ Imaging according to symptoms
- Chest X-ray
- CT scan
- Endoscopy
- PET scan
- Bone scan

→ Biopsy/resection → Histological diagnosis → **Staging**

Tumour histology
1 Grade
2 Histological subtype

Tumour spread
T size of tumour
N lymph node involvment
M distant metastases

Functional class
Performance score
0 = Asymptomatic
1 = Symptomatic, able to do light work
2 = Inactive for < half the day
3 = Inactive for > half the day
4 = Moribund

Biochemical derangement
- Albumin
- Haemoglobin
- Renal function
- Calcium
- Sodium

→ Treatment

Surgery

May be curative

or allow palliation

However, many cancers have spread before surgery

Radiotherapy

Early effects
Skin erythema
Inflammation to any dividing cells, e.g. GI tract
Oedema
Vasculitis
Cancer cells may be more sensitive than normal cells

Late effects
Poor wound healing if further surgery
Poor blood supply
Fibrosis

Chemotherapy

Tumour size (kg)
Slow growth Gompertzian curve
A
B
C
Rapid growth
Detection
Usually < 2 yrs
Chemotherapy
Years
Diagnosis

Cycles of chemotherapy
Given at 3-week intervals (to allow bone marrow recovery)
A = little response (static or progressive disease)
B = partial response → resistance
C = complete response

Resistance due to
1 ↑Expression of target enzyme, e.g. tetrahydrofolate reductase in methotrexate resistance
2 Multidrug resistance, e.g. *MDR-1* gene → ↑glycoprotein P → ↓cytotoxic drug accumulation in cells

Important diagnostic strategies

Cancer needs to be diagnosed, staged and then the effects of treatment monitored.

- **Diagnosis** is made by histological (tissue) or cytological (cells) examination. Cells (fine needle aspiration) or small tissue samples (needle biopsy) are usually sufficient, although in lymphomas the architectural pattern (lymph node) should be examined.
- **Staging** reflects the mechanisms of spread of the tumour (local invasion, lymph or blood spread), determines treatment and, along with histological subtype and grade, is the most powerful determinant of outcome. Tumour staging is occasionally done surgically but more often radiologically and may require other tests such as bone marrow examination (haematological malignancy).
- **Pathology**: histological characteristics define the 'aggressiveness' of the tumour, based on grade, mitotic rate, nuclear pleomorphism,

Medicine at a Glance, Fifth Edition. Edited by Patrick Davey and Alex Pitcher.

Companion website: www.wiley.com/go/medicine5e

tubule formation, etc. Specific tumour histological markers may have prognostic significance and may influence treatment. For example, HER2 receptor and the use of trastuzumab and hormone receptor expression and endocrine treatment (breast cancer).

- **Tumour genetics**: karyotyping and cytogenetics may be used in the diagnosis of both haematological (e.g. leukaemia and lymphoma's) and solid malignancies (e.g. testicular cancer [extra copies of Chromosome 12p]). Molecular profiling (e.g. next generation sequencing) of cancer is being increasingly employed both to provide diagnostic information and as predictive biomarkers to influence therapeutic options (for example, epidermal growth factor receptor (EGFR) mutations in lung cancer).
- **Tumour markers**, particularly in ovarian cancer (CA-125), germ cell tumours (α-fetoprotein, β-human chorionic gonadotrophin) and lymphoma (lactate dehydrogenase) are used in evaluating treatment response and surveillance, and may relate to tumour burden. The polymerase chain reaction (PCR) amplifies specific molecular markers of malignant cells and detects residual disease in chronic myeloid leukaemia (CML) and follicular lymphoma.
- **Measures** of age, performance score, activity and physiological function are important determinants of both appropriate treatment selection and treatment response, as are laboratory measures (e.g. albumin).

Principles of surgical oncology

Surgery is used for both diagnosis and staging of the tumour. Historically, radical surgery gave the optimal chance of cure. It still remains an important modality and can be the primary treatment in breast, ovarian cancer, sarcomas, melanomas, head and neck tumours, lung cancer, colon cancer and, when appropriate, resection of oligo- (one or few) metastatic deposits. Surgical resection should, for local control, extend to a clear (cancer-free) margin of 1 cm in most cancers. Resection margins can be classified pathologically as R0 (no cancer cells seen microscopically at the margin), R1 (no visible tumour but microscopic evidence of cancer cells at the margin) or R2 (tumour seen macroscopically at resection margin, i.e. visible residual tumour). With modern adjuvant and neoadjuvant therapies (radiation or chemotherapy) to complement surgery, more conservative surgical operations with reduced morbidity are possible.

Surgery can have an important role in palliation and local control of tumours when complete excision is not possible. For example, surgical fixation of a pathological fracture or, in obstructing bowel tumours, surgery may be used to bypass the lesion to relieve symptoms.

Basic principles of radiotherapy

Radiotherapy plays an essential role in the treatment of many cancers. It may be used for curative or adjuvant treatment (e.g. radiotherapy to the breast and lymph nodes following surgery for breast cancer). It is also used for palliative treatment where the aim is for local control and symptom management, such as pain control in bone metastasis and control of haemoptysis in lung cancer.

Ionizing radiation induces DNA damage, which triggers apoptosis (programmed cell death). Radiation doses are divided (fractionated) to allow for recovery of normal tissue and thus reduce side-effects. Certain tissues (e.g. the lens, nervous and cardiac tissue) are particularly radiosensitive and mandate careful radiation planning. The concurrent use of chemotherapy is increasingly improving the outcome of radiotherapy, as in cervical carcinoma.

Computed tomography (CT) planning, conformal (shaped beam) radiotherapy and intensity-modulated radiotherapy enable tailored radiotherapy with minimal irradiation of adjacent tissues. Brachytherapy (the use of seeds, wires or implants, applied close to the malignancy), radioimmunotherapy and stereotactic radiotherapy are techniques that exploit this principle further.

Systemic anticancer therapy

Systemic anticancer therapy is the term used to describe medicines used to treat malignancy. These treatments include cytoxic drugs (chemotherapy), endocrine therapy, targeted treatments and immunotherapy. These treatments can be given in the following settings.

- Curative – given with the aim of curing the malignancy.
- Neoadjuvant – therapy given prior to any definitive treatment (e.g. prior to surgical resection) with the aim of reducing the size of the tumour prior to resection.
- Adjuvant – therapy given following definitive treatment (usually surgery) with the aim of reducing recurrence of the cancer.
- Palliative (non-curative) – with the aim of alleviating symptoms and prolonging life.

Basic principles of chemotherapy

Chemotherapy works by:

- damaging the DNA of rapidly dividing cells, which is detected by the *p53/Rb* pathway, thus triggering apoptosis
- damaging the cellular spindle apparatus, preventing cell division
- inhibiting DNA synthesis.

Chemotherapy can lead to cure, either when given alone (choriocarcinoma, childhood acute lymphoblastic leukaemia, some lymphomas and leukaemias, germ cell tumours) or in combination with surgery (osteosarcoma, adenocarcinoma of the breast and ovary, colorectal cancer, squamous cell carcinoma of the upper gastrointestinal [GI] tract). Chemotherapy can be given prior to surgery (neoadjuvant) or following surgery (adjuvant chemotherapy) with the aim of reducing cancer relapse. It may prolong life and improve symptoms without producing cure (palliative chemotherapy), as in acute myeloid leukaemia, small cell carcinoma of the lung and ovarian cancer. Increased understanding of cancer cell biology has improved current treatments.

Chemotherapy includes the following classes.

- **Folate antagonists, purine and pyrimidine analogues**: these drugs (methotrexate, 5-fluorouracil, hydroxyurea) inhibit DNA synthesis.
- **Alkylating agents**: these damage DNA. They include cyclophosphamide (breast cancer, lymphoma), melphalan (myeloma) and platinum-based drugs like cisplatin/carboplatin (testicular cancer, lymphoma, squamous cell carcinoma, ovarian and bladder cancer).
- **Topoisomerase I and II interacting drugs** intercalate double-stranded DNA (dsDNA) and form a cleavable complex with topoisomerase II, an essential nuclear enzyme that causes dsDNA breaks. Examples include the anthracyclines (breast cancer, lymphoma) and etoposide (teratoma, lung cancer). Related drugs,

including topotecan and irinotecan, associate with topoisomerase I to cause reversible single-stranded DNA breaks.

- **Alkaloids and taxanes**: inhibit microtubule function and disrupt mitosis. Examples include the vinca alkaloids (leukaemia, lymphoma, bladder cancer) and the taxanes (ovarian cancer, breast cancer).

Side-effects of chemotherapy

Chemotherapy causes myelosuppression and so risks infection (neutropenia) (see Chapter 54) and bleeding (thrombocytopenia). Damage to mucous membranes causes a sore mouth and diarrhoea and stimulation of the chemoreceptor trigger zone (area postrema) produces nausea and vomiting. Any rapidly dividing tissues, such as the hair follicles (alopecia) and germinal epithelium (infertility), are vulnerable to the effects of chemotherapy and late effects such as secondary malignancies are increasingly recognized. All chemotherapy drugs should be considered teratogenic. Some drugs cause specific organ toxicity, such as to the kidney (cisplatin) and nerves (vincristine). Supportive care with the 5-hydroxytryptamine (serotonin) 5-HT_3 antagonists, neurokinin-1 receptor antagonists and steroids has improved the control of nausea. Several recombinant human proteins are in routine use to support the effects of myelosuppression, e.g. granulocyte colony-stimulating factor reduces the depth and duration of neutropenia.

There has been rapid development in our understanding of cancer biology and, as technology has advanced, new and more specific therapies have been developed which are transforming the way malignancy is treated. Treatment is being tailored to specific characteristics seen in each specific cancer (precision/personalized medicine). Chemotherapy continues to have a major role in treating many malignancies, but other more 'targeted' therapies are increasingly being used. It is important to realize that each treatment may have a different spectrum of side-effects.

Other therapies

- **Monoclonal antibodies**: several monoclonal antibodies are used successfully, including trastuzumab (breast cancer: anti-HER-2), rituximab (lymphoma: anti-CD20) and cetuximab (EGFR inhibitor: colorectal cancer). Bevacizumab is a monoclonal antibody against vascular endothelial growth factor receptor that inhibits angiogenesis. It has a role in ovarian and colorectal cancer.
- **Tyrosine kinase inhibitors**: as an example imatinib, an oral tyrosine kinase (bcr/Abl gene product) inhibitor, has revolutionized the treatment of CML. Osimertinib, used in non-small cell lung cancer, targets the EGFR.
- **Immunotherapy**: the principle behind these treatments is to harness the immune system to target the cancer. This is a rapidly developing field and has transformed the management of some malignancies (including malignant melanoma and non-small cell lung cancer). Immune checkpoint inhibitors (for example, CTLA4 or PD-L1/PD1 inhibitors) are now the standard of care in several malignancies and are being investigated in others. Other approaches to target the immune system include the use of cytokines (IL-2, TNF-α) and manipulation of T cells (CAR T cells, particularly in haematological malignancies).
- **Others**: multiple different treatments are being developed that exploit known mutations within cancer cells. For example, inhibitors of poly (adenosine diphosphate ribose) polymerase (PARP) target cancer cells with defects within the homologous recombination DNA repair pathway (for example, patients with *BRCA* mutations). This treatment is now standard of care for patients with breast and ovarian cancer. Genomic profiling of tumours is increasingly being performed to identify clinically relevant mutations in tumour DNA which may help identify personalized treatments.

Hormonal therapy: some tumours (e.g. breast, prostate) are hormone responsive. The removal of endogenous hormones in some cases improves prognosis, e.g. one-third of premenopausal women with advanced breast cancer have a remission with oophorectomy. Drugs interfere with hormone action within cancer cells, e.g. tamoxifen, a competitive inhibitor of the oestrogen receptor, with some oestrogenic activity, and aromatase inhibitors (block oestrogen synthesis) are used in breast cancer. Androgens are important for the growth and malignant transformation of prostatic tissue. Androgen deprivation therapy is the primary treatment for metastatic prostate cancer and can be produced by castration or by medical means with gonadotrophin-releasing hormone (GnRH) analogues.

Germline genetic testing: most cancers are sporadic, but some may be the result of germline pathogenic mutations. Hereditary cancers are important to identify as this has important consequences for both the patient (treatment implications and further cancer risk) and family members. Appropriate genetic counselling and genetic testing are vital, as advice can then be given to help detect cancer at an earlier stage (through screening) or even prevent the development of certain cancers in the first place (prophylactic surgery).

Resistance to therapies is a major challenge in the management of patients with cancer and is an area of ongoing and active research.

Figure 190.1 Examples of needs of individuals living with cancer

Psychological
• self-worth
• body image
• coping
Physical
• pain
• nausea
• vomiting
• fatigue
Social
• family
• relationships
• school, work
Emotional
• anger
• despair
• fear
• hopelessness
Spiritual
• meaning of life
• suffering
• pain
Practical
• finances
• child care
• housekeeping
• legal
Informational
• disease
• procedures
• coping skills
• symptoms
• treatment
• services

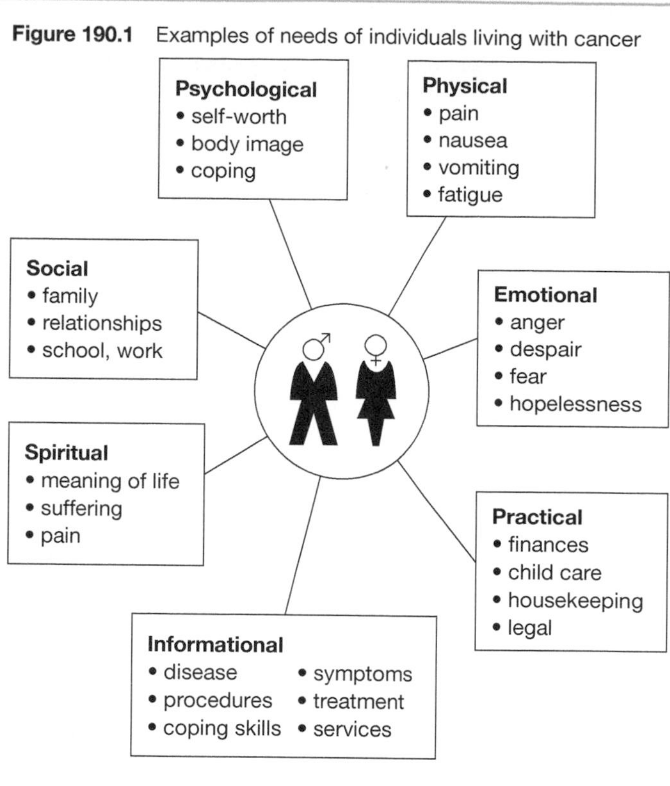

Figure 190.2 Service provision based on proportion of patients requiring assistance

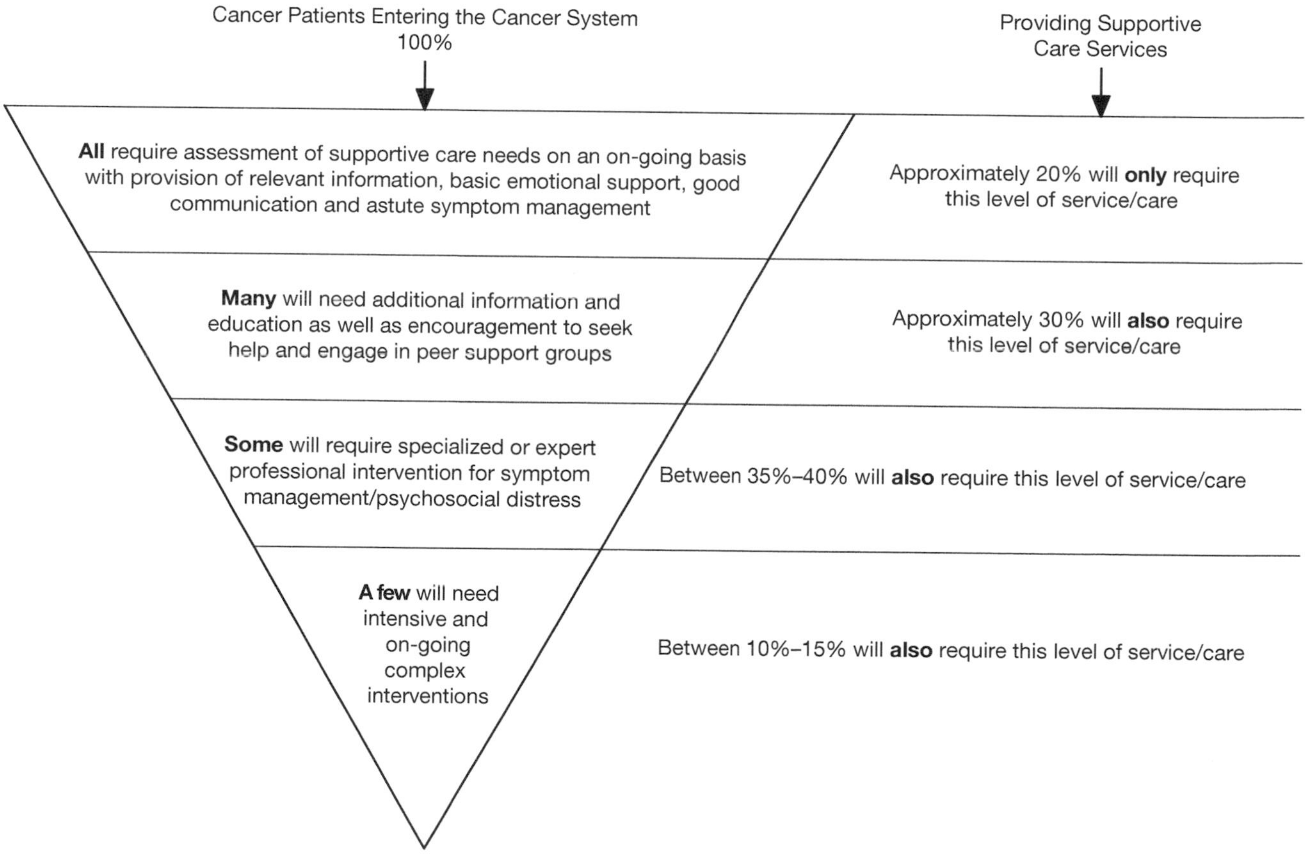

Cancer Patients Entering the Cancer System
100%
Providing Supportive
Care Services
All require assessment of supportive care needs on an on-going basis with provision of relevant information, basic emotional support, good communication and astute symptom management
Approximately 20% will only require this level of service/care
Many will need additional information and education as well as encouragement to seek help and engage in peer support groups
Approximately 30% will also require this level of service/care
Some will require specialized or expert professional intervention for symptom management/psychosocial distress
Between 35%–40% will also require this level of service/care
A few will need intensive and on-going complex interventions
Between 10%–15% will also require this level of service/care

Cancer screening and early detection

Cancer screening

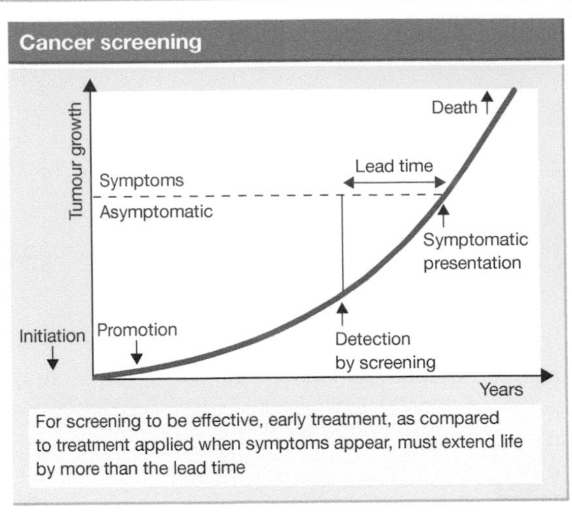

For screening to be effective, early treatment, as compared to treatment applied when symptoms appear, must extend life by more than the lead time

Breast cancer screening

Symptomatic presentation	Screening presentation (mammography)
50% have regional lymph node (LN) metastases	20% regional LN metastases
Average size = 2.5 cm	Detects more <1 cm cancers (good prognosis)
	60% palpable lumps 40% normal physical exam

Guidelines

Age (years)	Imaging
<40	If high risk (i.e. strong family history of breast cancer): MRI
> 40	If at high risk: yearly mammograms/MRI
50–70	Mammogram every 3 years
Previous breast cancer	Yearly mammogram

Cervical cancer screening

Clinically Important Human papillomavirus (HPV) Genotype

Genotype	Pathogenesis
High risk (oncogenic)	
Type 16	Causes 50% of all squamous cell carcinomas of the cervix and 55% to 60% of cervical cancers worldwide
Type 18	Causes 20% of cervical adenocarcinomas
Other: types 31, 33, 35, 39, 45, 51, 52, 56, 58, 59, (66), 68	All types combined cause 25% of cervical cancers
Low risk (wart-causing)	
Types 6 and 11	Cause 90% to 95% of ano-genital warts

Principles of screening

Early disease detection offers the best hope for cure with the least intervention. Treatment success is often dependent on the spread (stage) and biology (grade and behaviour) of disease, both of which worsen with time. Successful screening strategies should:

- address a common and dangerous disease
- use a simple, safe, inexpensive and valid screening test
- be acceptable to all social groups
- enable curative treatment, which when instituted earlier has a significant impact on survival.

Although observational, cohort and randomized controlled trials have shown the advantage of some screening programmes, there are problems. Screening may:

1 lead to anxiety
2 only increase the lead time (before development of symptoms) but not increase survival
3 only increase the detection of indolent cancers, which never become clinically apparent. When added to clinically relevant cancers, these apparently increase the number of early cases and overall survival. In screening, one of the earliest indicators of a future decrease in mortality is a decrease in the **absolute rate** (not percentage) of cases of advanced disease.

The impact of screening has been limited by the huge size of target populations, the difficulty of follow-up, poor compliance and poor test sensitivity with high false-positive rates.

Breast cancer

In 1963, the first randomized cancer screening trial investigating mammography in breast cancer was undertaken, using mortality as an endpoint. Subsequently, several studies have supported this approach and show that screening 50–69-year-old women with mammography decreases the breast cancer mortality.

Extending breast cancer screening to women aged 40–49 has been controversial because:

- although breast cancer is the leading cause of death in such women, breast cancer incidence and mortality rates are lower in this age group
- to date, the randomized controlled trials have been too small to be definitive
- the sensitivity of mammography is lower in denser breast tissue
- there is a higher relative rate of ductal carcinoma *in situ*.

The current guidelines in the UK recommend the following.

- A two-view mammography for ages 50–70 every three years.
- Yearly mammograms for those with previous breast cancer.
- Screening should start yearly at the age of 40 for those with a strong family history of breast cancer.
- Screening if required <40 years of age, by yearly MRI.

- Screening age for women at very high risk of breast cancer (e.g. gene mutation or previous irradiation to breast tissue) is determined by genetic mutation and calculated risk e.g. yearly MRI screening from age 30 for women with a *BRCA1* or *BRCA2* mutation and age 20 for women with a TP53 mutation (Li-Fraumeni syndrome).
- Women should be breast aware and follow the NHS five-point plan (see below).

As a result of the UK breast screening programme, 4% of women are recalled for further tests, and one in four of these women will be found to have cancer (therefore three out of four will have benign disease). Overall, cancer is found in eight out of 1000 women and overall deaths from breast cancer in the UK are reduced by 1300. The UK NHS is currently investigating extending breast screening to women aged 47–50 and 70–73.

The finding that some breast cancer is genetically inherited has opened the question of genetic screening. Assessment of family history of cancer and referral to a genetics service is important for women with a strong family history of cancer (particularly breast, ovarian and other cancers such as prostate and pancreatic cancer). This will ensure that testing of appropriate genes is performed (for example, *BRCA-1* and *-2*) and other family members are assessed if required. The best management of those found to carry these genes is unclear although prophylactic surgery (mastectomy and oophorectomy) and tamoxifen (anastrazole and/or raloxifene if postmenopausal) may be options. Fully informed disscussion and genetic couselling are paramount.

Colorectal cancer

Colorectal cancer is the second leading cause of cancer death. For localized disease, the five-year survival rate is 90%, for node-positive (Dukes' stage C) disease it is 70%, and for patients presenting with metastatic disease it is 10%. Many screening studies show early cases can be detected by colonoscopy, sigmoidoscopy, digital rectal examination and faecal blood examination. Of asymptomatic patients aged >50 years, 1–5% have positive faecal occult bloods, of whom 10% have cancer and 20–30% have adenomas. Bowel cancer screening has reduced overall mortality from colorectal cancer and is recommended routinely. The current UK guidelines for colorectal screening advise the following.

- Screening using the faecal immunochemical test (FIT) as the primary screening test (this has replaced the guaiac test), and is now implemented throughout the UK. This programme is aimed at men and women aged 60–74 years, every two years.
- Those with a very high incidence of colon and/or rectal cancer (e.g. familial polyposis coli, Lynch syndrome or ulcerative pancolitis) should have colonoscopies every 1–2 years (depending on risk).
- Rectal examination should be included in routine check-ups.

Some cancer societies recommend sigmoidoscopy or colonoscopy at age 50 years, for all. However, this is not routine practice in the UK.

Cervical cancer

The mortality rate for cervical cancer has decreased in several countries, following the introduction of screening programmes based on Papanicolaou (Pap) smears. Although there are no randomized controlled trials, the introduction of Pap smear screening in Finland and Iceland was associated with a 50% and 80% reduced mortality rate respectively over a 20-year period. The current UK guidelines recommend the following.

- Screening all women between 25 and 64 every 3–5 years.
- The newer technique of liquid-based cytology (LBC) is now the preferred technique for cervical screening.
- Central to the pathogenesis of cervical cancer is the presence of high-risk strains of human papillomavirus (hrHPV) in the cervical epithelium. hrHPV testing should now be performed on all cervical screening samples. Cytology is then performed on those samples positive for hrHPV. If abnormal cells are seen, colposcopy is the next investigation. If no abnormality is seen on cytology but the sample is HPV positive, a further cervical screening test should be performed after one year.
- The HPV vaccine is now offered for girls and boys aged 12–13 in the UK. Screening should still continue in those vaccinated.

The future for screening

In the last 10 years, the incidence of prostate cancer has increased. The average age of presentation with prostate cancer is 70 years, close to life expectancy, and competing causes of death influence both the epidemiology and management of the disease. Furthermore, the negative impact of treatment (impotence/incontinence) limits potential utility. Finally, no study has yet shown conclusively that the benefit from screening outweighs the harm from the possible investigation and overtreatment. Studies are, however, ongoing, investigating the role of transrectal ultrasonography (TRUS), prostate-specific antigen (PSA) and digital rectal examination in screening. The role of bi-parametric MRI scan is also being investigated as an initial screening test. It may be appropriate to screen high-risk patients (men with a family history of prostate cancer, or those who carry a high-risk genetic mutation, e.g. *BRCA2*).

There is increasing evidence to support a lung cancer screening programme, and work is currently underway in the UK investigating computed tomography screening for lung cancer.

The UK Collaborative Trial of Ovarian Cancer Screening is currently an ongoing trial assessing the effectiveness of two possible methods of ovarian cancer screening: an annual CA125 test and an annual transvaginal ultrasound.

Screening may differ significantly by country. In South Korea and Japan, for example, which have higher incidences of gastric cancer, population-based cancer screening by endoscopy or radiological examination is offered.

Education and awareness

There are tumours where the screener should be the patient.

- **Testicular tumours**: typically detected by accident or self-examination, although rare is the commonest tumour in young men. Education, increased awareness reduce delays in diagnosis.
- **Skin tumours**: education about the dangers of excess sun (ultraviolet) exposure, especially for fair-skinned individuals and those with a personal/family history of melanoma or dysplastic naevi syndrome, has decreased the incidence of sun-related cancers and improved early diagnosis. A high-profile public education programme in Scotland decreased the proportion of thick, poor-prognosis lesions from 34% to 15%.
- **Breast cancer** (see above): women should follow the NHS five-point plan.

1. Know what's normal for you.
2. Look at your breasts and feel them.
3. Know what changes to look for: changes in size, shape of the breast or changes to the skin (dimpling/puckering), new breast or axillary lump, changes to the nipple (inversion/skin changes/discharge) or any persistent breast pain.
4. Report any changes straight away.
5. Attend screening if you are eligible.

192 Breast cancer

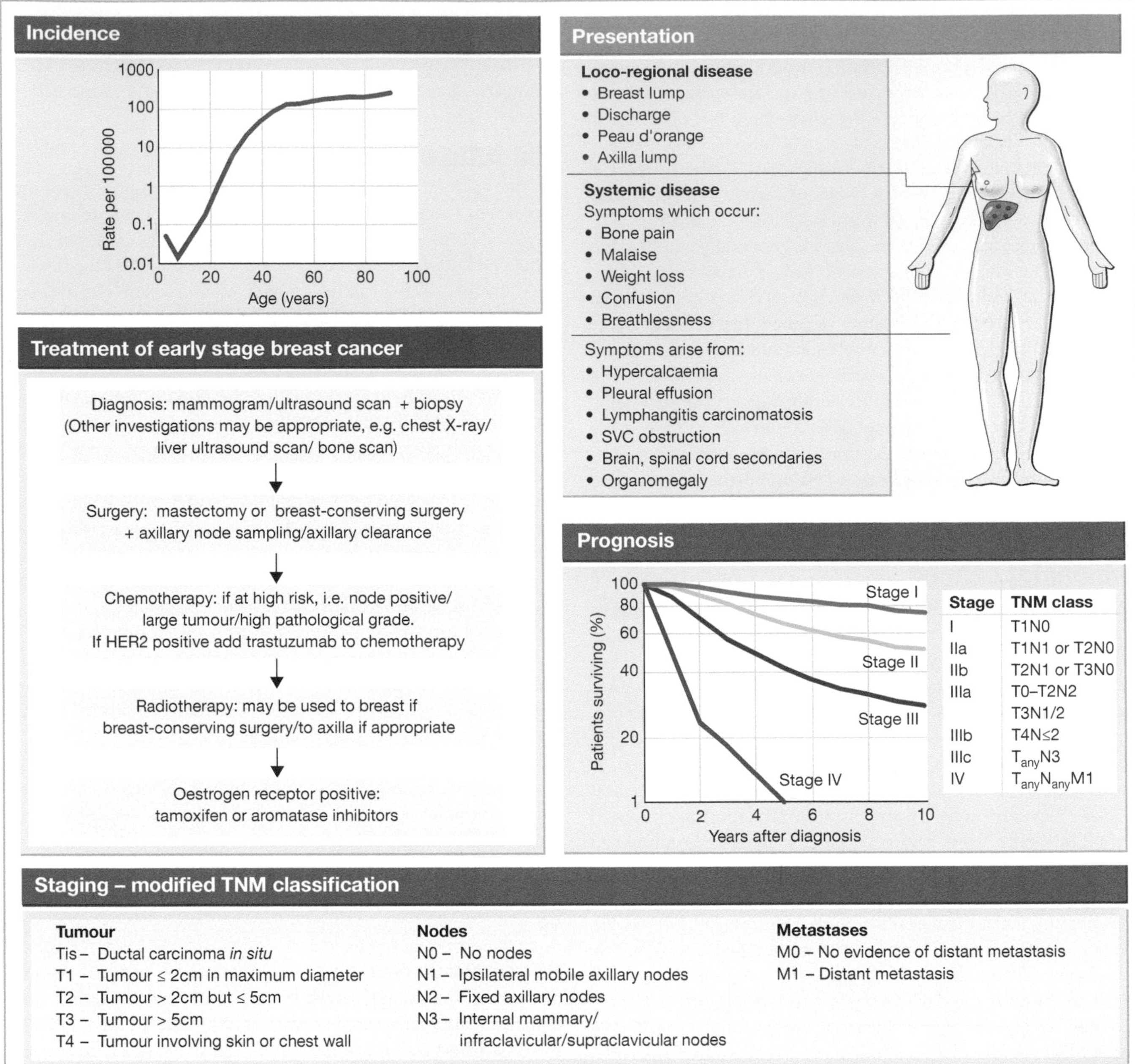

Incidence
1000
100
10
1
0.1
0.01
Rate per 100 000
0
20
40
60
80
100
Age (years)
Presentation
Loco-regional disease
• Breast lump
• Discharge
• Peau d'orange
• Axilla lump
Systemic disease
Symptoms which occur:
• Bone pain
• Malaise
• Weight loss
• Confusion
• Breathlessness
Symptoms arise from:
• Hypercalcaemia
• Pleural effusion
• Lymphangitis carcinomatosis
• SVC obstruction
• Brain, spinal cord secondaries
• Organomegaly
Treatment of early stage breast cancer
Diagnosis: mammogram/ultrasound scan + biopsy
(Other investigations may be appropriate, e.g. chest X-ray/
liver ultrasound scan/ bone scan)
Surgery: mastectomy or breast-conserving surgery
+ axillary node sampling/axillary clearance
Chemotherapy: if at high risk, i.e. node positive/
large tumour/high pathological grade.
If HER2 positive add trastuzumab to chemotherapy
Radiotherapy: may be used to breast if
breast-conserving surgery/to axilla if appropriate
Oestrogen receptor positive:
tamoxifen or aromatase inhibitors
Prognosis
100
80
60
40
20
1
Patients surviving (%)
0
2
4
6
8
10
Years after diagnosis
Stage I
Stage II
Stage III
Stage IV
Stage
TNM class
I
T1N0
IIa
T1N1 or T2N0
IIb
T2N1 or T3N0
IIIa
T0–T2N2
T3N1/2
IIIb
T4N≤2
IIIc
$T_{any}N3$
IV
$T_{any}N_{any}M1$
Staging – modified TNM classification
Tumour
Tis – Ductal carcinoma in situ
T1 – Tumour ≤ 2cm in maximum diameter
T2 – Tumour > 2cm but ≤ 5cm
T3 – Tumour > 5cm
T4 – Tumour involving skin or chest wall
Nodes
N0 – No nodes
N1 – Ipsilateral mobile axillary nodes
N2 – Fixed axillary nodes
N3 – Internal mammary/
infraclavicular/supraclavicular nodes
Metastases
M0 – No evidence of distant metastasis
M1 – Distant metastasis

Epidemiology and aetiology

Breast cancer is the most common tumour in women, with around 55 000 women diagnosed in the UK each year and 11 500 dying of the disease. The lifetime risk to a woman of developing breast cancer is one in seven. Most breast cancer occurs without an obvious cause, although several predisposing factors are recognized.

- **Oestrogen exposure**: particularly unopposed by progestogens, explaining the association with early menarche, late menopause and nulliparity.
- **Family and personal history**: 10% of breast cancer is genetically determined with links to the highly penetrant genes *BRCA-1*, *BRCA-2* and *p53*. A previous history of breast, endometrial or ovarian cancer indicates a genetically determined

Medicine at a Glance, Fifth Edition. Edited by Patrick Davey and Alex Pitcher.

Companion website: www.wiley.com/go/medicine5e

increased risk. Chest irradiation and specific types of previous benign breast disease are also risk factors.

- High socioeconomic status is associated with increased risk.
- Risk of breast cancer is increased by age, obesity and alcohol intake.

Molecular genetics

The autosomal dominant *BRCA-1* or *-2* genes occur in 2–5% of all breast cancer patients, but in a much higher proportion of young patients aged <40 years with a strong family history (i.e. more than one affected first-degree relative) of breast and ovarian cancer. Other familial syndromes associated with breast cancer include gene mutations in *PALB2*, *PTEN* (Cowden syndrome) and Li–Fraumeni syndrome (TP53 mutation),

Pathology

- **Invasive carcinoma of the breast** (ductal carcinoma) accounts for >70% of all breast cancers. Lobular carcinoma is the next most common pathological diagnosis. Medullary, mucinous, papillary or tubular carcinomas are rarer subtypes.
- **Ductal carcinoma *in situ*** is a malignant cell proliferation within the ducts without stromal invasion, usually unilateral and occasionally multifocal. It is often detectable on mammography due to the presence of calcification. Without treatment, 14–53% of patients develop invasive breast cancer.
- Breast cancer can also present as **Paget's disease** of the nipple (tumour of main excretory ducts involving overlying nipple and skin) and rarely as lymphoma, sarcoma, squamous or clear cell carcinomas.

Histological grading and pathology

Breast adenocarcinomas are graded histologically using the 'modified Bloom and Richardson' scoring scheme to categorize aggressiveness and probable behaviour, on the basis of tubule formation, nuclear pleomorphism and mitotic rate (Ki-67). Other important histological findings are as follows.

- Receptor status: breast cancer cells may express oestrogen and/or progestogen receptors (ER/PR receptors). Their presence or absence affects prognosis and treatment.
- Twenty-five percent of breast cancers overexpress HER-2/neu and these have a worse prognosis.
- Invasive breast cancers are grouped into subtypes based on histology and immunohistochemistry (IHC). These groups influence treatment decision and prognosis.
    - Luminal A: ER positive, HER2 negative, Ki-67 low, PR high.
    - Luminal B: ER positive, HER2 positive or negative, Ki-67 high or PR low.
    - HER 2 overexpression: HER2 positive, ER and PR absent.
    - Basal-like: HER2 negative, ER and PR absent (triple negative breast cancer) often associated with germline BRCA 1 or BRCA 2 mutations.

Investigations

Initial diagnosis of a breast mass or breast abnormality detected by breast screening should involve a 'triple assessment' approach.

1 Clinical examination and a full history (including menopause staus and family history).

2 Imaging.

- Two-view mammography (oblique/craniocaudal): rarely useful in women <40 years old (breasts are radiodense).
- Breast ultrasonography: useful if there is a palpable mass and can distinguish cystic from solid lesions. Malignant lesions have indistinct edges. Not useful for screening.
- Magnetic resonance imaging (MRI) is increasingly used.

3 Biopsy: core biopsy with or without fine needle aspiration: manual or stereotactic (if indicated).

Staging

- Routine haematological and biochemical tests (including liver function tests and calcium).
- Other tests including (i) chest radiograph; (ii) ultrasonography of liver; (iii) computed tomography (CT) scan of the chest, abdomen and pelvis; and (iv) isotope bone scan, which may be indicated for high-risk patients. Further tests include the use of PET CT and imaging of brain and spinal cord if indicated. Additional tests such as cardiac assessment prior to therapy may be required.

Treatment of early-stage breast cancer

- **Surgery**: for most patients the primary surgical treatment aims to remove the tumour and to obtain staging and prognostic information from the tumour and axillary nodes. Surgery may be modified radical mastectomy or breast-conserving (lumpectomy with postoperative radiotherapy). Local excision of the tumour (with a histologically confirmed margin of normal tissue), combined with postoperative radical radiotherapy, achieves as good local control as total mastectomy, though the latter is indicated for large (>4 cm), multicentric tumours or if there is extensive ductal carcinoma *in situ*. Axillary management depends on whether there is known lymph node involvement or not; if there is, then axillary node clearance/dissection is performed. Otherwise sentinel lymph node biopsy/axillary node sampling is performed. This more limited procedure limits postoperative morbidity. If, however, subsequent histology confirms the presence of nodal involvement, patients need to undergo either completion clearance or radiotherapy.
- **Radiotherapy**: adjuvant radiotherapy to the breast remnant reduces the risk of local tumour recurrence following breast-conserving surgery. Radiotherapy to the axilla is given if axillary node sampling has revealed positive nodes, although not if full axillary dissection has been performed, because it adds little to local control and has an unacceptably high incidence of lymphoedema.
- **Adjuvant (and neoadjuvant) systemic therapy**: 30–50% of patients with apparently resectable breast cancer subsequently die of their disease, suggesting that micrometastases were present at diagnosis. Systemic adjuvant therapy reduces the risk of disease relapse and improves overall survival. Systemic treatment may be given prior to surgery (neoadjuvant) and/or following sugery (adjuvant).
- **Endocrine therapy**: tamoxifen, an antioestrogen, reduces the risk of disease relapse in women with hormone receptor-positive disease. It is given for 5–10 years and is the treatment of choice for premenopausal women. For postmenopausal women, aromatase inhibitors (e.g. anastrozole, letrozole) are being used as first-line treatment. Recent clinical trials have shown benefit of combining

drugs that block the cell cycle (cyclin-dependent kinase [CDK] 4 and 6 inhibitor) to adjuvant endocrine treatment in those with hormone receptor positive (and HER2 negative) breast cancers at high risk of relapse.

- **Chemotherapy**: most patients (not small [<1 cm], low-grade, node-negative disease) with moderate- to high-risk disease benefit from adjuvant chemotherapy. Equivalent relative benefit is seen in post- and premenopausal women. Combination chemotherapy is used (typically an anthracycline-containing regimen, e.g. epirubicin in combination with or followed by a taxane [docetaxel and paclitaxel]). In patients where the benefit of adjuvant chemotherapy is unclear, genomic tests are increasingly being used to gain additional prognostic/predictive information to identify patients at high risk for relapse (and who would therefore benefit from the addition of chemotherapy).
- **Targeted therapy**, e.g. trastuzumab. This is a humanized monoclonal antibody to the HER2 receptor used in the (neo) adjuvant treatment of HER2-positive breast cancer. It has been shown to improve both relapse-free and overall survival. Other HER2-targeting agents (e.g. pertuzumab) and anti-HER2 antibody drug conjugates have been investigated.
- **Bisphosphonates**: prophylactic bisphosphonates have been shown to improve cancer-specific survival in patients with low oestrogen status (i.e. postmenopausal women or women undergoing ovarian suppression).

Follow-up

Follow-up is used to detect disease recurrence, manage treatment-related toxicity, and screen for a new primary lesion and for psychological support, but it does not improve survival. The cancer risk to the second breast is increased four-fold. Mammography should be performed yearly, bilaterally if the patient had breast-conserving treatment.

Locally advanced breast cancer

This is defined as tumours >5 cm in size or showing evidence of skin or chest wall invasion (i.e. 'fixed') or inflammatory breast cancer (erythematous with lymphatic permeation). A response to primary treatment with chemotherapy may facilitate surgery and in some instances may allow breast-conserving surgery.

Metastatic/advanced breast cancer

The treatment depends upon a number of factors including endocrine and HER2 status, the age of the patient and extent of disease. Treatment options include the following.

- **Endocrine treatment**: in some patients with hormone receptor-positive disease, endocrine therapy is the treatment of choice (e.g. tamoxifen or aromatase inhibitors). This treatment is now often given with the addition of cyclin-dependent kinase (CDK) 4/6 inhibitors (e.g. palbociclib). Other options include combining endocrine treatment with an mTOR inhibitor (everolimus) or PI3K (phosphatidylinositol 3-kinase) inhibitor (in those with PIK3CA [phosphatidylinositol-4,5, bisphosphate 3-kinase catalytic subunit alpha] mutation).
- **Chemotherapy** is considered in young, healthy patients with rapidly progressive, visceral disease, particularly if relapse has occurred early after surgery or in oestrogen receptor (ER)-negative disease that is unlikely to respond to hormonal therapy. The same regimens used in the adjuvant setting are given. The first line of treatment includes anthracyclines (but not if already used adjuvantly), with taxanes being used as second line. Third- and fourth-line agents include capecitabine, eribulin and vinorelbine. Pathology may influence the types of chemotherapy agents given, for example, the use of platinum agents in *BRCA* mutated/basal-like (triple negative) breast cancers.
- **Anti-HER2 therapy** such as trastuzumab for HER2-positive women is most often given together with chemotherapy (but should not be used with anthracycline chemotherapy because of the increased risk of cardiotoxicity). Antibody drug conjugates (ADCs) that target HER2 are further options in the metastatic setting.
- **Other treatments** include the use of poly (ADP ribose) polymerase (PARP) inhibitors in patients with *BRCA* mutated breast cancer, and the use of immune checkpoint inhibitors in triple negative breast cancer.
- **Bisphosphonates** (e.g. zolendronic acid) or a RANKL inhibitor (denosumab) are routinely used in the management of bony metastases.
- Other treatment modalities such as **surgery** and **radiotherapy** can be considered for palliation and are also used in the management of single (oligo) metastatic disease.

193 Prostate cancer

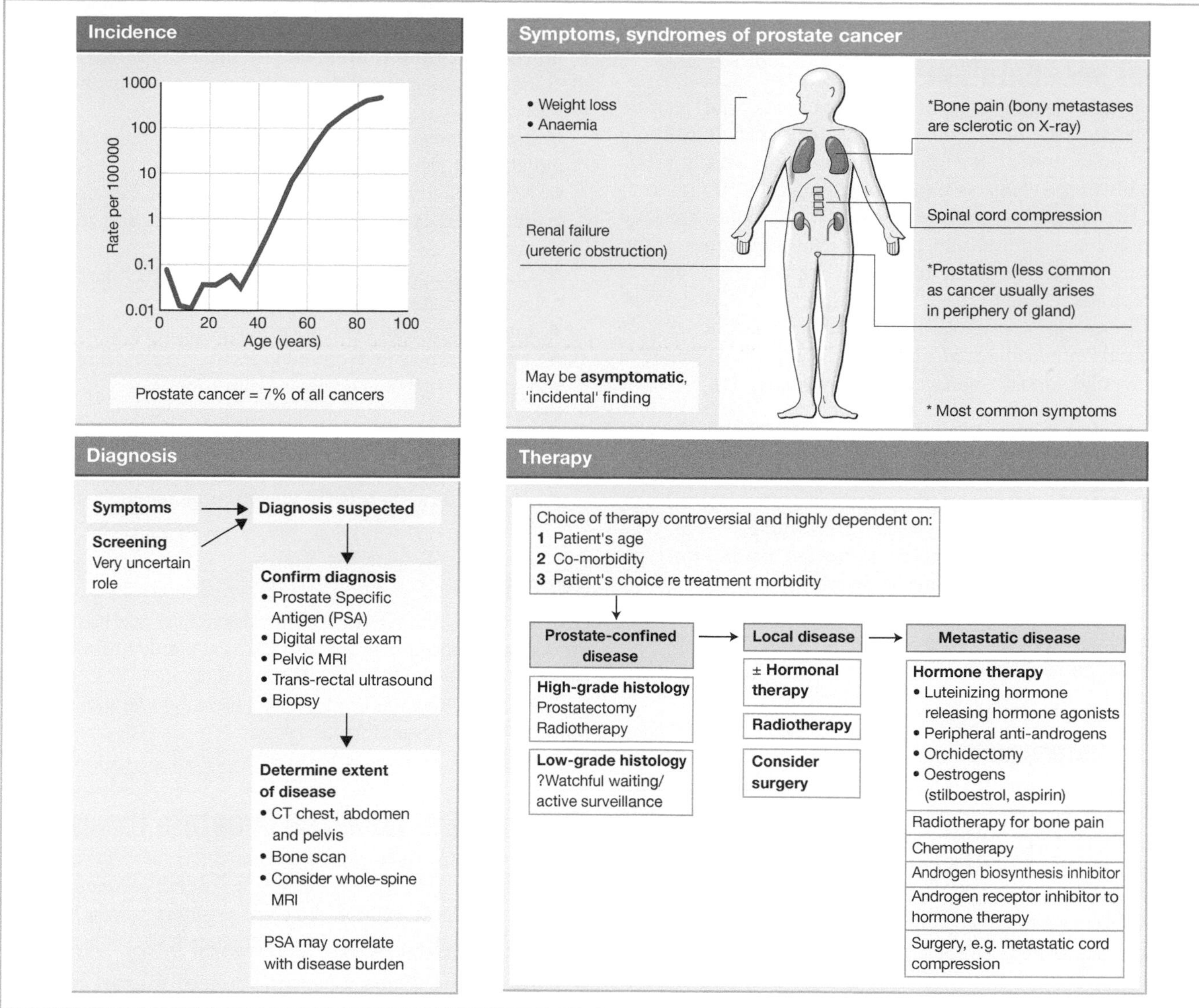

Prostate cancer is the most common malignancy in men and it may soon exceed lung cancer as the most frequent cause of male cancer death. Many patients have small, indolent cancers that will never be clinically significant, so the older age of patients, co-morbidities and the adverse impact of surgery on quality of life make screening with prostate-specific antigen (PSA) and treatment decisions about early stage disease particularly controversial.

Aetiology

Malignant transformation is a common complication of the ageing prostate (in men over the age of 80, postmortem studies have shown foci of prostate cancer in up to 70%). Age, ethnicity, family history, radiation exposure, diet and environmental pollutants contribute to the risk.

Pathology

- Adenocarcinoma is the most common pathology. It arises in the acinar epithelium in the peripheral region of the gland. Cells stain for acid phosphatase and PSA. Various grading systems predict the biological behaviour of the tumour. The most commonly used of these is the Gleason system, where the tumour is graded histologically between grade I (well differentiated, uniform gland formation) and grade V (very poorly differentiated, minimal gland formation). The overall Gleason score is the addition of the

Medicine at a Glance, Fifth Edition. Edited by Patrick Davey and Alex Pitcher.

Companion website: www.wiley.com/go/medicine5e

highest grade to the most predominant grade seen in the tumour biopsy for a total score out of 10.

- Rarer tumours (<2%) include neuroendocrine carcinoma, transitional cell carcinoma arising in the ductal epithelium, stromal sarcomas and lymphomas (these are treated differently to adenocarcinomas).

Clinical presentation

Early prostatic cancer is typically asymptomatic and may be detectable clinically only by the presence of a rectally palpable mass or induration of the gland. The tumour usually arises peripherally in the gland, so obstructive symptoms ('prostatism') happen late unless secondary to associated benign prostatic hypertrophy. Haematuria and perineal pain sometimes occur. Patients may have metastatic disease at diagnosis, and present with symptoms related to these, such as the constitutional symptoms of weight loss, anaemia, bone pain, lymphadenopathy or neurological complications including cord compression (requires urgent investigation and management; see Chapter 54).

Staging (see Table 193.1)

Localized prostate cancers are also classified as low, intermediate or high risk based on staging, Gleason score and PSA. This classification informs treatment decisions. Prostate cancer most typically metastasizes to bone. It may, however, spread through the lymphatics to regional pelvic nodes and then to abdominal nodes. Visceral metastases may also occur (most commonly seen with poorly differentiated tumours).

Clinical approach

Investigations in suspected prostate cancer aim to confirm the diagnosis histologically and determine whether nodal disease or metastases are present (typically inferred from a higher PSA, larger tumours, high Gleason score). If disease is confined to the prostate, local therapy such as radical prostatectomy or radiotherapy may be appropriate. These treatments may have similar outcomes (>30% incontinence and >80% impotence). Early disease can be overtreated with devastating complications, and active surveillance/watchful waiting may be an appropriate option in some patients.

Table 193.1 TNM staging of prostate cancer.

T1	Tumour neither palpable nor imageable, identified only in resected specimens or by biopsy
T2	Tumour confined to the prostate
T3	Tumour extending through the prostate capsule
T4	Tumour is fixed or invading adjacent structures other than the seminal vesicles (bladder, rectum or pelvic side wall, etc.)
N0	No regional lymph node metastasis
N1	Metastasis in regional lymph node
M0	No evidence of distant metastases
M1	Distant metastases present

Investigations

- **Full history** including family history and co-morbidities. Full examination including digital rectal examination (DRE) should be performed. Bone metastases can be the first presentation of prostate cancer, so any man over the age of 50 presenting with persistent bone pain should have investigations including a DRE and PSA.
- **Biochemistry and routine bloods**: including serum PSA levels. Raised alkaline phosphatase may suggest bone involvement.
- **Radiology**.
  - *Multiparametric MRI*: this is increasingly being used as an initial investigation in men with a high PSA.
  - *Computed tomography* (CT) of the chest abdomen and pelvis may identify pelvic or abdominal nodes and metastatic disease.
  - *Choline positron emission tomography* (PET) may be used to look for metastasis.
  - *Isotope bone scan* to identify bone metastasis.
  - *MRI spine* may be required to identify vertebral metastasis and spinal cord/cauda equina compression.
- **Prostate biopsy**.
  - *Transrectal ultrasonography* (TRUS): most common route; 12 cores are often taken.
  - *Transperineal route* (MRI guided) is increasingly used.

Genetics

Genetic testing (and referral to clinical genetics) may be indicated for young patients and those with a strong family history of cancer (particularly looking for *BRCA* mutations). Screening for prostate cancer remains controversial but might be indicated for those at high risk (see Chapter 191).

Treatment of localized prostate cancer

The principal treatment approaches include surgery, radiotherapy and active surveillance. There is no overall consensus about the benefit of intervention in early prostatic cancer. Patients should be informed and involved in treatment decisions.

- **Surgery** is an option for organ-confined disease, and often preferred in younger patients although this has never been tested against radiotherapy in a randomized clinical trial.
- **Radical radiotherapy** has similar survival figures; new initiatives are investigating increasing the radiation dose using more targeted (conformal) radiotherapy and combining radiotherapy with hormonal therapy. Patients with low-risk tumours survive for an equally long period (five-year survival rate is 85%) whether they receive radical radiotherapy or are simply kept under observation (active surveillance).
- **Brachytherapy** using radioactive palladium or iodine seeds implanted directly into the prostate gland can be performed on an outpatient basis, and is used for small low-grade tumours with excellent results in carefully selected patients.
- **High-intensity focused ultrasound** (HIFU) offers an alternative approach and may be appropriate for some localized prostate cancers.
- Active **surveillance** is an option for men with low- or intermediate-risk prostate cancer who wish to defer treatment (and therefore avoid unnecessary side-effects). These men are

monitored by serial PSA measurements, imaging and repeat prostate biopsy. If there is evidence of disease progression, these patients can then be offered curative treatment.

- **Hormone treatment** (androgen ablation): prostate cancer cell growth shows a striking dependence on androgens. Hormonal therapy directed at interfering with this association typically produces disease response in both metastatic and locoregional disease. Bilateral orchidectomy or gonadotrophin-releasing hormone (GnRH) agonists (which block pituitary-driven testicular androgen production) (e.g. goserelin) can mediate this. Complete androgen blockade requires the concomitant use of a peripheral antiandrogen (bicalutamide) and GnRH agonist and has minimal extra efficacy, so these agents are typically used sequentially. Synthetic oestrogens such as diethylstilboestrol produce similar effects but are associated with significant cardiovascular and thromboembolic morbidity. Neoadjuvant hormone therapy before radiotherapy can reduce the size of the prostate gland, hence also reducing the radiation treatment volume and lowering toxicity; there is also improved local control and disease-free survival. Adjuvant hormone therapy is recommended for men receiving neoadjuvant treatment and radical radiotherapy who are at high risk of prostate cancer mortality. Antiandrogen side-effects include hot flushes, weakness, impotence and loss of sexual drive.

Metastatic prostate cancer

- **Hormonal treatment**: widespread metastatic disease is often initially very responsive to hormone therapy (castrate sensitive); it is the first line of therapy in many cases, and is associated with a considerable symptomatic improvement and clinical response. An LHRH analogue (such as goserelin) is given with antiandrogen cover (e.g. bicalutamide) to prevent testosterone surge and tumour flare (which can result in complications such as spinal cord compression or hydronephrosis). Bilateral orchidectomy is an alternative to continuous LHRH analogues. Selective gonadotrophin releasing-hormone (GnRH) antagonists, such as degarelix can also be considered. Combining androgen blockade with additional treatments such as abiraterone (androgen biosynthesis inhibitor) or androgen receptor inhibitors has shown additional benefit in first-line treatment.
- The response to initial treatment should be followed closely and accurately by regular assessment of PSA levels and clinical review. Patients may continue to respond to hormone therapy for several years, but on average the disease escapes hormonal control after about 18 months (castrate resistant).
- **Chemotherapy**: in patients with high-volume disease, using chemotherapy (docetaxel) in the castrate-sensitive setting has been shown to improve outcomes. It is therefore an option for first-line treatment if the patient is fit enough.
- **Castrate-resistant prostate cancer**: treatment options include abiraterone (androgen biosynthesis inhibitor) and enzalutamide (androgen receptor inhibitor) or chemotherapy.
- **Other treatment**: the addition of abiraterone or androgen receptor inhibitors to androgen ablation has shown benefit in the first-line metastatic setting. Poly (ADP-ribose) polymerase (PARP) inhibitors are being investigated for those with mutations in DNA repair genes, including *BRCA* mutations.
- **Radiotherapy** has a role to play in the palliation of symptoms either from the primary tumour or from troublesome sites of metastases.
- **Osteoclast inhibition** using bisphosphonates or antibodies against the RANK ligand decrease skeletal morbidity.
- Bone-seeking **radioisotopes** such as radium-223 may have a role in some patients with extensive bony metastases.

194 Cancer with an unknown primary

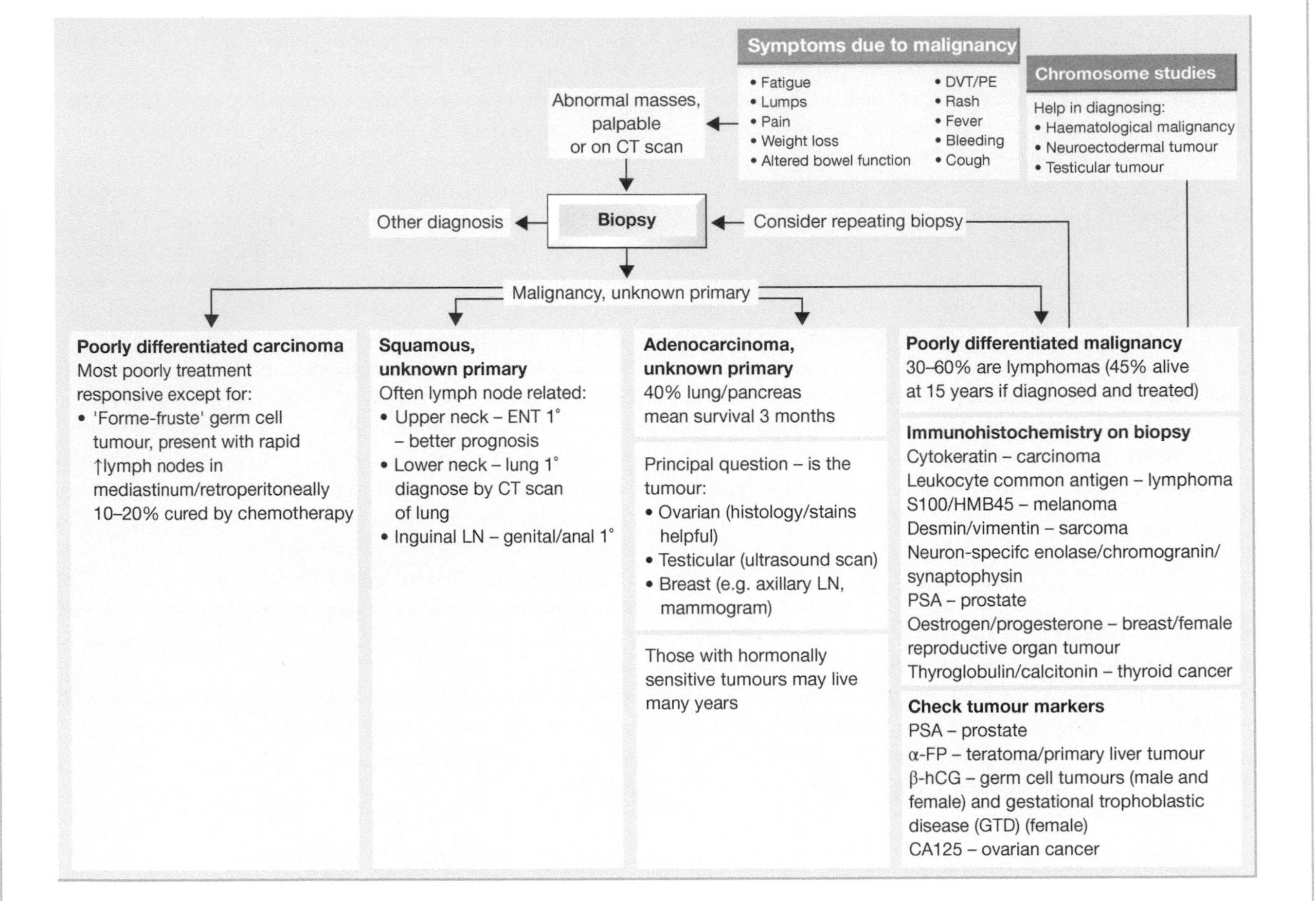

Cancer is present without a clear primary source in 3–5% of cases. This represents a heterogeneous group of cancers containing treatable and in some cases curable subtypes. The typical spectrum of neoplasms of unknown primary site can be divided into the following pathological groups.

1 Adenocarcinoma (well or moderately differentiated)
2 Squamous cell carcinoma
3 Carcinomas with neuroendocrine differentiation (well or poorly differentiated)
4 Poorly differentiated carcinoma
5 Undifferentiated neoplasm

Initial work-up

The initial evaluation and work-up of patients presenting with a presumed cancer of unknown primary (CUP) should focus on identifying subsets which may benefit from specific treatments (such as lymphomas and germ cell tumours). An adequate biopsy (often radiologically guided) and use of immunohistochemistry analysis are essential to establish the tissue of origin.

Assessment includes:

- **History and physical examination**: full history (including family history) and comprehensive physical examination (including head and neck, rectal, pelvic and breast examination) should be performed.
- **Imaging**: CT scan of the thorax, abdomen and pelvis forms the foundation of any cancer assessment. A mammogram should be considered in female patients. A CT PET can be very useful to delineate disease pattern/spread (such as squamous cell carcinoma or identifying single-site disease).
- **Endoscopic investigation**: colonoscopy, oesophagogastroduodenoscopy or bronchoscopy can provide useful diagnostic and histological information if suggestive of a gastrointestinal or lung cancer respectively.
- **Tumour markers**: initial panel should include α-fetoprotein (AFP), human chorionic gonadotrophin (HCG), and prostate specific antigen (PSA) should be considered in male patients. Other tumour markers should be considered based on history, examination, radiological and biopsy information. Assessment of LDH (once CUP is confirmed) is an important prognostic factor.

Other investigations are based on information gleaned from the primary screen/investigations. If a neuroendocrine cancer is suspected, then Octreotide® scan, dotatate-PET and fasting gut hormones (including chromogranins) should be performed. The use of gene expression profiles is under investigation.

Neoplasms of unknown primary site

Poorly differentiated malignancy

Poorly differentiated carcinomas and poorly differentiated neoplasms represent 30% of all CUPs and are now less common due to advances in diagnosis and immunohistochemistry techniques. Of the poorly differentiated neoplasms that are hard to identify histologically, the most important (due to treatability) of the non-epithelial cancers are melanoma, sarcoma and lymphomas.

Between 30% and 60% of undifferentiated neoplasms are lymphomas and eminently treatable and potentially curable with chemotherapy and radiotherapy. Following treatment, >45% of these patients are alive and disease free after 15 years.

It is important to determine whether a poorly differentiated tumour is a variant of a germ cell tumour, as these are highly responsive and curative with chemotherapy. These typically present with lymphadenopathy involving the mediastinum or retroperitoneum as rapidly progressive tumours in younger adults (20–50 years old). There may be chromosomal abnormalities i(12p), or AFP staining of histological samples.

The most common cause for diagnostic uncertainty is an inadequate biopsy sample. This is particularly true with fine needle aspiration (FNA) due to the small volume and frequently under-represented areas of malignant abnormality. A repeat biopsy combined with immunohistochemistry can be very useful in this situation.

Karyotyping and cytogenetic analysis can identify chromosomal translocations which can be helpful in diagnosis particularly for a number of haematological diagnoses (such as leukaemias and lymphoma). They are also proving increasingly useful in diagnosing solid tumours such as testicular cancer.

Molecular profiling of cancers is being invaluable in providing diagnostic information and influencing therapeutic options.

Adenocarcinoma of unknown primary

Adenocarcinoma of unknown primary is the most common type of cancer presenting with an unknown primary (60%) and has the poorest prognosis. 40% are the result of lung or upper gastrointestinal (e.g. hepatic, pancreatic and biliary) cancer. The diagnosis is achieved from certain histological features, e.g.:

- papillary formation suggests an ovarian or thyroid origin
- mucinous signet rings suggest gastric in origin.

History and examination (including rectal, vaginal and breast examination) along with tumour markers and imaging should be performed.

- Mammography and CT of the abdomen (finds a primary in up to 30% of patients).
- Upper or lower GI endoscopy has a very low sensitivity in patients without relevant symptoms.
- In male patients, testicular ultrasonography is important.

Treatable adenocarcinomas (important to identify)

- **Papillary serous ovarian cancer**: suggested by psammoma body formation in women with malignant ascites and a pelvic mass. Serum CA-125 antigen levels may be raised. Surgical cytoreduction and platinum-based chemotherapy along with other targeted treatment prolong survival, with some long-term survivors. Genetic testing (germline *BRCA* testing) is also indicated in this group.
- **Occult breast cancer**: serum CA-15.3 antigen levels may be raised. Women with axillary node metastasis usually (40–80% of cases) have a locally advanced breast primary that should be treated surgically. Further options for treatment include endocrine treatment (e.g. tamoxifen/aromatase inhibitors) if oestrogen receptor positive, or chemotherapy or other targeted agents such as trastuzumab if HER2 positive (see Chapter 192).
- **Prostate cancer** in men: can present with osteoblastic bone metastases. Serum PSA levels are usually elevated. Androgen deprivation therapy may provide prolonged remissions (see Chapter 193). Other cancers that commonly spread to bone include lung, breast, thyroid, renal and multiple myeloma.
- **Single-site adenocarcinoma of unknown primary**: may warrant an aggressive approach with surgical excision +/- chemotherapy or radiotherapy.

Squamous cell carcinomas

Patients with squamous cell histology typically present with lymphadenopathy. It is the site of the lymphadenopathy that suggests the location of the underlying primary.

- Upper cervical lymphadenopathy is commonly the result of an ear, nose, throat (ENT) primary, whereas involvement of lower cervical nodes more commonly represents metastases from lung cancer. In young patients with lymphadenopathy and poorly differentiated squamous cell carcinoma (SCC), it is important to determine whether tissue polymerase chain reaction reveals Epstein–Barr virus. This may suggest a nasopharyngeal carcinoma which has a more favourable prognosis, being sensitive to chemotherapy combined with radiotherapy.
- Inguinal nodes containing SCC typically arise from a genital or anal primary.
- Skin SCC is rarely metastatic unless immunocompromised.

Neuroendocrine carcinoma

This is a diverse tumour group, representing a continuum between more indolent carcinoid or low-grade neuroendocrine carcinoma and highly aggressive high-grade neuroendocrine carcinoma, including small cell carcinoma. Diagnosis of these cancers depends on immunohistochemical staining for chromogranin and/or synaptophysin. Low-grade neuroendocrine cancers are generally managed initially with somastostatin analogues (such as octreotide), with chemotherapy being reserved only for refractory disease. High-grade neuroendocrine carcinomas are highly aggressive but are very sensitive to platinum-based chemotherapy. However, they frequently relapse quickly after treatment cessation.

General approach to management

Specific treatments are based on the subset to which the patient belongs and should follow a similar pathway to those with the primary disease. The majority of patients with CUP (80–85%), however, do not belong to a specific subset. Combination chemotherapy using a platinum agent (e.g. cisplatin/carboplatin) is the most commonly used regime for this group. Sensitivity to anticancer treatment, however, is modest and overall prognosis is poor. The role of targeted treatment is being investigated and entry in clinical trials is important.

The decision to treat relates to both the disease and the patient (overall performance status is particularly important). Referral to an oncologist is appropriate for every patient with cancer. Patients should be discussed at multidisciplinary team meetings to explore management options. In all patients with cancer, or indeed any terminal illness, a holistic approach with compassion and support, both emotional and physical (e.g. planning terminal care in conjunction with the local hospice), is vital and the measure of a good physician. Modern approaches to the management of cancer change rapidly and caring for patients with life-threatening diseases is challenging.

195 Paraneoplastic cancer syndromes and hormone-producing cancers

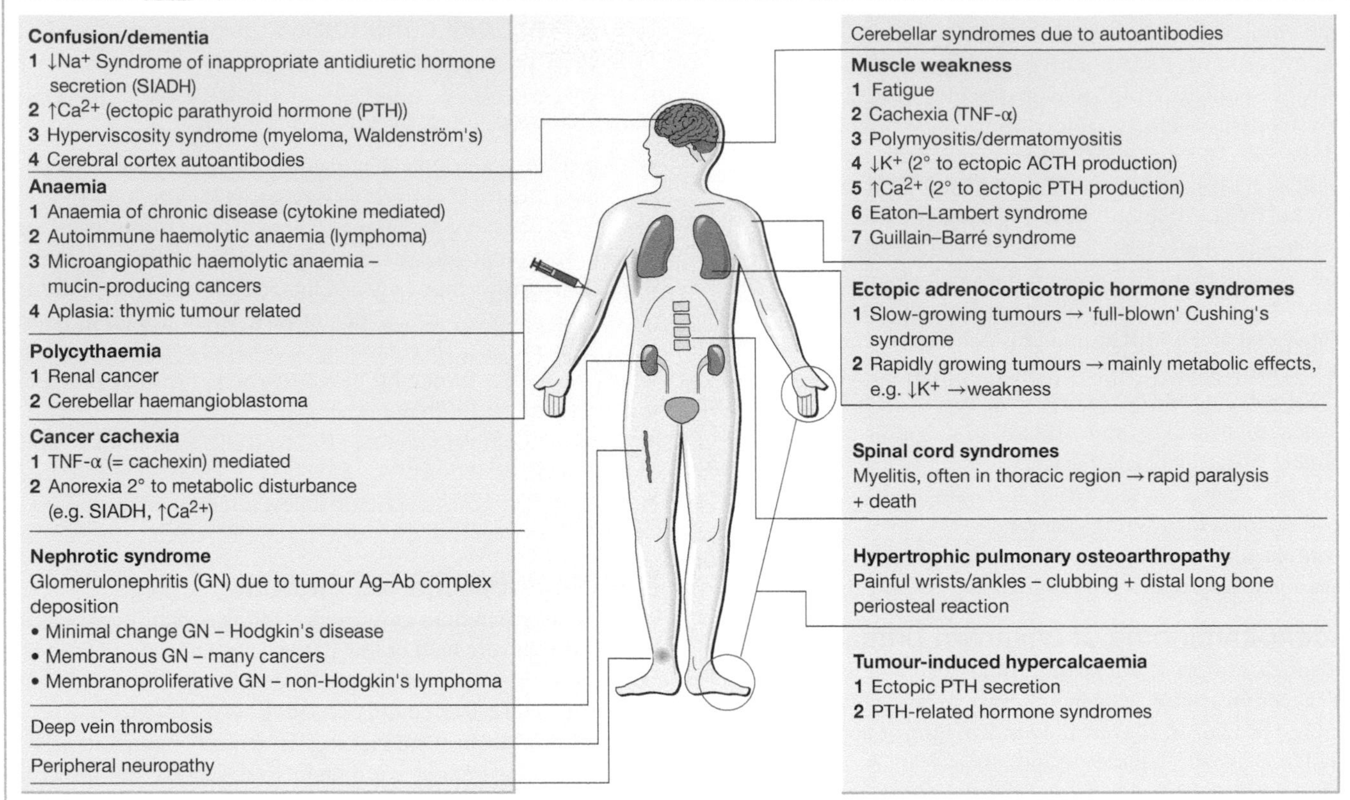

Cancers produce illness through direct effects (e.g. local invasion) and the release of biologically active substances. Diseases produced by the latter are termed 'paraneoplastic syndromes', the most common of which are anaemia, cachexia and fatigue, tumour-induced hypercalcaemia, syndrome of inappropriate antidiuretic hormone secretion (SIADH), Cushing syndrome from ectopic adrenocorticotrophic hormone (ACTH) and hypoglycaemia associated with the production of insulin-like growth factors (IGFs).

Pathogenesis

Paraneoplastic syndromes arise from a variety of mechanisms, many of which are still unknown: (i) through the release of normal cellular proteins, in increased amounts (e.g. ectopic hormone production); (ii) through cytokine production; (iii) via autoantibody production, which typically results in neurological disorders; and (iv) via abnormal metabolism of steroids, the production of enzymes or the expression of fetal proteins.

Anaemia

Anaemia in cancer can relate to many factors, including iron deficiency (especially in gastrointestinal tumours) and folate deficiency (in malnourished patients, and those with very rapidly dividing tumours). However, much anaemia relates to the 'anaemia of chronic disease', whereby the inflammatory response associated with malignancy leads to the production of a number of cytokines that suppress the bone marrow. These include the following.

- Disturbance of normal iron metabolism by transforming growth factor β, interleukin (IL)-1, IL-6 and interferon γ. These may act through increasing the levels of hepcidin, which suppresses iron uptake and utilization.
- Tumour necrosis factor (TNF)-α (whose levels can be greatly increased in patients with cancer) antagonizing the effects of erythropoietin on the bone marrow. Satisfactory haemoglobin levels can be achieved in about 50% of such patients by giving synthetic recombinant erythropoietin.
- Rarely, a patient's malignancy induces an autoimmune haemolytic anaemia.
- Rarer still, malignancy can induce red cell aplasia.

Cachexia

The weight loss and malaise associated with cancer relate to the tumour burden but also, importantly, to the production of cytokines such as TNF-α or cachexin. Steroids and progesterones may have a useful symptomatic role.

Medicine at a Glance, Fifth Edition. Edited by Patrick Davey and Alex Pitcher.

Companion website: www.wiley.com/go/medicine5e

Syndrome of inappropriate ADH secretion

The inappropriate secretion of vasopressin or antidiuretic hormone (ADH) results in hyponatraemia, renal sodium loss, hypervolaemia and inappropriately high urine osmolality. Clinically, this may only produce biochemical disease, but it may also produce symptoms relating to the hyponatraemia: tiredness, mental clouding, delirium and coma. The mechanism for SIADH in cancer is twofold: (i) reflex release, by central nervous system tumours, drugs or co-existing lung disease; and (ii) ectopic hormone release by the tumour, as in small cell lung cancer (SCLC), and more rarely tumours of the duodenum, pancreas, thymus and lymphomas. A precursor molecule is split to produce ADH and neurophysin.

The underlying disease should be aggressively treated; fluid restriction is the mainstay of management. Refractory cases may respond to demeclocycline, which induces nephrogenic diabetes insipidus.

Hypercalcaemia

The most common clinical presentation of an ectopic hormone syndrome is tumour-induced hypercalcaemia (TIH), typically associated with the production of parathyroid hormone-related protein (PTHrP), which shares structural similarities with PTH (shares the 6 out of 7 amino acids at the N-terminal) and may activate the PTH receptor. The solid tumours causing ectopic PTH-like secretion are those of squamous cell (e.g. lung), genitourinary or gynaecological origin. The differential diagnosis is hypercalcaemia from bony metastases, usually from lung, breast, prostate, thyroid or renal cell primaries, which develop in 10–20% of patients with disseminated malignancy. Bony metastases, which are the most common cause of malignancy-associated hypercalcaemia, cause hypercalcaemia by causing the release of TNF-α, various prostaglandins and other paracrine agents that activate local osteoclasts. Multiple myeloma and human T-cell leukaemia virus (HTLV)-associated lymphoma are the most common haematological malignancies associated with TIH, the latter being, in part, the result of the production of vitamin D within the tumour.

Treatment involves correcting the volume depletion that all hypercalcaemic individuals have (caused by calcium-induced diabetes insipidus). Bisphosphonates have revolutionized management of TIH, but PTHrP-related hypercalcaemia is often refractory. Bisphosphonates inhibit osteoclast function, reduce raised levels of calcium quickly, slow the development of bone metastases, and reduce both the associated symptoms and complications. Steroids are used for steroid-responsive tumours, e.g. multiple myeloma and lymphoma. Further options for treatment of hypercalaemia of malignancy include denosumab and calcitonin.

Cushing syndrome

Tumours can produce bizarre syndromes of metabolic upset related to ectopic hormone production. The most common of these is Cushing syndrome in SCLC, caused by ectopic ACTH production, first reported by Brown in 1928. Overall, 40% of patients with SCLC secrete polypeptides, most of which are not functional, e.g. the precursor molecule to ACTH (proopiomelanocortin) is often present in these tumours but only possesses 4% of the biological activity of ACTH. Overall, only 2–3% of patients with SCLC have Cushing syndrome. When the syndrome is acute and prominent, it is typically associated with hirsutism, acne and hypokalaemia, and warrants medical control (see Chapter 161) both in its own right and because it increases the toxicity of chemotherapeutic regimens.

Hypoglycaemia

Hypoglycaemia in cancer occurs through three mechanisms.

1 Massive size of a slow-growing tumour; for example, mesenchymal sarcomas, lymphomas or mesotheliomas often secrete 'big' IGF factor II.
2 IGF typically from hepatic or adrenal carcinomas.
3 Insulin secretion by insulinomas, with the rare but classic presentation of fasting hypoglycaemia, commonly associated with neuropsychiatric sequelae and relentless weight gain.

Neurological paraneoplastic syndromes

Paraneoplastic neurological degeneration-associated tumours may be difficult to detect. Diagnosis also relies on identification of paraneoplastic neuronal autoantibodies. Management centres around the identification and treatment of the primary tumour. There are a number of paraneoplastic syndromes that can affect the nervous system.

- **Cerebellar syndrome**: antineuronal antibodies (anti-Yo, -Hu, -Ri and -Tr) are associated with this syndrome of cerebellar–cortical degeneration, most commonly seen with carcinoma of the lung, breast or ovary. The cerebellar syndrome has prominent involvement of eye movements, is extremely disabling and precedes the diagnosis of the underlying cancer. The prognosis is poor and is not reversible with successful treatment of the malignancy. Magnetic resonance imaging is typically normal and the diagnosis is often one of exclusion. Toxic, metabolic, degenerative and rare differentials such as Creutzfeldt–Jakob disease and HIV should be considered.
- **Lambert–Eaton myasthenic syndrome**: most often occurs with SCLC. It is characterized by symmetrical muscle weakness, hyporeflexia and autonomic dysfunction, with improvement in strength on reinforcement. Eye involvement (unlike in myasthenia gravis) is rare. Nerve-evoked acetylcholine release at the neuromuscular junction is reduced. Serum antibodies against voltage-gated calcium channels occur.
- **Encephalomyelitis**: commonly limbic (associated with SCLC) and associated with dementia or acute behavioural disturbance with hallucination and delusions.
- A **subacute sensory neuropathy** producing a sensory ataxia is associated with lymphoma, SCLC and the presence of anti-Hu antibodies.

Dermatological paraneoplastic syndromes

There are many dermatological paraneoplastic syndromes, all of which are associated with stomach or other intra-abdominal malignancies.

- Trousseau's sign of superficial migratory thrombophlebitis.
- The sign of Leser–Trelat (prominent seborrhoeic keratosis).
- Acanthosis nigricans: hyperpigmented velvety plaques found in the axillae and flexural areas.

After the age of 50, half of dermatomyositis cases are associated with an occult malignancy. Pemphigus is associated with malignancy. Gynaecomastia is associated with the production of human chorionic gonadotrophin by hepatomas or germ cell tumours.

Rare syndromes

These include polymyositis, glomerulonephritis, thrombocytosis, erythrocytosis and pseudo-obstruction.

196 Palliative care

Pain

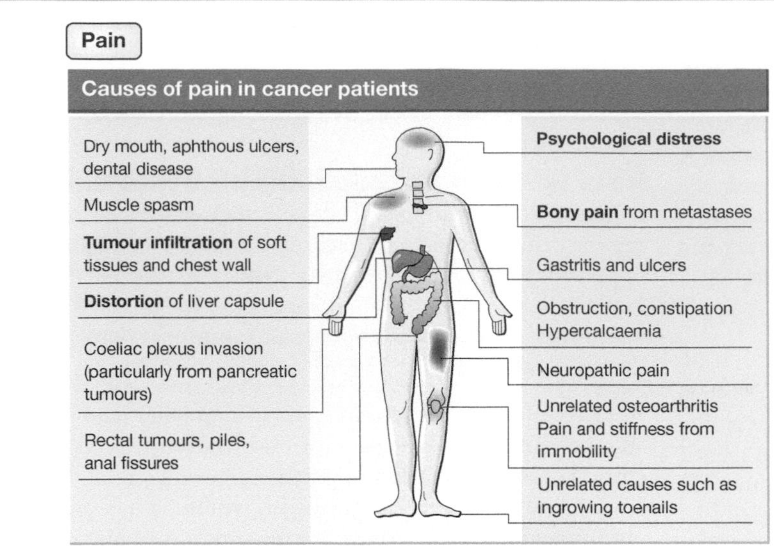

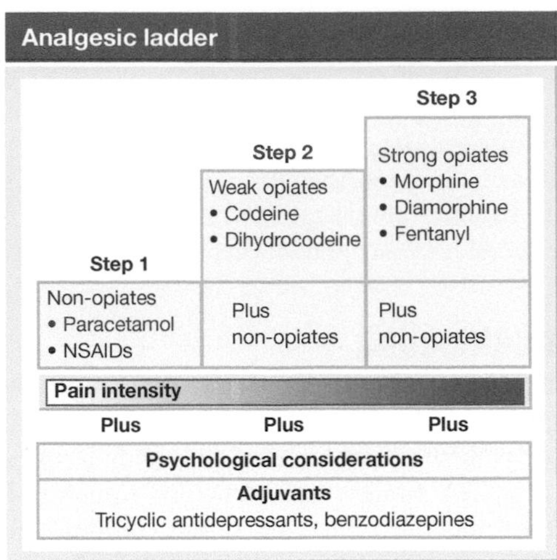

Analgesic ladder
Step 3
Strong opiates
• Morphine
• Diamorphine
• Fentanyl
Step 2
Weak opiates
• Codeine
• Dihydrocodeine
Step 1
Non-opiates
• Paracetamol
• NSAIDs
Plus non-opiates
Plus non-opiates
Pain intensity
Plus
Plus
Plus
Psychological considerations
Adjuvants
Tricyclic antidepressants, benzodiazepines

Palliative care is an approach that improves the quality of life of patients and their families facing the problems associated with life-threatening illness, through the prevention and relief of suffering by means of early identification and impeccable assessment and treatment of pain and other problems, physical, psychosocial and spiritual. (World Health Organization definition of palliative care)

There is a perception that palliation should be reserved only for patients who are imminently dying. However, palliative care enhances quality of life, and may also positively influence the course of illness and can be applicable early in the course of illness in conjunction with other therapies that are intended to prolong life. Palliative care can be delivered alongside active treatment. Palliative care is appropriate for any advanced progressive malignant and non-malignant illness. All clinicians need skills in palliative management; however, some patients, particularly those with complex needs, need referral to a specialist palliative care service. This chapter will deal with two key symptom control issues: management of pain and of the dying process.

Pain

Assessment

A proper pain assessment is the cornerstone of effective pain control. Pain in progressive illness is complex and multifactorial. Focusing exclusively on the physical causes of pain can sometimes explain why pain relief may be inadequate. When assessing the physical cause, consider that pain may relate to the cancer, e.g. local infiltration (visceral, nerve and bone pain), to disabilities relating to chronic illness, e.g. musculoskeletal problems, or to co-morbidities. Consequently, there are often many causes and sites of pain and each of these must be assessed. A careful history should be taken, noting the following.

- Where the pain is, and where it radiates to.
- The type and severity of pain.
- The onset of pain.
- Response to analgesics.
- Exacerbating and alleviating factors.

History and physical examination often establishes the cause of pain, though it may be necessary to perform investigations such as X-rays, isotope bone scans, computed tomography scans, etc. A complete assessment should also include the following aspects.

- **Emotional pain**: when faced with advanced illness, patients frequently experience depression, uncertainty, despair, anger and fear.
- **Social pain**: socially isolated patients can feel unsafe, and those who are financially insecure can feel threatened.
- **Spiritual pain**: patients with advanced illness often search for meaning. For some, this meaning may be embedded in a religious framework. Spiritual distress can occur during this search and can significantly affect a patient's perception of pain.

Treatment of pain

A good history will guide management. Specific types of pain may respond to specific treatments (see Table 196.1).

Analgesics

The World Health Organization advocates a three-step ladder for prescribing analgesics (see figure above). Analgesics should be prescribed regularly. Inadequate pain control at one step requires a move to the next step. Adjuvant co-analgesics can be used at each step for treating that element of the pain that is opioid insensitive.

Opioids

The correct use of opioids has made a major impact on the management of pain in patients with advanced disease. Unfortunately, fears by professionals and patients about the use of strong opioids, lack of understanding about how opioids should be prescribed and an inability to recognize pain that is opioid resistant can lead to ineffective prescribing.

Prescribing opioids: Morphine continues to be the 'gold standard' analgesic. Oral morphine is available in two forms: immediate-acting (four-hourly) and slow-release (12- and 24-hourly) preparations. When prescribed correctly, it is a safe, predictable and reliable drug. Correct prescribing of morphine requires that:

Table 196.1 Treatment for different types of pain.

Cause of pain	Opioid sensitivity	Management	Examples of other options
Large infiltrating tumour mass	Partial	Opioids NSAIDs Steroids	Treat tumour bulk, e.g. radiotherapy
Musculoskeletal pain	Partial	Peripherally acting analgesics (paracetamol, NSAIDs) Physiotherapy Massage	Benzodiazepines
Colic	Insensitive	Treat underlying cause, e.g. side-effect from opioids or anticholinergic drugs	In bowel obstruction, consider reversal, e.g. with surgery or anticancer therapy. Steroids and/or octreotide if reversal is not possible
Bone pain	Partial	NSAIDs Opioids	Radiotherapy Orthopaedic surgery – especially if a metastasis has caused an unstable joint or long bone at risk of fracture; Bisphosphonates
Capsular stretching, e.g. liver capsule pain	Partial	Opioids Steroids; NSAIDs	Anticancer therapy
Nerve pain – symptoms include pain that is described as burning, stabbing or shooting in nature and there may be altered sensation	Usually insensitive	Tricyclic antidepressants Antiepileptics (gabapentin) Opioids (might be partially opioid sensitive)	Steroids Nerve blocks Radiotherapy
Muscle spasm	Partial	Benzodiazepines	Baclofen

- morphine should be given orally if possible
- it must be prescribed regularly to pre-empt pain
- in acute pain, rapid titration of the dose is best achieved using regular immediate-release opioid
- extra doses for breakthrough and incident pain must be co-prescribed and used as necessary
- side-effects, e.g. constipation, anticipated and prevented
- pain should be continuously reassessed.

Failure of opioid therapy may be due to incorrect prescription (wrong dose, interval, route of administration, e.g. unable to absorb), poor compliance or the pain being opioid insensitive.

Side-effects of morphine

- Constipation is virtually universal. It is essential to co-prescribe an appropriate laxative (e.g. sodium docusate) at initiation.
- Nausea and vomiting (less common).
- Drowsiness in 50% of patients. This often wears off after a week on a stable dose. Explanation and reassurance are usually all that is necessary.
- Other side-effects include confusion, sweating, dry mouth, itch, hallucinations and myoclonus.

Alternative opioids: Morphine metabolites can be responsible for side-effects. Morphine is dependent on the kidney for excretion. Deterioration in renal function may result in accumulation of metabolites and increasing side-effects. Alternative opioids, e.g. fentanyl (transdermal preparation) and oxycodone, may be used when opioid-sensitive pain exists but morphine causes excessive side-effects or is contraindicated.

The terminal phase of illness and end-of-life care

When a patient has an advanced, progressive illness, it is important to assess for preferences and wishes about how they want their care to be managed when they deteriorate. This process is known as 'advance care planning'. It gives confidence to the patient that their professional carers will manage them appropriately in the future if they are not in a position to participate in decision making. It is important for cancer patients and their relatives to be engaged in open discussion about resuscitation status. Best practice includes recording this discussion and completing a Do Not Attempt Cardiopulmonary Resuscitation (DNA-CPR) document for patients for whom CPR is likely to be futile.

Healthcare professionals should do their best to ensure that the dying patient has a 'good death'. To facilitate this, the professional must be aware of the complex problems occurring round this time. Physical symptoms, including pain, must be controlled and wider issues (e.g. the needs of the family) should be appreciated. Anticipating symptoms and good communication with relatives are fundamental. The needs of the patient may continuously change and should be assessed regularly to ensure optimal care. The three most common symptoms are as follows.

1 **Pain**: where possible ask about pain and check for easily reversible causes. Some patients may need to start opioids, and those on regular opioids, who cannot take oral medication, will need parenteral (often subcutaneous) therapy.

2 **Breathing**: when a patient's condition deteriorates there are likely to be changes in respiration that can be predicted. Often, the pattern of breathing alters and it is reassuring to the relatives to be warned of these potential changes. As the patient weakens, the ability to cough up secretions is lost, this results in noisy breathing. It can usually be relieved by anticholinergic drugs.

3 **Restlessness and distress**: terminal distress, preterminal agitation, terminal restlessness and terminal anguish are all terms used to describe agitation and distress in patients close to death. Terminal restlessness reflects significant suffering on the part of the patient and causes considerable distress to the relatives who witness it. It is particularly important to assess the patient and rule out easily reversible causes, e.g. catheterization for urinary retention. Sedation should be offered to ease a patient's distress and midazolam is often the drug of choice.

197 Head computed tomography cases

Extradural haemorrhage (EDH): axial CT

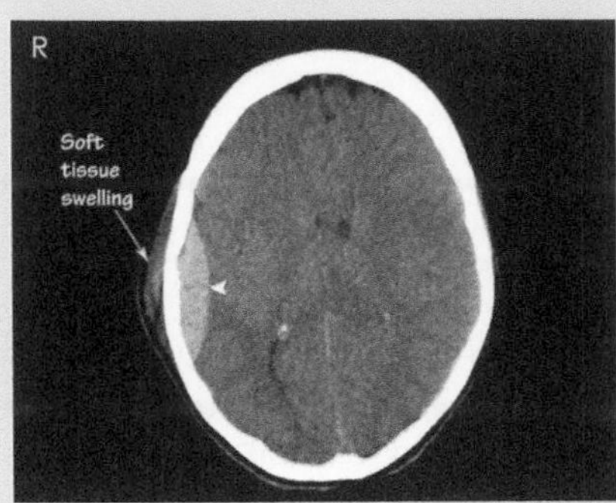

A lens-shaped area of high density is seen within the skull on the right (arrowhead). This is the typical appearance of an extradural haemorrhage which usually arises following injury to the middle meningeal artery. There was an underlying fracture of the temporal bone in this patient seen on bone window settings.

Subdural haematoma (SDH): axial CT

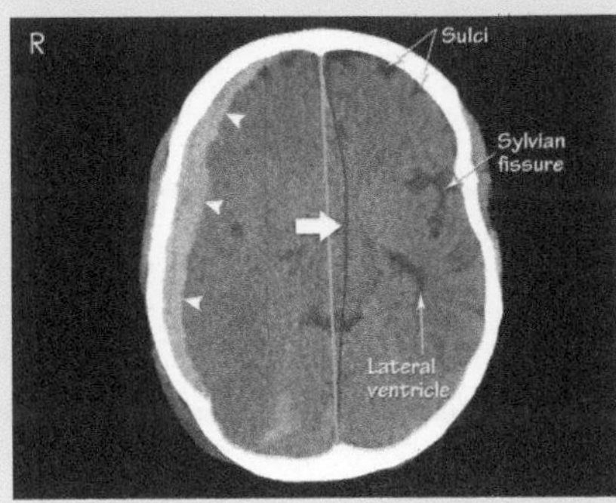

A crescentic rim of high-density material (acute blood) is seen over the surface of the right cerebral hemisphere (arrowheads). There is evidence of mass effect with effacement of the sulci, Sylvian fissure, and lateral ventricle (compare with left), with shift of midline structures (green to red line).

Subarachnoid haemorrhage (SAH): axial CT

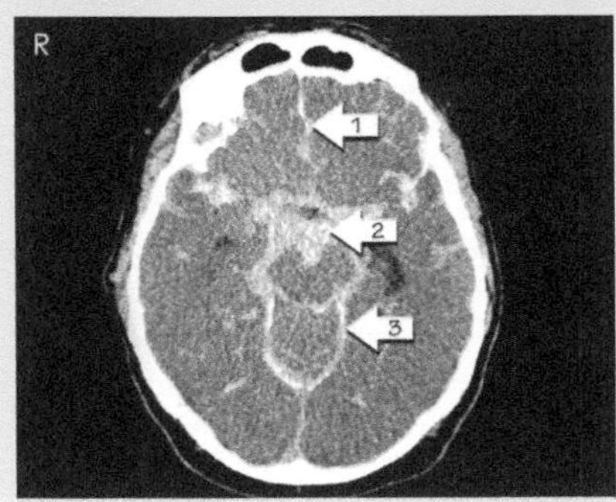

There is widespread high-density material (acute blood) within the subarachnoid space. The blood is seen in the interhemispheric fissure (1), the suprasellar cistern (2), and is layered over the tentorium cerebelli (3). The underlying cause was an aneurysm found on CT angiography.

Intracerebral haemorrhage (ICH): axial CT

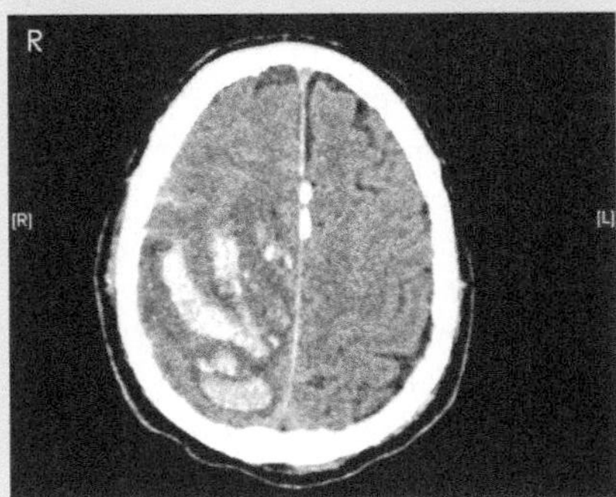

Areas of high density represent acute intracerebral haemorrhage of the right cerebral hemisphere. The high-density areas (blood) are surrounded by low-density areas (oedema). Mass effect is seen with loss of sulci on this side and slight midline shift.

Cerebral infarction: axial CT

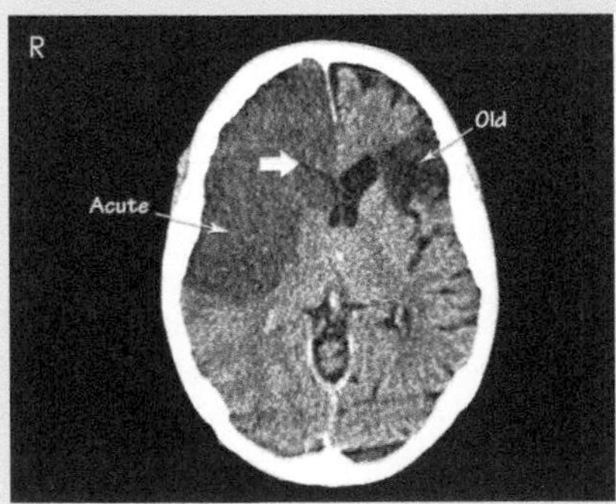

On the right there is a large low-density area indicating an acute infarction of the right middle cerebral artery (MCA) territory. This is causing mass effect with loss of sulci, effacement of the right lateral ventricle anterior horn (arrow) and some midline shift. For comparison an old low-density infarct is seen on the left.

Cerebral tumour: axial CT post-contrast

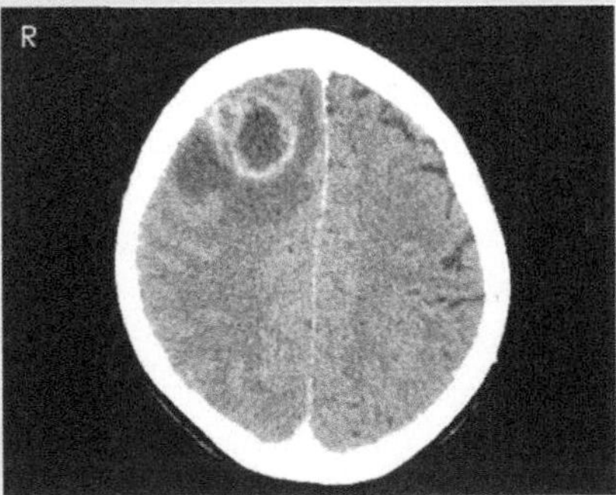

A peripherally enhancing lesion is seen in the right cerebral hemisphere. Note its central low-density area (necrosis) and the surrounding low density (oedema). Mass effect is seen with sulcal effacement on this side and slight deviation of the falx cerebri. Biopsy proved this to be a malignant tumour.

Medicine at a Glance, Fifth Edition. Edited by Patrick Davey and Alex Pitcher.

Companion website: www.wiley.com/go/medicine5e

Intracranial haemorrhage

A head computed tomography (CT) scan is performed without an intravenous (IV) contrast agent to detect acute bleeding. This is because blood is dense and therefore difficult to distinguish from the IV contrast agent. The appearance of a haemorrhage on CT imaging changes with time, and so correlation with the onset of clinical symptoms and signs is essential.

Acute blood is bright but becomes darker over the next few days. After one month, a haematoma becomes the same density as cerebrospinal fluid (CSF).

Extradural haematoma

An extradural haematoma (EDH) is a collection of blood between the skull and dura mater. It is most often due to arterial bleeding following head trauma. The majority are located in the temporoparietal region and are caused by bleeding from the middle meningeal artery secondary to a skull fracture, which is present in up to 90% of cases. CT imaging features of acute EDH include the following.

- Well-demarcated, 'lentiform' (biconvex), high-density extra-axial (outside the brain) collection.
- Rarely crosses suture lines between cranial bones because the dura mater is firmly attached to the skull at the sutures.
- Air within an EDH suggests an open fracture, or a fracture of the paranasal sinuses or mastoid air cells.

Subdural haematoma

A subdural haematoma (SDH) is a collection of extra-axial blood between the dura mater and arachnoid mater. It is most often due to venous bleeding from bridging veins that traverse the subdural space following head trauma and deceleration injuries. It may also be seen in shaken baby syndrome, patients with coagulopathy and in cerebral atrophy (where minimal trauma can cause significant bleeding due to increased tension on the bridging veins). An SDH may lead to raised intracranial pressure and cause displacement of midline structures to the contralateral side. CT imaging features of acute SDH include the following.

- 'Crescentic', high-density, extra-axial collection conforming to the cerebral convexity (although it can become lentiform).
- Crosses suture lines as the collection is subdural.
- Moderate and large SDHs can cause midline shift.
- Falx cerebri appears dense, thickened and irregular with interhemispheric SDH (associated with non-accidental injury in children).

Subarachnoid haemorrhage

A subarachnoic haemorrhage (SAH) is bleeding into the subarachnoid space (the space between the arachnoid mater and pia mater, which contains CSF). It most often occurs spontaneously from a ruptured aneurysm in the circle of Willis and patients typically complain of sudden-onset, extremely severe headache. CT imaging typically reveals high-density blood in the CSF spaces (ventricular system, over cerebral hemispheres, Sylvian fissure, basal cisterns). If SAH is confirmed, a CT angiogram or a conventional cerebral angiogram is performed. If CT imaging is negative but the clinical suspicion is high and there are no contraindications, lumbar puncture can be performed for the detection of xanthochromia.

Intracerebral haemorrhage

Intracerebral haemorrhage (ICH) is bleeding into the brain parenchyma (intra-axial). It is also known as haemorrhagic stroke and is the second most common cause of a cerebrovascular event after ischaemic stroke. CT imaging allows differentiation of a haemorrhagic event from an ischaemic event, which dictates subsequent management of these conditions. The greatest risk factors are hypertension and anticoagulation therapy. Other causes include penetrating trauma, deceleration injuries, rupture of an intracerebral aneurysm or bleeding from an arteriovenous malformation or tumour. Patients usually present with neurological deficit.

Cerebral infarction

Cerebral infarction is caused by a sudden perfusion deficit to an area of the brain, resulting in a corresponding loss of neurological function. This is known as ischaemic stroke, which is the most common cause of a cerebrovascular event. If the neurological deficit lasts less than 24 hours, the event is termed a transient ischaemic attack (TIA). Thromboembolic events are by far the most common cause. Thrombosis most often occurs at cerebral artery branch points and is related to vascular wall damage and hypercoagulable states. Emboli may arise from atherosclerotic plaques of extracranial arteries or thrombus originating from the heart.

CT imaging features of cerebral infarction evolve over time. Within the first three hours of symptom onset, a faint low-density area may be seen affecting a vascular territory of the brain parenchyma. Between six and 12 hours, there is usually sufficient cell swelling (cytotoxic oedema) to produce a CT-identifiable region of low density affecting both the grey and white matter. Subsequent bleeding into the area of infarction may occur from the damaged blood vessels, which causes high density within the low-density infarct. Infarction is often accompanied by oedema, which may cause a mass effect ranging from minor sulcal effacement to shift of midline structures. In the following weeks to months, the infarct is resorbed by macrophages, leaving it appearing as an area of low density (dark) affecting both grey and white matter.

Intracranial tumours

Intracranial tumours may be primary or metastatic. Most are solitary primary tumours arising from the brain parenchyma or other related tissues (vessels, nerves, meninges, pituitary, lymphatics, skull). Metastatic tumours are often multiple and typically from cancers such as lung, breast, melanoma and renal cancers. The clinical presentation of brain tumours varies with their site and size but includes headaches, seizures, focal neurological deficits and signs of raised intracranial pressure (e.g. papilloedema). CT imaging is initially performed without a contrast agent and then with a contrast agent if a space-occupying lesion is suspected radiologically or clinically. Brain tumours usually cause disruption of the blood–brain barrier, resulting in vasogenic oedema from capillary leakage, which spares the grey matter. Most tumours enhance on contrast agent CT imaging and are often surrounded by a halo of low-density subcortical oedema with varying degrees of mass effect.

Classic CT head features

- **Haemorrhage** High density (acute), density drops over few days, CSF density after one month (chronic)
- **Extradural haematoma** 'Lentiform', rarely crosses sutures, usually associated with skull fracture
- **Subdural haematoma** 'Crescentic', usually crosses sutures
- **Subarachnoid haemorrhage** Blood in CSF spaces, e.g. sulci and ventricles
- **Intracranial haemorrhage** Intra-axial/parenchymal blood
- **Infarct** Low density in vascular territory, grey and white matter affected, cytotoxic oedema
- **Tumour** Typically enhancing focal parenchymal lesion, vasogenic oedema

198 Head magnetic resonance imaging cases

Sagittal brain MRI : T_1 (left) and T_2 (right)

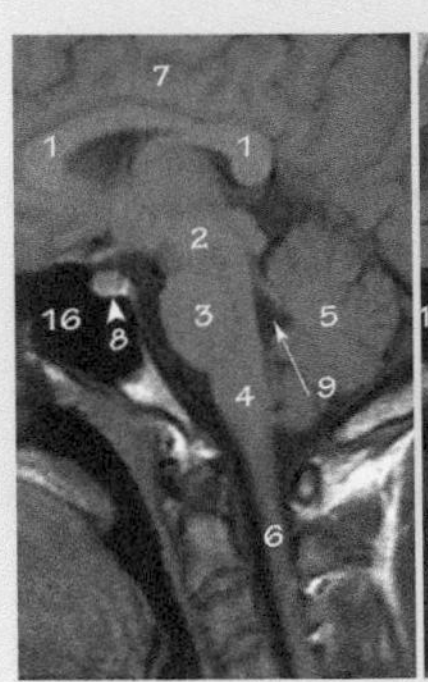

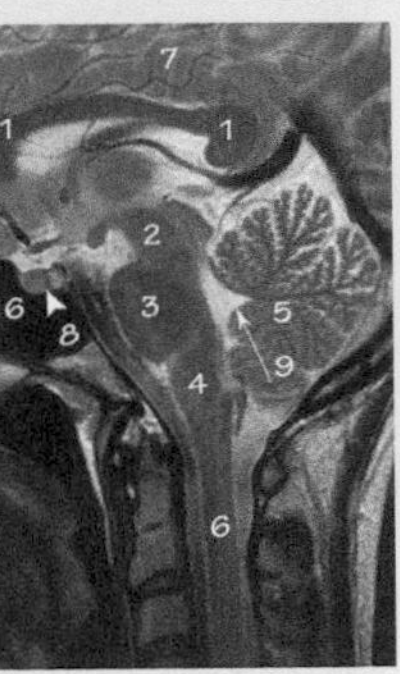

Axial brain MRI: T_2 at level of lateral ventricles (left) and T_2 at level of cerebellum (right)

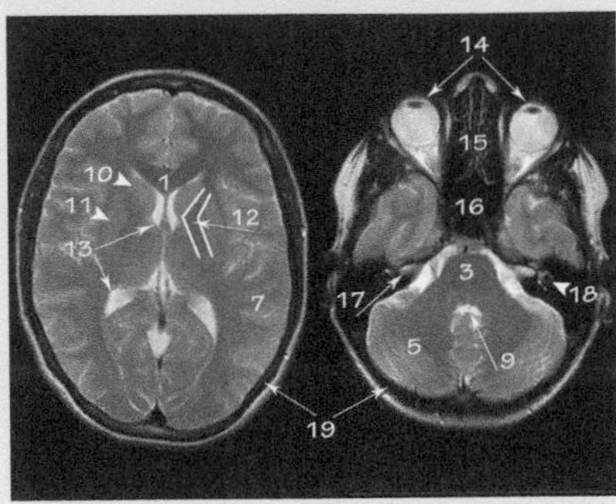

Key

1 Corpus callosum
2 Midbrain
3 Pons
4 Medulla oblongata
5 Cerebellum
6 Spinal cord
7 Cerebrum
8 Pituitary gland
9 Fourth ventricle
10 Caudate nucleus
11 Lentiform nucleus
12 Internal capsule
13 Lateral ventricle
14 Eyes
15 Ethmoid air cells
16 Sphenoid sinus
17 Internal auditory meatus
18 Cochlea
19 Skull

Multiple sclerosis: axial T_2 at level above lateral ventricles

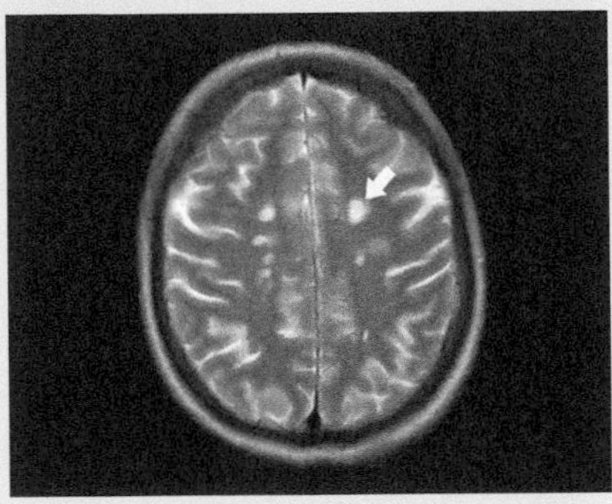

Bilateral foci of high signal (arrow) are present within the white matter which should be dark on T_2. These lesions lie immediately above and to the side of the lateral ventricles. The periventricular white matter is a typical location for multiple sclerosis lesions.

Cerebral infarction: DWI (left) and ADC (right)

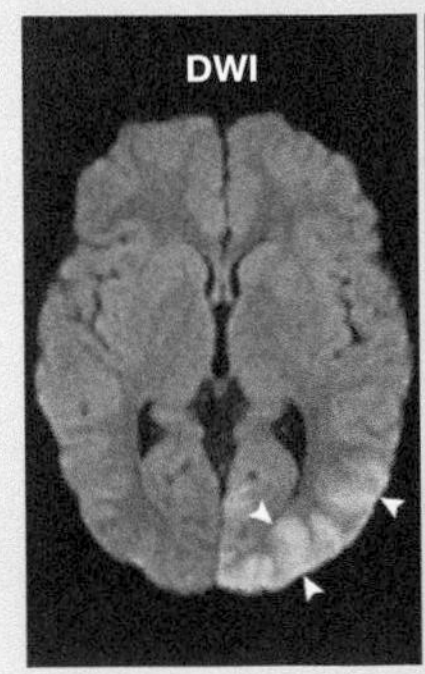

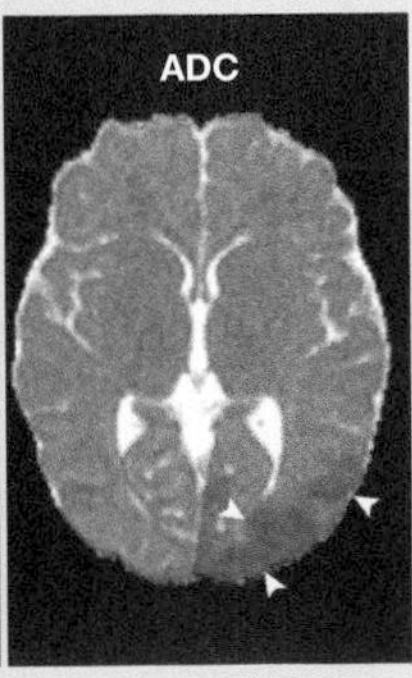

The DWI shows bright signal (arrowheads) in the distribution of the left posterior cerebral artery. The ADC image shows this area as low signal and therefore it is not due to T_2 signal (note the bright ventricles). This is evidence of restricted diffusion which is a sign of infarction. DWI is the most sensitive investigation for acute cerebral infarction.

Pituitary tumour: sagittal T_1 images pre- and post-gadolinium injection

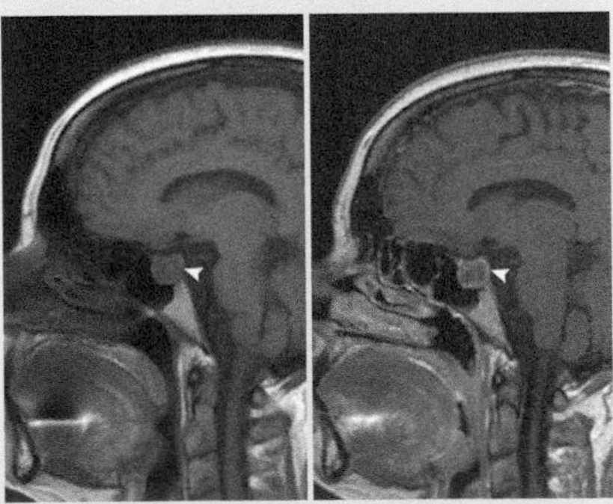

This patient presented with headaches and visual field disturbance (bitemporal hemianopia). The pre-contrast image (left) shows a pituitary adenoma (arrowhead) which demonstrates abnormal enhancement on the post-contrast scan (right). This is classified as a macroadenoma (>1 cm). The bigger a pituitary lesion becomes the more likely it is to cause visual disturbance due to compression of the optic chiasm which lies immediately above the pituitary gland.

Medicine at a Glance, Fifth Edition. Edited by Patrick Davey and Alex Pitcher.

Companion website: www.wiley.com/go/medicine5e

The neuroanatomy seen on magnetic resonance imaging (MRI) is similar to that seen on computer tomography (CT) imaging (see Chapter 197). However, MRI allows visualization of structures with greater differentiation and detail even without the use of contrast agent enhancement. The MRI series of the brain are viewed in a similar format to CT images (axial, sagittal and coronal planes). MRI also has the advantage of viewing the brainstem without the significant artefact limitations of CT images. The standard MRI investigation of the brain includes T1-weighted, T2-weighted, proton density (PD)-weighted and fluid-attenuated inversion recovery (FLAIR) sequences. T1-weighted images with gadolinium enhancement may also be acquired. Each of these acquisition sequences demonstrates different patterns of tissue signal characteristics, which commonly form the basis of interpretation and diagnosis.

- **T1-weighted acquisition sequences**: the signal intensity on T1-weighted acquisitions depends on the fat content of the tissues in question. Subcutaneous fat appears very bright and the myelin sheaths of white matter appear brighter than grey matter. Cerebrospinal fluid (CSF) and pathological fluid appear dark. T1-weighted images are best at defining anatomy due to their excellent spatial resolution. In the brain, however, they are also useful in conjunction with T2-weighted images to distinguish blood from other pathology, estimate the age of a haemorrhage and differentiate fatty lesions from other pathology.
- **T2-weighted acquisition sequences**: the signal intensity on T2-weighted acquisitions depends on the water content of the tissues in question. CSF is very bright and can be easily identified within the different components of the ventricular system and subarachnoid space. Fat is darker than on T1-weighted acquisitions, so white matter appears darker than grey matter. T2-weighted images are often the best sequence for evaluating pathology. This is because pathological lesions often contain water and are therefore bright and easily seen on T2. This is true for infective processes, tumours and inflammatory conditions such as multiple sclerosis, which typically reveals bright plaques on T2-weighted images.
- **PD acquisition sequences**: this sequence is acquired at the same time as the T2 sequence. The signal intensity on PD-weighted acquisitions depends on the number of protons per unit tissue. Tissues with a high number of protons are bright (e.g. CSF) and those with a low number of protons are dark. PD sequences are often helpful, but pathological fluid is usually more easily differentiated from other structures on different sequences, such as FLAIR.
- **FLAIR acquisition sequences**: these are similar to $T2_2$ except the bright signal from CSF is suppressed. This allows clearer evaluation of T2 bright lesions, especially those near CSF-filled spaces (e.g. white matter plaque adjacent to the ventricular system).

Intracranial haemorrhage

Intracranial haemorrhage may be diagnosed and evaluated by MRI. MRI is superior to CT imaging for detecting haemorrhage in the subacute and chronic phases. However, CT imaging remains the preferred modality in the acute setting because it is much faster. The signal intensity of haemorrhage changes with time on both T1- and T2-weighted sequences. This is because the breakdown products of blood clots induce various artefacts. Initially, artefact is due to the presence of oxygenated haemoglobin, which is dark on T1 and bright on T2. After several hours, deoxyhaemoglobin is predominant and this is dark on both T1 and T2. After approximately three days, there is an increasing amount of intracellular methaemoglobin, which is bright on T1 but dark on T2, and then free methaemoglobin which is bright on both. Eventually, over months, methaemoglobin is exchanged for haemosiderin, which is dark on both sequences.

In order to accurately direct management, the timing of any haemorrhagic event should be established from the history.

Cerebral infarction and diffusion-weighted MRI

When there is a sudden perfusion deficit to the brain, the glial cells undergo ischaemic change, which causes malfunction of their cell membrane sodium pump. This results in an influx of sodium and water into cells, and restricted diffusion of intracellular water molecules out of the cells by the cell membranes. The net effect is cell swelling, known as cytotoxic oedema.

Diffusion-weighted imaging (DWI), a specialized form of MRI, makes use of the Brownian motion of water molecules in the brain to generate a signal. Therefore, a high magnitude of molecular diffusion generates a high-intensity signal. While classic Brownian motion refers to free movement of molecules, there is restricted movement in biological tissues due to tissue architecture (e.g. cell membranes) and therefore water diffusion is referred to as apparent diffusion. This phenomenon is represented by an image map of the apparent diffusion coefficient (ADC), whereby restricted diffusion generates a low-intensity signal. In the acute ischaemic setting, the restricted diffusion causing cytotoxic oedema results in a low ADC and high DWI signal intensity. This method of diagnostic imaging is very helpful to distinguish acute infarction from old established infarcts.

Intracranial tumours

Magnetic resonance imaging is more sensitive and specific than CT in detecting and evaluating brain tumours. Intracranial tumours such as meningioma, ependymoma, astrocytoma and metastases are appreciated as being isointense or low signal intensity on T1-weighted images and high signal intensity on T2-weighted images, with high signal secondary to the surrounding vasogenic oedema. Imaging after injection of gadolinium is a mainstay of imaging intracranial tumours with MRI as most brain tumours cause disruption of the blood–brain barrier and readily take up the contrast agent.

199 Stroke

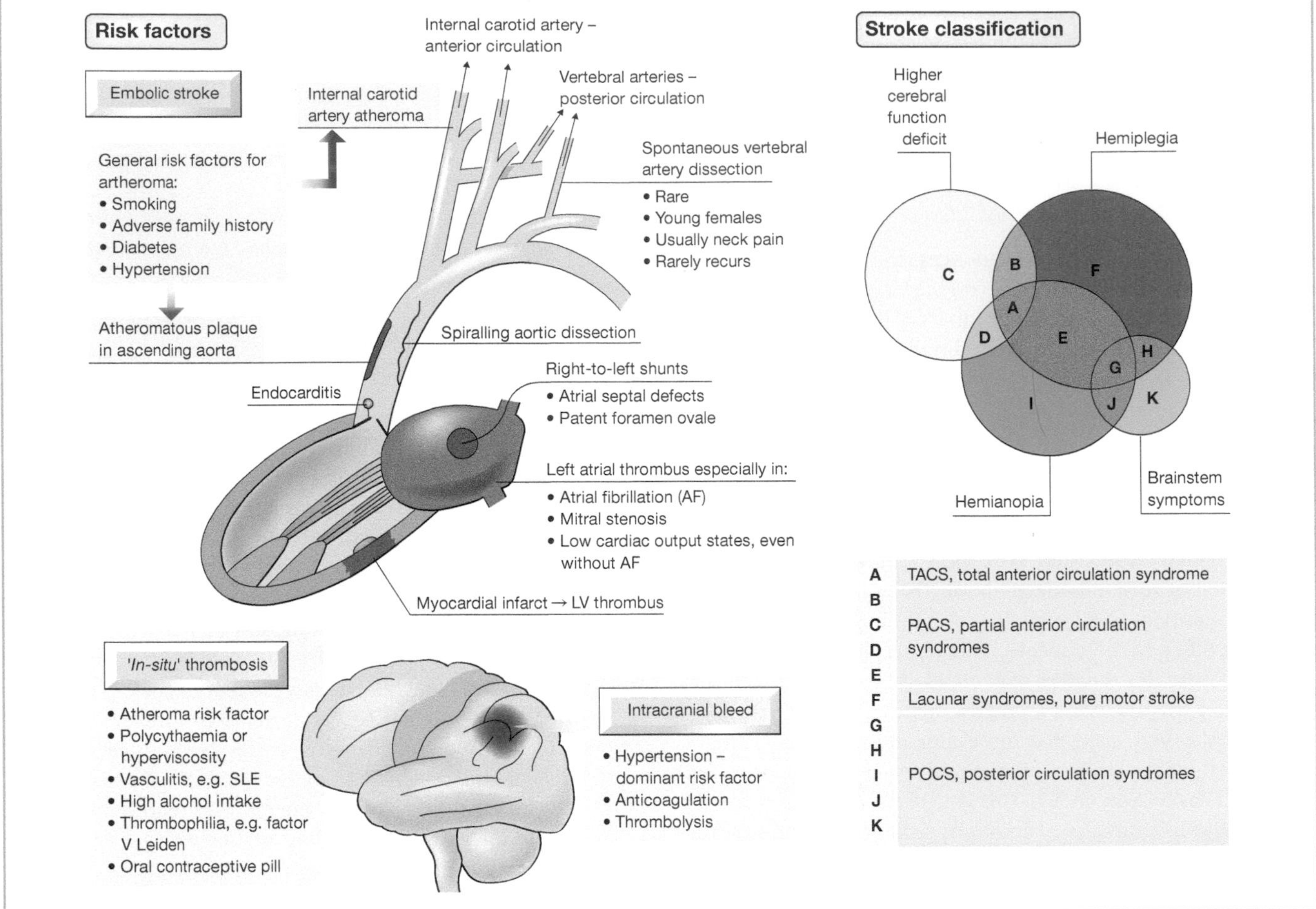

Stroke is the most common condition affecting the brain, with approximately 150 000 new strokes per year in the UK. The burden of mortality and morbidity is high: 30% of people with acute stroke die, 25% are rendered severely disabled.

Key features

Neurological symptoms resulting from cerebrovascular disease are:

- **of sudden onset**: very occasionally, other neurological diseases present suddenly, e.g. brain tumours, demyelination and hypoglycaemia. Evolving neurological signs are not usually the result of vascular pathology, although occasionally major vessel occlusion (e.g. internal carotid artery) presents as a stuttering stroke
- **focal**: referable to a specific anatomical site and associated with loss of function
- **usually vaso-occlusive**, either thromboembolic (emboli from the heart in 20% of cases or from atheromatous plaques in the aorta, extra- or intracranial circulation in the remaining 80%), leading to major vessel occlusion, or *in situ* vascular blockage, usually small vessel and leading to lacunar syndromes
- **occasionally caused by haemorrhage** (10% of all strokes), which should be considered in those with marked hypertension, on anticoagulants or presenting with prominent headache.

There are a small number of very common stroke syndromes and a very large number of rare stroke syndromes.

Time course of strokes

- **Transient ischaemic attacks** (TIAs) by definition can last up to 24 hours although usually they last less than a few minutes. TIAs can affect all vascular territories, causing any pattern of neurological dysfunction. The most characteristic is amaurosis fugax, where embolic atherogenic debris from the carotid artery travels to the ophthalmic branch of the internal carotid, causing unilateral blindness, lasting less than a few minutes.
- **Significance**: TIAs imply an active intravascular plaque, i.e. one on which thrombosis is actively occurring and embolizing distally. They are a major risk factor for subsequent disabling stroke; 50% of strokes occurring after a TIA do so within a week, so preventing these strokes is a medical emergency.

Medicine at a Glance, Fifth Edition. Edited by Patrick Davey and Alex Pitcher.

Companion website: www.wiley.com/go/medicine5e

- **Investigation**: urgent investigation (carotid ultrasonography and magnetic resonance angiography) to determine whether a high-grade lesion (i.e. >70% stenosis in the symptomatic internal carotid artery) is present should be undertaken because surgical resection (carotid endarterectomy) significantly reduces the rate of disabling stroke.
- **Minor strokes** have small neurological deficits. Their importance is the same as TIAs – they may be a harbinger of more severe strokes. Sufferers have established vascular disease and need vigorous antiatherogenic therapy.
- **Completed stroke** implies that the deficit is major, persistent and does not subsequently deteriorate. Unless recovery is good, 'the horse has bolted' and investigations as a prelude to carotid endarterectomy are not indicated.

Anatomy of strokes

An important distinction is between stroke in the anterior (carotid) or the posterior (vertebrobasilar) circulation, because this relates to prognosis (see Table 199.1) and determines the nature of the investigations. Constitutional differences in the cerebral circulation, and the effects of diffuse atheroma on the circle of Willis, mean that it is not always possible to give an accurate clinical determination of the site of occlusion.

Anatomy of stroke 'syndromes'

Carotid territory stroke

Carotid territory stroke presents with a combination of hemiplegia and language dysfunction (dominant hemisphere) or dyspraxia (inability to carry out complex tasks not caused by motor deficits) or denial of the existence (neglect) of the left side (non-dominant hemisphere). Middle cerebral artery (MCA) occlusion has in addition hemianaesthesia and hemianopia (total anterior circulation syndrome [TACS]). An MCA infarct is often large and extensive brain damage may occur, resulting in coma and even death. Recovery is often very poor. Partial anterior circulation presents with a less extensive motor deficit and not all elements of TACS.

Vertebrobasilar (posterior circulation) stroke

There are many eponymous brainstem vascular syndromes of dubious relevance. The combination of any of the following with sudden onset suggests a posterior circulation stroke.

- Diplopia.
- Dysarthria.
- Unsteadiness.
- Dysphagia.
- Unilateral weakness with contralateral facial weakness.
- Bilateral visual loss.
- Amnesia.

Posterior strokes, unlike anterior circulation ones, may have a stuttering evolution. Basilar artery occlusion is frequently catastrophic and fatal. Pontine strokes cause coma, pinpoint pupils, paresis, pyrexia and frequently death.

Lacunar syndromes

Lacunar syndromes are by definition small (<1.5 cm^3). They may cause internal capsule strokes, which are usually either pure motor or pure sensory. Neither of these has an ocular field defect. Recovery is typically more complete than in MCA occlusive syndromes.

Summary of causes of hemiplegia

(see Chapter 59)

- **MCA cortical infarct** (hemiplegia + hemianaesthesia + hemianopia): haemorrhage into the internal capsule produces a similar triad of signs. Alteration of consciousness is common.
- **Internal capsule lesions**: usually produce rather discrete neurological deficits, such as a 'pure' motor hemiplegia/monoplegia or 'pure' sensory hemianaesthesia.
- **Basis pontis**: dysarthria but not dysphasia may occur, i.e. clumsy hand–dysarthria syndrome.
- **Brainstem lesions**: associated with nystagmus, ocular palsies and cerebellar signs.

Table 199.1 Stroke prognosis (%).

	TAC	PAC	LAC	POC
Thirty days				
Dead	40	5	5	5
Dependent	55	40	30	30
Independent	5	55	65	65
One year				
Dead	60	15	10	20
Dependent	35	30	30	20
Independent	5	55	60	60

LAC, lacunar infarction; PAC, partial anterior circulation; POC, posterior circulation; TAC, total anterior circulation.

Risk factors for stroke

These are as for arterial disease, i.e. increasing age, male sex, family history of vascular disease, hypertension, smoking and diabetes. Structural heart disease predisposes to stroke, especially recent myocardial infarction (MI) (±1% of patients have a stroke during an MI) or atrial fibrillation (especially in those >65 years or with left ventricular [LV] dysfunction). Excess alcohol is a substantial risk factor, particularly in young men. Polycythaemia underlies a few strokes. It has not been established that high cholesterol is a strong primary risk factor for stroke, though lowering cholesterol does appear to reduce the risk of first stroke in trials and it is an important measure in secondary prevention. Neurosyphilis is now very rare, but 45% of cases present as a stroke. For intracerebral haemorrhage, the strongest risk factor is hypertension or vascular abnormality, e.g. arteriovenous malformation or aneurysm, a bleeding diathesis or thrombolytic therapy.

'Young stroke'

Most people aged under 40 years who have had a stroke have the same risk factors as older patients. Consider also:

- Infective endocarditis.
- Antiphospholipid syndrome.
- Paradoxical embolism through a patent foramen ovale.
- Cerebral vasculitis (including systemic lupus erythematosus).
- Carotid/vertebral/aortic dissection.
- Mitochondrial diseases such as MELAS (mitochondrial encephalopathy, lactic acidosis, stroke-like episodes).
- Inherited thrombophilias, such as protein C and S deficiency, usually produce venous thrombosis in the deep veins of the calf, but occasionally cause stroke, particularly venous sinus thrombosis.
- Structural abnormalities of the extracranial vessels (e.g. moya moya disease, angiographic diagnosis of bilateral distal occlusion/multiple stenosis of the internal carotid artery, with net-like collaterals around the brain base).
- Drug induced, e.g. cocaine.

Management of stroke

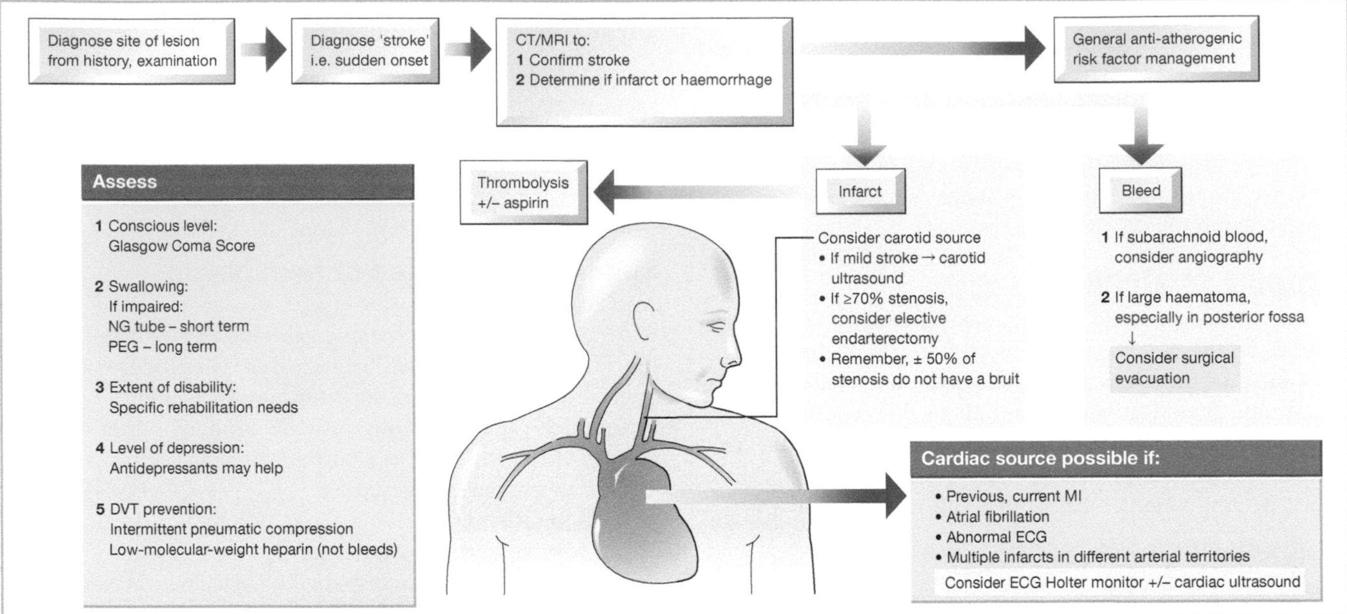

The mechanism of stroke (infarct or bleed) must be determined by computed tomography (CT) or magnetic resonance imaging (MRI).

- **Infarct**: the origin of thrombus must be worked out, i.e. from *in situ* thrombosis or emboli originating more proximally, either from the heart or atheromatous plaques in:
  - the carotid artery, which are diagnosed by ultrasonography
  - the aortic arch found by transoesophageal echocardiography; management is unclear.
- **Haemorrhage**: if the clinical condition of the patient is not poor, and especially if there is any suggestion that the bleed is the result of a subarachnoid haemorrhage, it may be appropriate to undertake angiography (conventional or magnetic resonance) to exclude an aneurysm/arteriovenous malformation that might benefit from surgery/intervention.

Acute management

A realistic assessment of prognosis should be sympathetically communicated to relatives. Patients should, if possible, be nursed in dedicated stroke units because these improve outcome.

Cerebral infarcts

- Blood pressure in the long term should be low, but should not be decreased acutely because this may provoke watershed infarcts.
- Aspirin (300 mg, then 75–100 mg per day) and other antiplatelet agents are used to decrease the incidence of further strokes. Current evidence suggests that disability is reduced if thrombolysis (recombinant tissue plasminogen activator) is given <4.5 hours from symptom onset. Thrombectomy can be beneficial for large vessel occlusion.

Intracerebral haemorrhage

- Blood pressure should probably be lowered more rapidly in cerebral haemorrhage.
- Posterior fossa bleeds may need neurosurgical evacuation to prevent coning of the brain. Likewise, large intracerebral bleeds with mass effects in young people may benefit from evacuation.

All strokes

- Swallowing dysfunction should be assessed. If the risk of aspiration is not low, feeding should be by nasogastric (NG) tube or, in the longer term, by percutaneous endoscopic gastrostomy (PEG) feeding tube.
- Prevention of deep venous thrombosis (DVT): using intermittent pneumatic compression or possibly low-dose heparin (not cerebral bleeds).
- Good nursing care is the most important factor in outcome.
- Physiotherapy to prevent contractures and help in mobilization.
- Depression occurs in 50–75% of patients. Antidepressants may help.

Long-term management (see Table 200.1)

- **General vascular risk protection**: the annual stroke recurrence rate of 10% is reduced by meticulous control of vascular risk factors (secondary prevention), especially smoking, diabetes and blood pressure (aim for ≤140/85). Cholesterol reduction reduces the rate of further strokes, and statins are indicated for most patients with ischaemic stroke for secondary prevention.
- **Carotid endarterectomy**: most patients ≤75 years with small anterior circulation stroke syndromes should have carotid imaging. Those with high-grade lesions (≥70% stenosis) may benefit from carotid endarterectomy.
- **Anticoagulation**: in patients with atrial fibrillation, long-term treatment with warfarin or novel oral anticoagulants is more effective than antiplatelets for prevention of further strokes.
- **Management and prevention of disability**: after a first stroke, 25–50% do not re-achieve independence and require extensive nursing support. Financial and physical aids help.
- **Multidisciplinary management of home environment** can restore independence.

Table 200.1 The management of stroke.

Problem	Frequency	Importance	Preventive measures	Interventions for established problem
Fever	Common	Associated with worse outcome	Routine antipyretics	Fanning, antipyretics, treat underlying cause
Low Po_2	Common	↑ Brain ischaemia	Positioning to avoid cardiorespiratory problems	Supplementary O_2
Low BP	Uncommon – may reflect dehydration	May ↑ brain ischaemia	Avoid cause	Treat cause
High BP	Very common	May reflect long-standing ↑ BP, or reaction to CVA; may ↑ brain oedema/bleeding		BP lowering – but these may ↑ brain ischaemia – often required pre-thrombolysis
↑ Blood glucose	20–40%	Associated with ↓ outcome	Avoid dextrose infusions	Insulin
↑ Intracranial pressure (ICP)	↓ Consciousness in most CVAs reflects ↑ ICP	Most common cause of death ≤1 week	Raising end of bed; avoid overhydration	Anti-oedema drugs, ventilation, decompressive surgery
Sleep disordered breathing	65% of patients	Unknown	Avoid sedatives	Continuous positive airway pressure
Dysphagia	50% of patients	Prevents feeding; increases risk of chest infection	Routine screening (speech and language therapy – SALT)	Nil by mouth, parenteral or enteral feeding
Epileptic seizures	5% of patients	Leads to neurological deterioration	None	Anticonvulsants
Spasticity and contractures	Depends on preventive measures	Limits function and predisposes to bed sores	Positioning, relief muscle tone (anxiety, pain, overuse)	Physiotherapy, splinting, tone-modifying drugs, botulinum toxin
Emotionalism	20%	Interrupts therapy, social isolation		Antidepressants
Urinary infection	25% in first month	Unwell → ↓ functional level	Maintain hydration, avoid catheters	Antibiotics, fluids
Chest infection	25% in first month	↓ Po_2; → ↓ functional level	Early mobilization, chest physiotherapy, SALT	Antibiotics, chest physiotherapy
Undernutrition	20%	Associated with worse outcome	Nutritional screening; oral supplementation	Oral supplementation, enteral tube feeding
Electrolyte imbalance	Common	May → confusion, seizures	Monitor biochemistry	Supplements, etc.
Deep venous thrombosis (DVT)	50%	May progress to lethal PE; pain, fever	Early mobilization, good hydration, antiplatelet drugs, intermittent pneumatic compression	Anticoagulation
Pulmonary embolism (PE)	5%	May → death	As above	As above
Urinary and/or faecal incontinence	50%	Demeaning, bed sores	Avoid exacerbating factors, e.g. diuretics	Treat cause if found; bladder retraining, pads, catheters
Pressure sores	<3% with good nursing	Painful, distressing, can → death	Good nursing	Relieve pressure, antibiotics, vitamins
Falls and fractures	Falls common in 35%; fractures rare	Pain, ↓ functional level	Careful supervision; anti-osteoporosis drugs	Standard orthopaedic care for fractures
Painful shoulder	Common	↓ Function and mood	Avoid traction injury	Physiotherapy, analgesics, local steroid injections
Low mood	Very common	Associated with worse outcome	Positive attitude in stroke unit staff	Antidepressants, cognitive behavioural therapy

BP, blood pressure; CVA, cerebrovascular accident.

201 Other vascular disorders of the brain

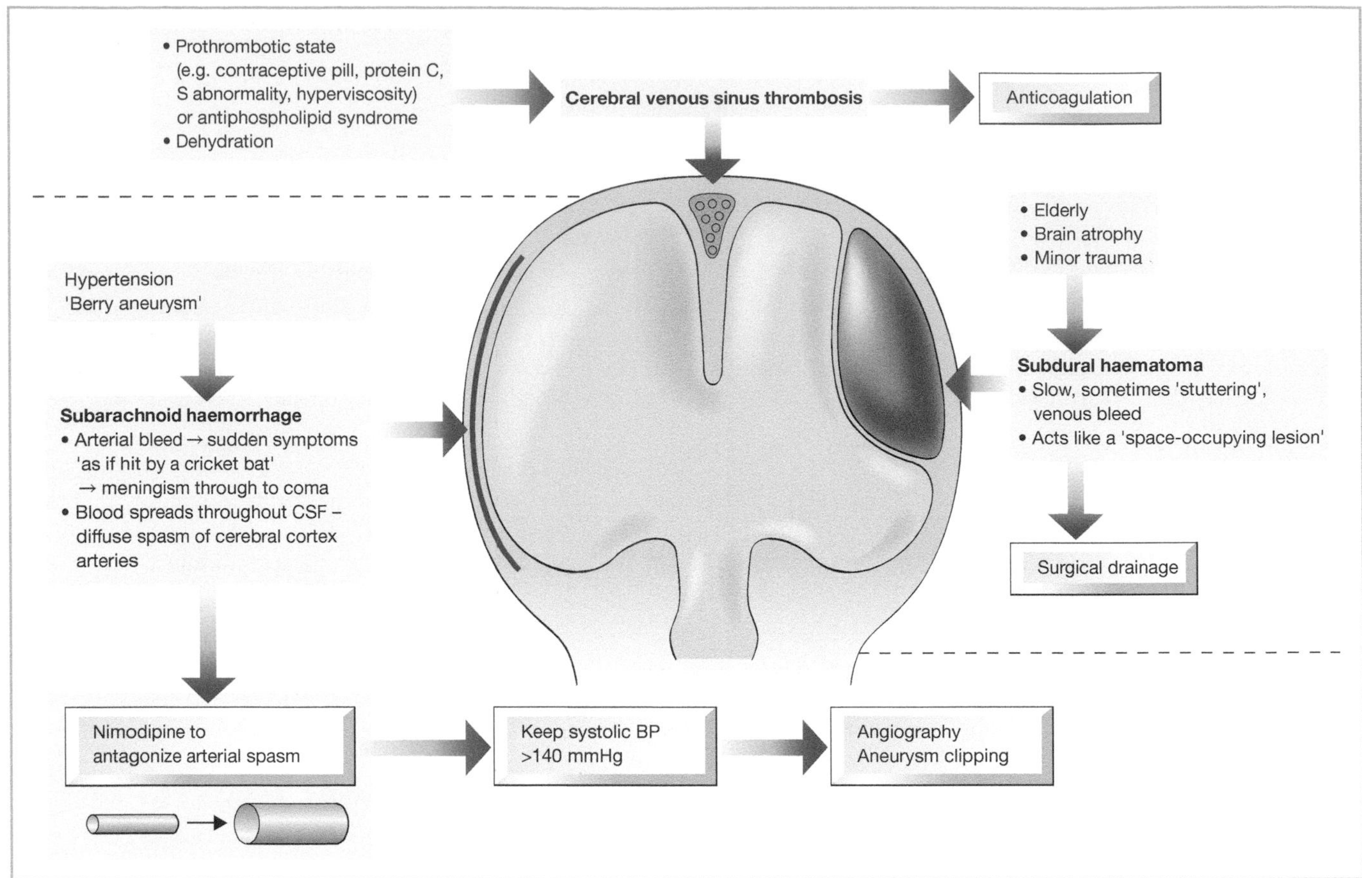

Subarachnoid haemorrhage

Subarachnoid haemorrhage (SAH) is an arterial bleed from a ruptured berry aneurysm (70% of cases) or arteriovenous malformation (10% of cases). There are 3000 cases per year in the UK.

Clinical features and diagnosis

Classic presentation is with a thunderclap headache, often in the occiput. The signs range from none (headache only), through mild meningism to coma. Focal neurological signs are uncommon. Thirty percent of patients die of the acute bleed: if a rebleed occurs, the mortality rate is ≥60%. A computed tomography (CT) scan should be performed in all suspected cases of SAH. If this is not diagnostic then a delayed (≥12 h after symptom onset) lumbar puncture, looking for xanthochromia (bilirubin on spectrophotometry), should be undertaken.

Treatment

Acutely, hypotension should be avoided (with intravenous fluids/inotropes if blood pressure [BP] is too low), although more chronically BP should be lowered to <140/85. Subarachnoid blood induces damaging cerebral artery spasm, which can be antagonized by nimodipine to improve outcome. The responsible aneurysms can be detected by angiography and treated by endovascular occlusion with platinum coils or by surgical clipping (open craniotomy) if not accessible by the endovascular route.

Prognosis

Prognosis is poor once coma or a major neurological defect has developed – intervention should therefore occur early on. Overall, <40% of cases have a good outcome.

The prevalence of an unruptured intracranial aneurysm on magnetic resonance imaging (MRI) is about 2% and the overall risk of rupture is about 1% per year. The decision whether to treat these asymptomatic lesions is complex and based on size and location.

Subdural haemorrhage

Subdural haemorrhage is a venous bleed, often occurring in the context of brain shrinkage (from age, dementia, chronic alcoholism, etc.). Blood slowly oozes into the subdural space. As this

Medicine at a Glance, Fifth Edition. Edited by Patrick Davey and Alex Pitcher.

Companion website: www.wiley.com/go/medicine5e

breaks down, osmotically active degradation products are formed, sucking in fluid from the extracellular space. Thus subdural haemorrhages act as space-occupying lesions, expanding slowly over several weeks. Clinically, there may be a history of trauma, although this is often absent. Subsequently, there is the slow (a few weeks or more) progression of a focal neurological deficit; equally, elderly patients may present rather non-specifically with decreased mobility ('off legs') or decreased mental agility. Focal neurological signs are not invariably present. CT scanning is diagnostic, although a diagnostic trap for the unwary is that 'old' blood (i.e. of the age found in many subdural haemorrhages) may be isodense with the brain.

Surgical evacuation should be considered in all affected patients, however elderly.

Venous sinus thrombosis

Cerebral venous sinus thrombosis is a life-threatening condition with an extremely broad range of clinical neurological presentations and a large differential diagnosis.

Demographics

Cerebral vein thrombosis is a rare event, there being estimated to be only some 250–500 cases/year in the UK (60 in peri-/postpartum women). Seventy-five percent of patients are female and younger ages predominate.

Clinical features

Cerebral vein thrombosis must be considered in acute or subacute headache, seizures and disorders of consciousness or papilloedema. The condition can mimic stroke, abscess, tumour, encephalitis or idiopathic intracranial hypertension. The presenting symptoms depend on which vein is occluded. The pathophysiology can be traced to one of the following two causes.

1 Due to local cerebral vein occlusion leading to local effects – so producing focal signs (e.g. cortical signs – weakness, etc.) or from deep structures (e.g. dysfunction of the thalamus produces confusion, amnesia, mutism; brainstem dysfunction leads to coma). Occlusion of small cortical veins leads to venous infarction which is highly epileptogenic and may present with seizures.

2 Due to occlusion of cerebral sinuses, leading to intracranial hypertension (so producing headache, found in 90%; the only symptom in 20%; while 80% have focal defects).

Aetiology

There is a wide range of underlying aetiologies, including inherited thrombophilias, oral contraception, pregnancy, local intracranial sepsis and systemic inflammatory diseases, such as sarcoidosis and Behçet disease. It occurs very rarely following lumbar puncture. A predisposing illness is found in 85% of patients. Very rarely, cerebral vein thrombosis occurs following COVID vaccination, sometimes as a complication of vaccine-induced thrombotic thrombocytopenia (VITT).

Diagnosis

The diagnosis can usually be reliably made with MRI with contrast angiography, which shows the thrombus and the venous infarct which, in 40%, can undergo haemorrhagic transformation.

Treatment

Treatment with heparin may improve survival and disability, and patients who continue to deteriorate may be suitable for local thrombolysis. If the intracranial pressure is high, mannitol ± acetazolamide are sometimes used. Surgical removal of the brain infarct has been recommended by some for high intracranial pressures with deteriorating neurological condition.

202 Dementias

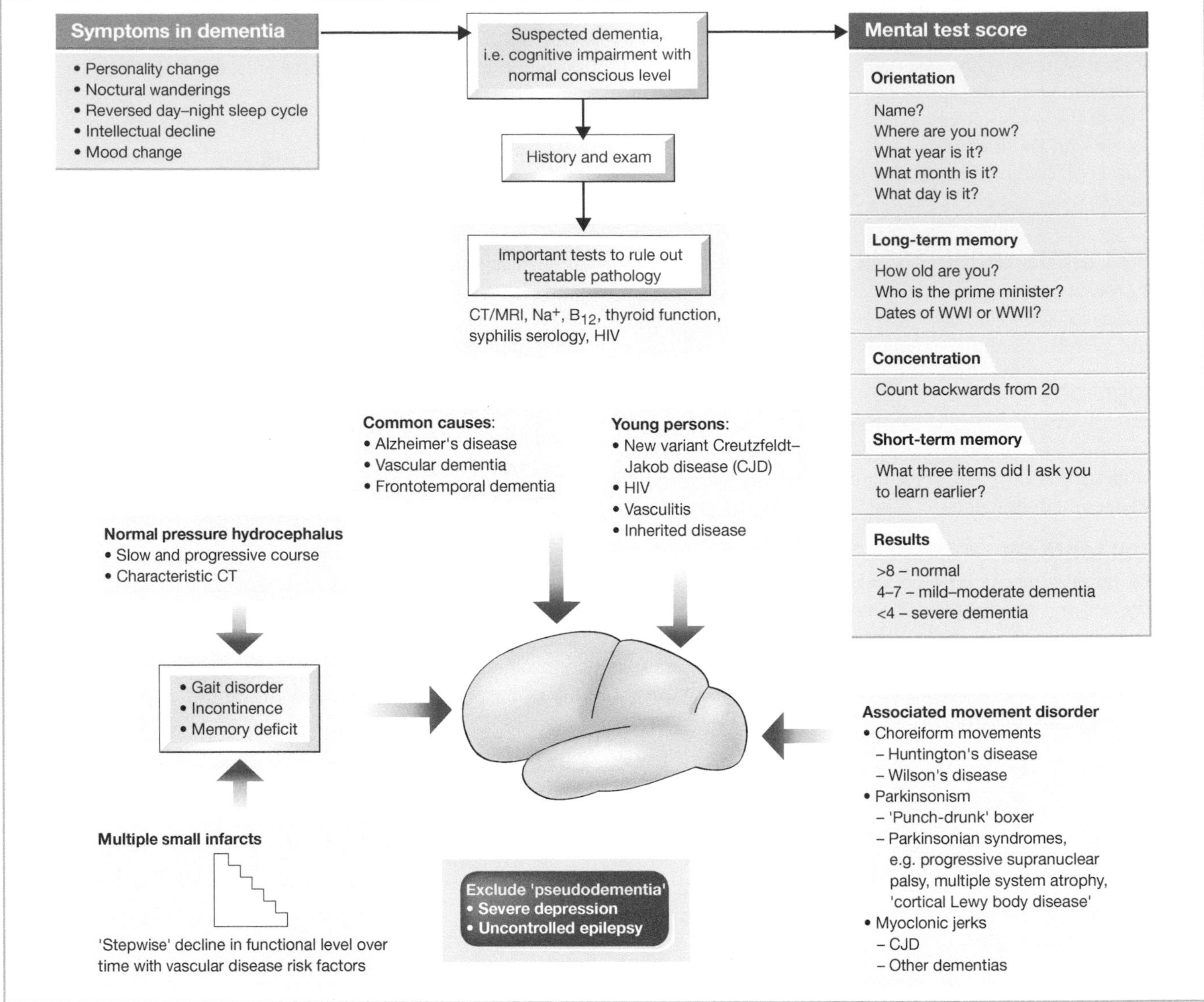

Dementia is 'the global impairment of cognition with normal levels of consciousness', in contrast to an acute confusional state, in which conscious level is impaired. The incidence is 5% in those aged ≥65 years and 20% in those aged ≥85 years. With emerging therapies, it is important to attempt a specific diagnosis, although this is not easy because clinical tools are not accurate. Many people labelled as having Alzheimer disease have a different postmortem diagnosis. Patients who complain of memory disturbance are far more likely to be suffering from anxiety, because those with genuine dementia usually have no insight. Potentially treatable causes of cognitive impairment include the following.

- Depression: all patients with dementia should have a mental state examination to exclude depressive pseudodementia. However, it should be remembered that depressive symptomatology is a feature of all dementias.
- Normal pressure hydrocephalus may be the result of a diffuse abnormality affecting cerebrospinal fluid uptake; it causes ventricular dilation, and is suggested by the triad of dementia, incontinence and gait disturbance. Therapeutic lumbar puncture can lead to overt improvement and is used to select patients suitable for shunting.
- Subdural haematoma may present without any antecedent history of trauma as a subacute change in cognitive function with gait disturbance.
- Intracranial tumours are a common cause of subacute cognitive decline. Focal symptoms/signs are usually present.
- Hypothyroidism may produce mild to moderate cognitive impairment.

Medicine at a Glance, Fifth Edition. Edited by Patrick Davey and Alex Pitcher.

Companion website: www.wiley.com/go/medicine5e

- Chronic severe hyponatraemia.
- Vitamin B_{12} deficiency.
- HIV.
- Neurosyphilis or general paralysis of the insane.
- Vasculitis.
- Paraneoplastic syndromes (see Chapter 195) rarely cause pure dementia, e.g. tumour-associated limbic encephalitis can present with personality changes.
- Autoimmune encephalopathy due to antivoltage-gated potassium channel antibodies.
- Whipple disease is associated with cognitive impairment, which may improve with antibiotics.

All patients should therefore have computed tomography (CT) head scans, and vitamin B_{12}, thyroid function, HIV and syphilis serology checked, as well as a full blood count, biochemical tests of renal and hepatic function and an erythrocyte sedimentation rate to look for systemic diseases producing cognitive impairment.

Alzheimer disease

Alzheimer disease begins most frequently with gradual impairment of episodic memory, but eventually produces global cognitive decline, i.e. early on, new memory cannot be laid down, although childhood memories remain accessible. Later on, no memory can be recalled. Although it may be normal early in the disease, volumetric magnetic resonance imaging (MRI) shows specific atrophy of the temporal lobes. Of the cases of Alzheimer disease, 5% are familial and usually of earlier onset. Mutations have been identified in the *Presenilin 1* and *2* genes and in the amyloid precursor protein gene (*APP*). Certain apolipoprotein E polymorphisms, specifically ε4, predispose to Alzheimer disease.

- **Pathologically** there is cortical neuron loss, including loss of cholinergic neurons. These form the basis of the usage of acetylcholinesterase inhibitors, which have small but definite beneficial effects.
- **Outlook**: the disease progresses relentlessly, causing death from pneumonia or inanition after 8–10 years. The key to management is to care for the sufferer on a 'symptom-by-symptom' basis and to provide good support and relief for the caregiver.

Frontotemporal dementia

Frontotemporal dementia (FTD) is a heterogeneous form of dementia with a spectrum of clinical and pathological features. In behavioural variant FTD, there is prominent personality change and a dysexecutive syndrome develops, i.e. sufferers are reluctant to initiate any actions or they may be frankly disinhibited. Semantic dementia and progressive non-fluent aphasia are forms of FTD associated with specific language disorders and sometimes parkinsonism. Preserved areas of ability such as memory are key diagnostic features that distinguish FTD from Alzheimer disease. Onset is usually at age 65 years or older. MRI shows frontal and/or temporal atrophy.

The FTDs are pathologically heterogeneous and include forms with tau pathology (FTD-τ) or ubiquitin pathology (FTD-U) and Pick disease, in which characteristic neuropathology occurs. Some of the FTD-τ cases are the result of mutations in the microtubule-associated tau protein. Of patients with motor neuron disease (MND), 30% develop a mild dysexecutive syndrome and occasionally (3–4%) frank FTD as the predominant clinical finding, with denervation atrophy and fasciculations appearing later. In both FTD-U and MND-associated dementia, ubiquitinated inclusions stain for the nuclear protein TDP-43. A significant number of patients with MND/FTD overlap syndromes characterized by ubiquitin pathology carry a common mutation, a hexanucleotide repeat expansion on chromosome 9.

Vascular dementia

The history is of stepwise evolution of cognitive impairment and focal neurological signs, in someone with the appropriate risk factors. A small stepping gait is characteristic. Memory may be less impaired in relation to defects in visuoperceptual tasking. MRI shows atrophy with diffuse white and grey matter vascular lesions (Binswanger encephalopathy is CT evidence of white matter infarction, with dementia, in hypertensive patients with a stroke). The diagnostic accuracy is often hampered by finding cerebrovascular disease in Alzheimer disease patients. Treating vascular disease risk factors and administering aspirin may slow progression.

Dementia with Lewy bodies

This causes parkinsonism (see Chapter 210). Typical features are fluctuating cognition, nocturnal visual hallucinations and disordered rapid eye movement (REM) sleep. Imaging is normal or shows diffuse atrophy. L-dopa may dramatically exacerbate the psychiatric symptoms, while treatment with antipsychotics can lead to a catastrophic and potentially fatal decline in motor performance.

Prion diseases

In prion disease, mutated forms of the prion protein (PrP) induce a conformational change in other PrP molecules ('permissive templating'), so producing non-functional, non-metabolizable forms which are cytotoxic. Sporadic and inherited forms of Creutzfeldt–Jakob disease (CJD) cause a rapidly progressive dementia with myoclonus, ataxia and cortical blindness progressing over weeks to months. The electroencephalograph (EEG) shows characteristic repetitive complexes. Variant CJD (transmitted from cattle infected with the bovine spongiform encephalopathy agent) seems to occur in younger patients, has a slower evolution and is associated with psychiatric symptoms as the earliest feature, though the initial epidemic in the UK has now come to an end.

Cognitive impairment in younger patients

The distinction between young and old in terms of causation is potentially artificial, and consideration of the conditions listed below should be driven by the presence of specific neurological symptoms and signs, such as dystonia, and the presence of specific risk factors.

- Use of 'recreational' drugs, especially alcohol, and also glue.
- Human immunodeficiency virus (HIV)-related dementia occurs as a late feature. Infections and structural lesions must be ruled out (lymphoma, toxoplasmosis, progressive multifocal leukoencephalopathy).
- Cerebral vasculitis.
- End-stage multiple sclerosis.
- Adrenoleukodystrophies resulting from fatty acid dysmetabolism cause a 'multiple sclerosis-type' pattern with prominent dementia.
- CADASIL: a white matter disease associated with mutations in the notch-3 gene – presents as hemiplegic migraine, encephalopathy or a progressive dementia.
- Wilson disease: the majority of cases present before the age of 30 with neuropsychiatric problems and dystonia of the mouth and tongue associated with a high-amplitude limb tremor.
- Uncontrolled epilepsy may produce a 'twilight' state, in which seizures are so frequent as to disallow full recovery in between. Rarely, so-called 'non-convulsive status' – in which patients appear vacant and are seen to perform repetitive movements – may be misinterpreted as a rapidly progressive dementia. The EEG is diagnostic.

203 Epilepsy

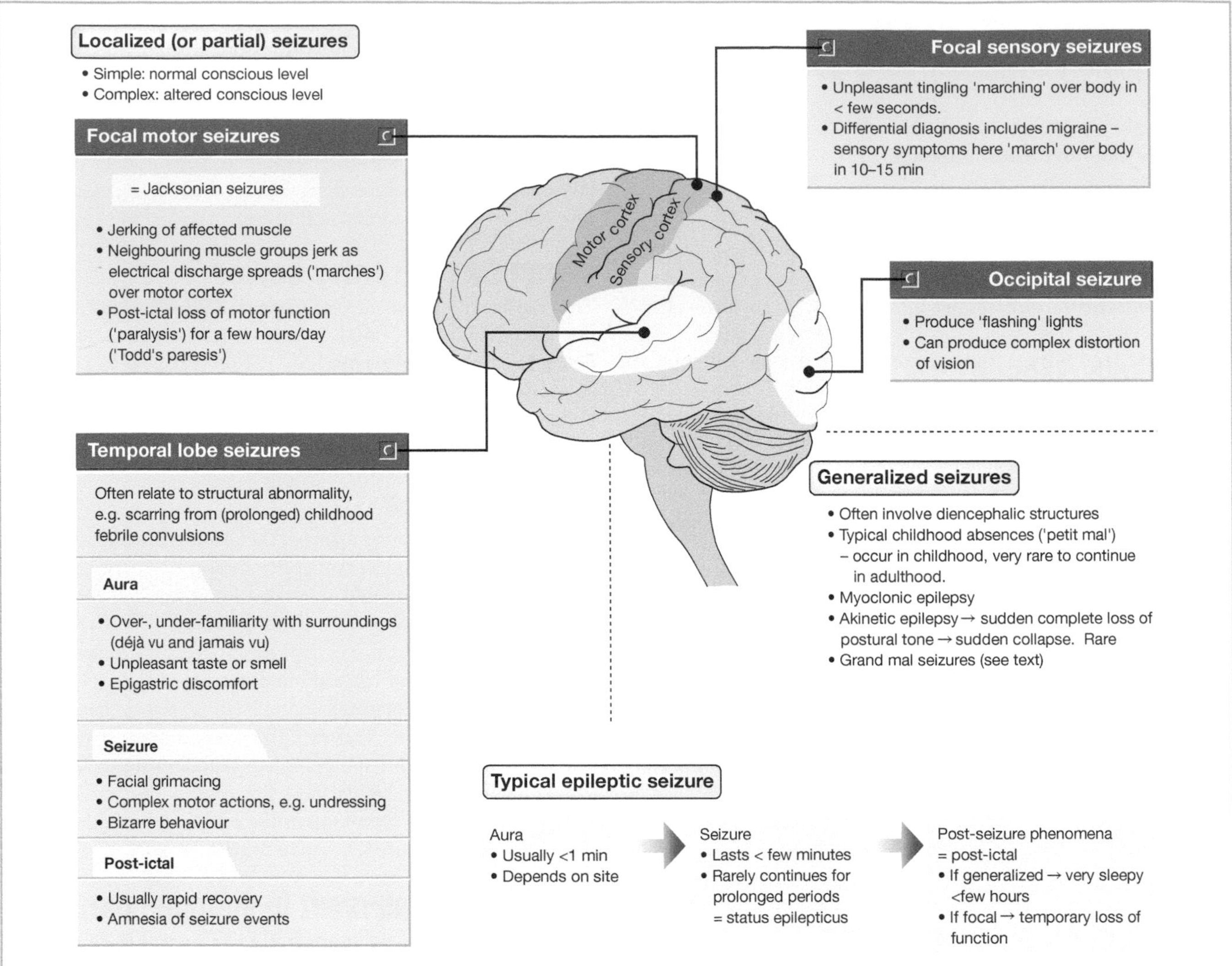

Localized (or partial) seizures
• Simple: normal conscious level
• Complex: altered conscious level
Focal motor seizures
= Jacksonian seizures
• Jerking of affected muscle
• Neighbouring muscle groups jerk as electrical discharge spreads ('marches') over motor cortex
• Post-ictal loss of motor function ('paralysis') for a few hours/day ('Todd's paresis')
Temporal lobe seizures
Often relate to structural abnormality, e.g. scarring from (prolonged) childhood febrile convulsions
Aura
• Over-, under-familiarity with surroundings (déjà vu and jamais vu)
• Unpleasant taste or smell
• Epigastric discomfort
Seizure
• Facial grimacing
• Complex motor actions, e.g. undressing
• Bizarre behaviour
Post-ictal
• Usually rapid recovery
• Amnesia of seizure events
Motor cortex
Sensory cortex
Focal sensory seizures
• Unpleasant tingling 'marching' over body in < few seconds.
• Differential diagnosis includes migraine – sensory symptoms here 'march' over body in 10–15 min
Occipital seizure
• Produce 'flashing' lights
• Can produce complex distortion of vision
Generalized seizures
• Often involve diencephalic structures
• Typical childhood absences ('petit mal') – occur in childhood, very rare to continue in adulthood.
• Myoclonic epilepsy
• Akinetic epilepsy → sudden complete loss of postural tone → sudden collapse. Rare
• Grand mal seizures (see text)
Typical epileptic seizure
Aura
• Usually <1 min
• Depends on site
Seizure
• Lasts < few minutes
• Rarely continues for prolonged periods = status epilepticus
Post-seizure phenomena = post-ictal
• If generalized → very sleepy <few hours
• If focal → temporary loss of function

Epilepsy is 'the recurrent tendency to spontaneous, disordered electrical discharge in the brain manifesting as alteration in motor, sensory or psychological function'. Generalized seizures arise in the brain of anyone subjected to the appropriate stimulus, e.g. hypoxia or electroconvulsive therapy. Therefore a single seizure does not make the diagnosis of epilepsy.

Causes of seizures

- Metabolic, especially ↓ Na^+ or ↓ glucose; liver failure, renal failure.
- Drugs, especially alcohol (particularly chronic alcohol excess and alcohol withdrawal), 'street' drugs, penicillins, antipsychotics, antidepressants.
- Cerebrovascular disease.
- Tumours.
- Intracranial infections, especially meningitis, encephalitis, syphilis.
- Cerebral anoxia, especially arrhythmia related.
- Developmental brain abnormalities.
- Degenerative brain disease.
- Hippocampal sclerosis.
- Primary epilepsy syndromes, genetic (e.g. 'channelopathies') or sporadic.

Treatment of the underlying cause, if it can be identified, is the preferred management option; anticonvulsants may also be required.

Epidemiology

The lifetime risk of a generalized convulsion is 3–4%, with peaks at the beginning (neonatal convulsions) and end of life

Medicine at a Glance, Fifth Edition. Edited by Patrick Davey and Alex Pitcher.

Companion website: www.wiley.com/go/medicine5e

(tumours, stroke). The incidence is 0.7%. There are 300 000 people in the UK with active seizures; 15–20% attend hospital each year.

Simplified classification

The simplest way to divide seizures is whether on the electroencephalograph (EEG) electrical activity is focal or generalized.

Primary generalized epilepsy

Primary generalized (grand mal) epilepsy refers to electrical seizure activity on the EEG arising in both hemispheres simultaneously. It usually begins in childhood or adolescence; there may be a family history. Brain imaging (computed tomography, magnetic resonance imaging) is normal. It is often photosensitive (triggered by flashing lights). There are three common manifestations.

1 **Typical childhood absences** ('petit mal').
2 **Myoclonic jerks.**
3 **Generalized tonic–clonic seizures**: a brief tonic stiffening of the limbs associated with sudden loss of consciousness followed by a variable period of clonic jerking.

Differential diagnosis of generalized tonic–clonic seizures

- All causes of seizures.
- Loss of cardiac output, e.g. arrhythmias, vasovagal, postural hypotension, etc.
- Psychogenic: seizures usually occur in public places, often hospitals; eyes are held tightly shut; bizarre movements are common. May also occur in those with genuine epilepsy.

Localization-related epilepsy

There is a clear electrical focus on the EEG from which the seizure activity arises. Often an abnormality is identified on imaging (hippocampal sclerosis, benign tumours, arteriovenous malformations, cortical dysplasia). There is usually no family history.

The common forms are as follows.

- Simple partial seizures.
- Complex partial seizures (the term 'complex' denotes altered awareness).
- If electrical activity spreads, a secondary generalized seizure occurs.

Diagnosis

The diagnosis of epilepsy is clinical, based on the history from the patient and reliable observers. The EEG supports the clinical diagnosis and differentiates between primary generalized seizures (3 Hz spike and wave discharge triggered by flashing lights) and localization-related seizures (focal spike discharges). Of patients with true seizures, 50% have a normal interictal EEG, emphasizing the importance of the history in making the diagnosis. Similarly, imaging findings must be interpreted in the context of the appropriate history of seizures.

Specific syndromes

Typical childhood absences

This was previously called 'petit mal' epilepsy. Onset is at age 3–6 years. It is associated with brief interruptions of 3–5 seconds in awareness, with minimal or no motor manifestation. Attacks can be provoked by hyperventilation. There is a characteristic EEG pattern of 3 Hz spike and wave activity. It responds to sodium valproate or ethosuximide and is likely to remit fully by adolescence.

Juvenile myoclonic epilepsy

This develops later in childhood, though a history of typical childhood absences is common. It is associated with early morning myoclonic jerks, which may be reported as clumsiness. Generalized tonic–clonic seizures occur in most. The epilepsy responds to levetiracetam. In most, the tendency to seizures is life-long.

Complex partial seizures with secondary generalization

These are common. Seizures arising from the temporal lobes are typically heralded by an aura, which can take the form of abdominal rising sensations, altered taste and, more rarely, visual and auditory hallucinations. Patients appear 'blank' during an attack and may make repetitive movements, e.g. lip smacking. Of cases, 70% are controlled on monotherapy, although a significant number have drug-resistant seizures and are socially and economically handicapped. Approximately 30% of complex partial seizures arise outside the temporal lobe, usually from the frontal lobe.

Frontal lobe seizures

These present a diagnostic challenge because the EEG is often normal, even during an attack, and the seizure semiology may be bizarre. Patients may appear to remain awake, but to thrash their limbs about uncontrollably and yell. Instantaneous recovery often occurs and patients may be labelled as having non-epileptic attacks.

Jacksonian seizures

These are simple partial seizures arising in the motor cortex. The onset is with rhythmical twitching of the face, which spreads down through the arms and into the legs in a characteristic march-like fashion. There is a high likelihood of finding a structural lesion, so imaging is mandatory.

Treatment

Primary generalized epilepsy responds well to levetiracetam or lamotrigine; it may be worse on carbamazepine. There is little evidence for any other anticonvulsant specificity by seizure type, so drugs are selected on patient characteristics and cost.

- Side-effect profile: phenytoin is avoided in young people because it causes gingival hyperplasia and androgenizes the face.
- Potential for teratogenicity: all the older drugs, particularly sodium valproate, are teratogenic, as are the newer agents, though probably to a lesser degree. Preconception counselling is vital.
- Effect on other drugs: particularly the oral contraceptive pill.

Monotherapy is preferred. Any changes should be made gradually and in the context of an overall seizure pattern, not in response to single seizures.

Status epilepticus (common causes: poor compliance in a known epileptic, sudden anticonvulsant withdrawal, alcohol withdrawal, drug overdose, hypoglycaemia) is defined as continuous seizure activity (arbitrarily for 30 min) or frequent seizures without recovery. This is a medical emergency with a high morbidity. Continuous seizure activity eventually results in cerebral oedema and cardiorespiratory arrest. Management involves the following.

- **A**irway, **B**reathing and **C**irculation (ABC).
- Urgent glucose (fingerprick testing), electrolytes and toxicology screen.
- 10 mg diazepam intravenously: terminates most seizures and can be repeated once.
- Phenytoin or fosphenytoin intravenous infusion.
- Phenobarbital with intensive care support (can cause severe respiratory depression).
- Intubation and transfer to the intensive care unit for propofol infusion.

204 Multiple sclerosis

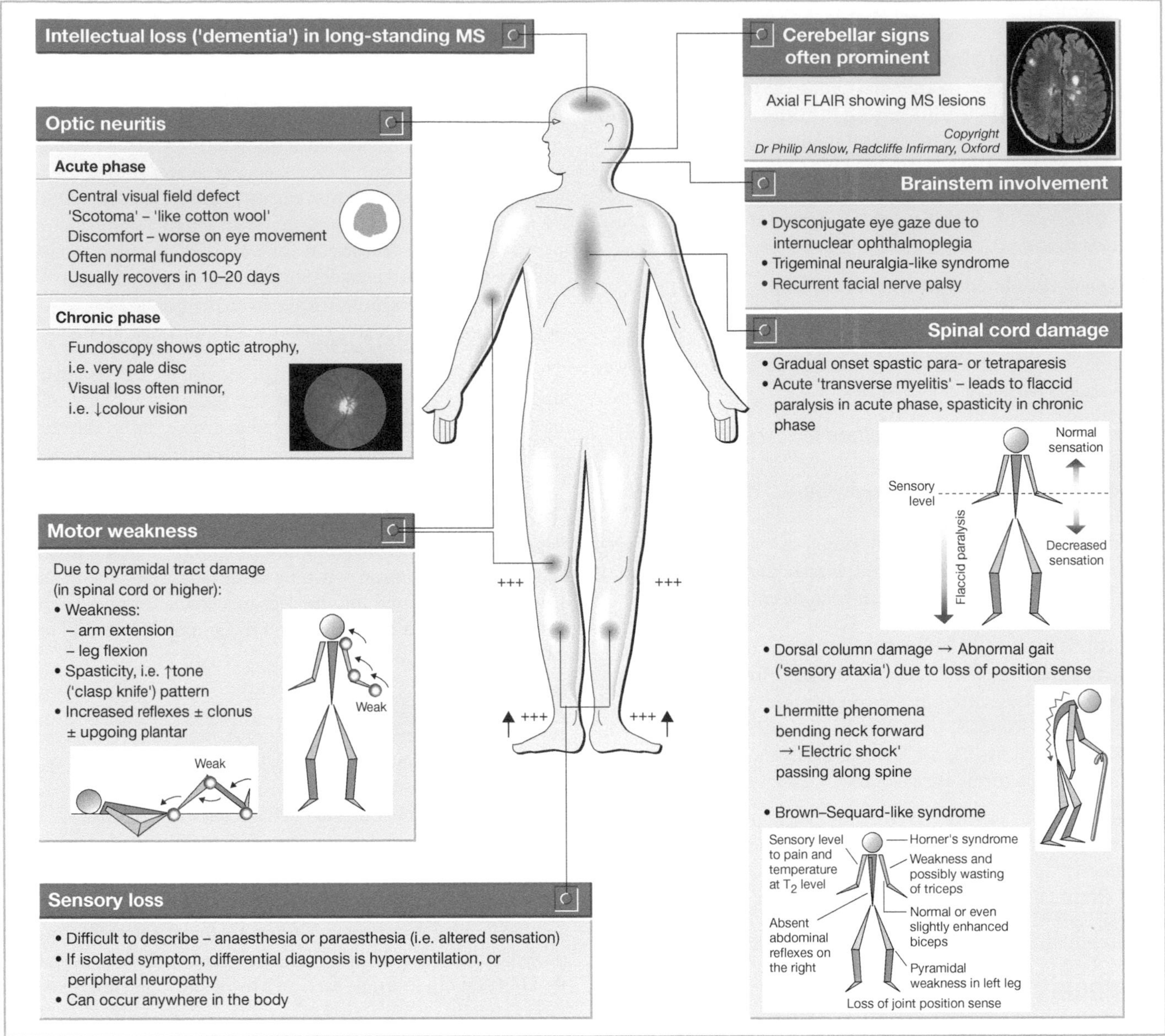

Intellectual loss ('dementia') in long-standing MS
Cerebellar signs often prominent
Axial FLAIR showing MS lesions
Copyright Dr Philip Anslow, Radcliffe Infirmary, Oxford
Optic neuritis
Acute phase
Central visual field defect
'Scotoma' – 'like cotton wool'
Discomfort – worse on eye movement
Often normal fundoscopy
Usually recovers in 10–20 days
Chronic phase
Fundoscopy shows optic atrophy, i.e. very pale disc
Visual loss often minor, i.e. ↓colour vision
Brainstem involvement
• Dysconjugate eye gaze due to internuclear ophthalmoplegia
• Trigeminal neuralgia-like syndrome
• Recurrent facial nerve palsy
Spinal cord damage
• Gradual onset spastic para- or tetraparesis
• Acute 'transverse myelitis' – leads to flaccid paralysis in acute phase, spasticity in chronic phase
Normal sensation
Sensory level
Flaccid paralysis
Decreased sensation
• Dorsal column damage → Abnormal gait ('sensory ataxia') due to loss of position sense
• Lhermitte phenomena bending neck forward → 'Electric shock' passing along spine
• Brown–Sequard-like syndrome
Sensory level to pain and temperature at T_2 level
Horner's syndrome
Weakness and possibly wasting of triceps
Normal or even slightly enhanced biceps
Absent abdominal reflexes on the right
Pyramidal weakness in left leg
Loss of joint position sense
Motor weakness
Due to pyramidal tract damage (in spinal cord or higher):
• Weakness:
– arm extension
– leg flexion
• Spasticity, i.e. ↑tone ('clasp knife') pattern
• Increased reflexes ± clonus ± upgoing plantar
Weak
Weak
+++
+++
+++
+++
Sensory loss
• Difficult to describe – anaesthesia or paraesthesia (i.e. altered sensation)
• If isolated symptom, differential diagnosis is hyperventilation, or peripheral neuropathy
• Can occur anywhere in the body

Multiple sclerosis (MS) is the most common of a group of inflammatory conditions in which the basic pathological process is loss of myelin in the brain and spinal cord. This leads initially to a relapsing and remitting neurological disturbance, but ultimately, in all but a few patients, to permanent and progressive disability as a result of loss of axons. It is a common disease (50 000 sufferers in the UK, lifetime risk in the UK 2–5/1000) affecting young people, for whom currently there is no proven treatment that alters long-term disability. It is presumed to be a disorder of altered immune responsiveness to targets in the central nervous system (CNS), in which there is a genetic susceptibility and a series of environmentally determined triggers, the nature of which (viral, toxic, etc.) remains obscure, although it also shows some features of a primary degenerative process.

The relative risk of developing MS in first-degree relatives is 15, although the absolute risk is still low. There is marked geographical variation (common in people of Scandinavian origin, rare in Japan and Africa).

Medicine at a Glance, Fifth Edition. Edited by Patrick Davey and Alex Pitcher.

Companion website: www.wiley.com/go/medicine5e

Clinical spectrum

There are a number of typical patterns of disease.

- **Relapsing and remitting**: initially the patient presents with episodes of monophasic neurological disturbance with return to normal function in between attacks. Thereafter, the patient may not return to normality, so there is a background of progressive dysfunction with superimposed relapses (termed secondary progressive MS). This accounts for most patients with MS.
- **Relapsing progressive**: there is a progressive course with superimposed relapses but no recovery in between episodes.
- **Primary progressive**: there is relentless progression from the outset. This subtype is associated with males, later onset and a paucity of imaging changes, a presentation with progressive spastic paraparesis, and an overall poorer prognosis. There is rarely any response to steroids.

Clinical features

The most common clinical features are as follows.

- Optic neuritis and subsequent optic atrophy: patients experience blurring of vision through to more profound visual loss, with restoration of eyesight over several months. Colour vision may be permanently lost.
- Cerebellar ataxia (see Chapter 62).
- Spastic paraparesis (see Chapter 207).
- Internuclear ophthalmoplegia: the internuclear tracts are nerve fibres linking the nuclei of the nerves controlling the external ocular muscles. MS plaques commonly disrupt them. There is failure of conjugate eye movements, with slow adduction in the ipsilateral eye usually associated with contralateral nystagmus.
- Patchy sensory disturbance.

The clinical signs most commonly associated with MS are shown in the figure above.

Diagnosis

- Magnetic resonance imaging (MRI) shows typical changes in most patients (with white matter hyperintensities usually around the ventricles or in the brainstem) although a spinal cord presentation can be associated with normal imaging.
- Visual evoked potentials (VEPs) to document slowing of optic nerve conduction caused by demyelination are a useful adjunct if the MRI cannot distinguish the changes of vascular disease.
- Lumbar puncture to look for oligoclonal bands is much less frequently performed than in the past but is of use when the MRI changes are not diagnostic, particularly early in the disease or if it is confined to the spinal cord. Oligoclonal bands in the cerebrospinal fluid occur in 97% of MS patients, but also in other conditions: paraneoplastic cerebellar degeneration, Behçet disease, neurosarcoid and CNS infections.

Differential diagnosis

A first attack of demyelination can be caused by parainfectious immune-mediated damage (acute disseminated encephalomyelitis). To make a diagnosis of MS, demonstration of dissemination in space (i.e. lesions in different parts of the CNS) and time is required through history, examination and investigations. A number of rarer conditions can look like MS.

- Progressive cerebrovascular disease can occasionally be difficult to distinguish on clinical and imaging grounds, but is associated with negative oligoclonal bands and usually normal VEPs.
- Cerebral vasculitis.
- Neuromyelitis optica.
- Similar white matter changes to those seen in MS can occur in Sjögren syndrome, sarcoidosis and Behçet disease of the nervous system, and occasionally in cerebral lymphoma.

Prognosis

Occasional patients run a relentlessly progressive course from the beginning of the disease and may die within a few years of the first symptoms. In most patients, however, MS does not significantly shorten life. The disease runs a course over decades, during which time there will in most patients be an increasing burden of disability. However, some patients experience a relapsing and remitting course with good functional recovery for many years.

Treatment

- **Overall approach**: this is vital. The patient requires psychological support, with accurate advice about work, home life (and adaptations) and prognosis, and a balanced view on therapy – the last sometimes being particularly difficult. A multidisciplinary approach involving general practitioners, social workers, relatives, physiotherapists, occupational therapists and sometimes psychiatrists is crucial. This approach is true for all diseases but is particularly important in MS.
- **Acute relapses**: corticosteroids (high dose intravenously or orally) have been shown to reduce the severity and duration of acute relapses, although not in every patient. There is no effect on relapse rate or long-term disability. In general, steroids become less effective after repeated attacks.
- **Disease process and progression**: a number of drugs (β-interferon, copaxone, natalizumab) appear to reduce the number of clinical relapses in selected patients and the number of new lesions on MRI. The effect on long-term disability is less clear but a focus of much current research. Two drugs (ocrelizumab and siponimod) have recently been shown to be effective in reducing the accrual of disability in progressive MS.

Symptomatic treatment

- Unpleasant sensory phenomena such as shooting pains and paraesthesiae can be treated with anticonvulsants such as carbamazepine and gabapentin.
- Bladder spasticity can be treated with oxybutynin or intermittent self-catheterization – although this risks frequent urinary tract infections. Such infections are common in MS; fever may (temporarily) dramatically worsen weakness.
- Sexual dysfunction in men may respond to sildenafil (Viagra®).
- Constipation is common and requires laxatives, and sometimes manual evacuation.
- Muscle spasticity can be treated with baclofen.
- Depression severe enough to require medication occurs in 30% of patients.

Neuromyelitis optica

Neuromyelitis optica (NMO) presents as attacks of optic neuritis with 'longitudinally extensive transverse myelitis'. Each can occur in isolation, giving rise to the concept of 'NMO spectrum' disorders. In the past, NMO was considered to be a variant of MS but is now recognized to be a specific disease entity characterized by antibodies to aquaporin 4 (AQP) or myelin oligodendrocyte glycoprotein (MOG), a distinct pathology of complement-mediated destruction and perivascular astrocytosis and a different response from MS to immunotherapy.

205 Infections of the central nervous system

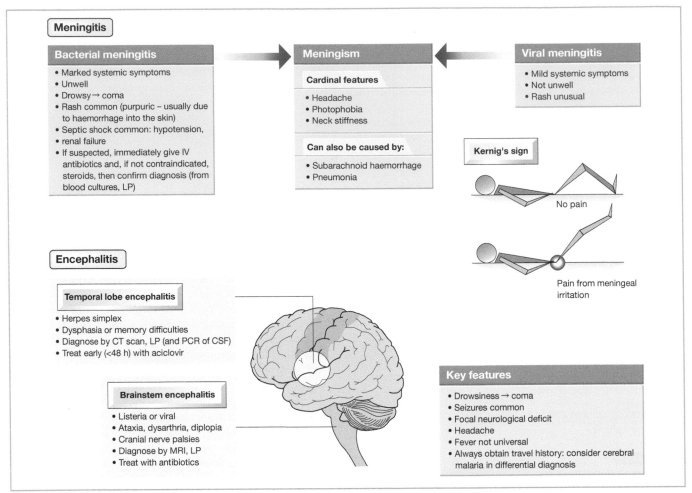

Meningitis

Bacterial meningitis
- Marked systemic symptoms
- Unwell
- Drowsy → coma
- Rash common (purpuric – usually due to haemorrhage into the skin)
- Septic shock common: hypotension,
- renal failure
- If suspected, immediately give IV antibiotics and, if not contraindicated, steroids, then confirm diagnosis (from blood cultures, LP)

Meningism

Cardinal features
- Headache
- Photophobia
- Neck stiffness

Can also be caused by:
- Subarachnoid haemorrhage
- Pneumonia

Viral meningitis
- Mild systemic symptoms
- Not unwell
- Rash unusual

Kernig's sign

No pain

Pain from meningeal irritation

Encephalitis

Temporal lobe encephalitis
- Herpes simplex
- Dysphasia or memory difficulties
- Diagnose by CT scan, LP (and PCR of CSF)
- Treat early (<48 h) with aciclovir

Brainstem encephalitis
- Listeria or viral
- Ataxia, dysarthria, diplopia
- Cranial nerve palsies
- Diagnose by MRI, LP
- Treat with antibiotics

Key features
- Drowsiness → coma
- Seizures common
- Focal neurological deficit
- Headache
- Fever not universal
- Always obtain travel history: consider cerebral malaria in differential diagnosis

A number of infectious processes may affect the central nervous system (CNS), including meningitis, encephalitis and cerebral abscess. The range of bacteria, viruses, fungi and parasites that can be responsible is broad, especially in the immunocompromised such as transplant recipients or those with HIV disease.

Meningitis

Acute meningitis presents with fever, headache, stiff neck and photophobia, and can be caused by bacteria or viruses.

- **Bacterial meningitis**: often associated with a septic syndrome (fever, tachycardia, hypotension or shock; see Chapter 164), complicated by septicaemia-induced disseminated intravascular coagulation (see Chapter 186). The two most common organisms are *Neisseria meningitidis* and *Streptococcus pneumoniae* (more common in elderly people and those who abuse alcohol or with damaged dura – skull fracture, ear sepsis, sinus disease). Once bacterial meningitis is suspected, broad-spectrum antibiotics (e.g. high-dose ceftriaxone) must be given immediately (i.e. in the community if necessary). Steroids have been shown to improve outcome in streptococcal meningitis and so should be administered early. The diagnosis is confirmed by identifying the organism using blood culture, cerebrospinal fluid (CSF) (see Table 205.1), microscopy, culture and polymerase chain reaction (PCR) or blood serology. The prognosis is variable. In meningococcal meningitis, 5–10% die, and a significant proportion have permanent sequelae, including loss of digits (infarction secondary to hypotension), deafness, blindness and intellectual impairment. Immunization against meningococcal serotype A and C is effective (but serotype B, against which there is no vaccine, now accounts for 90% of cases in the UK).
- ***Listeria monocytogenes***: causes meningitis in susceptible individuals (pregnant women, people with alcohol problems, immunocompromised individuals), with a rapidly progressive picture resembling brainstem encephalitis with focal signs and meningism. Treatment is with ampicillin.
- **Viral meningitis**: presents with prominent headache and less obvious signs of meningeal irritation than in bacterial infections.

Medicine at a Glance, Fifth Edition. Edited by Patrick Davey and Alex Pitcher.

Companion website: www.wiley.com/go/medicine5e

Table 205.1 Cerebrospinal fluid (CSF) findings in different infections.

Disease	CSF pressure	Protein	Cell count	Glucose
Bacterial meningitis	Raised	Moderately to severely elevated	>50 polymorphs	Low
Viral meningitis	Normal	Mildly elevated or normal	Lymphocytes	Normal
Tubercular meningitis	Raised or normal	Moderately elevated	Pleocytosis or lymphocytosis	Low
Encephalitis	Raised or normal	Mildly elevated or normal	Lymphocytosis	Normal
Malignant meningitis	Mildly raised or normal	Raised	Raised: either reactive lymphocytes or malignant cells	Low

The responsible organism is identified (CSF, PCR or serology) in only 50% of cases, and is often an enterovirus. Many of the common exanthemata of childhood, including measles and chickenpox, may be accompanied by a meningitic illness which, although usually mild, can rarely be life-threatening. Management is symptomatic with rehydration and analgesia.

- **Non-infectious causes** of meningism (i.e. headache, photophobia and stiff neck) include subarachnoid haemorrhage and migraine (although this requires exclusion of more serious diagnoses). Malignant meningitis usually presents with sequential cranial nerve palsies, initially painless, later painful, but can cause meningism. Spinal nerve root involvement also occurs.
- **Meningoencephalitis** is meningitis plus some parenchymal involvement.
- **Tubercular meningitis or cryptococcal meningitis**: a chronic presentation may occur; these are more common in the immunocompromised. Tubercular meningitis is increasing in frequency in the West (see Chapter 170).

Encephalitis

Encephalitis implies infection of the brain substance itself. This is rare. The clinical picture is of fever, headache and a diffuse (i.e. confusion, drowsiness up to coma) rather than focal disturbance of cerebral function. The onset may be very dramatic over just a few hours, although more usually the history extends back several days. Other features include seizures, wandering, behavioural change and frank psychiatric syndromes.

The diagnosis is made from the combination of suggestive clinical features and a lymphocytosis in the CSF. Supportive data come from finding focal inflammation on magnetic resonance imaging (MRI), focal slow wave activity on an electroencephalograph (EEG) and detection of the organism (culture, PCR, serology). There are a large number of viruses responsible, with a marked geographical variation (e.g. Japanese B in the Far East, West Nile in the USA) so a travel history is vital. A cause is only identified in 30% of cases. The prognosis is variable.

The principal treatable cause is herpes simplex encephalitis (HSV), which has the following features.

- Rare: causes 20% of viral encephalitis.
- Presents with a viral prodrome followed by behavioural changes with amnesia and sometimes dysphasia.
- Rapid evolution to coma may occur.
- EEG shows repetitive epileptic discharges localized to the temporal lobes. CT/MRI shows necrotizing inflammation in the temporal lobes.
- Treatment: immediate high-dose aciclovir. The prognosis is poor and long-term sequelae are common: 10% die acutely, 10% are so severely impaired as to be rendered institutionalized, 20% are left dependent, and 60% recover but in the majority formal neuropsychological testing reveals residual deficits and most do not function at their premorbid occupational level.

Cerebral abscess

Cerebral abscess is rare and presents with headache, fever and focal neurological signs. Infection arises from direct spread (e.g. infected ears, sinuses) or from infected emboli (endocarditis or cyanotic congenital heart disease). First-line investigation is CT/ MRI. Lumbar puncture (LP) must not be performed because the risk of 'coning' (i.e. herniation of the brain through the foramen magnum, precipitating coma and death) is high. Organisms are cultured from the blood or pus aspirated from the abscess. Echocardiography to exclude cardiac infection (see Chapter 93) should be undertaken. Treatment is with prolonged antibiotics and sometimes neurosurgical drainage. The mortality rate is 25%.

Prion diseases

The biologically unique features of these diseases are that they can be simultaneously inherited and infectious. The agent of transmission is thought to be a protein (a 'prion') only, rather than an 'organism' containing DNA or RNA. Prion diseases principally result in dementia (see Chapter 202) and include the following.

- Sporadic Creutzfeldt–Jakob disease (CJD): rare ($1/10^6$), causes rapid dementia with myoclonus and a characteristic EEG.
- Variant CJD: ≤200 cases in total in UK to date, and the incidence appears to be declining. Occurs in younger people with a slower course than sporadic CJD. Characteristic pathological features. A psychiatric presentation (depression, personality changes) is frequently seen.
- Autosomal dominant CJD: familial form of classic CJD.
- Gerstmann–Straussler–Scheinker syndrome: familial spongiform encephalopathy with prominent ataxia.
- Fatal familial insomnia.
- Kuru: endemic in New Guinea highlanders who performed ritual cannibalism. Now very rare.

Parasitic diseases

A number of parasitic diseases may cause neurological problems, ranging from the coma associated with cerebral malaria (see Chapter 169) to fits occurring with cysticercosis.

Neurological consequences of HIV disease

Neurological problems are common in HIV (see Chapter 166) and include the consequences of direct viral infection of the CNS (AIDS dementia, seroconversion meningitis, Guillain–Barré syndrome-like polyneuropathy), opportunistic infections (toxoplasmosis, cryptococcal meningitis, progressive multifocal leukoencephalopathy), primary cerebral lymphoma and drug toxicity (antiretrovirals: nucleoside analogues and protease inhibitors).

206 Tumours and the nervous system

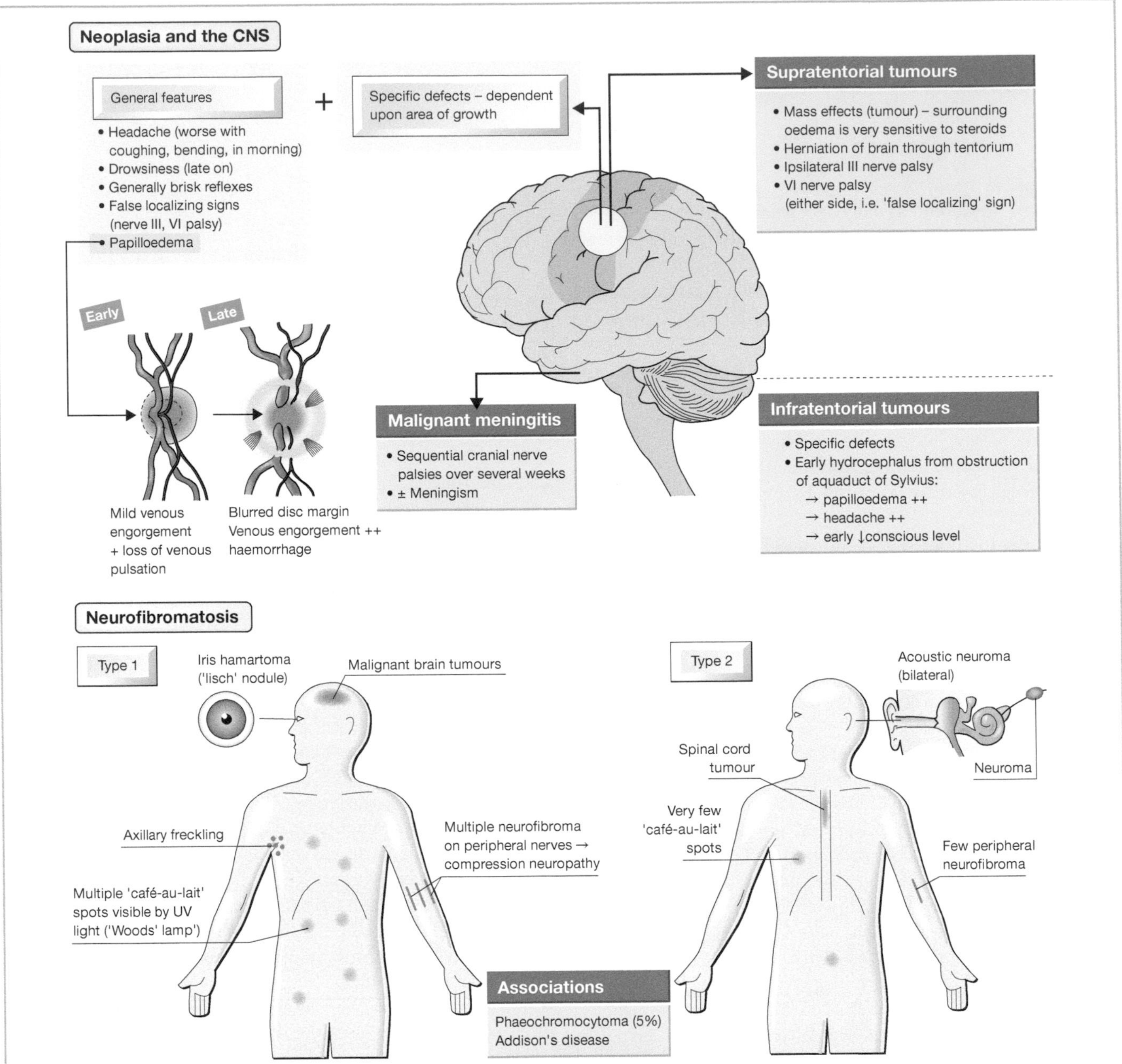

Neoplasia and the CNS

Central nervous system (CNS) neoplasia may present with the following.

- Epilepsy.
- Symptoms of raised intracranial pressure (headache, intellectual deterioration, vomiting) with papilloedema. Posterior fossa (e.g. cerebellar) metastases produce a rapid rise in intracranial pressure and rapid onset of symptoms.
- Focal deficits, the onset of which is often slow, but occasionally sudden (i.e. stroke-like). The deficit relates to damage caused by the expansion of the tumour (which acts as a space-occupying lesion) and the surrounding oedema. Focal signs usually reflect the site of the tumour, but occasionally false localizing signs occur

Medicine at a Glance, Fifth Edition. Edited by Patrick Davey and Alex Pitcher.

Companion website: www.wiley.com/go/medicine5e

from the tumour shifting brain contents and damaging distant nervous structures (e.g. VIth nerve palsy). These false localizing signs are rare but important because they indicate that the tumour is extensive enough to damage distant brain tissue, i.e. death is imminent unless urgent intervention occurs.

Diagnosis is usually straightforward, using computed tomography (CT) or magnetic resonance imaging (MRI) and stereotactic guided biopsy. Occasionally, tumours are difficult to see on an unenhanced CT scan; accordingly, once a tumour is suspected, CT scanning must be contrast enhanced. Electroencephalography, although not indicated, may during the course of epilepsy investigations suggest an underlying neoplasm (focal slow-wave activity). Lumbar puncture must not be undertaken because of the risk of 'coning' the brain into the foramen magnum.

Specific tumours

Fifty percent of CNS tumours are secondary deposits from extracranial malignancies, commonly breast, lung, kidney, thyroid, stomach, prostate and melanoma. Accordingly, many patients with brain tumours should be investigated for an extracranial primary (breast examination, chest X-ray, prostate specific antigen, abdominal imaging). A quarter of patients with carcinomatosis have brain involvement.

Primary tumours may be malignant or benign. However, the clinical effects of histologically non-malignant tumours may not be benign because pressure effects from expansion within the cranial cavity may lead to disability and death.

- **Astrocytoma**: the most common primary brain tumour, prevalent in the 50–60-year age range. They are divided into four types (I–IV) depending on the degree of malignancy. Glioblastoma multiforme is so undifferentiated as to make the cell of origin impossible to define. Growth is rapid and attempts at surgical excision result in disability and do not improve survival. Dexamethasone results in rapid reduction in neurological deficit as a result of reduction in oedema. Radiotherapy and temozolomide chemotherapy improve quality of life in selected cases and may extend survival by a few months. Mutations in *IDH1* are associated with a better prognosis.
- **Oligodendroglioma**: a slow-growing tumour, which may thus show calcification on CT scanning. Oligodendrogliomas occur in a younger population than astrocytomas.
- **Ependymoma**: occurs anywhere throughout the ventricular system and infiltrates into surrounding tissues.
- **Primary CNS lymphoma**: may be single or multifocal and is more common in immunocompromised patients, such as those with HIV, where the Epstein–Barr virus drives tumour growth. Metastatic spread from systemic lymphoma is uncommon and is usually meningeal rather than parenchymal. Primary CNS lymphoma may be exquisitely sensitive to steroids, which should therefore be avoided before a tissue diagnosis has been achieved.
- **Meningiomas**: these account for 20% of intracranial tumours; they arise from the arachnoid granulations and are usually closely related to the venous sinuses. They exert their clinical effects by direct compression of the brain and, although presentation is usually slow, it may be surprisingly acute, leading to the view that there is an inflammatory component. A reactive hyperostosis may occur in the overlying bone. The aim of treatment is complete surgical excision, but the recurrence rate is 30% at 10 years.
- **Acoustic neuroma/schwannoma**: the most common infratentorial tumour. They arise from the vestibular portion of nerve VIII and lie in the cerebellopontine angle, giving rise to symptoms referable to cranial nerves VIII, VII and VI.

Malignant meningitis

The spread of tumours to the nervous system may be via the bloodstream to the meninges. This can cause a diffuse subacute meningitis with headache, stiff neck and vomiting, or a multifocal neurological syndrome of deafness and other, typically lower, cranial nerve palsies. Examination of the cerebrospinal fluid (CSF) reveals a reactive lymphocytosis, a low glucose and a high protein. CSF cytology may reveal tumour cells. Occasionally, severe limb weakness can result from diffuse infiltration of the nerve root with tumour. Treatment is usually unsuccessful, except in the case of lymphoma.

Paraneoplastic disorders

The loss of normal expression and regulation of genes in malignant tumours may lead to the cell surface expression of proteins normally only found in neurons (onconeuronal antigens). These may initiate an immune response, provoking damage of the nervous system. Antineuronal antibodies can be detected but these may not be pathogenic. Each of the syndromes has in common:

- an evolution over weeks to months
- a relentlessly progressive course
- a failure to respond to treatment of the primary tumour or of the immune response (steroids, intravenous immunoglobulin or plasma exchange). The exceptions are Eaton–Lambert myasthenic syndrome and anti-*N*-methyl-D-aspartic acid receptor antibody-associated limbic encephalitis
- oligoclonal bands in the CSF
- specific antibodies (anti-Hu, anti-Yo, etc.)
- relatively normal CNS imaging.

Specific syndromes are described in Chapter 195.

Neurocutaneous syndromes

These are dominantly inherited and are the result of mutations in tumour suppressor genes. They lead to benign and malignant tumours.

- **Neurofibromatosis** has an incidence of one in 3000, occurs in several patterns and may have an associated phaeochromocytoma (which should be suspected if hypertension occurs).
  - Type 1 (peripheral type) is characterized by multiple neurofibromas, café-au-lait patches, axillary freckling, Lisch nodule in the iris, meningiomas and malignant brain tumours, usually astrocytomas of the optic pathway. It is caused by mutations in the neurofibromin gene and has a very high new mutation rate.
  - Type 2 (central type) is the result of mutations in a gene called *Merlin*. Although the hallmark of this disease is the occurrence of bilateral vestibular schwannomas, most patients develop benign or malignant tumours in the spinal cord and elsewhere in the brain. There are also cutaneous manifestations.
- **Von Hippel–Lindau disease** involves tumours in multiple organ systems. As well as cerebellar and spinal cord haemangioblastomas and ocular angiomas, von Hippel–Lindau disease causes renal angiolipomatosis and renal cell carcinoma, phaeochromocytoma and islet cell tumours.

207 Spinal cord disease

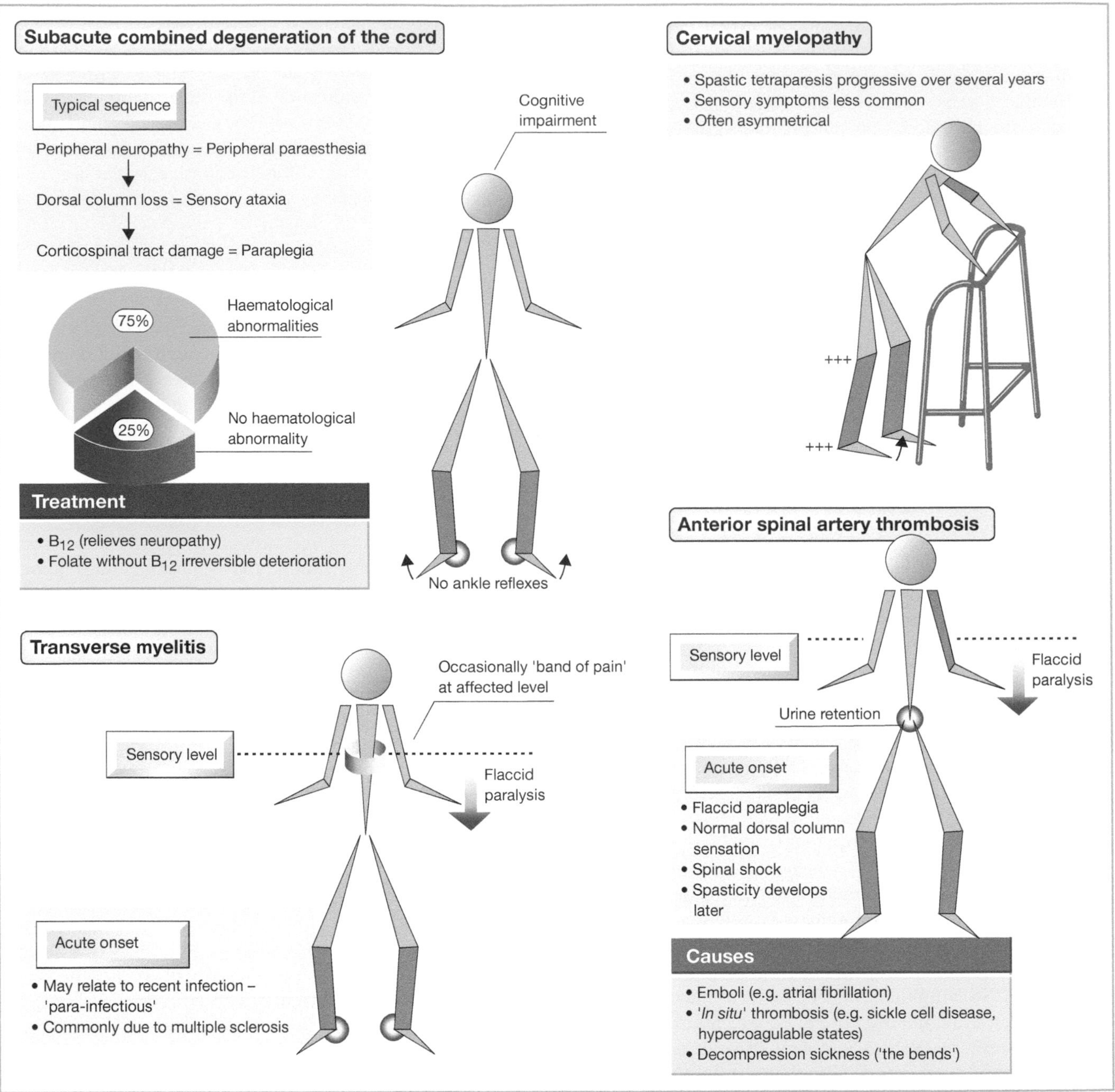

Subacute combined degeneration of the cord
Typical sequence
Peripheral neuropathy = Peripheral paraesthesia
Dorsal column loss = Sensory ataxia
Corticospinal tract damage = Paraplegia
75%
Haematological abnormalities
25%
No haematological abnormality
Treatment
• B12 (relieves neuropathy)
• Folate without B12 irreversible deterioration
Cognitive impairment
No ankle reflexes
Cervical myelopathy
• Spastic tetraparesis progressive over several years
• Sensory symptoms less common
• Often asymmetrical
+++
+++
Anterior spinal artery thrombosis
Sensory level
Flaccid paralysis
Urine retention
Acute onset
• Flaccid paraplegia
• Normal dorsal column sensation
• Spinal shock
• Spasticity develops later
Causes
• Emboli (e.g. atrial fibrillation)
• 'In situ' thrombosis (e.g. sickle cell disease, hypercoagulable states)
• Decompression sickness ('the bends')
Transverse myelitis
Occasionally 'band of pain' at affected level
Sensory level
Flaccid paralysis
Acute onset
• May relate to recent infection – 'para-infectious'
• Commonly due to multiple sclerosis

Acute spinal cord compression

Spinal cord compression presents with motor dysfunction predominantly affecting the lower limb, *whatever the level of the lesion*. This is associated with a sensory level and upper motor neuron signs below the level of the lesion. Abdominal reflexes are lost when the lesion is above T9. This is a medical emergency whatever the cause – urgent magnetic resonance imaging (MRI) is mandatory, and the results of such imaging dictate management. The spinal cord is most often compressed by:

- secondary tumours from the breast, prostate and lung
- prolapsed intervertebral discs, which usually herniate laterally, causing asymmetrical signs, although central disc prolapse can also occur.

Medicine at a Glance, Fifth Edition. Edited by Patrick Davey and Alex Pitcher.

Companion website: www.wiley.com/go/medicine5e

Abscess and other inflammatory lesions can also compress the spinal cord. The treatment usually involves surgical decompression or radiotherapy for malignant tumours.

Progressive spastic paraparesis

Bilateral weakness with marked spasticity of the lower limbs and extensor plantar responses can be subacute or chronic. It is always investigated by MRI of the spine, and has a number of important causes.

- **Vitamin B_{12} deficiency**: this causes corticospinal tract damage (spastic paraparesis) associated with a peripheral neuropathy (absent ankle jerks) and dorsal column dysfunction (a high stepping gait, rombergism and pseudoathetosis of the outstretched fingers). This syndrome complex is termed subacute combined degeneration of the cord (SACD). It is important to appreciate that neurological dysfunction in isolation can occur before a rise in mean cell volume (MCV) or anaemia (see Chapter 174). In SACD, folic acid alone may exacerbate the neurological deficit. Accordingly, in megaloblastic anaemias with any suggestion of spinal cord involvement, it is crucial to measure vitamin B_{12} and replace it if deficient. 'Low normal' B_{12} levels with an appropriate clinical picture suggestive of SACD should prompt measurement of methylmalonic acid and homocystine levels, which are a more accurate measure of B_{12} functionality than crude levels of the vitamin.
- **Copper deficiency**: this can cause a clinical picture identical to SACD but with a normal B_{12}. Deficiency can occur as part of a generalized malabsorption syndrome or occasionally as a consequence of zinc supplementation.
- **Cervical spondylotic myelopathy**: this is a condition of middle-aged and elderly people, in which degenerative changes in the vertebrae cause slowly progressive constriction of the cervical cord and sometimes the nerve roots at the exit foramina, producing a 'radiculopathy' (wasting, weakness, sensory loss, decreased reflexes). It can present with various combinations of neck pain, tingling of the upper limbs, sphincter dysfunction and gait disturbance. Reflexes in the arms and legs (except those supplied by compressed nerve roots) are very brisk, and often show clonus. Diagnosis is by MRI. The aim of surgery is to prevent worsening because only rarely does it improve symptoms.
- **Hereditary spastic paraparesis**: a genetically heterogeneous disease that can be autosomal dominant or recessive. It selectively affects the long motor tracts and characteristically produces more spasticity than weakness. It is very slowly progressive and typically comes on in early adult life, although cases may present into the fifties.
- **Motor neuron disease**: 1% of cases present with an indolent form called primary lateral sclerosis, in which upper motor neuron signs predominate until late in the illness. Survival may be prolonged (10–15 years as opposed to 2–3 years for amyotrophic lateral sclerosis).
- **Primary progressive multiple sclerosis.**

Transverse myelitis

This is an inflammatory illness localized to the middle of the spinal cord, which presents as acute weakness with an ascending sensory level, i.e. rather similar to acute cord compression (which must be excluded by urgent MRI). A proportion of patients have had a recent flu-like illness and this condition may occur as a parainfectious complication of *Mycoplasma* or *Legionella* spp., Epstein–Barr virus infections, herpes simplex and zoster, and others. Imaging may show a focal lesion in the spinal cord or be normal. In a proportion of patients, transverse myelitis is the first manifestation of multiple sclerosis. A related autoimmune form of cord demyelination ('longitudinally extensive transverse myelitis') is associated with aquaporin-4 antibodies.

Anterior spinal artery thrombosis

The particular anatomical arrangement of the blood supply to the spinal cord makes the middle and upper thoracic regions vulnerable to vascular insufficiency. Two posterior spinal arteries, which provide good collateral circulation, supply the posterior portion of the spinal cord. The anterior part of the cord (spinothalamic tracts, corticospinal tracts), however, is supplied by a solitary anterior spinal artery formed by the anastomosis of a branch from each vertebral artery at the level of the medulla. At a variable level (typically T4), there is a paucity of collateral circulation. If the blood supply here is compromised (e.g. by *in situ* thrombosis or an embolus), this leads to ischaemia in the anterior spinal artery territory which presents as a sudden (maximally over a few hours) flaccid paraparesis and loss of bladder function. Dorsal column function is preserved. Autonomic instability from spinal shock may ensue.

Imaging is often normal acutely. There is no treatment and the prognosis for recovery is poor. An embolic source should be sought (e.g. atrial fibrillation, recent myocardial infarction), vasculitis excluded, and general antiatherogenic measures undertaken.

Disc prolapse

The prolapse may be central or lateral, so compressing the exit foramina of the nerves, producing radicular pain. The most common example of this is a L4–5 or L5–S1 disc prolapse, resulting in pain radiating down the buttock and lower limb (sciatica). The signs are of decreased straight leg raising and diminished reflexes. Recovery is usually spontaneous – occasionally laminectomy is required.

Syringomyelia

This is an exceptionally rare illness, in which the central canal in the cervical spinal cord enlarges into a large fluid-filled cavity (the syrinx). This is predisposed to by mild (or more severe) herniation of the cerebellar tonsils into (or beyond) the foramen magnum (the Arnold–Chiari malformation) or previous trauma. The expanding syrinx damages local structures, especially the decussating spinothalamic tracts (producing loss of pain and temperature sensation and, distressingly, severe pain in the same distribution), the corticospinal tracts (spastic weakness) and anterior horn cells (muscle wasting). Cranial nerve signs follow extension of the syrinx into the medulla. Diagnosis is by MRI. Neurosurgical drainage may have a role.

Spinal shock

Sudden transsection of the spinal cord at a cervical or upper thoracic level (often traumatic) can lead to loss of autonomic vasomotor control of blood pressure, which leads to catastrophic hypotension. Substantial fluid replacement is needed.

208 Neuromuscular disease

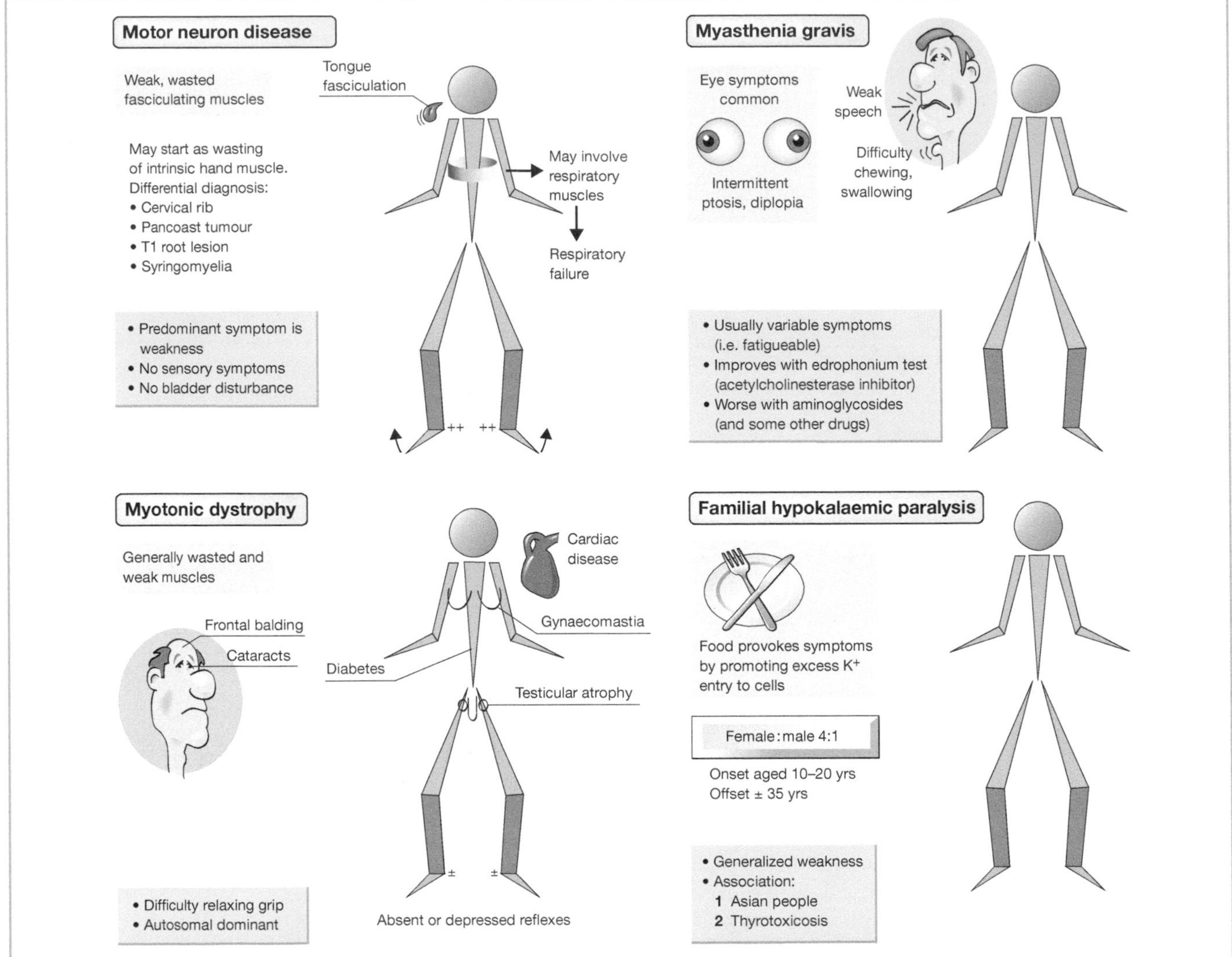

The motor unit

There are four possible sites at which pathological processes of the neuromuscular unit may act.

1 The anterior horn cell or lower motor neuron.
2 The peripheral nerve.
3 The neuromuscular junction.
4 The muscle.

Peripheral neuropathies are dealt with in Chapter 209.

Motor neuron disease

Motor neuron disease (MND) is a disorder of complex aetiology, which leads to selective, but not exclusive, degeneration of upper and lower motor neurons. It is characterized by the deposition of ubiquitinated intraneuronal inclusions which stain for the nuclear protein TDP-43. It is relatively rare (2/100 000 per year) and malignant in behaviour – the average time from diagnosis to death is 2.5 years. Of cases of MND, 5% show familial inheritance (autosomal dominant), but 5% of sporadic cases also have gene mutations (due to low penetrance rare variants). The most common mutation is a hexanucleotide repeat in a gene of unknown function (*C9orf72*) on chromosome 9, which can also cause frontotemporal dementia. Other genes in which mutations are associated with MND are *TDP-43*, *FUS* and *SOD1*.

Clinical features

The most common presentation (70%) is with wasting and weakness of one limb. Examination shows mixed upper and lower motor signs in several limbs – a combination of fasciculation,

Medicine at a Glance, Fifth Edition. Edited by Patrick Davey and Alex Pitcher.

Companion website: www.wiley.com/go/medicine5e

wasting, weakness, extensor plantar responses and brisk reflexes (amyotrophic lateral sclerosis). Tongue fasciculation is a useful sign because it makes a compressive lesion of the spinal cord an unlikely explanation for the observed neurological dysfunction.

Other patients (20%) present with prominent bulbar symptoms before developing signs in the limbs (progressive bulbar palsy) or a pure lower motor neuron picture of symmetrical weakness, wasting and areflexia (progressive muscular atrophy). Similarly, the disease may appear to be restricted to the upper motor neurons and presents a picture of progressive spastic paraparesis. This variant, known as primary lateral sclerosis, is more indolent and survival may be prolonged. Approximately 5% of patients have co-existing frontotemporal dementia and up to 40% have more subtle executive dysfunction.

Diagnosis

Diagnosis is clinical but supported by electromyographic demonstration of denervation in all four limbs. There are no specific treatments and management aims to preserve nutritional status and provide supportive respiratory and terminal care. The glutamate antagonist riluzole prolongs time to ventilation and tracheostomy by three months.

Poliomyelitis

Poliomyelitis is rarely seen in countries with effective immunization programmes. It produces asymmetrical motor weakness with bulbar and respiratory compromise in the context of an acute febrile illness. Some patients undergo late deterioration in function decades after the acute illness (post-polio syndrome).

Myasthenia gravis

Myasthenia gravis is an autoimmune disease – antibodies are directed against the acetylcholine receptor in the majority of patients and against the neuromuscular junction protein MUSK in a minority of others. The clinical features are variable, but include the following.

- Symmetrical proximal muscle weakness, which fatigues on exertion.
- Prominent involvement of the extraocular muscles, producing diplopia and ptosis. Significant limb weakness without eye involvement is rare. In contrast, myasthenia confined to the eyes (ocular myasthenia) is a distinct condition in which many patients do not have acetylcholine receptor antibodies and whose course is more benign.
- Bulbar involvement with dysphagia, dysarthria and a risk of aspiration.
- Myasthenic crises with a rapid evolution of neuromuscular weakness, leading to emergency ventilation.
- An association with thymoma in older patients, and thymic hyperplasia in younger patients.

Treatment is with immunomodulatory therapy (corticosteroids, azathioprine, plasma exchange), thymectomy and drugs that prolong the action of acetylcholine in the neuromuscular junction.

Inflammatory myopathies

Inflammatory myopathies are of presumed autoimmune aetiology, although usually without specific antibodies, where muscle is involved in isolation or in the context of a more diffuse connective tissue disease. They can be painful. The creatine phosphokinase level is elevated by several thousand. There is a clinical and pathological spectrum from polymyositis to dermatomyositis (see Chapter 220). The latter is associated in elderly people with malignancy and more often involves swallowing dysfunction. Therapy is with steroids, intravenous immunoglobulin and occasionally plasma exchange.

Inclusion body myositis affects middle-aged to elderly people and presents with the insidious onset of slowly progressive, asymmetrical, painless wasting and weakness of muscles, especially the quadriceps. There is no effective treatment.

Muscular dystrophies

Muscular dystrophies are inherited diseases leading to progressive wasting and weakness. The nosology of the dystrophies is being redefined according to specific genetic mutations and associated molecular deficits.

- Dystrophinopathies are caused by mutations in the gene encoding the very large membrane-associated protein dystrophin, thought to have a function in anchoring the muscle cytoskeleton to the extracellular matrix. Duchenne muscular dystrophy is caused by mutations that lead to complete loss of functional protein and a severe muscle disease, with onset in early childhood, loss of ambulation by adolescence and death in the twenties or thirties from cardiorespiratory failure. Becker dystrophy is caused by mutations in dystrophin, which produce a truncated and partially functional protein. Onset can be at any time from infancy to late adult life and the prognosis is much more favourable.
- Sarcoglycanopathies are rarer disorders resulting from mutations in genes encoding a variety of other membrane-associated proteins.
- Limb girdle muscular dystrophies.
- Facioscapulohumeral muscular dystrophy.
- Oculopharyngeal muscular dystrophy.

Myotonic dystrophy

Myotonic dystrophy is a multisystem disorder characterized by distal weakness and wasting, male-pattern balding, increased incidence of diabetes mellitus, cardiac conduction defects, cataract and excessive daytime somnolence. It is caused by mutations in the non-coding part of the myotonin protein kinase gene, which contains a triplet repeat (CTG) and undergoes dynamic expansion. Successive generations are progressively more severely affected (genetic anticipation). In one pedigree, the phenotype may range from cataract to congenital myotonic dystrophy with death in infancy. Genetic testing usually makes diagnosis by electromyography unnecessary.

Metabolic myopathies

Metabolic myopathies are rare disorders caused by specific enzyme defects in pathways important for muscle function. There is a wide spectrum of clinical presentation, but suggestive features are exertional muscle pain and myoglobinuria.

- Mitochondrial diseases: myopathy is associated with a variable phenotype, including glucose intolerance, pigmentary retinopathy, seizures, stroke-like episodes and deafness. One form is chronic progressive external ophthalmoplegia.
- Disorders of fatty acid metabolism, e.g. carnitine palmitoyl transferase deficiency.
- Disorders of carbohydrate metabolism, e.g. glycogen storage diseases such as acid maltase deficiency.
- Periodic paralysis occurs in a hypokalaemic and a rarer hyperkalaemic form. These are the result of mutations in ion channels (channelopathies). Patients present with attacks of generalized weakness lasting for several hours. Precipitants include large meals, alcohol and cold weather.

209 Peripheral neuropathy

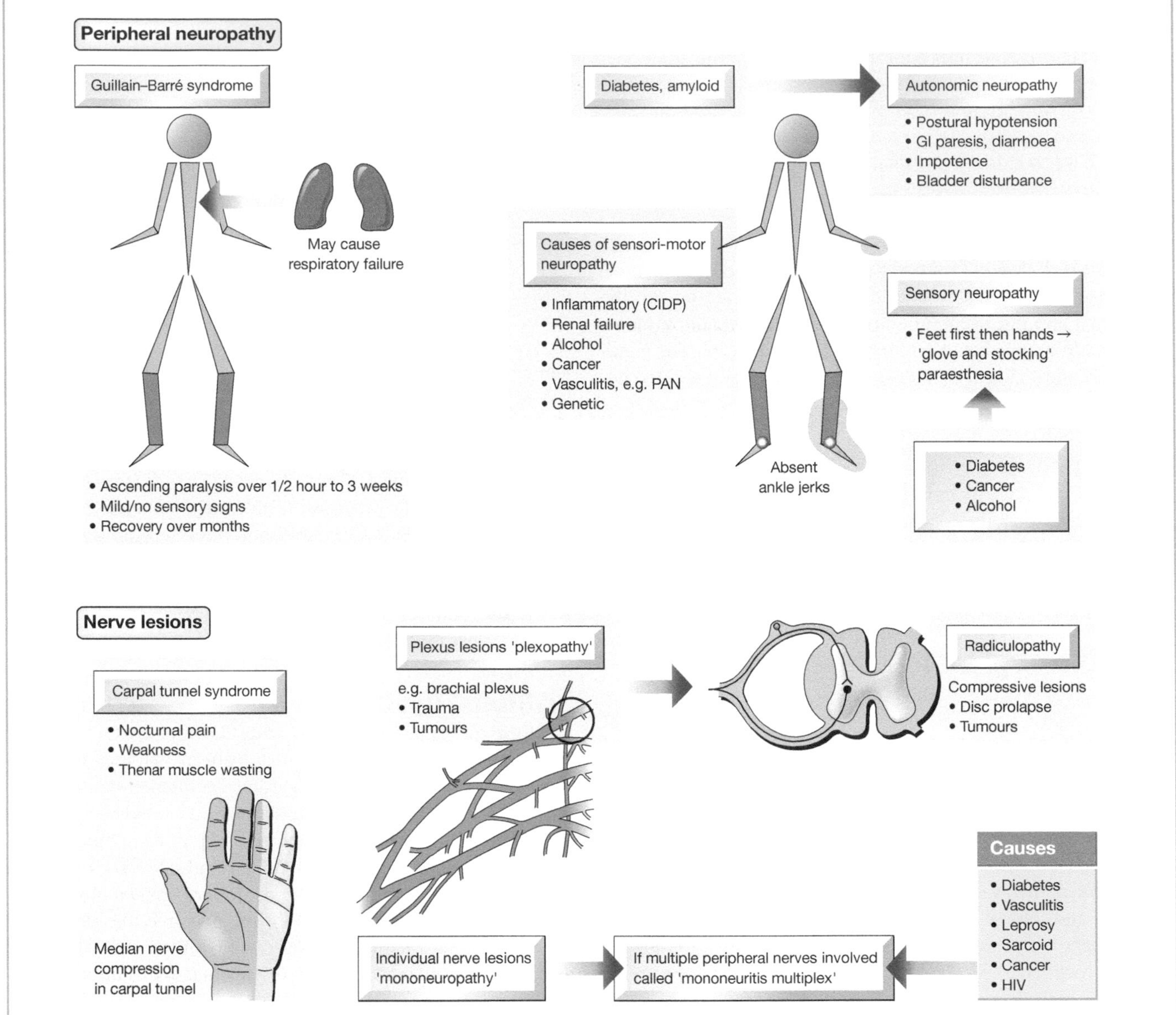

Clinical approach

Accurate diagnosis of a peripheral neuropathy requires an understanding of neuropathy classification and the speed of onset of symptoms, and a knowledge of which diseases commonly cause neuropathy.

Neuropathy classification

- **Polyneuropathies**: diffuse damage to peripheral nerves. The longest nerves (i.e. supplying the hand and foot) are most vulnerable to damage and are usually affected earliest. Polyneuropathies may be:
  - pure motor or pure sensory
  - sensorimotor: the most common pattern. Damage is symmetrical. Paraesthesiae and dysaesthesiae are early symptoms. Cramps and spasms commonly occur later. Examination shows diminution of reflexes, weakness, variable wasting and sensory loss. Sensory ataxia is manifest by rombergism and pseudoathetosis. Trophic changes such as ulcers and joint deformity are found in long-standing neuropathies
  - autonomic.
- **Radiculopathy**: a disorder of the nerve roots; if present at multiple levels, it is termed a polyradiculopathy.

Medicine at a Glance, Fifth Edition. Edited by Patrick Davey and Alex Pitcher.

Companion website: www.wiley.com/go/medicine5e

- **Plexopathy**: affecting the nerves of the brachial or lumbosacral plexus.
- **Mononeuropathy**: isolated to a single peripheral nerve, or if a number of anatomically discrete nerves are affected, it is called a mononeuritis multiplex.

Consider the evolution of the problem (although there is considerable overlap).

- Acute: vascular, inflammatory, toxic.
- Subacute: inflammatory, toxic, nutritional, systemic illness.
- Chronic: hereditary, metabolic.

Investigation of peripheral nerve disease

Initial screening blood tests should include full blood count, erythrocyte sedimentation rate, electrolytes and liver function tests to look for any evidence of systemic disease. Specific causes of neuropathy should be excluded with blood glucose, vitamin B_{12}, thyroid function, serum electrophoresis (for a paraprotein) and autoantibodies (especially antineutrophil cytoplasmic antibody and antinuclear antibody). Neuropathy is confirmed and classified (i.e. demyelinating vs axonal) by nerve conduction studies and electromyography (EMG). Parameters measured include (i) nerve conduction velocity; (ii) amplitude of nerve and muscle response to stimulation; and (iii) denervation of muscle, i.e. spontaneous electrical activity (fibrillation).

In demyelinating neuropathies (e.g. Guillain–Barré syndrome), there is slowing of conduction velocity and little evidence of denervation. In axonal neuropathy (e.g. caused by drugs such as vincristine), there is normal motor conduction velocity with decreased compound muscle action potential and evidence of denervation on EMG.

Nerve biopsy is not performed frequently. It is most useful to confirm vasculitis before commencing therapy.

Polyneuropathies

Inherited

Peripheral neuropathy occurs as part of many complex neurogenetic disorders. The most common cause of inherited, isolated, peripheral neuropathy is hereditary motor and sensory neuropathy or Charcot–Marie–Tooth disease. The most common genetic subtype is a duplication of part of the short arm of chromosome 17, which causes a very slowly progressive demyelinating neuropathy with wasting below the knees, pes cavus and hand involvement.

Metabolic derangement

- Diabetes mellitus is the most common cause of peripheral neuropathy in the developed world. The usual picture is a progressive, predominantly sensory neuropathy. Loss of vibration sense is the earliest sign. Over time, if diabetes is poorly controlled, autonomic involvement becomes universal. Pain can be difficult to manage. Vitamin deficiencies (vitamin B_{12}, thiamine, vitamin E) all cause neuropathy as part of a broader neurological syndrome.
- Chronic renal failure and liver failure can produce peripheral neuropathy.
- Hypothyroidism is a rare cause.

Toxic and drug induced

Alcohol is a very common cause, as are drugs: amiodarone, metronidazole, cytotoxics, pyridoxine, isoniazid, dapsone, lithium, antiretrovirals.

Inflammatory/immune polyneuropathy

- Guillain–Barré syndrome: incidence 1–2 per 100 000. It is an autoimmune response occuring typically 1–3 weeks after an infection (cytomegalovirus and *Campylobacter* sp. are most common). Mild sensory symptoms are often present. Weakness, which is usually a mixture of proximal and distal, ascends proximally over a few days. Respiratory failure requiring ventilation may occur (vital capacity should be frequently measured). Spontaneous recovery – sometimes full, occasionally incomplete – is usual, although 5% die. Autonomic imbalance can produce cardiac arrhythmias. Illness duration is shortened with γ-globulin or plasma exchange, but steroids are ineffective.
- Chronic idiopathic demyelinating polyneuropathy (CIDP) runs a waxing–waning course. Nerve conduction studies are diagnostic. Steroids or γ-globulin help.
- Other neuropathies: vasculitis, critical illness polyneuropathy, infective (leprosy, Lyme disease, HIV, diphtheria), traumatic (entrapment or crush injuries) and paraneoplastic.

Common mononeuropathies

Nerve entrapment is generally the result of local factors, but in some conditions it is much more common and sometimes multiple: (i) hypothyroidism; (ii) acromegaly; (iii) Paget disease; (iv) rheumatoid disease; and (v) hereditary neuropathy with susceptibility to pressure palsies caused by deletion of the *PMP-22* gene.

In mononeuropathies, it is important to consider the possibility that the apparently isolated nerve lesion is part of a mononeuritis multiplex syndrome.

- **Median nerve**: by far the most common mononeuropathy is carpal tunnel syndrome. Lifetime incidence is 6% in women, 0.6% in men (especially manual workers using vibrating machinery). Typical symptoms are of pain, discomfort and tingling in the hand radiating to the forearm and occasionally the shoulder. These commonly wake the patient from sleep and are relieved by shaking the wrist. Symptoms are also precipitated by repetitive flexion at the wrist, e.g. when steering a car. Treatment is by surgical release. Wrist splints are occasionally helpful.
- **Ulnar nerve**: this nerve is vulnerable to compression and injury at the elbow (e.g. arthritis, fracture) where it is superficially located. Patients present with numbness of the little and ring fingers and ulnar border of the hand, wasting and weakness of the first dorsal interosseous, and weakness of the abductor digiti minimi.
- **Lateral popliteal (common peroneal) nerve**: this is very vulnerable to compressive injury at the head of the fibula (e.g. by a plaster cast). Lesions cause painless foot drop as a result of weakness of tibialis anterior. The ankle jerk is retained.

Rarer mononeuropathies

Radial nerve damage is the result of nerve compression in the axilla (e.g. by a chair: 'Saturday night' palsy) or as the nerve winds round the head of the humerus. Patients present with wrist drop.

Femoral nerve damage relates to diabetes, pelvic lesions, particularly inflammation or haematoma (in anticoagulated patients), iliopsoas pathology or, more rarely, lesions in the femoral canal. The quadriceps wastes, extension at the knee is weak, and there is variable sensory loss over the anterior thigh.

Mononeuritis multiplex

This occurs in diabetes, systemic vasculitis, leprosy, sarcoidosis, non-metastatic manifestation of malignancy and HIV. Investigation and treatment are of the underlying disease.

210 Movement disorders

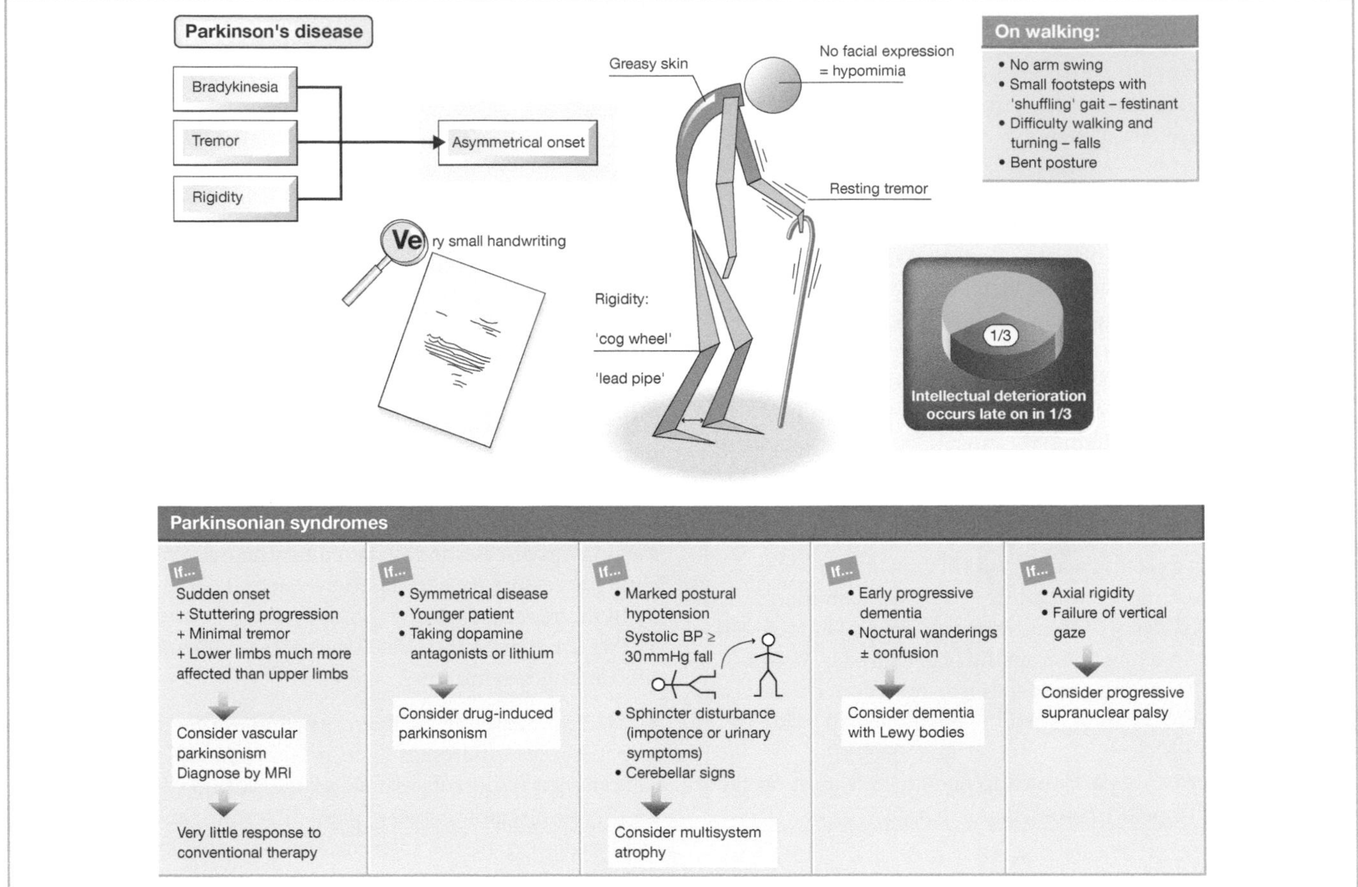

Parkinsonism

The term 'parkinsonism' describes a syndrome of poverty of movement, resting tremor, rigidity and varying degrees of postural instability.

Parkinson disease is characterized by asymmetrical onset, slow progression and good response to L-dopa therapy. Only 60% develop tremor. The pathology is loss of dopamine-producing cells of the substantia nigra and Lewy bodies (intraneuronal inclusions). The aetiology, except in genetic cases, is poorly understood. Although predominantly an age-dependent sporadic disease, about 5% of patients have mutations in a range of genes. Onset in young adulthood (<30 years) is associated with a recessive mutation in the *Parkin* gene. Mutations in *LRRK2* cause the disease and the common *Gly2019Ser* mutation is present in 1% of patients with sporadic and 4% of patients with hereditary Parkinson disease.

Diagnosis

The diagnosis is clinical – structural imaging is normal. Helpful signs are asymmetrical loss of arm swing, micrographia (small handwriting) and facial hypomimia, and the more 'classic' signs of 'cogwheel' stiffness and resting tremor. Bradykinesia is best tested for by checking repetitive finger or foot tapping, which shows degradation in amplitude and interruptions in Parkinson disease. Other neurodegenerative conditions are included in the differential diagnosis and are suspected if there are:

- early falls
- early cognitive impairment
- symmetrical onset
- prominent autonomic disturbance including sphincter involvement
- pyramidal tract or cerebellar signs.

Treatment and prognosis

Parkinson disease is progressive and pharmacological manipulation changes as the condition advances. At onset, it is usually a problem of poverty of movement. Later on, troublesome dyskinesia, unpredictable freezing and 'on–off' phenomena dominate the picture. Ten percent of patients develop these problems for each year from diagnosis. Most patients ultimately develop detectable cognitive impairment, with frank dementia in about one-third.

Medicine at a Glance, Fifth Edition. Edited by Patrick Davey and Alex Pitcher.

Companion website: www.wiley.com/go/medicine5e

Drug therapy involves increasing dopamine levels in the central nervous system (CNS), by giving either L-dopa with a peripheral decarboxylase inhibitor, or drugs that stimulate CNS dopamine receptors (dopamine agonists, e.g. pramipexole, ropinorole, cabergoline, apomorphine) or inhibit the breakdown of CNS dopamine. Drug side-effects are common and include dyskinesias and 'on–off' phenomena. Dopamine agonists should be used with caution and are associated with rare but devastating side-effects in susceptible individuals, such as pathological gambling and hypersexuality. In complex disease, dominated by unintended side-effects of medication, deep brain stimulation, especially of the subthalamic nucleus, is used.

Drug-induced parkinsonism

Neuroleptics, antiemetics and occasionally calcium channel blockers and lithium can all produce parkinsonism. This is typically an early side-effect and is more common with ageing. In contrast to Parkinson disease, it is symmetrical in onset, tremor is less prominent and improvement occurs on withdrawal of the offending agent. Sometimes drugs unmask idiopathic Parkinson disease.

Vascular parkinsonism

This rare disorder is characterized by bradykinesia and rigidity of the lower limbs, with marked sparing of the upper limbs. There will usually be a history of stuttering evolution, vascular risk factors and an abnormal magnetic resonance image.

Neurodegenerative akinetic–rigid syndromes mimicking Parkinson disease

- **Multiple system atrophy** (MSA): formerly known as Shy–Drager syndrome, nigrostriatal degeneration or olivopontocerebellar atrophy, depending on the predominant clinical features, until it was realized that all these conditions are linked by the same pathology (specific glial inclusions that stain for α-synuclein) and that they overlap clinically. Current classification divides the condition into MSA-P if parkinsonian features predominate, or MSA-C if cerebellar features dominate. Patients have the insidious onset of parkinsonism with sphincter disturbance, postural hypotension, cerebellar signs and, characteristically but less commonly, stridor. Cognition is unaffected. The prognosis is poor (death within 2–8 years) and the response to L-dopa is absent or rapidly wanes.
- **Progressive supranuclear palsy**: characterized by prominent axial rigidity, loss of postural reflexes leading to early falls, progressive loss of downgaze and upgaze, dystonia of eyelid opening and facial dystonia imparting a characteristic expression of frowning and surprise. Cognitive impairment occurs later in the condition, which leads to death within 5–7 years.
- **Dementia with Lewy bodies**: parkinsonism with prominent nocturnal wanderings and hallucinations, early and progressive cognitive impairment and myoclonus. Poor response to L-dopa and idiosyncratic but severe reactions to neuroleptics.
- **Corticobasal degeneration**: the picture is of a stuttering evolution of parkinsonism plus parietal lobe abnormalities, including, characteristically, an alien limb abnormality of the arm, dysphasia, extensor plantars, myoclonus and dystonia, and dementia. It is rare. Death occurs in 5–7 years.

Dystonia

Dystonic tremor can mimic Parkinson disease and typically manifests as a jerky, irregular tremor often alleviated when the patient adopts particular positions (the 'null' point) or aggravated by specific tasks. Focal dystonias such as writer's cramp and hemifacial spasm (see Chapter 62) can be treated with injections of botulinum toxin. It is a presynaptic blocker of neuromuscular transmission, causing weakness of the injected muscles for up to three months, relieving the symptoms over that period.

Huntington disease

Huntington disease is caused by an expanded trinucleotide repeat mutation in the *Huntingtin* gene and is inherited as an autosomal dominant. This is a disorder of insidious onset and inexorable progression, in which the first changes are often in personality (poor impulse control, irritability); the subsequent development of chorea, dementia and immobility occurs over 10–15 years.

Drug-induced movement disorders

The neuroleptic class of drugs (e.g. haloperidol), including antiemetics (e.g. prochlorperazine), are dopamine receptor antagonists and, in addition to parkinsonism, can induce acute dystonias, including oculogyric crisis, akathisia (motor restlessness) and tardive dyskinesias. The last are involuntary writhing movements of the face (especially mouth) and limbs, commonly seen in patients treated for schizophrenia.

Movement disorders in young people

The main condition to consider is Wilson disease because it is treatable. This is an autosomal recessive disease caused by mutations in a gene coding for a copper-transporting protein. It can present as:

- fulminant hepatic failure in childhood
- progressive neuropsychiatric disturbance in adolescence
- focal dystonia, dysarthria and drooling.

Diagnosis is by finding a low level of ceruloplasmin and free copper in serum. Patients with neurological Wilson disease all have Kayser–Fleischer rings visible on slit-lamp examination of the cornea. The condition is treated by copper chelation therapy, usually with penicillamine.

Movement disorders relating to infection

A variety of movement disorders occur as an immune reaction to infections, especially *Streptococcus*. Patients can present with chorea, parkinsonism or some combination including mild psychiatric symptoms such as obsessionality or tics. In a significant proportion of patients, it is possible to identify antibasal ganglia antibodies, though the association is still uncertain.

Gilles de la Tourette syndrome

Gilles de la Tourette syndrome presents with a combination of multiple motor and vocal tics (i.e. involuntary vocalizations), both of varying complexity, with onset in childhood usually between seven and 11 years of age. The prevalence is 1/2000 with a very wide range of severity. Involuntary swearing (coprolalia) is a feature in a minority of cases. Obsessive–compulsive disorder is often also present. The tics can be treated with neuroleptics, e.g. sulpiride, or clomipramine.

Dopa-responsive dystonia

Dopa-responsive dystonia is another rare but treatable genetic disorder caused by mutations in a gene in the pathway of dopa synthesis. It presents with lower limb dystonia, which fluctuates throughout the day. Treatment with L-dopa can result in dramatic improvement.

211 Osteoarthritis

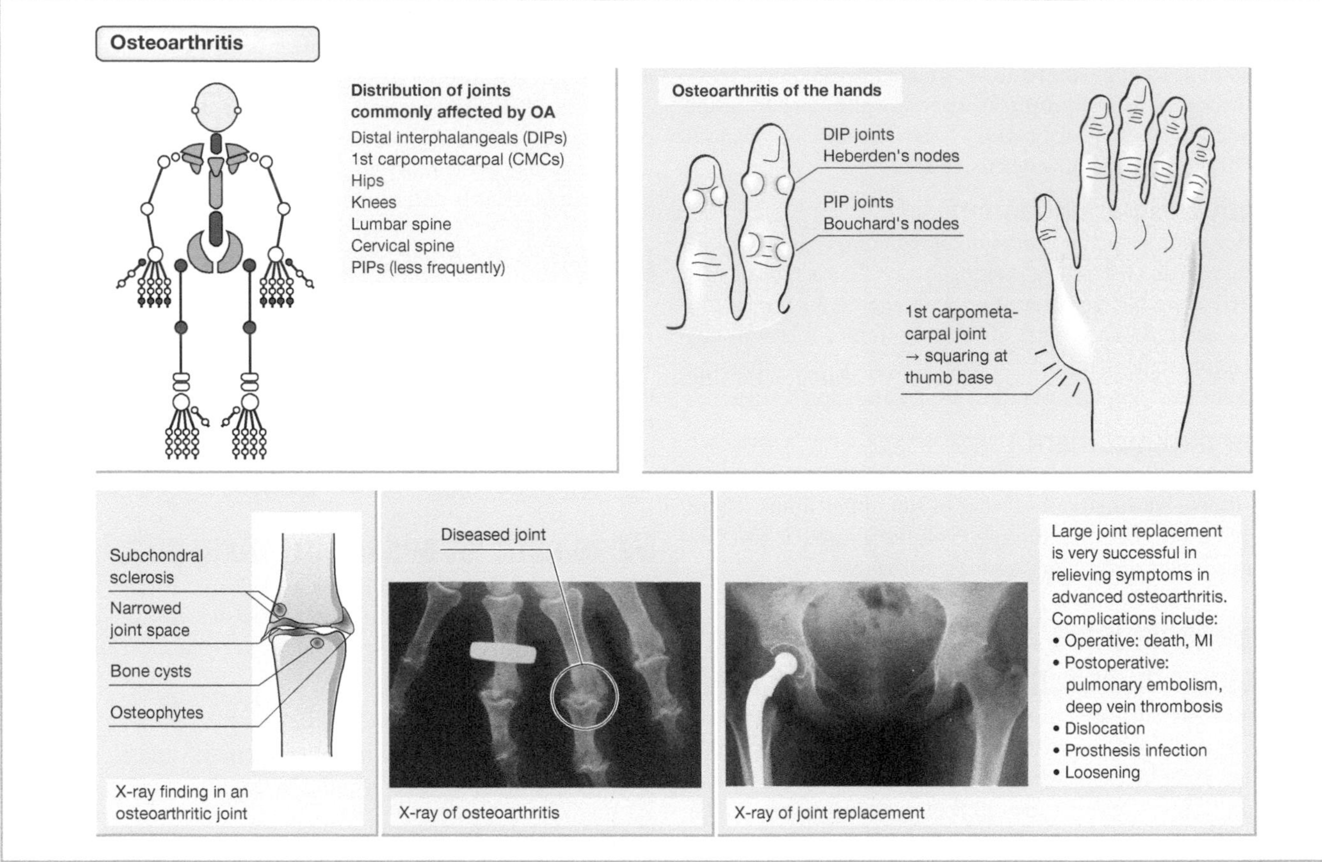

Osteoarthritis (OA) is the most common arthropathy of adults. Its aetiology is multifactorial, and it is characterized by progressive cartilage loss and hypertrophic changes in surrounding bone (osteophytosis), resulting in progressive joint disease. Inflammation is now considered to contribute to pathogenesis but is not a marked clinical feature.

Epidemiology

The overall prevalence of OA is 12–15% in at least one joint, and is much higher in the >65 year age group. The prevalence continually increases with advancing age, such that more than 80% of >75 year olds have radiographic evidence of OA. There is a slight female preponderance overall, particularly in interphalangeal joint disease.

Aetiology and pathogenesis

The cause is unknown but familial aggregation of cases is consistent with an important genetic contribution. Siblings of patients undergoing major lower limb joint replacement for OA are three times more likely than the general population to require similar surgery themselves.

Pathological features are primarily those of progressive cartilage damage and loss, but it is increasingly recognized that pathological changes may also occur in the subchondral bone, joint capsule and surrounding structures. There is also increasing evidence that inflammation plays a role in pathogenesis. Matrix metalloproteinases and cytokines released into the joint may mediate cartilage damage and loss via accelerated matrix degradation. Reactive bony hypertrophy next to cartilage loss results in characteristic 'osteophyte' development. There is subchondral bone sclerosis and cyst formation which is evident on plain X-rays (see figure above).

Classification

1 **Primary or idiopathic OA.**
2 **Secondary OA**: this arises from the following causes.
   - Trauma, including repetitive use in some occupations associated with heavy loading of the joints. OA may also develop as a late complication of trauma, particularly if osteochondral fracture or meniseal injury has occurred in the knee.
   - Obesity increases the risk of knee OA.

Medicine at a Glance, Fifth Edition. Edited by Patrick Davey and Alex Pitcher.

Companion website: www.wiley.com/go/medicine5e

- Congenital conditions, e.g. hip dislocation or underlying joint dysplasia.
- Inflammatory arthritis (rheumatoid arthritis, gout).
- A late complication following bacterial infection of a joint.
- Acromegaly.
- Haemophilia.

Clinical features

The following are distinguishing features in the history.

- Joint pain tends to be insidious in onset. Typically, there is slow stepwise deterioration in symptoms.
- Pain is aggravated by activity, relieved by rest, is worst at the end of the day and as the condition progresses, and becomes increasingly severe, occurring on minimal movement. Sleep disturbance may exacerbate fatigue and be associated with secondary fibromyalgia.
- Stiffness is minor in the morning but recurs throughout the day with periods of rest, and is described as 'gelling' following inactivity.
- Bony swelling may be noted particularly in the hands (see figure above) as Heberden's nodes (distal interphalangeal [DIP] joint involvement) and Bouchard's nodes (proximal interphalangeal [PIP] joint involvement). Variable symmetry of large joint involvement occurs that often impairs gait and mobility.

Physical findings

The distribution of joints affected in OA is shown in the figure. Examination reveals the following.

- Bony prominence due to a combination of marginal osteophytes and joint deformities (occasionally OA can cause effusions, particularly if it is associated with intra-articular calcium crystal deposition).
- Malalignment, e.g. varus deformity due to medial compartment OA at the knee.
- Reduction in range of movement in affected joints with 'end of range' pain and limitation, and palpable 'crepitus'.
- Instability in later stages, particularly where there is associated muscle wasting around the joint and substantial cartilage loss.

Subsets of osteoarthritis

- **Primary generalized OA**: predominantly in middle-aged women, affecting the first carpometacarpal (CMC) joint, PIP joint, distal DIP joint, knee, hips and spine.
- **Chondromalacia patellae**: limited patellofemoral joint OA, causing pain on climbing stairs, running or squatting.
- **Inflammatory/erosive OA**: this affects predominantly postmenopausal women in the distal DIP and/or PIP joints of the hand. Episodes of pain and clinical inflammation may mimic rheumatoid or psoriatic arthritis. X-rays often show erosions as well as the classic hallmarks of OA. It is probably associated with crystal deposition (calcium pyrophosphate, hydroxyapatite).

Investigations

Inflammatory markers (erythrocyte sedimentation rate, C-reactive protein) are normal; serology for antinuclear antibody and rheumatoid factor is unnecessary except in cases with symptoms suggestive of clinical inflammation. Synovial fluid from joint aspiration is clear with normal viscosity and is non-inflammatory (low white cell count) on microscopy; the fluid should be examined for calcium pyrophosphate crystals. Plain X-ray reveals characteristic features of joint space narrowing, bony sclerosis, subchondral cysts and osteophytes (the radiological hallmark) (see figure). Consider iron and calcium studies in those with atypical distribution or age of onset (to exclude haemochromatosis or hyperparathyroidism).

The differential diagnosis may include arthropathy of psoriasis, reactive arthritis or crystal deposition disease, indicating tests for these conditions where clinically indicated.

Management

The goals of therapy are to relieve pain and maintain function. Management is multifaceted and should include non-pharmacological approaches. These include education, risk factor assessment and modification (e.g. weight loss); activity modification (flexibility, strength and resistance/endurance training); consideration of assistive devices (stick or mobilization aid); physiotherapy and occupational therapy.

Pharmacological management

- There is currently no disease-modifying treatment for osteoarthritis, so pharmacological management relies largely on analgesia. Choice of analgesia should take into account the patient's severity of symptoms, any co-morbidities and risk of adverse event.
- A stepwise approach begins with the lowest effective dose of simple analgesia such as paracetamol, and topical therapies such as ice, heat or locally applied analgesic creams or gels such as topical non-steroidal anti-inflammatory drugs (NSAIDs) or capsaicin.
- Oral low-dose NSAIDs may be used in those without contraindication or adverse risk profile.
- Unresponsive or progressive pain may necessitate full-dose NSAID therapy or other analgesia. Opioid analgesia should be avoided in hip or knee OA and reserved only for exceptional circumstances.
- Intra-articular injection of corticosteroid sometimes gives relief of pain, though this may be short-lived. Repeated injections six months apart may be beneficial in symptom control, usually to a maximum of three injections into a single joint. Periarticular injection of painful soft tissues may also be of benefit. In a small number of patients, a course of intra-articular injections of hyaluronan (a component of synovial fluid) may be useful.

Physical therapy and activity modification

- Weight reduction substantially reduces the loading of lower limb load-bearing joints, which may be up to six times body weight during exercise.
- Low-impact aerobic exercise regimens (cycling/swimming) and weight loss programmes are particularly associated with symptomatic improvement and may reduce progression and the requirement for surgery.
- 'Unloading' of the joint using an 'assistive device' (e.g. stick) or mobilization aid may reduce pain. Of note, these may increase load and provoke symptoms on the contralateral side.
- Knee braces and foot orthoses may be helpful for lower limb problems. Small joint splints, e.g. 'thumb splints', may be useful for hand OA.

Surgical therapy

- Joint replacement surgery (arthroplasty) dramatically improves pain, function and quality of life in those with advanced disease. Outcome following hip or knee surgery is good or excellent in 95% of patients. The prostheses may be expected to function satisfactorily for 15 years. The main complications are sepsis and aseptic loosening. Revision surgery may subsequently be required and still provides good results in 80% of cases.
- 'Joint preservation surgery' may be helpful in addressing labral tears or femoroacetabular impingement (hip).

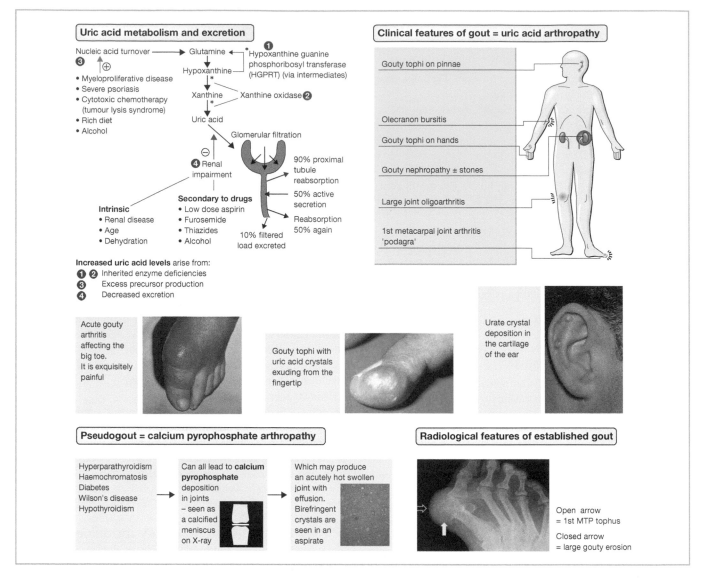

212 Gout and pseudogout (calcium pyrophosphate dihydrate arthropathy)

Uric acid metabolism and excretion

Nucleic acid turnover → Glutamine ← *Hypoxanthine guanine phosphoribosyl transferase (HGPRT) (via intermediates) ❶

❸ ⊕
- Myeloproliferative disease
- Severe psoriasis
- Cytotoxic chemotherapy (tumour lysis syndrome)
- Rich diet
- Alcohol

Hypoxanthine → * Xanthine → * Uric acid

Xanthine oxidase ❷

Glomerular filtration

⊖ ❹ Renal impairment

Intrinsic
- Renal disease
- Age
- Dehydration

Secondary to drugs
- Low dose aspirin
- Furosemide
- Thiazides
- Alcohol

90% proximal tubule reabsorption

50% active secretion

Reabsorption 50% again

10% filtered load excreted

Increased uric acid levels arise from:

❶ ❷ Inherited enzyme deficiencies

❸ Excess precursor production

❹ Decreased excretion

Clinical features of gout = uric acid arthropathy

Gouty tophi on pinnae

Olecranon bursitis

Gouty tophi on hands

Gouty nephropathy ± stones

Large joint oligoarthritis

1st metacarpal joint arthritis 'podagra'

Acute gouty arthritis affecting the big toe. It is exquisitely painful

Gouty tophi with uric acid crystals exuding from the fingertip

Urate crystal deposition in the cartilage of the ear

Pseudogout = calcium pyrophosphate arthropathy

Hyperparathyroidism
Haemochromatosis
Diabetes
Wilson's disease
Hypothyroidism

→ Can all lead to **calcium pyrophosphate** deposition in joints – seen as a calcified meniscus on X-ray

→ Which may produce an acutely hot swollen joint with effusion. Birefringent crystals are seen in an aspirate

Radiological features of established gout

Open arrow = 1st MTP tophus

Closed arrow = large gouty erosion

Crystal-related arthropathy defines a syndrome of synovitis (synovial inflammation) in response to crystal deposition/formation in the joint. Two types of crystals are commonly implicated: monosodium urate (gout) and calcium pyrophosphate dihydrate (pseudogout). The resulting synovitis may be limited to a single joint (monoarticular) or become more widespread (polyarticular). Gout is the more common entity.

Gout

Epidemiology

Gout is the most common form of inflammatory arthritis, affecting up to 3.9% of the adult population in the USA and up to 2.5% in Europe. The age standardized prevalence rate increased annually from 1990 to 2017, with highest increases in countries with a high sociodemographic index. The age standardized prevalence rate in 2017 for males (790/100 000) was >3× that for females (253/100 000). Gout almost never occurs in premenopausal females and increases in both sexes with age. Disability associated with gout is also increasing annually. Factors contributing to the global burden of gout include high BMI and impaired kidney function. Environmental factors such as dietary purine intake, alcohol consumption and the use of drugs such as diuretics contribute. Inherited metabolic abnormalities contribute by causing overproduction or underexcretion of uric acid.

Hyperuricaemia: pathogenesis and measurement

Uric acid is the end-product of purine metabolism and is produced and excreted as shown in the figure. Hyperuricemia = serum uric

Medicine at a Glance, Fifth Edition. Edited by Patrick Davey and Alex Pitcher.

Companion website: www.wiley.com/go/medicine5e

acid (SUA) >416 μmol/L (>339 μmol/L in premenopausal women). Any factor causing overproduction or underexcretion will raise SUA. Gout may occur with normal range SUA and raised SUA is not *diagnostic* of gout (see below). The risk of developing acute gout increases as SUA increases.

- Levels <420 μmol/l are associated with an incidence of 0.8/1000.
- Levels of >540 μmol/l increase this to 49/1000.

Serial SUA measurement guides treatment of gout (treat to SUA target approach).

Clinical features

Hyperuricaemia is associated with gouty arthropathy, kidney disease and metabolic syndrome (a cluster of risk factors for cardiovascular disease and events).

The spectrum of clinical features of gouty arthropathy is shown in the figure.

- Classic gout gives rise to a monoarthritis: 50% start in the first metatarsophalangeal (MTP) joint. Ten percent of first episodes are polyarticular. Crystal arthritis characteristically gives rise to severe pain, redness, swelling and tenderness, usually with a peak intensity within 12 hours of onset. Attacks are agonizing and may last 7–10 days.
- Acute episodes of gout may be triggered by trauma (including surgery), exercise, alcohol excess, volume depletion (including diuretic use) or starvation.
- Acute gout may progress to chronic gout. Chronic gout usually requires uric acid-lowering therapy.
- Chronic gout may be associated with characteristic subcutaneous deposits of urate (tophi – 'tophaceous gout') and may become polyarticular in nature.
- Urate crystals may precipitate in the renal parenchyma, giving rise to gouty nephropathy and renal stones. This may worsen pre-existing renal impairment which is in turn a risk factor for hyperuricaemia.

Differential diagnosis

The differential diagnosis of monoarticular gout includes septic arthritis, trauma and cellulitis, as there is often significant swelling and erythema of the surrounding tissues. The patient may also be febrile. The differential of asymmetrical, large joint, polyarticular gout includes the seronegative arthropathies and osteoarthritis.

Investigations

The clinical picture is often highly suggestive (see Clinical features). However, definitive diagnosis requires demonstration of intracellular monosodium urate crystals in synovial fluid neutrophils aspirated from the inflamed joint. These are seen as negatively birefringent needle-shaped crystals on polarized light microscopy. Crystals may also be obtained from a tophus. As joint sepsis may co-exist with gout, microscopy and culture of synovial fluid should also be undertaken.

- Measurement of SUA is *not diagnostic*. Uric acid levels may be normal in 20% of acute attacks and abnormal in asymptomatic individuals.
- Patients without clear risk factors (e.g. premenopausal females or young males with no family history) should have a full blood count to rule out haemolysis or occult haematological malignancy (increased DNA turnover generates purines and may give rise to gout). Determination of renal excretion of uric acid may also be indicated in those without clear risk factors and is mandatory if renal calculi are present.
- Plain radiographs in established gout show punched-out cortical erosions (see figure), often away from the joint margin, unlike the erosions found in rheumatoid arthritis.
- Plain radiographs in pseudogout sometimes show calcification of the fibrocartilage (e.g. knee menisci, triangular cartilage in wrist) and hyaline cartilage (knee, glenohumeral joint). The structural changes are similar to those of osteroarthritis, with cartilage loss, sclerosis, cysts and osteophytes, which may be prominent and exuberant.
- Given the association between gout and the metabolic syndrome (obesity, hyperglycaemia, hyperlipidaemia, hypertension), these co-morbid conditions should be sought and treated to reduce cardiovascular risk.

Management

Treatment of the acute attack

European Alliance of Associations for Rheumatology (EULAR) guidelines for gout advise early treatment with oral colchicine and/or non-steroidal anti-inflammatory drugs (NSAIDs) as first-line agents for the acute attack. Where colchicine and/or NSAIDs are contraindicated, a 3–5-day course of oral prednisolone may be preferable and is the treatment of choice for severe polyarticular flares. Intra-articular aspiration and injection of long-acting steroid are both safe and effective in the acute attack.

Prophylaxis against further attacks

All patients should be educated on risk reduction (avoidance of alcohol, sugar-sweetened drinks, excessive meat and seafood intake; weight loss). Urate-lowering therapy (ULT) is indicated in all patients with recurrent flares, erosive arthropathy, tophi and/or renal stones and recommended following the first attack for those under 40, with co-morbidities or high SUA >480 mmol/l. This is achieved by pharmacological inhibition of xanthine oxidase (allopurinol or febuxostat) or promotion of uric acid excretion (probenicid). A 'treat to SUA target' approach is recommended with gradual uptitration of ULT to achieve a target SUA level of 360 mmol/l (most) or 300 mmol/l (chronic erosive arthropathy/tophi/polyarticular flares).

Colchicine (or NSAID if colchicine cannot be used) should be maintained for the first six months of ULT to reduce the risk of flares. Patients with crystal proven, severe tophaceous gout in whom target SUA cannot be reached with ULT can be offered rasburicase. Doses of colchicine and allopurinol should be adjusted in renal impairment and NSAIDs avoided.

Patients commencing certain cancer chemotherapy regimes may be at risk of hyperuricaemia due to tumour lysis syndrome. Those deemed at risk should be pretreated with fluids and allopurinol (or recombinant rasburicase) to prevent gout and crystal-induced renal tubular injury.

Pseudogout (CPPD arthropathy)

Calcium pyrophosphate deposits (CPPD) in joint cartilage are a common age-related phenomenon which may be present in one-quarter of those >60 years old. Less commonly, it is related to a familial predisposition (activating mutations in Ank, a trans-membrane transporter of inorganic pyrophosphate), hyperparathyroidism, haemochromatosis or magnesium. When CPPD crystals are released into the joint, they induce an inflammatory response resulting in synovitis, presenting as an acute monoarthritis. Diagnosis is by joint aspiration and the demonstration of characteristic positively birefringent rhomboidal crystals in the synovial fluid on polarized light microscopy. Treatment is with NSAIDs or intra-articular steroids. Pyrophosphate arthropathy often has a chronic course, which may mimic rheumatoid arthritis or osteoarthritis. Fifty percent of such cases are punctuated by episodes of acute pseudogout. Pseudogout is the most common cause of monoarthritis in the elderly.

Arthritis associated with infectious agents

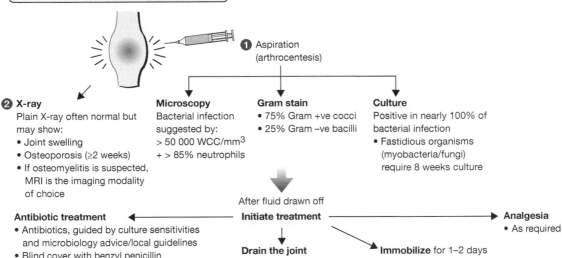

Routes by which infection can reach a joint

1. Haematogenous spread from remote site
2. Local spread from adjacent osteomyelitis
3. Local spread from adjacent skin/soft tissue infection, e.g. cellulitis, bursitis
4. Iatrogenic spread from diagnostic/ therapeutic measure
5. Trauma including puncture, cutting, intravenous drug abuse

Management of septic arthritis

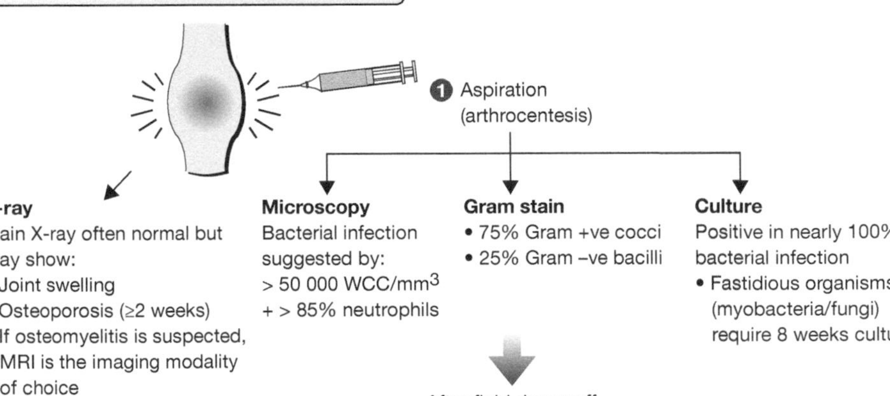

2 X-ray
Plain X-ray often normal but may show:
- Joint swelling
- Osteoporosis (≥2 weeks)
- If osteomyelitis is suspected, MRI is the imaging modality of choice

Microscopy
Bacterial infection suggested by:
> 50 000 WCC/mm^3
+ > 85% neutrophils

Gram stain
- 75% Gram +ve cocci
- 25% Gram –ve bacilli

Culture
Positive in nearly 100% of bacterial infection
- Fastidious organisms (myobacteria/fungi) require 8 weeks culture

After fluid drawn off

Initiate treatment

Antibiotic treatment
- Antibiotics, guided by culture sensitivities and microbiology advice/local guidelines
- Blind cover with benzyl penicillin + flucloxacillin unless unusual organisms are suspected
- Treat according to sensitivities, once they become available

Drain the joint
- Aspiration/arthroscopy
- Joints such as the hip should be aspirated under imaging guidance
- Hip and prosthetic joints – refer for early orthopaedic intervention
- Consider arthroscopic washout in all cases

Immobilize for 1–2 days
- Then passive range of mobile exercises
- Then active/weight bearing as infection resolves

Analgesia
- As required

Medicine at a Glance, Fifth Edition. Edited by Patrick Davey and Alex Pitcher.

Companion website: www.wiley.com/go/medicine5e

Definitions

Three distinct clinical patterns are recognized.

1 Septic arthritis from colonization with pathogenic organisms.
2 Arthritis as a significant clinical feature of systemic infection, e.g. rubella, parvovirus B19 infection, Lyme disease.
3 Reactive arthritis: a sterile joint inflammation that develops as an immunologically mediated reaction to infection at a distant site. Triggering infections most commonly arise in the urogenital or gastrointestinal tract. Reactive arthritis is considered in Chapter 217.

Epidemiology of joint infection

Annual incidence varies widely and is related to the prevalence of the underlying predisposing conditions.

Septic arthritis

Pathogenesis and aetiology

Pathogenic organisms may reach a joint by several routes (see figure). Predisposing factors include the following.

- **Impaired host defences.**
  - Inherited impairment of host defences, e.g. complement deficiency, hypogammaglobulinaemia.
  - Immunosuppressive illness or therapy, e.g. HIV, steroids, cytotoxics.
  - Chronic illness, e.g. diabetes mellitus, renal failure, cirrhosis, leg ulcers.
  - Elderly or very young.
- The presence of a **prosthetic or damaged joint** (osteoarthritis/rheumatoid arthritis/gout).

Notably, septic arthritis is usually a disease of the very young, the elderly or those with damaged joints. Young adults with disseminated gonococcal infection may present with septic arthritis.

Clinical features

Septic arthritis affects the knee, hip, shoulder, wrist, ankle and elbow most commonly. Twenty percent of presentations are polyarticular. Symptoms are usually sudden in onset and progressive, usually with florid systemic features. The joint(s) is red, swollen, tender and hot. It is usually held in flexion, avoiding movement and weight bearing. Disseminated gonococcal infection may feature urogenital or CNS symptoms and a pustular rash. Prosthetic joint infection in the early postoperative period is usually self-evident with high fever and a wound discharging pus. Later infection is associated with low-grade fever, recurrent pain, impaired function and less impressive local signs. Infection should always be considered in those with loosening of the prosthesis.

Organisms responsible for septic arthritis

In healthy adults the range of pathogens is narrow.

- *Staphylococcus aureus* is the most frequent joint pathogen in adults.
- About 25% of infections overall are due to Gram-negative bacilli.
- 15% are due to β-haemolytic streptococci.

In the immunocompromised subject, consider less typical organisms.

- Gram-negative bacilli and *Streptococcus pneumoniae* in the debilitated patient (malignancy, chronic alcohol use, diabetes, etc.).
- *Pseudomonas* in people who inject drugs.
- Under two years of age: high incidence of *Haemophilus influenzae* infection.

Management

A management algorithm of joint sepsis is shown in the figure. Antibiotic therapy should be selected depending on joint aspirate culture and sensitivity. There is no evidence base on which to advise duration of therapy or route of administration, but antibiotic therapy is traditionally continued for at least two weeks parenterally and a further four weeks orally. Close consultation with infectious disease or clinical microbiology experts is vital. Arthrocentesis followed by regular aspiration or open drainage of the joint is essential because of the destructive effects of pus on joint cartilage. Joints such as the hip should be aspirated under imaging guidance. Hip and prosthetic joints should be referred for early orthopaedic intervention. Consider arthroscopic washout in all cases. Progression to chronic infection has decreased from 10–20% to <2% of acute infections with early antibiotic therapy and appropriate surgical intervention.

Arthritis as a feature of systemic infection

Viral agents such as parvovirus B19, rubella and other acute viral syndromes (hepatitis, mumps) may have arthritis as a predominant feature. The presentation may be indistinguishable in joint distribution from acute-onset rheumatoid arthritis. Characteristic features of the underlying infection are usually present, and the joint symptoms usually subside without sequelae within six weeks of onset. Serology is useful when the result influences management.

214 Vasculitis

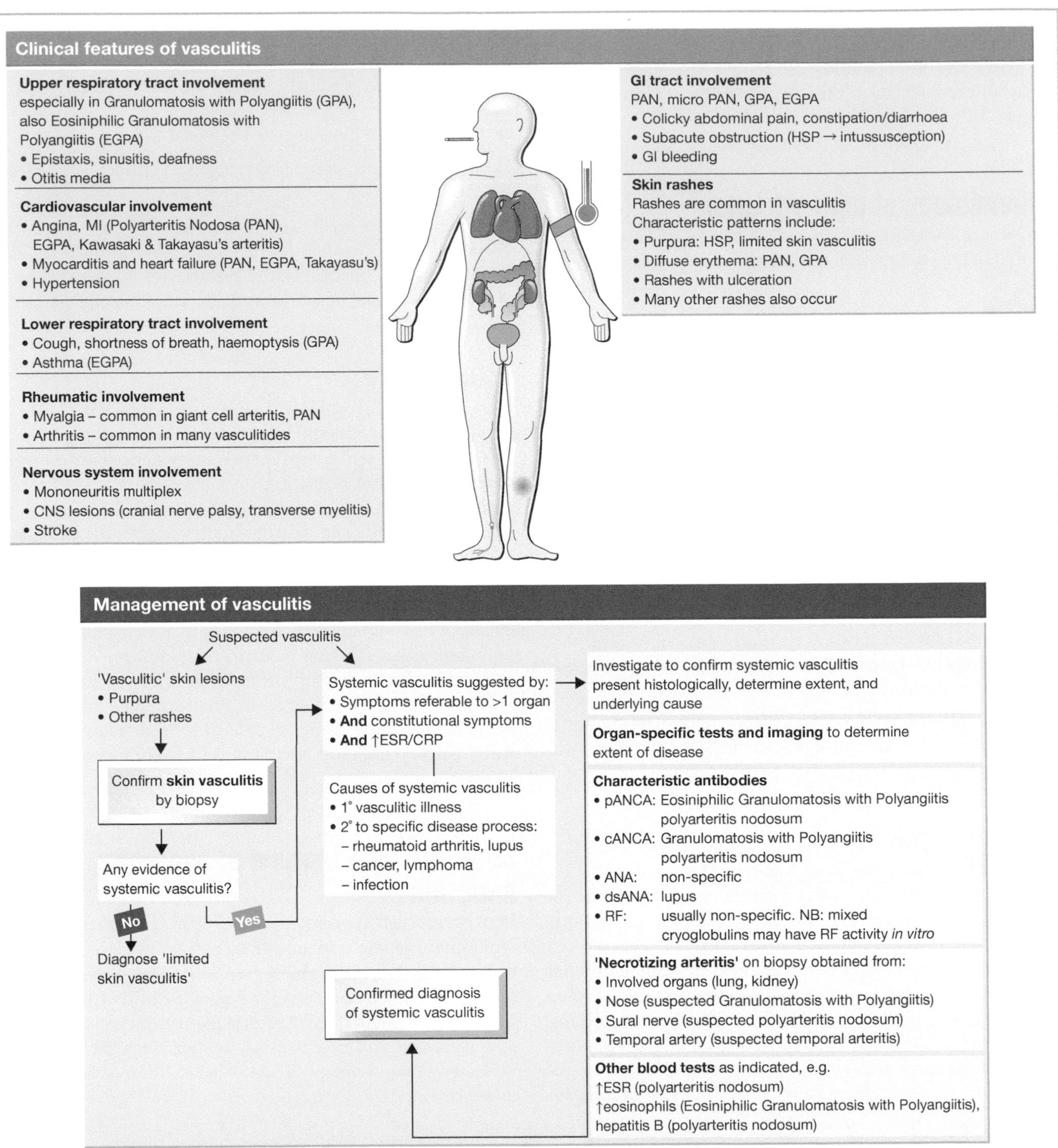

Clinical features of vasculitis
Upper respiratory tract involvement
especially in Granulomatosis with Polyangiitis (GPA), also Eosiniphilic Granulomatosis with Polyangiitis (EGPA)
• Epistaxis, sinusitis, deafness
• Otitis media
Cardiovascular involvement
• Angina, MI (Polyarteritis Nodosa (PAN), EGPA, Kawasaki & Takayasu's arteritis)
• Myocarditis and heart failure (PAN, EGPA, Takayasu's)
• Hypertension
Lower respiratory tract involvement
• Cough, shortness of breath, haemoptysis (GPA)
• Asthma (EGPA)
Rheumatic involvement
• Myalgia – common in giant cell arteritis, PAN
• Arthritis – common in many vasculitides
Nervous system involvement
• Mononeuritis multiplex
• CNS lesions (cranial nerve palsy, transverse myelitis)
• Stroke
GI tract involvement
PAN, micro PAN, GPA, EGPA
• Colicky abdominal pain, constipation/diarrhoea
• Subacute obstruction (HSP → intussusception)
• GI bleeding
Skin rashes
Rashes are common in vasculitis
Characteristic patterns include:
• Purpura: HSP, limited skin vasculitis
• Diffuse erythema: PAN, GPA
• Rashes with ulceration
• Many other rashes also occur
Management of vasculitis
Suspected vasculitis
'Vasculitic' skin lesions
• Purpura
• Other rashes
Confirm skin vasculitis by biopsy
Any evidence of systemic vasculitis?
No
Yes
Diagnose 'limited skin vasculitis'
Systemic vasculitis suggested by:
• Symptoms referable to >1 organ
• And constitutional symptoms
• And ↑ESR/CRP
Causes of systemic vasculitis
• 1° vasculitic illness
• 2° to specific disease process:
– rheumatoid arthritis, lupus
– cancer, lymphoma
– infection
Confirmed diagnosis of systemic vasculitis
Investigate to confirm systemic vasculitis present histologically, determine extent, and underlying cause
Organ-specific tests and imaging to determine extent of disease
Characteristic antibodies
• pANCA: Eosiniphilic Granulomatosis with Polyangiitis polyarteritis nodosum
• cANCA: Granulomatosis with Polyangiitis polyarteritis nodosum
• ANA: non-specific
• dsANA: lupus
• RF: usually non-specific. NB: mixed cryoglobulins may have RF activity in vitro
'Necrotizing arteritis' on biopsy obtained from:
• Involved organs (lung, kidney)
• Nose (suspected Granulomatosis with Polyangiitis)
• Sural nerve (suspected polyarteritis nodosum)
• Temporal artery (suspected temporal arteritis)
Other blood tests as indicated, e.g.
↑ESR (polyarteritis nodosum)
↑eosinophils (Eosiniphilic Granulomatosis with Polyangiitis), hepatitis B (polyarteritis nodosum)

Definition

The vasculitides are a group of conditions characterized by inflammation of the arterial wall and are usefully classified according to the size of the vessel involved (see Table 214.1). They may arise as a primary process or secondary to other conditions such as drug reactions, infection or neoplasia. Diagnosis is based upon clinical features, confirmation of the pathological lesion on tissue biopsy, and the presence of autoantibodies found in association with certain types of vasculitis.

Key points

- Clinical features of systemic vasculitis result from ischaemic damage in the affected organ(s) and the severity of the vasculitis is reflected by the extent or amount of tissue damage. Inflammation is widespread in systemic vasculitis and there may be involvement of several organs.
- Systemic features (fever, weight loss, malaise, anorexia) associated with high inflammatory markers (ESR, CRP, fibrinogen) are common and indicate widespread inflammation.

Table 214.1 Classification of the vasculitides.

Size of vessel affected	Primary	Secondary
Large arteries	Giant cell arteritis Takayasu arteritis	Rheumatoid arthritis (aortitis) Ankylosing spondylitis, Behçet syndrome Infection: syphilis
Medium arteries	Kawasaki disease Classic polyarteritis nodosa	Infection: hepatitis B and C
Medium and small arteries	ANCA-associated vasculitides (AAV): 1. granulomatosis with polyangiitis (GPA) 2. Eosinophilic granulomatosis with polyangiitis (EGPA) 3. Microscopic polyangiitis (MPA)	Rheumatoid arthritis, systemic lupus erythematosus (SLE), Sjögren syndrome Drugs (see below) Infection, e.g. HIV
Small arteries (leukocytoclastic/ hypersensitivity)	Henoch–Schönlein purpura (IgA vasculitis) Essential mixed cryoglobulinaemia	Drugs, e.g. sulfonamides, penicillins, thiazides Infection, e.g. tuberculosis, group A streptococci Malignancy, lymphoma Rheumatoid arthritis, SLE, Sjögren syndrome

- A thorough evaluation of organs potentially involved is necessary to determine the extent and severity of disease. This requires thorough history taking and examination of the patient, followed by laboratory investigations and imaging or biopsy of all target organs.
- Diagnosis of specific forms of vasculitis is made on the basis of clinical, laboratory, radiology and histological findings.

Epidemiology and pathogenesis

Giant cell arteritis is common, with an annual incidence of 18/100 000, mainly affecting those >60 years old (annual incidence 10–25/100 000). Other systemic vasculitides are much less common (3/100 000 in the UK). Vasculitis is particularly prevalent at the extremes of age. For example, Kawasaki disease is almost exclusively paediatric whereas giant cell arteritis generally occurs after the sixth decade. Some vasculitides are clearly associated with viral infections, e.g. hepatitis B with polyarteritis nodosa. Takayasu arteritis is a rare large vessel vasculitis of the major large arteries (e.g. the aorta and its major branches), occurring particularly in young females. It has a higher prevalence in Asia than elsewhere.

There is no exclusive pathology, but the following are frequently found.

- 'Leukocytoclastic vasculitis': a characteristic histological appearance with vessel wall inflammation, fibrinoid necrosis and 'leukocytoclasis' resulting from dissolution of leukocytes.
- Necrosis of medium and small arterial walls: found in the systemic necrotizing vasculitides (granulomatosis with polyangiitis [GPA], eosinophilic granulomatosis with polyangiitis [EGPA] and polyarteritis nodosa [PAN]). Lesions are focal and segmental within vessels so tissue diagnosis may be elusive. Granulomata and eosinophilic infiltrates characterize GPA and EGPA respectively.
- Giant cell arteritis (GCA): arterial wall inflammation (including 'giant cells') on temporal artery biopsy (TAB).

History and examination

- Systemic features often predominate: weight loss, fatigue and fever (see Chapter 45), particularly in the large vessel vasculitides.
- Involvement of more than one organ in an inflammatory process is a key clue to the presence of an underlying vasculitis, particularly ANCA-associated vasculitis. Specific symptoms and signs are dependent on the end-organs involved. Renal, respiratory (upper and/or lower tract inflammation), skin and peripheral nerve involvement should be sought.
- Giant cell arteritis often presents with severe, unremitting headache associated with scalp tenderness (lying the head on a pillow is painful, as is combing hair). Transient visual disturbance (amaurosis fugax) or blindness can occur due to inflammation of the retinal arteries and is a medical emergency. Masseter muscle (jaw) claudication may occur on eating. Patients are at increased risk of stroke.
- Takayasu arteritis often presents with non-specific features and/or systemic illness (fever, malaise). There may be tenderness over any palpable arteries. Bruits occur and peripheral pulses may disappear (hence its synonym, 'pulseless' disease). Inflammation of intracranial vessels is associated with increased risk of stroke. Aortitis may result in aortic regurgitation and/or involvement of the coronary os and contiguous arteries causing angina and/or infarction.

Investigations (See also Table 66.1)

The aims of investigation are to confirm the diagnosis and determine the extent of disease (which organs are involved?), its current activity and the extent of damage that has already occurred. Laboratory findings in vasculitic syndromes are shown in the figure.

Immunology

- Antineutrophil cytoplasmic antibodies (ANCAs) are circulating antibodies directed against cytoplasmic components of neutrophils. These are classified according to the pattern of neutrophil staining: (i) cytoplasmic (cANCA) associated with antibodies to proteinase-3 (PR3-ANCA), which are strongly associated with GPA; and (ii) perinuclear (pANCA) directed commonly against myeloperoxidase, associated with other primary small vessel arteritides. Titres of ANCA antibodies may vary during the disease course but it is not currently recommended that these are used to guide therapeutic decision making.
- Rheumatoid factors (RFs) are antibodies directed against the Fc component of immunoglobulin (Ig). They occur in many patients with rheumatoid arthritis, and are also found in many other vasculitides (systemic lupus erythematosus [SLE], cryoglobulinaemia, PAN) and chronic infections.
- Antinuclear antibodies (ANAs) are classified according to the pattern of nuclear staining. A diffuse pattern is found with anti-DNA antibodies, characteristic of SLE, though found also in other conditions. Anti-double-stranded DNA antibodies are specific for active SLE. Staining restricted to the centromere suggests

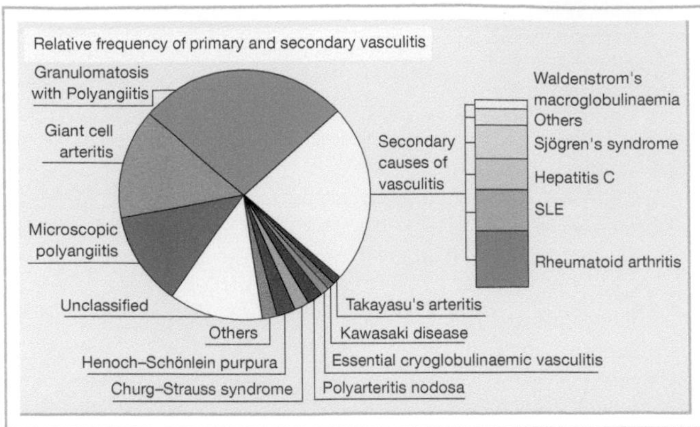

systemic sclerosis. A speckled staining pattern is found with antibodies against extractable nuclear antigens. There are several different forms, common in SLE (anti-Ro, Sm) and Sjögren syndrome (anti-Ro, La).

Radiology

Plain chest radiographs may show pulmonary infiltrates (small and medium vessel vasculitides). Computed tomography and magnetic resonance imaging are useful in investigation of the upper respiratory tract and sinuses (GPA). Suspicion of large vessel vasculitis should be investigated with ultrasound or MRI for temporal arteries and either PET-CT or MRI/MR angiography (MRA) for aorta and extracranial arteries. Coeliac axis angiography may show clusters of small aneurysms, 'bunches of grapes', in some vasculitides (especially PAN).

Histology

Tissue biopsy is often undertaken for definitive diagnosis. Suitable sites for biopsy are accessible blood vessels (e.g. superficial temporal arteries in suspected GCA), involved skin or other organs such as kidney, muscle, nerve and lung in small/medium vessel vasculitis. Findings are as above but as lesions may be patchy, a negative biopsy does not rule out vasculitis; 70% of GCA are biopsy positive. Diagnostic yield is increased using ultrasound findings.

Assessing other organ involvement

Screening for involvement of major organs in the medium and small vessel vasculitides is by routine biochemical tests (kidney, liver) or radiology (lung) in the first instance. Characterization of the extent and severity of this involvement requires more invasive investigation and may include biopsy. Imaging of the aorta (abdominal, thoracic, intra- and extracranial branches) is undertaken in large vessel vasculitis.

Prognosis and treatment

These diseases retain a significant morbidity and mortality despite recent therapeutic advances. Immunosuppression is the mainstay of therapy. All patients with vasculitis should be managed in a specialist centre and receive regular disease assessment and surveillance.

1 **Large vessel vasculitides** are generally responsive to steroids. All patients should be assessed and managed with respect to safety risks of glucocorticoids. High-dose glucocorticoid therapy (40–60 mg/day prednisolone) should be initiated immediately for induction of remission in GCA or Takayasu arteritis. When disease is controlled, steroids should be reduced to a target of 15 mg/day at 2–3 months and approximately 5 mg/day for GCA and approximately 10 mg/day for Takayasu at one year. Sight-threatening GCA should be treated with pulse IV steroid immediately. Where prednisolone is high risk and/or remission is not achieved and/or relapses are not responsive to short increases in steroids, tocilizumab (anti-IL-6) may be added as adjunct therapy to achieve the target of remission. Methotrexate is an alternative, though evidence for its efficacy is limited. Patients with Takayasu arteritis should have a slower glucocorticoid taper *and* co-prescription of a traditional DMARD, e.g. methotrexate. Anti-TNF biologics are indicated for severe, relapsing or refractory disease. Major relapse in Takayasu, e.g. with vascular symptoms or event, requires reintroduction of high-dose steroid as for new disease. Antiplatelet therapy is no longer recommended for large vessel vasculitis but should be considered where vascular ischaemic complications accrue.

2 **ANCA-associated vasculitides** (GPA, Churg–Strauss syndrome EGPA, microscopic polyangiitis) may present with life- or organ-threatening damage, e.g. renal, respiratory or neurological, in which case systemic corticosteroid plus rituximab (see Chapter 217) or intravenous pulse dose cyclophosphamide are indicated for induction of remission. Plasma exchange should be added if response is inadequate or for severe pulmonary haemorrhage or rapidly progressive glomerulonephritis. For active, non-life/organ-threatening disease, e.g. limited upper respiratory tract GPA, methotrexate or mycophenolate mofetil plus oral prednisolone are recommended. When remission is attained, glucocorticoids should be tapered and methotrexate, azathioprine or rituximab introduced as maintenance therapy for approximately two years. Relapses should be assessed (major or limited) and treated/retreated as above. Disease which is refractory (non-responsive) should be treated with cyclophosphamide or rituximab (crossover) if the patient has already failed to respond to one of these agents. Refractory disease should also prompt a reconsideration of the diagnosis.

3 Primary small vessel vasculitis is typically self-limiting in nature (e.g. Henoch–Schönlein purpura [IgAV]). In systemic small vessel vasculitis, the prognosis is worse for those with renal or other major organ involvement. A comprehensive evaluation of the extent and severity of multiorgan involvement is vital to prevent potentially fatal complications, and to avoid unnecessary use of toxic agents in limited small vessel vasculitis. An algorithm for management and treatment is shown in the figure.

Kawasaki arteritis

This syndrome, essentially only occurring in childhood, is important in adult medicine as it may underlie cases of myocardial infarction/acute coronary syndromes in teenagers and young adults. Predominantly male children (M:F 16:1) present with a systemic illness comprising prolonged high fever and a rash with erythema of the hands/feet, progressing to peeling a few days later. The conjunctiva becomes infected, and the lips and oral cavity are typically inflamed with sloughing of the mucosa. Any other organs may be involved; a carditis is particularly common. Coronary dilation (seen by transthoracic echocardiography) occurs early, and in the absence of treatment, 20% develop aneurysms of the coronary arteries. The illness is self-limiting (mortality <0.1% in the acute phase); the main therapeutic issue is to prevent the formation of coronary aneurysms which predispose to later myocardial ischaemia. IV immunoglobulin reduces the risk of coronary aneurysms and should be given promptly in Kawasaki arteritis.

215 Metabolic bone disease

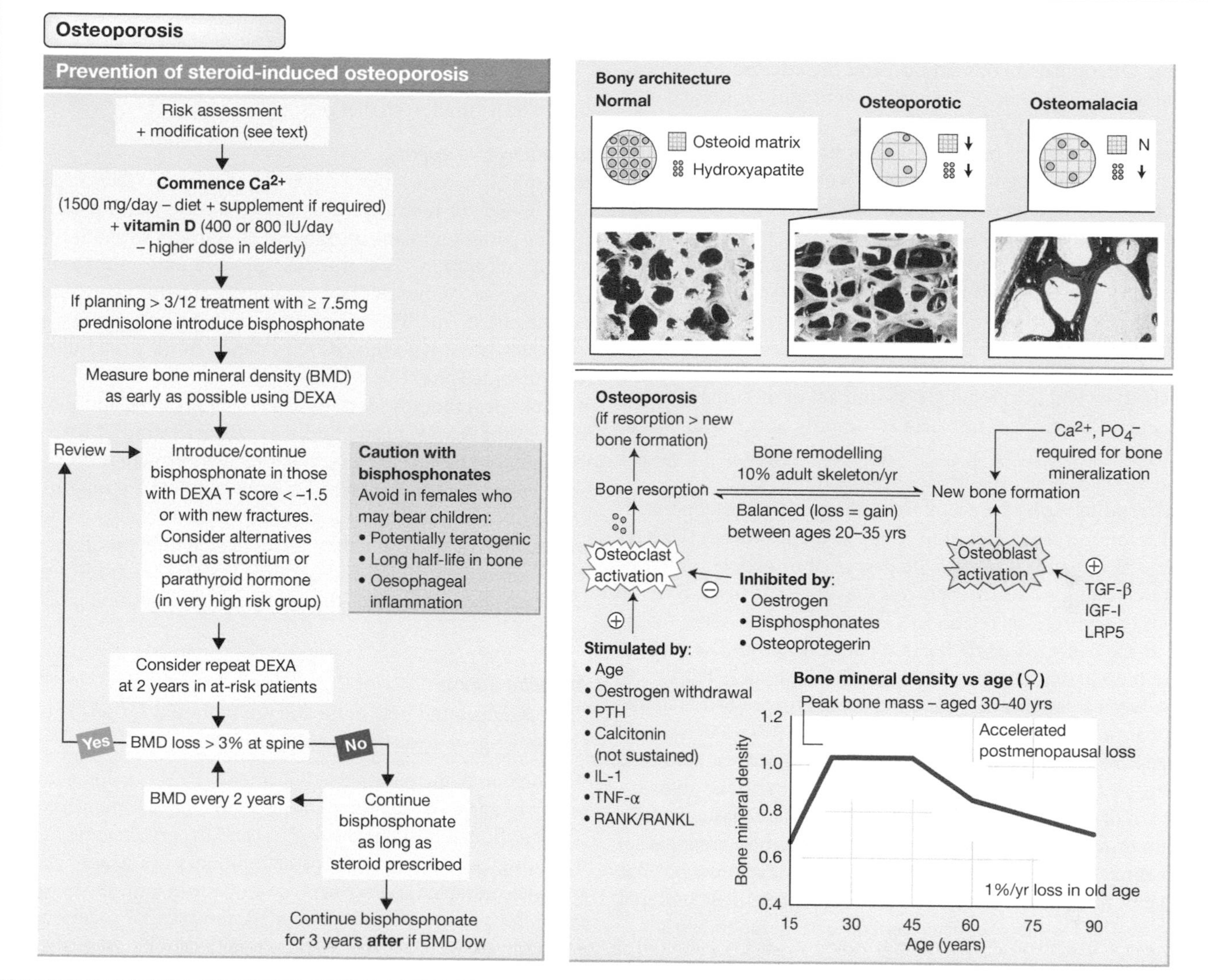

Osteoporosis

Osteoporosis is very common and predisposes to skeletal fractures from a quantitative decrease in bone matrix components (osteoid and hydroxyapatite) of bone. Fifty percent of women and 15% of men sustain an osteoporosis-related fracture by age 90. Osteoporosis may be primary or secondary to a specific disease. Osteoporosis is common in elderly women, especially those with a late menarche, early menopause or long history of oligomenorrhoea (e.g. athletes, anorexia nervosa). Other important risk factors include smoking, alcohol, steroid use, sedentary lifestyle (or non-weight-bearing exercise), positive family history (peak bone mass is under strong genetic control) and lean body type. Secondary osteoporosis occurs in the following.

- Endocrine disease: thyrotoxicosis, Cushing disease, hypogonadism, hyperparathyroidism, secondary amennorrhoea.
- Rheumatological and systemic inflammatory disease: rheumatoid arthritis or any inflammatory arthropathy, inflammatory bowel disease.
- Gastroenterological disease: malabsorption syndromes, chronic active hepatitis, alcohol related liver disease.
- Organ transplantation.
- Neoplasia.
- Drugs: steroids, unfractionated heparin, aromatase inhibitors, antiepileptic drugs (phenytoin, carbamazepine), alcohol.
- A variety of rare genetic disorders, including osteogenesis imperfecta and hypophosphatasia.

Medicine at a Glance, Fifth Edition. Edited by Patrick Davey and Alex Pitcher.

Companion website: www.wiley.com/go/medicine5e

Patient assessment and clinical features

Evaluation includes a detailed patient history, physical exam (including BMI) and plain radiographs (if fracture suspected). Osteoporosis is asymptomatic unless fracture occurs. Pain, loss of height and increasing thoracic kyphosis are features of thoracic vertebral fractures. Measurement of bone mineral density (BMD) is undertaken according to national or international guidelines (e.g. American Association of Clinical Endocrinologists or National Osteoporosis Foundation), and includes peri/postmenopausal women, those on ≥ 7.5 mg/day of prednisolone, and others at high risk.

The 10-year *clinical fracture risk* can be calculated using the Fracture Risk Assessment (FRAX®) tool which is available online. FRAX is a validated algorithm for fracture risk assessment. Inputs include BMD measurements and risk factors, both modifiable (e.g. alcohol, smoking) and unmodifiable (e.g. age, parental history), and supports patient-centred decision making.

Diagnosis

Diagnosis of osteoporosis is made on the basis of BMD T-score (see below) or where a fragility (low-impact or atraumatic) fracture occurs. Low-impact fractures commonly occur at the distal radius (Colles fracture) or femoral neck. Atraumatic (wedge) fractures of vertebrae usually occur in the thoracic region.

Plain radiographs are useful for demonstrating osteoporosis-related fractures. **Dual-emission X-ray absorptiometry** (DEXA) measures BMD and quantifies the degree of osteopenia (mild to moderate bone loss) or osteoporosis (severe bone loss). BMD is commonly reported in relation to two norms: a Z-score (compared to the expected BMD for that patient's age and sex) and a T-score (compared to young adults of the same sex). The difference between a patient's score and the norm is expressed as standard deviations above and below the mean. The WHO definitions of osteoporosis and osteopenia relate to these scores: a T-score between −1.0 and −2.5 defines osteopenia (low bone mass); a T-score of or less than −2.5 defines osteoporosis. Measurement is useful in those at risk (e.g. steroid therapy, premature menopause) and in those aged <70 years with low-impact fractures. BMD is one component of the FRAX fracture risk assessment tool and change in BMD is a key reported outcome of therapeutic trials.

Prevention and management

Prevention of osteoporosis and fractures is a major public health goal. Fracture risk is related to BMD and risk of falls in an individual. The WHO recommends that treatment decisions are based on the 10-year fracture risk (FRAX) rather than measured BMD. Recommendations for prevention of osteoporosis and fragility fractures include the following.

- **Maximization of peak adult bone mass**: young females should be advised of the effect of lifestyle and dietary modifications on peak adult bone mass. These include minimizing alcohol and caffeine intake, not smoking cigarettes, adequate dietary calcium intake and regular weight-bearing exercise throughout life.
- **Reducing the rate of bone loss**: bone loss occurs with increasing age and accelerates in the postmenopausal period. Increased fracture risk can be mitigated by lifestyle modification (as above) and pharmacological therapy. Pharmacological therapy falls into two main classes: antiresorptive (prevents bone breakdown) and anabolic (promotes bone formation). Traditional and newer 'biological' agents are available in these two treatment categories (see below).
- **Prevention of fractures**: those with established osteoporosis should be assessed for factors that may cause falls (e.g. drugs causing postural hypotension, poor visual acuity). Extrinsic devices such as mobility or stability aids and padded hip protectors (to protect against hip fractures) may be useful.

Pharmacological therapy

General measures apply to all patients. Adequate calcium (1000–1200 mg/day) and vitamin D (1000 IU/day or sufficient to ensure measured serum levels are within the normal range) should be assured from diet or supplements.

Antiresorptive agents

- **Bisphosphonates**: these agents bind to bone. They are taken orally weekly or monthly on an empty stomach with plain water and the patient remains upright for 30 minutes to avoid the risk of GI ulceration. Intravenous preparations are available. Osteonecrosis of the jaw (ONJ) and atypical femoral fractures are rare adverse events. The optimal duration of therapy with bisphosphonates is not determined by evidence, but a 'drug holiday' is recommended after five years.
- **Biological therapy**: denosumab is a monoclonal antibody that binds to the RANK ligand and prevents activation of RANK on the surface of osteoclasts and their precursors, thereby decreasing bone resorption and increasing bone mass and strength. It is licensed for osteoporosis range BMD. Denosumab is associated with a small increase in risk of infection and of hypocalcaemia in renal impairment. ONJ and atypical femoral fractures are rare adverse events. It is given by subcutaneous injection every six months.

Anabolic agents

These agents build new bone and are indicated for severe osteoporosis with, or at very high risk of, fracture.

- **Hormonal**: the parathyroid hormone (PTH) analogue teriparatide is injected subcutaneously daily for 24 months. It is contraindicated in skeletal neoplasia and hypercalcaemia.
- **Biological therapy**: sclerostin inhibitors are a new class of anabolic therapies. Sclerostins are proteins produced by osteocytes which inhibit bone formation. Romosozumab is a monoclonal antibody which binds sclerostin and may be prescribed for severe osteoporosis. It is injected subcutaneously once monthly for 12 months. It is contraindicated in patients with previous myocardial infarction or stroke. Hypocalcaemia may occur. ONJ and atypical femoral fracture are rare adverse effects.

Steroid therapy and osteoporosis

Steroid therapy is associated with an increase in fracture risk which is not well assessed by change in BMD alone as it is also related to bone quality and increased falls risk (e.g. poor vision due to cataracts). Rapid loss of bone occurs early on initiation of steroid therapy and is greatest for the first three months, thereafter slowing to a rate 2–3× normal loss. Osteoporosis risk is related to steroid dose and treatment duration (total cumulative dose). Highly significant bone loss occurs with prednisolone doses ≥7.5 mg/day for three months, but there is no safe steroid dose for bone loss and *any steroid exposure* is significant in those with an existing fragility fracture, who should all receive prophylaxis. Many conditions requiring steroids are themselves associated with osteoporosis, e.g. rheumatoid arthritis, systemic lupus erythematosus and inflammatory bowel disease.

The figure shows an approach to prevention of bone loss in those taking steroids. Other adverse effects, e.g. cataracts increasing falls risk, should also be corrected.

Osteomalacia/rickets

Osteomalacia results from impaired mineralization of the osteoid matrix. It causes skeletal deformity in the young (rickets) and bone pain, non-specific aches, fractures and proximal muscle weakness in adults (osteomalacia). The causes include the following.

- **Vitamin D deficiency**: dietary inadequacy, lack of sunshine or malabsorption are the most common causes in clinical practice, e.g. osteomalacia is relatively common in Asian women who dress traditionally, vegetarians and those (children and the elderly) with poor diets. It also results from coeliac disease.
- **Vitamin D metabolic abnormality**: reduced liver 25-hydroxylation (cirrhosis), reduced renal hydroxylation (renal failure) or increased hepatic metabolism (anticonvulsants).
- **Very rare causes** include vitamin D receptor mutations causing defective vitamin D-mediated calcium absorption, 1α-hydroxylase deficiency and familial (X-linked) hypophosphataemic rickets.

Clinical features and investigations

Delay or deficiency in bone mineralization in childhood (rickets) leads to structural skeletal deformities, including enlargement of the ends of the long bones, widened cranial sutures and frontal bossing in those aged over one year and tibial bowing and genu varum/valgum (knock or bow knees) in older children. Adults experience non-specific pains and aches, predominantly in the proximal limb girdles and lower back. Pressure over the long bones or the rib cage may elicit tenderness. Significant osteomalacia may cause pathological fractures and results in secondary hyperparathyroidism which may complicate the picture biochemically and radiologically. This diagnosis must be considered in at-risk individuals with musculoskeletal symptoms.

- Diagnosis is sometimes evident from plain radiographs showing Looser's zones or pseudofractures (translucent bands occur at sites of stress, e.g. the ribs, axillary borders of the scapulae and pubic rami).
- Characteristic biochemistry: low phosphate (early), low calcium (variable) and raised alkaline phosphatase (late due to secondary hyperparathyroidism).
- Low vitamin D and high parathyroid hormone (PTH).

Treatment

- Treat any underlying cause (e.g. coeliac disease).
- Give oral daily vitamin D supplementation according to the degree of depletion and bony abnormality.
- Malabsorption states require high doses.
- Deficiency of vitamin D due to renal or hepatic disease may be overcome by using hydroxylated forms such as alfacalcidol or calcitriol.

Therapy relieves symptoms and corrects bony abnormalities within 3–4 months. Occasionally, hyperparathroidism becomes autonomous in long-standing osteomalacia (tertiary hyperparathyroidism).

Parathyroid and renal bone disease

See Chapters 150 and 160.

216 Other bone disease

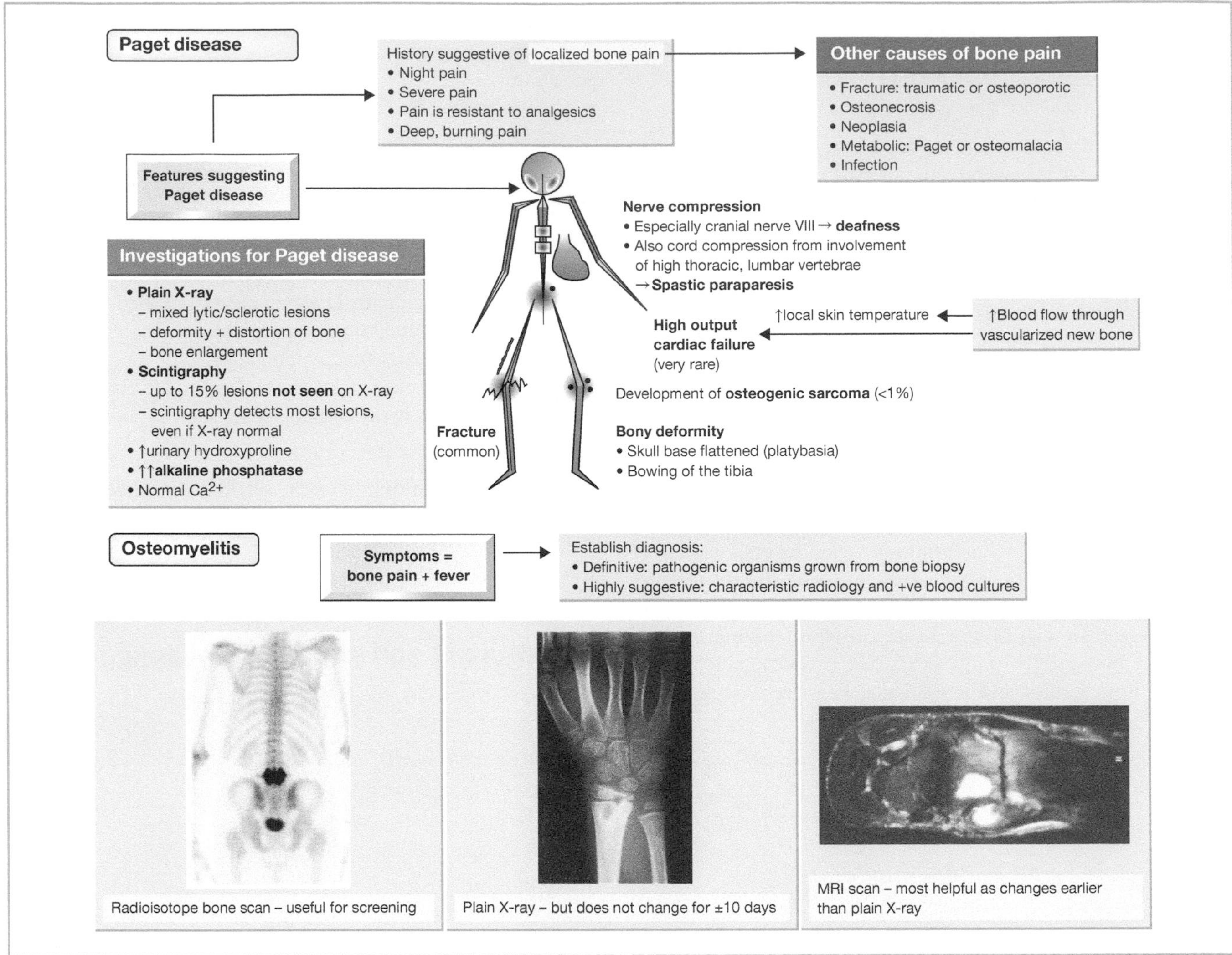

Paget disease
History suggestive of localized bone pain
• Night pain
• Severe pain
• Pain is resistant to analgesics
• Deep, burning pain
Other causes of bone pain
• Fracture: traumatic or osteoporotic
• Osteonecrosis
• Neoplasia
• Metabolic: Paget or osteomalacia
• Infection
Features suggesting Paget disease
Nerve compression
• Especially cranial nerve VIII → deafness
• Also cord compression from involvement of high thoracic, lumbar vertebrae → Spastic paraparesis
Investigations for Paget disease
• Plain X-ray
– mixed lytic/sclerotic lesions
– deformity + distortion of bone
– bone enlargement
• Scintigraphy
– up to 15% lesions not seen on X-ray
– scintigraphy detects most lesions, even if X-ray normal
• ↑urinary hydroxyproline
• ↑↑alkaline phosphatase
• Normal Ca2+
↑local skin temperature
↑Blood flow through vascularized new bone
High output cardiac failure (very rare)
Development of osteogenic sarcoma (<1%)
Fracture (common)
Bony deformity
• Skull base flattened (platybasia)
• Bowing of the tibia
Osteomyelitis
Symptoms = bone pain + fever
Establish diagnosis:
• Definitive: pathogenic organisms grown from bone biopsy
• Highly suggestive: characteristic radiology and +ve blood cultures

Radioisotope bone scan – useful for screening

Plain X-ray – but does not change for ±10 days

MRI scan – most helpful as changes earlier than plain X-ray

Paget disease

This is associated with abnormal remodelling of bone, often in a monostolic pattern, but may be widespread. Up to 40% of cases may have an identifiable affected relative, indicating a significant genetic contribution. It is primarily a disorder of osteoclasts, which become highly activated, altering the normal homeostasis of bone remodelling.

- **Early stages**: increased bone resorption occurs, so producing lytic lesions (osteoporosis circumscripta, resorption front).
- **Later stages**: disproportionate stimulation of new bone formation occurs in a disorganized fashion, resulting in areas of bone sclerosis.

Cycles of resorption and formation result in a huge increase in bone turnover and ultimately grossly disorganized bone, which is weak and prone to fracture.

Epidemiology

The incidence of Paget disease in many countries is reported to have declined dramatically (by up to 50%) in the last few decades. Paget disease occurs mainly in the elderly (>70 years). Prevalence is approximately 2–3% of the over-55 population in the USA, slightly higher in Britain and rare in most of Asia and Africa. Male preponderance is 1.4:1, with a marked increased prevalence in relatives. Mutations in the sequestosome gene are found in 30% of familial and 10% of sporadic Paget and probably cause disease through osteoclast activation via the NF-κB pathway. Such germline mutations are not always associated with clinical disease and it is not clear how they cause disease with such a patchy and often limited skeletal distribution.

Clinical features

Paget disease is often asymptomatic, with the only abnormality being an isolated raised alkaline phosphatase. Between 5% and

Medicine at a Glance, Fifth Edition. Edited by Patrick Davey and Alex Pitcher.

Companion website: www.wiley.com/go/medicine5e

10% develop symptoms bringing them to medical care. Symptomatic presentation depends on the sites and extent of bony involvement. Twenty percent of patients have a single bone lesion. The pelvis, spine, long bones and skull are most commonly affected. Common symptoms include bone pain, bone deformities and increased warmth over an affected area. Important bony complications are fractures (10%), deformity and osteogenic sarcoma (rare <1%). A sudden increase in pain, deformity or serum alkaline phosphatase should alert the clinician to one of these possibilities. Other complications are very rare, and include the following.

- Neurological (compressive) complications: cranial nerve palsy, conductive hearing loss (or sensorineural) and spinal stenosis.
- Other: including hypercalcaemia, or hypercalciuria, which in turn may lead to renal stones.

Investigations

- **Raised alkaline phosphatase** reflects increased metabolic (osteoblastic) activity, which is linked to increased osteoclast activity.
- **Radiology**: targeted X-rays show gross bony distortion and deformity and mixed osteolytic and sclerotic areas, with abnormal trabecular architecture. It is unique in causing enlargement of the affected bones. An area of sharply demarcated osteolysis may be apparent, particularly in early disease. This may appear as a 'flame-shaped resorbing front' in a long bone or an area of osteoporosis circumscripta. **Isotope bone scintigraphy** (radionucletide bone scan) is recommended to define the extent and metabolic activity of skeletal involvement accurately (15% of lesions, usually early active areas, are not visible on plain film).
- **Bone biopsy** if imaging cannot exclude tumour.
- **Calcium** in Paget disease is normal but may rise with a fracture or prolonged inactivity.

Management

Treatment aimed at improving symptoms is recommended over 'treatment to target' aimed at normalizing total alkaline phosphatase. Asymptomatic disease does not require treatment. **Indications for treatment** include:

- active disease at the skull base or in the spine above L2 or any neurological compromise (cranial or spinal nerves)
- pain
- progressive deformity
- the very rare complications of either immobilization hypercalcaemia or high-output cardiac failure.

Treatment of symptomatic patients

Bisphosphonates are recommended for the treatment of bone pain. Bisphosphonates inhibit bone resorption and dramatically reduce bone turnover. Zoledronic acid (by infusion) is the recommended bisphosphonate.

- Analgesia.
- Calcitonin is occasionally useful for severe pain or extensive lytic disease but has been largely replaced by bisphosphonates. Side-effects include troublesome flushing, nausea and hypocalcaemia.
- Surgery is used to relieve compression neuropathy or joint involvement leading to disability.

Osteonecrosis (avascular necrosis)

Avascular necrosis is the death of cellular elements of bone, occurring in all ages and both sexes, which potentially causes structural collapse.

Aetiology and pathogenesis

Avascular necrosis is associated with pregnancy, corticosteroid therapy, radiotherapy and cytotoxic chemotherapy. It may also occur in sickle cell disease and other haemoglobinopathies and decompression sickness, though many cases are idiopathic. It commonly affects the femoral head and the scaphoid after fracture of these bones.

Clinical features

- The characteristic feature is bone pain.
- Initially pain occurs on weight bearing, subsequently at rest and at night.
- Increasing severity of pain, becoming resistant to escalating analgesia.

Management

Radiographs are frequently normal early on; subsequently, patchy osteopenia and osteosclerosis develop, and later still a characteristic 'crescent sign' demarcates viable and dead bone. In advanced disease, there is destruction and collapse of the articular surface. Magnetic resonance imaging (MRI) is the imaging technique of choice in early disease and is highly sensitive.

Treatment includes the following.

- Conservative with analgesia and muscle strengthening early in the course, with reduced weight and load bearing until recovery occurs (may be protracted, *c.* 12 months).
- Surgical 'core decompression'.
- May require joint replacement if severe and associated with structural collapse.

Osteomyelitis

Osteomyelitis is infection of the bone arising either from direct inoculation with infecting organisms, e.g. an 'open' fracture, or from haematogenous spread. Though common in children, it is relatively rare in adults.

Underlying conditions and responsible organisms

- Diabetes leads to Gram-negative and/or *Staphylococcus aureus* foot infection.
- 90% of adult osteomyelitis is due to *Staphylococcus* infection.
- *Staphylococcus aureus* septicaemia (e.g. a complication of intravenous cannulation in hospitalized patients) is complicated by osteomyelitis in 1% of cases.
- Sickle cell disease (80% of infections are due to *Salmonella* species).
- Immunosuppression predisposes to many different infections.
- Spinal tuberculosis is relatively common in countries with a high prevalence of tuberculosis. In some areas, infection with atypical mycobacteria is common.

Clinical features

Osteomyelitis presents with systemic symptoms (fever, malaise) and local pain. Vertebral osteomyelitis can lead to vertebral collapse and cord compression. Osteomyelitis in patients with diabetes is often painless. Sterile and occasionally septic arthritis can complicate the picture.

Diagnosis and treatment

Magnetic resonance imaging is the investigation of choice for early disease since X-rays often show no abnormalities. Diagnostic ultrasound also has a potential role. Treatment is with prolonged antibiotics (initially intravenously), debridement of dead bone and stabilization when necessary. Occasionally, it proves impossible to eradicate the infection, and lifelong antibiotics are required.

217 Rheumatoid arthritis

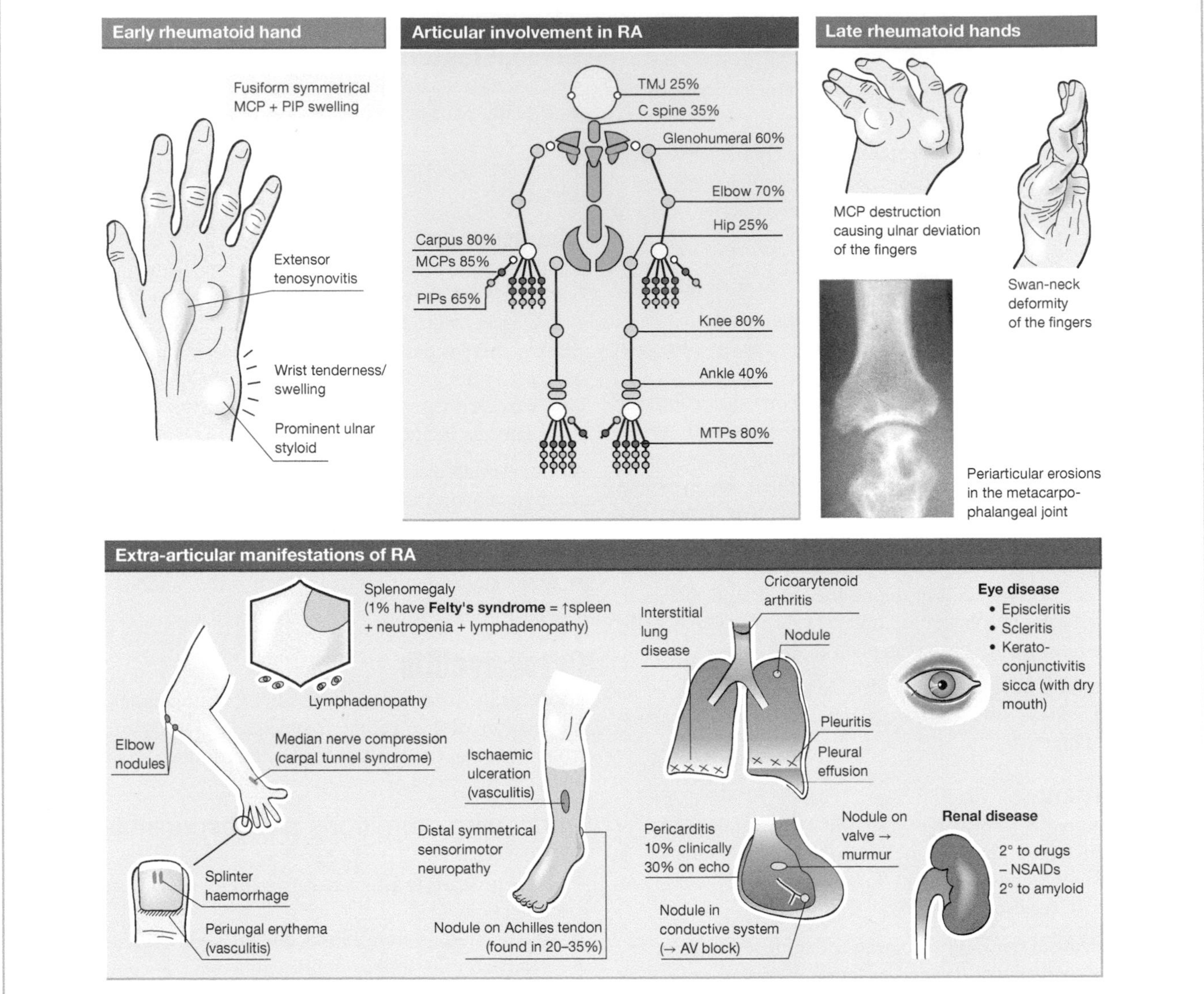

Rheumatoid arthritis (RA) is a systemic autoimmune disorder characterized by a chronic, symmetrical and erosive arthritis of synovial joints, which may result in major disability and handicap. Autoantibodies to immunoglobulin (rheumatoid factor, RF) and/or cyclic citrullinated peptides (anti-CCP antibodies or ACPA) are found. Extra-articular manifestations are common, occurring in up to 40% of patients over the lifetime of their disease, though this may be diminishing in the modern treatment era. Life expectancy may be reduced, largely due to excess cardiovascular mortality and infection. The introduction of biologic agents, particularly those directed against TNF, fundamentally changed the treatment and outcomes of RA in the 2000s.

Epidemiology

Worldwide prevalence is 1% and the peak age of onset is the early 40s, although it may present at any stage. Women are 2–3 times more commonly affected than men, but the sex ratio varies with age (at 30 years, F:M ratio is 10:1, at 65 years, 1:1). The genetic contribution to the disease is emphasized by familial aggregation of cases (sibling recurrence risk is 2–5%) and the association with HLA-DR4 (70% of cases).

Aetiology and pathogenesis

Rheumatoid arthritis (RA) is characterized by an immune-mediated response to an undefined antigen in a genetically predisposed individual. This process triggers inflammation,

Medicine at a Glance, Fifth Edition. Edited by Patrick Davey and Alex Pitcher.

Companion website: www.wiley.com/go/medicine5e

endothelial cell activation and recruitment of specific inflammatory cells to the joint, facilitated by the upregulation of adhesion molecules on synovial vascular endothelium and on circulating inflammatory cells. Amplification of inflammation occurs in response to the local production of inflammatory cytokines (tumour necrosis factor [TNF]-α, interleukin [IL]-1 and IL-6).

Synovial tissue proliferates and becomes locally invasive in the joints. Pannus, a thickened inflammatory granulation tissue, is the characteristic pathological lesion in RA. Activated macrophages within the pannus produce destructive collagenases and proteases. These enzymes mediate the erosion of cartilage at the subchondral bone/cartilage junction and inwards until the articular cartilage is destroyed. Cartilage destruction causes instability of joints, resulting in the characteristic deformities and radiological destruction of RA.

Recent epidemiological studies highlight an association between RA and cigarette smoking (increases with pack-years smoked) and periodontal disease.

Clinical features at onset/early

- Joint swelling, tenderness, pain and stiffness. Stiffness which is particularly troublesome in the morning and improves as the day goes on is characteristic of joint inflammation.
- Small joints of the hands, feet and wrists tend to be affected symmetrically, followed by involvement of larger joints such as knees and elbows where effusions occur.
- Onset is often subacute or insidious, and may be asymmetrical with fluctuating joint symptoms.
- Fatigue and lassitude are common.

Clinical examination at onset may be normal, but more usually reveals the characteristic features of synovitis, i.e. warmth, swelling and tenderness of the metacarpophalangeals (MCPs) and proximal interphalangeals (PIPs), the wrists and metatarsophalangeal (MTP) joints of the feet in a strikingly symmetrical distribution.

- NB: Inability to make a tight closed fist or reduced power grip strength may precede clinically detectable synovitis in early RA.
- Tenosynovitis is a prominent early feature, often affecting the extensor tendon sheaths on the dorsum of the hand.

Alternative presentations of RA include the following.

- **Explosive onset** in 5–10% (e.g. 'waking up' with acute inflammation in multiple joints).
- **Systemic onset** in 5%, usually in middle-aged men. Systemic, non-articular manifestations (e.g. weight loss) dominate. Arthritis may be relatively minor but elevated inflammatory markers and rheumatoid factor (RF) titres are usual.
- **Palindromic onset** in 5%, comprising irregular episodes of transient though possibly severe synovitis. Attacks come on suddenly, may be debilitating and resolve fully within 48 hours. 50% of these evolve into typical RA (typically RF positive).
- **Polymyalgic onset** in 5%: diffuse proximal limb girdle stiffness without joint inflammation; associated with the presence of RF. Shows a less dramatic response to steroids than classic polymyalgia and progresses to typical RA in time.

Classification (See Chapter 66) criteria for RA are shown in Table 217.1. Clinical detection of synovitis is key and training in this skill is encouraged. The differential diagnosis of RA includes the following.

- Infection-related transient arthritis, e.g. parvovirus B19, hepatitis B, rubella infection; these typically last <6 weeks.
- Reactive arthritis.
- Small joint arthritis associated with psoriasis (RF negative).
- Non-erosive arthritis of systemic lupus erythematosus or other connective tissue disease.

Clinical features: established/chronic RA

The **natural course** of RA is unpredictable. It is characterized by acute 'flares' of involved joints and variable systemic and extra-articular symptoms. Acute flares give rise to joint stiffness, pain, discomfort and functional impairment as a result of active synovitis (e.g. inability to grip due to MCP and PIP swelling and stiffness). This fluctuating clinical picture may be accompanied by ongoing slowly progressive structural joint damage which, if unchecked, ultimately leads to severe loss of function; historically (before biologic therapies), only 50% of patients were able to work full time after 10 years of disease. Extra-articular manifestations and co-morbidities contribute significantly to the morbidity and mortality of RA.

Extra-articular manifestations of RA

These are decreasing in prevalence in the era of early diagnosis and effective treatment but remain significant contributors to morbitity and mortality.

- Rheumatoid vasculitis ranges from bland to severe (skin ulceration, necrosis or mononeuritis). It affects up to one in nine males and one in 30 female patients.
- RA-associated interstitial lung disease (RA-ILD) may be present at or around diagnosis; screening with pulmonary function tests and/or CT thorax is recommended. A pattern of usual interstitial pneumonitis (UIP) with subpleural and basal honeycombing is most commonly found. RA is associated with other lung manifestations. Methotrexate may be associated with a hypersensitivity pneumonitis in approximately 0.4% of treated RA patients but evidence now suggests that it is not a cause of ILD. Up to one-third of ILD patients with APCA antibodies may go on to develop clinical RA and should be referred for assessment.
- Ocular manifestations of RA range from the mild (episcleritis) to severe and sight-threatening (scleritis). Scleritis is less commonly found in the modern era.

Co-morbidities

- Infections are at least three times more common than in the general population, particularly in those on steroids or biologic therapy. At-risk patients (>10 mg prednisolone or biologic therapy) should undergo screening (TB, viral hepatitis) and vaccination against pneumococcus, influenza, SARS-CoV-2 and herpes zoster (over-50s is recommended).
- Cardiovascular disease risk is significantly increased in RA mainly due to chronic systemic inflammation. Chronic use of NSAIDs or steroids may contribute. Control of inflammation has been shown to mitigate the risk and tight management of traditional cardiovascular risk factors is strongly advised.

Investigations

- An acute inflammatory response (raised erythrocyte sedimentation rate [ESR] and/or C-reactive protein [CRP]) is found in active inflammation.
- RF testing in RA has a reported pooled sensitivity of 69% and specificity of 85%. Other causes of positive RF include infective

Table 217.1 2010 ACR-EULAR classification criteria for rheumatoid arthritis. This classification system facilitates early diagnosis of RA in an era of widely available effective treatments. It is focused on features present in early RA that predict persistent or erosive disease, is score based and can be applied in newly presenting patients who have at least one joint with clinical synovitis (detectable inflammation) which is not explained by another condition. This eligibility condition MUST be fulfilled – it cannot be applied to patients with arthralgia only. A total score (sum score for four domains) of ≥ 6/10 classifies as 'definite RA'. 'Small joints' means MCP, PIP joints, second through fifth MTP joints, thumb IP joints and wrists. Large joints include hips, knees, ankles, elbows and shoulders.

Domain	Criterion	Definition	Score
A	Joint involvement Swollen or tender on clinical examination, may be confirmed by ultrasound	1 large joint	0
		2–10 large joints	1
		1–3 small joints (± involvement of large joints)	2
		4–10 small joints (± involvement of large joints)	3
		>10 joints (at least 1 small joint)	5
		1 large joint	0
B	Serology (at least 1 test result is needed)	Negative RF *and* negative ACPA	0
		Low-positive RF *or* low-positive ACPA	2
		High-positive RF *or* high-positive ACPA (>3× upper limit of normal)	3
C	Acute-phase reactants (at least one test needed)	Normal CRP and normal ESR	0
		Abnormal CRP or abnormal ESR	1
D	Duration of symptoms	<6 weeks	0
		>6 weeks	1

Source: © ACR.

endocarditis, hepatitis C, cryoglobulinaemia, lymphoma, viral infection and TB.

- Anti-CCP antibodies (ACPA) have higher (pooled) specificity (95%) but similar sensitivity (67%) to RF; sensitivity is higher with newer ACPA assays. The positive likelihood ratio (LR+) is greater for APCA than RF (12.46 vs 4.86) while negative likelihood ratios (LR–) are similar (0.38–0.36). Dual positive RF *and* CCP has a LR+ of 27.
- X-rays typically reveal only soft tissue swelling at presentation. Erosive changes often occur within two years of onset, usually first in the feet.
- Ultrasonography (particularly power Doppler) or MRI may be useful in confirming inflammatory synovitis prior to radiographic change.

Assessment of disease activity is undertaken clinically and should include tender and swollen joint count. These, together with ESR or CRP, are used in the generation of a commonly used disease activity score (DAS-28 or other) which also includes the patient's global assessment of disease activity. Patient-reported validated scores of functional status/health-related quality of life should be sought annually to inform patient-centred decision making.

Management

The goal of management is to suppress active disease, maximize function and participation and avoid deformity and disability. All patients should be managed in specialist rheumatology units in a partnership model of care within the framework of a multidisciplinary team. In the last 10 years, a growing armoury of pharmacological agents has been developed against six precise inflammatory targets (see below). Monitoring of the patient for the presence or development of co-morbidities (see above), extra-articular manifestations, articular damage and disability is carried out concurrently. Surgery (orthopaedic or plastic) and rehabilitation are required for a minority of patients with severe debilitating disease in the modern era. Patients with co-morbidities relevant to therapy (e.g. co-existent hepatitis B) should be co-managed with the relevant specialists. Regular clinical assessment and comprehensive patient education, including in strategies for self-management, are central to achievement of best outcomes for patients.

See figure below for therapy.

Pharmacological therapy (Table 217.2)

The goal of modern therapy is disease remission, characterized by absence of inflammatory symptoms or clinical synovitis. Specialist clinicians achieve this via a 'treat to target' approach, the target being a validated disease activity score (DAS) indicative of remission. While this may not be possible in all, significant improvement in symptoms, function and long-term outcomes is achievable in the majority of patients.

Disease-modifying antirheumatic drugs (DMARDs) should be offered to all. There are three broad categories.

- **Traditional or conventional disease-modifying antirheumatic drugs (cDMARDs)** include methotrexate, sulfasalazine and leflunomide. Methotrexate (MTX) is recommended at diagnosis and is regarded as the 'anchor drug' in RA. If MTX in full dose fails to suppress disease, other cDMARDs may be added as dual or triple combination therapy.
- **Biologic DMARDs (bDMARDs)** may be added to MTX for inadequate response. Biologic therapies are targeted against specific inflammatory mediators in RA and include anti-TNF, anti-IL-6, B-cell depleting agents and an inhibitor of T-cell co-stimulation. They are given by subcutaneous injection or intravenous infusion.
- Small molecule, orally administered **targeted synthetic tsDMARDs** which inhibit janus kinases (JAK-inhibitors).

Details of the key DMARDS in each category can be found in Table 217.2.

An algorithmic approach to therapy which deploys sequential or combined prescription of DMARDs is recommended by the

Table 217.2 Pharmacological therapy.

Category	Drug	Administration	Adverse effects NB: Allergic reactions, rashes and infections can occur with all	Monitoring/safety issues NB: Live vaccinations contraindicated in all
Traditional/conventional DMARDS (cDMARDS)				
	Methotrexate	Oral or subcut *plus* folic acid 48 h post MTX dose	Mucosal (oral ulcers, mucositis), hair fall, transaminitis, myelosuppression hypersensitivity, pneumonitis, hepatic fibrosis, teratogenic	Frequent FBC, renal and LFTs, baseline CXR and PFTs recommended Contraception required
	Leflunomide	Oral	Ulcerative stomatitis Paraesthesia Drug reaction with eosinophilia and systemic symptoms (DRESS) Infections Long half-life: cholestyramine 'washout' may be required for ADRs Teratogenic	Frequent FBC, renal, LFTs Screen for latent TB Check BP and weight at each clinic visit Contraception required
	Sulfasalazine	Oral	See figure below	As MTX
Biologic DMARDS (bDMARDS)				
Anti-TNF (neutralizing ab)	Infliximab	IV	Injection site reaction (mild) Infections: including unusual and severe infections Reactivation of latent TB Heart failure worsening Only certolizumab licensed for all three trimesters of pregnancy	Prior to commencement, screen for infection (hepatitis B, C, TB [IGRA and CXR]) and anti-dsDNA antibodies Screening for TB annually if continued risk
	Adalimumab Certolizumab Golimumab	Subcut		
Anti-TNF (receptor blockade)	Etanercept	Subcut		Tocilizumab: prior to therapy all should be screened for infection (hepatitis B, C, TB [IGRA and CXR]) Lipids at baseline and 8 weeks FBC and LFTs
Anti-IL6	Tocilizumab	Subcut	Transient neutropenia Infections Hyperlipidaemia Intestinal perforation	
B-cell depletion	Rituximab	IV	Infusion-related reactions (can administer IV steroid, paracetamol and antihistamine pre infusion) Hypogammaglobulinaemia	Monitor IgM; Gamma globulins Screen for latent TB and viral hepatitis PML (very rare but fatal)
Anti-cd28 co-stimulatory blocker	Abtacept	Subcut	Similar profile to anti-TNF	Screen for latent TB and viral hepatitis
Targeted synthetic biologics				
Janus Kinase (JAK) inhibitors	Tofacitinib	Oral	Infections (serious) including reactivation of TB and herpes zoster Cytopenias (esp. neutropenia) Venous thromboembolism Hyperlipidaemia	Prior to therapy: screen for TB and viral hepatitis Renal, liver function and FBC (dose reduction in renal and hepatic impairment; contraindicated in viral hepatitis) at baseline and thereafter 3 monthly Check lipids at 8 weeks Do not use in pregnancy
	Baricitinib	Oral		
	Upadacitinib	Oral		

major specialist rheumatological associations in Europe (EULAR) and the USA (ACR) and guidelines are updated regularly. Medications should be initiated and managed by specialists. Overview of the pharmacological approach to patients who are DMARD naive (including at diagnosis) and those with an incomplete response to DMARD (moderate or high disease activity score) is provided in the figure below.

Adjunctive therapy with corticosteroids: for polyarticular flares, severe systemic illness, intermittent troublesome (mono- or pauciarticular) inflammation and/or vasculitis, steroids may be helpful. A short course of low-dose oral prednisolone (7.5–10 mg/day) is usually sufficient for management of flares or to control symptoms while DMARDs are taking effect. Methylprednisolone may be given IV as intermittent 'pulses' for severe systemic disease. Intra-articular injection of depot steroids and local anaesthetic may be useful for recalcitrant joint inflammation.

Prognosis and outcome

The course and outcome of RA in an individual patient are unpredictable but very much improved by modern 'treat to target' strategies. No disease-specific biomarkers have been identified to guide therapy. Known poor prognostic factors include the following.

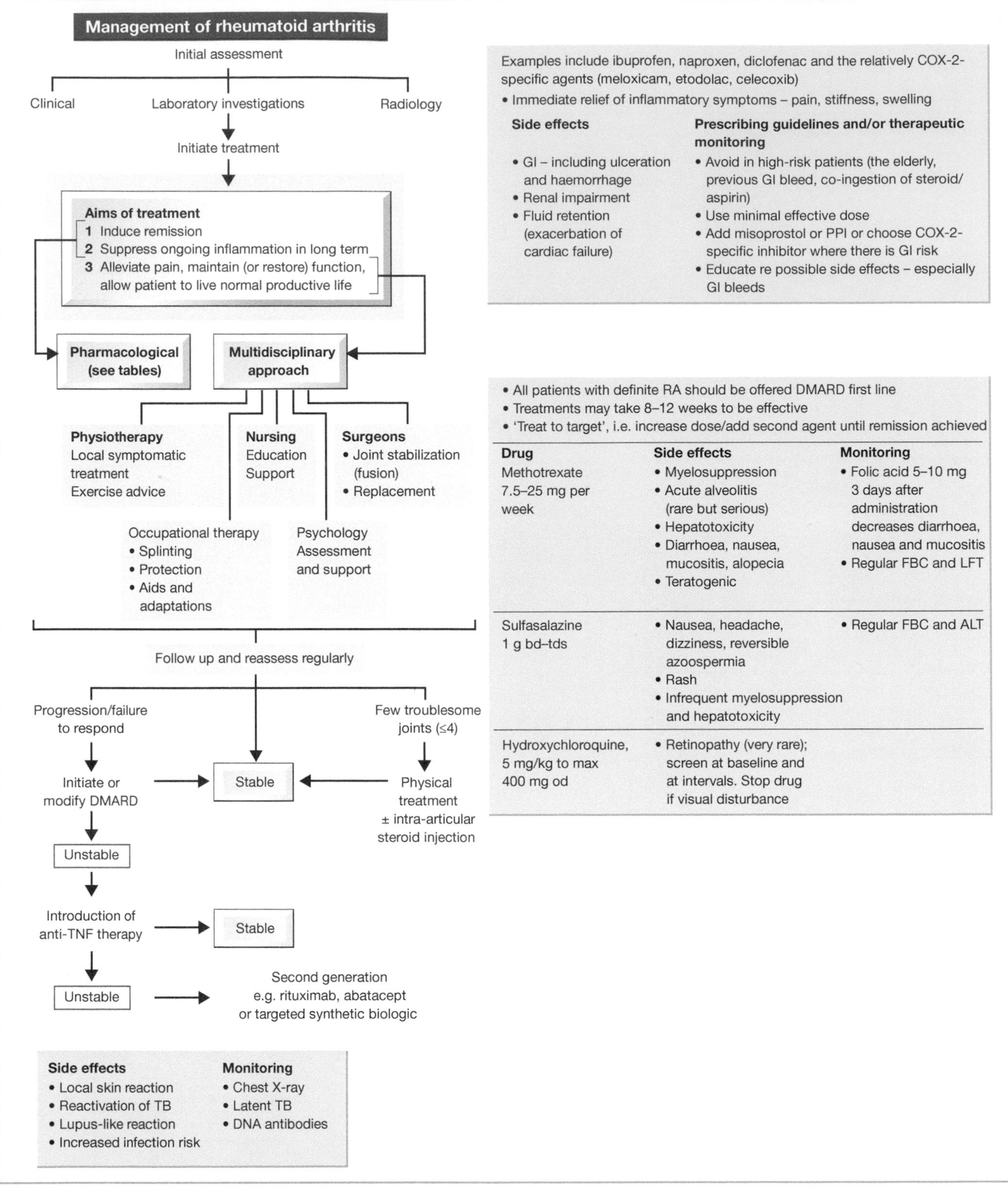

Drug	Side effects	Monitoring
Methotrexate 7.5–25 mg per week	• Myelosuppression • Acute alveolitis (rare but serious) • Hepatotoxicity • Diarrhoea, nausea, mucositis, alopecia • Teratogenic	• Folic acid 5–10 mg 3 days after administration decreases diarrhoea, nausea and mucositis • Regular FBC and LFT
Sulfasalazine 1 g bd–tds	• Nausea, headache, dizziness, reversible azoospermia • Rash • Infrequent myelosuppression and hepatotoxicity	• Regular FBC and ALT
Hydroxychloroquine, 5 mg/kg to max 400 mg od	• Retinopathy (very rare); screen at baseline and at intervals. Stop drug if visual disturbance	

- Persistent active RA despite traditional DMARD therapy.
- High ESR and CRP despite therapy.
- Extra-articular features, e.g. nodules/vasculitis.
- Rheumatoid factor and/or anti-CCP antibody positivity (especially if high titre).
- Erosions on plain radiographs within two years of onset.
- Failure of two or more conventional DMARDs.

The spectrum of severity of RA ranges from mild or subclinical to aggressive and destructive forms, associated with excess mortality. These outcomes are improved in the modern therapeutic era, though adverse effects of DMARD medications (particularly infection) are a cause of morbidity. Long-term major complications of RA include the following.

- Neurological: cervical myelopathy and peripheral neuropathy.
- Cardiac involvement: ischaemic, nodular valve and pericarditis.
- Amyloidosis (causing renal failure and the nephrotic syndrome).
- Rheumatoid arthritis-interstitial lung disease.
- Vasculitis causing skin ulcers, distal ischaemia and mononeuritis.

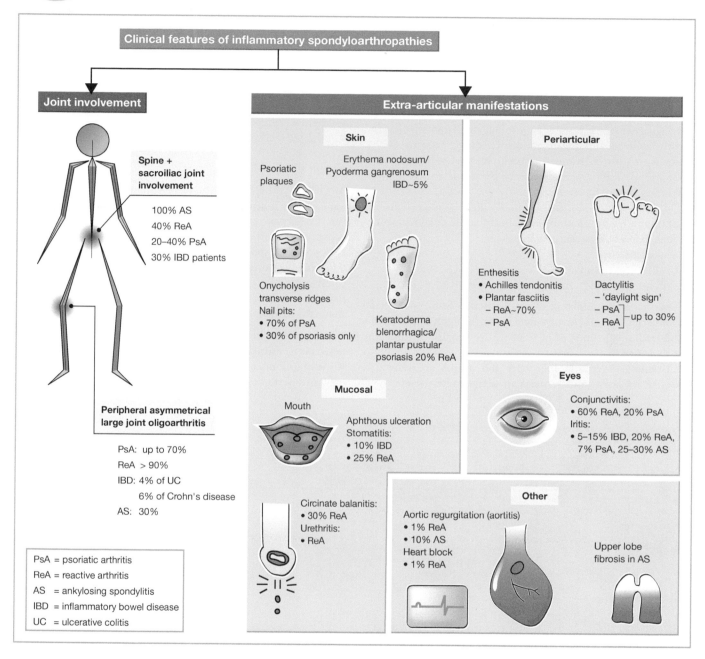

Inflammatory spondyloarthropathies

Clinical features of inflammatory spondyloarthropathies

Joint involvement

Spine + sacroiliac joint involvement
100% AS
40% ReA
20–40% PsA
30% IBD patients

Peripheral asymmetrical large joint oligoarthritis
PsA: up to 70%
ReA > 90%
IBD: 4% of UC
6% of Crohn's disease
AS: 30%

PsA = psoriatic arthritis
ReA = reactive arthritis
AS = ankylosing spondylitis
IBD = inflammatory bowel disease
UC = ulcerative colitis

Extra-articular manifestations

Skin
Psoriatic plaques
Erythema nodosum/ Pyoderma gangrenosum IBD~5%
Onycholysis transverse ridges
Nail pits:
• 70% of PsA
• 30% of psoriasis only
Keratoderma blenorrhagica/ plantar pustular psoriasis 20% ReA

Periarticular
Enthesitis
• Achilles tendonitis
• Plantar fasciitis
– ReA~70%
– PsA
Dactylitis
– 'daylight sign'
– PsA
– ReA
up to 30%

Mucosal
Mouth
Aphthous ulceration
Stomatitis:
• 10% IBD
• 25% ReA
Circinate balanitis:
• 30% ReA
Urethritis:
• ReA

Eyes
Conjunctivitis:
• 60% ReA, 20% PsA
Iritis:
• 5–15% IBD, 20% ReA, 7% PsA, 25–30% AS

Other
Aortic regurgitation (aortitis)
• 1% ReA
• 10% AS
Heart block
• 1% ReA
Upper lobe fibrosis in AS

The spondyloarthropathies (SpA) are a group of chronic inflammatory arthritides which share similar clinical, pathological and radiological features and a strong association with the histocompatibility antigen HLA-B27. They are categorized as axial (axSpA, involving predominantly the axial spine) or peripheral (pSpA, involving mainly the peripheral joints) with some overlap. AxSpA is further subdivided into two groups according to radiographic findings of spinal inflammation: non-radiographic (nr-axSpA) and radiographic axial SpA (r-axSpA), also known as ankylosing spondylitis.

The spondyloarthropathies comprise conditions previously considered under the umbrella term 'seronegative spondyloarthropathy' and include:

- ankylosing spondylitis (AS)
- psoriatic arthropathy (PsA)
- reactive arthritis (ReA) following infection; sexually acquired reactive arthritis (SARA) follows a sexually acquired infection; enteric reactive arthritis (ERA) follows an enteric infection
- enteropathic arthritis (inflammatory bowel disease [IBD]).

Medicine at a Glance, Fifth Edition. Edited by Patrick Davey and Alex Pitcher.

Companion website: www.wiley.com/go/medicine5e

Epidemiology

These conditions may present at any age, though they most frequently affect young adults. Males are consistently affected more commonly than females (3:1 for SARA, 2.5:1 for AS), except for the peripheral arthritis of IBD, which is more commonly found in females. The prevalence ranges from 150–500/100 000 for AS to 20/100 000 for SARA/ERA.

Clinical features

The following clinical features may occur in all SpAs (see Table 218.1).

- Peripheral arthritis (joint inflammation, usually asymmetrical and oligoarticular medium or large joints; small joints are less frequently involved, with the exception of psoriatic arthritis).
- Axial arthritis; inflammatory back pain and stiffness characterize axSpA; radiographic evidence of this is consistent with ankylosing spondylitis (r-AxSpA).
- Dactylitis (general inflammation of a digit, 'sausage digits').
- Enthesitis (inflammation and pain at the site of attachment of tendons to joints, especially Achilles).
- Tendonitis.
- Uveitis (also conjunctivitis).
- Skin (psoriasis rash, nails).

The particular combination of extra-articular features and axial and/or peripheral joint involvement is usually highly characteristic of the traditional subtypes of seronegative spondyloarthropathy (see Table 218.1).

Classification criteria for pSpA and axSpA are shown in Table 218.2. Classification criteria are designed for use in clinical trials and have high specificity and low sensitivity. In clinical practice, the expert clinical judgement of a specialist rheumatologist is required for diagnosis.

Ankylosing spondylitis (r-AxSpA)

The onset is usually in late teens or early adulthood. First-degree relatives are affected in 10% of cases. The male:female ratio is 2.5:1. AS usually presents with insidious onset of inflammatory-type pain in the lower back/buttock and/or thoracic region. Features of back pain suggesting inflammation include:

- young age (<40 years)
- significant early morning stiffness (>20 min)
- improvement on exercise
- localized tenderness over the sacroiliac joints (stiffness usually in buttock[s])
- pain at night.

Any level of the spine may be involved, but characteristically the lumbar spine is involved early on and the cervical spine relatively late. Chest pain may arise from the thoracic spine itself, the costovertebral joints or the costochondral junctions.

Ankylosing spondylitis may affect the spine at any level but thoracolumbar disease is more common than neck involvement. Chest expansion (<2.5 cm) and thoracic spine rotation are greatly reduced (see Figure 218.2). Examination of the lumbar spine shows the following.

- A decrease in flexibility in all three planes. Reduction in forward flexion is measured by Schober's test (see Figure 218.3).
- Advanced disease results in bony ankylosis and the development of deformities characteristic of AS (see Figure 218.2). As the

Table 218.1 Typical findings in the spondyloarthritides.

	Ankylosing spondylitis	**Reactive arthropathy**	**Inflammatory bowel disease associated**	**Psoriatic arthropathy**
Sex	M > F	M > F	M = F	F = M
Age at onset	<30 years	<30 years	Any age	Any age
Joints	axSpA: bilateral SIJ Approx. 40% pSpA	>90% pSpA 20% axSpA (unilateral SIJ)	>90% pSpA 30% axSpA (unilateral SIJ)	>90% pSpA 30% axSpA (unilateral SIJ)
MSK Extra-articular feature				
Sausage digits (dactylitis)	–	+	–	+
Enthesitis, tendonitis (Achilles tendonitis, plantar fasciitis)	++	+++	+	+++
Non-MSK extra-articular features				
Uveitis	+++	++	+	+
Conjunctivitis	0	+++	+	++
Skin and mucous membranes	0	++ (keratoderma blenorrhagica) + circinate balanitis	+ (pyoderma gangrenosum, erythema nodosum)	+++ (psoriasis)
Aortic incompetence	+	+	0	0
Urethritis	0	++	0	0
Prostatitis	++	++	0	0

Table 218.2 Spondyloarthritis International Society classification criteria for SpA.

Peripheral spondyloarthritis (pSpA)			**Axial spondyloarthritis (axSpA)**
Entry criteria: **One of**	**Arthritis** **OR** **Enthesitis** **OR** **Dactylitis**	Either	Sacroiliitis on imaging plus ≥1 SpA features OR HLA-B27 plus ≥ SpA features
Plus ≥1 SpA feature	Uveitis Psoriasis Crohn's/ulcerative colitis preceding infection HLA-B27 + sacroiliitis on imaging	SpA features for axSpA	Inflammatory back pain (IBP) Arthritis Enthesitis (often at the heel) Uveitis Dactylitis Psoriasis Crohn's/ulcerative colitis Good response to NSAIDs Family history for SpA HLA-B27 Elevated CRP
OR			
Plus ≥2 SpA feature	Arthritis Dactylitis Enthesitis Positive family history of SpA Inflammatory back pain ever		

Figure 218.2

Ankylosing spondylitis: Clinical features

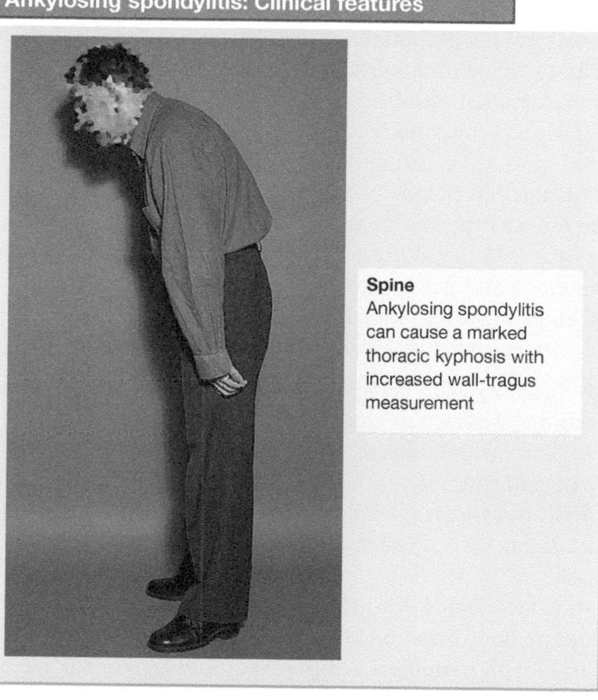

Spine
Ankylosing spondylitis can cause a marked thoracic kyphosis with increased wall-tragus measurement

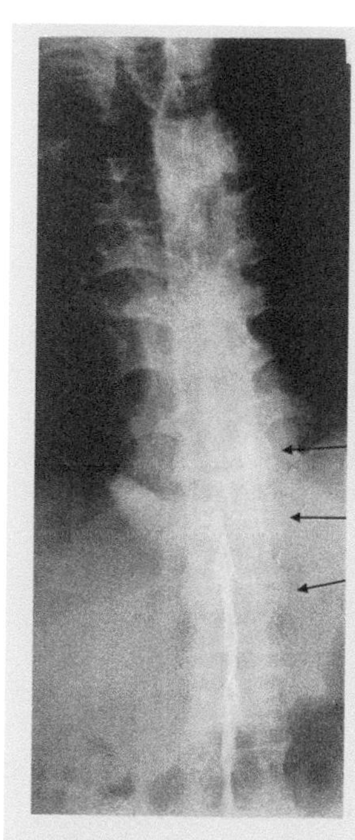

Thoracic and lumbar spine radiograph
There is fusion of the vertical bodies in the thoracic and lumbar spine. Widespread syndesmophyte formation has resulted in the typical bamboo spine appearance (arrowed)

disease progresses and ankylosis develops, the symptoms of active inflammation recede and those of disability predominate.

Investigations

- Inflammatory markers (erythrocyte sedimentation rate, C-reactive protein) are raised in under 50% of cases. Rheumatoid factor is negative.
- HLA-B27 is present in >90% compared with 8% of the general population. However, only about one in 20 of HLA-B27-positive individuals will develop AS. HLA typing for B27 should only be carried out where there is a relatively high pretest probability on clinical grounds.
- Plain radiographs may show juxta-articular sclerosis, erosions and widening of the sacroiliac joints and eventually ankylosis (fusion), but they are insensitive to early disease. Magnetic resonance imaging is the investigation of choice for early disease, because it can detect inflammatory change as well as erosions. Sagittal views of the thoracolumbar spine may show typical 'shiny corners' in the vertebrae, facet joint disease and costovertebritis. Computed tomography is also very sensitive at detecting small erosions.

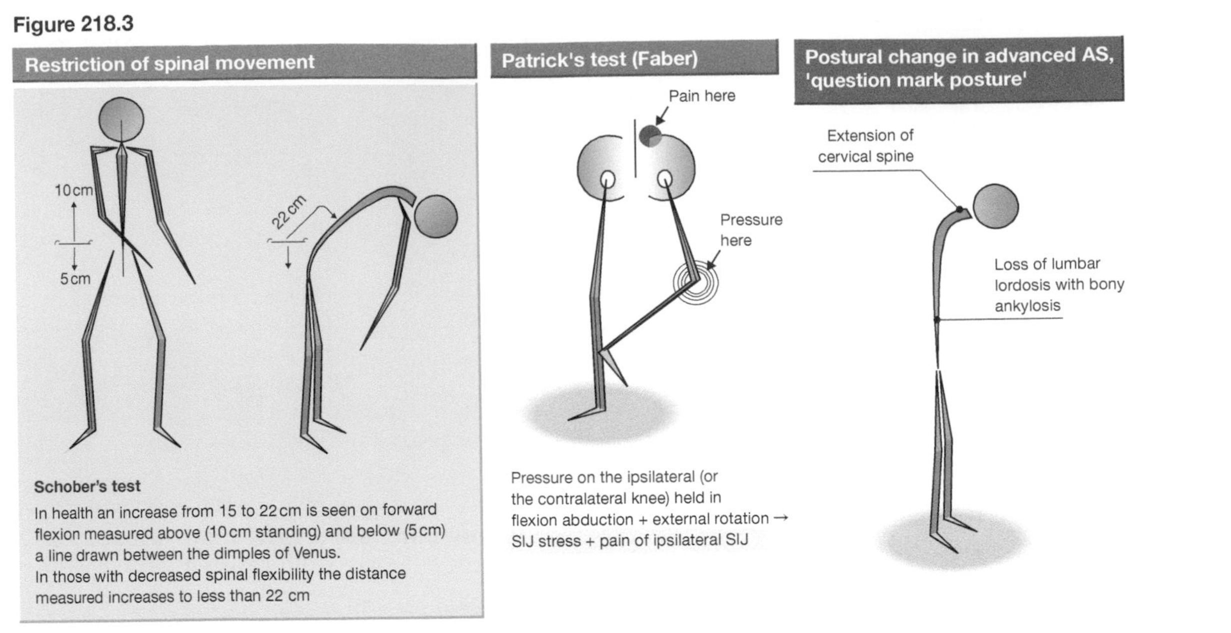

Figure 218.3
Restriction of spinal movement
10cm
5cm
22cm
Schober's test
In health an increase from 15 to 22cm is seen on forward flexion measured above (10cm standing) and below (5cm) a line drawn between the dimples of Venus.
In those with decreased spinal flexibility the distance measured increases to less than 22 cm
Patrick's test (Faber)
Pain here
Pressure here
Pressure on the ipsilateral (or the contralateral knee) held in flexion abduction + external rotation → SIJ stress + pain of ipsilateral SIJ
Postural change in advanced AS, 'question mark posture'
Extension of cervical spine
Loss of lumbar lordosis with bony ankylosis

- AS may be complicated by osteoporosis, and in selected patients a dual-emission X-ray absorptiometry (DEXA) scan of the hips may be indicated (lumbar spine measurements are unreliable because of new bone growth).

Psoriatic arthritis (pPsA ± axSpA)

Ten percent of those with psoriasis (plaque, guttate, pustular) develop arthritis, which may precede skin lesions or begin simultaneously (33%). It is important to enquire about a family history of psoriasis in anyone presenting with a mono- or oligoarticular arthritis. Psoriatic nail changes (pitting, onycholysis) occur in 70% of those with arthritis. Occult psoriasis may be apparent only in the scalp, natal cleft or umbilicus. Overall morbidity is less than in rheumatoid arthritis, but the arthritis tends to be relentlessly progressive.

Clinical patterns of psoriasis-associated spondyloarthritis

- pSpA: asymmetrical large/medium joint oligoarthritis in 50–70%.
- Peripheral small joint arthritis in 15–25% (indistinguishable from rheumatoid arthritis; negative rheumatoid factor and ACPA).
- Distal interphalangeal arthritis is associated with dystrophic changes in adjacent nails in 5–10%.
- Arthritis mutilans is a destructive arthritis of the small joints of the hands that rapidly results in joint destruction of such severity as to cause the fingers to collapse and lose length or 'telescope' (so-called 'opera glass hands') in <5%.
- AxSpA: axial arthritis/sacroiliitis: asymmetrical and isolated in 5%, or with peripheral joints involvement in 20–40%.
- Dactylitis ('sausage digits') are common and diagnostic.

Management of psoriatic arthritis and ankylosing spondylitis

As in other chronic inflammatory conditions, diagnosis and management should be specialist led, in partnership with the patient, in a multidisciplinary setting and following a 'treat to target' approach. The goal of treatment is to maximize health-related quality of life (symptom control, prevention of deformity and disability, maximize participation and function) by controlling inflammation. Treatment should be individualized according to signs and symptoms of the disease (axial, peripheral, periarticular and non-MSK manifestations); co-morbidities (cardiovascular risk and depression); and functional status/health-related quality of life, all of which should be regularly assessed. Disease activity scores (DAS) specific to p/axSpA include clinical examination findings and patient-reported outcomes and are used to guide therapeutic decision making.

Management includes the following factors.

- Intense physiotherapy, hydrotherapy and self-directed exercise/self-management programmes.
- Non-steroidal anti-inflammatory drugs (NSAIDs) first line for pain and stiffness.
- Intra-articular steroids may be useful, including for sacroiliac joints (SIJs). Systemic steroid therapy should be short term only.
- Conventional synthetic DMARDs (csDMARDs), e.g. methotrexate or sulfasalazine (see Chapter 217) should be initiated in those with peripheral arthritis and poor prognostic factors, e.g. high inflammatory markers, dactylitis, significant skin/nail involvement or radiographic damage.
- Targeted biologic therapies (bDMARDs) directed against TNF-α, IL-17 and IL-23 are recommended for persistently active disease in patients not responsive to/who cannot take DMARD where the risk/benefit profile is favourable. Safety screening (TB and hepatitis B) and monitoring are required. Given by subcutaneous injection or infusion.
- Biologics targeting TNF-α (anti-TNF-α/TNFi) are highly effective for AS and for skin and arthritis in PsA (see Chapter 217 for agents).
- Biologics targeting IL-17 or IL-23 proinflammatory pathways include the following.
  - IL-17A inhibitor therapy (sekukinumab, ixekizumab) has proven efficacy in PsA and AS (nr- and r-AxSpA). Associated

with an increased rate of non-serious infections and should not be used in inflammatory bowel disease. Screen for TB and hepatitis B.

- Anti-IL-23 (guselkumab) and anti-IL-12/IL-23 (ustekinumab) therapies have proven efficacy in active psoriatic arthritis. Ustekinumab is also licensed for inflammatory bowel disease. Associated with an increased rate of non-serious infections.

- Targeted synthetic DMARDs include the following.
  - Janus kinase (JAK) inhibitors (tofacitinib) and selective JAK inhibitors (upadacitinib) are efficacious in spondyloarthropathy. Tofacitinib (EU and USA) and upadacitinib (EU) are licensed for psoriatic arthritis. Upadacitinib is also licensed (EU) for ankylosing spondylitis (r-axSpA). JAK inhibitors are variably associated with infection, including TB (screen prior to use) and zoster, increases in lipid parameters, intestinal perforation and venous thromboembolism (VTE). Monitoring of FBC, LFTs and lipids is advised.
  - The phosphodiesterase-4 (PDE4) inhibitor apremilast is licensed for PsA (EU and USA). GI upset is common.

Reactive arthritis

Aseptic inflammation of the joints (typically lower limb oligoarticular) may complicate a range of infections at distant sites; typically, genital tract and enteric infections are responsible. Seventy percent of patients are HLA-B27 positive. *Chlamydia*, *Salmonella*, *Shigella*, *Yersinia* and *Campylobacter* species are well-recognized triggers. Although bacterial proteins and DNA can be isolated from the joints, sometimes viable organisms are never cultured.

Non-MSK features are common, including conjunctivitis, aseptic urethritis, mucosal ulceration (circinate balanitis, hard palate) and psoriaform rash on the hands and feet (keratoderma blennorrhagica). The differential diagnosis includes other spondyloarthritides, septic arthritis/trauma and gout. The diagnosis is clinical, but the following investigations may be useful.

- Inflammatory markers are raised. Rheumatoid factor/ACPA negative. Synovial fluid analysis is indicated primarily to exclude sepsis or crystals (sterile leukocytosis).
- Urinalysis: pyuria (usually sterile). Culture: urine/stool/synovial fluid/high urethral or vaginal swab, and serology for *Chlamydia* and *Yersinia*. Referral to an ID clinic may be appropriate.
- HLA-B27 testing may be helpful.

Management

Establish the diagnosis and rule out sepsis. Initiate bed rest, intra-articular steroids and splinting in the acute attack, followed by passive strengthening exercises at about 10 days. NSAIDs are useful for symptom control but some patients (<5%) may need systemic corticosteroids.

Recurrent or chronic symptoms may require disease-modifying antirheumatic drugs (DMARDs, e.g. sulfasalazine or methotrexate) and, exceptionally, anti-TNF agents are indicated. Remission is usual at 2–6 months, but persistence of symptoms and recurrent flares are common (*c.* 30%). Long-term follow-up of more severe forms of reactive arthritis suggests that up to 20% may develop axSpA over 20 years. Severe systemic features with weight loss, fevers and deranged liver function tests may mimic deep sepsis or malignancy in some cases. The role of antibiotic therapy in limiting arthritic complications is controversial. However, in sexually acquired forms of the disease, contact tracing and eradication of *Chlamydia* are clearly important.

Enteropathic arthritis

- Peripheral and/or axial joint involvement occur. Axial is more common (up to 30% of Crohn's); 100% of B27-positive IBD patients develop sacroiliitis.
- Extra-articular/extraintestinal manifestations occur in the eye (5%) and the skin (pyoderma gangrenosum <5% and erythema nodosum <10%).
- Type I peripheral enteropathic arthritis is oligoarticular, self-limiting and associated with flares of IBD. Type II peripheral enteropathic arthritis is polyarticular, protracted and not related to disease activity in the gut.
- Both types of arthropathy may respond to sulfasalazine or methotrexate. Anti-TNF-α therapy is also highly effective. UC arthropathy is also responsive to bowel resection.

Systemic lupus erythematosus

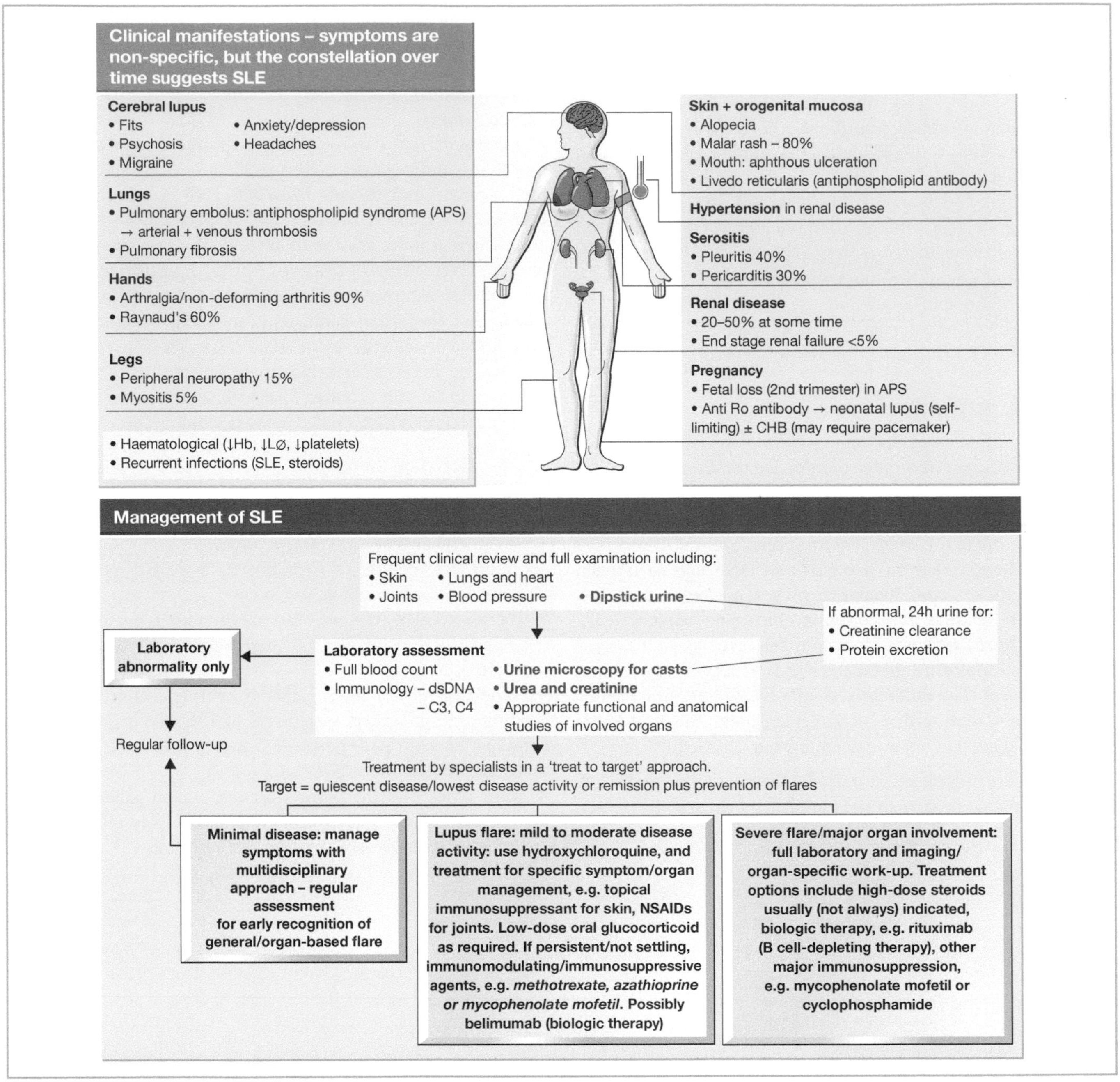

Clinical manifestations – symptoms are non-specific, but the constellation over time suggests SLE

Cerebral lupus
- Fits
- Psychosis
- Migraine
- Anxiety/depression
- Headaches

Lungs
- Pulmonary embolus: antiphospholipid syndrome (APS) → arterial + venous thrombosis
- Pulmonary fibrosis

Hands
- Arthralgia/non-deforming arthritis 90%
- Raynaud's 60%

Legs
- Peripheral neuropathy 15%
- Myositis 5%

- Haematological (↓Hb, ↓LØ, ↓platelets)
- Recurrent infections (SLE, steroids)

Skin + orogenital mucosa
- Alopecia
- Malar rash – 80%
- Mouth: aphthous ulceration
- Livedo reticularis (antiphospholipid antibody)

Hypertension in renal disease

Serositis
- Pleuritis 40%
- Pericarditis 30%

Renal disease
- 20–50% at some time
- End stage renal failure <5%

Pregnancy
- Fetal loss (2nd trimester) in APS
- Anti Ro antibody → neonatal lupus (self-limiting) ± CHB (may require pacemaker)

Management of SLE

Frequent clinical review and full examination including:
- Skin
- Joints
- Lungs and heart
- Blood pressure
- **Dipstick urine**

If abnormal, 24h urine for:
- Creatinine clearance
- Protein excretion

Laboratory assessment
- Full blood count
- Immunology – dsDNA – C3, C4
- **Urine microscopy for casts**
- **Urea and creatinine**
- Appropriate functional and anatomical studies of involved organs

Laboratory abnormality only → Regular follow-up

Treatment by specialists in a 'treat to target' approach.
Target = quiescent disease/lowest disease activity or remission plus prevention of flares

Minimal disease: manage symptoms with multidisciplinary approach – regular assessment for early recognition of general/organ-based flare

Lupus flare: mild to moderate disease activity: use hydroxychloroquine, and treatment for specific symptom/organ management, e.g. topical immunosuppressant for skin, NSAIDs for joints. Low-dose oral glucocorticoid as required. If persistent/not settling, immunomodulating/immunosuppressive agents, e.g. *methotrexate, azathioprine or mycophenolate mofetil*. Possibly belimumab (biologic therapy)

Severe flare/major organ involvement: full laboratory and imaging/organ-specific work-up. Treatment options include high-dose steroids usually (not always) indicated, biologic therapy, e.g. rituximab (B cell-depleting therapy), other major immunosuppression, e.g. mycophenolate mofetil or cyclophosphamide

Systemic lupus erythematosus (SLE) is a multisystem disease characterized by inflammation involving many systems, and exhibits a relapsing and remitting course. It is strongly associated with autoantibodies to components of the cell nucleus (antinuclear antibodies [ANAs]). Its protean manifestations lead to its inclusion in the differential diagnosis of many 'difficult to diagnose' cases in clinical practice and patients may have had symptoms for some time before a diagnosis is made.

Medicine at a Glance, Fifth Edition. Edited by Patrick Davey and Alex Pitcher.

Companion website: www.wiley.com/go/medicine5e

Aetiology and epidemiology

The aetiology of SLE is unknown, but multiple genetic and environmental factors are probably involved. Concordance is 25% in monozygotic twins, but only 2% in non-twin siblings indicating strong genetic influences. The HLA-DR3 association is thought to reflect complement null alleles on these haplotypes. Inherited deficiencies of early complement cascade components (e.g. C1q and C2) are extremely strongly associated with SLE. It is particularly prevalent in the African-American female population of the USA (one in 250), in contrast to the low prevalence in similar ethnic groups in West Africa. In mixed-ethnicity UK populations, the prevalence is 45–50/100 000 females. Females are 10 times more commonly affected than males. Peak onset is 15–40 years.

A range of drugs (e.g. minocycline, procainamide, hydralazine) can induce a lupus-like syndrome, particularly in those with certain metabolic polymorphisms of the cytochrome P450 system (e.g. slow acetylators) which usually resolves on discontinuation of the drug.

There is no single immunopathological feature. Vasculitis, coagulopathy, tissue inflammation and immune complex deposition may all occur. There are abnormalities in cellular and humoral immunity; the complement system, which may underlie abnormal clearance of immune complexes; apoptosis, which may lead to the generation of characteristic antinuclear and antiphospholipid antibodies.

Renal pathology is well studied and five histological groups of glomerulonephritis are recognized (WHO criteria), from minimal change to proliferative and sclerosing glomerulonephritis. Anti-DNA antibodies may be involved in the pathogenesis of lupus nephritis.

Clinical features and classification criteria

Non-specific constitutional features include joint pains, extreme lethargy/fatigue, weight loss and lymphadenopathy. Systemic upset (fever and extreme malaise) is usually very marked in active lupus and is often the dominant presenting feature. The best recognized clinical feature of lupus is the 'butterfly'/malar facial rash, commonly following sun exposure. Other rashes, mouth ulcers and a non-deforming arthritis are common. Vital organ involvement, such as renal or central nervous system (CNS), determines prognosis and treatment. Renal involvement may manifest as nephrotic syndrome or covertly with proteinuria, active renal sediment and progressive loss of renal function. CNS manifestations, such as headaches, seizures, strokes, cognitive decline and altered behaviour, are common. Encephalopathy occasionally occurs.

Formal classification criteria for lupus have been defined by the American College of Rheumatology and the European Alliance of Associations for Rheumatology (EULAR) (see Table 219.1).These are primarily intended for use in clinical trials but may be used in clinical practice, in which case they are highly specific but lack sensitivity and may miss early or mild disease. Lupus should be diagnosed and managed by clinical specialists in multidisciplinary units.

Table 219.1 2019 ACR/EULAR classification criteria[a] for SLE

Obligatory entry criterion: ANA ≥1:80 (HEp-2 cells or equivalent)		**Weighted score**
Additive criteria: clinical domains		
Constitutional	Fever	2
Haematological	Leukopenia	3
	Thrombocytopenia	4
	Autoimmune haemolysis	4
Neuropsychiatric	Delirium	2
	Psychosis	3
	Seizure	5
Mucocutaneous	Non-scarring alopecia	2
	Oral ulcers	2
	Subacute cutaneous OR discoid lupus	4
	Acute cutaneous lupus	6
Renal	Proteinuria >0.5 g/24h	4
	Renal biopsy WHO Class II or V lupus nephritis	8
	Renal biopsy WHO Class III or IV lupus nephritis	10
Serosal	Pleural or pericardial effusion	5
	Acute pericarditis	6
Musculoskeletal	Joint involvement	6
Additive criteria: clinical immunology domains and criteria		
Antiphospholipid antibodies	Anticardiolipin antibodies OR Anti-β2GP1 antibodies OR Lupus anticoagulant	2
Complements	Low C3 OR low C4	3
	Low C3 AND low C4	4
SLE-specific antibodies	Anti-dsDNA antibody OR Anti-Smith antibody	6

Classify as systemic lupus erythematosus with a score of 10 or more if entry criterion fulfilled.

[a]See note on applicability to diagnosis in text.

Immunology and other investigations in SLE

- **Immunology**: ANA testing: a positive ANA test is required as an entry criterion in the ACR/EULAR 2019 classification criteria for SLE (see Table 219.1). Laboratory testing for ANA is indicated where there are clinical features suggestive of SLE or a connective tissue disease and should not be undertaken otherwise. Approximately 10% of the elderly population will test positive for ANA. See Chapter 66 for additional immunological tests.

Double-stranded DNA (dsDNA) antibodies tested by *Crithidia luciliae* immunofluorescence are more specific but less sensitive for SLE; titres also correspond only loosely to activity (see Tables 219.2 and 219.3). Antibodies to Smith antibody are similarly specific to SLE. Antibodies to the extractable nuclear antigens Ro (SSA) and La (SSB) are found in SLE and in primary Sjögren syndrome. Maternal anti-Ro antibodies are associated with neonatal lupus and fetal congenital heart block in a very small percentage of Ro-positive mothers. Antihistone antibodies are associated with drug-induced lupus. Complement components C3 and C4 are typically low due to consumption in active SLE but are unreliable as a routine guide to disease activity. In contrast to other inflammatory disorders, C-reactive protein may be normal in active SLE; a raised level raises the suspicion of complicating infection.

- **Lupus band test (biopsy of uninvolved skin)**: specific for lupus, demonstrating a characteristic band of IgG and/or IgM

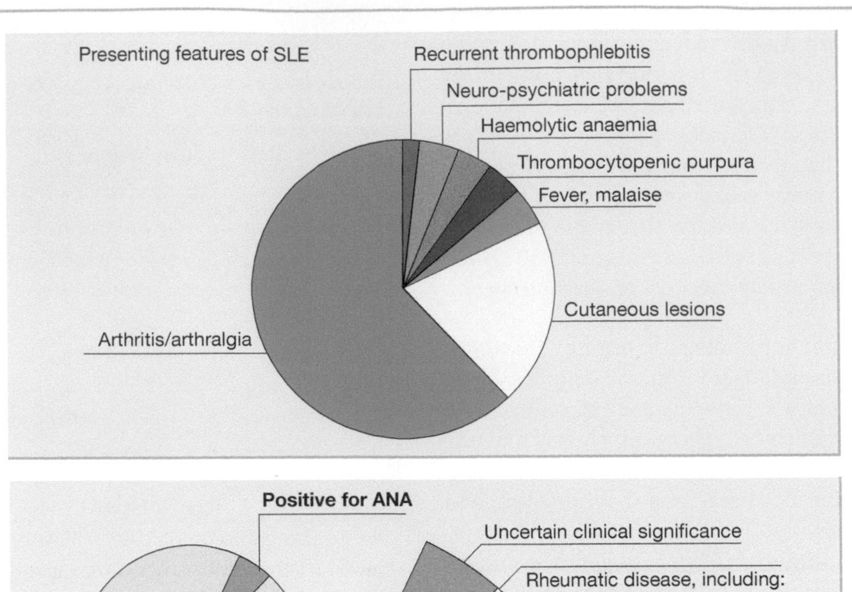

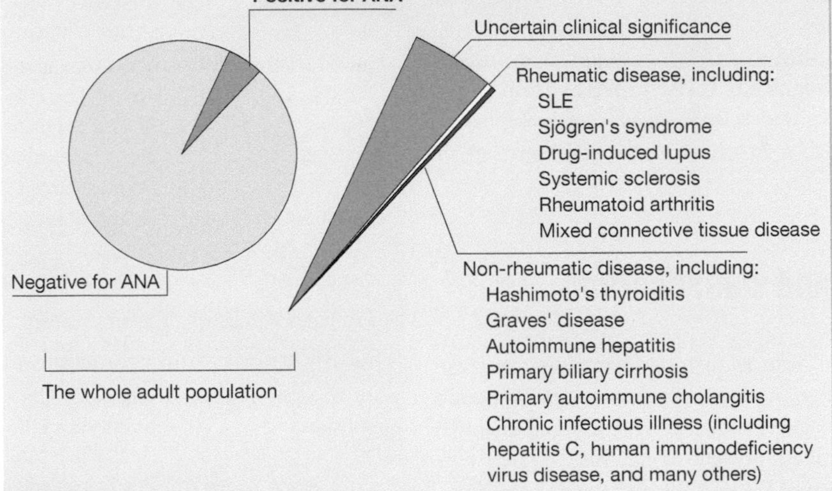

deposition at the dermo-epidermal junction in involved and uninvolved skin.

- **Haematology**: leukopenia/lymphopenia occur in active SLE. Anaemia may be due to chronic disease or Coombs-positive haemolysis. Immune thrombocytopenia can occur, and can predate lupus by many years.
- **Renal function**: renal impairment (decreased glomerular filtration rate) or proteinuria (>3+ dipstick, >0.5 g/24 h) are common in SLE, and of major therapeutic importance. An 'active renal sediment' with red cell and/or granular casts may be the *only* indication of serious renal disease. Renal biopsy should be performed to guide treatment in lupus nephritis.
- **Clotting abnormalities**: venous and arterial thromboses may occur due to autoantibodies found in **antiphospholipid syndrome** (APS). These activate *in vivo* clotting but *in vitro* cause a *prolonged* activated partial thromboplastin time (APTT) or 'lupus anticoagulant' effect. Full laboratory screen for APS includes (i) APTT or lupus anticoagulant, detected with the dilute Russell viper venom test, dRVVT and (ii) IgG/IgM antiphospholipid (aPL) antibodies against anticardiolipin and β2-glycoprotein I-(β2GPI-Ab) (see also Chapter 66). Only the antibody tests are informative if a patient is anticoagulated. If positive, the screen should be repeated at 12 weeks. Triple positivity (two positive IgG aPL antibodies plus one positive lupus anticoagulant test) is associated with high VTE risk.

In the appropriate clinical context, one such laboratory abnormality can suggest the presence of the APS and haematological opinion and management advice should be sought. Clinical features of APS include pregnancy morbidity and arterial and/or venous thromboses, including CVA.

Management and therapy

Lupus is a chronic unpredictable disease that relapses and remits. Clinical management aims to reduce/minimize disease activity or induce remission and prevent flares. Preventive strategies include protection against ultraviolet radiation and prompt evaluation and treatment of infection. Close clinical supervision, with regular assessment of the disease, is vital to determine the need for immunosuppressive therapy, particularly to minimize long-term organ damage.

A number of internationally validated disease activity scores are utilized in clinical trials to 'measure' general or organ-specific activity. These are not widely used in clinical practice but their scores broadly map to 'mild', 'moderate' and 'severe' disease classifications which guide treatment decisions.

Pharmacological options for treatment include the following.

- **NSAIDs**: short term for musculoskeletal manifestations, avoid in renal lupus or hypertension.

Table 219.2 Immunological and other tests for SLE.

Test	% positive (approx.)
dsDNA binding	65–75%
Antinuclear antibodies (high titre, IgG class)	95
Raised serum IgG level	65
Low serum complement (C3/C4 levels)	60
Platelet autoantibodies	60
Cryoglobulinaemia	20
Antibodies to extractable nuclear antigen:	
• Sm	5–30
• RNP	35
• Ro	30
• La	15
Antibodies to phospholipids	30
Rheumatoid factor (low titre)	30
Skin biopsy of normal skin +ve for IgG, C3 and C4 deposits	75–85
Raised ESR	60
Leukopenia	45
Direct Coombs test +ve	40
Lupus anticoagulant	10–20
C-reactive protein	May indicate infection
Proteinuria	30

Table 219.3 Interpretation of changes in complement and dsDNA in SLE.

dsDNA	C3	C4	Interpretation dsDNA antibodies
↑	→	→	↑ Activity: watch for change in clinical state
↓/→	↓	↓	Renal involvement should be suspected
↑/→	↑	↑	Look for infection: measure C-reactive protein (not usually increased unless infection present)

- **Antimalarials**: hydroxychloroquine is currently recommended for all patients as it improves overall disease outcomes in epidemiological studies. It is particularly helpful for musculoskeletal and cutaneous manifestations. Side-effects include rare cardiac and retinal toxicity. A 5 mg/kg daily dose regimen is recommended as is regular ophthalmological screening.
- **Systemic immunosuppression** is used for acute lupus flares and major organ involvement.
  - Corticosteroids: used topically for inflammatory rashes and orally for active disease, such as serositis and constitutional upset. May be given intravenously for acute severe or organ-threatening manifestations such as CNS lupus. Beware of cumulative steroid toxicity and mitigate risks via, e.g., co-prescription of bone protection.
  - Azathioprine, methotrexate, calcineurin inhibitors (e.g. tacrolimus) and mycophenolate mofetil are useful immunomodulatory agents for moderate or persistent disease activity. They also reduce overall steroid burden/exposure which is a key priority.
  - Cyclophosphamide is a potent agent which may be indicated in severe organ-threatening lupus activity, e.g. renal or CNS in specialist care settings. High-dose mycophenolate mofetil (2–3 g/day) is an alternative (not for CNS).
  - Rituximab is a monoclonal antibody therapy which depletes B cells. It is given intravenously at six-monthly dose intervals. It is mostly used in refractory severe disease, e.g. renal and haematological.
  - SLE-specific biological therapies: belimumab (anti BLyS, B lymphocyte stimulator) was approved in 2011 and newer agents are in development/clinical trials. Add-on belimumab may be useful for persistently active or flaring non-renal (mild-to-moderate) disease or to maintain disease control when steroid reduction is not tolerated. Therapeutic targets for the drugs in development are specific to lupus and target B cells, complement and interferon pathways that have been shown to be important in SLE activity and progression. Their place in therapeutic strategies for SLE is not yet known.
- **Anticoagulation** is used in the APS: life-long warfarin is used in patients who have experienced thrombosis. Target INR is determined by the severity of APS and conferred VTE risk. Direct-acting oral anticoagulants are not recommended in APS, and specifically not for patients who are 'triple positive' (see above) or who have experienced arterial thrombosis.
- **Symptomatic treatment** as appropriate, e.g. depression, epilepsy, Raynaud phenomenon and mouth ulcers.
- **Adjunct therapy**: scrupulous attention should be paid to correcting traditional adverse cardiovascular risk factors, e.g. hypertension, dyslipidaemia, BMI, exercise, smoking, and to the prevention of infection, including by vaccination. Daily sunblock (UVA + B) is recommended. Angiotensin-converting enzyme inhibitors (ACEi) have a role in reducing proteinuria and blood pressure in renal lupus.

Prognosis

Historically, SLE was associated with poor outcomes but survival is now >90% at 10 years. There is an excess all-cause mortality in those with severe vs mild disease at diagnosis. Lupus also carries an increased cardiovascular disease risk, much of which is related to chronic inflammation and steroid use. End-organ involvement differs widely between individuals and influences outcomes. Patient access to healthcare and education, approaches to disease control and new therapeutic strategies all improve prognosis. Attention to co-morbidities prevention (particularly cardiovascular risk factors and infection) plus minimization of long-term steroid exposure are also key.

220 Myositis syndromes, polymyalgia rheumatica and systemic sclerosis

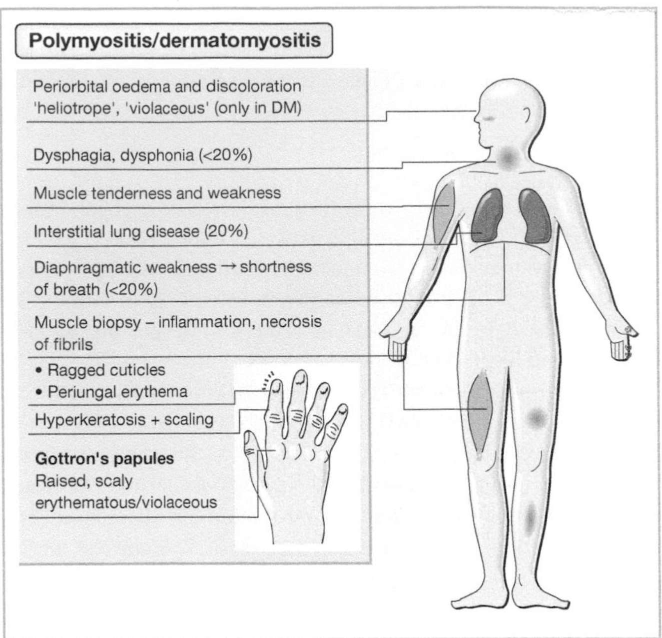

Myositis

Myositis is an inflammation of muscles and presents with aching, tender, weak muscles, sometimes in a characteristic distribution. Muscle enzymes (creatine phosphokinase [CK or CPK]) are raised and levels may be used to monitor treatment. Where inflammation is suspected, magnetic resonance imaging (MRI) may be diagnostic or is used to guide biopsy. Electromyography (EMG) findings are also characteristic. Immune-mediated myositis may be characterized by myositis-*specific* autoantibodies (MSA, e.g. anti-jo-1) which act as biomarkers for specific myositis diseases: MSAs are associated with characteristic phenotypes, prognosis and therapeutic response (see Table 220.1). Myositis-*associated* autoantibodies (MAA, e.g. U1RNP) are also predictive of clinical myositis and are usually found in conditions such as systemic lupus erythematosus (SLE) or undifferentiated connective tissue disease.

Immune-mediated myositis syndromes

These conditions have autoantibody production and myositis as key pathological features. The recent discovery of novel myositis-specific autoantibodies and the characterization of associated clinical features have changed the approach to myositis in clinical practice.

Polymyositis (PM) and dermatomyositis (DM) are the main immune-mediated inflammatory myopathies of unknown aetiology. The peak incidence of PM is 40–60 years. DM also occurs in childhood. Overall prevalence is 5–10 per million. Pathological findings are of inflammation in muscles (and skin in DM) and in the vessels that supply them.

Clinical features and classification

Both PM and DM are characterized by a subacute onset of proximal arm and leg weakness. Classic DM is associated with a rash, most commonly affecting the face and trunk but also on the dorsum of the hands (Gottron's papules). Table 220.1 shows characteristic adult myositis phenotypes and autoantibody associations. Childhood-onset (juvenile) DM is an inflammatory myopathy resulting in muscle atrophy and contractures or limb/regional growth restriction, skin involvement, subcutaneous calcification and vasculitis affecting the skin, muscle and gut.

Investigations

The most helpful tests are markers of muscle damage (biochemical, electrical, histological). CK is raised in >70% cases; EMG is abnormal in almost all polymyositis, with characteristic findings. Muscle biopsy shows inflammatory cellular infiltrate with necrosis of muscle fibres. MRI findings are characteristic, show the extent of myositis, and guide choice of site for biopsy. Myositis autoantibodies are positive in approximately 50–75% (see Table 220.1). As myositis syndromes may be associated with malignancy (anti-TIF1-γ), a screening history and full physical examination are required to search for underlying malignancy. Further investigations are guided by risk factors and clinical findings.

Management and outcome

Early diagnosis is important to preserve muscle function and avoid major organ involvement.

- High-dose prednisolone initially to achieve disease control. Tapering of steroids occurs according to symptoms and CK level.
- 10–15% may not respond to steroids or relapse on steroid taper. Second-line agents such as methotrexate, azathioprine or mycophenolate are then initiated.
- Intravenous immunoglobulin can be useful, particularly in skin disease.
- In the absence of underlying malignancy, up to 85% of patients have a good or partial response to steroids.

Polymyalgia rheumatica

Polymyalgia rheumatica is a relatively common (*c*.1% prevalence in those aged >60 years) inflammatory disorder of unknown aetiology affecting older adults, resulting in pain and stiffness of the proximal muscle groups. The disease is more common in females (2:1) and uncommon in non-Caucasians. The pathophysiology is unclear and no histological lesion is diagnostic. There is no myositis but there may be synovitis. Polymyalgia rheumatica may be disabling in older adults but is not life-threatening. Response to steroids is characteristic. Morbidity may arise due to long-term steroid therapy and second-line agents may be required to limit steroid exposure.

Medicine at a Glance, Fifth Edition. Edited by Patrick Davey and Alex Pitcher.

Companion website: www.wiley.com/go/medicine5e

Table 220.1 Characteristic adult myositis phenotypes and autoantibody associations.

Autoantibodies	Typical clinical features
Anti-aminoacyl-tRNA synthetase; antisynthetase syndrome	Moderate to severe proximal myositis (CK usually in 1000s). Fever, synovitis, 'mechanic's hands' and interstitial lung disease (ILD). May also involve oesophageal muscles (-> dysphagia) and respiratory muscles (->respiratory failure)
Anti-Jo-1	Similar to antisynthetase syndrome. Usually a more chronic course and higher frequency of ILD
Anti-Mi-2	Classic dermatomyositis with skin findings (lilac-coloured rash, oedema of the upper eyelids and a scaly violaceous eruption over the extensor surfaces of the joints – knuckles, elbows, knees; Gottron's papules). Myositis usually mild. Usually good response to therapy
Anti-TIF1-γ	Cancer-associated dermatomyositis (most commonly lung, ovary, breast, gastrointestinal tract and myeloproliferative disorders). Severe skin disease. Guarded prognosis due to association with malignancy
Anti-MDA5	Clinically amyopathic dermatomyositis. Associated with rapidly progressive ILD, often poor response to treatment
Anti-HMGCR	Associated with statin use. Severe proximal muscle weakness. Usually responsive to intravenous immunoglobulin

Clinical and investigative features

- Pronounced early morning stiffness in the limb girdles with ache and weakness, which leads to difficulty rising from squat or raising arms above head.
- Systemic features of weight loss, fatigue and lassitude may occur.
- Up to one-fifth have concurrent giant cell arteritis (see Chapter 218).
- Erythrocyte sedimentation rate (ESR) is usually >60. Fibrinogen and C-reactive protein (CRP) are also raised.
- Other laboratory investigations, including muscle enzymes, are usually normal.
- Normochromic anaemia and/or raised alkaline phosphatase may be found. There is no diagnostic radiology.

Management

- Oral prednisolone therapy gives prompt and dramatic improvement in symptoms, initially 15 mg/day (typically for two months), tapering slowly by 1 mg per month as symptoms resolve and inflammatory markers fall. Steroid therapy can usually be stopped after 12–18 months but up to 20% of patients require long-term low-dose maintenance. Immunosuppressive agents, including methotrexate, may be useful as steroid-sparing drugs.
- Relapses in symptoms are managed by increasing up to the last effective dose of prednisolone.
- Bone protection with calcium/vitamin D preparations or bisphosphonates is usually indicated due to steroid requirement.

Systemic sclerosis

Systemic sclerosis (scleroderma) is a chronic inflammatory condition involving skin and, variably, internal organs. It is characterized by pathological features of fibrosis (skin and e.g. lungs) and vasculopathy (Raynaud phenomenon), gastric antral vascular ectasia (GAVE) and pulmonary arterial hypertension (PAH). Two clinical phenotypes are recognized with classification based on extent of skin involvement: diffuse cutaneous (dcSSc, skin involvement extends proximally above knees and elbows) and limited cutaneous SSc (lcSSc, skin involvement limited to below knees and elbows). Limited cutaneous SSc is often referred to as CREST syndrome, the mnemonic CREST representing the major clinical features of: calcinosis; Raynaud syndrome; (o)esophagitis; scleroderma; and telangiectasia. Characteristically, small ulcers and pits may develop on the tips of digits and risk infection and necrosis with pulp loss. Progressive sclerodactyly may result in flexion contractures and loss of hand function. A spectrum of chronic disease severity from mild to severe is observed in clinical practice.

Immunology

Systemic sclerosis is characteristically associated with antitopoisomerase 1/Scl-70 (dcSSc) and anticentromere (lcSSc) autoantibody formation, noting that there may be overlap. Other autoantibodies, e.g. anti-RNA polymerase III, may be found. Characterization of the typical phenotype associated with this is ongoing. Secondary antiphospholipid syndrome (see Table 66.1) may be associated with an increased risk of tissue necrosis in association with Raynaud and digital tip ulceration.

Prevalence and outcome

Epidemiological studies report an overall prevalence of 7.2–33.9 (Europe) and 13.5–44.3 (North America) per 100 000; differences may reflect case finding. Age at diagnosis is usually 30–55 years and women are affected 4–10 times as commonly as men. Up to 50% are reported to develop interstitial lung disease. The prevalence of SSc-associated PAH is approximately 5–15%. Morbidity and mortality data reflect an era in which both diagnostic and therapeutic options were limited, for a reported 10-year survival of approximately 75% (Europe) and 80% (USA). Cardiorespiratory involvement, particularly ILD and PAH, is associated with poor prognosis.

Pathology

The key pathological processes underlying systemic sclerosis are inflammatory with resultant fibrosis and vasculopathy. Recent research into pathways of immune activation in SSc have led to clinical trials of therapeutic strategies targeting cytokines important in fibrosis, with promising results. There is not as yet a targeted molecular therapeutic pathway but there is some evidence for an immunomodulatory approach, particularly in the early stages of diffuse cutaneous disease.

Clinical features, investigation and management

If characteristic skin features are present, the diagnosis is usually easily made. These include skin thickening (scleroderma) and tightening (sclerodactyly of fingers) with loss of usual skin markings, progressing to hand contractures in severe disease. These are often accompanied by telangiectasia, subcutaneous calcinosis and ulceration of the digits. Facial features of reduced oral aperture, skin tightness and facial telangiectasia may be prominent. Early disease presents with more subtle features including new-onset Raynaud phenomenon (cold-triggered peripheral vasospasm with triphasic colour change), which may be asymmetrical and prolonged, and 'puffy hands' with inability to press palms and fingers together fully (prayer sign). In addition, a full history is required to uncover symptoms of internal organ involvement requiring further investigation and management.

The clinical features include the following.

- **Upper GI tract**: oesophagitis (dyspepsia, reflux, heartburn), dysmotility (dysphagia, regurgitation), GAVE (iron deficiency anaemia, melaena).
- **Lower GI tract**: bacterial overgrowth (large intestinal dysmotility and wide-mouthed diverticulae) leading to diarrhoea/steatorrhoea and malabsorption of iron, B_{12} and fat-soluble vitamins, anal sphincter dysmotility producing faecal incontinence.
- **Cardiorespiratory**: cardiac conduction disturbances; diastolic dysfunction. Hypertension (accelerated/malignant HT in SSc renal crisis). Peripheral ulceration. Venous thromboembolism (check antiphospholipid screen).
- **Respiratory**: ILD causing breathlessness, pulmonary arterial hypertension causing progressive breathlessness, right ventricular failure.
- **Skin**: scleroderma (any skin); sclerodactyly (fingers), Raynaud phenomenon, may be associated with skin ulceration (can be slow to heal) and secondary infection and/or tissue loss/autoamputation, may be painful.

Management

A key principle of management in SSc is the early detection of significant internal organ involvement through regular screening. This is especially important for poor prognosis features such as PAH and ILD. *Symptomatic* PAH and ILD are poor prognostic factors and screening is recommended to detect these conditions in their early (treatable) pathological phases. In addition to full history and physical examination at each visit, serial echocardiograms and lung diffusion capacity (DLCO) should be carried out annually in asymptomatic patients. Where pulmonary arterial pressure is elevated per echocardiographic criteria, referral to a specialist centre for right heart catheterization ± PAH treatment is indicated as a matter of urgency. PAH in SSc is confirmed on right heart catheterization by the recording of a mean pulmonary artery pressure >20 mmHg at rest with pulmonary capillary wedge pressure ≤15 mmHg and pulmonary vascular resistance ≥2 Wood units.

A fall in serial DLCO measurement or six-minute walk test may alternatively signal the development of ILD. Prompt evaluation with CT thorax imaging and specialist pulmonology review and treatment should be undertaken.

The last decade has seen the more routine use of immunomodulation in early diffuse cutaneous SSc and this approach, combined with improved screening and therapies of PAH and ILD, has led to an improvement in overall disease outcomes and morbidity. In addition, therapies for specific internal organ manifestations such as ILD and PAH have progressed significantly and offer much hope, particularly for very early organ involvement found on screening. SSc renal crisis (accelerated hypertension and acute renal failure) was previously the primary cause of mortality but this is no longer the case, largely due to the efficacy of ACEi which should be used first line for hypertension in SSc.

221 Eczema and urticaria

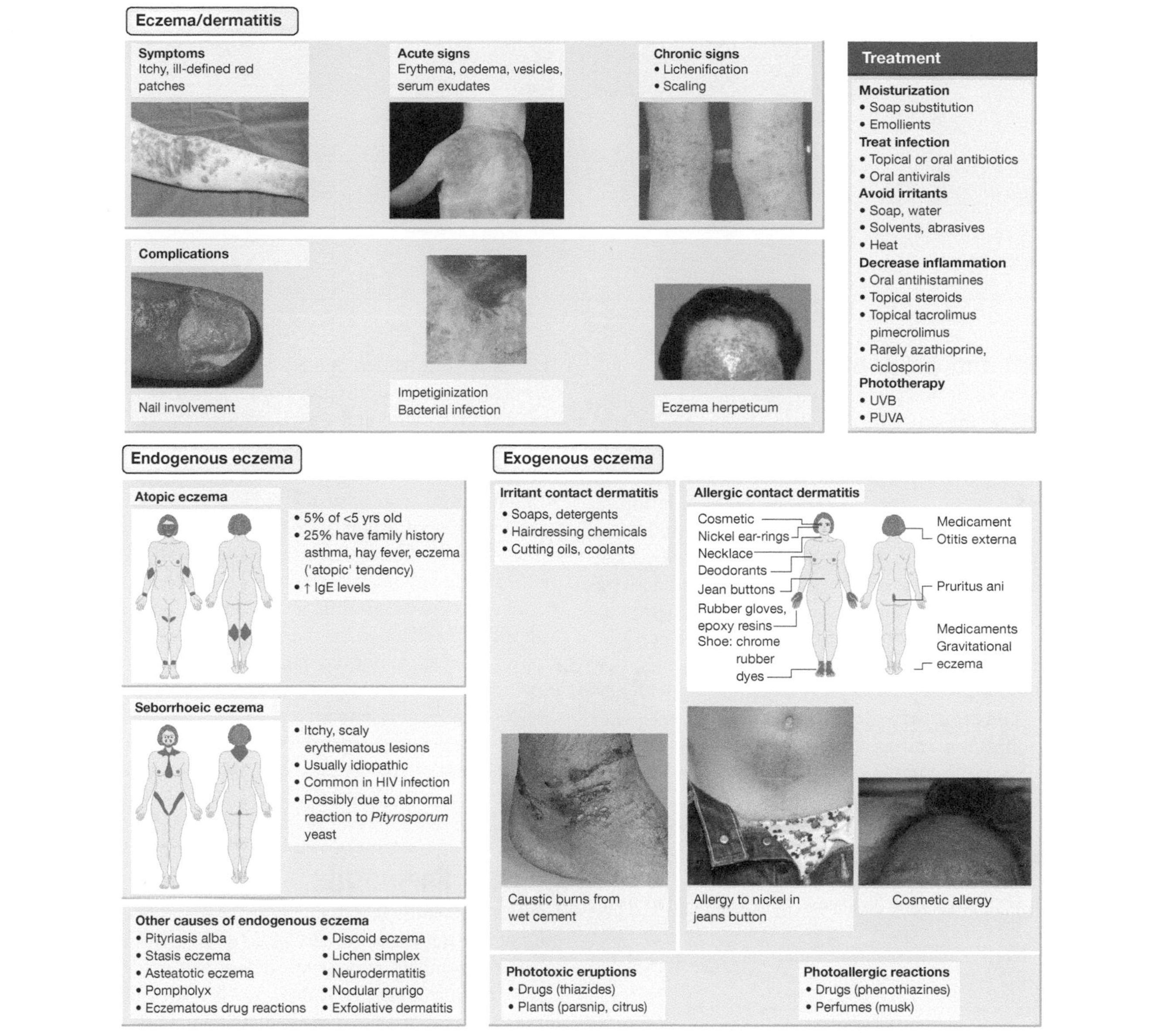

Eczema/dermatitis
Symptoms
Itchy, ill-defined red patches
Acute signs
Erythema, oedema, vesicles, serum exudates
Chronic signs
• Lichenification
• Scaling
Treatment
Moisturization
• Soap substitution
• Emollients
Treat infection
• Topical or oral antibiotics
• Oral antivirals
Avoid irritants
• Soap, water
• Solvents, abrasives
• Heat
Decrease inflammation
• Oral antihistamines
• Topical steroids
• Topical tacrolimus pimecrolimus
• Rarely azathioprine, ciclosporin
Phototherapy
• UVB
• PUVA
Complications
Nail involvement
Impetiginization
Bacterial infection
Eczema herpeticum
Endogenous eczema
Atopic eczema
• 5% of <5 yrs old
• 25% have family history asthma, hay fever, eczema ('atopic' tendency)
• ↑ IgE levels
Seborrhoeic eczema
• Itchy, scaly erythematous lesions
• Usually idiopathic
• Common in HIV infection
• Possibly due to abnormal reaction to Pityrosporum yeast
Other causes of endogenous eczema
• Pityriasis alba
• Stasis eczema
• Asteatotic eczema
• Pompholyx
• Eczematous drug reactions
• Discoid eczema
• Lichen simplex
• Neurodermatitis
• Nodular prurigo
• Exfoliative dermatitis
Exogenous eczema
Irritant contact dermatitis
• Soaps, detergents
• Hairdressing chemicals
• Cutting oils, coolants
Allergic contact dermatitis
Cosmetic
Nickel ear-rings
Necklace
Deodorants
Jean buttons
Rubber gloves, epoxy resins
Shoe: chrome rubber dyes
Medicament
Otitis externa
Pruritus ani
Medicaments
Gravitational eczema
Caustic burns from wet cement
Allergy to nickel in jeans button
Cosmetic allergy
Phototoxic eruptions
• Drugs (thiazides)
• Plants (parsnip, citrus)
Photoallergic reactions
• Drugs (phenothiazines)
• Perfumes (musk)

Eczema and dermatitis are practically synonymous. They are subdivided aetiologically and clinically. Lesions are very itchy, with ill-defined edges. Histologically, intercellular epidermal oedema (spongiosis) is seen.

Atopic dermatitis

Atopic dermatitis is a relapsing condition beginning in infancy and sometimes continuing into later life. Atopy is an inherited tendency to develop an altered state of immune reactivity (type I and other hypersensitivity reactions). Patients who have a personal or first-degree family history of asthma, hay fever, conjunctivitis or eczema have the atopic diathesis (25% of the population). Atopic patients have elevated serum IgE levels.

Clinical features

Ill-defined erythematous scaly patches occur on the face and in flexural sites. Scratching and rubbing lead to infection, skin thickening and lichenification. Atopic dermatitis is a clinical diagnosis. Infection is common and skin swabs may be indicated. IgE may be elevated.

Medicine at a Glance, Fifth Edition. Edited by Patrick Davey and Alex Pitcher.

Companion website: www.wiley.com/go/medicine5e

Urticaria and angioedema

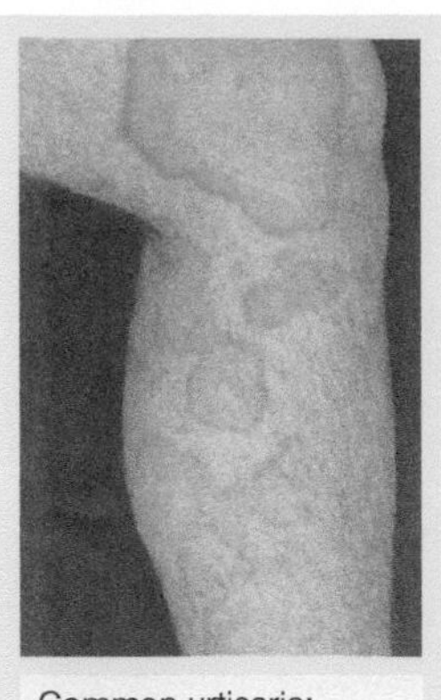

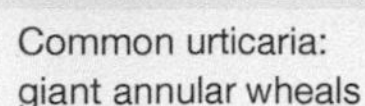

Common urticaria: giant annular wheals

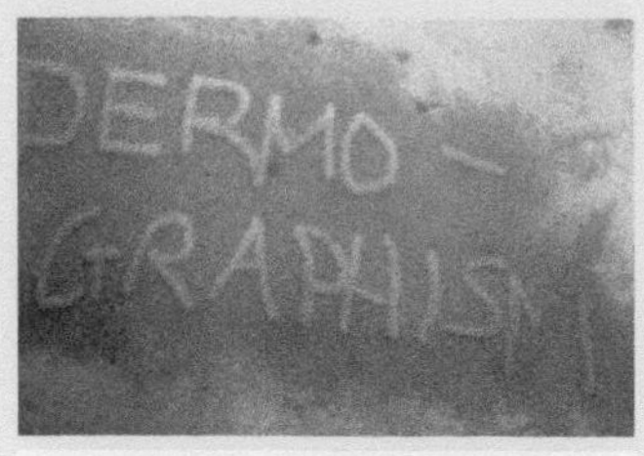

Dermographism: linear wheals after scratching

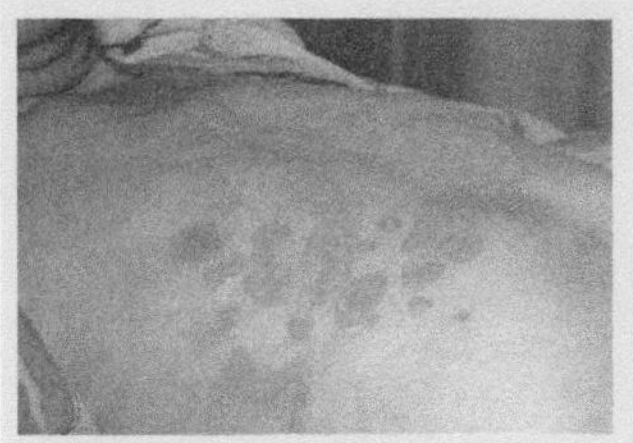

Drug induced urticaria: penicillin allergy

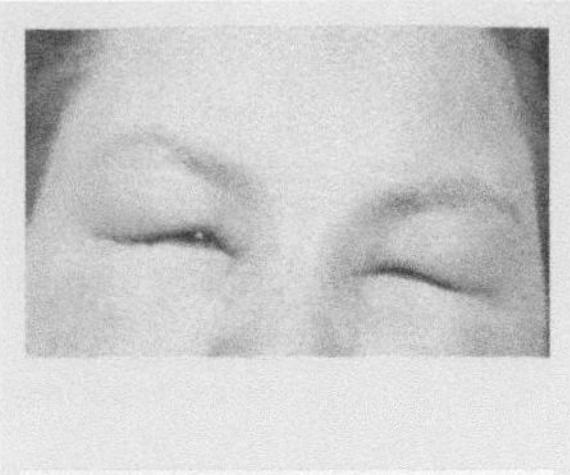

Angioedema of the face: marked eyelid swelling

Management and prognosis

Atopic eczema can be difficult to manage. The principles of therapy are to moisturize the skin with emollients and minimize itching with oral antihistamines. Irritants such as soap, chronic wet work, heat and solvents should be avoided. House-dust mite avoidance may be helpful. Specific treatments include topical therapy with tar, steroids or calcineurin inhibitors and antibiotics for complicating infection. A sunny, dry climate is beneficial. Systemic therapy with oral/intravenous antibiotics and antiviral agents may be indicated. Phototherapy with ultraviolet light, conventional immunosuppressive drugs (such as azathioprine, ciclosporin or methotrexate) or biologic agents (e.g. dupilumab) may be indicated in more severe cases. Secondary infection with herpes simplex virus (eczema herpeticum) constitutes an emergency requiring hospitalization and treatment with systemic aciclovir. The major features of the condition resolve in 40% after five years of age and 90% by 15–20 years of age.

Other types of endogenous eczema

- **Lichen simplex**: eczema in response to repeated trauma or scratching.
- **Nodular prurigo**: a widespread nodular manifestation of the above.
- **Stasis eczema** (varicose eczema, lipodermatosclerosis): results from venous hypertension (which may relate to venous valvular damage from deep venous thrombosis, pregnancy, etc.). Leakage of blood from the capillaries into the surrounding tissue deposits fibrin and haemosiderin around the capillaries, so diminishing tissue perfusion and predisposing to skin ulceration. It occurs over the inner shin and medial malleolus, and is itchy, indurated, scaly and purpuric. It can be complicated by contact dermatitis caused by topically applied drugs, and diagnosed by patch testing or by 'autosensitization' (secondary generalization of chronic stasis eczema supposedly resulting from 'sensitization' to epidermal antigens). Autosensitization affects the face, neck and extensor regions of the arms and thighs.
- **Asteatotic eczema**: occurs on the legs of elderly patients where there is dry skin. There is a glazed 'crazy-paving' effect. It responds to emollients and topical steroids.
- **Discoid eczema**: characterized by itchy, symmetrical, coin-shaped lesions on the extensor surfaces of the limbs and feet. The lesions are differentiated from those of ringworm/tinea corporis (which have an active border), psoriasis (often non-itchy with a silvery scale) and mycosis fungoides (asymmetrical and persistent). Discoid eczema is treated with emollients, topical steroids, antibiotics and systemic antihistamines.
- **Pompholyx**: acute vesicular eczema of the palms and soles. It is treated with potassium permanganate soaks, and topical or systemic steroids. Concomitant fungal infection of the foot (tinea pedis) should be sought. Pompholyx often recurs.
- **Seborrhoeic dermatitis**: a common, mildly itchy, scaly, red rash with a predilection for the scalp, face, chest, back, axillae and groins. It is an abnormal cutaneous reaction to commensal *Pityrosporum* yeasts. It may occur in HIV infection and Parkinson disease. Treatment is with topical steroids plus an anti-yeast agent (e.g. imidazole) and topical calcineruin inhibitors. When the scalp is affected (dandruff), ketoconazole or selenium sulfide shampoo can be helpful.

Contact dermatitis

Contact dermatitis is a major industrial and occupational category of disease. It may be allergic or an irritant. Almost anything in the environment may be an irritant and many substances are sensitizers, including medicaments. Allergic contact dermatitis is the archetypal type IV cell-mediated immunological reaction. Patch testing is the principal investigation. A battery of common allergens is applied to the non-inflamed back. The patches are removed at 48 hours and the reactions read. The patient is seen again at 72 hours and late responses recorded. Interpretation (false negatives, false positives and significance of positives) is a specialist activity. Treatment: withdrawal of the offending agent is vital, but prophylaxis is important in industry because, once initiated, allergic contact dermatitis may persist despite removal of the responsible allergen(s).

Prevention of hand eczema

Hand eczema may be a diagnostic and management problem. Often atopic, irritant and allergic factors co-exist. The use of cotton gloves inside rubber gloves for all wet and dirty tasks is recommended. Consider prophylaxis with barrier preparations where there is industrial/occupational risk.

Table 221.1 Causes and exacerbating factors of common urticaria (most cases are idiopathic).

Drugs	Aspirin, codeine, morphine, non-steroidal anti-inflammatory drugs
Foods	Fish and shellfish, eggs, nuts, tomatoes
Additives	Tartrazine, benzoates
Inhalants	Pollen, spores, house dust
Infections	Focal sepsis (e.g. urinary tract infection, upper respiratory tract infection, hepatitis, *Candida* spp., protozoa, helminths)
Systemic	Systemic lupus erythematosus, reticuloses and carcinoma

Urticaria

Urticaria (hives) describes itchy red (erythematous) wheals (i.e. skin swellings resulting from leaky capillaries). Management aims to exclude an underlying cause, identify and remove precipitants or provocatants (see Table 221.1), and provide effective symptomatic treatment.

Epidemiology, aetiology and pathogenesis

Urticaria is very common and results from mast cell degranulation (a type I immunological reaction) in response to an antigen, with the release of histamine and other vasoactive mediators, leading to erythema and oedema. Of patients with this condition, 70% have idiopathic urticaria (where the antigen is not known) and the remainder have other forms (see Table 221.2). The differential diagnosis includes insect bites, prodromal pemphigoid, toxic erythema and erythema multiforme.

Urticaria, when severe, can also affect subcutaneous tissues, so producing angioedema (swelling in the hands, lips and around the eyes, and less commonly but more importantly of the tongue or larynx).

- Angioedema may be idiopathic.
- It may occur in individuals exposed to food antigens to which they have been sensitized, e.g. peanuts.
- Angioedema may occur in those with congenitally deficient C1 esterase levels (hereditary angioedema).

Investigations and management

If something other than acute idiopathic urticaria is suspected (e.g. symptoms for >2 months), a full blood count, eosinophil count and erythrocyte sedimentation rate, thyroid autoantibodies, thyroid function, renal and liver function and complement levels should be examined, and a stool sample taken for ova, cysts and parasites. Counselling and reassurance are the mainstays of treatment. Itching may be exacerbated by psychological factors. High doses of non-sedating anti-H_1-receptor histamines by day (up to four times licensed dose) are supplemented by sedating antihistamines at night. The patient should be warned about drowsiness, alcohol and driving. Sometimes the addition of high doses of an anti-H_2-receptor agent such as cimetidine is helpful, as well as leukotriene receptor antagonist (montelukast). Systemic steroids are generally eschewed but have a role in severe cases. Dapsone, conventional immunosuppressive drugs and the anti-IgE agent omalizumab are used for refractory cases.

Acute laryngeal angioedema and anaphylaxis can be life-threatening, but are not usually a feature of idiopathic or physical urticarias. An intramuscular injection of 0.5 ml of 1:1000 adrenaline (epinephrine) (500 μg) is the recommended treatment in adults. Fixed dose (300 μg) 'pen' injections are available for at-risk individuals.

Table 221.2 Types of urticaria.

Type	Features
Common urticaria	Lesions last for several hours
Angioedema	Deeper dermal and subdermal involvement
Contact urticaria	Immediate response to allergens (e.g. foods)
Physical urticaria	Lesions last several minutes, but <1 h
Dermographism:	In response to scratching or trauma
Cholinergic	In response to heat/exercise
Cold/aquagenic	In response to cold/water
Heat/solar	In response to heat/sun
Urticarial vasculitis	Lesions last several days or longer; purpuric
Hereditary angioedema	C1 esterase inhibitor deficiency
Autoinflammatory syndromes:	
Cryopyrin periodic syndromes	Fever, chills, arthralgia, eye pain and redness
Schnitzler syndrome	Fever, bone pain, arthralgia, IgM gammopathy

Urticarial vasculitis

Urticarial vasculitis (5% of all urticarias) is a leukocytoclastic vasculitis and is suspected if urticarial lesions last >48 hours and resolve with purpura. It is associated with diseases such as systemic lupus erythematosus and hepatitis B and C. Treatment depends on the cause, but oral corticosteroids or other immunosuppressants are sometimes needed.

Hereditary angioedema

Hereditary angioedema (HAE) caused by congenital (autosomal dominant) deficiency of C1 esterase inhibitor (C1-inh) is suspected when there is a family history and angioedema, often spontaneously or in response to infection/trauma. Type I HAE is due to mutations causing premature stop codons in the C1-inh gene, while Type II HAE have mutations in the enzymatic site in C1-inh, reducing or abolishing function. A third type of HAE is associated with gain-of-function mutations in clotting factor XII. Urticaria is virtually never present. Patients may present with abdominal pain, mimicking an acute abdomen. Angioedema may affect any part of the body and may affect the larynx, causing respiratory obstruction. The finding of a normal C3 and absent C4 during an attack is highly suspicious of HAE, which can be confirmed by measurement of total and functional C1 esterase inhibitor levels. Modified androgens such as oxandrolone and danazol or an antifibrinolytic such as tranexamic acid can be used for prophylaxis. Purified C1 esterase inhibitor may be used as prophylaxis before surgery and when attacks are very frequent. Lanadelumab is a monoclonal antibody against kallikrein which is used as prophylaxis. Acute attacks can be treated with purified C1 esterase inhibitor or with icatibant, a bradykinin antagonist. The latter can be self-administered at home as it is given by subcutaneous injection. In emergencies, fresh frozen plasma may be used but may cause a deterioration rather than improvement in symptoms. Respiratory obstruction should be managed by intubation or tracheostomy. Adrenaline and hydrocortisone are relatively ineffective. All patients with HAE should be under the care of an immunologist.

222 Psoriasis

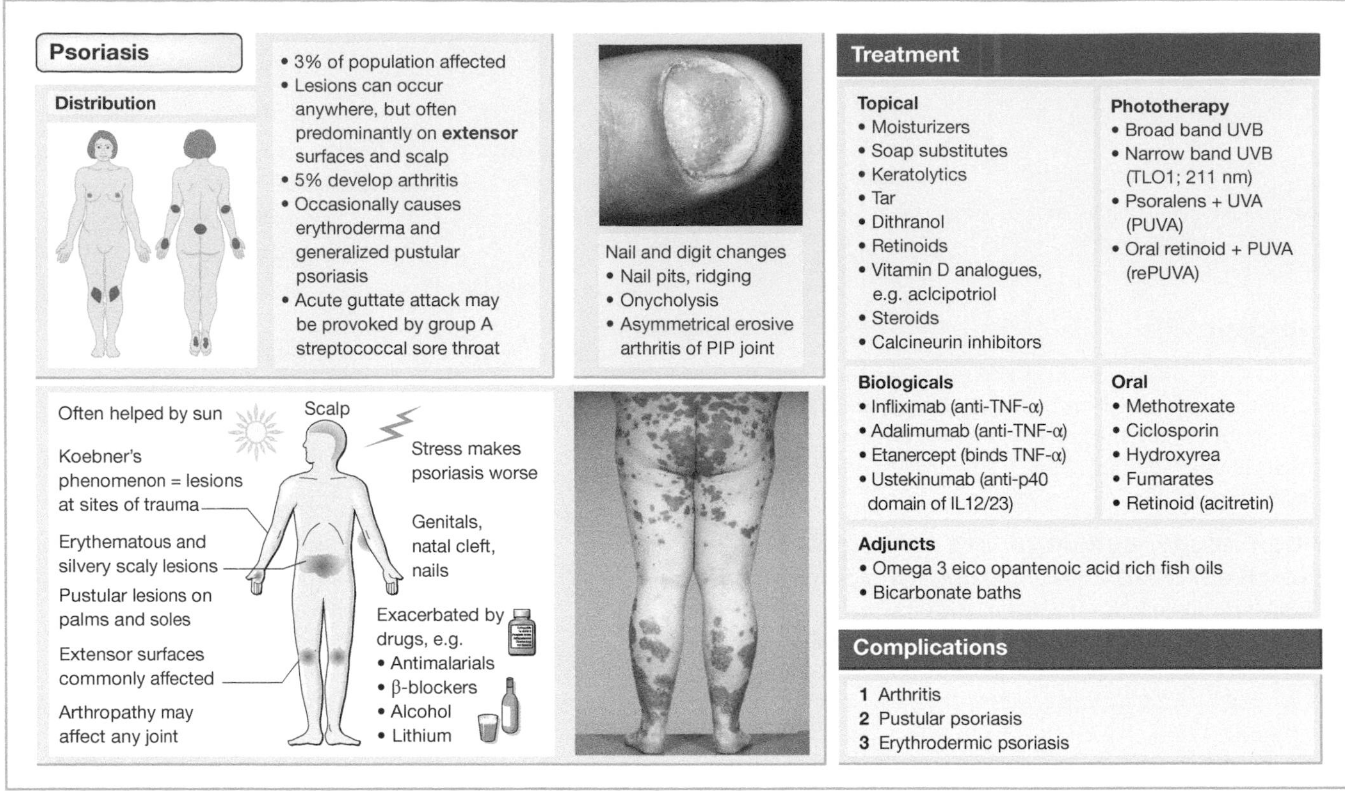

Psoriasis
Distribution
• 3% of population affected
• Lesions can occur anywhere, but often predominantly on **extensor** surfaces and scalp
• 5% develop arthritis
• Occasionally causes erythroderma and generalized pustular psoriasis
• Acute guttate attack may be provoked by group A streptococcal sore throat
Nail and digit changes
• Nail pits, ridging
• Onycholysis
• Asymmetrical erosive arthritis of PIP joint
Often helped by sun
Scalp
Stress makes psoriasis worse
Koebner's phenomenon = lesions at sites of trauma
Genitals, natal cleft, nails
Erythematous and silvery scaly lesions
Pustular lesions on palms and soles
Exacerbated by drugs, e.g.
• Antimalarials
• β-blockers
• Alcohol
• Lithium
Extensor surfaces commonly affected
Arthropathy may affect any joint
Treatment
Topical
• Moisturizers
• Soap substitutes
• Keratolytics
• Tar
• Dithranol
• Retinoids
• Vitamin D analogues, e.g. aclcipotriol
• Steroids
• Calcineurin inhibitors
Phototherapy
• Broad band UVB
• Narrow band UVB (TLO1; 211 nm)
• Psoralens + UVA (PUVA)
• Oral retinoid + PUVA (rePUVA)
Biologicals
• Infliximab (anti-TNF-α)
• Adalimumab (anti-TNF-α)
• Etanercept (binds TNF-α)
• Ustekinumab (anti-p40 domain of IL12/23)
Oral
• Methotrexate
• Ciclosporin
• Hydroxyrea
• Fumarates
• Retinoid (acitretin)
Adjuncts
• Omega 3 eico opantenoic acid rich fish oils
• Bicarbonate baths
Complications
1 Arthritis
2 Pustular psoriasis
3 Erythrodermic psoriasis

Aetiology, pathogenesis and clinical features

A polygenic susceptibility exists. Some human leukocyte antigen (HLA) types (Cw6) are associated with skin disease alone, whereas others (e.g. B27) are associated with additional joint disease. The PSORS1 cluster of genes on chromosome 6 are involved, but other genes implicated are for IL-12 and IL-23R. Infections, stress or drugs may precipitate attacks of psoriasis. A Th2 cytokine profile of activation occurs involving tumour necrosis factor (TNF)-α. Psoriatic plaques are characterized by the dual pathological features of epidermal hyperproliferation and cutaneous inflammation.

Psoriasis manifests as red, silver-scaled lesions, which may be guttate or nummular, or plaques. The scalp is frequently involved, as are the nails. Pustulosis may occur, particularly in the palms and soles, and occasionally psoriasis causes erythroderma. Arthritis, which can be severe, can complicate the disease. The common subtypes of psoriasis are as follows.

- **Chronic plaque psoriasis**: the differential diagnosis includes atopic dermatitis, seborrhoeic dermatitis, mycosis fungoides and tinea.
- **Guttate psoriasis**: this form of psoriasis may be precipitated by a streptococcal sore throat or other infection. Lesions are small (<1 cm), scaly and widespread. Spontaneous resolution usually occurs after a few months. The differential diagnosis includes secondary syphilis and pityriasis rosea.
- **Erythrodermic psoriasis**: widespread erythema occurs, with 'skin failure', which may lead to failure of thermoregulation, infection, fluid and protein loss, and a high output form of heart failure. Other causes of erythroderma include eczema, mycosis fungoides (cutaneous T-cell lymphoma) and drug eruption (e.g. toxic epidermal necrolysis).
- **Pustular psoriasis**: this severe form results in a sudden crop of widespread small pustules throughout the skin, with considerable systemic upset.

The chronic inflammation of psoriasis is associated with the metabolic syndrome, a combination of medical disorders that, when occurring together, increase the risk of developing cardiovascular disease and diabetes.

Investigations, management and prognosis

A skin biopsy, if necessary, shows irregular epidermal hyperplasia, suprapapillary thinning, clubbing of rete pegs, leukocyte infiltration and epidermal pustulosis.

Management and prognosis

Treatment is hierarchical and depends on severity, site, age, sex and occupation. Topical steroids, calcineurin inhibitors, tar, dithranol and vitamin D analogues are used for mild to moderate disease. Phototherapy and systemic drugs are used for more severe cases. These include retinoids, conventional immunosuppressive drugs and biologic agents. The facets of the metabolic syndrome require prevention and management.

Reactive arthritis

The reactive arthritis syndrome (arthritis, urethritis, conjunctivitis) occurs in response to urinary or gastrointestinal tract infection in genetically predisposed individuals, and is part of the same disease continuum as psoriasis. Skin lesions in reactive arthritis syndrome are similar to psoriasis. In reactive arthritis, thickened yellow palms and soles with a cobblestone appearance, with or without pustular lesions (keratoderma blennorrhagicum) and involvement of the penis (circinate balanitis), are found. Other features of psoriasis may be present.

Blistering diseases

Autoimmune blistering diseases

	Bullous pemphigoid	Pemphigus vulgaris	Dermatitis herpetiformis
Incidence	Common	Rare	Very rare
Age	Elderly	40–50 years	Young adults Elderly
Antibody attack target	Basement membrane hemidesmosome	Interepidermal cell desmosomal structure	Not characterized
Diagnosis	Biopsy	Biopsy Serum antibodies	Biopsy (skin and gut) Demonstration of villous atrophy
Treatment	Topical steroid Prednisolone 40–60 mg/day	Topical steroid Prednisolone 80–120 mg/day	Topical steroid Dapsone Gluten-free diet
Underlying malignancy	Possible	Rarely	GI Lymphoma risk
Prognosis	Excellent	Variable	Good

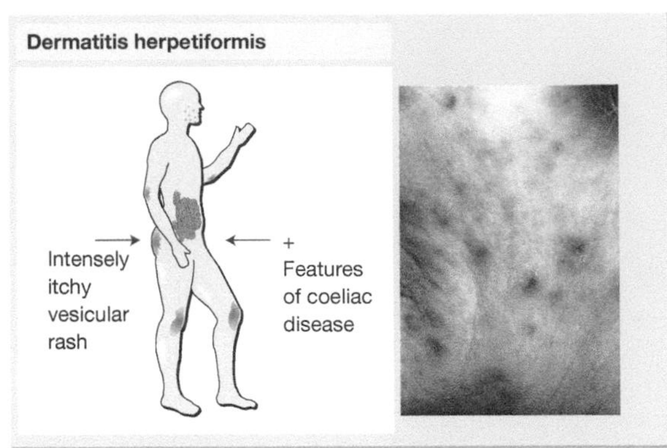

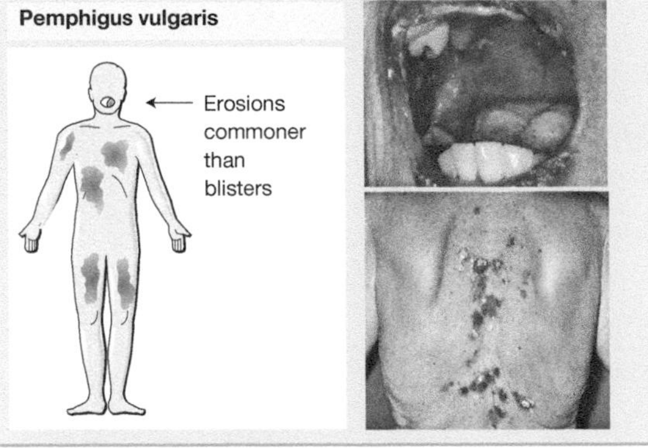

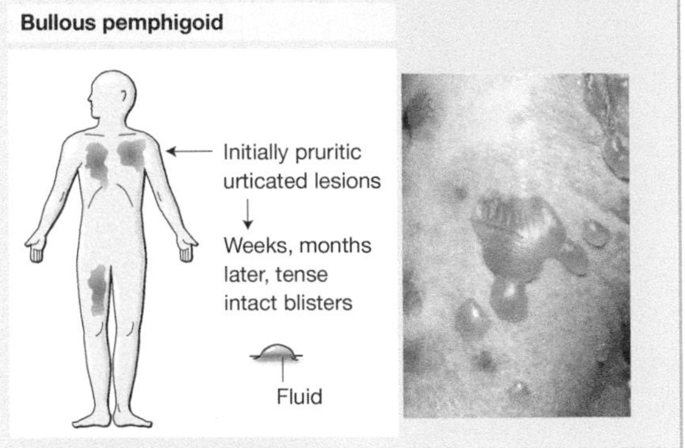

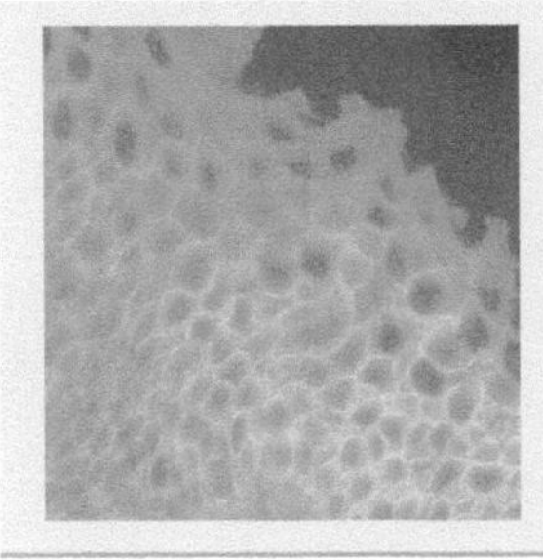

Bright green immunofluorescence of IgG in the intercellular space in a patient with pemphigus vulgaris

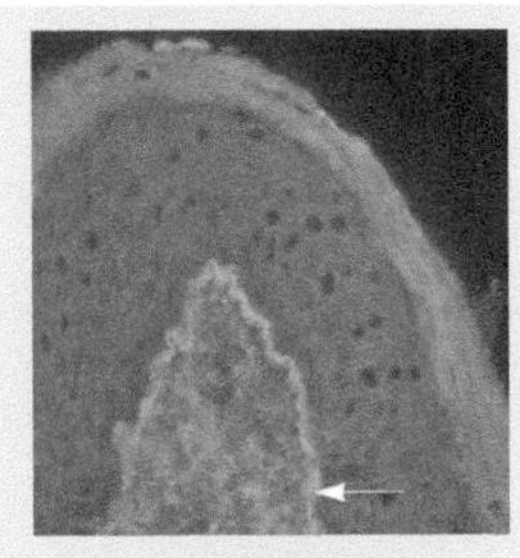

Bright green immunofluorescence of IgG at the BMZ (arrow) in a patient with pemphigoid

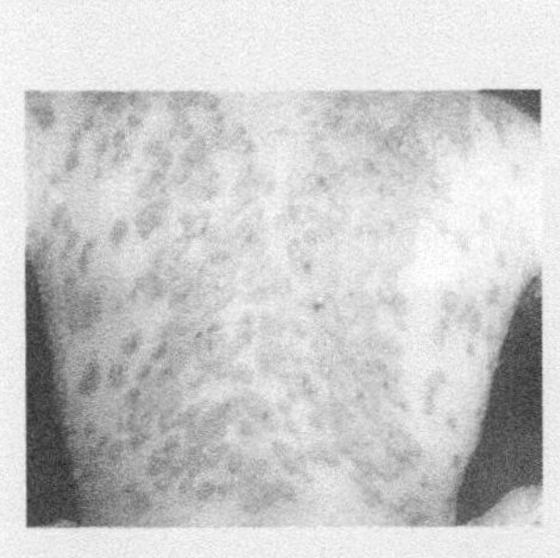

Pemphigus vulgaris: widespread superficial blisters and erosions

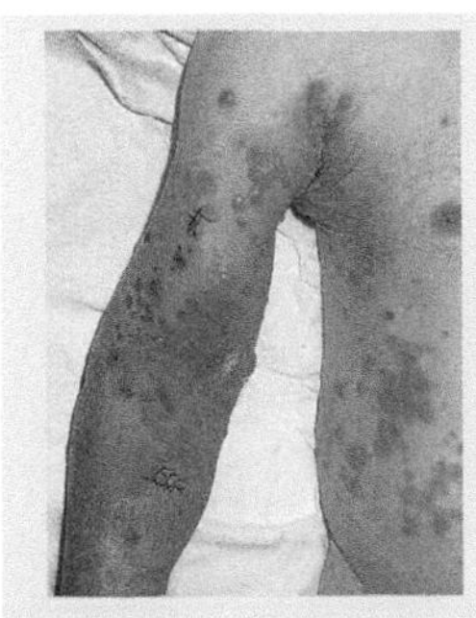

Bullous pemphigoid: tense blisters (bullae) on an erythematosus and urticated base

Medicine at a Glance, Fifth Edition. Edited by Patrick Davey and Alex Pitcher.

Companion website: www.wiley.com/go/medicine5e

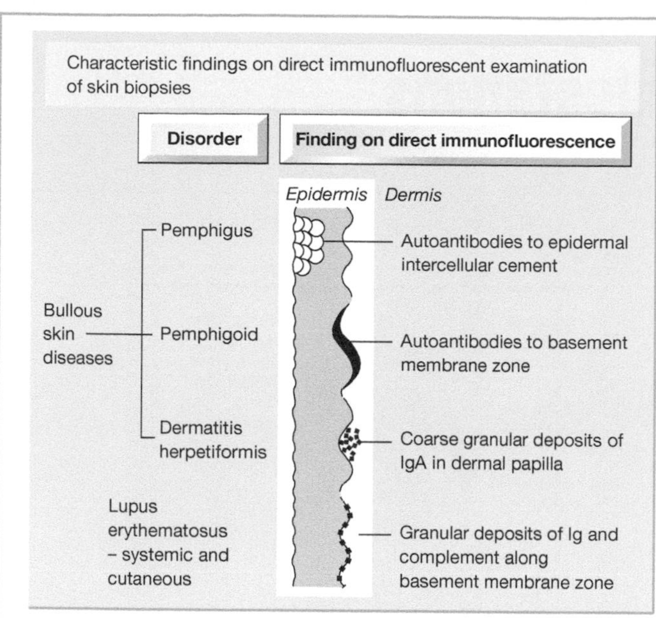

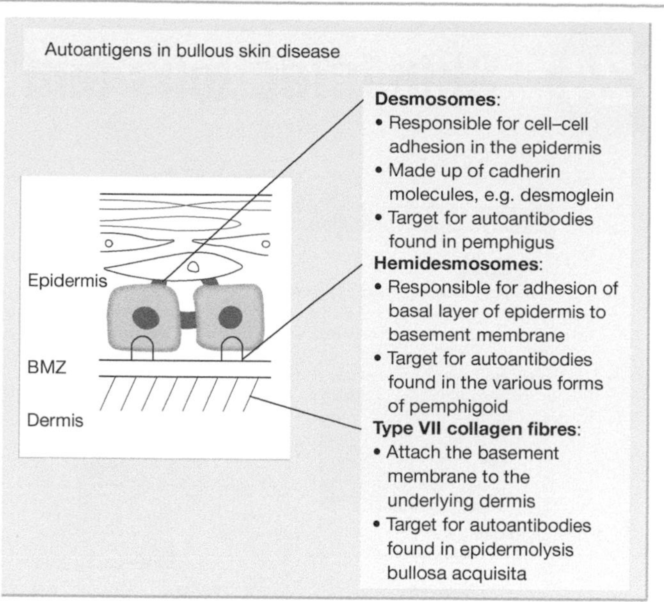

Autoantigens in bullous skin disease
Epidermis
BMZ
Dermis
Desmosomes:
• Responsible for cell–cell adhesion in the epidermis
• Made up of cadherin molecules, e.g. desmoglein
• Target for autoantibodies found in pemphigus
Hemidesmosomes:
• Responsible for adhesion of basal layer of epidermis to basement membrane
• Target for autoantibodies found in the various forms of pemphigoid
Type VII collagen fibres:
• Attach the basement membrane to the underlying dermis
• Target for autoantibodies found in epidermolysis bullosa acquisita

Blisters are common, e.g. acute eczema, herpes, impetigo or insect bites. Some drug eruptions are bullous, e.g. toxic epidermal necrolysis, as are some systemic diseases, e.g. porphyria cutanea tarda and amyloid. There are also primary bullous skin diseases.

Congenital blistering diseases

Several very rare, non-infective diseases are associated with blisters from an early age (e.g. epidermolysis bullosa).

Toxic epidermal necrolysis: Lyell syndrome

This serious, life-threatening idiosyncratic reaction can be the result of a drug reaction or an intercurrent illness. The 'full-blown' disease is rare, but milder cases, usually caused by drug reactions, are much more common. Clinically, there is widespread skin loss, compromising cutaneous homeostasis. There is severe systemic upset. Cardiovascular collapse, infection and failure of thermoregulation contribute to a high mortality. Mucocutaneous involvement is common. Scarring may occur if the patient survives. Intravenous γ-globulins, ciclosporin, anti-TNF-α and granulocyte colony-stimulating factor can be used. The role of systemic steroids is controversial.

Bullous pemphigoid

Bullous pemphigoid is a common disease of elderly people, arising from an autoimmune attack on the hemidesmosome of the basement membrane. Circulating antibodies to the basement membrane zone (BMZ) are often found. There may be an association between seronegative disease, where mucosal lesions are more common, and malignancy. Clinically, the illness can start not as blisters but as erythematous, eczematous and urticated areas on the trunk and limbs. Tense blisters appear later in these sites. The diagnosis is confirmed by histology and tissue immunofluorescence. Most patients respond well to prednisolone 40–60 mg daily tapered and replaced by azathioprine longer term.

Pemphigus vulgaris

This is a rare disease, most common in the 45–50-year age group, resulting from antibody-mediated attack on the interepidermal cell desmosomal structure. Clinically, the presenting lesion may be confined to the oral mucosa, scalp, fingernails (paronychia) and genitalia. The blisters are intraepithelial and rupture readily, leaving raw erosions. Skin lesions may not appear for some months. Circulating antibodies are found in the serum. Histology shows an intraepidermal blister with acantholysis (rupture of prickle cells). Direct immunofluorescence demonstrates intercellular IgG and C3. Before the use of systemic corticosteroids, pemphigus vulgaris was fatal. High doses (80–120 mg) of prednisolone are life saving but often produce side-effects, which contribute to the mortality. Mycophenolate mofetil and rituximab (anti-CD20 antibody) are promising. Potent topical steroids are used for the mucocutaneous lesions.

Dermatitis herpetiformis

This is a very rare illness of young adults, with a second peak in old age. Patients almost always have a gluten-sensitive enteropathy (coeliac disease). It is strongly associated with certain human leukocyte antigen (HLA) haplotypes.

Clinically, intensely itchy groups of small blisters on an urticarial base occur over the elbows, knees, buttocks or face – often only excoriations may be seen. Investigations for coeliac disease may be positive: endomysial antibody, intestinal biopsy or tests for malabsorption (full blood count, serum iron and folate and red cell folate). Skin biopsy shows IgA deposition on the dermal papillae. The eruption responds to dapsone within a few days. A gluten-free diet allows most patients to discontinue dapsone. Follow-up requires awareness of the risk of agranulocytosis and haemolytic anaemia on dapsone and intestinal lymphoma complicating coeliac disease.

Skin infections and infestations

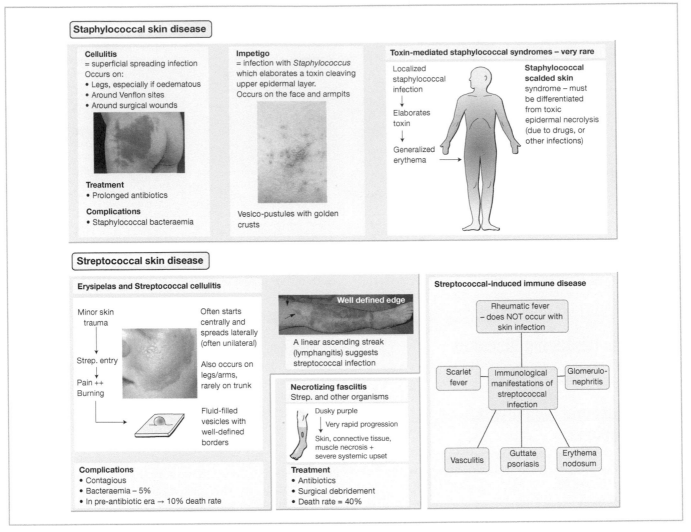

Staphylococcal skin disease

Cellulitis
= superficial spreading infection
Occurs on:
- Legs, especially if oedematous
- Around Venflon sites
- Around surgical wounds

Treatment
- Prolonged antibiotics

Complications
- Staphylococcal bacteraemia

Impetigo
= infection with *Staphylococcus* which elaborates a toxin cleaving upper epidermal layer.
Occurs on the face and armpits

Vesico-pustules with golden crusts

Toxin-mediated staphylococcal syndromes – very rare

Localized staphylococcal infection → Elaborates toxin → Generalized erythema

Staphylococcal scalded skin syndrome – must be differentiated from toxic epidermal necrolysis (due to drugs, or other infections)

Streptococcal skin disease

Erysipelas and Streptococcal cellulitis

Minor skin trauma → Strep. entry → Pain ++ Burning

Often starts centrally and spreads laterally (often unilateral)

Also occurs on legs/arms, rarely on trunk

Fluid-filled vesicles with well-defined borders

Well defined edge

A linear ascending streak (lymphangitis) suggests streptococcal infection

Complications
- Contagious
- Bacteraemia – 5%
- In pre-antibiotic era → 10% death rate

Necrotizing fasciitis
Strep. and other organisms

Dusky purple → Very rapid progression → Skin, connective tissue, muscle necrosis + severe systemic upset

Treatment
- Antibiotics
- Surgical debridement
- Death rate = 40%

Streptococcal-induced immune disease

Immunological manifestations of streptococcal infection:
- Rheumatic fever – does NOT occur with skin infection
- Scarlet fever
- Glomerulo-nephritis
- Vasculitis
- Guttate psoriasis
- Erythema nodosum

Staphylococci

Staphylococcal infection of the skin results in spreading superficial infections, deeper infection with abscesses or toxin-mediated damage. All suspected skin infections should be swabbed for microbiology. Advice from a microbiologist may be needed, e.g. to investigate for Panton–Valentine leucocidin toxin-producing strains.

- **Cellulitis**: often on the leg and unilateral (if bilateral, consider venous eczema as a diagnosis); it is predisposed by trauma, tinea pedis or chronic oedema. Acute episodes require intravenous (IV) antibiotics initially and some patients may need prophylactic low-dose penicillin. Risk factors such as tinea pedis, venous eczema and ulceration, and pelvic pathology should be sought and managed.
- **Impetigo**: caused by a toxin cleaving the upper layers of the epidermis; usually on the face and presenting as pustules and golden crusts. Treatment is with topical or oral antibiotics.
- **Abscesses**: may be small and localized to hair follicles (folliculitis) or larger and deeper in the skin, causing boils (furunculosis), which may be extensive (carbuncles). Boils/carbuncles require incision and drainage. If they recur, nasal carriage of staphylococci and/or diabetes should be considered.
- **MRSA** (methicillin-resistant *Staphylococcus aureus*): this is an increasing problem in dermatology. Treatment should be discussed with a dermatologist and/or microbiologist.
- **Staphylococcal scalded skin syndrome (SSSS)**: this is a reaction to a toxin produced by staphylococci, characterized by generalized erythema and exfoliation in an unwell child or immunocompromised adult. It must be distinguished from toxic epidermal necrolysis (a biopsy is informative); one helpful sign is lack of mucosal involvement in SSSS. The organism cannot be cultured from the skin. Systemic antistaphylococcal treatment and IV fluid replacement are given.

Medicine at a Glance, Fifth Edition. Edited by Patrick Davey and Alex Pitcher.

Companion website: www.wiley.com/go/medicine5e

Streptococci

Streptococci commonly produce skin and throat infection, and more rarely muscle, joint or heart infection. Damage may result directly or from toxin elaboration. Organisms may not always be cultured in streptococcal disease and diagnosis is clinical with retrospective rises in the antistreptolysin O and anti-DNAase titres. A portal of entry should be sought.

- **Erysipelas**: a superficial skin infection, of abrupt onset; it is painful and results in systemic upset. There is erythema, peeling and lymphangitis. IV antibiotics are indicated.
- **Scarlet fever**: caused by upper respiratory tract infection with streptococci which elaborate an erythrogenic toxin, resulting in cutaneous vasodilation.
- **Necrotizing fasciitis**: a serious, often mixed, infection involving streptococci, staphylococci, enterobacteriaceae and obligate anaerobes, or *Streptococcus pyogenes* alone. Often there is no obvious portal of entry in a healthy individual, although the infection may begin in a wound in an unwell patient. The first sign is dusky induration with rapid progressive painful necrosis of the skin, connective tissue and muscle. Prompt diagnosis is essential, IV antibiotics are rarely sufficient and surgical debridement is necessary. There is an appreciable mortality. The infection often occurs on a limb or the scrotum (Fournier's gangrene) or in a post-operative wound (Meleney's progressive synergistic gangrene).
- **Nephritis**, but not rheumatic fever, may follow streptococcal skin infections, so all such skin infections should be treated with systemic antibiotics.

Hypersensitivity reactions to streptococci are implicated in erythema nodosum, some vasculitis and guttate psoriasis.

Herpes skin infections

Herpes simplex

Any skin or mucosal site may be infected with, and show recurrence of, herpes simplex virus (HSV) infection. Herpetic lesions are painful vesicles and crusts on an erythematous base. They resolve over two weeks. Extragenital disease is usually caused by HSV1 and genital infections are usually caused by HSV2. The diagnosis is clinical, supported by viral culture, electron microscopy and serology. Management: aciclovir orally/intravenously and antibiotics for secondary infection. Long-term prophylaxis should be considered in some cases.

Herpes zoster (varicella) virus

This causes chickenpox or shingles. Shingles results from the reactivation of herpes zoster virus. Physical trauma to the involved dermatome may be the most common trigger. If immune deficiency is present (e.g. lymphoproliferative disorders), zoster may be severe and recurrent. Paraesthesiae and pain precede the eruption. Very rarely, there is pain and no eruption (zoster sine herpete). The rash is variable but usually asymmetrical. Erythematous oedematous papules and vesicles arise in one crop, become haemorrhagic and necrotic, and then scab and heal with superficial scarring. Outlying lesions are found in most patients. Recurrent zoster is rare and rarely at the same site.

Diagnosis is clinical but shingles can be confused with HSV, so viral culture, electron microscopy and serology are useful. Mild analgesics control the pain of the prodrome and the illness. A topical antibiotic is often needed for secondary infection and topical steroids suppress the cutaneous inflammation. Postherpetic neuralgia is a consequence of nerve involvement in zoster and is deservedly notorious for its intractability. A short course of oral prednisolone from the beginning of the disease may reduce the risk. Oral aciclovir reduces the time course of the cutaneous eruption if given within 72 hours, but does not prevent postherpetic neuralgia. Zoster affecting the ophthalmic branch of the trigeminal nerve may cause conjunctivitis or rarely optic neuritis, and expert advice should be sought. Zoster of S2 and below may cause acute retention of urine and constipation, and be complicated by haemorrhagic cystitis. Systemic aciclovir is indicated in these and immunosuppressed patients.

Varicella zoster immunoglobulin has no impact on established disease but may be given to those who have not had chickenpox but are at significant risk post exposure (e.g. pregnant women).

Warts

Warts are due to human papillomavirus (HPV), of which there are many types: HPV1–4, common warts and verrucas; HPV6 and -11 and genital warts; HPV16 and -18 and penile, vulval and cervical cancer. HPV has a fastidious requirement for human epidermal cells in a particular stage of differentiation. It causes a proliferation of keratinocytes, which partially keratinize and therefore sequester the virus from immunological elimination. Lesions may be sporadic, recurrent or persistent. Treatment is with keratolytics (such as salicylic acid or retinoic acid) or cryotherapy. Cautery and surgical excision may result in lower treatment success rates. Persistent warts can be treated by laser or intralesional bleomycin. Some types, in some sites (e.g. uterine cervix) and in predisposed individuals (e.g. HIV) can cause squamous cancer.

Mollusca

Mollusca are due to a poxvirus. The typical lesion is an umbilicated, dome-shaped papule or nodule. Lesions are common on the trunk in children and usually resolve spontaneously. Cryotherapy is the treatment of choice in adults but is only occasionally tolerated by a child, in which case topical 5% potassium hydroxide can be tried.

Fungal infections

- **Candidosis**: usually an intertriginous infection (i.e. affecting the axillae, submammary folds, crurae and digital clefts). It is a common cause of vulvovaginitis in women. In the immunoincompetent, it may also affect the mucosa and genitalia. It is a common concomitant opportunistic complication of dermatoses (e.g. eczema, psoriasis) at susceptible sites. It is treated with topical nystatin, imidazole or clioquinol, and occasionally with oral imidazole or triazole.
- **Pityriasis versicolor**: a superficial infection of the horny layer by the yeast *Pityrosporum orbiculare*. It is characterized by small, confluent, scaly, depigmented patches, which are often apparent for the first time after tanning. It can leave hypo- or hyperpigmented macules. Treatment is with a topical imidazole or selenium sulfide or occasionally with an oral triazole antifungal (e.g. itraconazole).
- **Dermatophytosis**: the term for ringworm infection (tinea). Lesions are red, scaly and itchy. The groins, feet and axillae are common sites; the lesions are then not necessarily circular and scaly, but are macerated and moist with a scaly edge. The nails may be involved (onychomyosis). Scarring may occur on the scalp due to an infected inflammatory plaque called a kerion. *Microsporum* spp. form spores around hairs (ectothrix) and fluoresce green under Wood's lamp, whereas *Trichophyton* spp. invade the hair shaft (endothrix) and do not fluoresce. Classic treatment is with a topical imidazole or griseofulvin orally. Systemic therapy is necessary for scalp or nail infections. Oral terbinafine or the triazole itraconazole are modern alternatives to griseofulvin.

Parasitosis

- **Scabies** must always enter the differential diagnosis of pruritus. Typically, the rash is symmetrical, involving the fingers, backs of hands, axillae, breasts and buttocks. Most lesions may be excoriated papules and nodules, but with care burrows are usually identified. Sites to examine carefully are digital clefts, around the nipples and the genitalia. By taking a skin scraping, burrow contents may be examined under a microscope. The presence of the female mite (*Sarcoptes scabiei*) or her eggs confirms the diagnosis. Only brief apposition of skin surfaces is needed to transmit the infestation; sexual contact is a common means of dissemination. Treatment: topical insecticides applied to cool, dry skin all over the body. Secondary eczema and infection should also be treated. In adult patients with scabies (without HIV), the head can be omitted. It is mandatory to treat partners and co-habitants at the same time. Concomitant sexually transmitted diseases should have been excluded.
- **Head lice** infestation is the result of *Pediculus humanus*, which feeds on perifollicular scalp blood vessels and lays eggs cemented to the hair shaft (nits).
- **Vagabond's disease** (a widespread itchy excoriated dermatosis) is caused by *Pediculus humanus corporis*, which lives in the seams of clothing and lays its eggs there.
- **Crab louse** (*Pthirus pubis*) is named because of its appearance and tenacious adherence to the hairy skin where it is feeding, causing pediculosis pubis.

Mycobacteria and the skin

- **Cutaneous tuberculosis**: common in the developing world but rare in the UK. It may be seen in elderly patients and in immigrants. A chest X-ray, tuberculin and ELISA (enzyme-linked immunosorbent assay), interferon-γ testing and skin biopsy with culture are needed.
- **Atypical mycobacterial infection**: a common cause of skin lesions in people with AIDS or who are immunologically suppressed.
- ***Mycobacterium marinum*** can result in an indolent granulomatous ulcer. If contracted in a swimming bath, it is called swimming pool granuloma; if seen in a pet fish keeper, it is called fish-tank granuloma.
- ***Mycobacterium ulcerans*** is an important cause of leg or arm ulceration in Africa (Buruli ulcer) or Australia (Searle's ulcer).
- ***Mycobacterium leprae***: see figure below.
- ***Mycobacterium chelonae*** is being seen increasingly after minor injury or skin surgery in mainly but not always immunocompromised people.

Leprosy	Tuberculoid TT	Borderline BT BB BL	Lepromatous LL
Immunological responsiveness	High (+ve lepromin test)	Intermediate	Low (–ve lepromin test)
Organisms in lesions	Few – hard to find	Some	Many – easy to find
Infectivity	Non-infectious	Slightly infectious	Infectious
Extent of lesions	Localized	Scattered	Generalized
Involvement	Skin & nerves only		Many tissues
Skin lesions	1–2 only; commonly on face		Innumerable & widespread

Tuberculoid leprosy: subtle depigmentation with a palpable erythematous rim at the upper edge

Borderline leprosy (BL). Borderline tuberculoid (BT) downgrading to BL. Showing typical well-defined hypopigmented macules of BT and many small lesions, some of which are papular

The 'leonine' facies of lepromatous leprosy

Nerve involvement	Thickened nerves in vicinity of skin lesions	Most peripheral nerves thickened
Anaesthesia distribution	Lesions hypoanaesthetic/no sweating	Lesions not hypoanaesthetic – but glove & stocking anaesthesia; trophic ulcers of periphery; muscle nerve paralysis
Clinical course	Disease localized; patients usually not very troubled by the disease – good prognosis, and spontaneous recovery may occur	Patients disabled by the disease with widespread organ involvement

General features of leprosy

Leprosy (Hansen's disease) results from infection (probably acquired through the respiratory tract) with *Mycobacterium leprae*.
Infected patients shed the bacillus from infected nasal secretions; only 1% of contacts develop the disease.
Incubation period 2–6 years. The clinical course depends on the host's immunity (see left); skin involvement is a prominent feature, as is peripheral nerve involvement, resulting in hypopigmented patches and anaesthesia.
Diagnosis: clinical, finding bacilli in skin smears, culturing bacilli in mice food pad. Lepromin test: intradermal injection of dead bacilli – early reaction (Fernandez) < 48 hours = sensitivity to leprosy protein, late reaction (Mitsuda) 4–5 weeks resistance of host to infection.
Treatment is with multiple drugs.
Treatment reactions include:
- Erythema nodosum leprosum – usually in LL leprosy, painful tender nodules on extensor surfaces
- Allergic response to mycobacteria, causing further nerve damage
- Iritis

Treatment reactions can result in permanent injury – treat promptly with thalidomide

225 Acne, rosacea and hidradenitis

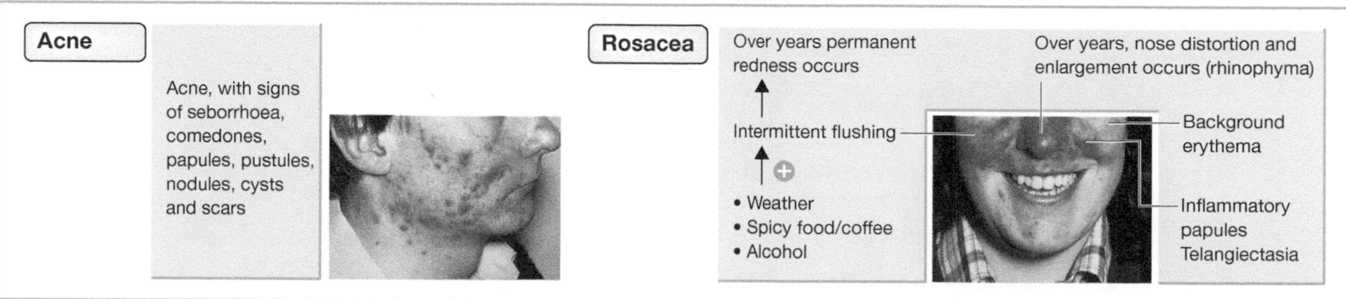

Acne vulgaris

Aetiology and pathogenesis

Acne vulgaris is universal in adolescence; 1% of men and 5% of women may require treatment up until the age of 40. Acne vulgaris is a chronic disorder of the pilosebaceous duct with increased sebum production, ductal hypercornification, a deranged symbiotic relationship with commensal micro-organisms (*Propionibacterium acnes*) and cutaneous inflammation. Increased sebum production is probably the fundamental abnormality.

The sebaceous glands are driven by androgens. Women with acne manifest a complex form of cutaneous androgenization. Many women with acne have polycystic ovaries on ultrasonography, although most do not have the other features of the polycystic ovary syndrome. There is no evidence for systemic endocrine abnormalities in men. Rarely, endocrine disorders, such as 'full-blown' polycystic ovary syndrome, Cushing syndrome, virilizing neoplasms or exogenous corticosteroids/androgens, underlie the acne.

Clinical features

The clinical features of acne are seborrhoea, comedones, papules, pustules, nodules, cysts and scars distributed on the face, neck, back and chest. Pyoderma faciale is acute severe facial acne. Acne fulminans is acute severe acne with fever, arthralgia and sterile lytic lesions of bone.

Investigations

Investigations are only indicated if Cushing syndrome or virilization is suspected. Pelvic ultrasonography can demonstrate polycystic ovaries, in addition to female hormone profile.

Management and prognosis

Treatment depends on the severity of the condition and an objective record of severity helps follow-up. The principles of therapy are to keep the skin clean, to discourage micro-organism growth and the use of keratolytics to relieve comedones.

- Mild acne: topical antibiotics, keratolytics and retinoids.
- Moderate to severe acne: both topical and systemic therapy, with oral antibiotics (which can result in failure of the oral contraceptive pill or teratogenicity) or antiandrogenic hormones (i.e. for women, a suitable contraceptive pill).
- Severe nodulocystic (conglobate) acne or failure to respond to other treatments is an indication for the oral retinoid (vitamin A derivative) isotretinoin (13-*cis*-retinoic acid). This highly effective drug affects all four aetiological factors operating in acne and reduces sebum production by 75–90%. Treatment lasts 6–8 months. Side-effects, which are essentially those of hypervitaminosis A, include teratogenesis (women must not get pregnant when on treatment), eczema, cheilitis (sore lips), conjunctivitis, benign intracranial hypertension, mood disturbance and biochemical hepatitis and hyperlipidaemia.

Acne is usually self-limiting. With the exception of isotretinoin, treatment does not alter the natural history, and thus should continue throughout the course of the disorder. Topical therapies are needed long term and antibiotics should be given for at least six months. Repeated courses or long-term treatment may be necessary. Maintenance topical treatment is needed after oral therapy is stopped. Combined therapy is rational because there are several pathogenic factors.

Rosacea

Rosacea is a disorder of unknown aetiology, associated with instability of the facial vasculature, facial flushing and the secondary development of inflamed papules and pustules, particularly affecting the cheeks, chin and central forehead. Coffee, spicy foods, alcohol and adverse weather are precipitants to avoid. It responds to oral antibiotics (e.g. tetracycline, erythromycin, metronidazole). Long-term cosmetic damage to the nose (enlargement with discoloration and rhinophyma) and facial telangiectasia can occur if not treated and usually require laser treatment.

Hidradenitis suppurativa

Hidradenitis suppurativa is the apocrine equivalent of acne vulgaris. In mild forms, patients have recurrent boils in apocrine areas (axillae, groins, breasts, behind the ears). Staphylococcal carriage and diabetes mellitus should be excluded. Chronic nodulocystic involvement of the groins with suppuration and fistula formation can occur. Hidradenitis can respond indifferently to oral antibiotics, hormonal manipulation and isotretinoin. Oral steroids may be necessary. Antitumour necrosis factor treatment with adalimumab shows promise. It may be necessary to resort to surgical excision.

Medicine at a Glance, Fifth Edition. Edited by Patrick Davey and Alex Pitcher.

Companion website: www.wiley.com/go/medicine5e

226 The skin and systemic disease

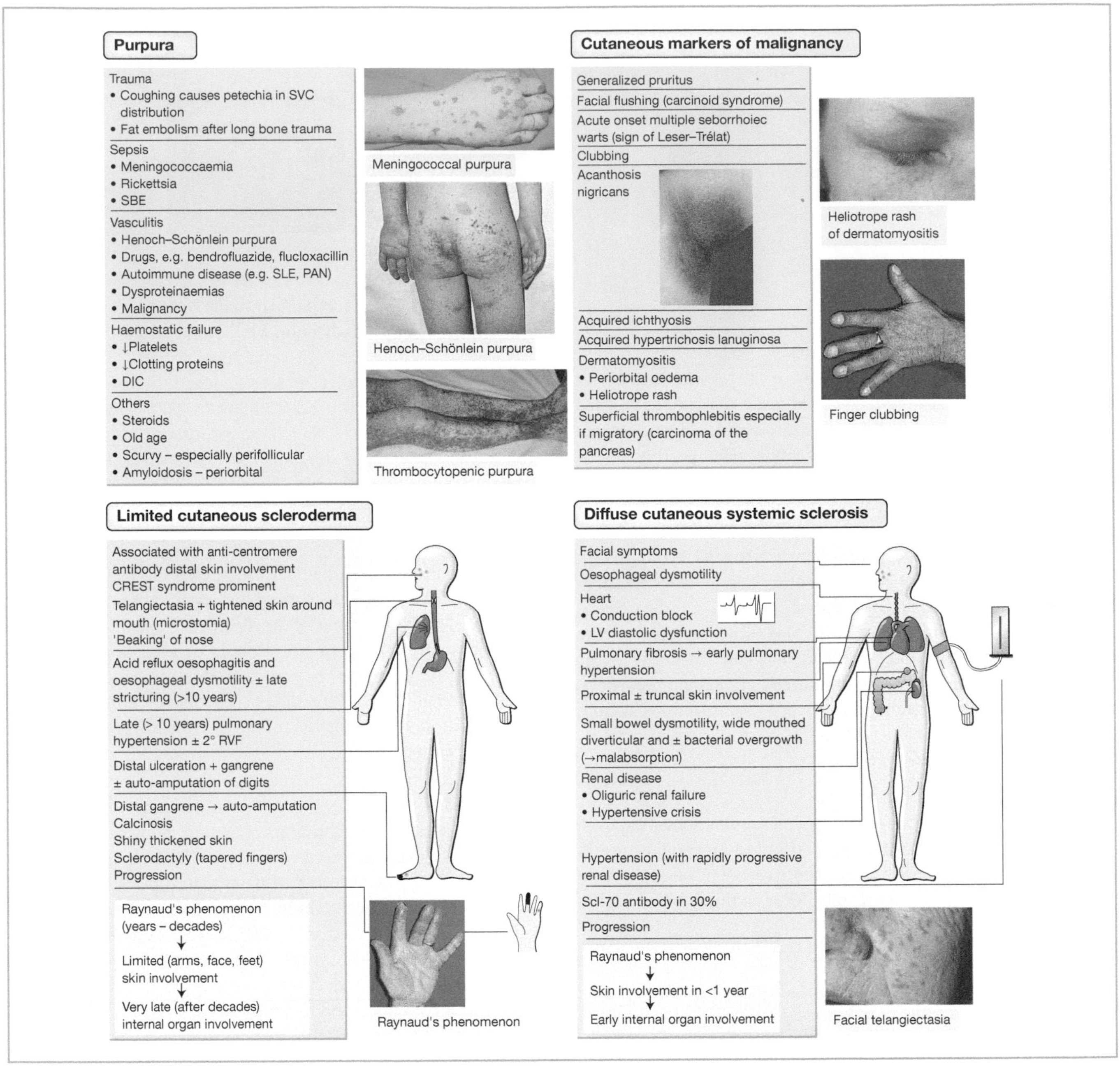

Purpura

Trauma
- Coughing causes petechia in SVC distribution
- Fat embolism after long bone trauma

Sepsis
- Meningococcaemia
- Rickettsia
- SBE

Vasculitis
- Henoch–Schönlein purpura
- Drugs, e.g. bendrofluazide, flucloxacillin
- Autoimmune disease (e.g. SLE, PAN)
- Dysproteinaemias
- Malignancy

Haemostatic failure
- ↓Platelets
- ↓Clotting proteins
- DIC

Others
- Steroids
- Old age
- Scurvy – especially perifollicular
- Amyloidosis – periorbital

Meningococcal purpura

Henoch–Schönlein purpura

Thrombocytopenic purpura

Cutaneous markers of malignancy

Generalized pruritus

Facial flushing (carcinoid syndrome)

Acute onset multiple seborrhoiec warts (sign of Leser–Trélat)

Clubbing

Acanthosis nigricans

Acquired ichthyosis

Acquired hypertrichosis lanuginosa

Dermatomyositis
- Periorbital oedema
- Heliotrope rash

Superficial thrombophlebitis especially if migratory (carcinoma of the pancreas)

Heliotrope rash of dermatomyositis

Finger clubbing

Limited cutaneous scleroderma

Associated with anti-centromere antibody distal skin involvement CREST syndrome prominent

Telangiectasia + tightened skin around mouth (microstomia)

'Beaking' of nose

Acid reflux oesophagitis and oesophageal dysmotility ± late stricturing (>10 years)

Late (> 10 years) pulmonary hypertension ± 2° RVF

Distal ulceration + gangrene ± auto-amputation of digits

Distal gangrene → auto-amputation

Calcinosis

Shiny thickened skin

Sclerodactyly (tapered fingers)

Progression

Raynaud's phenomenon (years – decades)
↓
Limited (arms, face, feet) skin involvement
↓
Very late (after decades) internal organ involvement

Raynaud's phenomenon

Diffuse cutaneous systemic sclerosis

Facial symptoms

Oesophageal dysmotility

Heart
- Conduction block
- LV diastolic dysfunction

Pulmonary fibrosis → early pulmonary hypertension

Proximal ± truncal skin involvement

Small bowel dysmotility, wide mouthed diverticular and ± bacterial overgrowth (→malabsorption)

Renal disease
- Oliguric renal failure
- Hypertensive crisis

Hypertension (with rapidly progressive renal disease)

Scl-70 antibody in 30%

Progression

Raynaud's phenomenon
↓
Skin involvement in <1 year
↓
Early internal organ involvement

Facial telangiectasia

The skin can be involved in, or react to, many systemic disease processes.

Raynaud phenomenon

Raynaud phenomenon is episodic, painful, digital ischaemia in response to cold or emotional stimuli, characterized by classic sequential colour changes of white to blue to red. The disorder may be primary and idiopathic or secondary to underlying disease (see Table 226.1).

- Idiopathic Raynaud phenomenon is diagnosed in young women who have no features of an underlying disorder on clinical evaluation or investigation.
- Raynaud phenomenon is more likely to be secondary, usually to systemic sclerosis, if it is especially severe (with digital skin changes) and persistent, or if it begins for the first time in early adulthood, in a male and is unilateral.

Investigations when indicated should include a chest X-ray (cervical rib), autoantibodies (antinuclear antibodies, double-stranded

Medicine at a Glance, Fifth Edition. Edited by Patrick Davey and Alex Pitcher.

Companion website: www.wiley.com/go/medicine5e

Table 226.1 Causes of Raynaud phenomenon.

- Cervical rib
- Vibrating tools
- Vasculitis and connective tissue diseases: systemic sclerosis, Sjögren syndrome, SLE, dermatomyositis, rheumatoid arthritis
- Cryoglobulinaemia
- Cold agglutinins
- Hyperviscosity syndromes
- Drugs (β-blockers, ergot alkaloids, cytotoxics)

DNA, antineutrophil cytoplasmic antibody), cryoglobulins, cold agglutinins and erythrocyte sedimentation rate. Treatment: heated gloves, oral nifedipine, angiotensin-converting enzyme (ACE) inhibitors and avoidance of cold. If severe, sympathectomy can be considered.

Human immunodeficiency virus

Skin disease is an important corollary of acquired immune deficiency syndrome (AIDS) and human immunodeficiency virus (HIV) infection (see Table 226.2). The incidence of several cutaneous diseases is increased in people who are HIV positive or who have AIDS. The percentage of people with HIV who have skin manifestations, and the number of manifestations, increase as HIV infection progresses. The incidence and severity sometimes correlate with the absolute numbers of T-helper cells, and the prognostic significance of some disorders is well recognized. HIV infection may affect the behaviour of other dermatological conditions such as psoriasis. Generally, HIV-related skin diseases improve with HAART (highly active antiretroviral therapy) although some patients may experience severe cutaneous immune restoration disease, e.g. due to herpes simplex or cytomegalovirus.

Drug eruptions

Drug reactions are very commonly seen in acute internal medicine and general practice. Regard any drug as capable of causing any cutaneous reaction. Some reactions are predictable (striae with steroids), some likely (photosensitivity with amiodarone, β-blockers exacerbating psoriasis) and some unpredictable or idiosyncratic (erythema multiforme with antibiotics).

Table 226.2 Cutaneous manifestations of HIV infection and AIDS.

Pruritus

Inflammatory dermatoses
- Seroconversion toxic erythema
- Psoriasis
- Seborrhoeic dermatitis
- Severe drug reactions
- Eosinophilic pustular folliculitis
- Papular pruritic eruption
- Vasculitis

Infections
- Folliculitis and cellulitis (including MRSA)
- Tinea and onychomycosis
- Candidosis
- Hairy leukoplakia (EBV)
- Atypical primary, secondary and late syphilis
- Bacillary haemangiomatosis
- Condyloma acuminata (viral warts)
- Molluscum contagiosum
- Cutaneous atypical mycobacterial infection
- Kaposi sarcoma (HHV8)
- Herpes simplex
- Herpes zoster
- Severe aphthous stomatitis

Other skin manifestations
- Cutaneous and nail hyperpigmentation
- Porphyria cutanea tarda
- Acquired ichthyosis and keratoderma
- Yellow nail syndrome
- Immune reconstitution disease

Neoplasia
- Kaposi sarcoma (HHV8)
- Cutaneous lymphoma
- Castleman disease (HHV8)
- Melanoma and non-melanoma skin cancer

EBV, Epstein–Barr virus; HHV, human herpes virus; MRSA, methicillin-resistant *Staphylococcus aureus*.

Vasculitis

Conditions producing a vasculitic reaction in the skin include the following.

- **Infection**: meningococcaemia, bacterial endocarditis and COVID-19.
- **Systemic vasculitis** (e.g. systemic lupus erythematosus [SLE], polyarteritis nodosa [PAN]): suspected when internal organs such as the kidneys and/or lungs are involved. Immunology and skin biopsy may be diagnostic, as may renal/lung histology.
- **Erythema nodosum** (EN): painful palpable lesions on the lower legs, arising from a vasculitis of the deep dermis. Although no cause may be found, EN is associated with infection (streptococcal sore throat, mycobacteria, etc.), drugs, sarcoidosis and inflammatory bowel disease. Resolution typically occurs over 5–6 weeks.
- **Other causes**, including drugs, connective tissue disease, paraneoplastic phenomena, clotting abnormalities and cryoglobulinaemia.
- **Skin infarcts**, affecting particularly the extremities, e.g. nailbed 'splinter haemorrhages' (caused by circulating immune complexes) occur in many acute and chronic infections, including bacterial endocarditis.
- **Purpura** has a wide differential diagnosis (see figure above). Two common causes are:
  - *Henoch–Schönlein purpura* (anaphylactoid purpura): occurs mainly in children as a result of an abnormal response to a viral infection. A purpuric rash occurs on the extensor aspects of the lower limbs. Nephritis may develop. It normally resolves without sequelae; very occasionally chronic renal damage occurs
  - *leukocytoclastic or allergic vasculitis*: may be confined to the skin (see figure below). The most common clinical pattern is acute, self-limiting, palpable purpura (other lesions may occur), which may be chronic or recurrent and usually affects the limbs with fever, malaise, arthralgia and gastrointestinal symptoms. The cause is often not discovered but infections, neoplasia and drugs should be excluded.

Skin markers of internal malignancy

There are a number of cutaneous stigmata of internal malignancy.

- **Pruritus**: lymphoma, polycythaemia rubra vera.
- **Ichthyosis**: dry skin with fish-like scales.
- **Acanthosis nigricans**: velvety hyperkeratotic plaques found in flexures and intertriginous areas; also caused by endocrine disorders (acromegaly, Cushing disease, Addison disease, hypothyroidism, insulin-resistant diabetes mellitus, polycystic ovary disease), drugs (steroids) or obesity, or rarely it is familial.
- **Dermatomyositis**: skin involvement consists of erythematous plaques over the knuckles, finger joints, elbows and knees. Nail cuticles are ragged. Eyelids are swollen and are discoloured violet (see Chapter 220). Of patients aged >50 years, 30% have an underlying cancer.
- **Migratory superficial thrombosis**: often relates to pancreatic cancer.
- **Secondary deposits in the skin**, e.g. Sister Joseph's nodule (periumbilical deposit from an intra-abdominal malignancy) or Virchow's node (left supraclavicular fossa lymph node deposit from gastric cancer). The scalp is a common site for cutaneous metastasis from internal solid cancers.

Systemic sclerosis

Systemic sclerosis is an autoimmune disease affecting the skin and internal organs that occurs in two forms: (i) limited cutaneous scleroderma localized to the skin; and (ii) diffuse cutaneous systemic sclerosis when internal viscera are involved. Scleroderma also occurs in a localized form (morphoea) and in malignancies (e.g. breast cancer), porphyria cutanea tarda, phenylketonuria and in the carcinoid syndrome.

- **Limited cutaneous scleroderma** (morphoea): skin lesions are circumscribed plaques. They can occur anywhere, or may involve the forehead (*en coup de sabre*). Systemic involvement is rare and occurs later.
- **Diffuse cutaneous systemic sclerosis**: female > male. Raynaud phenomenon precedes cutaneous sclerosis, with puffy swelling of the hands and feet, leading to atrophic thinning of ulcerated digital tips and nailfold involvement. Muscle weakness occurs (disuse atrophy or muscle involvement). Perioral involvement produces very tight skin around the mouth, restricting opening, and may require lateral release. Dry eyes and mouth (keratoconjunctivitis sicca and xerostomia – Sjögren syndrome) occur. Oesophageal involvement leads to difficulty swallowing, and small bowel disease produces abdominal pain and diarrhoea (caused by bacterial overgrowth). Pulmonary fibrosis produces shortness of breath (restrictive pattern on lung function testing). An erosive arthritis may cause joint pains. Renal failure occurs and is associated with a worse prognosis. Antinuclear antibodies are found in >90% and anticentromere antibodies in 70% with CREST (*C*alcinosis, *R*aynaud, o*E*sophagitis, *S*clerodactyly, *T*elangiectasia).
- No agent reliably arrests disease activity. Treatment is for symptom relief only. Digital vascular insufficiency is treated by cold avoidance, vasodilators (e.g. nifedipine, ACE inhibitors, intravenous prostacyclin, intravenous calcitonin gene-related peptide). In severe cases, digital amputation may be necessary. Oesophageal reflux responds to proton pump inhibitors. The prognosis is generally good, even with some organ involvement, although renal or pulmonary disease can be fatal.

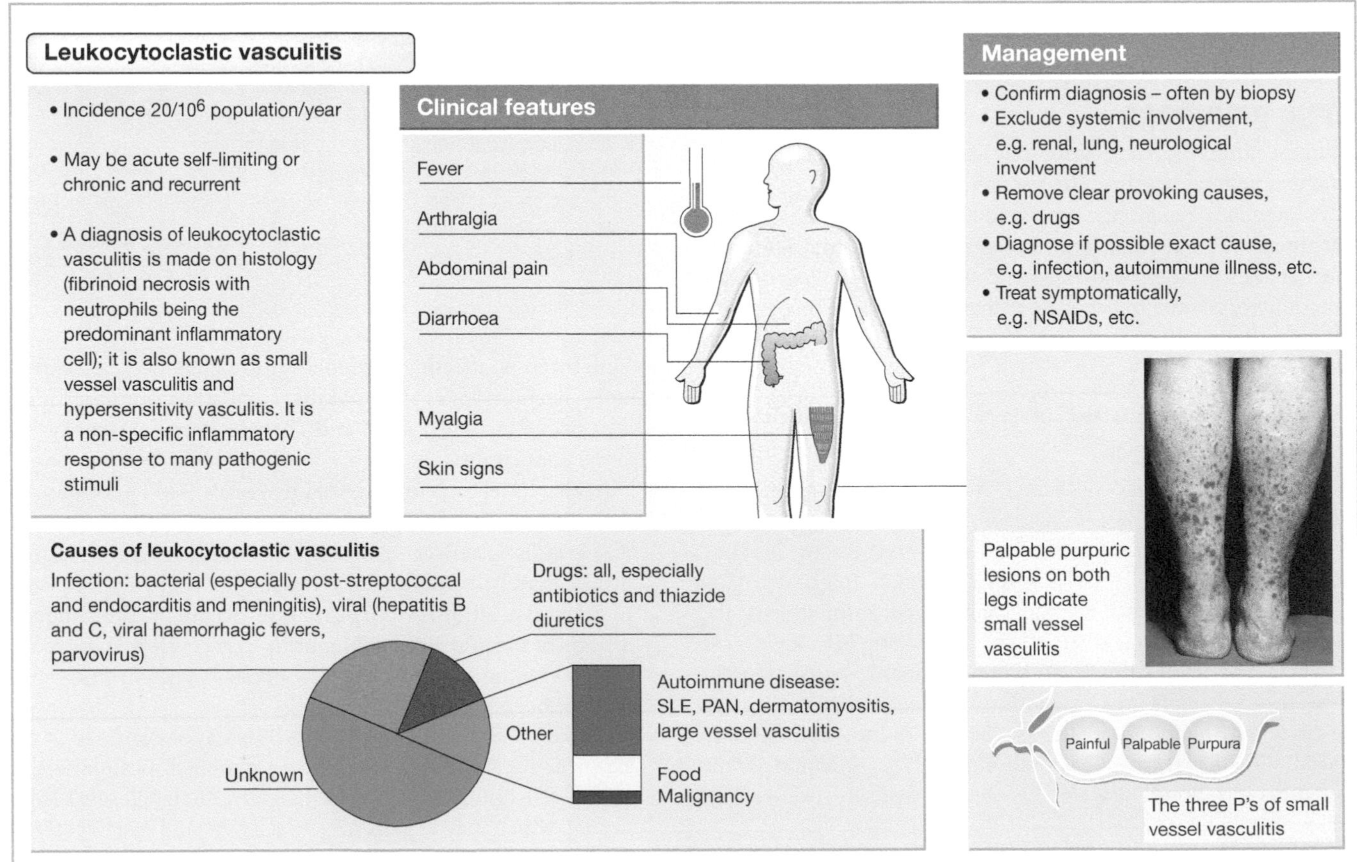

Leukocytoclastic vasculitis
• Incidence 20/10^6 population/year
• May be acute self-limiting or chronic and recurrent
• A diagnosis of leukocytoclastic vasculitis is made on histology (fibrinoid necrosis with neutrophils being the predominant inflammatory cell); it is also known as small vessel vasculitis and hypersensitivity vasculitis. It is a non-specific inflammatory response to many pathogenic stimuli
Clinical features
Fever
Arthralgia
Abdominal pain
Diarrhoea
Myalgia
Skin signs
Management
• Confirm diagnosis – often by biopsy
• Exclude systemic involvement, e.g. renal, lung, neurological involvement
• Remove clear provoking causes, e.g. drugs
• Diagnose if possible exact cause, e.g. infection, autoimmune illness, etc.
• Treat symptomatically, e.g. NSAIDs, etc.
Causes of leukocytoclastic vasculitis
Infection: bacterial (especially post-streptococcal and endocarditis and meningitis), viral (hepatitis B and C, viral haemorrhagic fevers, parvovirus)
Drugs: all, especially antibiotics and thiazide diuretics
Other
Autoimmune disease: SLE, PAN, dermatomyositis, large vessel vasculitis
Food
Malignancy
Unknown
Palpable purpuric lesions on both legs indicate small vessel vasculitis
Painful
Palpable
Purpura
The three P's of small vessel vasculitis

227 Disorders of skin pigmentation

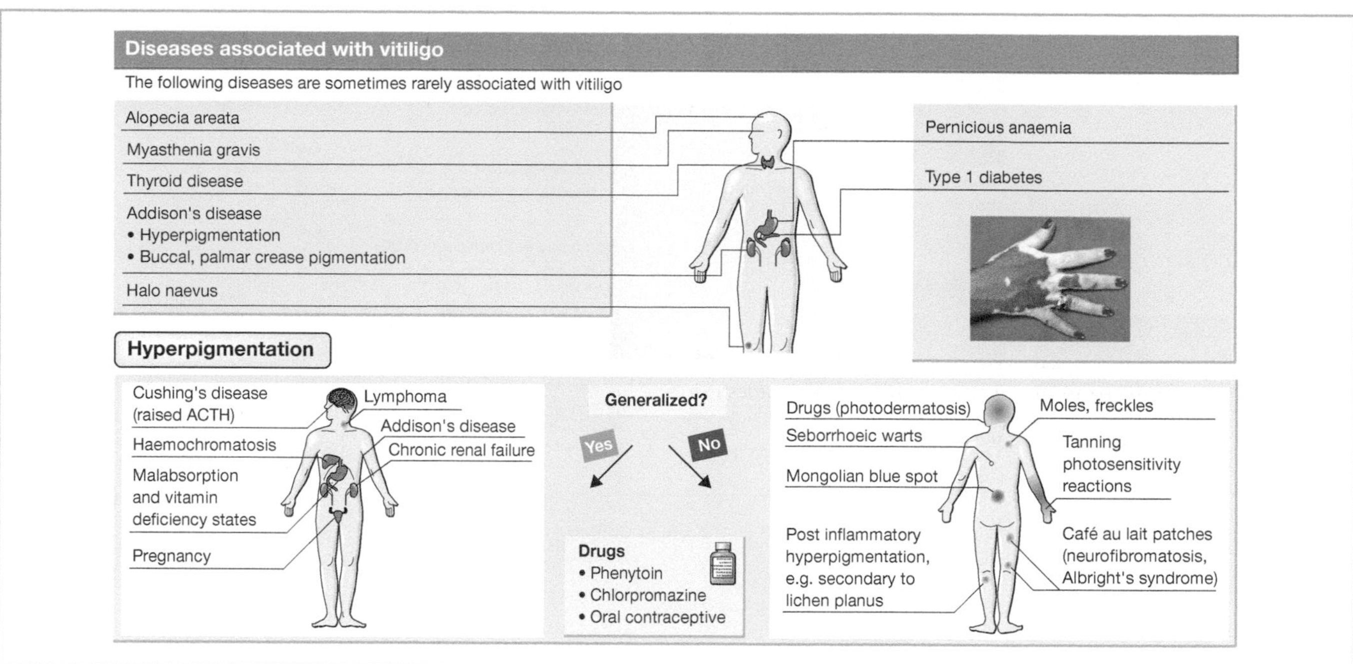

Excess or diminished pigmentation is usually due to excess or diminished melanocyte activity in the skin, although deposition of other pigments can be involved. Melanocyte activity is influenced by solar ultraviolet light. Both hypo- and hyperpigmentation are common complications of inflammatory dermatoses and are more pronounced in racially pigmented skin.

Hyperpigmentation

Congenital diseases associated with patches of hyperpigmented skin include melanocytic naevi and Fanconi and Albright syndromes. Café-au-lait patches are also found in neurofibromatosis but can be isolated.

Acquired diseases can give rise to localized or generalized hyperpigmentation.

- **Localized hyperpigmentation**: many inflammatory skin diseases can leave patches of hyperpigmentation. Chloasma (melasma) is patchy facial hyperpigmentation, due to endogenous or exogenous steroids, sunlight, drugs (e.g. antibiotics) and depilation.
- **Generalized hyperpigmentation**: can result from acquired endocrine or systemic illness or drugs, particularly photosensitive reactions to drugs, chemicals and plants.

Hypopigmentation

Hypopigmentation may be:

- congenital and generalized, as in the genetic disease of albinism, where melanization cannot occur as a result of tyrosinase deficiency, or localized, such as the hypopigmented ash leaf patches found in tuberous sclerosis
- acquired: postinflammatory hypopigmentation (common, can occur after any cause of skin inflammation, e.g. contact dermatitis) or with leprosy (depigmented anaesthetic areas). A common cause is vitiligo. A very rare cause is pituitary failure (generalized loss of skin pigment, often with loss of secondary sex characteristics).

Vitiligo

This is a common (1% of the population) autoimmune condition affecting all races, of unknown aetiology and associated with anti-melanocytic antibody production and organ-specific autoimmune disease.

Clinical features

Depigmented macules appear on sun-exposed areas, areas previously hyperpigmented (e.g. face, axillae, groins) and areas exposed to trauma or friction (an example of Koebner's phenomenon). Areas of vitiligo are readily demonstrated by an ultraviolet lamp (Wood's light). Hairs within a lesion become amelanotic (white).

Management and prognosis

Treatment is unsatisfactory, but the priorities are:

- protection from the sun to avoid skin cancer and to minimize the contrast between affected and unaffected skin
- cosmetic camouflage.

Of younger patients, 20% may repigment spontaneously, but it is usually unsatisfactorily patchy and perifollicular. Some patients respond to phototherapy.

Medicine at a Glance, Fifth Edition. Edited by Patrick Davey and Alex Pitcher.

Companion website: www.wiley.com/go/medicine5e

228 Skin tumours

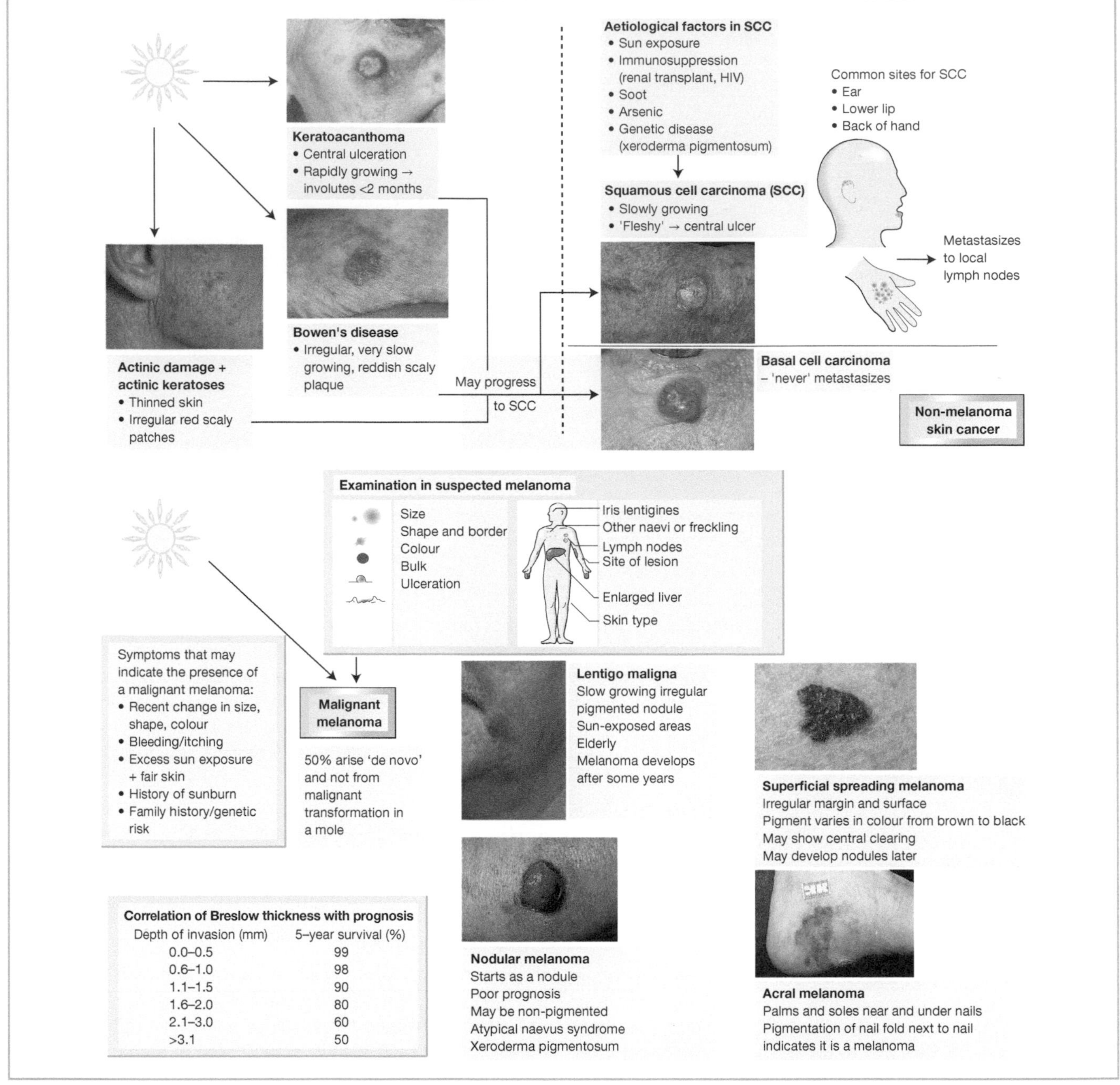

Keratoacanthoma
• Central ulceration
• Rapidly growing → involutes <2 months
Bowen's disease
• Irregular, very slow growing, reddish scaly plaque
Actinic damage + actinic keratoses
• Thinned skin
• Irregular red scaly patches
May progress to SCC
Aetiological factors in SCC
• Sun exposure
• Immunosuppression (renal transplant, HIV)
• Soot
• Arsenic
• Genetic disease (xeroderma pigmentosum)
Squamous cell carcinoma (SCC)
• Slowly growing
• 'Fleshy' → central ulcer
Common sites for SCC
• Ear
• Lower lip
• Back of hand
Metastasizes to local lymph nodes
Basal cell carcinoma
– 'never' metastasizes
Non-melanoma skin cancer
Examination in suspected melanoma
Size
Shape and border
Colour
Bulk
Ulceration
Iris lentigines
Other naevi or freckling
Lymph nodes
Site of lesion
Enlarged liver
Skin type
Symptoms that may indicate the presence of a malignant melanoma:
• Recent change in size, shape, colour
• Bleeding/itching
• Excess sun exposure + fair skin
• History of sunburn
• Family history/genetic risk
Malignant melanoma
50% arise 'de novo' and not from malignant transformation in a mole
Lentigo maligna
Slow growing irregular pigmented nodule
Sun-exposed areas
Elderly
Melanoma develops after some years
Superficial spreading melanoma
Irregular margin and surface
Pigment varies in colour from brown to black
May show central clearing
May develop nodules later
Nodular melanoma
Starts as a nodule
Poor prognosis
May be non-pigmented
Atypical naevus syndrome
Xeroderma pigmentosum
Acral melanoma
Palms and soles near and under nails
Pigmentation of nail fold next to nail indicates it is a melanoma

Correlation of Breslow thickness with prognosis

Depth of invasion (mm)	5-year survival (%)
0.0–0.5	99
0.6–1.0	98
1.1–1.5	90
1.6–2.0	80
2.1–3.0	60
>3.1	50

Skin cancers are the most common of all cancers, with over 100 000 cases per annum in the UK. Sun exposure is the unifying aetiological factor.

Premalignant disease

- **Solar or actinic keratoses**: flat, scaly, often erythematous lesions, which show partial-thickness epidermal dysplasia on histology and have a low risk of developing into Bowen disease or squamous cell carcinoma (SCC). They are usually associated with actinic (sun) damage. Treatment is with cryotherapy, curettage, topical 5-fluorouracil, diclofenac or imiquimod or photodynamic therapy.
- **Bowen disease** (intraepidermal carcinoma *in situ*): a single, red, scaly patch that may be mistaken for eczema or psoriasis, but neither itches nor responds to topical steroids. Sometimes there

Medicine at a Glance, Fifth Edition. Edited by Patrick Davey and Alex Pitcher.

Companion website: www.wiley.com/go/medicine5e

are multiple lesions. Aetiological factors and treatment are as above, but include surgical curettage or excision. The condition may progress to invasive SCC.

- **Keratoacanthoma**: a rapidly growing nodular lesion on the light-exposed skin of the hand or face but could be other parts of the skin. It reaches its maximum size at <1–2 months and appears as a smooth dome-shaped lesion with a central crater filled with keratinaceous material. It can spontaneously involute to leave scarring, but is best excised, as it is probably a form of SCC.
- **Congenital melanocytic naevi**: large pigmented lesions present from birth. They are common anywhere, but a bathing trunk distribution is recognized. There is a significant risk of malignant melanoma developing in very large lesions.
- **Dysplastic naevi**: may be associated with an increased risk of melanoma. The dysplastic naevus syndrome is the presence of many moles (dysplastic naevi), heterogeneous in size, shape, colour and surface, often abnormally distributed (scalp, buttocks, feet), usually larger than 0.5 cm, and iris lentigines in the context of a personal or family history of melanoma.

Malignant disease

- **Basal cell carcinoma/epithelioma** (BCC/BCE): an extremely common neoplasm, often on the face, head and neck of older people. BCEs 'never' metastasize, but indolent growth can lead to delayed presentation and deep invasion, leading to high rates of recurrence after conventional treatments. Sun damage is the greatest risk factor for BCE, but sometimes multiple BCEs are associated with previous X-ray treatment for ankylosing spondylitis (spine) and tinea capitis (scalp). Usual treatments are excision, curettage and cautery, or radiotherapy, all with a 5–10% recurrence rate. The superficial variant of BCCs can be successfully treated using topical imiquimod or photodynamic therapy. Tumours around the eye and nasal furrows have a 20% recurrence rate, as a result of infiltration along embryological fusion lines. A very high cure rate can be achieved using micrographic surgery (Mohs procedure) which is the treatment of choice for BCCs on the head and neck. Late presentation or failed treatment is complicated by fungation, involvement of other structures (such as the eye and lacrimal apparatus), and deep invasion with destruction of cartilage and bone, which may all represent incurable disease.
- **Squamous carcinoma**: occurs in sun-exposed areas in elderly people or as multiple tumours in very young people with xeroderma pigmentosum, a defect in DNA repair mechanisms. Other risk factors include smoking (lip tumours), human papillomavirus and chronic inflammation, e.g. associated with chronic venous ulceration (Marjolin's ulcer of the leg). The best known occupational cancer was cancer of the scrotum in chimney sweeps, which in the nineteenth century was related to exposure to the hydrocarbons in soot. SCC most commonly presents as an irregular ulcer or a slowly growing nodule. It may be very destructive locally, and can also metastasize to the lymph nodes. Treatment must therefore be ablative (i.e. excision, Mohs micrographic surgery or radiotherapy) and long-term follow-up is necessary.
- **Lentigo maligna** (Hutchinson's melanotic freckle): a slow-growing, pigmented macule on the face in older people. Histologically, it is an intraepidermal melanoma, but it can become invasive (lentigo maligna melanoma). Biopsy establishes the diagnosis. Treatment is by excision. Plastic repair may be necessary.
- **Malignant melanoma**: in the UK there are 8000 new cases and 2500 deaths per year, with rates doubling every decade. Predisposing factors include (susceptibility to) ultraviolet light exposure, congenital naevi, family history of melanoma, large numbers of acquired naevi, any number of atypical naevi, freckles, previous episodes of sunburn, and significant sun exposure before the age of 20 years.

  Melanoma is rare in African Caribbean and Asian individuals, and common in Scots and Australians. Four types of melanoma are recognized clinically: superficial spreading, nodular, acral lentiginous and lentigo maligna melanoma. Superficial spreading and nodular are the most common types and present in early adulthood. In men, the upper back is a common area, but in women it is the lower leg. Some melanomas (75%) do not arise from an existing mole. The earliest growth of superficial spreading melanoma is in the horizontal plane, so presentation is usually as a new or changing mole. Melanoma invades locally and metastasizes to lymph nodes early on. On examination, look for actinic damage, freckles, and numbers, types and distribution of moles (and iris lentigines – dark-brown macules), and check the local and distant lymph nodes and the liver. The crucial diagnostic and prognostic investigation is excisional histopathology and this also delivers definitive treatment. Multidisciplinary management is appropriate.

  The histological depth of the lesion on first presentation correlates with the prognosis (see figure). Melanoma is conventionally excised with wide margins. For extensive disease, surgical or laser debulking, amputation, isolated limb perfusion with chemotherapy, systemic chemotherapy, including with cytokines, and radiotherapy are used. Treatment of metastatic melanoma is not curative, but recent developments, particularly immunotherapy, have improved prognosis and survival significantly.
- **Kaposi sarcoma**: AIDS-related vascular neoplasm due to human herpes virus 8 (HHV8) infection.

Lymphoma

- **Mycosis fungoides**: a cutaneous T-cell lymphoma where there is slowly evolving infiltration of the skin with T lymphocytes. The cause is not known but human T-cell leukaemia virus 1 (HTLV-1) was first isolated from a patient with Sézary syndrome (erythroderma, lymphadenopathy and abnormal Sézary cells with cerebriform nuclei in the blood). The differential diagnosis of erythroderma is given in Chapter 69.

  The following stages are recognized.

  - Fixed itchy scaly patches (like eczema or psoriasis).
  - Fixed geographical plaques.
  - Nodules, tumours and ulcers.
  - Lymph node or systemic organ involvement.

It is possible that at an early stage, malignant change has not occurred and the prognosis with gentle treatment (topical steroids, PUVA [psoralens and ultraviolet A], topical nitrogen mustard, electron beam therapy) is good. With more advanced disease, therapy is more radical (radiotherapy, chemotherapy, extracorporeal photochemotherapy) and the outlook is bleak.

- **Adult T-cell lymphoma/leukaemia** (ATLL): may present with a cutaneous prodrome of granulomatous papules and nodules (from which proviral DNA can be recovered), and precedes and accompanies ATLL due to HTLV-1.
- **Hodgkin disease and non-Hodgkin lymphoma**: may involve the skin and, it is argued, may originate in the skin.

229 Orogenital disease

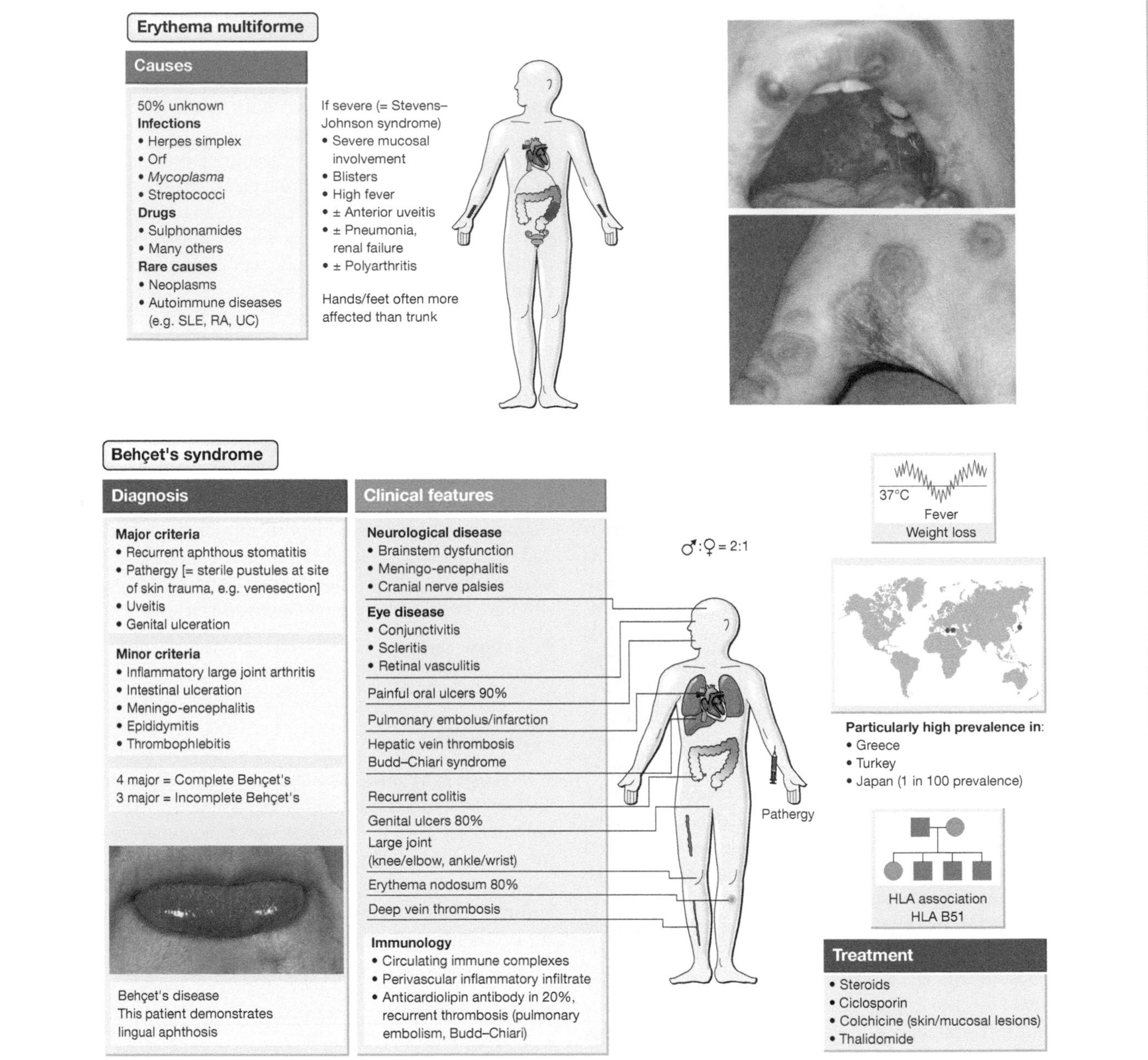

Erythema multiforme
Causes
50% unknown
Infections
• Herpes simplex
• Orf
• Mycoplasma
• Streptococci
Drugs
• Sulphonamides
• Many others
Rare causes
• Neoplasms
• Autoimmune diseases (e.g. SLE, RA, UC)
If severe (= Stevens–Johnson syndrome)
• Severe mucosal involvement
• Blisters
• High fever
• ± Anterior uveitis
• ± Pneumonia, renal failure
• ± Polyarthritis
Hands/feet often more affected than trunk
Behçet's syndrome
Diagnosis
Major criteria
• Recurrent aphthous stomatitis
• Pathergy [= sterile pustules at site of skin trauma, e.g. venesection]
• Uveitis
• Genital ulceration
Minor criteria
• Inflammatory large joint arthritis
• Intestinal ulceration
• Meningo-encephalitis
• Epididymitis
• Thrombophlebitis
4 major = Complete Behçet's
3 major = Incomplete Behçet's
Behçet's disease
This patient demonstrates lingual aphthosis
Clinical features
Neurological disease
• Brainstem dysfunction
• Meningo-encephalitis
• Cranial nerve palsies
Eye disease
• Conjunctivitis
• Scleritis
• Retinal vasculitis
Painful oral ulcers 90%
Pulmonary embolus/infarction
Hepatic vein thrombosis
Budd–Chiari syndrome
Recurrent colitis
Genital ulcers 80%
Large joint (knee/elbow, ankle/wrist)
Erythema nodosum 80%
Deep vein thrombosis
Immunology
• Circulating immune complexes
• Perivascular inflammatory infiltrate
• Anticardiolipin antibody in 20%, recurrent thrombosis (pulmonary embolism, Budd–Chiari)
♂:♀ = 2:1
Pathergy
37°C
Fever
Weight loss
Particularly high prevalence in:
• Greece
• Turkey
• Japan (1 in 100 prevalence)
HLA association
HLA B51
Treatment
• Steroids
• Ciclosporin
• Colchicine (skin/mucosal lesions)
• Thalidomide

Oral disorders

- **Oral ulceration**: the most common cause is idiopathic aphthous ulceration. Oral pemphigus is very rare but serious, and is frequently diagnosed late (see Chapter 225). Examination of all patients with oral ulcers should include examination of other mucocutaneous sites and a search for lymphadenopathy. Investigations include microbiology and virology, and a biopsy with immunofluorescence. Treatment of aphthae concentrates on improving oral hygiene, antibiotic and antifungal mouthwashes, and topical steroids.
- ***Candida***: an extremely common intraoral commensal, which acts as an opportunistic pathogen in those immunosuppressed from infection (e.g. HIV), disease (e.g. diabetes mellitus) or drugs (e.g. oral antibiotics, cytotoxics). White detachable deposits and plaques are the usual physical signs. Mouthwashes or nystatin lozenges and a systemic imidazole or triazole are effective treatments, but candidosis may recur depending on the context.
- **Leukoplakia**: a non-specific common disturbance of oral mucosal keratinization. Smoking and poor dental hygiene are

Medicine at a Glance, Fifth Edition. Edited by Patrick Davey and Alex Pitcher.

Companion website: www.wiley.com/go/medicine5e

associated factors. It may result from a syphilitic atrophic glossitis, but small, white mucus patches may occur anywhere in the oral cavity during secondary syphilis; 5% undergo malignant transformation.

- **Erythroplakia**: describes red patches in the mouth. They are more likely to be malignant than leukoplakia and should therefore be biopsied.
- **Lichen planus**: characterized by lilac erythematous patches topped by lacy white striae (Wickham's striae). It is more common on the buccal mucosa than the tongue, although all intraoral sites may be involved. Of patients with the condition, 30% have extraoral lichen planus, and 10–50% of all patients with lichen planus have oral lesions. Erosive or atrophic lichen planus may progress to malignancy.

Vulval disorders

The vulva can be affected by dermatoses such as seborrhoeic dermatitis, psoriasis, lichen sclerosus and lichen planus, or sexually transmitted diseases (STDs). Patients may be severely symptomatic with itch, irritation, dyspareunia and somatopsychic symptoms.

- **Vulval warts**: usually caused by human papillomavirus (HPV) types 6 and 11. All patients and their partners should be screened for STDs. Colposcopy and a cervical smear examination are indicated. Treatment is with liquid nitrogen therapy, topical podophyllin or topical imiquimod.
- **Lichen simplex**: refers to a chronic eczematous process exaggerated and propagated by scratching in response to itch. Treatment is with topical steroids and night-time sedation, possibly with tricyclic antidepressants. Additional causes of vulval itching include urinary incontinence and vaginal discharge, often as a result of candidosis. All women with pruritus vulvae should be screened for diabetes mellitus.
- **Lichen sclerosus**: an idiopathic, chronic, inflammatory dermatosis with subsequent atrophy, which can cause intense itching in the female. Lesions are shiny, white and red-rimmed with central telangiectasia, purpura and erosions. There may be loss of architecture of the labia and burying of the clitoris. Potent topical steroids relieve the itch and reverse the skin changes. Biopsy and continued monitoring are important because intraepithelial neoplasia and frank invasive carcinoma may develop.
- **Vulval intraepithelial neoplasia** (VIN): suspected when hard white plaques or erosions are seen. HPV may be involved. The invasive potential of VIN is small. Cryotherapy and topical imiquimod can be used. Multidisciplinary management (gynaecologists, oncologists, etc.) is desirable; 50% of vulval cancer is associated with HPV and 50% with lichen sclerosis with little overlap.
- **Extramammary Paget disease** presents as an irregular psoriasiform patch or plaque. It is adenocarcinoma *in situ*. There may be a subjacent epithelial neoplasm or an underlying gastrointestinal (GI), urological or gynaecological cancer.

Penile disorders

Uncircumcised men have more dermatological problems than those circumcised at birth. The penis is a common site for seborrhoeic dermatitis, psoriasis, lichen sclerosus, lichen planus and viral warts. Balanitis due to *Candida* or other microbials may be a presenting feature of diabetes mellitus.

- **Lichen sclerosus** of the penis may result in male dyspareunia, phimosis (inability to retract the foreskin) and even retention of urine. Chronic disease is associated with penile squamous cell carcinoma (SCC). Potent topical steroids help 50% of patients. Circumcision may be necessary.
- **Zoon balanitis**: an irritant mucositis of the uncircumcised male. It presents with moist raw patches and is treated by circumcision.
- **Erythroplasia of Queyrat** is the eponym for **Bowen disease** (SCC *in situ*) of the uncircumcised penis and is suspected if there are fixed red lesions of the penis. Biopsy is diagnostic. Treatment options include topical 5-fluorouracil, topical imiquimod, cryotherapy, radiotherapy or surgery. Oncogenic HPV is usually associated. Follow-up (for malignancy detection) is essential. As in the vulva, 50% of penis cancer is associated with HPV and 50% with lichen sclerosis with little overlap.
- **Extramammary Paget disease** presents as an irregular psoriasiform patch or plaque. It is adenocarcinoma *in situ*. There may be a subjacent epithelial neoplasm or an underlying GI or urological cancer.

Genital ulceration

Aetiology

Genital ulcers can be caused by dermatoses, STDs or other infections, Behçet disease, pyoderma gangrenosum, artefact or, most importantly, squamous carcinoma.

Investigations

These include microbiology (including mycology) and skin biopsy.

Treatment

Genital hygiene, emollient and topical antibiotic, antifungal and steroid applications.

Orogenital syndromes

Certain diseases result in simultaneous lesions in the mouth and genitalia.

- **Severe erythema multiforme**: the cause of erythema multiforme is often unknown, but includes herpes simplex infection, other infections such as those caused by *Mycoplasma* spp. and drug reactions. In mild to moderate disease, involvement is limited to the skin. Lesions characteristically start as pleomorphic red eruptions on the arms and legs, which spread centrally to the trunk. Spontaneous remission is usual, although topical steroids may improve itch. In severe disease (Stevens–Johnson syndrome) lesions occur in the mouth, conjunctiva and genitalia as well. Treatment is with systemic steroids and antimicrobials for any infection.
- **Behçet syndrome**: characterized by painful oral (90–100%) and genital (60–90%) ulceration and variable involvement of other systems as follows.
  - Ocular manifestations (keratitis, uveitis, optic neuritis) (50–90%).
  - Pustules, pyoderma gangrenosum, erythema nodosum and arthritis (20–50%).
  - Central nervous system involvement (e.g. vasculitis, thrombophlebitis) (10–20%).
  - Pulmonary infarction (10–40%).
  - Renal involvement (10%).
  - Budd–Chiari syndrome (10%).

There are no diagnostic tests for Behçet syndrome. Treatment is with systemic steroids; occasionally thalidomide is used. Many patients have mild disease and do well. However, cerebral/renal involvement is associated with severe treatment-resistant disease and a worse prognosis.

230 Endometriosis and adenomyosis

Common sites of endometriosis

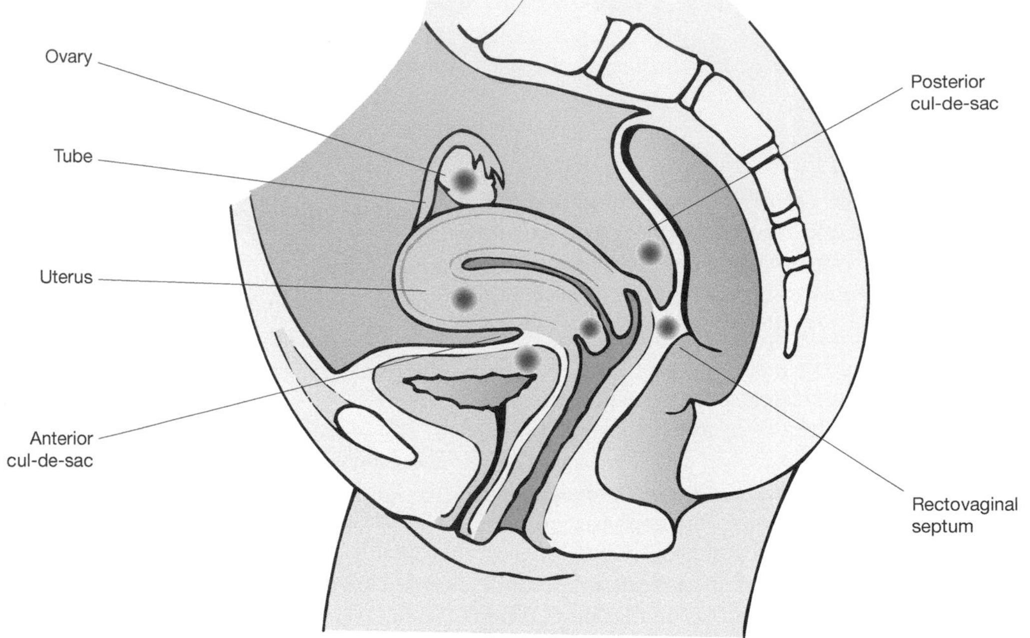

American Fertility Society (AFS) classification of endometriosis

Points assigned for each lesion visualized at surgery

		Endometriosis	<1 cm	1–3 cm	>3 cm
Peritoneum		Superficial	1	2	4
		Deep	2	4	6
Ovary	R	Superficial	1	2	4
		Deep	4	16	20
	L	Superficial	1	2	4
		Deep	4	16	20
		Posterior cul-de-sac obliteration	Partial		Complete
			4		40
		Adhesions	<1/3 enclosure	1/3–2/3 enclosure	>2/3 enclosure
Ovary	R	Filmy	1	2	4
		Dense	4	8	16
	L	Filmy	1	2	4
		Dense	4	8	16
Tube	R	Filmy	1	2	4
		Dense	4	8	16
	L	Filmy	1	2	4
		Dense	4	8	16

Endometriosis

Endometriosis typically causes pain and infertility, although some patients with endometriosis are asymptomatic. It can be detrimental to all aspects of life – physical, mental, intimate, education/work and recreation – for the sufferer and those close to them. It is chronic and incurable in some.

- **Definition**: a disease characterized by the presence of endometrium-like epithelium and/or stroma outside the endometrium and myometrium, usually associated with an inflammatory process.

Endometriotic lesions are usually on the pelvic peritoneum or serosal surface of pelvic organs. Ovarian lesions may form endometriomas (blood-filled ovarian cysts). Deep deposits may affect underlying structures (ureters, blood vessels, nerves). Adhesions often form between endometriotic lesions and peritoneal or serosal surfaces, tethering the affected organs to surrounding structures (pelvic side wall, uterus, fallopian tube, bowel). These adhesions can be filmy or very dense, extensive or limited to the site of one lesion. Extraperitoneal deposits may also occur but less frequently, such as within the umbilicus, nose, lung or the site of a laparotomy scar. Endometriosis is considered a steroid-dependent disease.

- **Prevalence**: occurs in 2–10% of women of reproductive age, up to 50% of infertile women and 80% of women with chronic pelvic pain.
- **Age**: the reproductive years, including in adolescence: not found before menarche and characteristically regresses after the menopause, although some may continue to have symptoms. Typically diagnosed in women during their twenties.
- **Pathogenesis**: unknown but theories include (i) *retrograde menstruation* (viable endometrial cells reflux through the tubes during menstruation and implant in the pelvis); (ii) *coelomic metaplasia* (multipotential cells of the coelomic epithelium are stimulated to transform into endometrium-like cells); (iii) *haematogenous dissemination* (endometrial cells are transported to distant sites); (iv) *autoimmune disease* (a disorder of immune surveillance that allows ectopic endometrial implants to grow); and (v) *genetic predisposition* (having a first-degree relative with endometriosis is a risk factor but it may not be a monogenic condition). Exposure to increased menstrual bleeding seems to be a risk factor: earlier menarche, long or heavier periods, shorter cycles (so more periods in any given time), fewer pregnancies. Lean body mass, diet low in fruits, vegetables, dairy, vitamin D and omega-3 polyunsaturated fats or high in red meats, coffee and transfats seem to be associated.

Symptoms and signs

- The most common symptoms are *pelvic pain* and *infertility*, but many patients are asymptomatic.
- *Cyclic pain* is the hallmark of endometriosis, including dysmenorrhoea (begins before or with menstruation and is maximal at the time of maximal flow), deep dyspareunia (pain with intercourse), pain with defaecation (dyschezia), pain on urinating (dysuria), and sacral backache with menses. It can also be noncyclical. Cyclical extrapelvic pain can suggest atypical deposits.
- *Cyclical extrauterine bleeding* can indicate endometriosis, e.g. rectal bleeding, haematuria, haemoptysis/coughing, nose bleeds.
- The severity of symptoms does not necessarily correlate with the degree of pelvic disease. Indeed, many women with minimal endometriosis complain of severe pelvic pain.
- Infertility may result from pelvic anatomical distortion due to extensive endometriosis and adhesions, but also occurs with minimal disease (rASRM stage I and II) for unknown reasons.
- Common physical findings include a fixed, retroverted uterus, uterosacral ligaments nodularity and enlarged, tender adnexa.

Diagnosis

- History and physical examination may suggest the diagnosis. Cyclical bleeding/pain from an unusual site should suggest the possibility. Understanding the effect of symptoms on all life domains should be established and fertility plans/contraceptive needs noted.
- Pelvic transvaginal ultrasonography or MRI may be used to look for evidence of endometriomas or deep endometriotic nodules. Ultrasound imaging has the advantage of being more accessible than MRI, and also can demonstrate indirect signs of endometriosis such as reduced visceral mobility or peritoneal cysts, both due to adhesions. However, it is dependent on operator abilities and the acceptability of the transvaginal approach. Skilled ultrasound assessment or MRI are about as sensitive as laparoscopy in detecting endometriomas and deep pelvic endometriosis, but not superficial endometriosis. Lack of evidence of endometriosis on imaging does not exclude the diagnosis.
- Diagnostic laparoscopy is no longer the gold standard investigation, but can be considered if imaging is negative or empirical treatment (see below) is unsuccessful or inappropriate. If performed, biopsy of suspected lesions for histological analysis is recommended, although negative histology may not completely rule out the diagnosis. Early lesions on the peritoneal surface are small and vesicular. Later lesions have a typical 'powder-burn' appearance, which refers to a puckered, black area surrounded by a stellate scar.

Classification

The revised American Fertility Society classification system (rASRM – see figure) is based on surgical findings with points subjectively assigned to each lesion depending on its size and depth. The presence and extent of adhesions are also scored. Stage I, 1–5 points, minimal disease; II, 6–15, mild; III 16–40, moderate; IV > 40, severe. Score does not correlate with symptoms.

Management

There are medical and surgical options for treatment, both of which have an estimated recurrence rate of 20–50% within five years. Medical treatments are predominantly for pain and without benefit for fertility (natural or assisted). In addition, most are mutually exclusive with conception whilst using. Surgery is invasive and expensive, but the overall complication rate is low, evidence supports its effectiveness for pain and it can be offered to women who are trying to conceive. It improves the chance of natural pregnancy in rASRM stage I or II disease, and possibly for those with endometriomas. The fertility benefit of surgery for deep endometriosis is less clear. Non-medical interventions (acupuncture, traditional Chinese medicine, nutrition and electro-, physio- or psychological therapy) may have a role for pain management but there is insufficient evidence to recommend any particular one, and some are not appropriate for those trying to conceive due to potential safety concerns.

Decisions about treatment should be made with patients after discussion of risks, benefits and consequences of the options, taking into account previous treatments and fertility wishes.

Medical management

The primary goal of medical therapy is suppression of ovulation and induction of amenorrhoea. This effect reverses on discontinuation of treatment, and it does not reduce ovarian reserve (over that associated with time). Improvement in pain scores is similar with all types of hormone treatments, as are recurrence rates. Medical therapy does not eradicate the lesions. 'Empirical' medical therapy is recommended when signs and symptoms support the diagnosis but definitive surgical diagnosis has not been achieved. Patients who do not respond to empirical therapy generally warrant diagnostic laparoscopy.

- **Non-steroidal anti-inflammatory drugs (NSAIDs)** not only reduce pain but also reduce menstrual flow. They are commonly used together with other therapy.
- **Combined hormonal contraceptives (CHCs)** (delivered orally, by transdermal patch or vaginal ring) reduce menstrual flow, or eliminate it if used continuously by omitting the routine monthly seven-day break (or discarding the seven placebo pills if included in a packet). Some will experience breakthrough bleeding with extended use and breaks can be planned every 2–3 packets if needed to prevent this.
- **Progestogens** inhibit growth of the endometrium and endometriotic lesions, reducing or eliminating menstruation. Treatment can be oral, including with the progestogen-only contraceptive pill (POP), or parenteral, with either a long-releasing subdermal implant (etonogestrel) or intrauterine system (levonorgestrel).
- **Gonadotropin-releasing hormone (GnRH) agonists** induce a reversible hypo-oestrogenic 'medical menopause' by downregulation of pituitary GnRH receptors. Delivery is usually by subcutaneous or intramuscular depot injections. Although effective, they induce unpleasant menopausal symptoms, and beyond six months may lead to osteoporosis. To prevent such side-effects, concomitant combined hormone replacement should be considered (add-back therapy); this does not compromise the reduction in pain achieved. GnRH agonists should usually be second-line treatments, after CHCs or progestogens. They appear to be less effective than the levonorgestrel-releasing intrauterine system.
- Other treatments that lower oestrogen levels may have a role for treating pain due to endometriosis, when other treatments (medical and/or surgical) have failed. There is some limited evidence to support the use of oral **GnRH antagonists** (acting at the level of the pituitary) and **aromatase inhibitors** (block ovarian oestrogen production). Both cause side-effects due to low oestrogen, which may require add-back therapy. Danazol, a steroid with strong androgenic properties, is no longer considered a treatment for endometriosis because of its severe side-effects.

Surgical management

- The aim is to excise (rather than ablate) endometriotic lesions, including for endometriomas (cystectomy), as this reduces recurrence of lesions and pain. The usual approach should be laparoscopic.
- Care must be taken to limit damage to the ovaries in women desiring future fertility; this may limit the extent of surgery and therefore the improvement in pain achieved.
- Deep endometriosis should be treated in specialist centres, with the appropriate specialist surgery when bladder, ureters or bowel are involved. Risks of organ damage are increased for deep deposits, with an complication rate of 6.8% for deep rectovaginal disease.
- Hysterectomy with excision of all visible endometriosis, with or without bilateral salpingo-oophorectomy, can be considered for those who do not want future pregnancy, but usually if other treatments have failed. Surgery may be complex with associated risks of visceral damage, and may not be curative.

Other considerations

- **Fertility preservation** (storage of oocytes or embryos: both are IVF procedures) should be discussed when there is extensive ovarian endometriosis, including that the long-term benefit is unclear and that it may only be available if self-funded.
- **Asymptomatic endometriosis** should not be treated. There are no proven preventive treatments.
- **Endometriosis and cancer**: risks of ovarian, breast and thyroid cancers are slightly increased (1.2%, 0.5% and 0.5% above the general population respectively). Additional monitoring above that for the general population is not recommended.
- **Hormone replacement treatment (HRT) and endometriosis**: endometriosis sufferers with premature ovarian insufficiency (POI – loss of ovarian function under the age of 40 years, evidenced by raised FSH and amenorrhoea of at least four months' duration) or early menopause (between 40 and 45 years), whether spontaneous or from pelvic surgery, require HRT to prevent long-term sequelae (osteoporosis, increased cardiovascular disease and diabetes) and menopausal symptoms. HRT can also be used in normal (peri-)menopause for the control of symptoms of low oestrogen. Oestrogen-only HRT should be avoided as it increases the risk of malignant transformation in endometriotic lesions. HRT for those with a history of endometriosis should therefore contain both oestrogen and progestogen. Tibolone can be considered at or beyond the average age of menopause for the control of menopausal symptoms, but not for younger women, whose HRT should be more physiological.

Adenomyosis

- **Adenomyosis** is defined as endometrial glands and stroma within the myometrium and is a separate entity to endometriosis, although the two may co-exist, as may fibroids. It occurs to some degree in 20% of women and gives rise to dysmenorrhoea, menorrhagia, dyspareunia and a smoothly enlarged boggy uterus on pelvic examination. It may be associated with infertility.
- **Diagnosis** is suggested by pelvic ultrasonography and/or magnetic resonance imaging, but it is currently still a histopathological diagnosis. There are no agreed diagnostic criteria for either imaging modality, or that have been correlated histologically. Advances in ultrasound technology are identifying features suggestive of adenomyosis in more and younger women. These include an enlarged globular uterus, asymmetrical thickening of the myometrium, myometrial cysts and/or hyperechoic islands, and changes to the appearance of the junctional zone (the layer

next to the endometrium). These features may be found in some asymptomatic women but may be associated with infertility in others, although the relevance in these women is unclear.

- **Treatment** may be medical, with non-steroidal anti-inflammatories (NSAIDs), or hormonal, as for endometriosis. Endometrial ablation and hysterectomy can be considered for those with refractory pain who have no wish for future pregnancy, the latter being curative. Uterine artery embolization (UAE), with the aim of reducing the blood supply to the area of adenomyosis, can be used to treat pain with a good safety profile. Although considered a fertility-sparing treatment, the effect on pregnancy outcome is unclear and ovarian reserve may be reduced as a result of disturbance to the pelvic blood supply. High-intensity focused ultrasound (HIFU) has been used successfully to ablate areas of adenomyosis. HIFU appears to preserve fertility and be without detriment to ovarian reserve.

231 Polycystic ovary syndrome

- **Definition**: polycystic ovary syndrome (PCOS) is a syndrome of ovarian dysfunction along with the cardinal features of hyperandrogenism and PCO morphology.
- **Diagnostic criteria**: two of the following three features are required:
  - polycystic ovaries
  - oligo/anovulation (infrequent/absent ovulation) or oligo/amenorrhoea (infrequent/absent periods)
  - clinical *or* biochemical hyperandrogenism

after exclusion of other aetiologies including, but not exclusively, thyroid disease, hyperprolactinaemia and other causes of hypogonadotrophic hypogonadism, hypergonadotrophic hypogonadism (severely diminished ovarian reverse/premature ovarian insufficiency), non-classic congenital adrenal hyperplasia, Cushing disease and androgen-secreting tumours.

- **Prevalence**: PCOS occurs in 8–13% of women of reproductive age, making it the most common hormonal disorder in women of this age. It has metabolic, reproductive and psychological consequences. Clinical presentation varies, often leading to delayed or missed diagnosis. It is the most common cause of irregular periods and of conception delay due to anovulation. It occurs in all ethnicities, and certain features are more pronounced in some.
- **Aetiology**: it is due to the inheritance of a combination of genes, which explains its variable phenotypes, although the genes responsible have not yet been identified.

Diagnosis

PCOS is a clinical diagnosis and investigations are there to exclude other causes of the symptoms. Around one-fifth of normal women will have polycystic ovarian morphology without any symptoms of the syndrome: these women do not have PCOS.

Four phenotypes of PCOS are recognized.

- Androgen excess + ovulatory dysfunction + polycystic ovarian morphology
- Androgen excess + ovulatory dysfunction
- Androgen excess + polycystic ovarian morphology (regular cycles/ovulation)
- Ovulatory dysfunction + polycystic ovarian morphology (without androgen excess)

Taking a detailed history is therefore important.

History

- **Menstrual history**: frequency and duration of menstrual bleeding, noting any changes to pattern and associated circumstances – weight changes, exercise, stress, medication. Anovulation can be associated with amenorrhoea, or very light or very heavy bleeding, or both, either of which can be of variable duration from days to weeks. Irregular periods are normal within the first year of menarche and most girls will have regular cycles which are ovulatory occurring between 21 and 35 days (or more than eight cycles a year) by the third year after menarche.
- **Androgenic symptoms**: often a source of distress, so sensitive enquiry is needed – symptoms may not be volunteered if they are not the given reason for presentation/referral. Time course of the appearance of androgenic symptoms is important and associated circumstances should be noted as for menstrual history. A short history may indicate an androgen-secreting tumour. Virilization and masculinization (severe androgenic symptoms including clitoromegaly and voice changes) are rarely seen in PCOS and should alert to other causes.
  - *Hirsutism* (unwanted growth of terminal hairs in a male pattern): these are longer (>5 mm if untreated), coarser and darker than vellus (normal body) hairs – upper lip, chin, neck, midline chest, around nipples, midline abdomen (typically below umbilicus, but may be above when more severe and extend laterally), sacrum, buttocks, thighs (extending laterally from pubic hair), arms. Document if hairs are removed, from where and method (waxing, threading, plucking, electrolysis, laser or bleaching) and frequency/time spent. This helps to direct treatment recommendations as well as measure response.
  - *Acne*: facial, chest, back.
  - *Scalp hair thinning* (alopecia): there are many other, non-androgenic causes and most women with alopecia do not have raised androgens.

Hirsutism rarely occurs without additional features of PCOS, whereas acne or alopecia alone may be less predictive of PCOS.

- **Fertility plans/contraceptive needs**: these will influence treatment choices.
- **Family history**: diabetes, high cholesterol, cardiovascular disease.

Examination

Blood pressure, height, weight and waist circumference should be recorded and BMI calculated.

Signs of hyperandrogenism should be recorded. Hirsutism can be documented using the modified Ferriman Gallwey score, although this is of limited usefulness when it has been treated, which is why a careful history is important. It is not necessary to request the patient to refrain from self-treatment. Acne should be documented (there is no agreed visual scoring) and hair loss can be recorded using the Ludwig visual score. It is not necessary to look for clitoromegaly unless masculinization is suspected.

Acanthosis nigricans should be looked for at the back of the neck and in the axillae.

Laboratory tests

- **Testosterone**: result within local laboratory normal ranges for total or free testosterone is sufficient to exclude other causes of biochemical hyperandrogenism, even though the routinely

Medicine at a Glance, Fifth Edition. Edited by Patrick Davey and Alex Pitcher.

Companion website: www.wiley.com/go/medicine5e

available assays are imprecise (radiometric or enzyme-linked). It should preferably be measured in the early follicular phase if menstrual cycles are regular (levels can rise around ovulation) and in the morning, due to diurnal variation. If the result is normal, more detailed analysis of androgens is not required for diagnosis of PCOS provided there are clinical signs of hyperandrogenism (especially hirsutism). If the result is normal, in the absence of hirsutism (the most reliable clinical sign of hyperandrogenism), free androgen index (100 × (total testosterone/sex hormone binding globulin) [SHBG]), calculated free testosterone or calculated bioavailable testosterone can be used to identify biochemical hyperandrogenism. Measuring other androgens (androstenedione, DHEAS) adds little to diagnostic accuracy for PCOS.

- **FSH and LH** to exclude hyper- or hypogonadotropic hypogonadism: these should be taken during the early follicular phase (days 2–5) in women with regular menstrual cycles, or randomly if cycles are irregular and longer than about 35 days. FSH should be within normal limits, although LH may be normal or raised. The concentration of LH may be raised relative to that of FSH, but this is not a diagnostic criterion as it is not sensitive enough. Slim women with PCOS tend to have higher LH:FSH ratios than those with obesity.
- **Prolactin**: to exclude hyperprolactinaemia (mildly raised levels under 1000 mIU/l are commonly seen in PCOS).
- **TSH/free T4**: to exclude thyroid disease.
- **17-Hydroxyprogesterone**: to exclude non-classical congenital adrenal hyperplasia.
- **Cholesterol** should be checked at baseline and thereafter according to other cardiovascular risk factors, e.g. cigarette smoking, obesity, family history.
- **HbA1c or an oral glucose tolerance test** (OGTT) should be performed at diagnosis and thereafter every 1–3 years depending on level of risk of diabetes, including weight/waist circumference/BMI, family history and ethnicity. Serum insulin, with or without glucose measurement, does not identify insulin resistance and should not be performed.

Pelvic ultrasound scan

Ideally transvaginal in order to accurately count the number of antral (growing) follicles in, and to measure the volume of, each ovary. If transvaginal is inappropriate or unacceptable, then transabdominal through a full bladder is the alternative, although antral follicles cannot be counted accurately. Ovarian ultrasound appearance should not be considered as part of the diagnosis for those who are less than eight years on from menarche (which is when gynaecological maturity is reached) as it is common for there to be a large number of ovarian follicles in this group. Polycystic ovaries are large and have a volume of 10 ml or more (assuming no dominant follicles, i.e. over 10 mm, corpora lutea or cysts).

The number of antral follicles required for diagnosis is more contentious: the 2003 PCOS guidelines gave a threshold of 12 or more follicles 9 mm or less in diameter in either ovary. This was questioned in the 2018 guidelines, as improved ultrasound technology has increased the detection of smaller antral follicles and the original threshold was based on only one paper. The threshold of 20 or more antral follicles (any diameter) was proposed by the 2018 guideline, acknowledging that this does not consider the impact of the ultrasonographer's skills, access to appropriately high-resolution equipment and antral follicles counts (AFC) declining with age. Those with AFC below 20 per ovary should not be discounted as having PCOS if the rest of their clinical picture is suggestive, especially if older.

Clinical consequences

Metabolic

Independent of BMI, PCOS is associated with insulin resistance (IR) due to a postreceptor defect, plus elevated insulin production by the islet cells of the pancreas. Other risk factors for insulin resistance – obesity, family history and ethnicity – compound that due to PCOS. In addition, annual weight gain in women with PCOS is increased, which predisposes to the risk of obesity. The mechanisms behind this weight gain are complex but include reduced postprandial heat loss (whereby fewer calories from a meal are burnt off as heat) and the energy-conserving actions of insulin. Another consequence of IR is the reduced hepatic production of SHBG – this results in a rise in unbound and thereby biologically active androgens. The risk of impaired glucose tolerance (IGT), gestational diabetes (GDM) and type 2 diabetes is three times higher in Europeans with PCOS, four times higher in those from the Americas and five times higher in Asians.

Women with PCOS are more likely to have raised lipid profiles and hypertension and obstructive sleep apnoea may be more common.

Whilst it is clear that women with PCOS have increased risk factors for cardiovascular disease (CVD), it is not clear if PCOS is an independent risk factor, or whether women with PCOS experience more CVD or have higher CVD morbidity. Published studies have not demonstrated that they do but that probably represents absence of data rather than absence of effect as there have been insufficient longitudinal studies including older women.

Reproductive

There are two stages in ovarian follicle development, both of which are abnormal in PCOS and contribute to irregular ovulation (and thereby irregular menstrual cycles) and reduced fertility. The first stage is known as preantral, during which follicles leave their resting state, when they are called primordial follicles, and enlarge, predominantly due to an increase in the number of cells in the granulosa cell layer. More preantral follicles are at the growing stage in PCO. The factors initiating primordial follicle growth are unknown, but it occurs independent of the hormones of the menstrual cycle (the gonadotrophins FSH and LH).

The second stage of follicle growth occurs once they have developed a fluid-filled cavity (an antrum). They are then called antral follicles and are visible on ultrasound scan. From this stage, their growth becomes dependent on the gonadotrophins. FSH causes antral follicles to enlarge and produce oestradiol from their granulosa cells and testosterone (a substrate for oestradiol) from their theca cells. LH is not normally released in significant quantities until there is a dominant follicle large enough to ovulate in response to a surge in LH level. When background LH levels are raised, as they are in PCOS, small antral follicles are exposed to LH and arrest their development in response. This leaves more antral follicles present than normal (visible as an increased antral follicle count with ultrasound) but few if any attain the size required for ovulation. Insulin has gonadotrophic actions on ovarian follicles and acts synergistically with LH, contributing to follicle arrest but also driving testosterone production.

The increased number of growing follicles of all stages results in normal or slightly raised oestradiol and testosterone, even though the peaks around ovulation are absent. Lack of ovulation means that the corpus luteum is not formed and the consequent peak of progesterone does not occur. This exposes the endometrium to oestrogen without the protective effect of progesterone and the risk of endometrial cancer in PCOS is increased up to six-fold because of this plus the additive effects of other risk factors – type 2 diabetes, obesity, nulliparity.

Psychological

A number of conditions are increased in women with PCOS: depression, anxiety, negative body image, sexual dysfunction, disordered eating and eating disorders. It is not clear how much these are the result of the clinical manifestations of PCOS or whether PCOS itself is an independent risk factor.

Management

The treatment of PCOS is symptomatic and likely to vary with life course. Weight management, whether reduction of weight or waist circumference, or maintenance of these within healthy parameters, is the most important holistic treatment and the one that will make all other interventions for any symptom more likely to succeed. There are no specific dietary interventions proven to be more successful in PCOS than others, including low-carbohydrate or low-glycaemic index diets, despite popular belief. Weight management requires calorie restriction plus increased activity.

Hyperandrogenism

Hair removal is an important component of treating hirsutism. Electrolysis and laser are the most effective methods, the former being more suitable for small areas (e.g. face). Both are expensive, involving repeated treatments, and most women will need to continue with top-up sessions to maintain the effect. Medical treatment should be seen as an adjunct to hair removal, as both are usually required for maximum effect. Medical interventions reduce androgenic drive and since the life cycle of a hair follicle is four months, significant results may not be seen for 6–12 months. Patient expectations must be managed accordingly and are often best judged by time spent on hair maintenance or frequency of removal, the aim of treatment being to minimize these.

Dermatological treatments for acne should be considered (topical, systemic) but antiandrogen therapies may be an adjunct and in some may replace the need for them. The use of Roaccutane® may be avoided or the recurrence of acne after a course reduced by introducing antiandrogen treatment.

Alopecia and scalp hair thinning are the most difficult to treat, and causes other than hyperandrogenism must be considered. Daily topical treatment with minoxidil solution can help promote new hair growth, but only does so whilst being used. Antiandrogen treatments may stabilize hair loss, but rarely promote new growth.

First-line treatment for hyperandrogenism is combined hormonal contraception (CHC). This acts to reduce ovarian production of sex steroids, including androgens. In addition, CHC increases hepatic production of SHBG, reducing biologically available androgens. There are some oral CHCs that contain a progestogen that will also act as a competitive inhibitor of the androgen receptor (e.g. drospirenone or cyproterone acetate – CPA). There have been no trials to demonstrate that these pills are more effective in treating symptoms of hyperandronism than other CHCs, but they are associated with an increased risk of venous thromboembolism. CHCs containing progestogens known to stimulate the androgen receptor (e.g. norethisterone and its derivatives) are best avoided on an empirical basis.

If CHCs are contraindicated or unacceptable to the patient, then an antiandrogen can be used. Reliable contraception must be used during antiandrogen treatment, as it can affect the development of the external genitalia of a male fetus.

Spironolactone (from which drospirenone is derived, see above) can be given orally in daily doses of 100–200 mg, or cyclical CPA given as 25 mg (half a tablet) daily for 10 days every calendar month (or for the first 10 days of a packet of pills if used with oral contraception). Spironolactone is generally well tolerated but it is a diuretic, so should be taken in the morning, and renal function should be monitored (especially serum potassium). It can cause irregular vaginal bleeding, especially in doses above 150 mg daily. The progestogenic actions of CPA are often sufficient to induce a fairly regular withdrawal bleed in those with irregular periods when taken cyclically. Prolonged or high-dose use is associated with an increased risk of a rare type of meningioma, the total dose of exposure being the risk factor.

Flutamide is another oral antiandrogen, but hepatoxicity limits its usefulness. Finasteride inhibits the peripheral conversion of biologically inactive testosterone into active dihydrotestosterone. The roles for flutamide and finasteride are limited and they should only be prescribed when other treatments have failed, and under the care of a clinician with experience in management options for hyperandrogenism.

Menstrual disturbance

Anovulation results in menstrual disturbance which can be inconvenient, distressing, a cause of anaemia and associated with increased risk of endometrial cancer. First-line treatment is CHC, but when this is unacceptable or contraindicated, cyclical progestogens can be used, e.g. medroxyprogesterone acetate 10 mg once a day for 10 days repeated every one or two calendar months. Other options include progesterone-only contraception, e.g. tablets, subdermal implants, depot injections or intrauterine systems. No trials have been performed to demonstrate the effectiveness of any preparation in providing protection against endometrial cancer in anovulatory women with PCOS.

Fertility

Anovulation due to PCOS can be treated with courses of ovulation induction (OI), a restorative treatment with the aim of allowing natural conception once ovulation has been achieved. Ovulation and pregnancy rates in response to all forms of OI are higher when the BMI is within the normal range for ethnicity. Antral follicle development can be stimulated with FSH. The negative feedback mechanism between oestradiol and the release of FSH from the pituitary can be manipulated by drugs that transiently lower pituitary exposure to oestradiol. Clomifene citrate (and its isomer tamoxifen) is a competitive antagonist of the oestrogen receptor. Letrozole is an aromatase inhibitor and blocks the production of oestradiol. Either drug when given orally in low dose for five days can raise endogenous FSH via negative feedback, resulting in the growth of a dominant follicle and ovulation.

Response to treatment must be monitored with ultrasound, as the main risk is to cause the development of more than one follicle, resulting in a multiple pregnancy. If pregnancy does not occur, there will be a menstrual period and the treatment can be repeated, usually for up to six cycles. Oral OI should be first-line treatment. Clomifene and letrozole have similar cumulative conception rates, which are close to those in naturally ovulating women. Only clomifene is licensed for ovulation induction in most countries. Letrozole may have the advantage over clomifene of being more likely to cause the growth of only one dominant follicle (and so have a lower risk of twins). In addition, more women may respond to it compared to clomifene.

When there is no response to letrozole or clomifene, daily injections of FSH can be given to induce follicle development (called gonadotrophin ovulation induction – GOI). This is also an option for women who have not conceived despite ovulating with an oral anti-oestrogen (about half of this group will conceive with a course of GOI). This is a more expensive treatment than oral OI due to the drug costs but also because more ultrasound scans are required.

Laparoscopic ovarian diathermy (LOD) is a surgical treatment for anovulation due to PCOS. It involves burning tiny holes into each ovary, usually with diathermy. The main effect of this is thought to be by raising endogenous FSH via the negative feedback pathway as a consequence of destroying ovarian follicles. Treatment may result in regular ovulation or may render the patient responsive to oral OI, if previously resistant. LOD has the advantage of being able to inspect the pelvis at the time of treatment (particularly useful if there is a concern about a possible pelvic cause for conception delay in addition to anovulation). However, it also has the surgical risks of the laparoscopy and of inducing premature ovarian insufficiency if too much ovarian tissue is destroyed during the procedure, although this risk is minimal in experienced hands and when the diagnosis of PCOS is secure. Its effect on inducing ovulation with consequent pregnancy wanes after 18–24 months. There is rarely justification in repeating the procedure because of the risk of excessive ovarian damage.

IVF is an option but is recommended as second or third line after OI.

Metformin

Metformin reduces insulin resistance and can be considered as a treatment for anovulation, although ovulation rates and conception rates per ovulation are lower than with anti-oestrogens or gonadotrophin injections. The advantage is that there is no increased risk of multiple pregnancy and so no monitoring ultrasound scans are needed and it is inexpensive. It may also have a place in weight management alongside lifestyle changes. It is not clear if it has a role in reducing risk of diabetes, above that identified in the non-PCOS population with high-risk features.

Hypertensive disorders of pregnancy

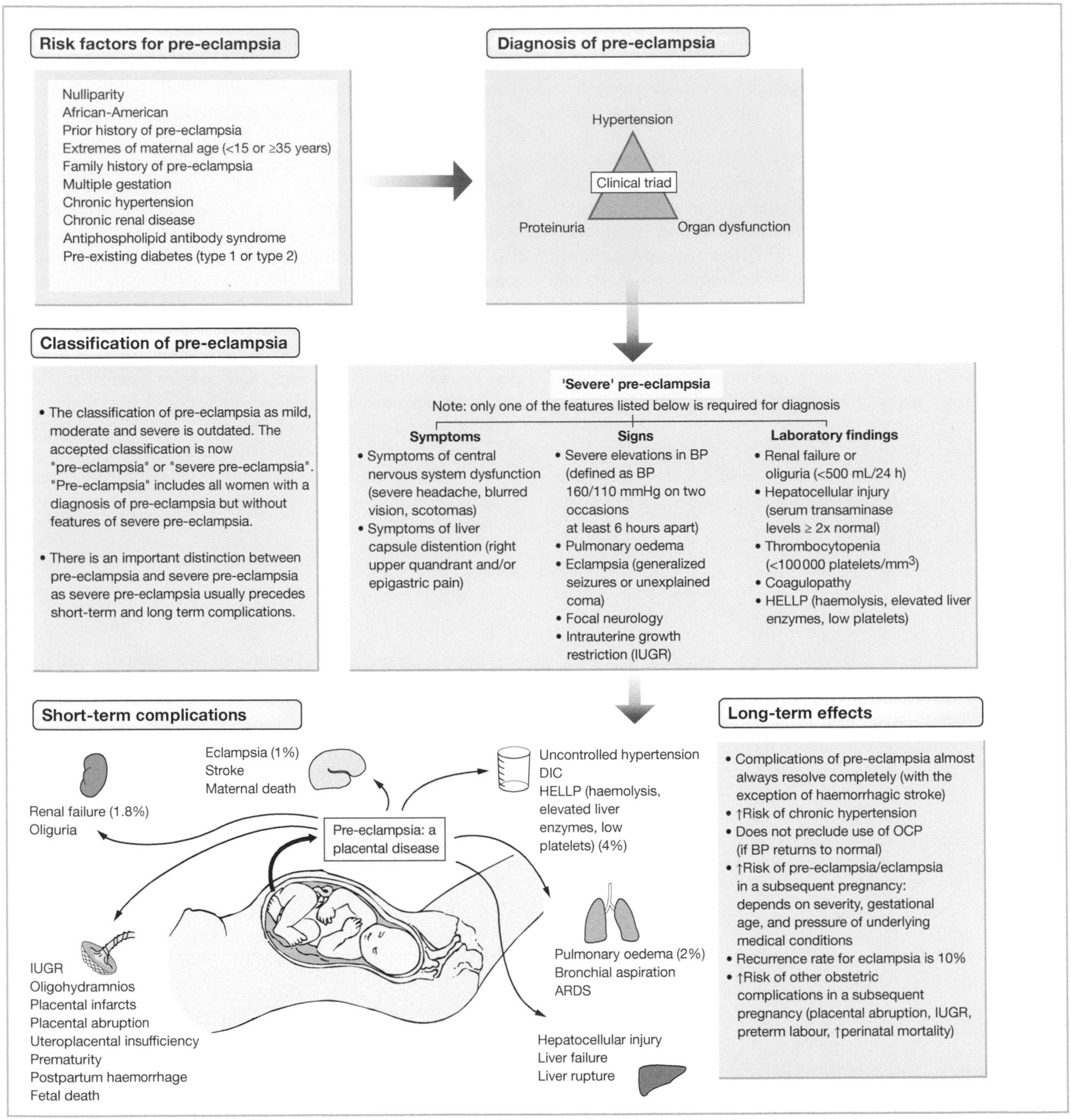

Risk factors for pre-eclampsia

Nulliparity
African-American
Prior history of pre-eclampsia
Extremes of maternal age (<15 or ≥35 years)
Family history of pre-eclampsia
Multiple gestation
Chronic hypertension
Chronic renal disease
Antiphospholipid antibody syndrome
Pre-existing diabetes (type 1 or type 2)

Diagnosis of pre-eclampsia

Clinical triad: Hypertension, Proteinuria, Organ dysfunction

Classification of pre-eclampsia

- The classification of pre-eclampsia as mild, moderate and severe is outdated. The accepted classification is now "pre-eclampsia" or "severe pre-eclampsia". "Pre-eclampsia" includes all women with a diagnosis of pre-eclampsia but without features of severe pre-eclampsia.
- There is an important distinction between pre-eclampsia and severe pre-eclampsia as severe pre-eclampsia usually precedes short-term and long term complications.

'Severe' pre-eclampsia

Note: only one of the features listed below is required for diagnosis

Symptoms

- Symptoms of central nervous system dysfunction (severe headache, blurred vision, scotomas)
- Symptoms of liver capsule distention (right upper quandrant and/or epigastric pain)

Signs

- Severe elevations in BP (defined as BP 160/110 mmHg on two occasions at least 6 hours apart)
- Pulmonary oedema
- Eclampsia (generalized seizures or unexplained coma)
- Focal neurology
- Intrauterine growth restriction (IUGR)

Laboratory findings

- Renal failure or oliguria (<500 mL/24 h)
- Hepatocellular injury (serum transaminase levels ≥ 2x normal)
- Thrombocytopenia (<100 000 platelets/mm^3)
- Coagulopathy
- HELLP (haemolysis, elevated liver enzymes, low platelets)

Short-term complications

Pre-eclampsia: a placental disease

Eclampsia (1%)
Stroke
Maternal death

Renal failure (1.8%)
Oliguria

Uncontrolled hypertension
DIC
HELLP (haemolysis, elevated liver enzymes, low platelets) (4%)

IUGR
Oligohydramnios
Placental infarcts
Placental abruption
Uteroplacental insufficiency
Prematurity
Postpartum haemorrhage
Fetal death

Pulmonary oedema (2%)
Bronchial aspiration
ARDS

Hepatocellular injury
Liver failure
Liver rupture

Long-term effects

- Complications of pre-eclampsia almost always resolve completely (with the exception of haemorrhagic stroke)
- ↑Risk of chronic hypertension
- Does not preclude use of OCP (if BP returns to normal)
- ↑Risk of pre-eclampsia/eclampsia in a subsequent pregnancy: depends on severity, gestational age, and pressure of underlying medical conditions
- Recurrence rate for eclampsia is 10%
- ↑Risk of other obstetric complications in a subsequent pregnancy (placental abruption, IUGR, preterm labour, ↑perinatal mortality)

Hypertensive disorders of pregnancy are a leading cause of maternal death globally, accounting for 14% of all direct maternal deaths.

Effects of pregnancy on maternal cardiovascular system

- Blood volume increases 800 ml by 12 weeks (1.5 l in twins).
- Blood pressure (BP) decreases in early pregnancy (due primarily to a decrease in systemic vascular resistance secondary to progesterone) and returns to baseline by term.

Classification

Chronic hypertension

- **Definition**: hypertension before pregnancy. The diagnosis should also be considered in women with BP ≥140/90 mmHg before 20 weeks' gestation.
- **Complications**: such pregnancies are at increased risk of superimposed pre-eclampsia, intrauterine fetal growth restriction (IUGR), placental abruption and stillbirth.
- **Management**: continue antihypertensive medications, except for angiotensin-converting enzyme (ACE) inhibitors as these are

associated with progressive and irreversible renal injury and possibly other structural anomalies in the fetus. Alternative antihypertensives include labetalol or modified-release nifedipine. Diuretic therapy is discouraged. Start 75–150 mg aspirin daily from 12 weeks of gestation.

- **Fetal monitoring:** serial ultrasound examinations for fetal growth, liquor and Dopplers should be initiated from 28 weeks' gestation. Delivery should be by 40 weeks.

Gestational hypertension

- **Diagnosis**: persistent elevation of BP ≥140/90 mmHg after 20 weeks of gestation without evidence of pre-eclampsia. It is a diagnosis of exclusion.
- **Aetiology**: it probably represents an exaggerated physiological response of the maternal cardiovascular system to pregnancy.
- Rarely associated with adverse maternal or fetal outcome.
- **Management**: First-line antihypertensives are labetalol or modified-release nifedipine. Target BP ≤135/85 mmHg.
- **Fetal monitoring**: ultrasound for growth, liquor and Dopplers at diagnosis, then serial growth scans as indicated.

Pre-eclampsia

- Also known as gestational proteinuric hypertension or pre-eclamptic toxaemia (PET).
- **Definition**: a multisystem disorder specific to pregnancy and the puerperium. More precisely, it is a disease of the placenta because it occurs in pregnancies where there is trophoblast but no fetal tissue (complete molar pregnancies).
- **Incidence**: occurs in 6–8% of all pregnancies.
- **Risk factors**: see figure.
- **Diagnosis**: the clinical diagnosis has two elements. *Hypertension*: defined as a sustained sitting BP ≥140/90 mmHg, and either:
    - *new-onset significant proteinuria*: defined as >300 mg/24 h or >30 mg/mmol urine PCR in the absence of urinary tract infection. Evidence of gestational proteinuric hypertension before 20 weeks should raise the possibility of an underlying molar pregnancy, drug withdrawal or (rarely) chromosomal abnormality in the fetus

or

- - *new-onset maternal organ dysfunction:* e.g. renal impairment, liver dysfunction, neurological complications, haematological complications or evidence of uteroplacental dysfunction (i.e. IUGR, abnormal Dopplers or stillbirth).
- **Placental growth factor (PlGF)** is involved in placental angiogenesis and can be measured in maternal blood. It aids in diagnosis or exclusion of pre-eclampsia (PET), and has some value in predicting whether PET will develop. In women with clinical suspicion of PET >20 weeks of gestation, the ratio of soluble FMS-like tyrosine kinase-1 (sFlt-1) to PlGF can be used, up to delivery. Between 20 and 34 weeks of gestation, an sFlt-1/PlGF ratio of under 33 excludes pre-eclampsia and a ratio of 85 or above is diagnostic. PlGF alone is also used in some centres.
- **Classification** (see figure): severe pre-eclampsia is classified as pre-eclampsia with severe hypertension (>160/110 mmHg), not responding to medication or involving other maternal organ systems. This can be life-threatening and close monitoring and magnesium sulfate may be required.
- **Aetiology**: the cause of pre-eclampsia is not known. Theories include an abnormal maternal immunological response to the fetal allograft, an underlying genetic abnormality, an imbalance in the prostanoid cascade, and the presence of circulating toxins and/or endogenous vasoconstrictors. The blueprint for the development of pre-eclampsia is laid down early in pregnancy. The primary event is a failure of the second wave of trophoblast invasion from 8 to 18 weeks, which is responsible for remodelling of the spiral arterioles in the myometrium adjacent to the developing placenta, and establishment of the definitive uteroplacental circulation. As pregnancy progresses and the metabolic demand of the fetoplacental unit increases, the spiral arterioles are now unable to accommodate the necessary increase in blood flow. This then leads to 'placental dysfunction', manifest clinically as pre-eclampsia. Although attractive, this hypothesis remains to be validated. Whatever the placental abnormality, the end result is widespread vasospasm and endothelial injury.
- **Complications**: eclampsia – defined as one or more generalized convulsions or coma in the setting of pre-eclampsia and in the absence of other neurological conditions – was thought to be the end stage of pre-eclampsia, hence the nomenclature. It is now clear, however, that seizures are but one clinical manifestation of 'severe' pre-eclampsia; 50% of eclampsia occurs preterm. Of those at term, 75% occur either intrapartum or within 48 hours of delivery.
- **Management**: delivery is the only effective treatment for pre-eclampsia, and is recommended:
    - in stable women with pre-eclampsia once a favourable gestational age has been reached (>37 weeks)
    - in all women with 'severe' pre-eclampsia regardless of gestational age, once stabilised (with the exception of 'severe' pre-eclampsia due to proteinuria alone or IUGR remote from term). Decision for delivery should be individualized and involve a senior obstetrician.
- There is no proven benefit to routine delivery by caesarean section. However, the probability of vaginal delivery in a patient with pre-eclampsia remote from term with an unfavourable cervix is only 15–20%.
- BP control is important to prevent haemorrhagic stroke (usually associated with BP ≥170/120 mmHg), but does not affect the natural course of pre-eclampsia.
- Intravenous magnesium sulfate should be given intrapartum and for at least 24 hours postpartum, in severe cases, to prevent eclampsia.
- **Prevention**: aspirin 75–150 mg once daily is recommended in all suitable women with one 'high-risk' factor or two 'moderate-risk' factors from 12 weeks of gestation.
- **Prognosis**: pre-eclampsia and its complications resolve after delivery (with the exception of haemorrhagic stroke). Fetal prognosis is dependent largely on gestational age at delivery and problems related to prematurity.

233 Cardiovascular disease in pregnancy

Management of specific cardiac lesions in pregnancy

Septal defects
- If lesions are small, patients are usually asymptomatic and require no specific treatment
- Large ventricular septal defects (VSD) are associated with aortic insufficiency, congestive cardiac failure, arrhythmias, pulmonary hypertension
- Air filters on all IV lines to prevent paradoxical air embolism

Right-to-left shunts
- Due to pulmonary hypertension with shunting of blood away from lungs
- In pregnancy, decreased systemic vascular resistance worsens shunt with increased hypoxia
- Management: avoid hypotension, maintain preload, oxygen, air filters on IV lines

Mitral/aortic valve stenosis
- Such lesions are particularly dangerous in pregnancy because of the fixed cardiac output and left atrial dilatation (which can result in arrhythmias and/or thrombus formation)
- Management: maintain preload, avoid tachycardia. Consider β-blockers for persistent heart rate ≥ 90–100 bpm. Adequate pain relief in labour to minimize tachycardia
- Autotransfusion immediately postpartum can precipitate pulmonary oedema

Mitral valve prolapse
- Patients are generally asymptomatic
- Treat symptomatic prolapse with β-blocker

RA
LA
RV
LV

Prosthetic valves
- Risks include embolization, valvular dysfunction, and infection (bacterial endocarditis)
- Management: therapeutic anticoagulation for any mechanical valve

Prophylaxis against bacterial endocarditis
- Vaginal delivery is associated with 2–3% risk of bacteraemia
- American Heart Association recommends endocarditis prophylaxis only for: (i) prosthetic heart valve/patch, (ii) prior infectious endocarditis, (iii) heart transplant, or (iv) unrepaired/partially repaired congenital heart disease

Cardiomyopathy
- Presents with left ventricular dysfunction and global dilatation
- Increased cardiac output in pregnancy may lead to decompensation
- Management: avoid hypotension, careful volume replacement, inotropic support to maximize cardiac output if needed

Aortic pathology
- Genetic aortopathies are high-risk pregnancies, e.g. Marfan syndrome, due to the risk of dissection
- Mortality is high in women with Marfan and aortic dilation >45 mm
- Family history, diameter of aorta and previous surgery predict risk of dissection

Diagnosis of deep vein thrombosis

Pregnancy predisposes to thromboembolism

Venous stasis — Virchow's triad — Vessel wall damage

Hypercoagulable state

Normal pregnancy contributes to venous stasis and a hypercoagulable state; the development of pre-eclampsia contributes to vessel wall damage

Clinical features of deep vein thrombosis

History:	Unilateral swelling and/or pain in the calf or thigh
Examination:	Unilateral leg swelling, erythema, pitting oedema and/or tenderness

Diagnosis
- Compression duplex ultrasound is the gold standard diagnostic test. If inconclusive and high clinical suspicion, this should be repeated

Diagnosis of pulmonary embolism

Clinical features

History:	Tachycardia, shortness of breath, tachypnoea, pleuritic chest pain, cough, and/or haemoptysis
Examination:	There may be tachypnoea, increased work of breathing and/or exertional desaturation, although this is a late sign
Labs:	ECG may show T wave inversion, sinus tachycardia, RBB or S1,Q3,T3. Chest X-ray (CXR) should be performed and is usually normal. Do not perform D-dimer. A normal ABG does not exclude PE

Ventilation/perfusion (V/Q) scan: Can be performed if CXR is normal.
If inconclusive, further imaging and anticoagulation are required
100% negative predictive value
Computed tomography pulmonary angiogram (CTPA): preferred if CXR is abnormal. Negative predictive value 99%
Choice of V/Q vs CTPA should be discussed with women

Maternal heart disease in pregnancy

Incidence

- Occurs in 1% of pregnancies.
- Remains the leading cause of maternal death in the UK.

Aetiology

- Congenital lesions account for >50% of heart disease in pregnancy.
- Other common causes include coronary artery disease, hypertension and thyroid dyfunction. Rare causes include myocarditis, cor pulmonale, cardiomyopathy, constrictive pericarditis and cardiac dysrhythmias. Historically, rheumatic fever accounted for 90% of heart disease in pregnancy, but is now rare.

Prognosis

Prognosis depends on four factors.

1 *Cardiac function*: a clinical classification was developed by the New York Heart Association (NYHA) in 1928 (see Table 87.1).
2 *Clinical conditions* that may further increase cardiac output (multiple pregnancy, anaemia, thyroid disease).

3 *Medications.*
4 The specific nature and severity of the *cardiac lesion* (see Table 233.1).

Management

- Should be individualized. Spontaneous labour at term is suitable for some women. Scheduled induction is indicated for women requiring invasive cardiac monitoring.
- Adequate pain relief (regional analgesia is preferred).
- Left lateral positioning.
- Maternal pulse oximetry and ECG monitoring.
- Fluid intake and output monitoring during labour and consider fluid restriction.
- Consider invasive haemodynamic monitoring for women with NYHA class III and IV disease.
- Uterotonics should be used with caution due to their effects on the cardiovascular system. Ergometrine causes vasoconstriction so should be avoided in most cases.

Table 233.1 Modified WHO classification of maternal cardiovascular risk.

WHO Class I risk (no detectable increased risk of maternal mortality)	• Small, mild or uncomplicated pulmonary stenosis, patent ductus arteriosis or mitral valve prolapse • Successfully repaired simple lesions • Isolated atrial/ventricular ectopic beats
WHO Class II risk (small increased risk of maternal mortality)	• Unrepaired atrial septal defect (ASD)/ ventricular septal defect (VSD) • Repaired tetralogy of Fallot • Most arrhythmias
WHO Class III (significantly increased risk of maternal mortality)	• Mechanical valves • Fontan circulation • Unrepaired cyanotic heart disease • Complex congenital heart disease • Marfan syndrome with aortic dilation 40–45 mm • Aortic dilation 45–50 mm with bicuspid aortic valve
WHO Class IV (high risk of maternal mortality – pregnancy contraindicated and termination should be discussed)	• Pulmonary arterial hypertension • Severe systemic ventricular dysfunction • Severe mitral or symptomatic aortic stenosis • Marfan syndrome with aortic dilatation >45 mm or bicuspid aorta with aortic dilation >50 mm • Severe coarctation

Thromboembolic disease in pregnancy

Incidence

- The leading direct obstetric cause of maternal mortality in the UK.
- Deep venous thrombosis (DVT) complicates 0.05–0.3% of all pregnancies. It is 3–5-fold more common in the puerperium, and 3–15-fold more common after caesarean section delivery. If untreated, 15–25% of patients with DVT will have a pulmonary embolus (PE) compared with 4–5% of treated patients.

Aetiology

Pregnancy is a thrombogenic state. Thromboembolic events are five-fold more common in pregnancy than in non-pregnant women. For other predisposing factors see Table 233.2.

Treatment

- **Low molecular weight heparin** (LMWH) is the treatment of choice for acute thromboembolism in pregnant women. Doses are calculated by weight and routine monitoring of anti-Xa levels is advised in women with a low or high BMI, renal impairment or previous events whilst anticoagulated. As a result of its long half-life and resistance to reversal by protamine sulfate, women are advised to omit their LMWH at the onset of labour, or 24 hours prior to planned induction.
- **Unfractionated heparin** is the initial treatment of choice in massive PE where there is cardiovascular compromise. It is given intravenously, aiming for a partial thromboplastin time (PTT) at 1.5–2.0 times normal. Heparin does not cross the placenta and, as such, is not teratogenic. Adverse effects include haemorrhage (5–10%), thrombocytopenia (2%) and osteoporosis (dose related). In the setting of acute haemorrhage, protamine sulfate can be given to reverse heparin action.
- Treatment should be continued for the duration of pregnancy and for 6 weeks postpartum, or for a total treatment duration of 3-6 months, whichever is longer.
- Alternative therapies (fibrinolytic agents, surgical intervention) are best avoided but considered in specific cases.

Table 233.2 Risk factors for VTE in pregnancy.

Pre-existing risk factors	Previous VTE, thrombophilia, medical co-morbidities (e.g heart failure, IBD, cancer, sickle cell, intravenous drug use, etc.), age >35 years, BMI >30 kg/m^2, parity ≥3, smoking, significant varicose veins, paraplegia
Obstetric risk factors	Multiple pregnancy, pre-eclampsia, caesarean section, prolonged labour (>24 hours), rotational or midcavity assisted birth, stillbirth, preterm birth, postpartum haemorrhage >1 litre, IVF
Transient/new risk factors	Surgical procedures, bone fracture, hyperemesis, dehydration, OHSS, immobility, hospital admission, systemic infection, long-distance travel

Prophylaxis

- Women with prior unexplained DVT have a 5–10% incidence of recurrence in a subsequent pregnancy.
- All pregnant women should undergo a VTE risk assessment whenever seen or if they develop new/transient risk factors and postnatally, to assess their need for prophylactic LMWH (see Table 233.2). In both the UK and USA, women with previous DVT, except relating to major surgery, are recommended *prophylactic* anticoagulation throughout pregnancy and for at least six weeks postpartum.
- Current UK guidance recommends prophylactic LMWH throughout pregnancy and for six weeks postpartum for women with four or more risk factors. Women with three or more risk factors are recommended LMWH prophylaxis from 28 weeks of gestation and for six weeks postnatally, and women with two or more are recommended at least 10 days postnatal LMWH.
- In women on long-term anticoagulation pre-pregnancy for a thrombophilia with or without a history of previous VTE, *therapeutic* anticoagulation is indicated throughout pregnancy. Consider monitoring anti-Xa levels.

234 Other medical and surgical conditions in pregnancy

Neurological diseases in pregnancy

Headache

Headache is common in pregnancy and causes include migraine and tension headache. Rarer causes include pre-eclampsia, sinusitis, idiopathic intracranial hypertension, cerebral tumours, infection (meningitis, encephalitis) and postdural puncture headache (seen in up to 30% of women within the first week after spinal analgesia, usually mild and self-limiting). Most headaches represent benign conditions. Headaches that disturb sleep, are exertional in nature or those associated with focal neurological findings are suggestive of an underlying structural lesion.

Seizure disorders

- **Incidence**: occurs in 0.3–0.6% of pregnancies; it is the most frequently encountered major neurological condition in pregnancy.
- **Classification**: primary (idiopathic, epilepsy) or secondary (to trauma, infection, tumours, cerebrovascular disease, drug withdrawal or metabolic disorders). New seizures in pregnancy should be regarded as pre-eclampsia/eclampsia until proven otherwise.
- **Effect of seizure disorder on pregnancy**: obstetric complications include an increased risk of hyperemesis gravidarum, preterm delivery, pre-eclampsia, caesarean section delivery, placental abruption and perinatal mortality. However, most women with seizure disorders will have an uneventful pregnancy.
- **Effect of pregnancy on seizure disorder**: this is variable. Seizure frequency is increased in 45% of pregnant women, reduced in 5% and unchanged in 50%. If seizures are well controlled before pregnancy, there is a low risk of deterioration. However, if poorly controlled, an increase in seizure frequency may occur. Due to a number of factors (delayed gastric emptying, increase in plasma volume, altered protein binding, accelerated hepatic metabolism), the pharmacokinetics of anticonvulsant drugs change during pregnancy. Poor sleep and pain in labour can both trigger seizures and women should be counselled on seizure in pregnancy to reduce risks.
- **Effects on fetus and neonates**: women with epilepsy should be recommended 5 mg folic acid daily, from three months prior to conception, to reduce the risk of fetal anomalies. Recent studies have shown that lamotrigine and levetiracitam are safe in pregnancy and women can be reassured that there is no increased risk of fetal anomalies on either of these agents.

Sodium valproate is associated with congenital malformations, including neural tube defects and neurodevelopmental disorders, so women on this agent should receive preconception counselling to reduce the chance of unplanned pregnancy. Valproate should not be given to women of child-bearing age without an adequate pregnancy prevention plan.

The risk of fetal anomalies increases with the number of different antiepileptic agents and the dose, so the lowest effective dose and fewest agents that maintain seizure control are preferred. However, preventing seizures is the priority and major changes to medication should not be made due to pregnancy alone. Specialist input should be sought and women should be advised not to stop antiepileptic drugs suddenly due to pregnancy.

Management of seizure disorder during pregnancy

Early referral to specialist services to optimise antiepileptic medication is recommended.

- Doses of anticonvulsants may require adjustment during pregnancy and postnatally.
- Seizures may cause maternal hypoxaemia with resultant fetal injury. The aim of therapy is to control convulsions with a single agent using the lowest possible dose.
- The chance of a seizure at delivery is low overall. Early delivery may be indicated in very poorly controlled epilepsy, and short-term use of benzodiazepines such as clobazam may be appropriate here.
- All anticonvulsant medications cross into breast milk to some degree. The amount of transmission varies with the drug, but the use of such medications is not a contraindication to breastfeeding.

Neurological emergencies in pregnancy

Status epilepticus

- **Definition**: repeated convulsions with no intervals of consciousness.
- It is a medical emergency for both mother and fetus.
- **Management**: as for non-pregnant women. Maintain maternal airway and vital functions, control convulsions and prevent subsequent seizures. Transient fetal bradycardia is common. Resuscitate the fetus *in utero* and stabilize the mother before making a decision about delivery. Prolonged seizure activity may be associated with placental abruption.

Disorders of consciousness

- Disorders of *content* (confusion) and *level* of consciousness (coma).
- **Differential diagnosis**: similar to that in non-pregnant women, but also includes eclampsia.
- **Management**: treat underlying aetiology. Supportive care.

Psychiatric disorders in pregnancy

Psychiatric medications should generally be continued in pregnancy, and assessed on an individual basis. In general, the risk of a clinical relapse poses a greater threat to the pregnancy than continued medication. Guidelines for drug treatment are: use the lowest effective dose, consider delaying treatment until after the first trimester to minimize the risk of teratogenicity, avoid sedating agents immediately before delivery to minimize neonatal sedation, electroconvulsant therapy (ECT) is generally avoided in pregnancy, but if required, is considered safe for the fetus.

- Postpartum depression occurs in 8–15% of all postpartum women, risk factors being prior depression (30% risk), prior postpartum depression (70–85% risk). Peak onset of symptoms is 2–3 months postpartum; symptoms usually resolve spontaneously within 6–12 months.
- Postpartum psychosis occurs in 1–2 per 1000 live births, risk factor are primiparity, personal or family history of mental illness, prior postpartum psychosis (25% risk). Peak onset of symptoms is 10–14 days postpartum, and management is hospitalization, pharmacological therapy, ECT as needed.

Pulmonary disease in pregnancy

Asthma

- Asthma occurs in 1–4% of pregnancies. During pregnancy the rule of thirds applies, a third improve, a third worsen, a third stay the same. Most women with mild well-controlled asthma tolerate pregnancy well, but women with severe asthma are at risk of deterioration. Management is the same as for non-pregnant women. Complications include intrauterine fetal growth retardation, stillbirth, and maternal death.

Amniotic fluid embolism

- Amniotic fluid embolism is an obstetric emergency with 85% maternal mortality. Risk factors include multiparity, prolonged labour, fetal demise, 'excessive' oxytocin augmentation, placental abruption, caesarean section delivery. Symptoms are of acute onset breathlessness, hypotension, cardiovascular collapse, coagulopathy, and hypoxaemia. Therapy is supportive

Pulmonary oedema

- Pulmonary oedema from non-cardiogenic causes, e.g. fluid overload, infection, pre-eclampsia, tocolytic therapy, or cardiogenic causes, e.g. arrhythmia or underlying heart disease. Managed as for non-pregnant women. High level care and cardiology input is vital.

Renal disease in pregnancy

Asymptomatic bacteriuria

- **Incidence**: occurs in 4–7% of all pregnancies, which is similar to that in non-pregnant women.
- In pregnancy, asymptomatic bacteriuria is more likely to progress to pyelonephritis (20–30%). Antibiotics should be given if urine culture is positive for significant growth of a pathogenic organism, or the woman has symptoms of infection.
- *Escherichia coli* is the most common causative organism.

Chronic renal failure

- **Complications**: miscarriage, pre-eclampsia, IUGR, stillbirth, preterm birth.
- Pregnancy outcome is dependent on baseline renal function (see Table 234.1) and presence and severity of hypertension. The degree of proteinuria does not correlate with pregnancy outcome.
- Renal function may deteriorate in pregnancy, requiring renal replacement therapy, and may not recover to baseline postpartum.
- In the case of significant deterioration of renal function, elective delivery should be considered.
- In women with end-stage renal disease, renal transplantation prior to conception offers the best chance of a successful pregnancy (especially if renal function is stable for 1–2 years and there is no hypertension). Immunosuppression (including ciclosporin, azathioprine and prednisolone) can be continued safely in pregnancy; however, mycophenolate mofetil is teratogenic and should be changed to an alternative agent in advance of conception.

Table 234.1 Pregnancy outcome in women with chronic renal disease.

	Category of chronic renal disease		
	Mild	**Moderate**	**Severe**
Serum creatinine (mmol/l)	120–150	150–250	>250
Serum creatinine (mg/dl)	<1.4	1.4–2.5	>2.5
Complications (%)	20	40	85
Viable delivery (%)	95	90	50
Long-term sequelae (%)	<5	25	55

Autoimmune diseases in pregnancy

Systemic lupus erythematosus

- Systemic lupus erythematosus does not generally worsen in pregnancy. Pregnancy outcome is related primarily to the severity of underlying renal disease.
- **Complications**: pre-eclampsia, IUGR, preterm birth.

Maternal anti-Ro and anti-La antibodies

Associated with complete fetal heart block in 2% of cases, so fetal echocardiography and regular fetal heart auscultation are required. There is also a 5% chance of neonatal lupus so the parents should be counselled about the possibility of a rash developing after birth.

Immune (idiopathic) thrombocytopenic purpura

- Immune thrombocytopenic purpura (ITP) is a maternal disease characterized by the presence of circulating antiplatelet antibodies.
- **Differential diagnosis**: pre-eclampsia, coagulopathy, drugs, gestational thrombocytopenia.
- **Complications**: IgG can cross the placenta and cause fetal thrombocytopenia. However, the correlation between maternal and fetal platelet count is poor. Fetal intraventricular haemorrhage in the setting of ITP is rare.
- **Management**: corticosteroids may be necessary if maternal thrombocytopenia is severe. Intravenous immunoglobulin, plasmapheresis and splenectomy are rarely necessary in pregnancy. Caesarean section delivery has not been shown to improve perinatal outcome. Avoidance at birth of difficult assisted vaginal births, fetal scalp electrodes, fetal blood sampling in labour and IM injection of vitamin K for the neonate should be considered.

Rheumatoid arthritis

- Improves in 75% of pregnancies, but >90% of women will relapse within six months of delivery.
- Corticosteroids are safe in pregnancy. Biological therapy can be continued in pregnancy, but discontinuation in the third trimester should be discussed to reduce the fetal levels of the agent at the time of delivery.

Surgical conditions in pregnancy

Surgical conditions complicate 2–3 per 1000 pregnancies and include appendicitis, biliary disease, ovarian disease. These can be complicated by haemorrhage, anaesthetic complications, infection, preterm delivery. Complications can be minimized if surgery is performed in the second trimester. Technical considerations include 1) left lateral tilt if ≥20 weeks to improve venous return; 2) continuous fetal monitoring ≥26 weeks' gestation; 3) avoidance of teratogenic agents; 4) specific anaesthetic considerations regarding fetus and mother.

Appendicitis

- **Incidence**: the incidence of appendicitis is not increased (1 in 1500 pregnancies), but an infected appendix is more likely to rupture in pregnancy.
- **Diagnosis**: diagnosis can be difficult as the appendix moves up in pregnancy and signs and symptoms can be vague. Ultrasound assessment of the appendix can be difficult and CT should be avoided.
- **Management**: surgical removal is generally recommended. A laparoscopic approach is appropriate in the first and second trimester.
- **Complications**: preterm birth, sepsis, abscess.

235 Fluid replacement therapy

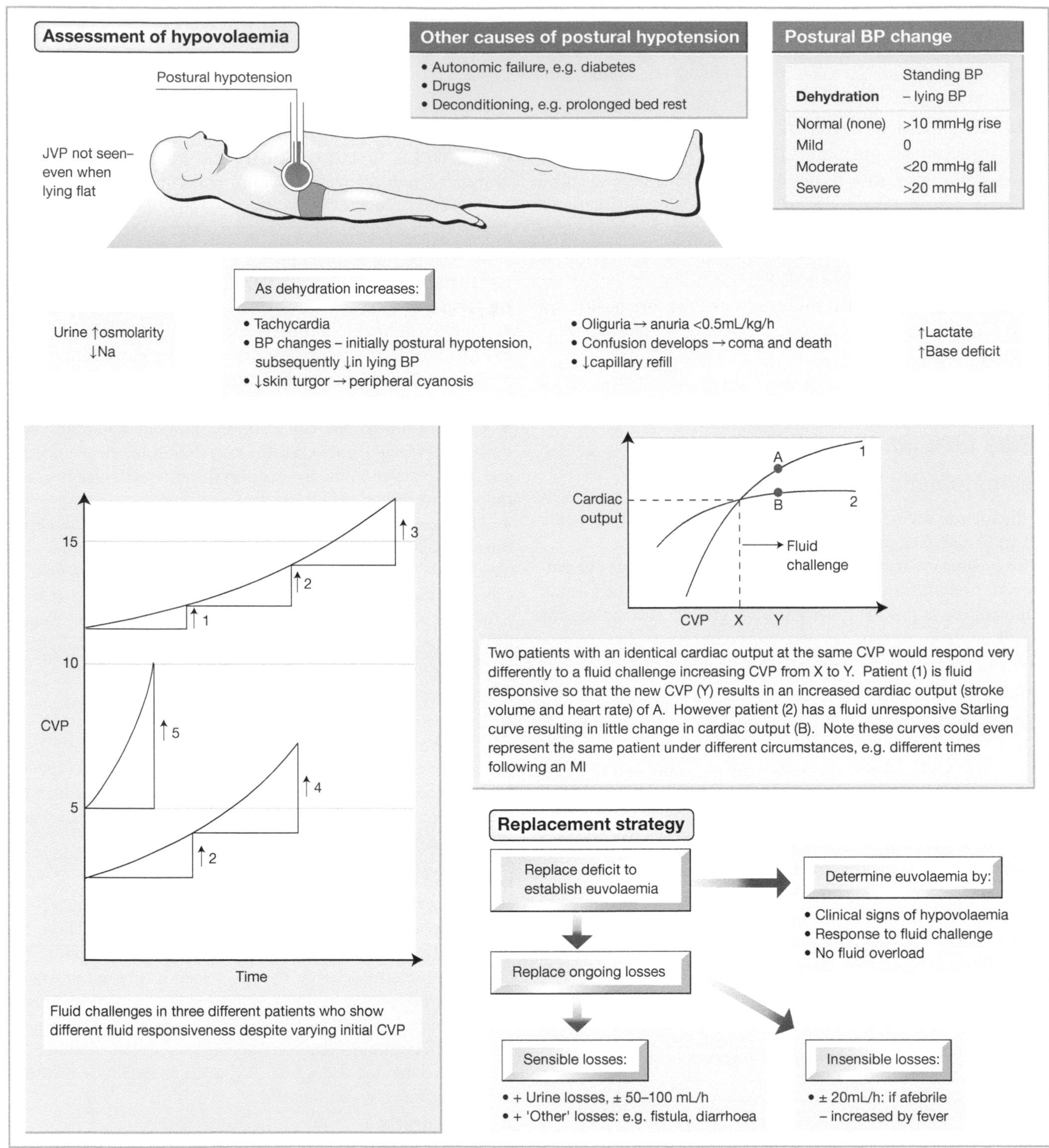

Fluid may be required either for the maintenance of euvolaemia or replacement of losses in hypovolaemic patients. The oral route is optimal for maintenance. Patients unable to eat and drink normally can be fed by a nasogastric, nasojejeunal or a percutaneous endoscopically placed gastric feeding tube. Occasionally, the enteral route is unavailable (recent gastrointestinal [GI] surgery, ileus);

Medicine at a Glance, Fifth Edition. Edited by Patrick Davey and Alex Pitcher.

Companion website: www.wiley.com/go/medicine5e

intravenous crystalloid may be administered for short periods to provide water and electrolytes, though parenteral nutrition needs to be considered if long-term maintenance is required.

Assessment of hypovolaemia

Profound hypovolaemia will eventually lead to tissue hypoperfusion and multiorgan failure. It may result from absolute losses (haemorrhage, diarrhoea, vomiting, burns, polyuria) or redistribution of fluid, sometimes known as 'third space' loss (sepsis, anaphylaxis, pancreatitis, trauma, spinal cord injury, ascites). The renin–angiotensin and sympathetic nervous systems are important in regulating the volume of the extracellular space. These compensatory mechanisms may make it difficult to detect mild hypovolaemia. Signs of hypovolaemia include the following.

- Reduced skin turgor, decreased capillary refill, tachycardia and low jugular venous pressure (JVP).
- Low urine output (<0.5 ml/kg/h) with high osmolality, low urine sodium and a urine urea creatinine ratio of <40, and eventual abnormal urea and creatinine levels in blood. Plasma urea is disproportionately high in dehydration and GI haemorrhage. It may be low in patients with liver disease even in the presence of substantial hypovolaemia.
- **Hypotension**: reduction in blood pressure (BP) is a late feature. An apparently 'normal' BP may be low if the patient suffers from untreated hypertension. Compensatory mechanisms mask significant hypovolaemia in the supine position, therefore hypotension may only become apparent on sitting or standing (postural hypotension). Such patients often complain of dizziness or syncope when erect. Hypovolaemia in the supine position may also be unmasked by raising the legs for 30 seconds (to increase venous return) and monitoring the effect on heart rate, BP and JVP (or central venous pressure [CVP]). This should not be performed if raising the legs is likely to be painful.
- Reduced weight.
- Lactate and base deficit rise when there is significant tissue hypoperfusion.

As with many critically ill patients, the signs above may be nonspecific and are not by themselves diagnostic, but taken together with the patient's history and diagnosis, one may make an assessment of volume status. In some patients, this is easy. For example, in a young man with four days of diarrhoea who has not been drinking, if examination shows tachycardia, reduced capillary refill, hypotension, reduced JVP and oliguria, there would be little doubt that the patient is severely dehydrated. However, if the patient is elderly with pre-existing heart failure and is admitted with acute pancreatitis, the assessment is far more complex. The fluid challenge is extremely useful in the diagnosis and treatment of hypovolaemia.

Fluid challenge

The response to a fluid challenge may be assessed by changes in stroke volume, cardiac output or CVP (reflecting right atrial pressure). The latter is most frequently used outside the intensive care unit. Traditionally, one is taught 'normal' values of right and left atrial pressures, but absolute values are of little use in guiding fluid therapy because they vary with ventricular compliance and venous tone. An absolute CVP value of 10 mmHg may represent hypovolaemia, euvolaemia or hypervolaemia in three different patients.

A fluid challenge involves giving a relatively small volume of crystalloid or colloid over a short period of time and monitoring the haemodynamic effects. Typically 250 ml of fluid is given over a period of 2–3 minutes. The change in CVP depends on the volume status of the patient. In a hypovolaemic patient, there is little increase in CVP following a fluid challenge (<3 mmHg), which may then be repeated. A rise of 3 mmHg in the CVP following a challenge implies an adequate circulating volume, whilst a rise >3 mmHg suggests hypervolaemia. The patient should also be monitored for improvements in other haemodynamic variables (↓ heart rate, ↑ BP, ↑ capillary refill) and tissue perfusion (↑ urine output, ↑ Glasgow Coma Score [GCS], reduction in acidosis/lactate), whilst avoiding signs of hypervolaemia.

Management of severely hypovolaemic patients

As with all critically ill patients, there needs to be good vascular access (ideally central venous) and appropriate monitoring, which should include electrocardiogram, pulse oximetry, hourly urine output, BP (arterial catheter if severe hypotension or shock), respiratory rate and GCS. An echocardiogram, pulmonary artery catheter, oesophageal Doppler or pulse contour analysis may be required in some patients.

Which fluid should be chosen?

Blood and plasma are required in acute haemorrhage, but judicious use of colloid or crystalloid may be required to maintain the circulation until this is available. In critically ill patients, the plasma volume-expanding effects of colloids and crystalloids are very similar.

- **Crystalloid-normal saline or a balanced salt solution such as lactated Ringer's solution** (Hartmann's solution): cheap compared to colloids. Its use avoids hyperchloraemic acidosis which may occur with large volumes of saline.
- **Colloid-albumin**: 4.5% or 20% salt poor (molecular weight 66.5 kDa). It is the most expensive colloid. There was some controversy over its use in the past, but a large multicentre trial showed no difference in safety compared to saline.
- **Colloids, including dextransgelatins** (Gelofusine®, Haemaccel®) and **hydroxyethyl starches** (HAES-Steril®, eloHAES®) have largely fallen out of favour because of cost, short- and long-term side-effects and efficacy.

Hyperchloraemic acidosis

Colloids contain osmotically active molecules which are usually in normal saline. The administration of large volumes of chloride-rich saline leads to a metabolic acidosis. This phenomenon is not observed with physiologically balanced salt solutions such as Hartmann's solution, containing much less chloride. Patients with dilutional hyperchloraemic acidosis suffer with nausea, abdominal pain and reduced urine output (hyperchloraemia reduces the glomerular filtration rate).

236 Illness in elderly people

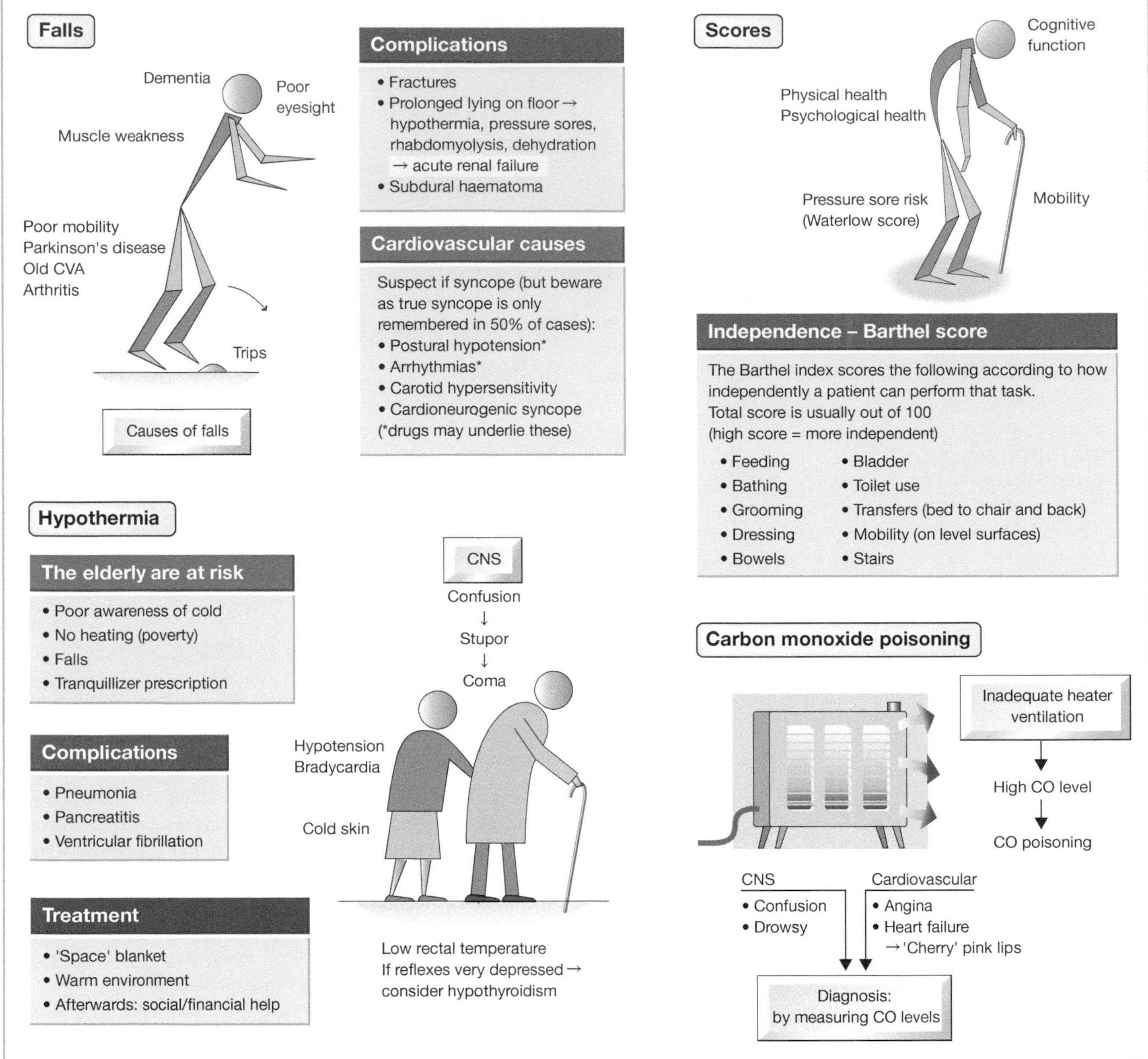

Falls
Dementia
Poor eyesight
Muscle weakness
Poor mobility
Parkinson's disease
Old CVA
Arthritis
Trips
Causes of falls
Complications
• Fractures
• Prolonged lying on floor → hypothermia, pressure sores, rhabdomyolysis, dehydration → acute renal failure
• Subdural haematoma
Cardiovascular causes
Suspect if syncope (but beware as true syncope is only remembered in 50% of cases):
• Postural hypotension*
• Arrhythmias*
• Carotid hypersensitivity
• Cardioneurogenic syncope
(*drugs may underlie these)
Scores
Cognitive function
Physical health
Psychological health
Pressure sore risk (Waterlow score)
Mobility
Independence – Barthel score
The Barthel index scores the following according to how independently a patient can perform that task.
Total score is usually out of 100
(high score = more independent)
• Feeding
• Bathing
• Grooming
• Dressing
• Bowels
• Bladder
• Toilet use
• Transfers (bed to chair and back)
• Mobility (on level surfaces)
• Stairs
Hypothermia
The elderly are at risk
• Poor awareness of cold
• No heating (poverty)
• Falls
• Tranquillizer prescription
Complications
• Pneumonia
• Pancreatitis
• Ventricular fibrillation
Treatment
• 'Space' blanket
• Warm environment
• Afterwards: social/financial help
CNS
Confusion
↓
Stupor
↓
Coma
Hypotension
Bradycardia
Cold skin
Low rectal temperature
If reflexes very depressed → consider hypothyroidism
Carbon monoxide poisoning
Inadequate heater ventilation
High CO level
CO poisoning
CNS
• Confusion
• Drowsy
Cardiovascular
• Angina
• Heart failure
→ 'Cherry' pink lips
Diagnosis: by measuring CO levels

Sick elderly people should in many respects be treated identically to young people, although there are important differences.

- Their premorbid condition is often worse due to multiple ongoing illnesses, multiple medications and varying degrees of dementia, poverty and social isolation. Thus, the rehabilitation potential following the acute illness may be more limited. Additional home support should be planned early on during hospital admission.
- The clinical presentation is often atypical and not classic.
- The differential diagnosis is usually broader.
- The risk to life from any illness is greater.
- Recovery is prolonged and may require substantial support.

Premorbid condition

It is vital to establish the premorbid condition, because this is the target to aim for in subsequent rehabilitation. How independent were they? Several scoring systems (e.g. activities of daily living) can be used to ascertain functional status; the Barthel score is commonly used to measure independence and thus rehabilitation potential and progress (see figure). Other scoring systems

Medicine at a Glance, Fifth Edition. Edited by Patrick Davey and Alex Pitcher.

Companion website: www.wiley.com/go/medicine5e

include the Clinical Fragility Score and the Edmonton Frailty Scale. For more extensive exploration of the clinical frailty score, look at www.criticalcarenice.org.uk/frailty

Polypharmacy

Elderly people are often prescribed multiple drugs for multiple pathologies. This leads to compliance issues (disease progression) and side-effects. Always consider whether the current illness can be explained by a side-effect of medication.

Differential diagnosis

In young patients, 'Occam's razor' applies: 'the least number of diagnoses needed to explain all the symptoms and signs establishes the correct diagnosis'. In elderly people, multiple pathologies often co-exist, e.g. heart failure, leg ulcers, diabetes and its complications, occult cancer, etc. A single unifying diagnosis is often not possible.

Clinical presentations and diseases

Presentations are often atypical, such as 'unwellness' without specific features or a decline in functional or cognitive capacity, rather than with organ-specific symptoms. The differential diagnosis is broader than in many younger patients.

- Acute confusion is a common presentation of many diseases. As the febrile response is diminished, infections often present with minor fever and minor constitutional upset, and major confusion. Abscesses, e.g. subphrenic and pelvic, may present as 'unwellness', without localizing symptoms/signs; delirium is a common presentation in elderly patients with COVID-19.
- Many diseases present with decreased function/cognition or apathy and weight loss, rather than more classically. Diseases that may present in this manner include thyrotoxicosis, depression, temporal arteritis and cancer.
- Tuberculosis is not uncommon in elderly people, and may present quite atypically, with non-specific 'unwellness', loss of appetite, etc.
- Diseases may relate to poverty: there are many examples, including accidental carbon monoxide (CO) poisoning resulting from ill-maintained heaters, which are underdiagnosed. CO binds to haemoglobin, decreasing oxygen transport. Presentation is with central nervous system (CNS) (headache, agitation, confusion, occasionally coma) and/or cardiac symptoms (heart failure, unstable angina) – common symptoms in elderly people that are often attributed to other pathology. Diagnosis is by measuring CO levels in the blood (HbCO levels are often available on point-of-care venous blood gas results). Treatment is with high-dose hyperbaric (i.e. high-pressure) oxygen in severe cases (contact Royal Navy diving centres) and, crucially, heater maintenance.
- Hypothermia: see figure.

Specific issues

Falls are common. The cause should always be sought, as specific therapy may be effective.

- Musculoskeletal conditions, such as osteoarthritis or age-related decline in muscle strength, are a common cause of falls. Sarcopenia is common. Physical rehabilitation, a Zimmer frame or other walking aid, and adjustment of the home environment may prevent falls and consequent fractures.
- Cardiovascular diseases causing recurrent falls include postural hypotension, cardioneurogenic syncope, carotid hypersensitivity syndrome and intermittent arrhythmias (bradyarrhythmias such as complete heart block, occasionally ventricular tachycardia). Carotid sinus massage, tilt-table testing and 24-hour electrocardiogram (ECG) taping may provide important clues to the presence of cardiovascular disease.
- Neurological disease, especially disability from a previous stroke, Parkinson disease, peripheral neuropathy (e.g. diabetic) or cervical myelopathy. Epilepsy rarely underlies recurrent falls.
- Dementia often underlies or contributes to falls and immobility.

The consequence of falls should also be considered.

- Fractures, which may be lessened by treating osteoporosis, providing hip protectors and adjusting the home environment.
- Assistance may be needed to get up – various alarms are available. Regular visits by friends and neighbours play a vital role.

Diagnostic issues

As clinical symptoms and signs may be less reliable, investigations should be broad. All elderly patients admitted acutely should have the following.

- Full blood count, electrolytes (K^+, Na^+, Ca^{2+}), renal and liver function, and inflammatory markers (both erythrocyte sedimentation rate and C-reactive protein).
- Chest X-ray and ECG.
- Blood and urine cultures unless infection has been ruled out by establishing an alternative diagnosis.

Special issues

- Special diagnostic multidisciplinary clinics for falls, dementia, syncope, etc. allow for optimal care and treatment.
- The threshold for 'blind' abdomen/pelvis computed tomography is low even without localizing symptoms/signs, because cancer and intra-abdominal/pelvic abscesses are common.
- Diagnosis of giant cell arteritis (GCA) should be made on history, examination, laboratory test, temporal artery biopsy/ultrasound. Steroids should be started without delay whilst awaiting results of these investigations. Forty percent to 60% of patients with GCA will have polymyalgia rheumatica (PMR) and 15–20% of patients with PMR have GCA.

Consequence and treatment of illness

The risk to life from any illness (e.g. pneumonia, myocardial infarction) is greater with increasing age, justifying aggressive medical therapy. Age alone is not a bar to high-technology intervention, such as cardiac surgery (aortic valve replacement is feasible in many aged 85 years or more), abdominal surgery, intensive care, etc. Aggressive treatments, although often having more benefit, equally often have greater risks. This calls for careful clinical judgement in deciding the most appropriate therapy. Cardiac arrest is associated with a poorer outcome in very elderly people (≥85 years). Decisions on the appropriateness of cardiopulmonary resuscitation and treatment escalation plans (TEPs) should be made on admission in conjunction with the patient or, if they lack capacity to make such decisions, with those people who have legal power of attorney for health and welfare, or after best interest decisions.

Rehabilitation

It is vital that, in order to optimize outcome, specialists in old age medicine, rather than general physicians, undertake rehabilitation, using multidisciplinary teams, including:

- physiotherapists
- occupational therapists
- social workers.

The aim should be to return the patient to a stable, long-term environment of their choice.

Chronic tiredness and other medically unexplained symptoms

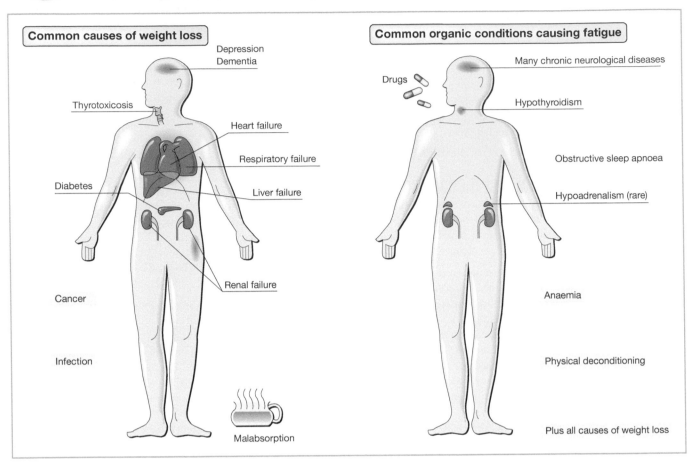

Common causes of weight loss

Depression
Dementia
Thyrotoxicosis
Heart failure
Respiratory failure
Diabetes
Liver failure
Renal failure
Cancer
Infection
Malabsorption

Common organic conditions causing fatigue

Many chronic neurological diseases
Drugs
Hypothyroidism
Obstructive sleep apnoea
Hypoadrenalism (rare)
Anaemia
Physical deconditioning
Plus all causes of weight loss

Chronic fatigue

Fatigue is a complex and common sensation accounting for 20% of general practitioner consultations. Tiredness results from:

- many (indeed most) organic diseases (see figure)
- psychological distress
- social stresses
- psychiatric illness: 20–80% of tired patients have a psychiatric disorder (depression, anxiety or somatic symptom disorder).

Tiredness may also be a medically unexplained symptom (MUS); the diagnoses applied may vary between this, chronic fatigue syndrome (CFS), postviral fatigue (especially if there have been symptoms in the past six months suggesting a viral infection) and myalgic encephalomyelitis (ME). The variation in the diagnosis made for long-standing fatigue largely follows medical and social styles, rather than reflecting any real change in the epidemiology of the aetiology of this symptom.

From this list, it can be seen that almost any illness or psychological distress can cause tiredness. Accordingly, the diagnosis of the cause of any fatigue rests on identifying the associated symptoms, as well as on the demographics (patient's age and sex: male sex and increasing age are associated with serious disease). Features suggestive of an underlying organic illness include the following.

- Weight loss: unintentional weight loss usually has a serious cause (see figure).
- Fevers, night sweats.
- Malaise.
- Persistent pains localized to one area.
- Persistent symptoms of new onset.
- Age ≥35 years.

It is important that serious organic or psychiatric pathology is diagnosed and treated; other causes of tiredness are usually diagnosed by exclusion (see Table 237.1). Accurate diagnosis relies on the history and examination, although investigations are also important. A normal full blood count, renal and liver function and inflammatory markers (C-reactive protein, erythrocyte sedimentation rate) are reassuring, but do not exclude all serious inflammatory/malignant disease (disseminated cancer can present as fatigue with normal blood tests – the diagnostic clue is often weight loss and age ≥50 years). One-third of patients with fatigue have no identifiable organic or psychiatric disorder (including CFS).

Medicine at a Glance, Fifth Edition. Edited by Patrick Davey and Alex Pitcher.

Companion website: www.wiley.com/go/medicine5e

Table 237.1 Physical disorders associated with fatigue.

- Vital organ failure (heart, lung, kidney, liver, bone marrow, skin)
- Chronic inflammation or infection
- Viral infections may cause *postviral fatigue* lasting <6 months. Symptoms can be prolonged following COVID infection, where they are called 'long COVID'
- Malignancy
- Endocrine disease (particularly thyroid disease, adrenal disease)
- Anaemia
- Sleep disorders (obstructive sleep apnoea)
- Neurological disease (multiple sclerosis, Parkinson disease)
- Drugs, e.g. β-blockers

Management and prognosis

These depend on the cause. If psychological stresses are significant, counselling may help. Of patients with non-specific fatigue, 25–50% still complain of fatigue a year later. Chronic fatigue for ≥6 months or associated with multiple associated somatic symptoms has a poorer long-term outlook. Most cases of fatigue are helped by physical reconditioning (a commonly advised exercise prescription is for 20 min sessions of aerobic exercise, suffciently intense to induce breathlessness, repeated three times a week); this is true whether or not organic illness is present, and so can be applied without prejudice as to the diagnosis.

Medically unexplained symptoms

These create an enormous workload for all doctors.

- Medically unexplained symptoms may account for up to 50% of new patient diagnoses in some specialties, such as gastroenterology or neurology.
- Some symptoms may be associated with physical or sexual abuse; in others, it may be a marker of family dysfunction.
- Any associated psychological disease should be rapidly diagnosed and treated.
- When a diagnosis of MUS is suspected, it is important to exclude serious illness using the minimum of tests.
- Equally, it is crucial to explain to patients, before the results of the test are known, that it is highly likely that these investigations will be normal; indeed, that they are primarily being done to reassure the patient, and not because the doctor believes they will be abnormal. This will avoid the patient believing that normal results mean that the physician should look harder for an underlying organic illness.
- It is best to acknowledge to the patient that the symptoms are medically unexplained, that these symptoms are frequently seen (thus the individual physician and profession have considerable experience and knowledge of them), and that they have a benign prognosis.
- It is not wise to offer mechanistic explanations that are based on guesswork, as these can often be disproved, leading to the patient losing confidence in their physician. Patients then seek help elsewhere; some patients seek large numbers of opinions (patients with MUSs in neurology clinics have been seen in about six previous specialties), and not surprisingly receive multiple different explanations for their symptoms, leading them to lose faith in doctors generally.
- There is some evidence that labelling these symptoms as functional, rather than medically unexplained, offends fewer patients.
- Dealing with symptoms, rather than seeking an underlying unifying interpretation, may help, e.g. drugs to help constipation or diarrhoea, exercise to help tiredness, anxiolytics to help anxiety, cognitive therapy to help worries about the future, etc., when patients are amenable.

Somatic symptom disorder (SSD, formerly known as somatization disorder)

Various specialties classify clusters of MUSs together: non-cardiac chest pain, fibromyalgia, irritable bowel syndrome, chronic fatigue syndrome and repetitive strain injury. There is evidence that it is best not to give patients' symptoms such a name, as, while it helps to legitimize their symptoms as an illness, it may also help perpetuate their symptoms. Cognitive therapy may help, as can treating any of the commonly associated depression and/or anxiety states.

Chronic fatigue syndrome

Many, if not most, patients with isolated tiredness do not have serious organic pathology – some have chronic fatigue syndrome (CFS), defined as 'new onset of persistent/relapsing, debilitating fatigue without previous fatigue, which does not resolve with bed rest and is severe enough to reduce daily activity to 50% of its premorbid level for ≥6 months'. It affects twice as many women as men and is very common – the overall incidence of tiredness in the general population is 1.5%. Such patients often have multiple other symptoms, each of which varies greatly from day to day.

Patients with CFS are often keen on an 'organic' diagnosis – this is almost a hallmark of the condition, and it is important not to be drawn into endless cycles of negative investigations. This is best done by explaining that the diagnosis is CFS before investigations are ordered, so that negative results come as a reassurance, not as a surprise or as a sign that the physician should look harder for any underlying pathology. Physical deconditioning often exacerbates symptoms, and regular exercise may have a role. Multidisciplinary individualized rehabilitation therapy may include counselling, cognitive behavioural therapy, supportive care, and exercise programmes. Antidepressants may be helpful for some people with CFS.

238 Psychiatric disorders

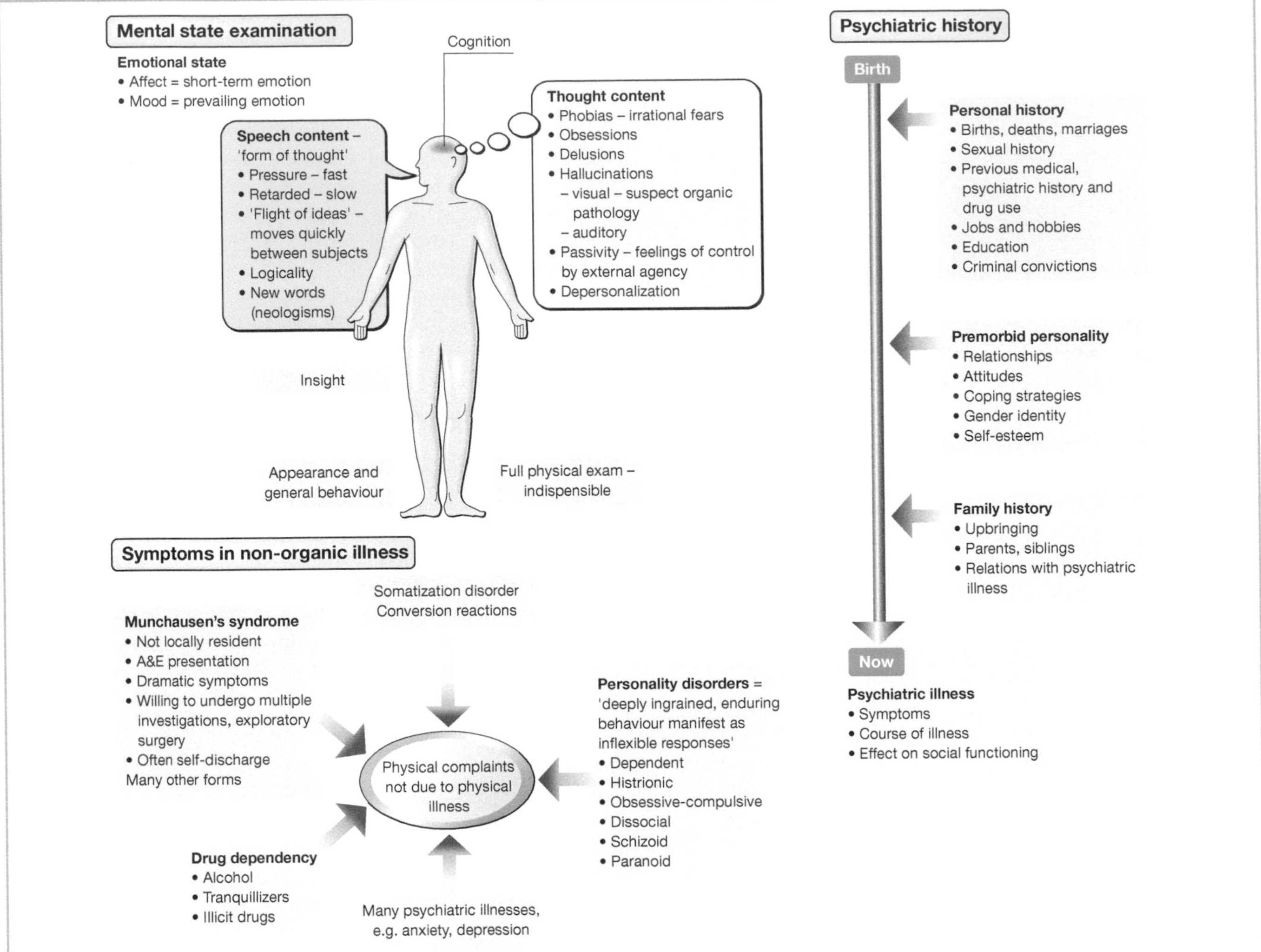

Psychological illnesses cause symptoms similar to those of organic disease, and may obscure an organic diagnosis or complicate its management. Of acute medical admissions, 5–10% require formal psychiatric review.

Neurotic diseases are an exaggeration of normal emotional responses. Psychotic illnesses have symptoms outside the range of normal human experience.

Common psychological illnesses seen in medical practice

Anxiety disorders

Anxiety disorders cause psychological symptoms (apprehension, fear of impending doom/disaster, irritability, depersonalization) and physical ones (sweating, tremor, palpitations, 'dizziness', inability to sleep, poor concentration) which can be confused with certain diseases (e.g. thyrotoxicosis, alcohol intoxication/withdrawal, hypoglycaemia and, extremely rarely, phaeochromocytoma). Symptoms may be situation dependent, e.g. phobic disorders (particular objects or animals trigger attacks) or more commonly free-floating, appearing without reason. Symptoms may appear in short overwhelming episodes ('panic attacks') – occasionally triggered by bad news, e.g. an untreatable diagnosis – or as longer, lower-intensity anxiety states. Treatment is psychological (explanation, reassurance, relaxation techniques). Short courses of benzodiazepines have a limited role.

Abnormal illness behaviour

Abnormal illness behaviour includes exaggerated anxiety, inappropriate adoption of the 'sick' role and prolonged illness denial. Abnormal psychological reactions need to be identified and treated in order to treat any underlying organic disease effectively.

Medicine at a Glance, Fifth Edition. Edited by Patrick Davey and Alex Pitcher.

Companion website: www.wiley.com/go/medicine5e

Somatic symptom and related disorders (formerly known as somatization disorders)

Somatic symptom and related disorders include the psychiatric conditions known as conversion disorder and somatic symptom disorder (SSD). People with these disorders experience significant physical symptoms (such as pain, weakness, breathlessness), that result in major distress and/or problems functioning. SSD and related disorders may or may not accompany other diagnosed medical conditions but the person's response is out of proportion to the symptoms experienced. People with these disorders are not faking their symptoms; the physical distress the person feels is real. The distress caused may lead to the person presenting to multiple healthcare providers and may result in many investigations and unnecessary procedures. Conversion disorder is characterized by voluntary motor or sensory function deficits, e.g. paralysis, pseudoseizures, blindness. SSD is characterized by somatic symptoms.

Treatment is intended to help control symptoms and help the person function as normally as possible. It typically involves the person having regular visits with a trusted healthcare professional, experienced in the management of SSD and related disorders. The healthcare professional can offer support and reassurance, as well as monitoring symptoms and avoiding unnecessary investigations and treatments. Psychotherapy may be helpful and in conversion disorders physiotherapy may be beneficial. Patients who are also experiencing depression and anxiety may benefit from appropriate medication.

Schizophrenia

This is characterized by a set of beliefs, symptoms and behaviour outside normal experience. Highly suggestive first-rank symptoms include the following.

- **Auditory hallucinations**, often abusive, repeating the patient's words, or commenting on their behaviour or personality.
- **Thought withdrawal, insertion and broadcasting**: external agencies or people can remove, insert or listen in to their thoughts.
- **Delusional beliefs**, i.e. ideas outside the social norms of that society. For example, a belief in a deity is often not delusional, but the belief that a deity can actually perform miracles can be.
- **External control** of thoughts, emotions or actions.

Symptoms are positive, when delusional beliefs and floridly abnormal behaviour predominate, or negative, when inaction, apathy and social withdrawal predominate. Schizophrenic patients come to the attention of acute medical services through:

- bizarre behaviour leading to accident and emergency attendance. Organic disease or drug intoxication may need to be excluded
- attempted (and successful) suicide which is common in psychosis – all self-harm cases should have psychotic illness excluded.

If schizophrenia is suspected, immediate psychiatric review should be requested. The diagnosis is made from the mental state examination (see figure). Treatment is with antipsychotic drugs, which inhibit dopamine subtype D1 and D2 receptors and/or central nervous system serotonin traffic. They improve positive symptoms but have less impact on negative ones. Similar symptoms occasionally arise from organic mental disorders, caused by drugs (e.g. 'street' drugs, steroids, rarely other drugs) or physical illness (e.g. temporal lobe epilepsy, brain tumours). These may need to be actively excluded.

Affective (mood) disorders

Depression

Depression results in a low mood and unhappiness. Conversation is slow, quiet and monotonous, with depressive ideation, low self-esteem, unworthiness and wretchedness. The intellect can be impaired. Physical symptoms can predominate. Somatic features of severe depression are early morning waking, appetite and weight loss, constipation and loss of libido/sexual prowess. In psychotic depression, symptoms are profound and derogatory or abusive auditory hallucinations can occur. Depression complicates most physical illnesses (especially stroke) and amplifies physical symptoms, resulting in great distress and frequent physician consultations. Treatment is psychological (mild–moderate cases) and with antidepressant drugs, which prolong the action of noradrenaline (norepinephrine) and/or serotonin in neuronal synapses. Electroconvulsive therapy acts quickly and is used for severe depression.

Mania

Mania results in mental restlessness with mood elevation, fast and disinhibited speech, 'flight of ideas' (never dwelling on one topic for long) and overconfident self-belief, with delusions about intellectual, physical, financial or sexual prowess or omnipotence. Sufferers are physically restless and may not eat or sleep. Hypomania, a mild form of mania, comprises mild euphoria, overactivity and disinhibition. Mania can alternate with depression – a bipolar illness. Severe mania is treated with major tranquillizers, and subsequent attacks can be prevented by the mood stabilizer lithium.

Personality disorders

Personality disorders (see figure), which manifest as lifelong inflexible responses, cause management difficulties.

Substance misuse

This results in medical, social and economic problems.

- **Cigarettes**: highly addictive. Smokers die some eight years before non-smokers (of ischaemic heart disease or cancer). Smoking ages skin (facial wrinkling). Counselling, nicotine replacement therapy and antidepressants have a minor role in cessation.
- **Alcohol**: can cause problem drinking (social disruption) or physical dependence (cessation leads to the withdrawal syndrome – tremor, sweating, tachycardia, anxiety, confusion, hallucinations and seizures, which are treated with chlordiazepoxide and vitamins).
- Minor or major **tranquillizers**.
- **Opiates**: common, often injected (HIV or hepatitis infection may result from shared needles). Premature death may result from infection or accidental overdose. Addicts may express opiate-seeking behaviour and commit petty larceny on hospital wards. Withdrawal causes sweating, shivering, tachycardia, hypertension and diarrhoea.
- **Ecstasy**: occasionally causes acute confusion, cardiac arrhythmias, memory loss or 'malignant' hyponatraemia and lethal cerebral oedema.

239 Substance misuse

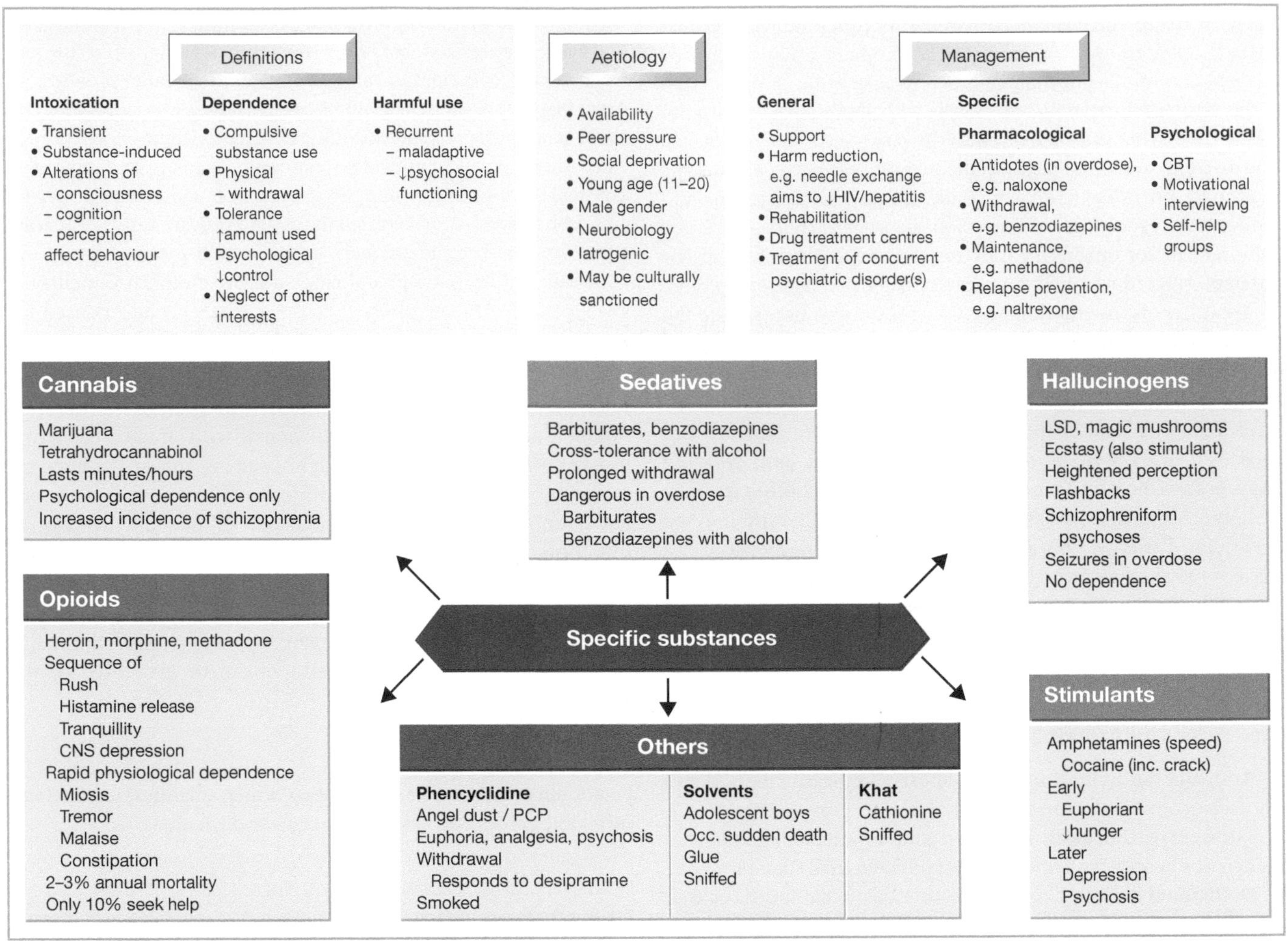

Definitions

Intoxication
- Transient
- Substance-induced
- Alterations of
  - consciousness
  - cognition
  - perception
  affect behaviour

Dependence
- Compulsive substance use
- Physical
  - withdrawal
- Tolerance
  ↑amount used
- Psychological
  ↓control
- Neglect of other interests

Harmful use
- Recurrent
  - maladaptive
  - ↓psychosocial functioning

Aetiology
- Availability
- Peer pressure
- Social deprivation
- Young age (11–20)
- Male gender
- Neurobiology
- Iatrogenic
- May be culturally sanctioned

Management

General
- Support
- Harm reduction, e.g. needle exchange aims to ↓HIV/hepatitis
- Rehabilitation
- Drug treatment centres
- Treatment of concurrent psychiatric disorder(s)

Specific

Pharmacological
- Antidotes (in overdose), e.g. naloxone
- Withdrawal, e.g. benzodiazepines
- Maintenance, e.g. methadone
- Relapse prevention, e.g. naltrexone

Psychological
- CBT
- Motivational interviewing
- Self-help groups

Specific substances

Cannabis
Marijuana
Tetrahydrocannabinol
Lasts minutes/hours
Psychological dependence only
Increased incidence of schizophrenia

Sedatives
Barbiturates, benzodiazepines
Cross-tolerance with alcohol
Prolonged withdrawal
Dangerous in overdose
  Barbiturates
  Benzodiazepines with alcohol

Hallucinogens
LSD, magic mushrooms
Ecstasy (also stimulant)
Heightened perception
Flashbacks
Schizophreniform psychoses
Seizures in overdose
No dependence

Opioids
Heroin, morphine, methadone
Sequence of
  Rush
  Histamine release
  Tranquillity
  CNS depression
Rapid physiological dependence
  Miosis
  Tremor
  Malaise
  Constipation
2–3% annual mortality
Only 10% seek help

Others

Phencyclidine	Solvents	Khat
Angel dust / PCP	Adolescent boys	Cathionine
Euphoria, analgesia, psychosis	Occ. sudden death	Sniffed
Withdrawal	Glue	
Responds to desipramine	Sniffed	
Smoked		

Stimulants
Amphetamines (speed)
  Cocaine (inc. crack)
Early
  Euphoriant
  ↓hunger
Later
  Depression
  Psychosis

Cannabis is the most common illicit drug used by the British general adult population (11% within the previous year), followed by cocaine (2.4%) and ecstasy (2%). In Britain, an estimated 500 000 people take ecstasy every weekend. Drugs are commonly used in combination. In ICD-10 (International Classification of Diseases version 10), substance use disorders are classified according to (i) substance and (ii) type of disorder. The latter include the following.

- **Acute intoxication**: transient disturbances of consciousness, cognition, perception, affect or behaviour following the administration of a psychoactive substance (PS).
- **Harmful use**: damage to the individual's health and adverse effects on family and society.
- **Dependence**: physiological dependence includes a withdrawal state, tolerance (increasing doses of PSs needed for the same effect) and consequently the PS being taken in larger amounts or for longer than intended. Psychological dependence involves a sense of compulsion to take the PS, difficulties in controlling its use, increasing time spent obtaining, ingesting or recovering from the PS, persistence with PS use despite awareness of harmful consequences, and a persistent but futile wish to cut down its use. There is usually a reduction or neglect of important social, occupational or recreational activities because of the PS use.
- **Withdrawal state**: physical and psychological symptoms occurring on absolute or relative withdrawal of a substance after repeated and usually prolonged and/or high-dose use of that substance. Onset and course of the withdrawal state are time limited and are related to the type of substance and the dose used before abstinence.
- **Psychotic disorder**: psychotic symptoms occurring during or immediately after PS use, characterized by vivid hallucinations, abnormal affect, psychomotor disturbances and persecutory delusions and delusions of reference.
- **Amnesic disorder**: memory and other cognitive impairments caused by substance use, most commonly alcohol.
- **Residual and late-onset psychotic disorders**: where effects on behaviour, affect, personality or cognition last beyond the period during which a direct PS effect might be expected (e.g. flashbacks).

Medicine at a Glance, Fifth Edition. Edited by Patrick Davey and Alex Pitcher.

Companion website: www.wiley.com/go/medicine5e

Aetiology and management

Availability and peer pressure are key aetiological factors; there is a strong association with younger age (11–24 years) and male gender. Neurobiological mechanisms, iatrogenic factors (e.g. prescribed benzodiazepines [BDZs]), a desire for the pleasurable effects of substances and the pharmacological properties of the PS may all also contribute. Substance misuse and psychiatric illness share several associations, including socioeconomic disadvantage. Substance misuse can exacerbate psychiatric symptoms (commonly depressed mood) or precipitate episodes of illness (e.g. psychosis). Conversely, certain psychiatric symptoms, such as impulsivity or anxiety, may increase drug use, and patients with certain psychiatric diagnoses (e.g. dissocial personality disorder) are much more likely to take illicit drugs.

Management of patients with psychiatric and substance misuse disorders (dual diagnosis) should ideally involve a multidisciplinary team trained to manage both disorders concurrently. As well as being obtained illicitly, some PSs may be acquired legally from chemists (codeine), shops (solvents) or doctors (benzodiazepines, ostensibly therapeutically). In the UK, illicit drugs are controlled under the Misuse of Drugs Act. Drugs are classified as Class A (the most harmful, e.g. opioids, hallucinogens, injected stimulants), Class B (e.g. oral stimulants, cannabis) and Class C (e.g. anabolic steroids, GHB, benzodiazepines).

Treatment can be in residential rehabilitation, hospital and community settings. Medication has several uses: short-term treatment as antidotes in overdose and alleviation or prevention of withdrawal, or longer-term treatment as substance replacement therapy (e.g. methadone) or relapse prevention (e.g. naltrexone, acamprosate). Psychological approaches such as cognitive behavioural therapy (CBT), motivational interviewing and self-help groups (such as Alcoholics Anonymous and Narcotics Anonymous) are effective.

Infection (HIV, hepatitis C) is the greatest risk associated with injected drug use; harm reduction strategies aim to minimize infection risk (e.g. needle exchange) and improve safety.

Specific substances

Opioids

Opioids include *heroin*, *morphine* and *methadone*. They may be smoked ('chasing the dragon'), sniffed ('snorting') or taken orally, intravenously ('mainlining'), intramuscularly or subcutaneously ('skin popping'). After an intensely pleasurable 'buzz' or 'rush' and release of histamine (itching, reddening of eyes), a sense of peace and detachment occurs, succeeded by central nervous system depression. Tolerance and withdrawal develop quickly. Ten percent of opioid misusers become dependent, but only 10% of these ever seek help; 2–3% die annually. Of the remainder, 25% are abstinent at five years and 40% at 10 years.

Miosis, tremor, malaise, apathy, constipation, weakness, impotence, neglect, malnutrition and evidence of HIV and other infection (e.g. hepatitis C) are signs of chronic dependence. Early withdrawal symptoms (24–48 h) include craving, flu-like symptoms, sweating and yawning. Mydriasis, abdominal cramps, diarrhoea, agitation, restlessness, piloerection ('gooseflesh') and tachycardia occur later (7–10 days).

Opioid dependence may be treated by replacement with methadone (opioid agonist) or buprenorphine (opioid partial agonist), which are less euphoriant and have a relatively long half-life. Methadone, lofexidine and buprenorphine are used for detoxification; naltrexone (opioid antagonist) blocks the euphoric effects and so can help prevent relapse. Signs of overdose (often accidental) include miosis and respiratory depression and may require naloxone.

Hallucinogens

Hallucinogens include *LSD* (lysergic acid diethylamide), which produces psychological (e.g. heightened perceptions) and physiological (dilated pupils, peripheral vasoconstriction, increased temperature) effects, but not dependence. Rare adverse effects include 'flashbacks', psychoses and (in overdose) seizures. *Ecstasy* (MDMA [3,4 methylenedioxymethamphetamine]) – a synthetic amphetamine analogue – has mixed stimulant and hallucinogenic effects and can induce hyperactivity and potentially fatal dehydration (or hyponatraemia from the resulting excess water consumption) and hyperpyrexia. *Magic mushrooms* (psilocybin) have effects similar to LSD but are less prolonged.

Stimulants

Amphetamines ('speed'), taken orally or intravenously, cause euphoria, increased concentration and energy, mydriasis, tachycardia and hyper-reflexia, followed by depression, fatigue and headache. Acute use may induce a schizophreniform psychosis. Methamphetamine is chemically related but more potent, long-lasting and harmful; it can be ingested, snorted or smoked (as 'crystal meth'). *Cocaine* may be sniffed, chewed or injected intravenously. Its effects (restlessness, increased energy, abolition of fatigue and hunger) resemble hypomania and last about 20 minutes. Visual/tactile hallucinations of insects (formication) and paranoid psychoses occur. Postcocaine dysphoria ('the crash'), with sleeplessness and intense depression, precedes withdrawal (depression, insomnia and craving). 'Crack' (a purified, very addictive form of cocaine) is smoked. The crack 'high' is extremely short and, on withdrawal, persecutory delusions are common.

Cannabis

The active compound of *marijuana* ('pot', 'grass', hashish, ganja) is tetrahydrocannabinol. The effects are psychological (euphoria, relaxation, well-being, omnipotence, hallucinations) and physiological (increased appetite, lowered body temperature). Substantial psychological dependence occurs. Adverse effects include conjunctival irritation, decreased spermatogenesis, lung disease, flashbacks, transient psychoses and apathy. Cannabis use is associated with increased incidence of depression and schizophrenia.

Sedatives and hypnotics

Overdose may cause respiratory depression. *BDZs* produce dependence, withdrawal (including seizures) and tolerance. BDZ dependence is often iatrogenic, although BDZs are also common street (illicit/recreational) drugs.

Others

Solvents are typically sniffed, principally by groups of boys aged 8–19 years (a red rash around the mouth and nose may be a sign of abuse). Initial euphoria is followed by drowsiness. Psychological dependence is common, but physical dependence is rare. Chronic abuse results in weight loss, nausea, vomiting, polyneuropathy and cognitive impairment. Toxic effects (sometimes fatal) include bronchospasm, arrhythmias, aplastic anaemia and hepatorenal or cerebral damage. *Phencyclidine* (PCP, 'angel dust') is usually smoked. Its effects include euphoria and peripheral analgesia and impaired consciousness or psychosis, which may require antipsychotics. *Khat*, used particularly by men from the Somali and Yemeni communities, contains cathinone, an amphetamine-like stimulant causing excitement and euphoria. It is not a controlled substance in the UK. *Nicotine*: around a quarter of British adults smoke. Counselling, nicotine replacement therapy, varenicline (partial nicotinic receptor agonist) and buproprion (noradrenaline and dopamine reuptake inhibitor) may aid smoking cessation.

240 Alcohol misuse

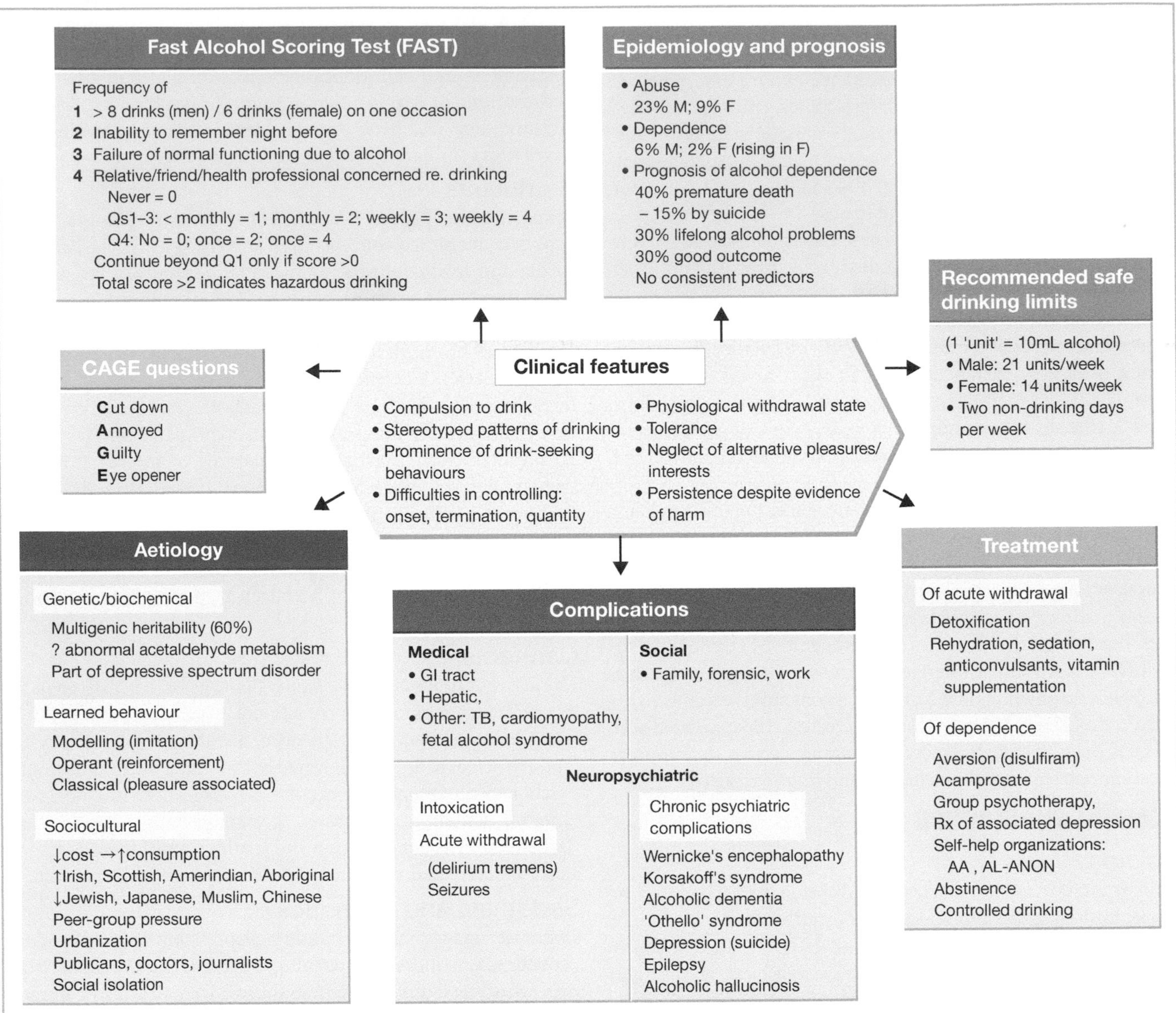

Fast Alcohol Scoring Test (FAST)
Frequency of
1 > 8 drinks (men) / 6 drinks (female) on one occasion
2 Inability to remember night before
3 Failure of normal functioning due to alcohol
4 Relative/friend/health professional concerned re. drinking
Never = 0
Qs1–3: < monthly = 1; monthly = 2; weekly = 3; weekly = 4
Q4: No = 0; once = 2; once = 4
Continue beyond Q1 only if score >0
Total score >2 indicates hazardous drinking
Epidemiology and prognosis
• Abuse
23% M; 9% F
• Dependence
6% M; 2% F (rising in F)
• Prognosis of alcohol dependence
40% premature death
– 15% by suicide
30% lifelong alcohol problems
30% good outcome
No consistent predictors
Recommended safe drinking limits
(1 'unit' = 10mL alcohol)
• Male: 21 units/week
• Female: 14 units/week
• Two non-drinking days per week
CAGE questions
Cut down
Annoyed
Guilty
Eye opener
Clinical features
• Compulsion to drink
• Stereotyped patterns of drinking
• Prominence of drink-seeking behaviours
• Difficulties in controlling: onset, termination, quantity
• Physiological withdrawal state
• Tolerance
• Neglect of alternative pleasures/ interests
• Persistence despite evidence of harm
Aetiology
Genetic/biochemical
Multigenic heritability (60%)
? abnormal acetaldehyde metabolism
Part of depressive spectrum disorder
Learned behaviour
Modelling (imitation)
Operant (reinforcement)
Classical (pleasure associated)
Sociocultural
↓cost →↑consumption
↑Irish, Scottish, Amerindian, Aboriginal
↓Jewish, Japanese, Muslim, Chinese
Peer-group pressure
Urbanization
Publicans, doctors, journalists
Social isolation
Complications
Medical
• GI tract
• Hepatic,
• Other: TB, cardiomyopathy, fetal alcohol syndrome
Social
• Family, forensic, work
Neuropsychiatric
Intoxication
Acute withdrawal
(delirium tremens)
Seizures
Chronic psychiatric complications
Wernicke's encephalopathy
Korsakoff's syndrome
Alcoholic dementia
'Othello' syndrome
Depression (suicide)
Epilepsy
Alcoholic hallucinosis
Treatment
Of acute withdrawal
Detoxification
Rehydration, sedation, anticonvulsants, vitamin supplementation
Of dependence
Aversion (disulfiram)
Acamprosate
Group psychotherapy,
Rx of associated depression
Self-help organizations:
AA , AL-ANON
Abstinence
Controlled drinking

Alcohol abuse is regular or binge consumption of alcohol sufficient to cause physical, neuropsychiatric or social damage.

Safe limits

- A 'unit' of alcohol (10 ml, 8 g) is roughly a small glass of wine, a pub single of spirits or a half pint of beer.
- The safe drinking limits are 21 units per week for men and 14 for women, with at least two drink-free days each week.
- The UK government guidelines for maximum daily use (<4 units a day for men, <3 units for women), reflecting concerns about binge drinking.
- Much smaller amounts may be hazardous to a fetus.

Classification

The ICD-10 (International Classification of Diseases version 10) classifies alcohol use disorders using the same system as for other psychoactive substances.

- **Acute intoxication** leads to slurred speech, impaired co-ordination and judgement, labile affect and, if severe, hypoglycaemia, stupor and coma. Differential diagnosis includes other causes of acute confusion, particularly head trauma.
- **Acute withdrawal** reflects the degree of previous dependence and usually occurs within one or two days of abstinence. It is characterized by malaise, nausea, autonomic hyperactivity, tremulousness, labile mood, insomnia and transient hallucinations or illusions (usually visual). Seizures are a recognized complication. Severe withdrawal, or 'delirium tremens' ('shaking delirium'), occurs in 5% of withdrawals and has a mortality of up to 15%, partly as a result of other medical complications.
- **Alcohol dependence**.
- **Psychotic disorders** related to alcohol use include the following. Alcoholic hallucinosis (usually threatening, second-person voices in a clear sensorium). Jealousy (paranoid delusions about infidelity). **Amnesic syndrome**: for example, Korsakoff psychosis.

- **Residual and late-onset disorders**: these include depression and dementia.

Epidemiology

- Prevalence rates worldwide vary widely and are related to overall consumption levels, availability and price.
- In the UK, heavy drinking (an average of 8 units/day for men and 6 units/day for women) is reported by 23% of men and 9% of women; younger people are more likely to exceed safe limits.
- The prevalence of alcohol dependence is 6% in men and 2% in women. Rates are particularly high in medical inpatients, and are increasing in women and adolescents.
- Alcohol abuse and dependence often begin in the early to mid twenties, at a time when most people begin to moderate their drinking as their responsibilities increase.

Detection and screening

- A fifth of primary care attenders have an alcohol use disorder.
- The detection of disorders can be difficult because they are not usually clinically obvious, but is crucial to:
  - enable appropriate treatment
  - avoid long-term complications
  - avoid withdrawal from unplanned abstinence (e.g. after surgery).
- Have a high index of suspicion in medical inpatients, and those with mental illness or two or more drink-driving offences.
- Many cases can be detected by documenting a typical drinking week.
- Screening questionnaires are also helpful (see figure).
- Collateral history can be revealing.
- Physical examination may reveal alcoholic stigmata, particularly signs of liver disease (jaundice, spider naevi, palmar erythema, gynaecomastia) and peripheral neuropathy.
- Macrocytosis without anaemia and raised γ-glutamyl transferase, alanine and aspartate aminotransferase or carbohydrate-deficient transferrin indicate recent harmful use.

Aetiology

This is multifactorial. Factors include the following.

- A strong genetic component (around 60%), which appears to be multigenic. Genetically determined alterations in alcohol metabolism may partially explain this, with those at low risk producing more (hangover-causing) acetaldehyde; 50% of Japanese people have an unpleasant 'flush reaction' on drinking alcohol due to a mutation in the acetaldehyde dehydrogenase 2 gene. There is often a positive family history of depression.
- **Occupation**: high-risk groups include the armed forces, doctors, publicans and journalists.
- **Cultural influences**: low rates are reported in Jews and Muslims, and high rates in Scottish and Irish people.
- The cost of alcoholic drinks.
- Behavioural models stress: learning by imitation (modelling), social reinforcement, the association between drinking and pleasure (classic conditioning), avoiding withdrawal symptoms (operant conditioning).
- Risk increases in the presence of chronic psychiatric or physical illness, particularly if complicated by chronic pain. There is an association with mood and anxiety disorders.

Complications

- **Neuropsychiatric complications.** Wernicke encephalopathy. Peripheral neuropathy. Erectile or ejaculatory impotence. Cerebellar degeneration. Dementia.
- **Other physical complications**: drinking damages almost every organ system in the body.
- **Social complications** include unemployment, marital difficulties, criminality, prostitution, homicides, domestic violence, accidental deaths, road accidents and suicides.
- **Psychiatric complications**: repeated heavy drinking is associated with: 40% risk of temporary depressive episodes, suicidal ideas and attempts, severe anxiety, insomnia.

  These often improve within 2–4 weeks of abstinence.
- **Fetal alcohol syndrome** (from drinking in pregnancy) is characterized by: decreased muscle tone, poor co-ordination, developmental delay, heart defects, a range of facial abnormalities.

Management

- Abstinence is the usual goal for treatment of dependence, although sometimes controlled drinking can be used.
- Achieving abstinence requires **acute detoxification**. This should be in a closely medically supervised environment if there is a risk of delirium tremens or withdrawal seizures, or the person is a child or vulnerable (e.g. cognitively impaired or lacking support).
  - This is initially high and a rapidly tailing sedation (e.g. a benzodiazepine, such as chlordiazepoxide or diazepam) to control withdrawal symptoms and prevent seizures. Monitor and adjust treatment using a scoring system such as the Clinical Institute Withdrawal Assessment for Alcohol (CIWA-AR) score.
  - Treatment of delirium tremens is usually with lorazepam or antipsychotics (e.g. haloperidol or olanzapine).
  - Treatment also includes rehydration, correction of electrolyte disturbance, and oral or parenteral thiamine.
- **Motivational interviewing** explores ambivalence to seeking treatment, drinking cessation, or both. It may help problem drinkers in denial to achieve insight and a desire to change.
- **Psychological therapies** (individually or in groups) may promote maintenance of abstinence or controlled drinking (i.e. within safe limits). They are useful for: sustaining motivation, learning relapse prevention strategies, developing social routines not reliant on alcohol, treating co-existent depression and anxiety.
- **Self-help groups** (e.g. Alcoholics Anonymous) are effective; they reduce pro-drinking activities and social ties.
- **Medication** may help maintain abstinence after detoxification. **Disulfiram** blocks alcohol metabolism, inducing acetaldehyde accumulation if alcohol is ingested, with resultant flushing, headache, anxiety and nausea. **Acamprosate** acts on the γ-aminobutyric acid system to reduce cravings and risk of relapse. **Naltrexone**, an opioid receptor antagonist, has similar therapeutic effects (licensed in the USA but not the UK).
- **Prevention measures** include: increasing taxation on alcohol, restricting its advertising or sale, school alcohol education: this reduces long-term alcohol use, risky alcohol-related behaviour and binge drinking.

Prognosis

- Continued alcohol problems increase the rate of early death by a factor of three or four. The most common causes are heart disease, stroke, cancers, liver cirrhosis, accidents and suicide.
- Only 15% of those with alcohol use disorder seek treatment; those who do have a better prognosis.

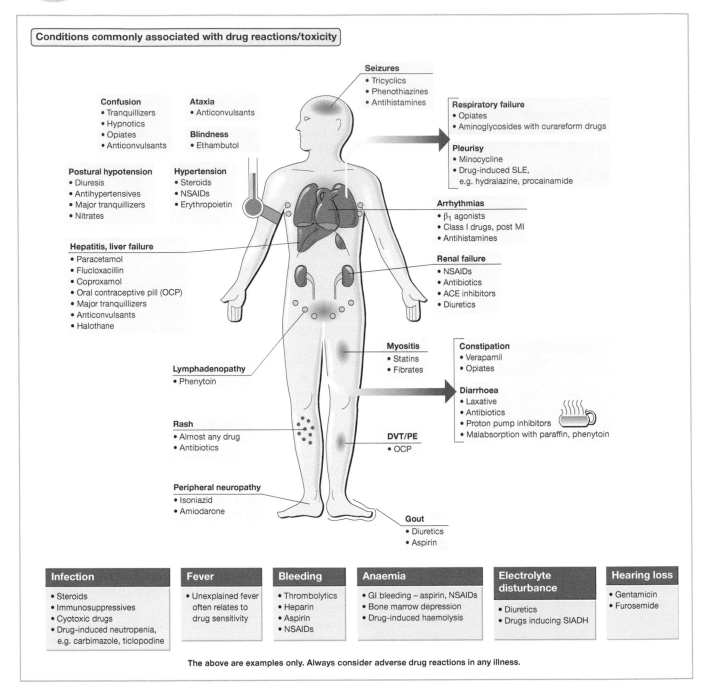

Drug toxicity (adverse drug reactions)

Conditions commonly associated with drug reactions/toxicity

Seizures
- Tricyclics
- Phenothiazines
- Antihistamines

Confusion
- Tranquillizers
- Hypnotics
- Opiates
- Anticonvulsants

Ataxia
- Anticonvulsants

Blindness
- Ethambutol

Respiratory failure
- Opiates
- Aminoglycosides with curareform drugs

Pleurisy
- Minocycline
- Drug-induced SLE, e.g. hydralazine, procainamide

Postural hypotension
- Diuresis
- Antihypertensives
- Major tranquillizers
- Nitrates

Hypertension
- Steroids
- NSAIDs
- Erythropoietin

Arrhythmias
- β_1 agonists
- Class I drugs, post MI
- Antihistamines

Hepatitis, liver failure
- Paracetamol
- Flucloxacillin
- Coproxamol
- Oral contraceptive pill (OCP)
- Major tranquillizers
- Anticonvulsants
- Halothane

Renal failure
- NSAIDs
- Antibiotics
- ACE inhibitors
- Diuretics

Myositis
- Statins
- Fibrates

Constipation
- Verapamil
- Opiates

Lymphadenopathy
- Phenytoin

Diarrhoea
- Laxative
- Antibiotics
- Proton pump inhibitors
- Malabsorption with paraffin, phenytoin

Rash
- Almost any drug
- Antibiotics

DVT/PE
- OCP

Peripheral neuropathy
- Isoniazid
- Amiodarone

Gout
- Diuretics
- Aspirin

Infection
- Steroids
- Immunosuppressives
- Cytotoxic drugs
- Drug-induced neutropenia, e.g. carbimazole, ticlopodine

Fever
- Unexplained fever often relates to drug sensitivity

Bleeding
- Thrombolytics
- Heparin
- Aspirin
- NSAIDs

Anaemia
- GI bleeding – aspirin, NSAIDs
- Bone marrow depression
- Drug-induced haemolysis

Electrolyte disturbance
- Diuretics
- Drugs inducing SIADH

Hearing loss
- Gentamicin
- Furosemide

The above are examples only. Always consider adverse drug reactions in any illness.

Adverse reactions to drugs are so common that it is crucial to determine whether any new symptom relates to a drug prescribed for another condition. Adverse reactions are classified as follows.

Predictable side-effects

Predictable side-effects at normal doses arise from those mechanisms responsible for therapeutic action. The following text is not comprehensive, but does give a number of different examples.

Medicine at a Glance, Fifth Edition. Edited by Patrick Davey and Alex Pitcher.

Companion website: www.wiley.com/go/medicine5e

Interference with normal physiological function: drugs used in normal doses

- β-receptor stimulation dilates peripheral blood vessels and β-blockade leads to vasoconstriction (cold peripheries).
- Bleeding with thrombolytic therapy.
- Immunosuppression from steroid therapy, presenting as severe/unusual infection: oral *Candida* infection with inhaled steroids for asthma; bone marrow suppression, with anaemia, infection and bleeding as a result of antineoplastic agents.
- Daytime sleepiness with nocturnal hypnotics.
- Movement disorders arising from long-term anti-parkinsonian drugs.
- Diarrhoea with broad-spectrum antibiotics, from altered bowel flora.

Interference with normal physiological function: drugs used in high concentrations (or when excretion is impaired)

- Excess inhaled β-receptor agonists in asthma leads to palpitations: β-receptor stimulation increases the strength and rate of cardiac contraction.
- Hypothyroidism from antithyroid drugs or thyrotoxicosis from excess thyroxine.
- Hypoglycaemia from insulin.
- Hypercalcaemia with vitamin D.

Diseases enhancing drug side-effects

There are a number of examples of this.

- Hyperglycaemia in patients given steroids – very common in clinical practice with COVID-19.
- β-blockade leading to bronchoconstriction in people with asthma; in phaeochromocytomas β-blockers lead to unopposed α-adrenergic stimulation, which produces intense vasoconstriction and increases peripheral resistance, so raising blood pressure, which may result in heart failure or stroke.
- Pre-existing heart failure may be exacerbated in those given verapamil, a negatively inotropic calcium channel blocker. Negative inotropism with calcium channel blockers partly correlates with negative chronotropism, i.e. the less they lower heart rate, the less negative inotropism occurs.
- Class I antiarrhythmics drugs can cause (lethal) ventricular arrhythmias in those with structural heart disease, e.g. previous myocardial infarction (MI).
- In bilateral renal artery stenosis, acute renal failure occurs if angiotensin-converting enzyme (ACE) inhibitors are given; constriction of the postglomerular arteriole is mediated by angiotensin II. In renal artery stenosis, this is critical in maintaining a high glomerular filtration pressure. If this vasoconstriction decreases, glomerular membrane filtration pressure is lost and renal excretory function falls; if both kidneys have stenosed renal arteries, acute renal failure results.
- Paracetamol is more toxic in those with chronic liver disease, e.g. alcoholism.

Electrolyte abnormalities increasing the likelihood of drug toxicity

- Hypokalaemia increases the action of digoxin (see section 'Increased tissue action due to renal failure'), and increases the likelihood of proarrhythmia occurring as a side-effect of antiarrhythmic, antidepressant or antihistamine drugs.
- Chronic hyponatraemia predisposes to saline-induced brainstem damage if corrected too rapidly (central pontine myelinosis).

Age increasing the side-effects of drugs

- Cardiovascular compensatory reflexes are diminished in elderly people, so postural hypotension is more common with antihypertensive therapy; this may present as fractured neck of femur or as recurrent falls.
- Renal tubular function declines in elderly people, so hyponatraemia from diuretics is more common; this may present as confusion.
- Increasing age diminishes brain reserves, so increasing the sensitivity to hypnotics and sedatives.

Sex increasing the possibility of side-effects

- Gynaecomastia in men treated with oestrogens.

Increased tissue action of the drug

Side-effects arising from increased tissue action of the drug, from increased tissue sensitivity or from overdosage may result from the following.

- A narrow therapeutic range: small changes in drug metabolism/dosage can easily produce toxic levels. Monitoring drug concentration where possible helps prevent this, e.g. digoxin, anticonvulsants, aminoglycosides.
- Renal or hepatic failure can slow metabolism of a drug or an active metabolite resulting in toxicity. In renal and/or hepatic failure, prescribe sparingly and always determine from the *British National Formulary* (BNF) whether the dose should be adjusted.

Increased tissue action due to renal failure

- **Digoxin** is renally excreted and is commonly given with diuretics to elderly people with heart failure. Old age, renal failure and hypokalaemia all predispose to toxicity, and manifest as (any) cardiac arrhythmia, visual disturbance (objects appear yellow), confusion, nausea and vomiting. The latter produces dehydration and pre-renal renal failure, further increasing digoxin levels and exacerbating toxicity. Treatment: wait for renal elimination and normalize potassium. If symptoms are life-threatening, give digoxin antibodies or dialyse.
- **Lithium** is renally excreted. If toxic levels develop (excess dosage, dehydration, deliberate overdose), ataxia, confusion (which may progress to coma), convulsions and nephrogenic diabetes insipidus occur. Circulating fluid is lost, producing pre-renal renal failure, so lithium levels rise further, exacerbating toxicity. Treatment: intravenous fluids and withholding lithium. Dialysis is occasionally needed.
- **Aminoglycosides** are renally excreted and used in severe infections, which themselves may cause renal failure. Dose should be calculated based on weight and creatinine clearance and drug levels should be very carefully monitored to avoid toxicity, which is manifest as vestibulocochlear nerve damage (deafness, difficulty with balance) and renal failure. Furosemide (frusemide) if given as a rapid, high-dose, intravenous 'push' can result in a similar ototoxicity.
- **Opioid poisoning** occurs in renal failure (most opioids are excreted renally), in cardiac failure (which impairs renal function), in elderly people (increased tissue sensitivity), in type II

respiratory failure (CO_2 retention increases the sensitivity of the respiratory centre to respiratory depression induced by opioids and other central nervous system [CNS] depressants), and with excess opioids (inadvertent or deliberate overdose). Opioid overdose impairs conscious level, which may lead to coma and depressed respiratory centre function, producing hypoventilation and leading to apnoea. Patients are often drowsy and hyperventilating with pinpoint pupils. Intravenous naloxone, a specific opioid receptor antagonist, rapidly improves conscious level and ventilatory function. Beware: as the half-life of naloxone in the circulation (±30 min) is less than that of opioids (up to several hours), naloxone administration may need to be repeated.

Toxicity arising from predictable drug–drug interactions

Often it is the way one drug interacts with another that results in toxicity.

- Altered drug concentration through inhibition/induction of cytochrome P450 (CYP): drugs inhibiting CYP isoforms increase the concentration of other drugs that depend on CYP for elimination. This may lead to toxicity, e.g. macrolide antibiotics inhibit CYP, slowing cisapride (a now withdrawn gut prokinetic agent) elimination, leading to toxic levels and ventricular arrhythmias. CYP induction by anticonvulsants decreases the effect of the oral contraceptive pill (OCP). Racial and familial differences in drug metabolism may be mediated by CYP isoform polymorphisms.
- Altered P-glycoprotein expression: P-glycoprotein decreases gastrointestinal (GI) drug absorption, increases CNS and kidney drug excretion, and extrudes drugs from cells, e.g. antineoplastic agents. Drugs that inhibit P-glycoprotein alter the concentration of other drugs, e.g. verapamil increases the concentration of ciclosporin.
- Altered protein binding: decreased protein binding increases levels of highly protein-bound drugs, e.g. antibiotics compete for the albumin binding of warfarin, increasing warfarin levels and the anticoagulant effect. Antibiotics also kill gut bacteria, decreasing vitamin K production (the natural antagonist to warfarin), so increasing warfarin's effect.
- Administration of drugs with complementary function. Antiplatelet agents promote bleeding in those on warfarin. Drowsiness results from polypharmacy with antipsychotics, nocturnal hypnotics and sedating antihistamines. Excessive bradycardia or asystole results from the combination of verapamil and β-blockers.
- Other interactions, e.g. amiodarone doubles the plasma levels of digoxin, and so may cause toxicity.

Toxicity arising from other predictable mechanisms

- Genetic interactions: factor V Leiden dramatically increases the risk of OCP-induced venous thrombosis. Glucose-6-phosphate dehydrogenase deficiency produces haemolysis with many drugs. Many drugs may precipitate acute porphyric attacks.
- Inhibition of related enzyme systems: non-steroidal anti-inflammatory drugs (NSAIDs) inhibit cyclo-oxygenase enzyme (COX) isoforms 1 and 2. COX-1 produces gastric mucosal protection factors, whereas COX-2 inhibition is responsible for the therapeutic efficacy of the drug. Early NSAIDs inhibited both isoforms, promoting GI bleeding. Recent NSAIDs are more selective and may cause fewer GI bleeds. NSAID-induced renal failure results from an inhibition of prostaglandin production and is more likely in those with pre-existing renal failure. Chronic NSAID consumption can produce chronic renal failure (with prominent tubular damage and a salt-wasting nephropathy), papillary necrosis and uroepithelial cancer.
- Toxicity from other drug constituents: thyroid dysfunction with amiodarone relates to the high levels of contained iodine. Amiodarone commonly induces hypothyroidism in areas with normal environmental iodine levels, and less commonly hyperthyroidism.
- Long-term toxicity is often predictable. Use of chronic high-dose steroids leads to Cushing syndrome, with osteoporosis, easy bruising and excess cardiovascular morbidity and mortality from hypertension and an adverse lipid profile. Anticancer drugs produce a significant late, i.e. 10-year, incidence of secondary tumours, often haematological, from the long-term effects of DNA damage.

Immune reactions

Immune reactions producing drug toxicity are subdivided according to the underlying mechanism.

- **Type I hypersensitivity reactions** usually occur after the third or fourth exposure to the drug. The sensitizing drug activates mast cell-bound IgE antibodies, causing degranulation, mild itching, urticaria and angioedema or anaphylaxis. Treatment: antihistamines, bronchodilators and steroids. The term 'anaphylactoid' is outdated; now called non-immunological anaphylaxis to ensure it is managed as per the Resuscitation Council UK anaphylaxis guideline. It results when drugs cause direct mast cell degranulation, e.g. opioids, contrast medium or aspirin. Reactions are not mediated by immunoglobulin, so previous exposure is not required. Some less severe reactions are sporadic, occur long after the start of treatment, and are difficult clinically to associate with drug therapy, e.g. intermittent angioedema with ACE inhibitors.
- **Type II hypersensitivity reactions** to drugs are rare. The most common example is penicillin-induced haemolytic anaemia, where red cell membrane-bound penicillin comes under IgG or IgM antibody-directed attack, so activating complement and producing cell lysis.
- **Type III hypersensitivity reactions** (serum sickness): offending drugs bind with specific IgG producing antigen–antibody complexes, e.g. penicillin, streptokinase, horse sera and sulfonamides. Immune complex deposition and subsequent inflammation within tissues cause the clinical features of fever, arthralgias, vasculitic skin rashes and renal impairment. Serum complement C3 and C4 are low. Eosinophilia may occur. Skin biopsies show a 'leukocytoclastic' vasculitis. No specific IgE to the antigen can be demonstrated, although specific IgG may be detected.
- **Type IV hypersensitivity reactions** are unusual causes of drug allergy. Frequent exposure sensitizes CD4+ T lymphocytes

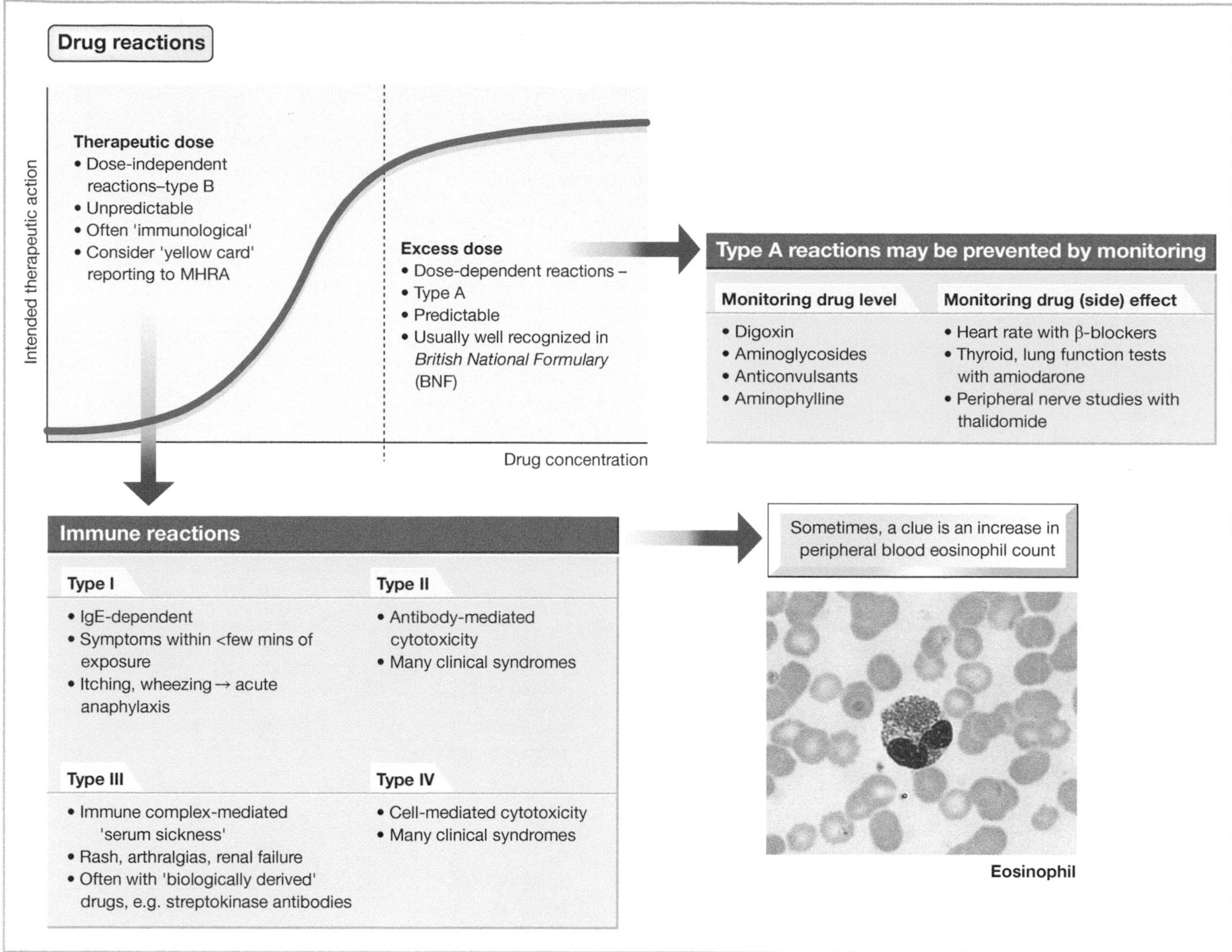

to a drug, e.g. topically applied penicillin. Lymphocytes migrate to the site of exposure and recruit other cells, including neutrophils and macrophages. Contact dermatitis occurs. This responds rapidly to steroids. Exposure to the offending agent via a patch test induces a diagnostic localized dermatitis after 48 hours.

Drug reactions
Intended therapeutic action
Therapeutic dose
• Dose-independent reactions–type B
• Unpredictable
• Often 'immunological'
• Consider 'yellow card' reporting to MHRA
Excess dose
• Dose-dependent reactions –
• Type A
• Predictable
• Usually well recognized in British National Formulary (BNF)
Drug concentration
Type A reactions may be prevented by monitoring
Monitoring drug level
• Digoxin
• Aminoglycosides
• Anticonvulsants
• Aminophylline
Monitoring drug (side) effect
• Heart rate with β-blockers
• Thyroid, lung function tests with amiodarone
• Peripheral nerve studies with thalidomide
Immune reactions
Type I
• IgE-dependent
• Symptoms within <few mins of exposure
• Itching, wheezing → acute anaphylaxis
Type II
• Antibody-mediated cytotoxicity
• Many clinical syndromes
Type III
• Immune complex-mediated 'serum sickness'
• Rash, arthralgias, renal failure
• Often with 'biologically derived' drugs, e.g. streptokinase antibodies
Type IV
• Cell-mediated cytotoxicity
• Many clinical syndromes
Sometimes, a clue is an increase in peripheral blood eosinophil count
Eosinophil

Unpredictable and other mechanisms giving rise to toxicity

Unfortunately, much drug toxicity falls into this category. The common ones should be learnt, but the clinician must always be aware of the potential for new and unexpected reactions. Examples include the following.

- Pneumonitis with high-dose (can occur with any dose) amiodarone manifests as breathlessness, sometimes with a nonproductive cough, and can be misinterpreted as worsening heart failure. Chest X-ray shows diffuse infiltrates. The carbon monoxide transfer factor is decreased. The diagnosis is confirmed by high-resolution computed tomography of the chest. Treatment: steroids (little evidence that they improve outcome) and time, because improvement is contemporaneous with amiodarone leaving the body, which, given its very long *in vivo* half-life of about 30 days, is often several months. Late diagnosis may lead to irreversible pulmonary fibrosis.
- Drug-induced skin rashes are often immunologically mediated, although other mechanisms also operate, e.g. β-blockers exacerbating psoriasis.
- Anticonvulsant hypersensitivity syndrome from carbamazepine or phenytoin presents as fever, rash, lymphadenopathy, malaise and hepatitis. Re-challenge with either drug is often fatal if the first illness involved hepatitis.
- Malabsorption with phenytoin.
- Myositis on statin therapy.
- The serotonin syndrome (see figure below).

Serotonin syndrome

Causes of serotonin syndrome	Clinical features
Any drug which increases serotonergic neuron activity, either administration or removal of serotonergic drugs; also if drugs which inhibit cytochromes CYP2D6/CYP3A4 are added to those already taking serotonergic drugs	Clinical triad of: • Mental state changes • Autonomic hyperactivity • Neuromuscular abnormalities
• Selective serotonin reuptake inhibitors (SSRIs): all • Antidepressant drugs: all • Monoamine oxidase inhibitors: all • Anticonvulsants: valproate • Antiemetics: ondansetron, metoclopramide • Analgesics: fentanyl, tramadol • Antitussives: dextromethorphan • Antibiotics: linezolide (MAO inhibitor), ritonavir • Some 'street' drugs: LSD, MDMA • Dietary supplements: St John's Wort, ginseng, tryptophan • Lithium	Incidence; 0.4 cases per 1000 patient-months for many serotonergic drugs Probably about 2–5000 cases/year in the UK, and 20–80 deaths Occurs in 15% of SSRI overdoses Pathophysiology: relates to ↑serotonergic neuron activity, possibly 5-HT_{2A}, and 5-HT_{1A}; also ↑CNS noradrenaline (norepinephrine) activity may be relevant
Severe serotonin syndrome is especially likely when combinations of the above drugs are taken	

Features of the serotonin syndrome – a spectrum, with subtle symptoms/signs in mild cases, usually occurring ≤ few minutes after new medication or change in dose

		Mild	Moderate	Severe
Mental state		Normal	Mild agitation, hypervigilance, pressured speech	Delirious, great agitation
Autonomic changes	Heart rate	↑	↑↑	↑↑↑
	Sweating	+	++	+++
	Pupil dilatation	+	++	+++
	Blood pressure	Normal – ↑	↑	↑↑ →frank shock
	GI tract		↑bowel sounds Diarrhoea	↑↑ bowel sounds
Temperature		Normal	↑to 40°C	High – up to 41°C
Neuromuscular changes	Muscle findings	Tremor	Inducible clonus	Rigid muscles (especially lower limbs)
	Reflexes	↑	↑↑	↑↑↑
Laboratory tests				Acidosis
Therapy	REMOVE PROVOKING DRUG(S)	Supportive Benzodiazepines	Rehydrate, cool; 5-HT_{2A} antagonists	↑Muscle enzymes If temp ± 41°C, neuromuscular paralysis and intubation/ventilation

Diagnosis; needs (1) knowledge that a serotonergic agent was given ≤ 5 weeks ago, (2) 1 or more of:
- Tremor with hyperflexia
- Spontaneous clonus
- Muscle rigidity and T°C ≥ 38; and ocular or inducible clonus
- Ocular clonus and agitation or sweating
- Inducible clonus and agitation or sweating

Differential diagnosis: anticholinergic syndrome, neuroleptic malignant syndrome (see Chapter 43), malignant hyperthermia (see Chapter 43)

Diagnosis

A full clinical history should be taken of the reaction and all drugs administered, including details about previous exposure and time from exposure to symptom onset. Eosinophils may be raised.

Management

- Discontinue the offending drug/agent. Avoid subsequently.
- Advise on any cross-reacting drugs.
- Use a MedicAlert bracelet for severe drug allergies.
- Inform the Medicines & Healthcare products Regulatory Agency (MHRA) (BNF yellow card).
- In immune reactions, initiate drug desensitization (exposure to escalating doses of the drug on multiple occasions) for essential agents, e.g. insulin, but not if alternative treatments are available.

242 COVID-19

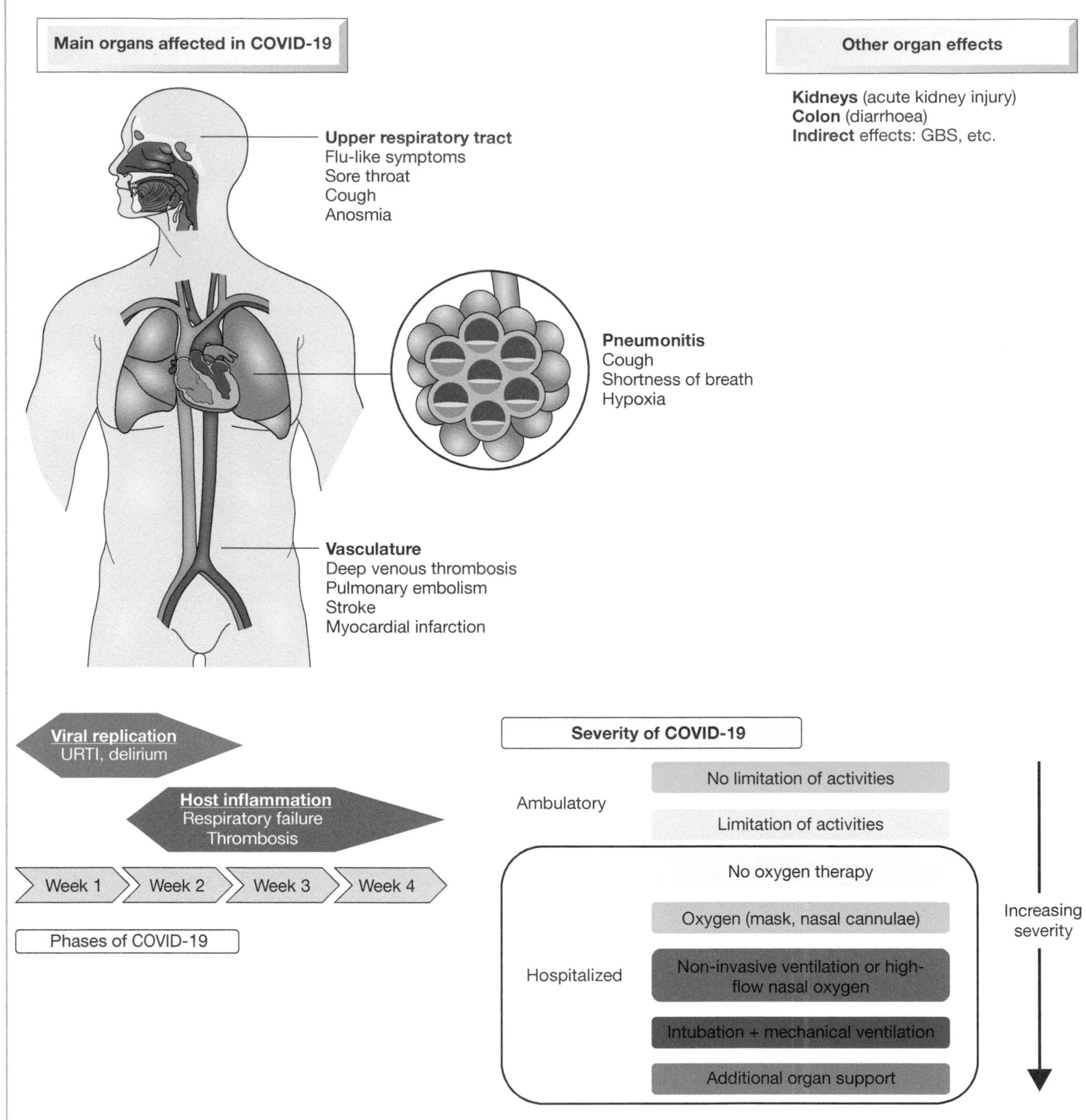

Medicine at a Glance, Fifth Edition. Edited by Patrick Davey and Alex Pitcher.

Companion website: www.wiley.com/go/medicine5e

Epidemiology

Transmission: COVID-19 is caused by SARS-CoV-2, a coronavirus that emerged from an animal reservoir (most likely bats) in late 2019 in China. Like many other upper respiratory tract pathogens, SARS-CoV-2 spreads between individuals via direct contact, droplets (particles of >5 μm diameter) and aerosols (≤5 μm). Droplets are thought to be the predominant form of spread, taking virus from the respiratory tract of one individual onto the mucosal surfaces of another, and into the upper respiratory tract, initially above the alveolar level. It is generally assumed that droplets do not travel more than 2 m from the index case, explaining the general 2 metre 'exclusion zone' used in social distancing. Aerosols travel much further but they tend to be produced more rarely than droplets.

- **Temporal dynamics**: the incubation period of around five days is slightly longer than for influenza. Peak infectivity occurs, on average, at the time of symptom onset, although a significant proportion of cases, particularly in children, are asymptomatic. The ability of the virus to be transmitted by both asymptomatic and presymptomatic individuals matches other infections that have recently produced pandemics (e.g. influenza, HIV) where transmission from an individual can also occur before they know that they are ill.
- **Outbreaks** are particularly common in healthcare institutions (care homes, hospitals) and confined spaces such as cruise ships and prisons, even with use of appropriate personal protective equipment.
- **Mutant variants** with different sequences to the original outbreak may be associated with altered phenotypes in terms of transmissibility and clinical features.

Pathogenesis

Infection of humans by SARS-CoV-2 depends critically on the molecular interaction between the SARS-CoV-2 spike protein and the human angiotensin-converting enzyme 2 (ACE2) that is expressed cells on epithelial (upper and lower respiratory tract, bowel) and endothelial surfaces (blood vessels, heart). In most cases, infection is limited to the upper respiratory tract, and symptoms are mild or even absent (around 30% of infections).

- **Severe disease** develops in a subset of COVID-19 patients after around 7–10 days of symptoms, due to a host hyperinflammatory response (by this stage viral levels are typically falling). Pathology is centred on alveolar cell damage with fluid build-up and localized immunothrombosis in the pulmonary vasculature, leading to respiratory failure. The accompanying 'cytokine storm' brings risk of vascular syndromes (arterial and venous) in other sites and multiorgan failure.
- **Risk factors** for severe COVID-19 overlap with known vascular disease risk factors. Age is unquestionably the primary determinant, with risk of death or critical illness rising with each decade of adulthood. Male gender, diabetes, obesity and hypertension are also associated with worse outcomes. Ethnicity, acting through these known vascular risk factors and other health inequalities, is also a strong risk factor for severe disease; so too is immunosuppression, presumably because of greater viral replication.

Clinical features

Mild disease

Clinical syndromes initially reflect the cellular distribution of ACE2. Common early symptoms reflect upper respiratory tract infection, with fever, cough, fatigue and myalgia, as well as loss of smell and taste due to infection in the olfactory epithelium. Lethargy, anorexia and diarrhoea (due to mild colitis) are also common, leading some patients to present with dehydration and weakness. Delirium is also a common problem in those with underlying risk factors (increasing age, dementia and other long-term conditions), requiring admission for nursing care alongside medical investigation.

Severe disease

Severe symptoms develop at around day 7–10 of illness in around 10–20% of those with mild symptoms.

- **Pneumonitis** with widespread alveolar involvement manifests as worsening cough and shortness of breath (moderate cases), followed by hypoxia and progressive respiratory failure (severe cases). A significant proportion of hypoxic patients simply report tiredness, leading on occasion to late presentation to hospital with established respiratory failure. The mortality of severe disease is very high without both specific and supportive treatment.
- **Deep venous thrombosis** and **pulmonary embolism** occur in around 25% of critically ill patients, reflecting endothelial activation and procoagulant changes within the blood. There is also an increased risk of arterial infarction spanning all stages of the illness, manifesting as stroke, myocardial infarction and peripheral ischaemia.
- **Multiorgan failure** may also occur, reflecting both direct infection of vital organs as well as the hyperinflammatory state.
- **Complications of critical illness** include secondary bacterial and fungal infection, polyneuropathy and post-traumatic stress disorder.

Other manifestations (not necessarily associated with severe illness)

- **Cardiac**: acute coronary syndrome, acute inflammatory cardiomyopathy with myocarditis, arrhythmia and heart block.
- **Kidney**: acute kidney injury.
- **Neurological**: brainstem encephalitis, transverse myelitis, Guillain–Barré syndrome, myasthenia gravis.
- **Haematological**: coagulopathy, immune thrombocytopaenic purpura, macrophage activation syndrome.
- **Paediatric inflammatory multisystem syndrome temporally associated with COVID-19 (PIMS-TS)**: a Kawasaki-like illness consisting of otherwise unexplained persistent fever and inflammation with evidence of single/multiorgan dysfunction.

Long-term complications

- **Lung fibrosis** may follow severe pneumonitis, although data on the frequency and clinical correlates of radiological findings remain sparse.
- **'Long COVID' syndrome**: even patients with relatively mild symptoms of COVID-19 may experience a range of symptoms, including fatigue, shortness of breath, palpitations and difficulty concentrating, for many months after infection, in the absence of demonstrable abnormalities in organ function. These symptoms appear broadly similar to those encountered after other viral infections such as dengue and EBV.

Immunity

The great majority of people experiencing symptomatic infection develop lasting immune responses (antibody- and cell-mediated) that appear to reduce the severity of subsequent infection. However, in individuals with chronic immunosuppression (e.g. transplant recipients, those on biologic therapy), the virus may be detectable for many weeks, potentially maintaining infectivity and ongoing clinical symptoms.

Diagnosis

The diagnosis of COVID-19 can be confirmed by a suggestive clinical story and the detection of SARS-CoV-2 by testing of respiratory tract samples (usually nose/throat swab).

- **RT-PCR** detects SARS-CoV-2 RNA and is the main method used because of its high sensitivity. The PCR test tends to remain positive for 10–14 days (although presence of viral RNA does not necessarily indicate infectivity).
- **Lateral flow antigen tests** detect the SARS-CoV-2 spike protein. They are significantly less sensitive but can be useful for immediate management/infection control decisions.
- **Serology**: prior SARS-CoV-2 infection (as well as successful vaccination) can be confirmed via detection of specific antibodies.

Other laboratory tests

Patients with COVID-19 tend to have significant lymphopenia and moderate neutrophilia (which is typically less than seen in invasive bacterial infections). High markers of inflammation including C-reactive protein (CRP), D-dimer and ferritin are associated with severe disease and overall outcome. It is also common to detect evidence of injury to the kidneys (raised creatinine), myocardium (troponin) and liver (mild rise in ALT).

Radiology

Patients with moderate or severe COVID-19 typically have patchy areas of bilateral lower zone shadowing on plain chest X-ray. CT scanning reveals wedge-shaped, subpleural areas of ground-glass opacification in the mid and lower zones. CT can also be used to detect pulmonary emboli in patients, particularly relevant when the degree of hypoxia is disproportionate to chest X-ray appearances.

Treatment and management

General principles

Infection control

Strict source isolation should be applied to suspected or confirmed COVID-19 cases, using either droplet or airborne precautions according to whether there are aerosol-generating procedures (AGPs) such as non-invasive ventilation. For all hospitalized patients, these precautions should continue for 14 days after an individual's first positive SARS-CoV-2 PCR test (provided there has been clinical improvement). This period may need to be extended for those with severe immunosuppression (as defined by the UK's Green Book on Immunization). Cohorting of patients with confirmed COVID-19 in bays is appropriate.

Planning for therapeutic escalation

Given the high probability of prolonged critical illness and death, there should be early discussions of goals and ceilings of care among clinicians, patients and their next of kin, taking into account the communication challenges associated with strict infection control.

Anti-inflammatory treatment

- **Corticosteroids** (most commonly dexamethasone 6 mg od oral or intravenous) substantially reduce mortality in patients with pneumonitis and hypoxia, via reduction of inflammation, as shown in the RECOVERY trial. The 'number needed to treat' appears particularly low in mechanically ventilated patients. However, steroids are not of benefit (and may be harmful) earlier in the course of infection (i.e. before the development of hypoxia).
- **Tocilizumab** (an IL-6 inhibtor) and **baricitinib** (a JAK-inhibitor) further reduce mortality in critically ill patients.

Antiviral treatment

Remdesivir is an adenosine nucleotide prodrug that is metabolized to the active substrate remdesivir triphosphate which inhibits SARS-CoV-2 RNA polymerase. Studies show significantly reduced mortality in patients admitted to hospital (e.g. on oxygen) but not in those already ventilated. Early administraion of **monoclonal antibodies** e.g. sotrovimab, or the protease inhibitor **nirmatrelvir** (given in combination with ritonavir) may reduce complications in those with underlying medical conditions.

Supportive treatment

- **Oxygen** should be prescribed and administered by nasal cannulae or Venturi mask to achieve a target saturation of 94–98% (88–92% or a patient-specific target range in those at risk of hypercapnic respiratory failure, e.g. COPD).
- **Non-invasive respiratory support** is generally used in patients who remain hypoxaemic despite standard flow oxygen therapy but do not yet require intubation, or where it has been decided that intubation would not be appropriate. Continuous positive airway pressure (**CPAP**) is generally considered to be the preferred form of therapy, with shorter periods on high-flow nasal oxygen (**HFNO**) also helpful. Both require an appropriate infection control environment as they are aerosol-generating procedures.
- In patients who are too unwell for, or intolerant of, non-invasive support, or who do not respond to a CPAP trial (deterioration in gas exchange, exhaustion), **intubation with invasive mechanical ventilation** is required.
- **Proning** (placing the patient on their front) can produce substantial improvements in oxygenation in both intubated and non-intubated patients.
- **Extracorporeal membrane oxygenation** (**ECMO**) may be considered in selected cases where there is poor progression with the above approaches.
- **Venous thromboembolism**: given the prothrombotic phenotype generally observed with COVID-19, prophylactic low molecular weight heparin is indicated, alongside maintenance of a low threshold for investigations of possible venous thromboembolism.
- **Antibiotics** should be considered if there is suspected bacterial superinfection. Pulmonary *Aspergillus* infection is also a recognized finding although isolation of the organism does not in itself confirm disease or the need for treatment. Standard forms of **renal support**, as well as nasogastric feeding, should be instituted according to standard guidelines.
- Possible cases of 'long COVID' should ideally be managed via a multidisciplinary approach involving medical, psychological and physiotherapeutic elements.

Preventing infection

- **Avoidance**: the infectiousness of presymptomatic/asymptomatic individuals means that preventing exponential spread through a population requires population-wide measures to reduce transmission. Non-pharmacological approaches, such as social distancing, hand-washing, facemasks in public places and mandating restrictions on freedom of movement and association, have been implemented in various countries at various times to try to control the spread of infection, and in many countries to avoid constrained healthcare systems being overwhelmed by large numbers of people requiring healthcare at the same time. Travel restrictions and bans have also been used. Vulnerable adults may need to take extra steps to avoid infection ('shielding'). Mass testing of well individuals via PCR or lateral flow devices (see Diagnosis, above) linked to 'track and trace' systems can in theory reduce the number of secondary cases arising from each index case ('R0') but requires extensive resources to execute at scale.

- **Vaccination**: Nucleic-acid based vaccines involving mRNA and viral vector platforms, all focusing on the SARS-CoV-2 spike protein, substantially reduce the severity of disease.

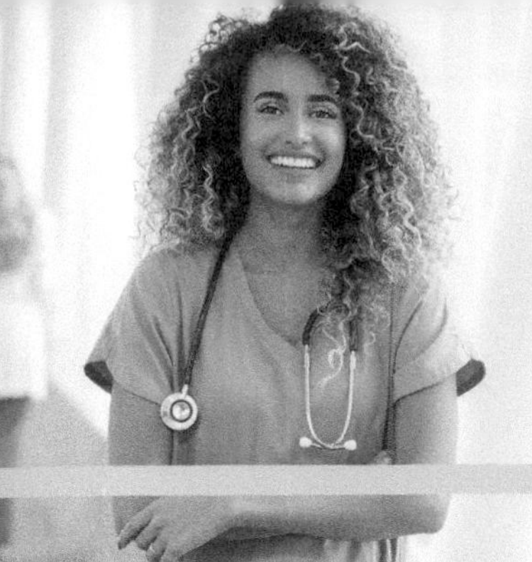

Index

Note: Page numbers in *italics* refer to figures, those in **bold** refer to tables.

Medicine at a Glance, Fifth Edition. Edited by Patrick Davey and Alex Pitcher.

Companion website: www.wiley.com/go/medicine5e